Fifth edition

Pinkus' Guide to Dermatohistopathology

Fifth edition

Pinkus' Guide to Dermatohistopathology

Amir H. Mehregan, MD
Clinical Professor
Department of Dermatology
Wayne State University School of Medicine
Detroit, Michigan

Ken Hashimoto, MD
Professor and Chairman
Department of Dermatology
Wayne State University School of Medicine
Detroit, Michigan

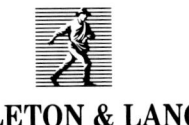

APPLETON & LANGE
Norwalk, Connecticut/San Mateo, California

0-8385-7902-7

Notice: Our knowledge in clinical sciences is constantly changing. As new information becomes available, changes in treatment and in the use of drugs become necessary. The authors and the publisher of this volume have taken care to make certain that the doses of drugs and schedules of treatment are correct and compatible with the standards generally accepted at the time of publication. The reader is advised to consult carefully the instruction and information material included in the package insert of each drug or therapeutic agent before administration. This advice is especially important when using new or infrequently used drugs.

Copyright © 1991 by Appleton & Lange
A Publishing Division of Prentice Hall
Copyright 1986, 1981, 1976 by Appleton-Century-Crofts

All rights reserved. This book, or any parts thereof, may not be used or reproduced in any manner without written permission. For information, address Appleton & Lange, 25 Van Zant Street, East Norwalk, Connecticut 06855.

91 92 93 94 95 / 10 9 8 7 6 5 4 3 2 1

Prentice Hall International (UK) Limited, *London*
Prentice Hall of Australia Pty. Limited, *Sydney*
Prentice Hall Canada, Inc., *Toronto*
Prentice Hall Hispanoamericana, S.A., *Mexico*
Prentice Hall of India Private Limited, *New Delhi*
Prentice Hall of Japan, Inc., *Tokyo*
Simon & Schuster Asia Pte. Ltd., *Singapore*
Editora Prentice Hall do Brasil Ltda., *Rio de Janeiro*
Prentice Hall, *Englewood Cliffs, New Jersey*

Library of Congress Cataloging-in-Publication Data

Mehregan, Amir H.
   Pinkus' guide to dermatohistopathology. — 5th ed. / Amir H. Mehregan, Ken Hashimoto.
     p.   cm.
   Includes bibliographical references and index.
   ISBN 0-8385-7902-7
   1. Skin—Histopathology. I. Hashimoto, Ken, 1931–
II. Title. III. Title: Guide to dermatohistopathology.
   [DNLM: 1. Skin Diseases—pathology. WR 105 M498p]
RL95.M44 1991
616.5'075—dc20
DNLM/DLC
for Library of Congress   91-4546
                                                       CIP

Acquisitions Editor: William Schmitt
Production Editor: Sandra K. Huggard
Production Assistant: Sasha Kintzler
Designer: S. Milo Byrum

PRINTED IN THE UNITED STATES OF AMERICA

This volume is dedicated to the memory of Drs. Felix and Hermann Pinkus. Their contributions to the progress of dermatology spanned nearly a century.

CONTENTS

Preface.. xv

SECTION I. FUNDAMENTALS AND TECHNIQUES................................... 1

1. Introduction and Aims 3
2. Normal Structure of Skin 5
   Developments 5
   Epidermis 8
   Epidermal Layers / Basal Cells / Prickle Cells and Granular Cells / Keratinized Cells / Epidermal Biology / Epidermal Architecture / Epidermal Symbiosis
   Dermoepidermal Junction..................... 16
   Dermis 18
   Pars Papillaris / Pars Reticularis / Subcutaneous Tissue
   The Pilar Apparatus 23
   Development / Structure of the Adult Follicle / Fibrous Root Sheath / Sebaceous Gland / Apocrine Gland / Arrector Muscle / Haarscheibe / Hair Cycle
   Eccrine Gland 35
   Intraepidermal Dendritic Cells............... 39
   Melanocytes / Langerhans Cells / Merkel Cells

3. Technical Data, Including Pitfalls and Artifacts 45
   Selection of Site and Lesion for Biopsy 45
   Biopsy Procedure............................. 47
   Punch Biopsy and Excisional Biopsy / Superficial and Deep Biopsy / Curette Biopsy
   Fixation 51
   Tissue Processing and Preparation of the Histologic Section 54
   Dehydration / Embedding / Cutting
   Stains 55
   Hematoxylin and Eosin Stain / Acid Orcein and Giemsa Stain (Pinkus and Hunter) / Other Elastic Fiber Stains / Periodic Acid–Schiff (PAS) Reaction of Hotchkiss and McManus / Alcian Blue Stain (Mowry) / Colloidal Iron Stain / Toluidine Blue Stain / Aldehyde Fuchsin Stain (Gomori) / Enzyme Digestion / Reticulum / Amyloid / Lipids / Iron / Melanin / Calcium / Silver and Other Metals / Silica / Stains for Fungi / Bacterial Stains
   Preparation of Tzanck Smear and Tissue Imprints...................................... 61
   Foreign Bodies 61
   Artifacts..................................... 63

4. Immunopathology of the Skin............. 65
   Direct Immunofluorescence 65
   Indirect Immunofluorescence.................. 66
   Immunoperoxidase and Other Immunohistochemical Methods 68
   Application of Direct and Indirect Immunofluorescence and Immunoperoxidase Methods
   Monoclonal Antibody Technique 69
   Diagnosis of Inflammatory Diseases of the Skin 69
   Pemphigus Vulgaris / Pemphigus Vegetans / Pemphigus Erythematosus (Senear-Usher Syndrome) / Pemphigus Foliaceus / Bullous Pemphigoid / Cicatricial Pemphigoid (Ocular or Benign Mucous Membrane Pemphigoid) / Herpes

Gestationis / Epidermolysis Bullosa Acquisita / Dermatitis Herpetiformis / Adult Linear IgA Bullous Dermatitis / Benign Chronic Bullous Dermatosis of Childhood / Discoid Lupus Erythematosus (DLE) / Systemic Lupus Erythematosus (SLE) / Subacute Cutaneous Lupus Erythematosus (SCLE) / Mixed Connective Tissue Disease (MCTD) / Scleroderma

5. **General Pathology: Terminology** **79**
    Epidermis 80
    General Configuration / Dyskeratosis, Dysplasia, Anaplasia / Cell Death / Transepithelial Elimination
    Dermis 88
    Basement Membrane / Pars Papillaris / Pars Reticularis

6. **Systematics of Histopathologic Interpretation** **95**
    Technique 95
    Categorizing 96
    Clinicopathologic Coordination 96

SECTION II. SUPERFICIAL INFLAMMATORY PROCESSES 99

7. **Eczematous Tissue Reactions** **101**
    Contact Dermatitis 101
    Primary Irritant Type / Sensitization Dermatitis / Acute Contact Dermatitis / Chronic Contact Dermatitis / Dermal Contact Sensitivity Reaction
    Dyshidrosiform Dermatitis 107
    Atopic Dermatitis 107
    Infantile Acropustulosis 108
    Erythema Toxicum Neonatorum 109
    Acrokeratosis Paraneoplastica 109
    Exfoliative Dermatitis 109
    Prurigo 110
    Lichen Simplex Chronicus 110
    Picker's Nodule and Prurigo Nodularis 111

8. **Psoriasiform Tissue Reactions** **115**
    Seborrheic Dermatitis 115
    Asteatotic Dermatitis 119
    Psoriasis 119
    Classic / Variants
    Reiter's Disease 126
    Nummular Eczema 127
    Sulzberger-Garbe Disease 128

9. **Lichenoid and Poikilodermatous Tissue Reactions** **131**
    Lichen Planus 131
    Histology / Atrophic Verrucous, and Follicular Lesions / Bullous Lesions / Pigmented Lichen Planus, Lichen Pigmentosus, and Erythema Dyschromicum Perstans
    Lichen Planus Actinicus 137
    Solitary Lichen Planuslike Keratosis 138
    Graft-vs-Host Disease 138
    Poikiloderma 138

Keratosis Lichenoides Chronica 139
Lichen Nitidus 139
Lichenoid Drug Eruptions and Other Lichenoid Lesions 141

10. **Toxic, Allergic, and Multiform Erythemas** **145**
    Urticaria 145
    Lichen Urticatus / Insect Bites
    Erythema Exudativum Multiforme 146
    Toxic Erythema 149
    Erythema Annulare Centrifugum / Erythema Chronicum Migrans / Erythema Gyratum Repens
    Acute Febrile Neutrophilic Dermatosis 150
    Cellulitis and Erysipelas 152
    Eosinophilic Cellulitis 152
    Hypereosinophilic Syndrome 152

11. **Vesicular and Bullous Diseases** **157**
    Acantholytic Disorders 157
    Pemphigus Vulgaris / Pemphigus Vegetans / Pemphigus Foliaceus, Pemphigus Erythematosus / Fogo Selvagem / Acrodermatitis Enteropathica
    Bullous Pemphigoid 162
    Cicatricial Pemphigoid 162
    Dermatitis Herpetiformis 163
    Chronic Bullous Dermatosis of Childhood 164
    Dermatoses of Pregnancy 164
    Toxic Epidermal Necrolysis 166
    Porphyria Cutanea Tarda 166
    Epidermolysis Bullosa 168
    Epidermolysis Bullosa Simplex / Epidermolysis Bullosa Letalis / Epidermolysis Bullous Dystrophica / Transient Bullous Dermolysis of the Newborn (Hashimoto et al)
    Impetigo and Subcorneal Pustular Dermatosis 174
    Necrolytic Migratory Erythema 175
    Other Bullous Lesions 175
    Mucous Membrane Lesions 177

12. **Inflammatory Virus Diseases** **181**
    Intranuclear Viruses 181
    Variola and Vaccinia 182
    Paravaccinia and Ecthyma Contagiosum 183
    Measles and German Measles 184
    Coxsackie and Echo Viruses 184
    Gianotti-Crosti Syndrome 187
    Pityriasis Rosea 187

13. **Miscellaneous Papulosquamous Eruptions** **189**
    Superficial Fungous Infections 189
    Noninflammatory Lesions / Tinea Superficialis
    Parapsoriasis 192
    Pityriasis Lichenoides / Parapsoriasis en Plaques / Parapsoriasis Lichenoides and Poikiloderma
    Pigmented Purpuric Eruptions 197
    Schamberg-Majocchi Eruption / Gougerot-Blum Eruption / Lichen Aureus (Purpuricus) / Differential Diagnosis

Lichen Striatus............................. 198
Scabies 199

SECTION III. DEEP INFLAMMATORY PROCESSES.................................. 203

14. Lupus Erythematosus and Related Conditions................................ 205
Histology of Lupus Erythematosus........... 205
Special Features / Variants
Jessner's Lymphocytic Infiltration 209
Photosensitivity Reactions 210
Pellagra
Dermatomyositis............................ 213

15. Dermal Vasculitides and Other Vascular Disorders 217
Necrotizing Angiitis......................... 217
Leukocytoclastic Vasculitis / Periarteritis Nodosa / Other Forms
Kawasaki's Disease 220
Embolism, Thrombosis, and Infarction....... 221
Embolism / Thrombosis / Livedo / Infarction
Chronic X-ray Dermatitis.................... 222
Erythema Elevatum Diutinum............... 223
Granuloma Faciale.......................... 223
Stasis Dermatitis............................ 224
Atrophie Blanche

16. Subcutaneous Inflammations: Panniculitis 231
Differential Diagnosis....................... 231
Individual Entities 232
Nodular Vasculitis / Erythema Nodosum / Erythema Induratum and Gummatous Syphilis / Panniculitis / Panniculitis in Diseases of Connective Tissue / Deep Fungous Infections / Other Inflammatory Entities / Equestrian Cold Panniculitis in Women / Noninflammatory Entities

17. Ulcers 241
Ulcers, Wounds, and Granulation Tissue 241
Generic Features of Ulcers
Specific Entities 242
Bacterial Infections / Disturbances of Immunity / Other Entities

18. Inflammation Involving the Pilosebaceous Complex 249
Staphylococcal Infections.................... 249
Acne Vulgaris and Related Conditions....... 249
Dermatophytic Folliculitis 250
Other Deep Follicular Inflammations......... 252
Perforating Folliculitis / Necrotizing Folliculitis and Pityrosporum Folliculitis / Disorders Associated with Hair of Blacks / Pilonidal Sinus
Superficial Lesions 254
Eosinophilic Pustular Folliculitis / Disseminate and Recurrent Infundibulofolliculitis / Folliculitis Decalvans
Follicular Keratoses......................... 256
Keratosis Pilaris and Related Conditions / Kyrle's Disease / Pityriasis Rubra Pilaris
Rosacea, Rhinophyma, and Lewandowsky's Disease 260

19. Alopecias Associated with Inflammation............................. 265
Alopecia Areata............................. 265
Alopecia Mucinosa 265
Scarring Alopecia 267
Pseudopelade of Brocq / Alopecia Neoplastica

20. Inflammation Involving Eccrine or Apocrine Glands 273
Eccrine Glands.............................. 273
Apocrine Glands............................ 274

SECTION IV. GRANULOMATOUS INFLAMMATION AND PROLIFERATION 279

21. Predominantly Mononuclear Granulomas 281
Tuberculosis................................. 281
Biology / Tuberculodermas / Tuberculids
Leprosy (Hansen's Disease).................. 287
Atypical Mycobacteria
Syphilis..................................... 290
Primary Lesion / Secondary Lesion / Tertiary Lesion / Other Treponematoses
Sarcoidosis and Sarcoid Reactions 293
Cutaneous Sarcoidosis / Sarcoidal Foreign Body Granulomas / Melkersson-Rosenthal Syndrome
Malakoplakia................................ 297
Histoplasmosis 297
Cutaneous Leishmaniasis.................... 298
Tularemia and Rhinoscleroma 300

22. Mixed Cell Granulomas 305
Fungal Granulomas......................... 305
Coccidioidomycosis / South American Blastomycosis / Chromomycosis (Chromoblastomycosis) / Actinomycosis, Nocardiosis, Botryomycosis / Cryptococcosis / Sporotrichosis / Opportunistic Fungi
Protothecosis 312
Worms and Larvae.......................... 312
Halogen Eruptions 314
Granuloma Gluteale Infantum
Foreign Body Granulomas 315
Granuloma Inguinale 316
Lymphogranuloma Venereum................. 317

23. Palisading Granulomas 321
Granuloma Annulare 321
Actinic Granuloma.......................... 324
Granulomatosis Disciformis (Miescher)

Necrobiosis Lipoidica	325
Rheumatic and Rheumatoid Nodes	326
Juxta-articular Nodes of Syphilis	
Granulomatous Slack Skin	326
Necrobiotic Xanthogranuloma	328
Cat-Scratch Disease	328

24. Predominantly Histiocytic Lesions 331
Xanthoma	331
Verruciform Xanthoma	
Juvenile Xanthogranuloma	332
Histiocytoma (Fibrous Histiocytoma)	333
Nature / Histology / Variants / Associated Epithelial Changes	
Reticulohistiocytoma	338
Generalized Eruptive Histiocytoma	340
Benign Cephalic Histiocytosis	340

25. Histiocytosis X (Langerhans Cell Granulomas) 343
Skin Manifestations	343
Histiopathology	343
Congenital Self-healing Reticulohistiocytosis	345

SECTION V. METABOLIC AND OTHER NONINFLAMMATORY DERMAL DISEASES 349

26. Changes of Collagen and Ground Substance 351
Scleroderma	351
Generalized / Morphea and Linear Scleroderma / Sclerodermoid Disorders / Eosinophilic Fasciitis	
Atrophodermas and Lipodystrophies	354
Atrophoderma of Pasini and Pierini / Senile Atrophy / Progeria / Corticosteroid Atrophy / Acrodermatitis Chronica Atrophicans / Lipodystrophy / Aplasis Cutis Congenita	
Lichen Sclerosus et Atrophicus	357
Reactive Perforating Collagenosis	358
Perforating Lesions in Chronic Renal Failure	
Ehlers-Danlos Syndrome	358
Scleredema, Lymphedema, and Myxedema	358
Mucopolysaccharidoses / Lichen Myxedematosus: Papular Mucinosis and Scleromyxedema / REM Syndrome	
Synovial Lesions and Myxoid Cysts	360
Affections of Ear Cartilage	361

27. Disorders of Elastic Fibers 369
Normal Properties	369
Disturbances	369
Congenital / Acquired	

28. Various Extracellular Deposits 383
Lipids	383
Calcium	383
Bone	385
Uric Acid	385
Hyalin	386
Amyloid	386
Skin Limited Types / Systemic Amyloidosis / Secondary Systemic Amyloidosis	
Blood and Blood Pigment	388
Foreign Bodies	389

SECTION VI. NONNEOPLASTIC EPITHELIAL AND PIGMENTARY DISORDERS 393

29. Darier's, Hailey-Hailey's, and Grover's Diseases 395
Keratosis Follicularis (Darier)	395
Warty Dyskeratoma	
Benign Familial Chronic Pemphigus (Hailey-Hailey)	399
Grover's Disease	

30. Ichthyosiform Dermatoses 403
Ichthyosis Vulgaris	403
X-Linked Ichthyosis	403
Lamellar Ichthyosis	404
Epidermolytic Hyperkeratosis	404
Ichthyosis Hystrix and Icthyosiform Nevi / Colloidion Baby / Harlequin Fetus / Rare Forms of Ichthyosis / Acquired Ichthyosis / Hyperkeratosis Lenticularis Perstans (Flegel's Disease)	

31. Pigmentary Disorders 413
Decrease and Increase of Epidermal Melanin	413
Depigmentation / Hyperpigmentation	
Increase of Subepidermal Melanin	415
Incontinentia Pigmenti	
Other Intradermal Colored Matter	416
Other Dermal Changes Affecting Color	418
Color Changes Due to Horny Layer	418

32. Virus Epidermoses 423
Molluscum Contagiosum	423
Virus Warts	424
Verruca Vulgaris / Verruca Plana / Verruca Filiformis and Verruca Digitata / Verrucae of Plantar Type / Condyloma Acuminatum / Epidermodysplasia Verruciformis / Focal Epithelial Hyperplasia (Heck's Disease)	

SECTION VII. MALFORMATION AND NEOPLASIA 435

Nevus	436
Benign Versus Malignant Tumors	436

33. Melanocytic Tumors and Malformations 439
How to Recognize Melanocytes, Nevus Cells, and Melanophages	439

Diagnosis of Specific Lesions................. 441
Lesions Involving Epidermal Melanocytes / Pigmented Nevus Cell Nevi / Congenital Nevi / Dermal Melanocytes / Lesions Related to Dermal Melanocytes

Malignant Melanoma 459
Biology / Lentigo Maligna / Lentigo Maligna Melanoma / Acral Lentiginous Melanoma / Superficial Spreading Malignant Melanoma / Nodular Malignant Melanoma

Criteria for Malignancy..................... 470
Histologic Grading of Malignant Melanoma and Prognosis 473

34. Epidermal Nevi and Benign Epidermoid Tumors.. 479

Epidermal Nevi 479
Verrucous Epidermal Nevus / Ichthyosis Hystrix / Inflammatory Linear Verrucous Epidermal Nevus (ILVEN) / Pigmented Hairy Epidermal Nevus / White Sponge Nevus / Epidermal Nevus Syndrome / Nevoid Hyperkeratosis of Nipples and Areolae / Acrokeratosis Verruciformis of Hopf / Acanthosis Nigricans / Reticulated and Confluent Papillomatosis (Gougerot and Carteaud) / Multiple Minute Digitate Hyperkeratoses / Stucco Keratosis

Seborrheic Verruca......................... 483
Activated Seborrheic Verruca / Clonal Seborrheic Verruca and Intraepidermal Nests

Clear Cell Acanthoma (Degos)............... 490
Palmar Pits 491
Porokeratosis.............................. 491
Porokeratotic Eccrine Ostial and Dermal Duct Nevus............................... 492
Large Cell Acanthoma 492
Acantholytic Acanthoma.................... 494
Keratoderma Palmare et Plantare........... 494
Callosities and Clavus 495
Pitted Keratolysis.......................... 496
Reticulated Pigmented Anomaly of the Flexures.................................. 496
Reticulate Acropigmentation................ 496

35. Epidermal Precancer, Squamous Cell Carcinoma, and Pseudocarcinoma 501

Precancerous Keratoses 501
Actinic Keratosis, Keratosis Senilis (Freudenthal) / Other Actinic Keratoses

Bowen's Precancerous Dermatosis (Carcinoma in Situ) and Erythroplasia of Queyrat 507
Cutaneous Horn........................... 509
Xeroderma Pigmentosum 509
Progression from Precancerosis to Cancer ... 510
Squamous Cell Carcinoma 512
Acantholytic Squamous Cell Carcinoma / Immature Tumors / Small-Cell Squamous Carcinomas / Spindle Cell Squamous Carcinomas / Verrucous Carcinoma of Skin

Pseudocarcinoma.......................... 516
Pseudoepitheliomatous Proliferation / Papillomatosis Cutis Carcinoides / Keratoacanthoma

36. Nevus Sebaceous and Sebaceous Tumors....................................... 523

Organoid Nevus (Nevus Sebaceus of Jadassohn) 523
Senile Sebaceous Hyperplasia............... 525
Sebaceous Trichofolliculoma 526
Sebaceous Adenoma....................... 526
Sebaceous Epithelioma..................... 527
Muir-Torre Syndrome 528

37. Hair Nevi and Hair Follicle Tumors 531

Hair Nevi 531
Nevus Comedonicus

Hair Follicle Tumors....................... 531
Trichofolliculoma / Trichoadenoma / Dilated Pore / Pilar Sheath Acanthoma / Tumor of Follicular Infundibulum / Inverted Follicular Keratosis / Trichilemmoma / Cowden's Disease "Multiple Hamartoma Syndrome" / Pilomatricoma

Trichoepithelioma......................... 536
Desmoplastic Trichoepithelioma / Basaloid Follicular Hamartoma / Atrophoderma Vermicularis and Other Follicular Hamartomas

Tumors of Perifollicular Connective Tissue... 542
Perifollicular Fibroma / Fibrofolliculoma / Trichodiscoma

38. Cysts Related to the Adnexa 549

Glandular Cysts........................... 549
Hidrocystomas / Mucinous Syringometaplasia / Steatocystoma Multiplex

Keratinous Cysts........................... 551
Epidermoid Cysts / Eruptive Vellus Hair Cysts / Pigmented Follicular Cyst / Trichilemmal Cysts / Proliferating Trichemmal Cyst (Pilar Tumor) / Other Types

39. Sweat Apparatus Tumors................. 563

Sweat Gland Nevi.......................... 563
Supernumerary Nipple

Apocrine Tumors 564
Apocrine Cystadenoma / Syringadenoma Papilliferum / Hidradenoma of Vulva (Hidradenoma Papilliferum) / Tubular Apocrine Adenoma / Erosive Adenomatosis of the Nipple / Cutaneous Cylindroma

Eccrine Tumors 569
Hidracanthoma Simplex (Syringoacanthoma) / Eccrine Poroma and Dermal Duct Tumor / Eccrine Syringofibroadenoma / Papillary Eccrine Adenoma / Syringoma / Eccrine Spiradenoma / Clear Cell Hidradenoma Eccrine Acrospiroma / Chondroid Syringoma (Mixed Tumor of the Skin) / Aggressive Digital Papillary Adenoma

40. Basal Cell Epithelioma 583

Terminology............................... 583
Histogenesis............................... 583
Epithelial Portion.......................... 585
Mesodermal Portion....................... 587
Premalignant Fibroepithelial Tumor 589
Superficial Basal Cell Epithelioma........... 589
Aggressive (Infiltrating) Basal Cell Epithelioma................................ 590

Sclerotic Basal Cell Epithelioma............. 591
Morphea-like Epithelioma 591
Nevoid Basal Cell Epithelioma Syndrome 596
Metastatic Basal Cell Epithelioma........... 596
Intraepidermal Epithelioma.................. 596

41. Adenocarcinoma and Metastatic Carcinoma.................................. **603**
    Sebaceous Adenocarcinoma 603
        Meibomian Carcinoma
    Adenocarcinoma of the Sweat Apparatus 603
        Eccrine Carcinoma / Malignant Transformation of Eccrine Tumors / Apocrine Adenocarcinoma and Paget's Disease / Pilomatrix Carcinoma / Undifferentiated Adnexal Carcinoma / Trabecular Carcinoma / Neuroendocrine Carcinoma (Merkel Cell Tumor)
    Metastatic Carcinoma........................ 615

42. Mesodermal Nevi and Tumors **619**
    Scar Versus Keloid Versus Fibroma Versus Connective Tissue Nevus..................... 619
        Normal Scar / Hypertrophic Scars and Keloids / Connective Tissue Nevi / Fibroma / Perifollicular Fibromas and Trichodiscomas / Acrochordon, Fibroma Pendulum, Acquired Fibrokeratoma, Myxoid Fibroma
    Lesions with Unusual Differentiation of Connective Tissue........................... 624
        Myxomas / Giant Cell Tumor of Tendon Sheath (Localized Nodular Tenosynovitis) / Juvenile Hyaline Fibromatosis / Fibrous Hamartoma of Infancy / Giant Cell Fibroblastoma / Osteoma and Chondroma
    Sarcoma Versus Histiocytoma Versus Pseudosarcoma............................. 627
        Spindle Cell Sarcoma / Epitheloid Sarcoma / Malignant Fibrous Histiocytoma and Atypical Fibroxanthoma / Dermatofibrosarcoma Protuberans / Pigmented Dermatofibrosarcoma Protuberans (Bodnar Tumor) / Nodular (Pseudosarcomatous) Fasciitis / Recurrent Digital Fibrous Tumor of Childhood
    Leiomyoma, Angioleiomyoma, and Leiomyosarcoma............................ 633
    Lipoma, Angiolipoma, and Liposarcoma 637
    Nevus Lipomatosus Superficialis and Focal Dermal Hypoplasia.......................... 637
        Hibernoma

43. Vascular Nevi and Tumors **645**
    Lesions Consisting of Vessels 645
        Hemangiomas / Telangiectasias / Cirsoid Aneurysm / Angiokeratoma / Lymphangioma
    Lesions due to Proliferation of Vessel-Associated Cells............................. 648
        Hemangiopericytoma / Acquired "Tufted" Angioma (Angioblastoma Nakagawa) / Malignant Proliferating Angioendotheliomatosis / Granuloma Pyogenicum / Bacillary (Epithelioid) Angiomatosis / Intravascular Papillary Endothelial Hyperplasia (IPEH) / Aneurysmal (Angiomatoid) Fibrous Histiocytoma

Epithelioid "Histiocytoid" Hemangiomas Angiolymphoid Hyperplasia with Eosinophilia.................................. 652
    Blue Rubber Bleb Nevus / Glomangioma / Malignant Angioendothelioma / Kaposi's Sarcoma

44. Neural Tumors............................ **663**
    Neuroma 663
    Neurofibroma................................ 663
    Neurilemmoma............................... 667
    Other Forms................................. 667
        Granular Cell Tumor

45. Lymphoproliferative Neoplasms......... **671**
    Cytologic Interpretation..................... 671
        Morphology of Cells / Involvement of Dermal Strata
    Structural Interpretation.................... 673
        Quantity of Infiltrate / Polymorphism Versus Monomorphism / Involvement of Epidermis and Adnexa
    Terminology and Classification 674
    Specific Disorders 674
        Leukemia Cutis / Extramedullary Plasmacytoma and Multiple Myeloma / Hodgkin's Disease / Malignant Lymphoma / Mycosis Fungoides / Sézary Syndrome / Lymphomatoid Papulosis / Pagetoid Reticulosis / Crosti's Reticulohistiocytoma of the Back / Benign Lymphoplasia / Arthropod Bite Reaction / Actinic Reticuloid / Angioimmunoblastic Lymphadenopathy / Sinus Histiocytosis with Massive Lymphadenopathy / Cutaneous Malignant Histiocytosis / Lymphomatoid Granulomatosis / Urticaria Pigmentosa and Mastocytosis

SECTION VIII. MUCOUS MEMBRANES, HAIR, AND NAIL 695

46. Lesions of Mucous Membranes **697**
    Inflammatory Lesions 697
        Plasmocytosis Mucosae / Psoriasis, Geographic Tongue, Balanitis Circinata / Lichen Planus and Lupus Erythematosus / Lichen Sclerosus et Atrophicus / Syphilis
    Bullous Lesions 699
        Pemphigus, Pemphigoid, Erythema Multiforme / Darier's and Hailey-Hailey's Diseases
    Ulcerative Lesions 700
        Aphthae and Aphthosis / Perlèche / Cheilitis Glandularis / Eosinophilic Ulcer of the Tongue / Mucous Retention Cyst / Infectious Granulomas / Noninfectious Granulomas
    White Lesions............................... 703
        Leukoplakia / Benign White Plaques / Oral Hairy Leukoplakia / Nevoid and Verrucous White Lesions
    Dark Lesions................................ 706
        Melanin Pigmentation / Vascular Lesions / Tattoos
    Neoplasms.................................. 707
        Epithelial Neoplasms / Mesodermal and Neural Neoplasms

47. Lesions of Hair and Nail **713**

    Disturbances of Hair 713

        Microscopic Examination of Hair / Pattern Alopecia / Acute Hair Loss / Hypertrichosis / Rhythmic and Discontinuous Disturbances—Hair Shaft Abnormalities / Unmanageable Hair / Hair in Congenital Disorders / Circumscribed Abnormalities / Pili Multigemini / Trichostasis Spinulosa / Trichonodosis / Disturbances of Hair Due to External Causes: Traction Alopecia and

        Trichotillomania / Trichosporosis and Trichomycosis / Extraneous Material on Hair / Hair Casts

    Disturbances of Nail 723

        Various Dermatoses / Hermorrhage / Pachyonychia Congenita / Pterygium Inversum Unguis

Index **731**

PREFACE

In the past decade we have witnessed great progress in dermatologic research. Enzyme histochemistry and immunopathology independent of or together with electron microscopy have provided avenues for further investigation of inflammatory skin diseases and reclassification of lymphoproliferative neoplasms and disorders of keratinization. Immunologic markers, applicable to fresh-frozen and formalin-fixed, paraffin-embedded tissue sections have given clues to cell differentiation and pathogenesis of various cutaneous tumors and have proved essential in differential diagnosis of some skin neoplasms. In this edition, a number of newly defined dermatologic entities have been included and all chapters have been updated with the information from over 800 recent publications. Outdated material has been eliminated in order to keep this edition as handy as previous ones. In keeping with the teaching of Pinkus, we have continued to place in each chapter those diseases that show a similar pattern of tissue reaction or tumors that resemble each other and must be differentiated under the microscope. We are offering the fifth edition as a complete textbook of dermatohistopathology, as well as a guide for further individual study.

Amir H. Mehregan
Ken Hashimoto

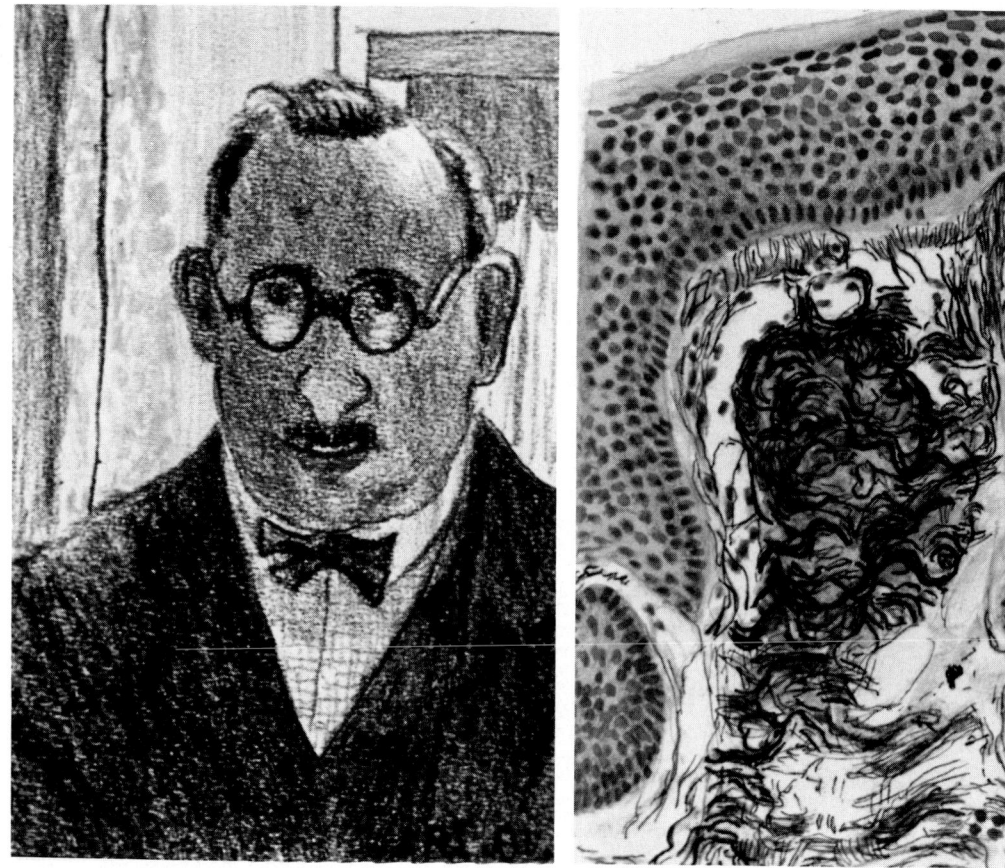
Felix Pinkus, self portrait (left). Elastic fibers in normal skin (right).

… SECTION

FUNDAMENTALS AND TECHNIQUES

1
INTRODUCTION AND AIMS

This book aims to be a guide to the interpretation of cutaneous biopsy sections and therefore is arranged according to histopathologic similarities and differences rather than in conformity with any clinical system of skin diseases.

It has been our experience that dermatologic residents need a guide beyond the information offered in textbooks. They have to be shown how to look at a section, how to analyze it, and how to tell important pathologic changes from insignificant and coincidental abnormalities. Even before that, they have to be taught normal skin structure and how it appears in haphazard and not always ideally prepared sections. They have to learn to recognize the pitfalls of technical artifacts. Histologic diagnosis of skin diseases usually does not result from looking for individual features and adding them up mechanically. Students must realize that they see one fleeting moment in the pathologic process fixed and that each stained section is a random, two-dimensional sample of a three-dimensional organ and may not be representative of all the changes present in the biopsy specimen. They must examine multiple sections and learn to interpret what they see in the three dimensions of space and the fourth dimension of time.

Some very good pathologists frown on too much interpretation: "Describe and diagnose on the basis of objective data" is the motto of many. All histopathologic examination includes interpretation, however, or we would be restricted to describing blue and red blotches rather than calling them epidermal cells, smooth muscle, or eosinophilic leukocytes. It is impossible to draw a distinct line between just enough and too much interpretation. What is called for is constant awareness of the distinction between observation and interpretation. One should not apply time-honored and worn expressions to histologic pictures but interpret them anew, when necessary, on the basis of lessons learned in many different fields: anatomy, experimental embryology, hematology, experimental pathology, biochemistry, and many others. The most profitable course is to observe first, then *consciously* to inject interpretation, and to point out to students as well as to readers of published articles why the interpretation is considered justified. Only then will we stimulate independent thinking and avoid being trapped in dogmatic statements.

All authors have personal opinions based on their education and training and the trend of their mental processes. This book, we feel sure, will be an outstanding example of such bias. We do not apologize, because all statements and interpretations are aimed at helping the student to make diagnoses by understanding what is going on in the tissue—or at least, what might be a reasonable explanation of the pathologic data in biologic terms.

We advise readers to consult other available texts frequently and to be elective in forming their own concepts. We hope that our specific aim in this book of showing students how to analyze their sections will be helpful for that purpose. Since publication of the fourth edition a number of books covering various fields in dermal pathology have been published.[1–6] A new edition of Lever and Schaumburg-Lever[7] appeared in 1989 and a new textbook, *Pathology of the Skin*, was edited by Drs. Farmer and Hood in 1991.[8] The annual *Year Book of Dermatology* provides abstracts of and comments on current publications.[9]

In this edition, we have revised the bibliography by including over 800 new articles and omitting others. Omission of many excellent publications was painful, but the *guide* is meant to inform and teach, not to give balanced credit to published work. A good number of new references concern the recent developments in immunopathology and application of various tissue specific markers in differential diagnosis of skin diseases and cutaneous neoplasms.

REFERENCES

1. Murphy GF, Mihm MC Jr: Lymphoproliferative Disorders of the Skin. Boston, Ma: Butterworths; 1986
2. Hashimoto K, Mehregan AH: Tumors of Skin Appendages. Boston, Ma: Butterworths, 1987
3. Hashimoto K, Mehregan AH: Tumors of the Epidermis. Boston, Ma: Butterworths, 1990
4. Rapini RP, Jordon RE: Atlas of Dermatopathology. Chicago: Year Book Medical Publishers, 1988
5. McKee PH: Pathology of the Skin with Clinical Correlations. Philadelphia: JB Lippincott Co., 1989
6. Gottlieb GJ, Ackerman AB: Kaposi's Sarcoma. Philadelphia: Lea & Febiger, 1988
7. Lever WF, Schaumburg-Lever G: Histopathology of the Skin, 7th ed. Philadelphia: JB Lippincott, 1989
8. Farmer E, Hood A: Pathology of the Skin. Norwalk, Conn: Appleton & Lange, 1991
9. Sober AJ, Fitzpatrick TB: The Year Book of Dermatology. Chicago: Year Book Medical Publishers, 1989

2
NORMAL STRUCTURE OF SKIN

The skin is a vitally important organ, has a complicated structure, and serves many functions.[1-3] "Normal skin," however, is an abstraction. Topography and differences of age, sex, and genetic constitution introduce so many variations that few general statements can be made. One has to have exact clinical information in order to adjudge a given section of skin normal or abnormal. Figure 2–1 illustrates four regions of skin photographed at identical magnification. Differences are obvious in the total dimensions of the organ, the absolute and relative thickness of epidermis and dermis, their architecture and structure, number and size of hair follicles and glands, and many other details.

Some major misconceptions and misnomers in dermatology have resulted from inadequate knowledge of normal development, structure, and function. Darier's division of skin cancers as basal cell, prickle cell, or mixed types was based on incomplete knowledge of epidermal biology and led to the strange misinterpretation that basal cells and prickle cells proliferate independently of each other.

The study of normal skin structure does not require an elaborate program of obtaining and preparing specimens of healthy skin. Many biopsy specimens submitted to the laboratory for diagnosis show normal features of some skin constituents. The student should establish a habit of examining all features of a skin section, not only those that are important for making a diagnosis. Effort thus expended will be repaid many-fold by the experience gained whenever a difficult point of interpretation arises. The better the anatomist and biologist, in due time, the better the dermatopathologist.

DEVELOPMENTS

The skin of the fetus[2,4,5] is derived from ectoderm and mesoderm. From the simple epithelial layer covering the surface of the embryo, the neuroectoderm is split off when the neural groove (neural crest) contributes to the skin by forming the sympathetic nervous system and furnishing melanoblasts. The secondary ectoderm (Fig. 2–2) soon becomes two-layered and later stratified (Fig. 2–3A) through mitotic activity greater than that needed to keep pace with general body growth. Ectoderm, in contrast to entoderm, has an inherent tendency toward stratification and expresses it even in tissue culture.[6] Glands derived from ectoderm are lined by at least two layers of epithelium.

Although mitotic activity occurs in both layers of the primitive epidermis, it soon is restricted to the basal layer, which thus becomes the germinal layer (stratum germinativum) from which cells move outward to become mature and exfoliated. The outer layer of embryonic epidermis is called the periderm and seems to fulfill a function of exchange between

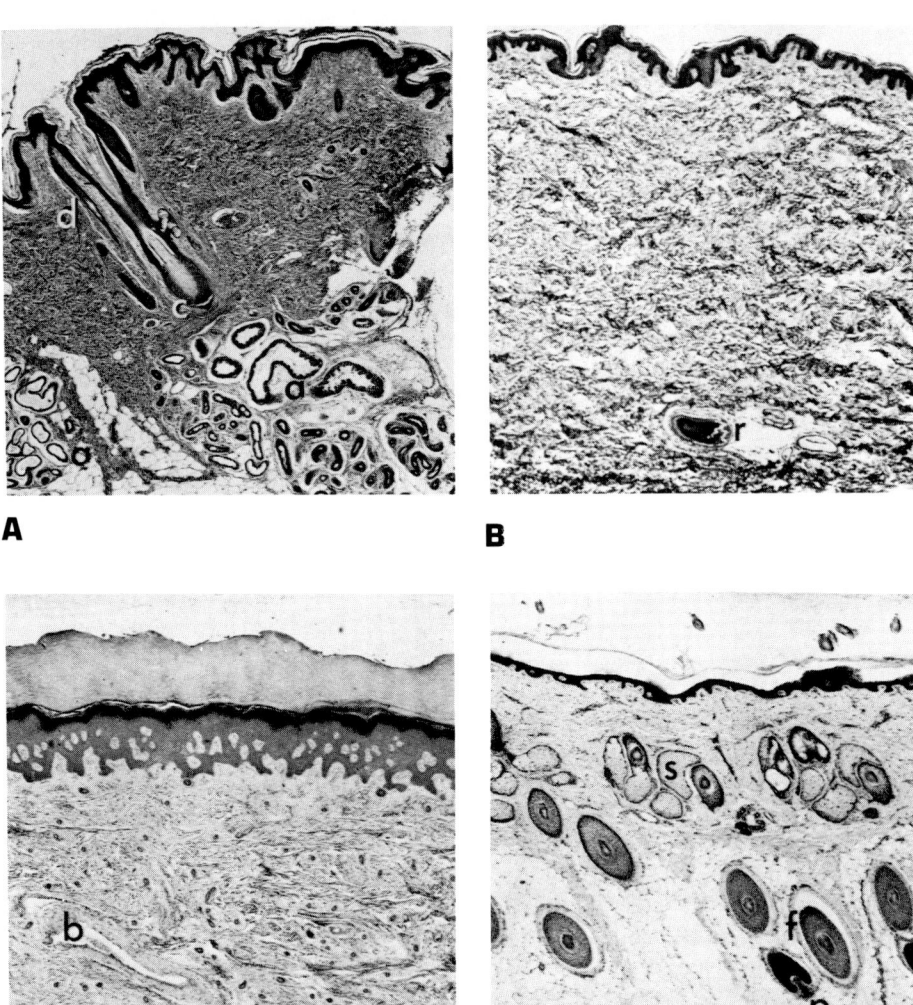

Figure 2–1.
Normal skin from four different body areas stained with H&E. X21. **A.** Axilla. **B.** Back of trunk. **C.** Sole. **D.** Scalp. a, apocrine coil; b, artery; c, catagen hair; d, apocrine duct; f, fibrous root sheath; p, hair papilla; r, hair root; s, sebaceous gland.

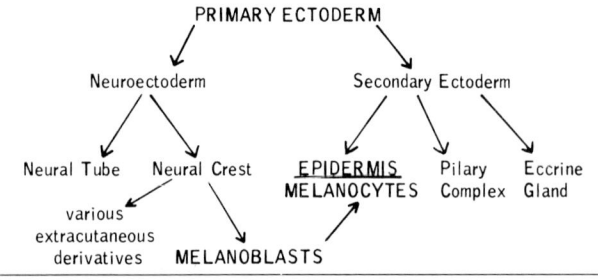

Figure 2–2.
Ectodermal derivatives. Note that the epidermis is but one of several ectodermal structures in the skin and that melanocytes reenter the skin secondarily as neuroectodermal derivatives and find their final location at the dermoepidermal junction.

body and amniotic fluid. Scanning electron microscopic studies have shown that the outer surfaces of periderm cells carry microvilli and fuzz, like those seen in exchange-active epithelia (Fig. 2–3B). After the 16th week, periderm is replaced by keratinizing cells, and the epidermis gradually assumes the characteristics of the stratified adult tissue. For diagnosis of fetal genetic disorders of keratinization such as the ichthyosis group of disorders, the best time is between weeks 16 and 24 of estimated age of gestation.[7]

The dermis (also called cutis and corium) is furnished by embryonic mesoderm.[8] Portions of the dermis are temporarily organized into somites and, thus, have metameral structure. Segmental organization, however, soon stops in the skin, and major portions of the dermis on the head, neck, and extremities are not derived from somites. So-called

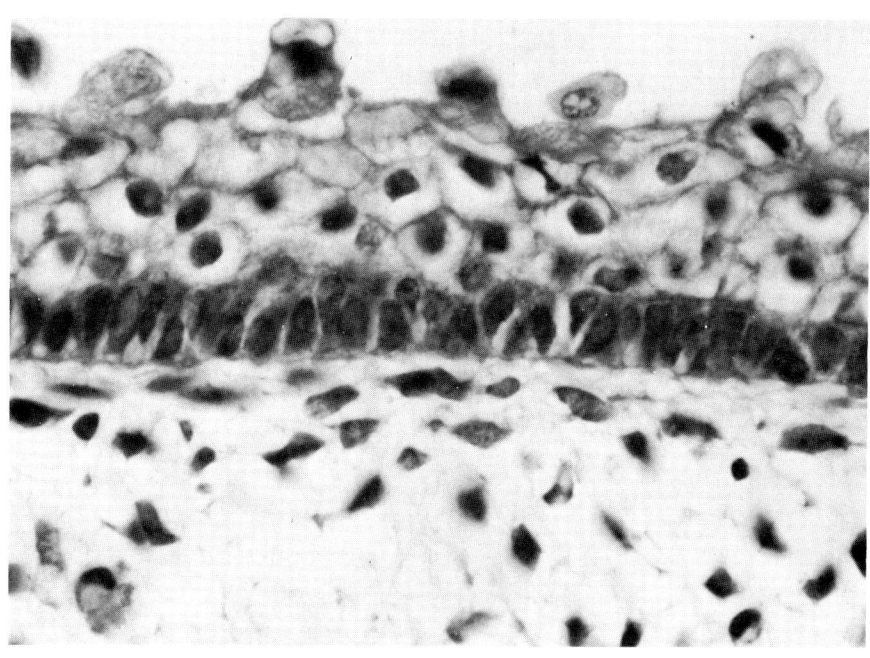

Figure 2–3.
A. Skin of fetal foot showing stratified epidermis, with columnar basal cells, pale (glycogenrich) prickle cells, and exfoliating periderm cells. Not all areas of body achieve this high degree of fetal differentiation. Dermis is relatively unstructured, consisting of stellate cells and few thin collagen fibers suspended in mucinous ground substance. H&E. X600. **B.** Scanning electron micrograph of surface of similar skin. Polygonal outline of uppermost prickle cells. Protruding periderm cells showing microvilli, some of which have exfoliated. X840. (Courtesy of Dr. W. H. Wilborn.)

dermatomes are established secondarily by the distribution of segmental nerves. Similarly, whereas some blood vessels are derived from segmental arteries, many form as a plexus in the local mesenchyme. In 40 to 45 days in the human embryo, a single plexus parallel to the skin surface exists at the dermal–subcutaneous interface, and the majority of blood vessels are discontinuous.[9] This suggests the formation of local cutaneous blood vessels rather than their developing from the main trunk. At certain times, the embryonic skin is a blood cell-forming organ, a function that can be revived under pathologic conditions. Connective tissue fibers are laid down gradually, reticulum and collagen first, then elastin.[10]

The two types of cutaneous adnexa—pilar com-

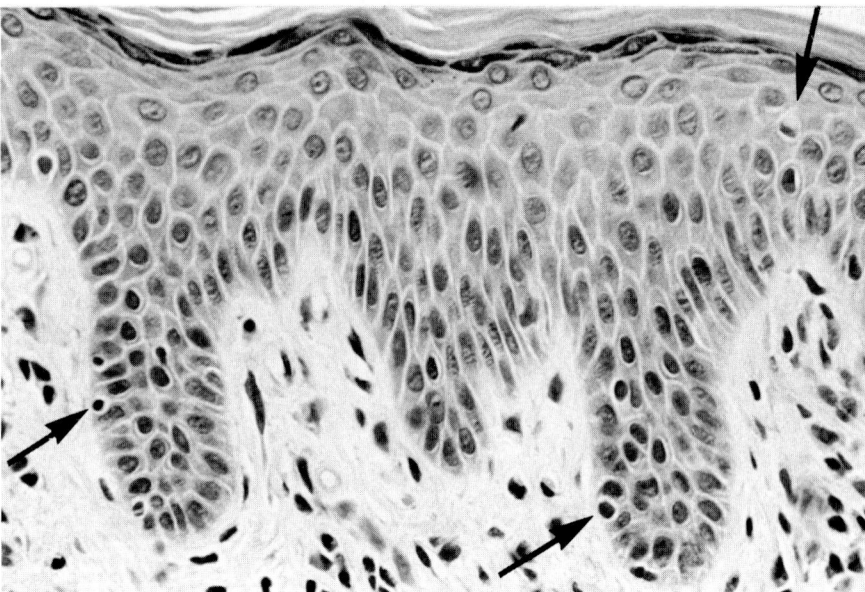

Figure 2-4.
Vertical section of adult epidermis. Well-developed ridges and papillae, thick stratum spinosum, and multiple stratum granulosum under the nonnucleated stratum corneum. Basal cells are more or less columnar. Two arrows point to junctional melanocytes. Arrow at right points to a high-level dendritic cell that may be a Langerhans cell. Papillae contain fixed tissue-type cells embedded in fibrillar connective tissue H&E. X370.

plexes and eccrine glands—differentiate individually from the epidermal basal layer in which ectoderm and mesoderm interact. The cells of hair germ and eccrine germ form a new biologic unit. They grow by mitotic division of their own elements and penetrate downward through the dermis. Hair canal and intraepidermal ducts of the eccrine gland (acrosyringium) are produced above the hair and eccrine germs by early keratinization of specialized units of epidermal cells.[11] Although the eccrine apparatus remains a simple tubular unit throughout life, the pilar germ becomes a complex miniature organ consisting of hair root, sebaceous gland, apocrine gland, arrector muscle, and haarscheibe. During growth and function, ectodermal and mesodermal components continuously interact, and the term "primary epithelial germ" should be abandoned in favor of either "older hair germ" or the more inclusive "hair apparatus germ." Many ultrastructural data on the embryology of human hair have been contributed by Hashimoto (reviewed by Holbrook[5]).

EPIDERMIS

The epidermis is a stratified epithelial tissue (Fig. 2–4) that renews itself continually through mitotic division of its basal cells. Daughter cells take suprabasal position and undergo a slow process of maturation during which they are described as prickle (spinous) cells, granular (keratohyalin) cells, and anuclear horny cells or corneocytes. All of these phases of the epidermal keratinocyte (Table 2–1) are comparable to the maturing stages of the erythropoietic series, from stem cell through erythroblast and normoblast to erythrocyte. The mature keratinized cell is the product of terminal differentiation of the daughter keratinocyte derived from germinative basal cell, just as the nonnucleated red cell is the all-important end product of hematopoiesis. Both are functionally active and biologically dead.

TABLE 2–1. BIOLOGY OF THE KERATINOCYTE

Common Name	Biologic Function	Hematologic Analog
Basal cell	Principal matrix (epidermal germinative cell) adhesion to dermis	Medullary stem cell
Prickle (malpighian) cell	Auxiliary matrix, early stage of keratinization, mechanical stability	Erythroblast
Granular (keratohyalin) cell	Progressing keratinization, part of physiologic barrier	Normoblast
Keratinized (horny) cell (corneocyte)	Functionally mature, biologically dead, mechanical and chemical barrier	Erythrocyte

Epidermal Layers

Precise terminology is a prerequisite for clear thinking and scientific communication. We, therefore, list various definitions in Table 2–2. The term basal cell means cell at the base in contact with the basal lamina (or lamina densa). Basal cells anywhere in the skin are the principal germinal cells for epidermis and adnexa, but under pathologic conditions, for example, in psoriatic epidermis, the anatomic basal cells are not synonymous with physiologic germinal cells. In psoriasis and in other conditions of rapid epidermal proliferation, one or more suprabasal layers may be part of the stratum germinativum.

Basal Cells

Epidermal basal cells may be flat, cuboidal, or columnar. In conformity with their shape, they contain a round or ovoid nucleus, although this depends

TABLE 2–2. DEFINITIONS AND RECOMMENDED TERMS IN EPIDERMAL AND ADNEXAL HISTOLOGY

Epidermis

Definition
Epithelial tissue derived from embryonic ectoderm and covering the outer surface of the skin. (See Fig. 2–2.) Sometimes inappropriately used in a wider sense for all ectodermal epithelia in the skin.

Recommended Terms
1. *Epidermis* for surface epithelium of skin.
2. *Mucosal epithelium* for surface epithelium of oral and other mucous membranes.
3. *Adnexal epithelium* (follicular, sebaceous, eccrine, and apocrine) for epithelial parts of hair follicles and cutaneous glands.
4. *Ectodermal epithelium* when two or all of the above are meant.
5. *Ectodermal modulated cell* for quasi-embryonic cell in wound healing or other emergency situations (see Fig. 2–14).
6. *Stratified* for any multilayered epithelium whether of ectodermal or entodermal origin.
7. *Squamous* for any multilayered epithelium in which cells flatten and usually keratinize toward the surface.
8. *Epidermoid* for any epithelium keratinizing in the epidermal (orthokeratotic) manner with keratohyalin formation.

The Ubiquitous and Confusing Basal Cell

Anatomic Definition
1. Lowest cell in epidermis in contact with dermis
2. Outermost cell of cutaneous adnexa in contact with dermis

Recommended Terms
1. *Epidermal basal cell*
2. *Adnexal basal cell*

Physiologic Definition
1. Immature matrix cell of epidermis
2. Immature matrix cell of adnexa

Recommended Terms
1. *Epidermal matrix (or germinal) cell*
2. *Adnexal matrix cell*

Pathologic Definition
1. Immature cell of benign tumors
2. Specific cell of basal cell epitheliomas (basal cell carcinomas)

Recommended Terms
1. *Basaloid cell*
2. *Basalioma cell*

Keratinocyte

Definition
Any epithelial cell that is part of a keratinizing tissue.

Recommended Terms
1. *Epidermal keratinocyte* (see Table 2–1).
2. *Adnexal keratinocytes* compose all parts of the hair and hair follicle, the sebaceous duct, and the intraepidermal sweat duct (acrosyringium).
3. *Prickle cell*, although actually a misnomer, remains the accepted term for cells between the basal and the granular or keratinized layers. *Spinous cell*, which has the same meaning, is less commonly used. *Squamous cell* implies that the cell either is or is expected to become a squame or flake. The term is applied mainly to the cells of epidermoid carcinomas.
4. *Keratinized cell* (*horny cell, corneocyte*) applies mainly to nonnucleated cells above the granular layer (orthokeratotic cells) but is also used for nucleated parakeratotic cells once they have reached the final stage of their development.

Nonkeratinocytes

Definition
Cells found in the epidermis that do not undergo keratinization.

Recommended Terms
1. *Dendritic cells* comprising *melanocytes, Langerhans cells*, and *Merkel cells*, all of which live in the epidermis as symbionts.
2. Mesodermal cells that have entered the epidermis by the process of exocytosis might be included in a wider sense but are better identified as small round cells, granulocytes, mast cells, and so on.
3. Nonkeratinizing tumor cells should be designated as nevus cells, malignant melanoma cells, Paget cells, and so on.

somewhat on the angle at which the section has been cut. Sections cut perpendicular to the skin surface and basal lamina reveal spindle-shaped basal cells with an oblong nucleus. The nucleus stains dark with hematoxylin and has a coarse chromatin network, usually without a prominent nucleolus. The tumor cells of basal cell epitheliomas (basal cell carcinomas, basaliomas) bear only a very superficial resemblance to normal basal cells. They are called basaloid cells, or in the case of basal cell epithelioma, basalioma cells. In addition to their role as germinal cells, basal cells maintain the connection between dermis and epidermis. Basal cells possess numerous pedicles or rootlets that greatly increase the contact surface with the basal lamina. Other surfaces of the basal cell are connected with neighboring basal cells and prickle cells by means of desmosomes on which intracellular tonofibrils attach. Thick bundles of the latter are known as Herxheimer spirals. Basal cells are connected to each other by desmosomes and gap junctions which are frequently seen in a series with desmosomes. They connect to the basal lamina by numerous fine filaments called anchoring filaments, which are particularly dense under the hemidesmosome.

Prickle Cells and Granular Cells

The multiple layers of prickle cells (spinous cells) constitute the rete malpighi. The term Prickle cell is a misnomer inasmuch as the cells do not have free-ending prickles or spines. Prickle cells that become separated from neighbors, as in pemphigus or other acantholytic dermatoses, show a smooth contour. The prickles appear during the dehydration procedure in specimens that are not well fixed. The tightly connected desmosomal areas are drawn out into bridges and, in transverse section, give the appearance of prickles. Early investigators chose condyloma acuminatum to study prickle cells because this hyperplastic and edematous epidermis shows cellular detail much better than normal tissue does. Figure 2–5 represents hyperplastic epidermis of chronic eczematous dermatitis. Electron microscopy has shown that intercellular spaces normally are very narrow and that cell contours are convoluted and interlocking. With intercellular edema or in specimens in which fixation caused some shrinkage (Fig. 2–6), cells pull away from each other but remain connected by the desmosomes, which now seem to sit as bridge nodules (Bizzozero's nodule) at the center of stretched out cell periphery. In spite of their complicated structure (Fig. 2–7), desmosomes break and reform with relative ease, probably within hours,[12] whenever keratinocytes move against each other or leukocytes migrate between them. The separated cell surfaces then have microvilli but these are submicroscopic and should not be confused with prickles.

Tonofibrils are largely responsible for the dense, somewhat bluish appearance of prickle cell cytoplasm in H&E section. Tonofibrils are demon-

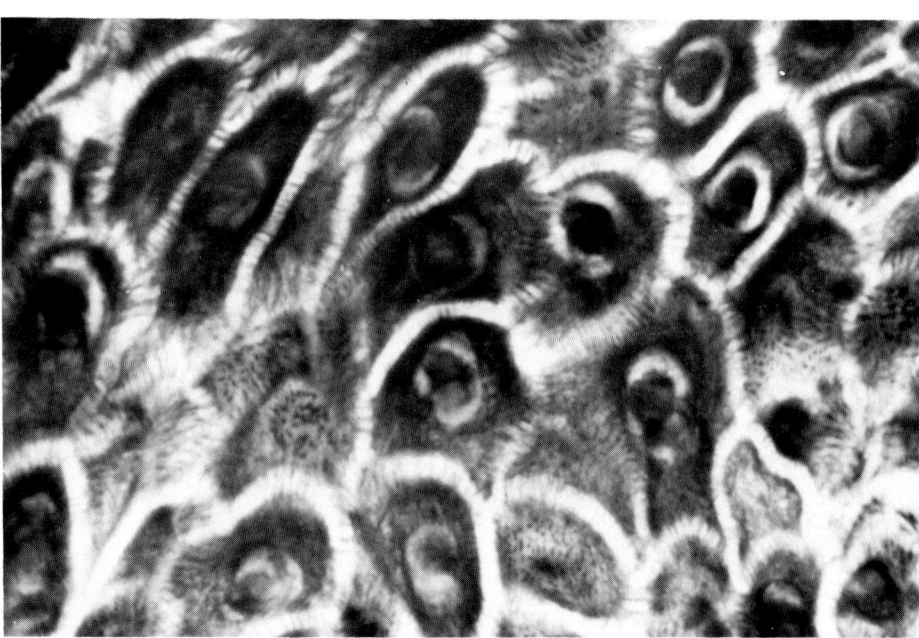

Figure 2–5.
Prickle cells in chronic eczematous dermatitis. Intercellular bridges are stretched across widened intercellular spaces. Bridges appear as dark dots where cut transversely, no free prickles. Slight thickening in center of some bridges represents Bizzozero's nodule (desmosome). Hematoxylin–Ponceau S–picric acid. ×900.

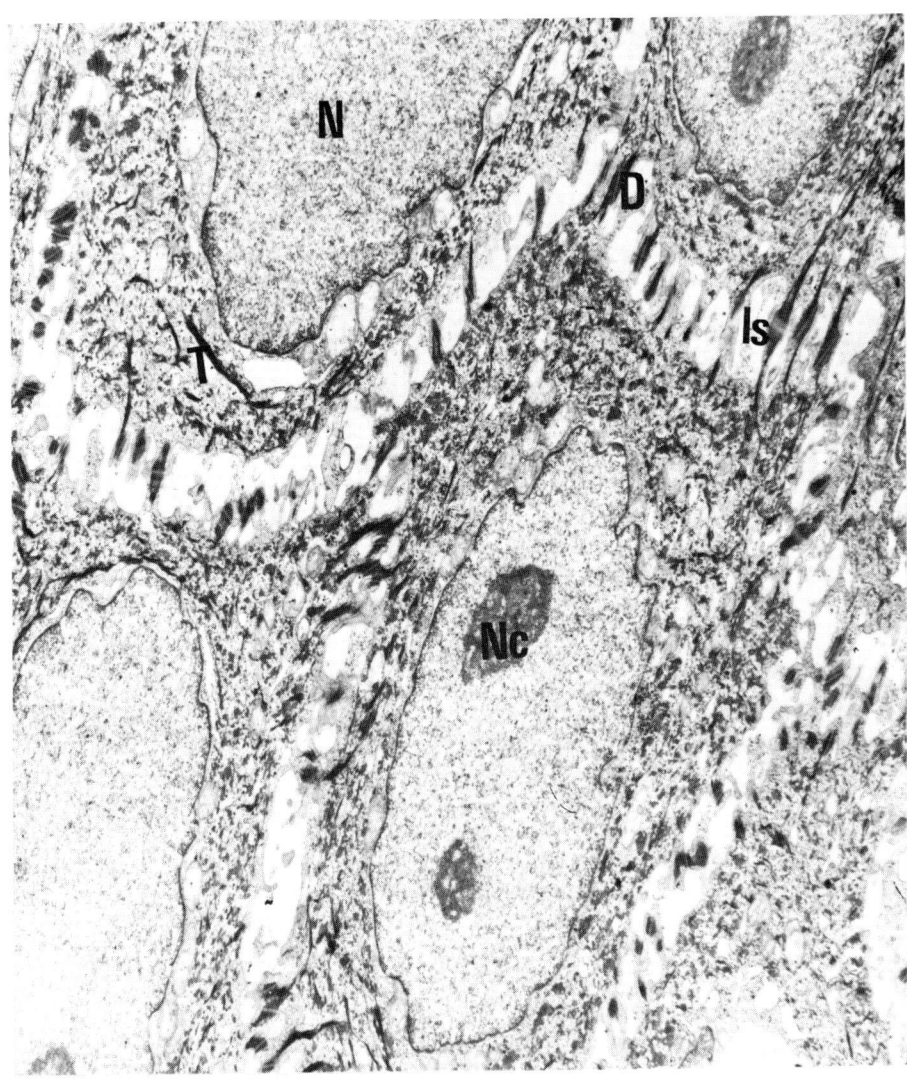

Figure 2–6.
Four prickle cells connected by stretched intercellular bridges in slightly edematous skin. Dark tonofilaments (T) in the cytoplasm extend into the bridges and are connected to desmosomes (D). Is, intercellular space; N, nuclei; Nc, nucleoli. Electron micrograph. X11,200. (Courtesy of Dr. A. P. Lupulescu.)

strable with monoclonal or polyclonal antikeratin antibodies using immunofluorescence or peroxidase methods.

Prickle cells are bulkier than basal cells, have vesicular nuclei with distinct membrane, and have one or several angular nucleoli (Fig. 2–6). Cells in the higher layers become flat and eventually acquire keratohyalin granules; the nucleus becomes pyknotic and then disappears. A cell normally goes through these stages in about 2 weeks, although individual variations exist.

Prickle cells usually contain glycogen. As the essential energy source for cellular metabolism, glycogen is found in all layers of the embryonic epidermis. It is first used up in the early hair germ and later is distributed in suprabasal layers, that is, glycogen disappears from basal cells, but it remains present in prickle cells until postnatal life.[4] In the adult, basal cells contain glycogen only under exceptional circumstances such as rapid proliferation after tape stripping. Prickle cells may contain glycogen in any acanthotic epidermis, either evenly distributed or, more frequently, concentrated in one part of the cytoplasm. Psoriatic epidermis contains it regularly.

The cells of the granular layer appear fusiform (Fig. 2–8A) in vertical sections of skin. Their true three-dimensional shape resembles that of a fried egg, which may be seen in tangential sections of thick epidermis (Fig. 2–8B). The degenerating nucleus produces a central bulge in the flattened cell body. Keratohyalin has a strong affinity for hematoxylin. Its chemical substance has been identified with filaggrin.[13] Keratohyalin granules are color-

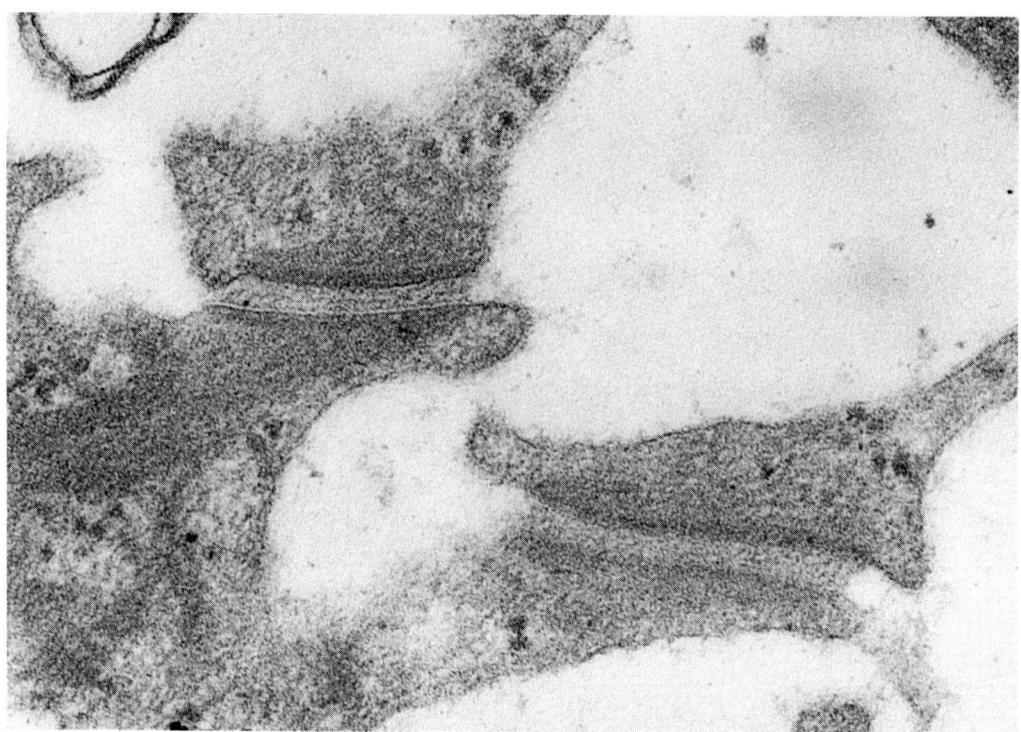

Figure 2–7.
High magnification of two desmosomes sitting at the center of stretched cytoplasmic bridges that contain dark tonofilaments. The desmosomes have several electron-dense and electron-lucent layers and a thickened plasma membrane at either side. (Courtesy of Dr. A. P. Lupulescu.)

less in living tissue, but their close arrangement and refractivity have an effect similar to that of glass beads on a projection screen, making the skin surface look white. They also diffuse all colors below them, so that black or brown material in the dermis appears gray. A blue tinge is added by the opaqueness of the white dermal collagen.[14] These effects assume clinical significance in several dermatoses, for example, lichen planus (Wickham's striae), leukoplakia, and certain pigmentary disorders.

Another organelle, first described by Selby and later by Odland, is produced in the uppermost layers of prickle cells.[15] It has been given a variety of names including lamellar body, membrane coating granule, keratinosome, cementosome, or Odland body. This body is visible only under the electron microscope (100–300 nm). It contains acid phosphatase and phospholipids in a laminated internal structure. After being discharged from the cell, these bodies or granules spread their contents in the intercellular spaces of the lower horny layer to produce intercellular adhesive cement, which simultaneously functions as a penetration barrier against foreign substances.

Also noted in the upper prickle cell layer to granular layer is a thickening of cell membrane. Initially it was thought that this occurred because the membrane coating granules that are discharged at this level of keratinization thicken the cell membrane from outside. It was later demonstrated, however, that this membrane thickening takes place from inside of the cells[16] by an addition of newly synthesized sulfur-rich protein called involucrin.[17] This layer is named the marginal band,[16] or the cellular envelope of cornified cell or cornified envelope.[18]

Keratinized Cells

Above the granular layer, the nuclei disappear. The cells assume the shape of pancakes and have dense membranes that are strengthened by the marginal band (Fig. 2–9). Because of the close adhesion of cell membranes between neighboring cells due to intercellular cement, splitting of cell body takes place in an irregular fashion when the outermost cells must

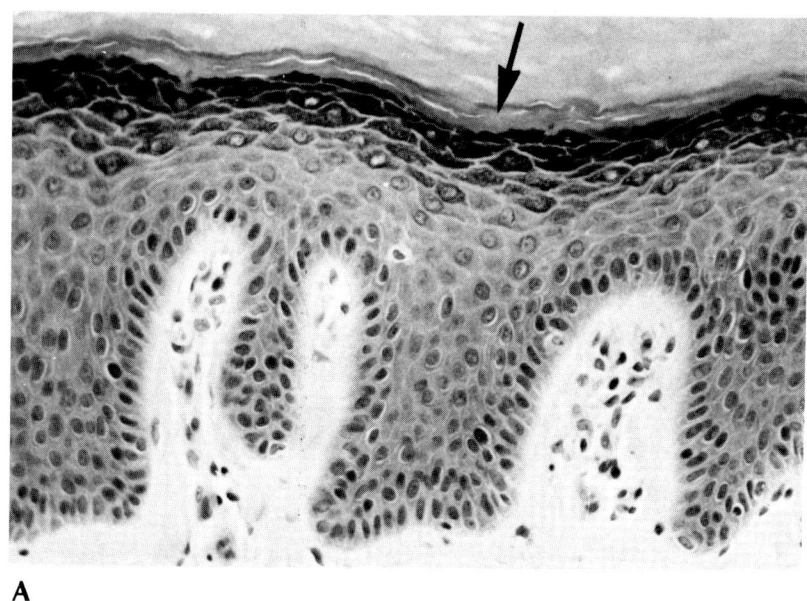

A

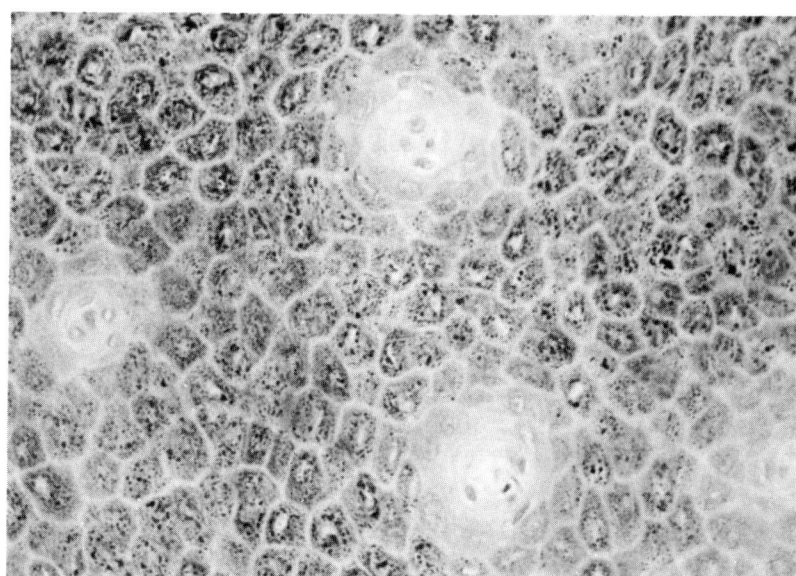

B

Figure 2–8.
A. Vertical section of thick epidermis of volar skin showing a thick stratum granulosum and stratum lucidum (arrow) that appears darker than the stratum corneum. Two cells in stratum spinosum, consisting of dark nucleus and light halo, may be Langerhans cells. H&E. X370. **B.** Tangential section through stratum granulosum with cross sections of three eccrine sweat ducts. The polygonal shape of granular cells is well depicted. H&E. X370.

shed. This produces the basketweave appearance of the stratum corneum. The apparently empty spaces are the cell bodies. The true shape of the corneocytes is best seen in scrapings such as the KOH fungus mount where the cells appear as symmetrical or elongated polygonal flakes with diameters varying from 30 μm to over 40 μm.[19] This type of examination reveals regional differences and shows characteristic alterations of horny cells in some dermatoses.[20,21] The transition zone between stratum granulosum and stratum corneum, if it is thick, can be recognized as stratum lucidum (Fig. 2–8A), the cells of which appear homogeneous and less eosinophilic (thus lucid) under the light microscope. The poor staining is due to immaturity of keratin in this layer.

Epidermal Biology

Figure 2–10 relates the changes of cell size and shape with epidermal biology. Nature's economy requires that only 4 broad and flat keratinized cells on the epidermal surface are needed to cover the area that is occupied by 100 columnar cells at the base. Thus, relatively infrequent mitoses in the basal germinal layer suffice to replace exfoliating surface lay-

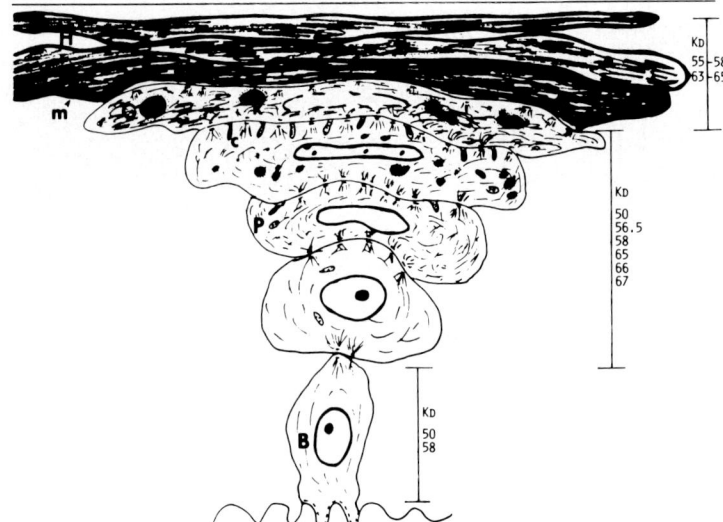

Figure 2–9.
Schematic representation of terminal differentiation of an epidermal basal cell (B) to prickle cell (P), granular cell (G) and horny cell (H). During this process keratohyalin granules (k), cementosomes or laminated bodies (c), and marginal band (m) are produced. Many different species of keratin designated by molecular weight (Kd) are synthesized in each layer, many of which disappear in the next layer, either by degradation or masking.

ers. Ordinarily, the presence of rete ridges makes the proportion of basal cells to keratinized cells much more favorable because the undulated basal surface can contain more cells per unit area of the skin surface, which is usually flat.

Mitotic indices of 0.1 to 1 per 1000, as determined by various investigators, are sufficient for average epidermal turnover in which the total lifespan of a keratinocyte is about 40 to 56 days.[22,23] This slow renewal of the epidermis can accelerate tremendously in emergencies, such as following removal of the stratum corneum by tape stripping or accidental trauma, and in disease, such as psoriasis.[24] The mitotic index may rise as high as 50 per 1000 viable cells. Under the reasonable assumption of 1 hour for mitotic duration, this makes complete renewal of the epidermis possible in 20 hours. It has been shown that in keeping with general biologic rules,[25] the epidermis needs 36 to 48 hours to retool for this speedup.

The direction of renewal (growth) in the human epidermis is outward under most circumstances except neoplasia or pseudoepitheliomatous proliferation.[26] The true biologic baseline for epidermal growth process is the epidermal–dermal interface. When the interlocking rete ridges and papillae elongate in psoriasis or lichen simplex, the suprapapillary portions of the epidermis are lifted up and moved farther away from this baseline. "Downgrowth" of the rete ridges does not exist in the sense that long ridges extend into a deeper level of the dermis.

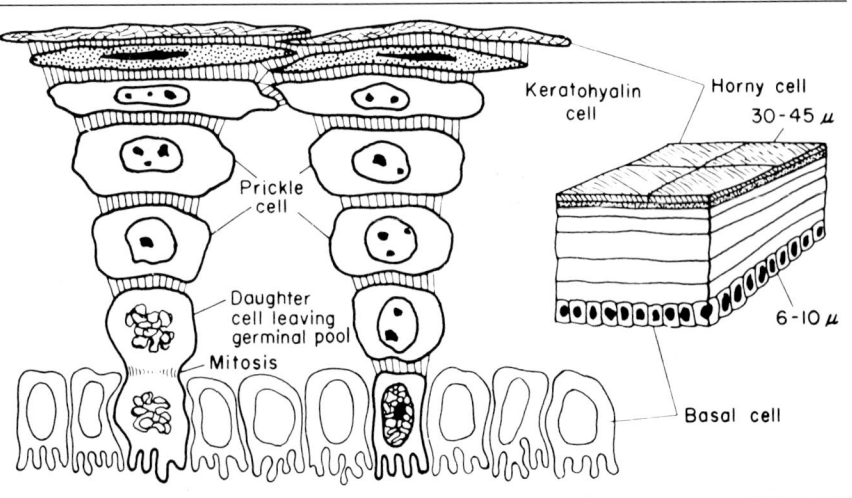

Figure 2–10.
Diagram of epidermal biology emphasizes changes in size and shape of keratinocytes from basal layer to horny layer. Insert shows 10 × 10 = 100 basal cells covering the same area as 2 × 2 = 4 keratinized cells. Mitotic division takes place in basal layer. (Adapted from Pinkus. In Handbuch der Haut- und Geschlechtskrankheiten, Ergänzungswerk, 1, 2, 1965. Courtesy of Springer-Verlag.)

Epidermal Architecture

The epidermis, a tissue consisting of living fragile cells in a state of steady biologic flux, forms a surprisingly tough outer coat without the benefit of extracellular skeletal substances. This is possible because the surface of the skin is tightly covered with tough cornified cells that contain keratin fibers and a strong cell membrane that is thickened by the formation marginal band. Filaggrin derived from keratohyaline granules embeds the keratin filaments. All these final products of keratinization are as much resistant to mechanical and chemical damages as hair and nail, also being keratin products. The individual horny cells are cemented together by the products of cementosomes or lamellar bodies that are also resistant to mechanical and chemical damages. Thus, the horny layer forms a very resistant outer barrier of the skin.

Inspection at low magnification[27,28] shows the surface of normal skin to be crisscrossed by both coarse and fine wrinkles that assume special configurations in the ridged skin of palms and soles (dermatoglyphics). In histopathologic examination, most surface wrinkles appear as relatively minor depressions between fairly straight or slightly rounded stretches. More pronounced serrations of the outer contour are pathologic (papillomatosis, see Chapter 5). The epidermal–dermal interface is straight only in atrophic skin, and on the face. The interface has a system of ridges between which the vascular papillae of the dermis are inserted. One might say that the epidermal ridges interdigitate with the projections of papillary dermis. This is illustrated in Figure 2–11, which also shows that rete pegs are a misinterpretation of transverse section of rete ridges. Oblique sections of thick normal skin (Fig. 2–12) furnish surprising but highly instructive pictures. This should be kept in mind in the interpretation of pathologic specimens because not all specimens are embedded and cut in the ideal manner.

Epidermal Symbiosis

The epidermis contains two independent structural units, the intraepidermal portions of pilar complex (acrotrichium) and the eccrine apparatus (acrosyringium). The epidermis may be considered a symbiosis because all the components maintain themselves in balance by mitotic division of their own germinal cells but they may act and react quite independently under pathologic conditions.

In adult life, acrosyringeal cells have several features by which they can be distinguished quite easily from epidermal keratinocytes.[29] They never contain melanin, even in the darkest black epidermis (Fig. 2–13), and do not contain microscopically visible tonofibrils (although electron microscopy reveals tonofilaments). These cells often have roundish nuclei with several small chromatin masses and begin to form keratohyalin and keratinize at a lower level in the epidermis than epidermal keratinocytes.

Acrotrichial keratinocytes, on the other hand, are practically indistinguishable from the epidermis

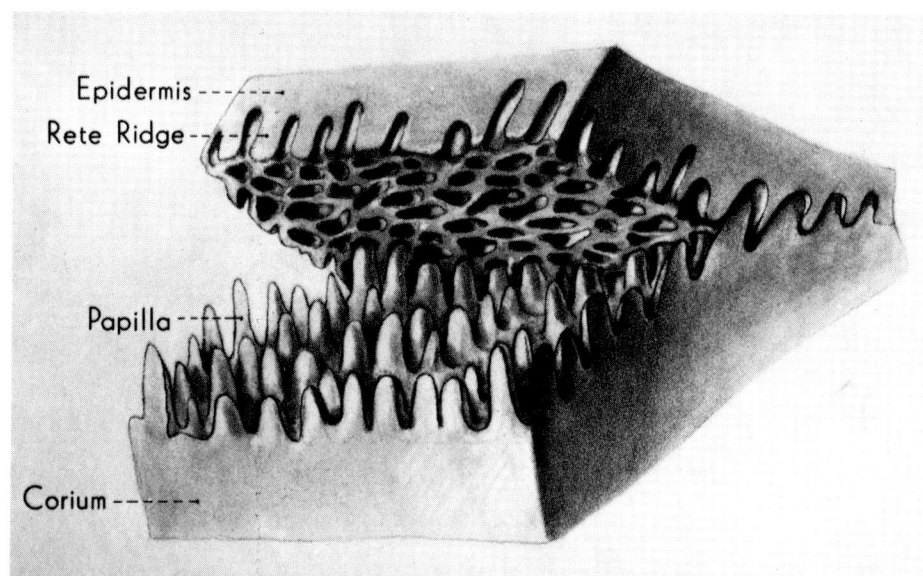

Figure 2–11.
Artist's drawing of dermoepidermal interface. This three-dimensional view illustrates the effect that would result if epidermis were lifted after pretreatment of fresh skin with dilute acetic acid or other agents. Dermal papillae are pulled out of reciprocating depressions between epidermal ridges. Front of tissue block shows peglike cross sections of rete ridges as seen in paraffin sections, as in Figure 2–4.

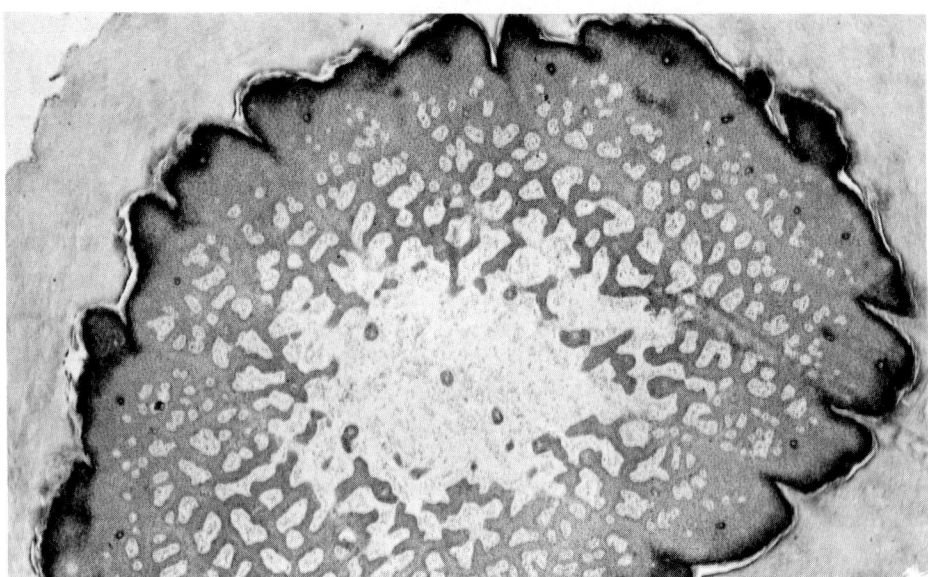

Figure 2–12.
Oblique section of finger skin. H&E. Pictures of this type, while confusing in histopathologic specimens (see Fig. 3–15), reveal three-dimensional architecture of epidermis and show regular spacing of cross-sectioned eccrine ducts.

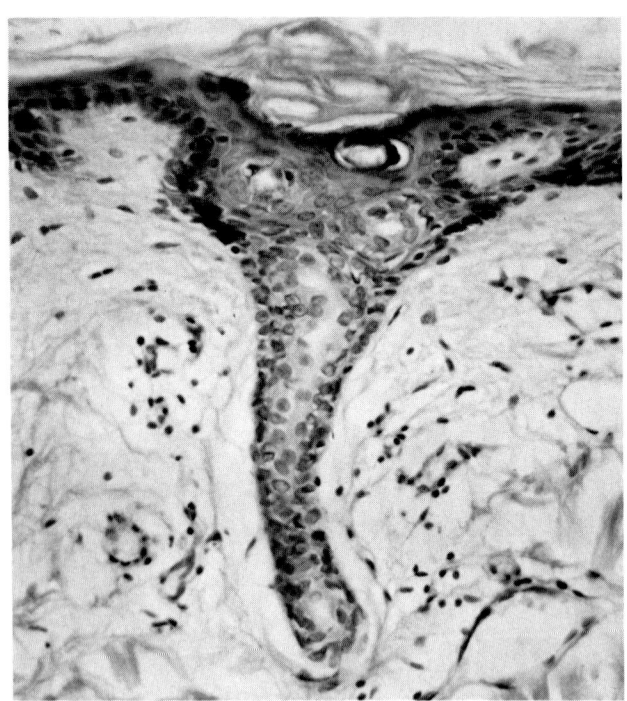

Figure 2–13.
Acrosyringium. Nonpigmented eccrine duct coils in relatively thin pigmented epidermis and is cut transversely six times in stratum malpighi and stratum corneum. Cells of intraepidermal eccrine unit contain keratohyalin in second and third turn and are fully keratinized in three upper turns. H&E. X180.

that surrounds them. This has been the reason for the often repeated but incorrect statement that the follicular infundibulum is an invagination of the epidermal layers. It is unnecessary to repeat at this point all the evidence for the existence of the intraepidermal follicular wall.[30] Once we accept the concept, however, many features of skin pathology, especially of epidermal and adnexal neoplasia can be explained.

Thus, acrosyringium and acrotrichium are biologically separate symbionts in the epidermis under normal and many abnormal conditions. In certain emergency situations, however, especially in wound healing, adnexal keratinocytes become modulated (Fig. 2–14), return to a quasi-embryonic state, and redifferentiate into epidermis indistinguishable from the one they replace. This ambivalence of adnexal cells must be kept in mind and will be referred to in later chapters.

DERMOEPIDERMAL JUNCTION

The dermoepidermal junction is a complicated structure in three dimension (Figs. 2–10 and 2–11). PAS stain (Fig. 2–15) reveals a sharply defined thin zone of neutral mucopolysaccharides, which is similarly prominent in immunofluorescent examinations in a number of diseases (Chapter 4). This zone is often referred to as basement membrane zone or BMZ. Electron microscopy (Fig. 2–16) has shown[29] that

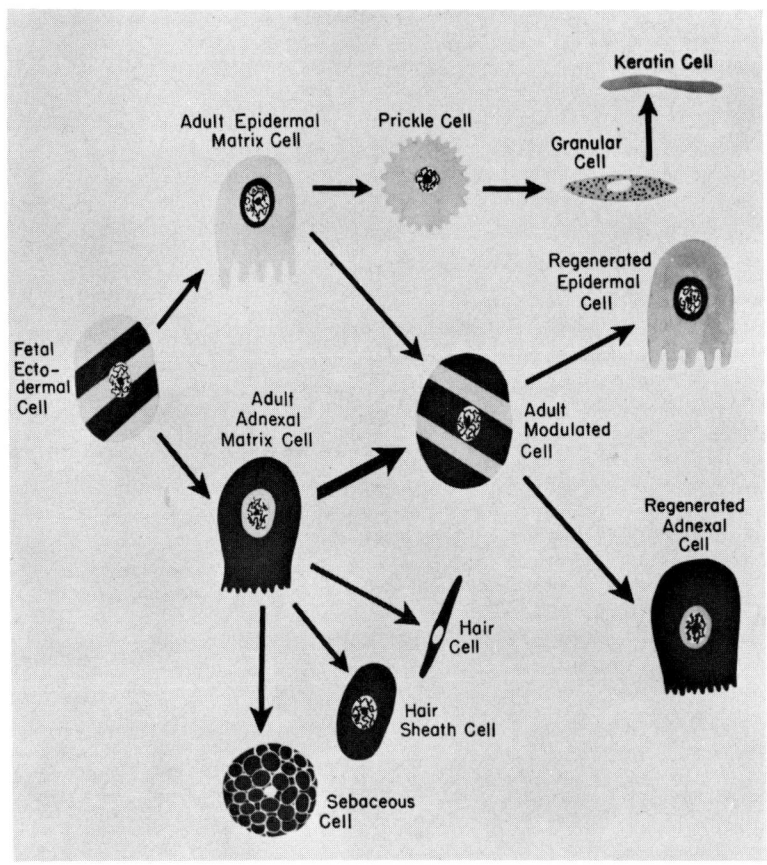

Figure 2–14.
Diagram of ectodermal pluripotentiality and modulation. Fetal ectodermal cell (left) has epidermal (light gray) and adnexal (dark) potential. Adult ectodermal cell, whether epidermal or adnexal matrix cell, preserves in latent form opposite potential (indicated by ring around nucleus), which becomes manifest in quasi-fetal modulated cell of healing wound. Modulated cells derived mainly from adnexal matrix cells redifferentiate in epidermal or adnexal direction.

PAS-positive BMZ is composed of several fine structures: the cell membrane of the basal cell and its rootlets are paralleled in all its convolutions by a thin (300 nm), electron-dense basal lamina (or lamina densa), which is separated from the cell membrane by an electron-lucent gap (lamina lucida). The cell carries hemidesmosomes to which intracellular tonofilaments converge. The dense basal lamina is connected to underlying collagen fibrils by special anchoring fibrils. Details are illustrated diagrammatically in Figure 2–17.

This basement membrane zone is what the term junction implies. It is a zone consisting of different materials that insure a firm cohesion between epidermis and dermis. How it is disrupted under pathologic conditions is found in the discussion of sub-

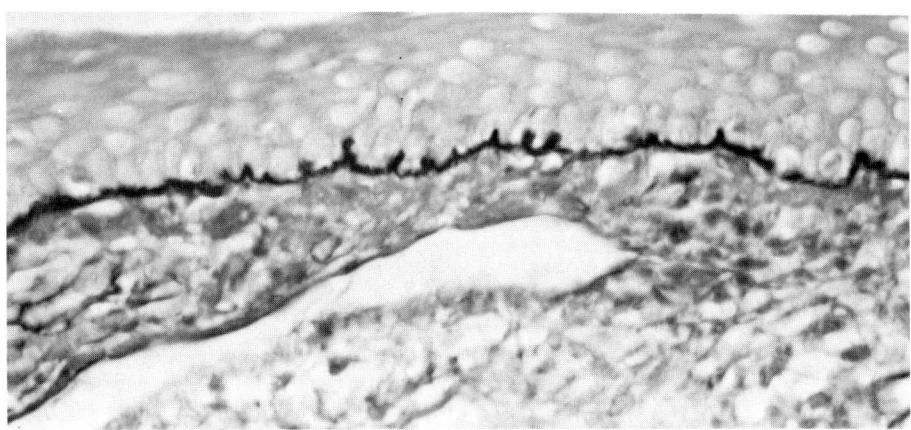

Figure 2–15.
PAS-positive basement membrane at dermoepidermal interface. Alcian blue–PAS–picric acid stain. X460.

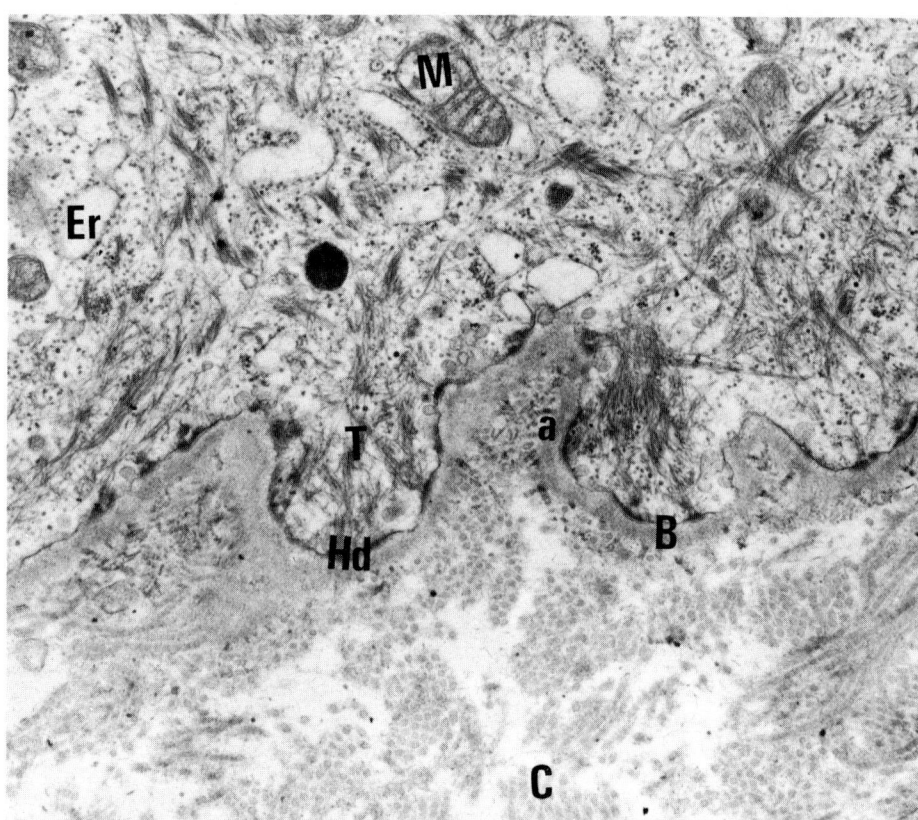

Figure 2–16.
Electron micrograph of dermoepidermal junction. Basal lamina (B) with anchoring fibrils (a) and hemidesmosomes (Hd) to which tonofilaments (T) extend. Mitochondrion (M) and rough endoplasmic reticulum (Er) in basal cell. Collagen fibrils (C) in dermis. X36,000. (Courtesy of Dr. A. P. Lupulescu.)

epidermal bullae (Chapter 11). The basement membrane zone is not a rigid immovable structure. It is probably constantly moving as basal cells divide, interact with dermis, or are pushed up by migrating dermal cells. Some of the constituents of the BMZ are contributed by the epidermis, others by the dermis, and basement membrane formation is the result of combined participation of the two tissues. Therefore, presence of basement membrane in a benign tumor or in basal cell epithelioma indicates that epithelium and mesenchyme are compatible and collaborating. Absence of basement membrane in a true carcinoma does not mean that it has been broken through and destroyed, but that its formation has ceased because of the malignant character of the epithelial cells. When epidermis undergoes pseudocarcinomatous proliferation, the benign but rapidly proliferating or migrating epithelium does not form a basement membrane until it returns to more normal conditions.

Basement membrane is also no physiologic barrier. Most substances injected into the dermis penetrate it easily. Neutrophils, lymphocytes, and Langerhans cells go through it from the dermis. Immunoglobulins collect on the membrane in many diseases, whereas the antibodies of pemphigus travel through it to bind to cell membranes.

DERMIS

The mesoderm of the skin is conveniently divided into three components: the pars papillaris consisting of papillae and subpapillary layer, the pars reticularis, and the subcutaneous fat tissue or hypoderm. In all layers we encounter cells, fibers, and ground substance, plus the more highly structured vessels and nerves. Embedded in the dermis are pilar and eccrine apparatuses, which are discussed later in this chapter.

Pars Papillaris

The pars papillaris contains relatively more cells and vessels than the pars reticularis. It is structurally and functionally associated with the epidermis, with which it forms the dermoepidermal junction, a unit junction that weighs a total of close to 900 g in the average adult. This estimate is based on the gen-

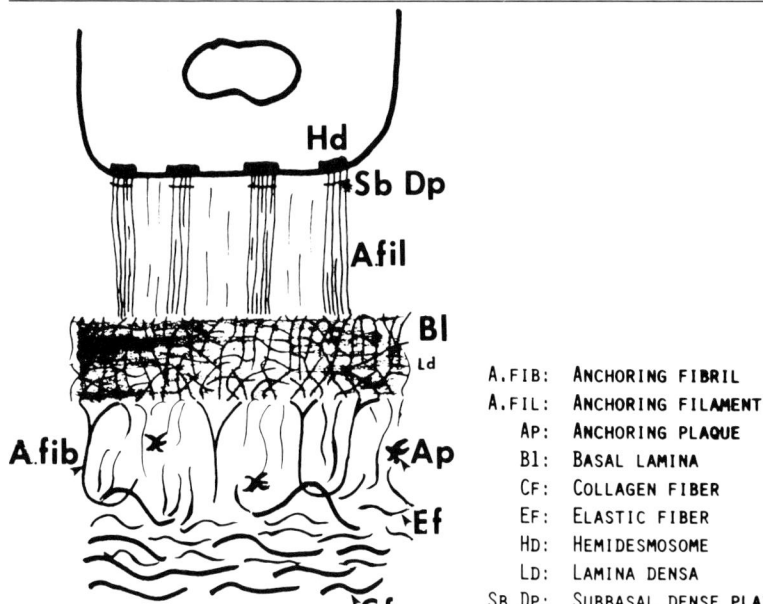

Figure 2-17.
Illustrations of various components of the basement membrane zone.

A.FIB: ANCHORING FIBRIL
A.FIL: ANCHORING FILAMENT
AP: ANCHORING PLAQUE
Bl: BASAL LAMINA
CF: COLLAGEN FIBER
EF: ELASTIC FIBER
HD: HEMIDESMOSOME
LD: LAMINA DENSA
SB DP: SUBBASAL DENSE PLATE

erally accepted values of 1.8 m² area for skin surface and 500 μm thickness of combined epidermis and pars papillaris. The pars papillaris, about one tenth of the entire skin, alone is involved in most of the common inflammatory dermatoses. Sweet[30] used the term "epidermal unit" with similar connotation, and Reed and Ackerman[31] unite papillary and periadnexal dermis under the term "adventitial dermis."

The frame of the pars papillaris is made of collagen fibers and thin bundles. Reticulum fibers are present in dense array just below the epidermis and are arranged vertical to the interface. Elastic fibers have a highly characteristic appearance and distribution. Thin fibers (Fig. 2–18) form a subpapillary baseline plexus at a variable distance from the epidermis. From this base, even finer fibers (elaunin fibers) rise vertically toward the epidermis without quite reaching it.[32] This brushwork of fine elastic fibers (oxytalan fibers) spreads like a fan toward the basal lamina. The baseline plexus and fine fibers shooting toward epidermis are valuable landmarks by which to judge the depth of inflammatory infiltrate and tumor cells. A special feature of face and extremities is the occurrence of elastic globes at the level of the basal plexus.[33] It is generally accepted that all fibers of the dermis and the ground substance are manufactured by fibroblasts, but the regulation of production process of each component is poorly understood.[34]

Blood vessels also form a subpapillary plexus from which capillary loops[35] enter the papillae. Lymph vessels are always present but not easily identified. They can be seen in O&G stain, their thin endothelial wall is accompanied by elastic fibers on the outside.[36] By electron microscopy the basal lamina is thin and discontinuous. Nerve fibers are not visible in routine stains, but Meissner's corpuscles (see Fig. 2–23) are identifiable in fingers and toes.

The pars papillaris contains fibrocytes, histiocytes, and some small round cells, presumably lymphocytes. It is difficult to separate fibrocytes from histiocytes in routinely stained normal skin. Only when histiocytes become macrophages and contain melanin or other substances can they be identified. We, therefore, often use the noncommittal term fixed-tissue-type cells in our descriptions. Small numbers of mast cells are a normal constituent of all portions of the dermis but they are more concentrated in perivascular spaces of upper dermis. Ground substance is present in the form of neutral and acid mucin substances. The former are represented by the PAS-positive basement membrane below the epidermis (see Fig. 2–15) and by similar membranes around blood vessels. The letter is detectable by alcian blue. It usually reveals small amounts of hyaluronic acid, but metachromatic acid mucopolysaccharides are not normally found in the pars papillaris.

Pars Reticularis

This portion constitutes the leather of hides and consists of a three-dimensional meshwork of collagen bundles that are accompanied by thick intercon-

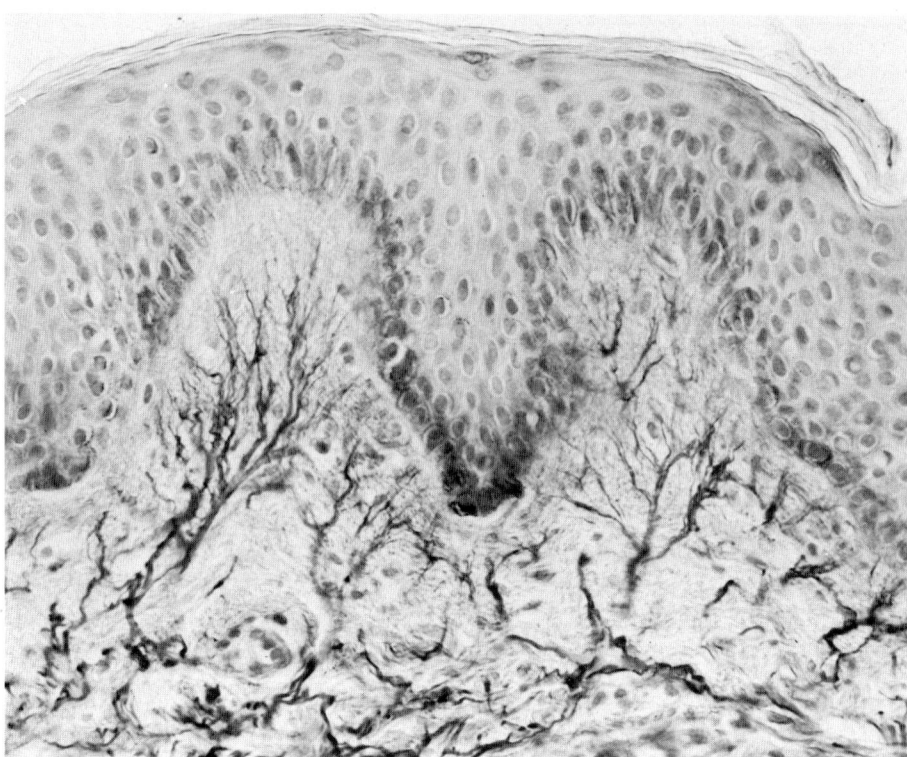

Figure 2–18.
Superficial elastic fibers of papillae and subpapillary layer. Brushlike thin fibrils ascend toward epidermis without quite reaching it. Slightly thicker fibers surround subpapillary vessels. O&G. X370.

nected elastic fibers and ribbons in similar three-dimensional arrangement. The orientation of collagen bundles is strikingly demonstrated by polarized light (Fig. 2–19) because they are birefringent. They have preferential direction in any particular region of the body surface. This is the basis of Langer's lines of cleavage, which guide the direction of surgical incisions. It also explains why randomly oriented sections may show many long bundles in some cases or many roundish blocks in others. The latter should not be interpreted as fragmented bundles, and similarly, cross sections of elastic fibers should not be mistaken for fragmented fibers. Electron microscopy shows longitudinal and transverse sections of collagen fibrils, approximately 100 nm thick. The longitudinal sections are periodically

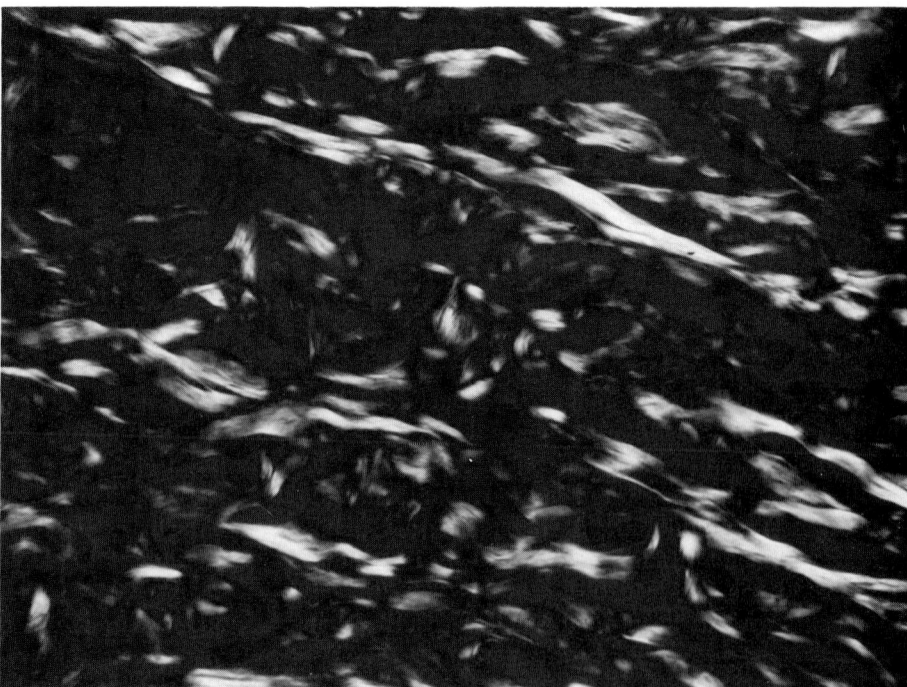

Figure 2–19.
Three-dimensional weave of collagen bundles is illustrated in this H&E-stained section photographed in polarized light. X180.

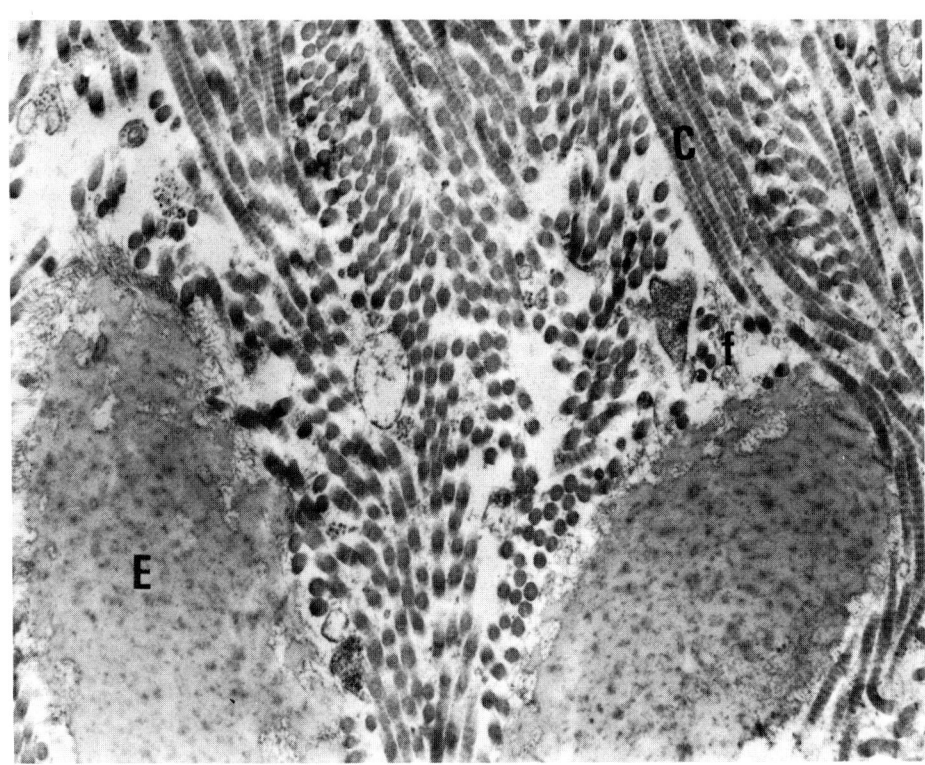

Figure 2–20.
Electron micrograph of collagen and elastic (E) fibers. Collagen fibers exhibit 68 nm cross striations. Elastic fibers consist of amorphous matrix and microfibrils, some of which occur free between collagen fibers. X18,600. (Courtesy of Dr. A. P. Lupulescu.)

banded. Elastic fibers, which consist of microfibrils (elastofibrils) embedded in an amorphous matrix of elastin, are much wider and irregularly contoured. Elastic microfibrils also occur free between the collagen fibrils (Fig. 2–20). Elastin is mainly composed of lysine-rich desmosine. Microfibril contains a cystein-rich glycoprotein called fibrillin.[37] The proportion of elastic fibers and collagen fibers varies with age. Relative quantity of collagen is highest in the third decade.[38] Ground substance is represented by relatively weak and diffuse reaction to alcian blue. Any more pronounced reaction is pathologic. Recently, fibronectin became detectable by its antibody. It is diffusely present between collagen bundles.

Fibrocytes, histiocytes, mast cells, and blood vessels are present in relatively small number, but no norms have been established. Veins, arteries, and nerves usually are found together in triads as in most other organs, a fact that makes it easier to identify nerves that are sizable only in the deep dermis and become tiny in higher strata. Although ar-

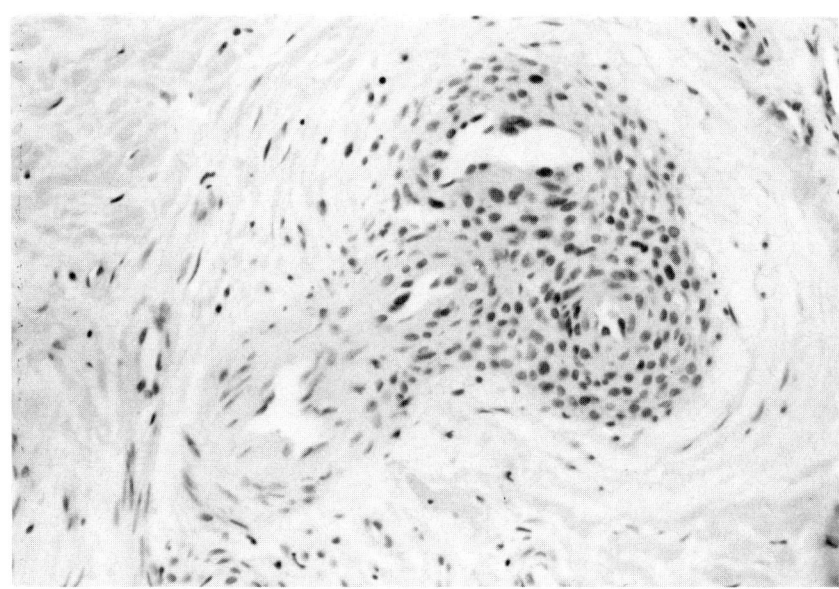

Figure 2–21.
Part of a neuromyoarterial glomus of Masson. Artery at left joins the Suquet–Hoyer canal, which is surrounded by multiple layers of glomus cells and thins out into a venous vessel at top. H&E. X400.

teriovenous anastomoses probably exist in all areas, the neuromyoarterial glomus of Masson is found most commonly on the volar surfaces of the hands and feet (Fig. 2–21).

Subcutaneous Tissue

Not a few skin diseases affect the hypoderm, and various forms of panniculitis are definitely in the realm of the dermatopathologist. The border between dermis and subcutis is never sharp. Individual fat lobes protrude higher, and connective tissue septa, very similar to dermis, are a regular constituent of the hypoderm, often forming retinacula between skin and fascia. Eccrine coils and the lower portions of hair follicles may be embedded in fat tissue in the midst of dermis as a reminder that in fetal life every hair root and sweat gland penetrates into the subcutaneous fat. Fetal fat tissue develops in the form of individual fat organs around small blood vessels, and adult tissue retains a lobular structure and rich vascularity. Each fat lobule is supplied by only one arteriole and therefore, blood supply is very limited, a fact that explains why transplanted tissue often necrotizes or becomes atrophic.[39] Fat cells, which have an average diameter of 94 μm,[40] have one feature worth looking for if there is doubt whether one is dealing with fat tissue or some form of vacuoles: The flat and ovoid nucleus often possesses a sharply defined central hole (Fig. 2–22).

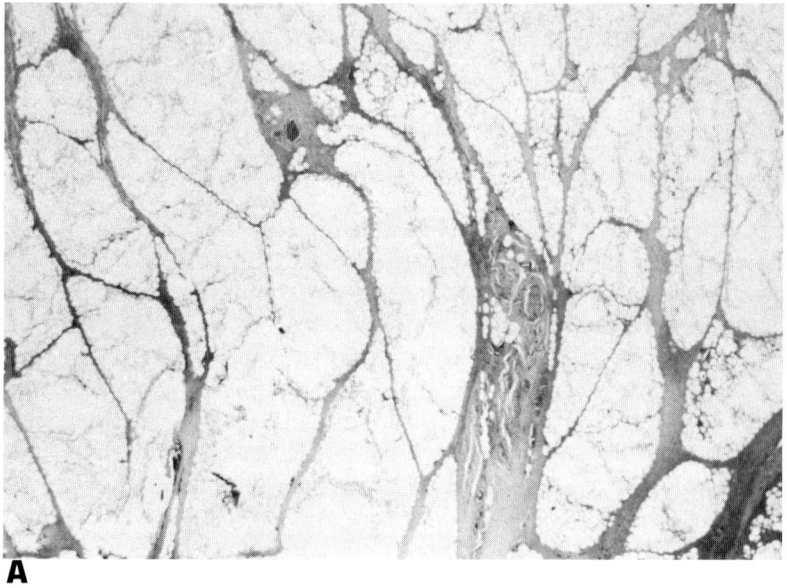

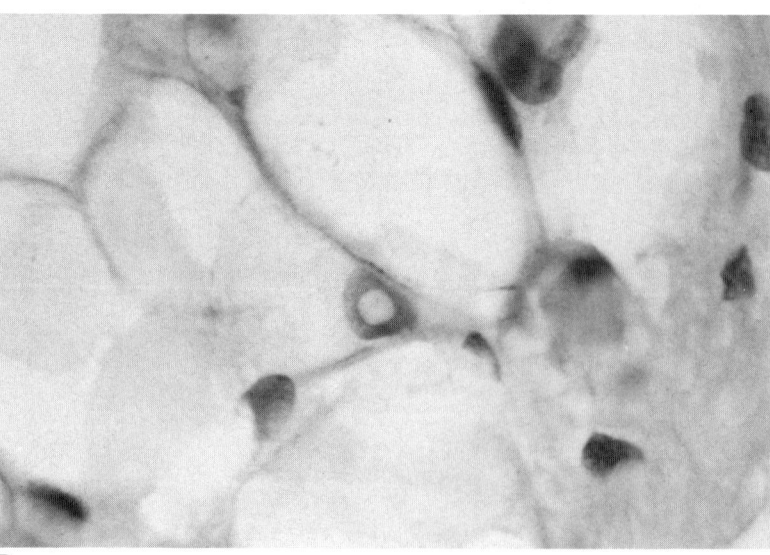

Figure 2–22.
Subcutaneous fat tissue. **A.** Low power shows fat lobules separated by thin and thicker fibrous septa carrying blood vessels. X14. **B.** High power shows several fat cells with thin cross sections of peripheral nuclei. One nucleus is shown in frontal view with the characteristic hole (or thin spot). X1100.

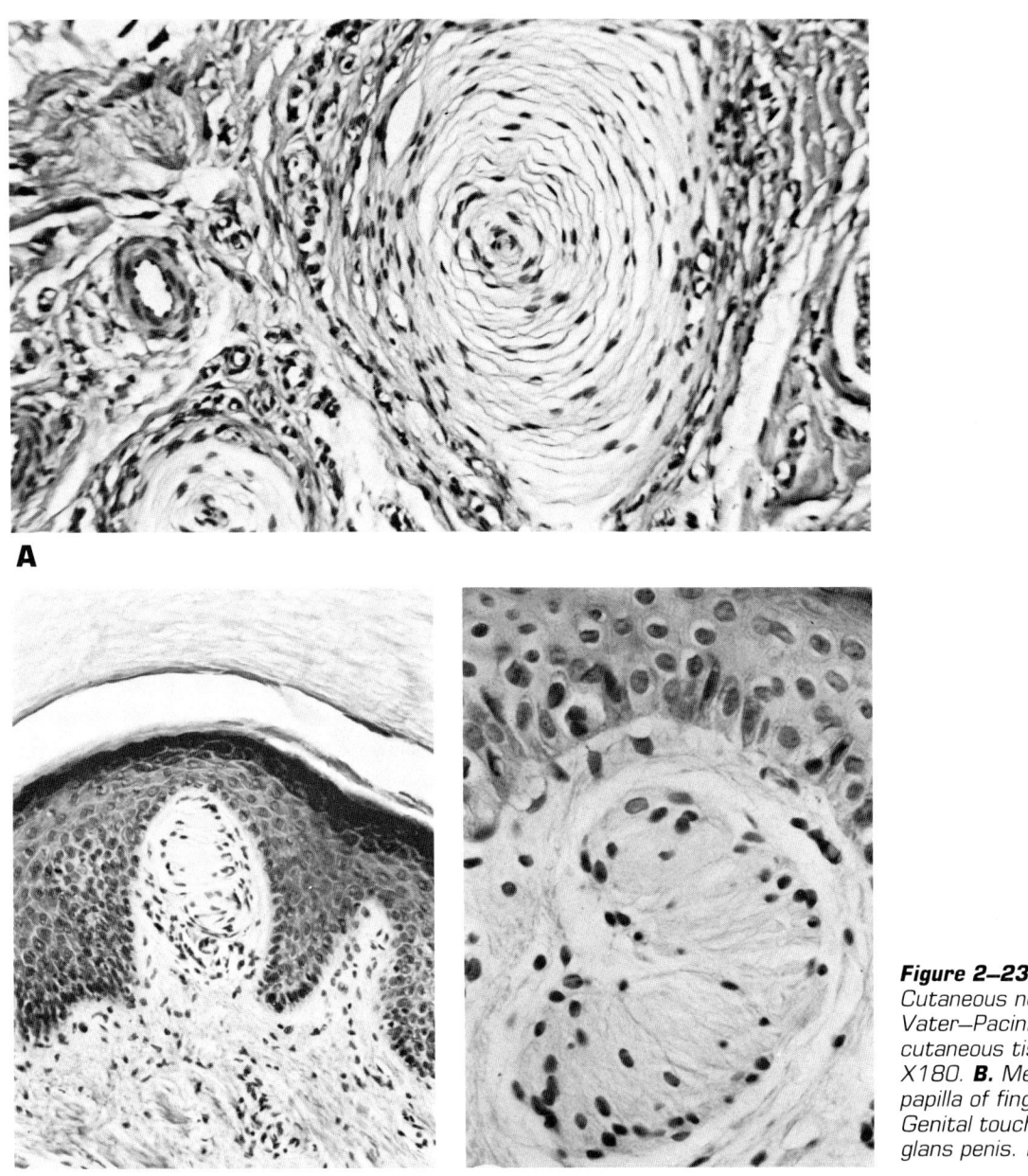

Figure 2–23.
Cutaneous nerve corpuscles. **A.** Vater–Pacini corpuscle in subcutaneous tissue of palm. H&E. X180. **B.** Meissner corpuscle in papilla of finger. H&E. X400. **C.** Genital touch corpuscle from glans penis. H&E. X600.

The largest nervous end organs found anywhere in the body are present in subcutaneous tissue of the acral parts of the extremities. They are Vater–Pacini corpuscles and consist of a central axon surrounded by multiple laminae of connective tissue that hold fluid ground substance between them to produce a hydrostatic balloon structure highly adapted to the perception of pressure changes in its surroundings (Fig. 2–23).

THE PILAR APPARATUS

Pilar complexes (Fig. 2–24) include hair follicle, sebaceous glands, hair muscle, and, in certain areas, apocrine gland. Moreover, pilar apparatuses often occur in groups of three (less commonly two, five, or more), and the biologic hairfield included the haarscheibe and associated eccrine glands. Thus, the skin may be thought of as being organized into many tiny districts, an intriguing idea discussed by dermatologists at various times.[41] The grouped arrangement of hairs is most obvious in the neck area of many women, where the relatively large sebaceous glands produce visible papules.[42] It is also visible in many sections of children's skin, and this should be kept in mind in many dermatoses affecting follicles. The previous presence of hair follicles can be deduced from the existence of an arrector

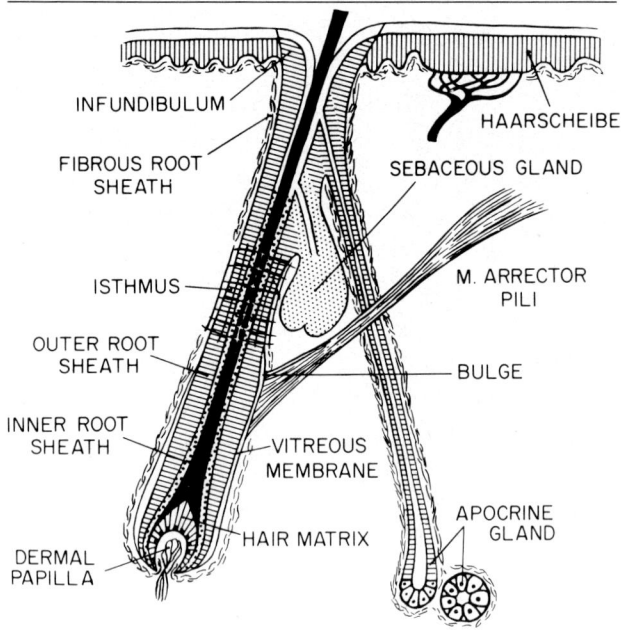

Figure 2–24.
Diagrammatic representation of pilar apparatus comprising hair follicle, sebaceous gland, apocrine gland, arrector muscle, and haarscheibe (hair disc). (From Pinkus. In Baccaredda-Boy, Moretti, and Frey (eds). Biopathology of Pattern Alopecia, 1968. Courtesy of S. Karger.)

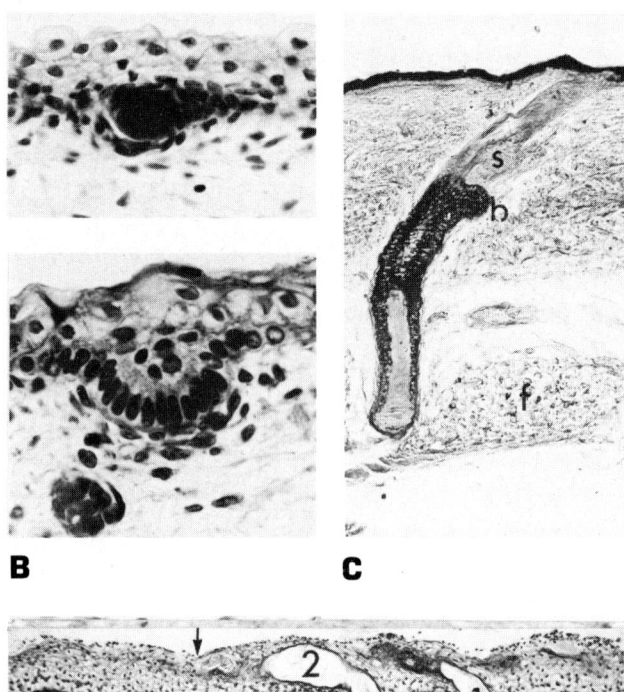

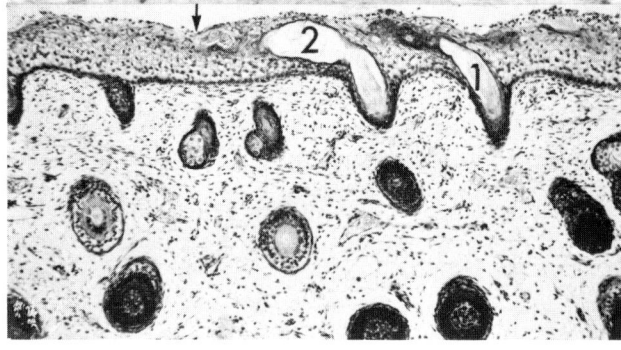

Figure 2–25.
*Fetal hair follicles. **A.** Sagittal. **B.** Frontal view of early hair germ showing bilateral symmetry. There is no invagination of the epidermis; ectodermal and mesodermal components are well shown. H&E. **C.** Curved follicle of black fetus. b, bulge; s, sebaceous gland; f, fat tissue lobe. Glycogen is absent from hair matrix and its products and from the upper follicle above the bulge. PAS–light green. **D.** Fetal eyebrow showing well-differentiated hair roots in dermis and curved, slanting, and keratinized hair canals (1 and 2) in nonkeratinized epidermis. Arrow indicates distal end of hair canal 2. H&E. (From Pinkus. In Montagna and Ellis (eds). The Biology of Hair Growth, 1958. Courtesy of Academic Press.)*

muscle, which often is the sole remnant of an atrophic pilar complex.

Development

Each pilar apparatus arises through an embryonic differentiation[43] of small groups of epidermal basal cells that are converted into prospective hair germ cells. They become associated with mesenchymal elements, the precursors of fibrous root sheath, and dermal papilla. The hair germ (Fig. 2–25) grows slantingly down through the developing dermis into the subcutaneous fat tissue. Follicles of genetically curled hairs acquire a curve during this process that may bring the hair matrix back under the site where the germ originated in the epidermis. At the same time, follicular cells grow upward at slant through the epidermis into the surface (Fig. 2–25D) and form the hair canal, the earliest site of keratinization in the fetal skin.[44] We can distinguish an anterior and posterior surface of the follicle; the latter forms a wider angle with the lower surface of the epidermis. Most hairs of animals and humans are directed toward the tail end of the body and, therefore, we can designate anterior (toward head and forming an acute angle with the epidermis), and posterior (toward the tail and forming an obtuse angle) surfaces.

Although the hair germ's anterior surface remains smooth, its posterior surface soon develops two or three buds. The two constant ones (Fig.

2–25C) develop into the bulge and the sebaceous gland, the inconstant one into the apocrine gland. Their arrangement never varies: the bulge is lowest; the sebaceous bud, above it; and the apocrine bud, highest. The arrector muscle differentiates within a field of metachromatic mesenchyme, obviously under the influence of the hair follicle but not in direct contact with it. The slender muscle fibers grow upward toward the epidermis and downward toward the bulge. The mesenchymal cells of the hair germ envelop the growing epithelial follicle in a fibrous sheath and form a terminal pad, part of which becomes enclosed in the hollow center of the hair matrix and develops into the dermal papilla (hair papilla).

Once matrix and papilla are united to form the bulbous lower end of the follicle, differentiation of the hair and its inner root sheath begins. Through intricate inductive processes, evidently originating in the dermal papilla, morphologically identical epithelial matrix cells begin to undergo differentiation along five different layers or sheaths (if viewed in three dimensions) and form the distinct end products of Henle's layer, Huxley's layer, root sheath cuticle, hair cuticle, and hair cortex. A sixth product of adult hair matrix, the medulla, is absent in fetal hairs. Inner root sheath is made first and keratinizes to form a protective cap over the fine tip of the hair (hair cone), similar to the enveloping bracts of a plant shoot piercing the ground. At this stage of hair cone formation the follicle is still growing downward and, in so doing, pushes the hair bulb down and away from the hair tip, which remains stationary. Only later are hair and inner sheath pushed upward into the hair canal. The hair becomes free when the inner root sheath and the roof of the hair canal disintegrate.

The first generation of hairs is called lanugo and is of similar quality all over the body surface. It usually completes its growth cycle before birth. The hairs of later generations differ in size and other attributes and are known by a variety of names. Tiny hairs are called vellus, stronger ones of the general body surface are known as terminal hairs.

Structure of the Adult Follicle

Strong hairs of scalp, beard, and genital regions have follicles extending into the hypoderm. The roots of smaller hairs lie in different levels of the dermis, and those of vellus hairs of the face are quite superficial. Sebaceous follicles of the face have tiny appendageal hair roots (Fig. 2–26).

Starting at the distal end of the follicle, we see

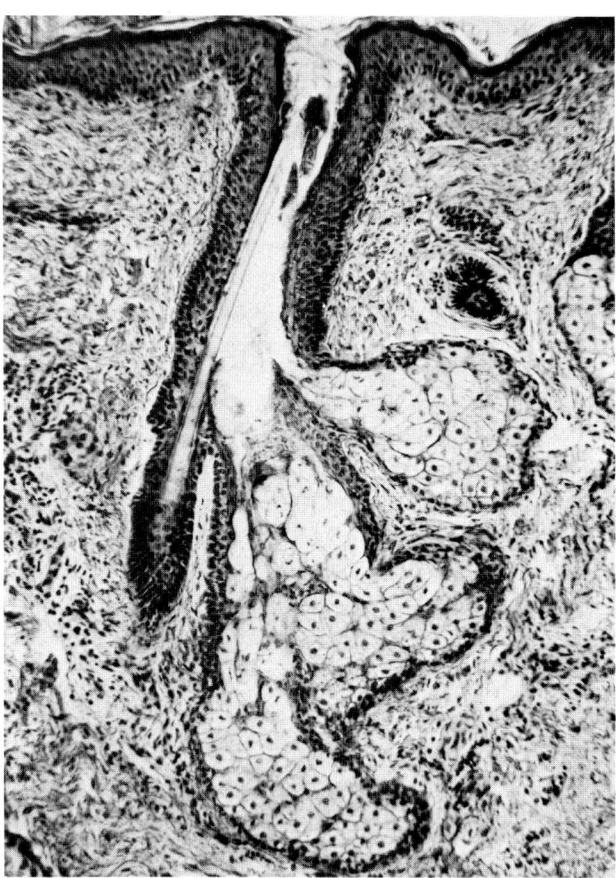

Figure 2–26.
Sebaceous follicle of facial skin. Hair root appears as an appendage. The two dark structures in the follicular canal are oblique sections of Demodex (see Fig. 18–22). H&E. X135.

a bulbous thickening (Fig. 2–27) formed by the egg-shaped dermal papilla around which the epithelial hair matrix is arranged like a shell. This portion is commonly called the hair bulb. The matrix and its division products add to the volume of the hair bulb, and the epithelial outer root sheath (trichilemma) forms a thin covering around the whole. The dermal papilla communicates with the subfollicular dermal pad and the fibrous root sheath by means of a narrow opening at the bottom through which capillaries enter and exit. The papilla of a growing (anagen) hair is strongly metachromatic and reactive for alkaline phosphatase.[45] Epithelial matrix cells have little cytoplasm and undergo mitotic division at a high rate, most of the activity being present in the lower half, whereas the cells of the inner two thirds of the upper bulb form hair cells (cortex) and medulla. The upper central portion of the hair bulb, where most of the hair cells are produced, are mingled with dendritic melanocytes that supply pigments to the keratinizing hair cells and medullary cells, which are soon vacuolated. The cells that are destined to form the hair cuticle may contain a small number of melanosomes. Nonpermanent structures such as the inner (Henle and Huxley layers) and outer root sheaths do not acquire melanosomes from hair bulb melanocytes. Albino hair roots have amelanotic melanocytes; senile white hairs lack melanocytes.

As cells are pushed upward from the matrix, they become slim and elongated, and the cross section of the follicle decreases even though the trichilemma (outer root sheath) becomes multilayered and thick. Matrix cells mature in six different ways depending on their distance from the base of the bulb (Fig. 2–28). The ring of cells closest to the base forms a single layer of quickly keratinizing elongated cells (Henle's layer), which establishes a firm coat around the soft central parts. The next several ranks of matrix cells produce the much thicker layer of Huxley, which keratinizes at a considerably higher level. Still further up along the periphery of the bulb, two interlocking layers of obliquely oriented cells, the cuticle of the inner root sheath and the cuticle of the hair, are formed. The largest portion of the matrix is used up in producing hair cortex, or the most important hair shaft, and the cells above the tip of the papilla give rise to the medulla, which is found only in thick hairs. Oblique sections of a large hair follicle at the level where Huxley's layer keratinizes (Fig. 2–29) are particularly instructive. Figures 2–28 and 2–29 show the hyaline (vitreous, glassy) membrane between the outer root sheath and perifollicular connective tissue. The fully keratinized inner root sheath stains very dark blue in O&G sections and has other specific staining reactions (yellow fluorescence with thioflavin T, acid fastness), that permit one to recognize small fragments or single cells under pathologic conditions.

The fully formed hair and inner root sheath (Henle, Huxley, and cuticle) are pushed upward through the relatively stationary tube of stratified epithelium, which is the trichilemma (outer root sheath). They enter the isthmus of the follicle above the bulge and the insertion of the arrector muscle. The bulge often is quite inconspicuous in adult hairs, but it may give rise to peculiar branching proliferations[46] resembling miniature trichoepitheliomas (Fig. 2–30), it may furnish an epithelial tendon (Fig. 2–31) for the muscle, or it may be the source of milia

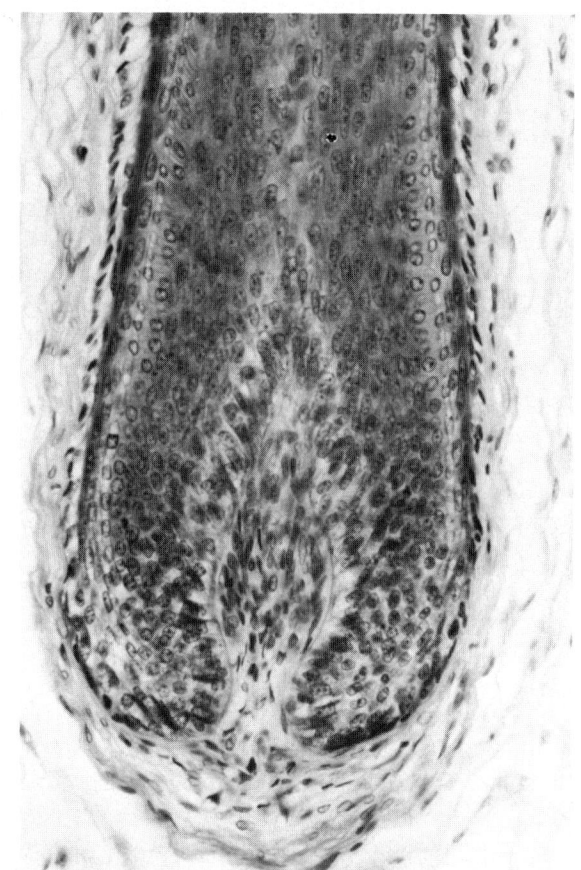

Figure 2–27.
Matrix region (bulb) of strong hair follicle. The fibrous root sheath surrounds the epithelial portion and inverts through a narrow neck into the roughly egg-shaped papilla, which has an elongated tip. The dermal papilla is connected to the epithelial matrix by a basement membrane. The lowest ranges of matrix cells give rise to three concentric layers of inner root sheath that are arranged on the outside of the thick hair cortex. The slanting nuclei between inner root sheath and fibrous root sheath constitute the outer root sheath (trichilemma) that starts at the lowest pole of the epithelial portion, surrounds the bulb as a thin single layer of cells, and begins to thicken at the upper border of the picture. The trichilemma has a thick basement membrane (the glassy or vitreous membrane of the follicle) tying it to the fibrous root sheath. The lighter staining cells in the center of the hair cortex are medulla, which spring from the uppermost matrix cells covering the tip of the papilla. H&E. X400.

through central keratinization. Its site marks the level to which the lower end of the club hair ascends in catagen, while the entire portion below disintegrates. The follicular isthmus, thus, is lower end of the permanent follicle. Its epithelial tube (see Fig. 2–32) is surrounded by an intricate net of elastic

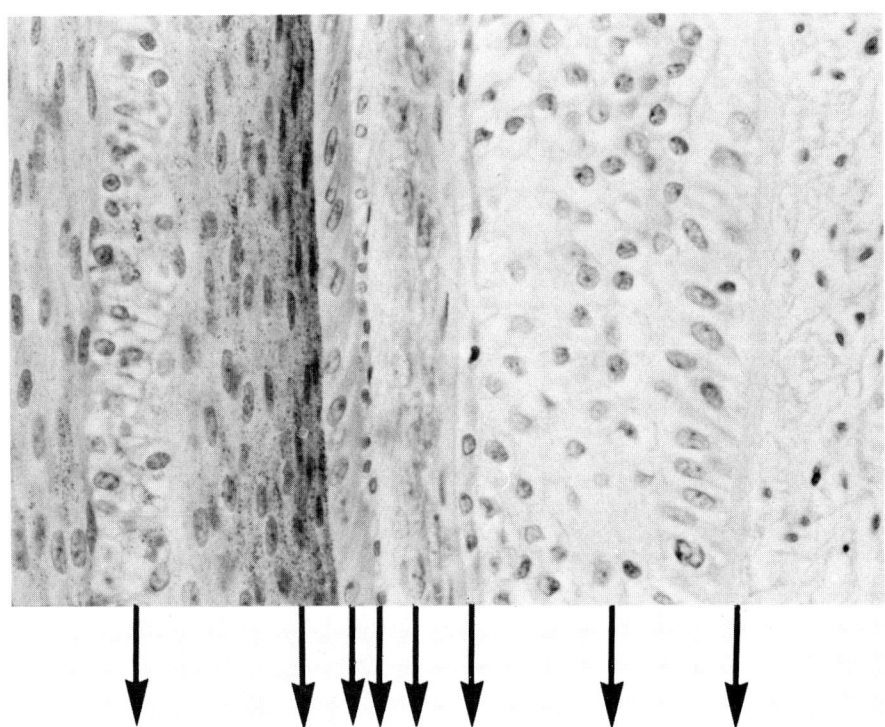

Figure 2–28.
Longitudinal section of keratogenous zone of hair and inner root sheath. Hair shaft at left shows medulla (A) within cortex (B). Nuclei of hair cuticle (C) have oblique direction, cell bodies interlock with cuticle of inner sheath (D) with small nuclei. Multiple Huxley's layer (E) and single Henle's layer (F) follow. Trichilemma (G) has large glycogen-filled cells. Its columnar basal cells rest on the vitreous membrane (H), to the right of which are fibers and cells of fibrous root sheath. H&E. X600.

fibers and cholinesterase-positive sensory nerve endings that respond to mechanical stimulation transmitted through the hair shaft. The isthmus is also the site where the inner root sheath disintegrates (Straile's zone of sloughing[47]) either at or below the level of the sebaceous duct. Disintegration seems to be due to programmed self-destruction, probably effected by proteases—the Henley's and Huxley's layers losing their staining characteristics before they break up. At the same time, the trichilemma (outer root sheath), which does not keratinize as long as it is in contact with Henle's layer, now begins to mature. Trichilemmal keratinization (Fig. 2–32) is a specific seventh form of follicular cell maturation,[48] mostly arising in the stratified epithelium of the outer sheath. The outer root sheath cells produced in the lower follicle migrate upward and inward and eventually keratinize in the lower isthmus area and shed into the hair canal. The outer root sheath matures with formation of bulky keratinized cells that contain no keratohyalin granules when examined under light microscope.

Electron microscopic examination of these cells, however, shows small sized keratohyalin granules. The innermost layer of the outer root sheath that abuts the Henle layer has its matrix cells in the hair bulb. These cells move upward and keratinize to form small keratohyalin and lysosomal vacules.[49] The keratinizing cells of the inner root sheath and hair medulla, on the other hand, form large eosinophilic droplets of trichohyalin, a substance related to keratohyalin. We shall discuss trichilemmal keratin formation again in the catagen stage of the hair cycle.

The entry of the sebaceous duct marks another change in follicular architecture and function. The duct itself, a short tube of stratified epithelium (Fig. 2–33), keratinizes in epidermoid fashion with formation of keratohyalin and pierces the follicular wall obliquely. Regardless of whether there is only one sebaceous duct or several, the follicular epithelium above this level produces regular keratohyalin and a loose lamellar epidermoid keratin layer, which differs from that of the epidermis on the ultrastructural level.[50] The pilar canal of this infundibular upper portion of the follicle, therefore, might better be termed pilosebaceous canal. It exists in sebaceous follicles with rudimentary hair roots as well as in free sebaceous glands of the oral mucosa (Fig. 2–34). The infundibulum extends through the epidermis to the surface and incorporates the remnant of the fetal hair canal. While indistinguishable morphologically from the epidermis with which it is fused, it is a biologic portion of the follicle (acrotrichium)[51] and

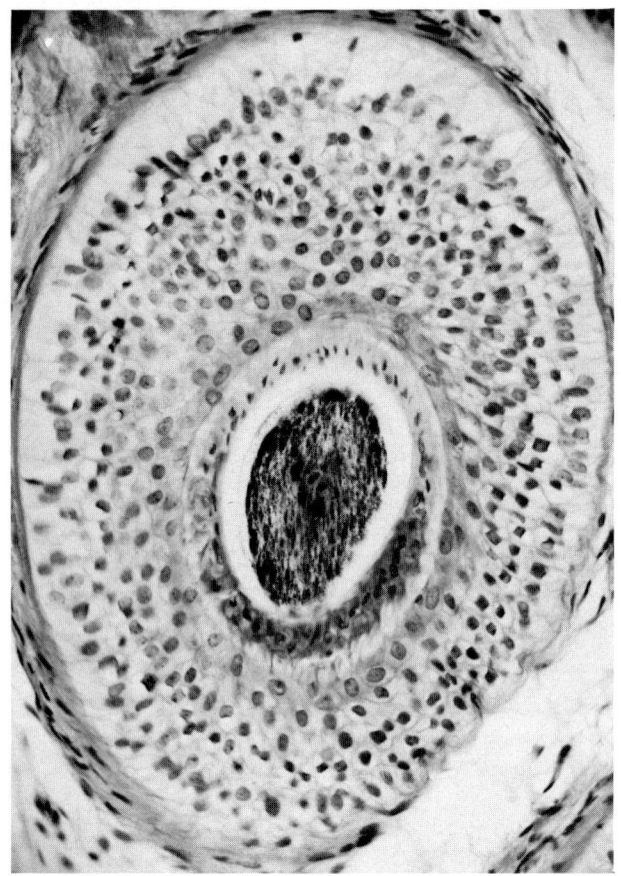

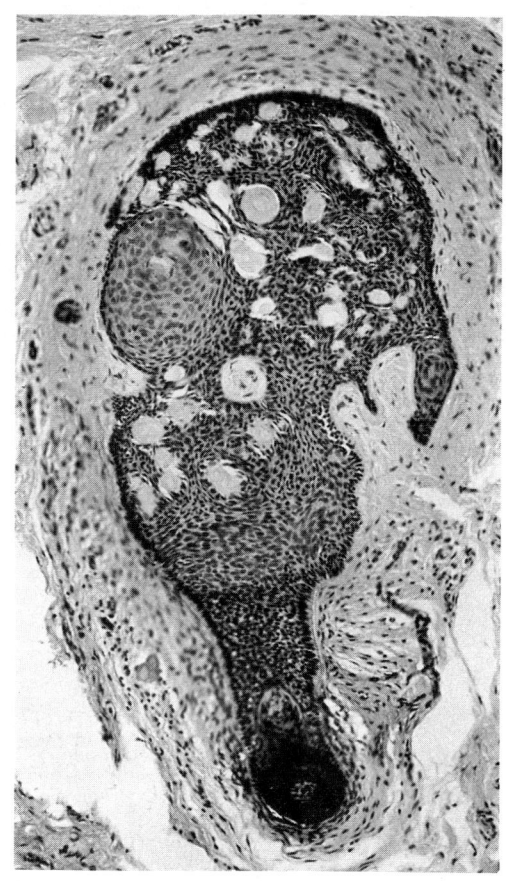

Figure 2–29.
Oblique section of scalp hair at level of keratinization of Huxley's layer. Hair with medulla, cortex, and fully keratinized (unstained) cuticle in center. Keratinized Henle's layer (striated) surrounds Huxley's layer, which shows nuclei and dark-staining trichohyaline granules in lower half, pyknotic nuclei only in upper half of picture. Basal cells of outer root sheath are columnar and appear light because they contain much glycogen; central cells are smaller and denser, showing no evidence of keratinization. Small dark nuclei between basal cells belong to amelanotic melanocytes. Direction of nuclei in fibrous root sheath indicates circular and longitudinal layers. H&E. X370.

Figure 2–30.
Bulge proliferation resembling a small trichoepithelioma. H&E X180.

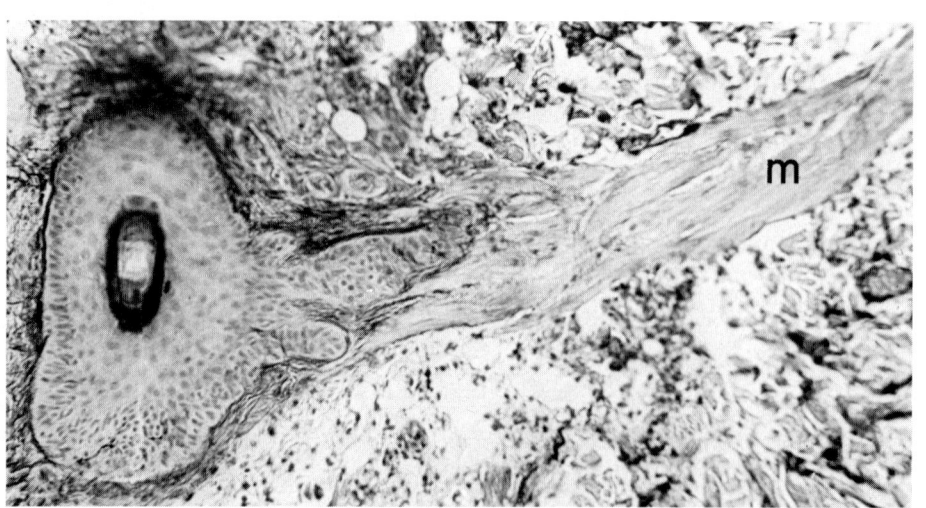

Figure 2–31.
Bulge area of a small follicle. Bulge proliferation forms an epithelial tendon for strong arrector muscle (m). Elastic fibers surround follicular isthmus and upper part of bulge and fade out below it. Inner root sheath is dark (blue). O&G.

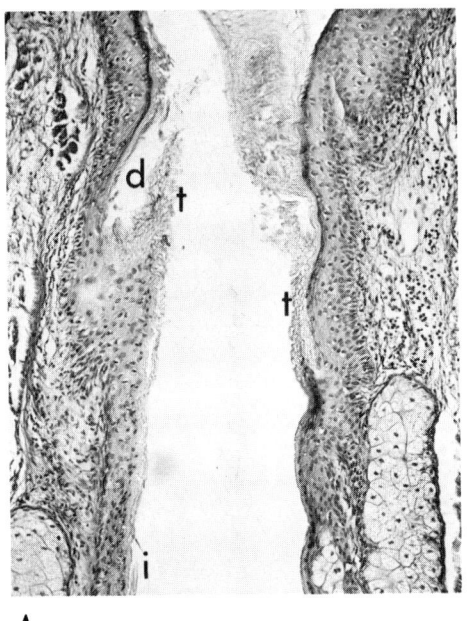
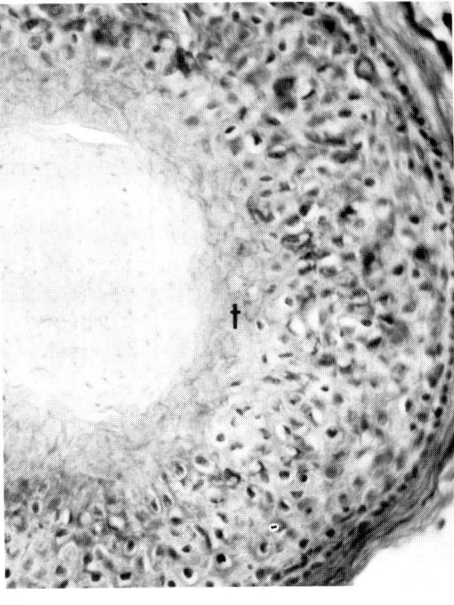

Figure 2–32.
Trichilemmal keratinization. **A.** Isthmus of anagen follicle. d, sebaceous duct; i, upper end of disintegrating inner root sheath; t, trichilemmal keratin forming a spur at lower circumference of sebaceous duct. Note, keratohyalin (dark) appears only above sebaceous duct level in infundibular portion of follicle. H&E. X86. **B.** Catagen club in transverse section. Light hair shaft is surrounded by darker trichilemmal keratin from which it has retracted in two places (artifactal cleft). Outer root sheath epithelium contains small amounts of glycogen (dark). Picture resembles a miniature trichilemmal cyst (see Fig. 38–8). PAS–hematoxylin–picric acid. X352. (From Pinkus. Arch Dermatol 99:544, 1969.)

consists of adnexal rather than epidermal keratinocytes, a fact that gains significance in wound healing and in neoplastic processes.

Fibrous Root Sheath

From its beginning, the entire hair follicle is enveloped in mesodermal stroma. Mesodermal cells accumulate below the early ectodermal germ (see Fig. 2–25) and accompany it downward through the dermis into the subcutaneous fat tissue, participating in the formation and growth of the hair germ. In adult life the dermal (hair) papilla is surrounded by the bell-shaped epithelial matrix, contains nourishing blood vessels, and seems to instruct the matrix cells to divide, rest, or retract.[52] It is connected to the fibrous root sheath through the neck of the papilla (see Fig. 2–27), which in strong hairs often contains an accumulation of fine elastic fibers, the Arao–Perkins body,[53] which has diagnostic significance in alopecia. The fibrous root sheath consists of circular and longitudinal collagen fibers along with fibroblasts and also carries capillary blood vessels. It varies in thickness and becomes very prominent in the catagen phase of the hair cycle as well as in some forms of alopecia. It is joined to the basal cells of the outer root sheath by a prominent basement membrane (see Figs. 2–27 and 2–28) that stains with PAS and often is metachromatic. This is the vitreous (glassy) membrane of the hair follicle and corresponds to a sticky, transparent substance ensheathing anagen hair that is visible when an anagen hair is pulled. The fibrous root sheath normally does not

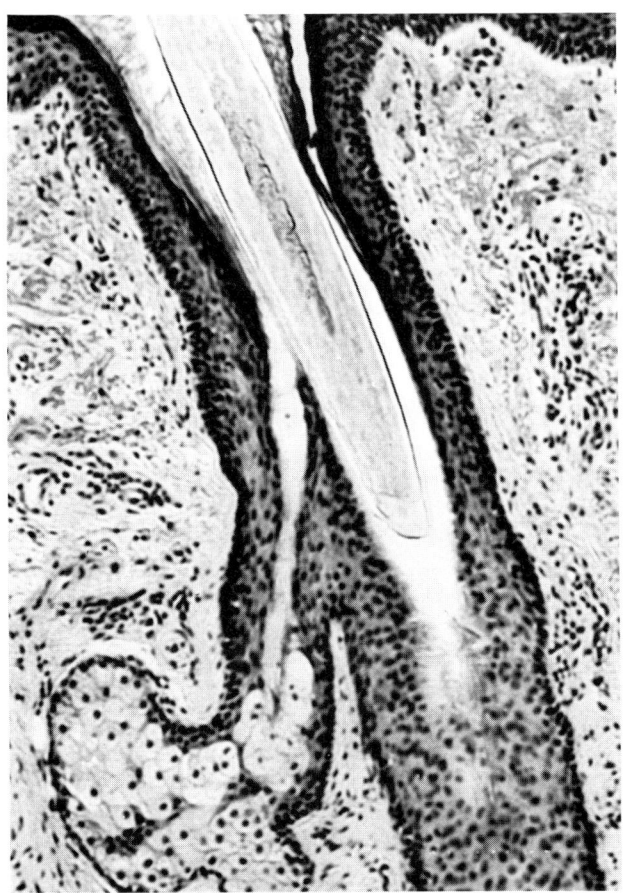

Figure 2–33.
Upper hair follicle with sebaceous gland and duct. Oblique section of medullated hair in pilosebaceous canal. Note loose epidermoid keratin in infundibulum. H&E. X135.

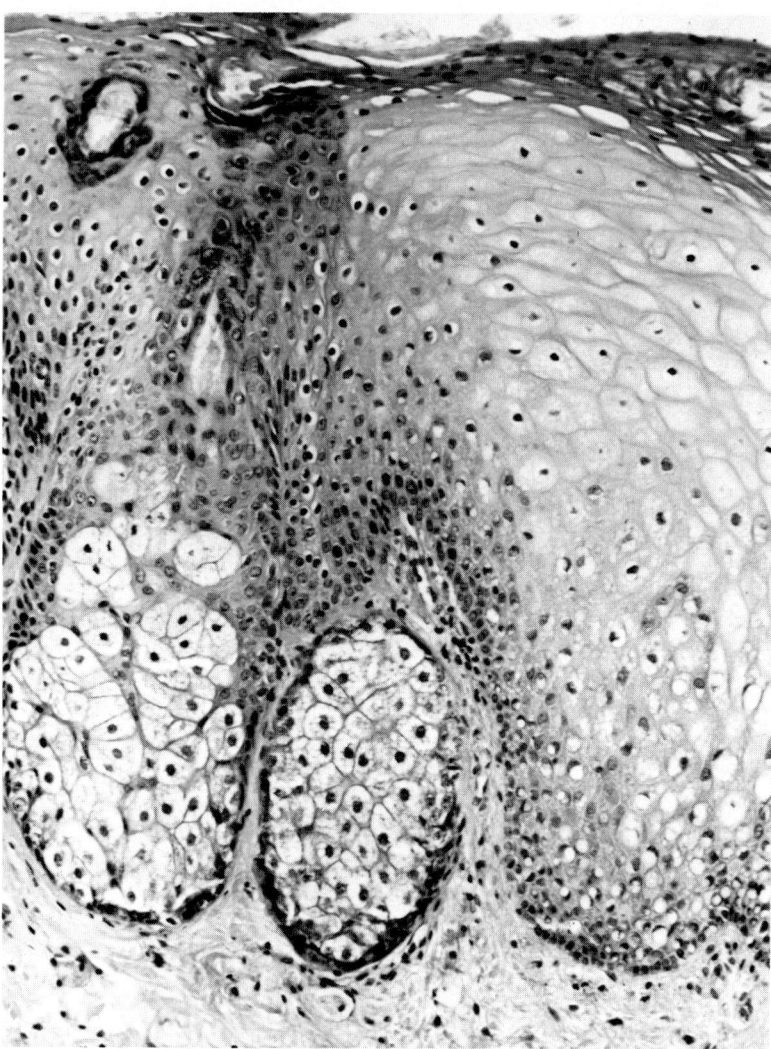

Figure 2–34.
Oral mucosa with free sebaceous glands. Note contrast between physiologic parakeratosis of oral surface epithelium and keratinization with keratohyalin of the sebaceous ducts traversing it. H&E. X135.

contain elastic fibers in the lower, transient portion of the follicle but shows a dense elastic component above the insertion of the hair muscle at the bulge (see Fig. 2–31). This elastic coat, mixed with nerve fibers, extends upward around the isthmus to the level of the sebaceous duct. Higher up, it is represented by loosely arranged fibers around the pilosebaceous canal. The relation of fibrous root sheath to follicular epithelium is quite different from the dermoepidermal junction. It is similar to the relation of stroma and epithelium in benign adnexal tumors and in basal cell epithelioma.

Sebaceous Gland

The normal gland (see Figs. 2–33 and 2–34)[54] has one peripheral basal layer of flat small cells, all inner layers being lipidized. Early atrophy is manifested by more bulky basal cells and smaller, less completely lipidized inner cells. Multiple layers of nonlipidized outer cells are definitely pathologic (e.g., sebaceous epithelioma). The contour of the gland is rounded, and continuous collapse of some lobes and formation of new ones give sebaceous glands a variety of shapes and cause vascular stroma to be enclosed deep in some glands. The most central cells of each lobe disintegrate (holocrine secretion), and the debris is extruded as sebum through the duct. The duct consists of stratified epithelium keratinizing in epidermoid fashion. The size of facial sebaceous glands increases with age,[55] but their proliferation activity decreases. Presence of demodex folliculorum deep in normal sebaceous glands is so common that one can discount its pathologic significance in most cases.

Many vellus hairs of the face are surrounded with a nonlipidized epithelial extension of the sebaceous gland, which appears like a skirt or cloak (mantle hair of F. Pinkus) and is seen in histologic sections as epithelial spurs flanking the isthmus (Fig. 2–35). According to Epstein and Kligman,[56] the epithelium of the mantle may give rise to milia through central keratinization. Felix Pinkus interpreted this as a malformation replacing sebaceous gland. Under this hoodlike epithelial cover however, one finds sensory nerve endings regularly spaced along the follicular circumference. Hashimoto described this as a protective epithelial cover for nerve endings.[57]

Apocrine Gland

The apocrine duct starts as a thin tube high in the follicular wall (Fig. 2–36A) or, occasionally, in the epidermis next to a follicle (displacement). The duct is short and inconspicuous and soon ends at the upper limit of the secretory tubule, which coils up in the deep dermis and subcutaneous fat tissue. The duct has two concentric layers of cuboidal cells and resembles the eccrine duct in routine sections. It also has a similar set of enzymes as shown in histochemical preparations[58,59] (Table 2–3). The secretory portion (Fig. 2–36B) consists of an inner layer of eosinophilic cells, which vary from flat to columnar according to the phase of the secretion cycle, and an outer layer of elongated myoepithelial cells. The apocrine tube has a much larger lumen than the eccrine gland and has a different set of enzymes (Table 2–3). It is encased in a network of reticulum and elastic fibers outside the PAS-positive basement membrane. Secretory cells have a round, vesicular nucleus near the base and copious cytoplasm containing a variety of granules. Projection of the apical cytoplasm into the lumen gives rise to the concept of apocrine secretion by decapitation. This was confirmed by electron microscopic studies (Fig. 2–36C); an apical cap balloons out like a mushroom and is decapitated at the base by the formation of a demarcation membrane.[60] Apocrine sweat contains corpuscular elements derived from the disintegrated apical cap that give it a milky or colored quality. The differences in size and morphology of apocrine and eccrine glands are shown in Figure 2–1A.

Apocrine glands are concentrated in the axillae and anogenital regions but are also found in other areas. Glands are encountered too commonly on the face, scalp, and anterior trunk to be considered abnormal (ectopic). The ceruminous glands of the ear canal[61] and the glands of Moll of the eyelids are modified apocrine glands.

Arrector Muscle

Musculus arrector pili (see Fig. 2–31) is a smooth muscle that may vary from one thin strand to several bulky cords. Under pathologic conditions, there seems to be an inverse relation between size of follicle and muscle. Skin with atrophic hair follicles, whether it be on scalp or lower legs, often contains surprisingly large muscles. Hypertrophy of the muscle is found in pityriasis rubra pilaris (Chapter 18). The arrector muscle typically contains elastic fibers that run parallel to the muscle fibers and form elastic tendons at both ends. Because students often have difficulty differentiating smooth muscle from nerves, we like to point out that muscle bundles usually appear straight in longitudinal section, whereas nerves appear wavy. Schwann cell nuclei are shorter than the long, rod-shaped nuclei of smooth muscle.

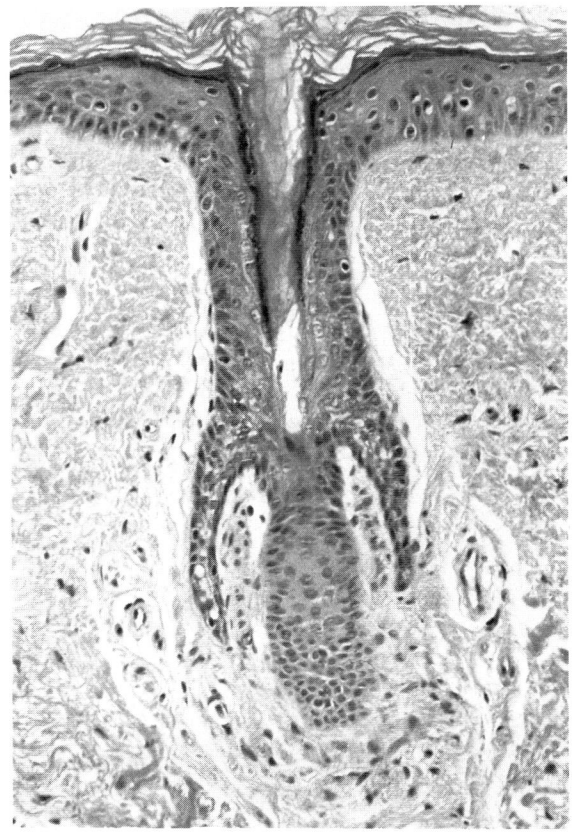

Figure 2–35.
Mantle hair (F. Pinkus) shows a vellus hair follicle surrounded by a skirt of atrophic sebaceous epithelium. H&E. ×180.

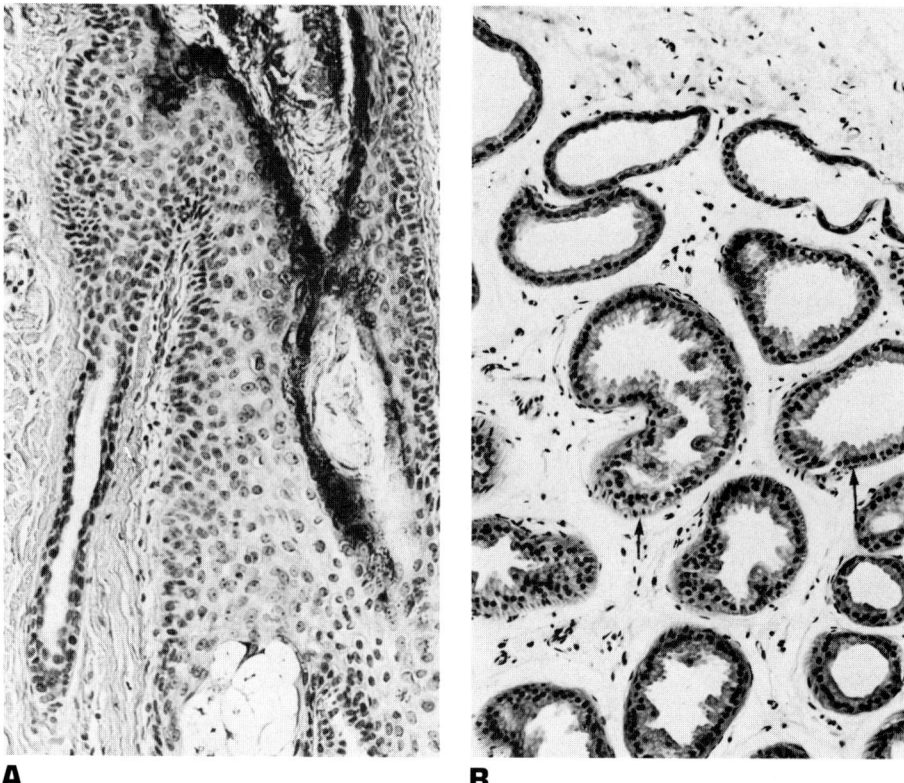

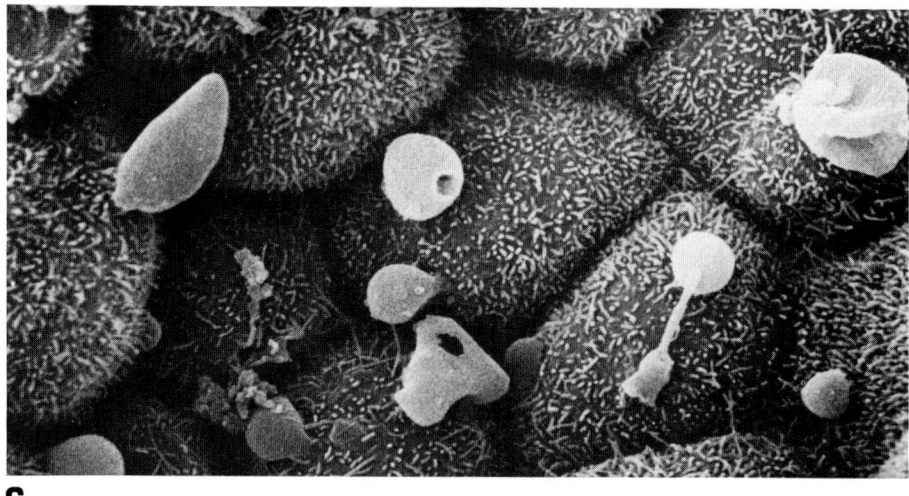

Figure 2–36.
Apocrine gland. **A.** Pilar complex of normal facial skin showing apocrine duct entering a hair follicle above sebaceous gland. Van Gieson. X135. **B.** Multiple sections of axillary apocrine coil showing that secretory cells may vary from flat to columnar in same unit. Nuclei of myoepithelial cells are visible wherever tubule is cut tangentially (arrows). **C.** Scanning electron micrograph of surface of apocrine secretory epithelium shows the bulging surface cap of the cells beset with microvilli. Some drops of secretion adhere to the cell surface. X4420. (Courtesy of Dr. W. H. Wilborn.)

Smooth muscle nuclear contours may assume a zigzag shape if the fiber is contracted during fixation. In cross section, both types of nuclei look small and round, but the muscle nucleus is in the center of the fiber, whereas the Schwann cell nucleus is located peripherally, particularly in large myelinated fibers surrounding the axons in center. The axon is seen as a tiny and faintly stained dot in the center of the empty-appearing myelin sheath. Acid orcein-giemsa (O&G) stain shows elastic fibers associated with muscle, but not with nerve, and shows muscular cytoplasm blue, whereas nerves appear pink. Other special stains are available if doubt persists. For example, desmin is demonstrable in smooth and striated muscles, while S-100 proteins are present in nerves. Both stains can be used in formalin-fixed,

TABLE 2–3. HISTOCHEMICALLY DEMONSTRATED ENZYME ACTIVITIES IN APOCRINE AND ECCRINE APPARATUSES

Enzyme	Intraepithelial Duct		Intradermal Duct		Secretory Portion	
	Apocrine*	Eccrine	Apocrine	Eccrine	Apocrine	Eccrine
Amylophosphorylase and branching enzyme	+++	+++	+++	+++	– to (±)	+++
Succinic and malic dehydrogenases	††	†	–	+++	+	+++
Leucine aminopeptidase	?†	?	+	+++	++	+++
Acid phosphatase	?	?	++	+++	++	+++
Alkaline phosphatase	?	?	–	–	+++ (in myoepithelial cells)	+++
Beta-glucuronidase	?	?	+	+	+++	+
Indoxyl esterase	–	–	–	+	++	+
Acetyl cholinesterase	–	–	–	–	– to ++ (in peripheral nerve fibers)	+++

* Refers to the portion embedded in the wall of the hair follicle.
† Indicates that no data are available.
Modified from Hashimoto and Lever[58] with additional data from Švob.[59]

paraffin-embedded tissue. In frozen section, myelin-basic proteins are positive in myelinated nerve, while neurofilament antibody can be used for both nonmyelinated and myelinated nerve fibers (Table 4–3).

Haarscheibe

Described by Pinkus[62] as a half-millimeter-round dermoepidermal disc in close vicinity to hairs and recognized as a nerve end organ, the hair disc (Fig.

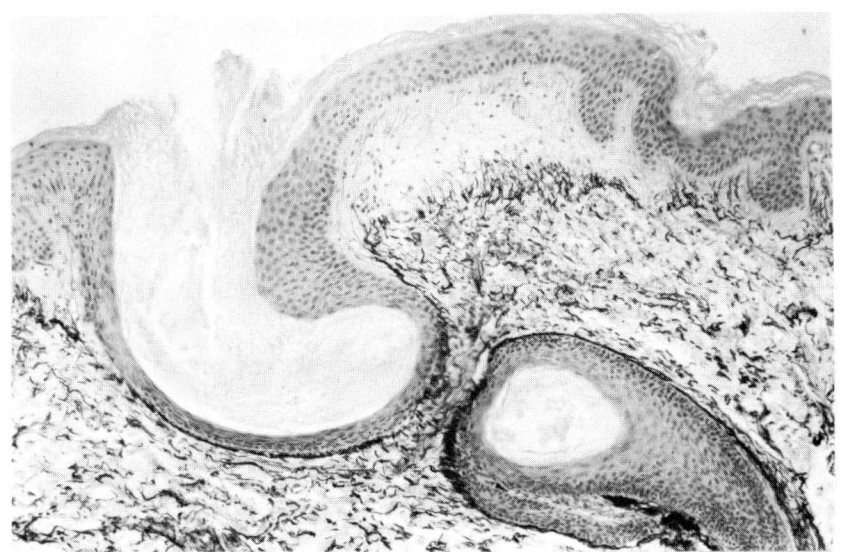

Figure 2–37.
Hair disc is a slight elevation adjacent to a hair follicle. Papillary dermis appears myxomatous. Acid orcein–Giemsa. ×125.

2–37) remained an anatomic curiosity until recent times, when neurophysiologists identified it as a slow-adapting touch receptor in mammalian skin. It is not easily recognized in routine sections but may be seen as a stretch of slightly elevated and thickened epidermis, limited by long epithelial ridges at either end. Electron microscopy has confirmed the existence of many tactile Merkel cells in the basal layer. The little organ has a well-vascularized dermal component in which a thick myelinated nerve aborizes and makes contact with the Merkel cells. Its Schwann cells contain melanin granules.[63]

Hair Cycle

No hair grows forever. The proliferative phase (anagen) lasts several years in vellus and terminal hairs, many years in long scalp hairs, but invariably it is followed by a resting phase (telogen). The intricate processes (Fig. 2–38) accompanying the period of subsiding growth (catagen) and the beginning of new hair growth at the end of telogen produce a great variety of histologic pictures, with which one has to become familiar so as not to misinterpret these in routine sections. The first sign of subsiding hair growth is loss of metachromasia of the dermal papilla, which can be recognized in O&G sections. Mitotic activity stops, and the hair matrix retracts from the papilla. The now-inactive melanocytes remain in the papilla except at the time when a hair changes to senile whiteness. At that crucial time, all melanocytes are caught in the dying, retracting hair and are lost to the next hair cycle.

The entire lower follicle collapses, its epithelial part becoming a thin cord, whereas the mesodermal part is transformed into thick fibrous sheath (Fig. 2–39). The hair itself escapes upward, formation of internal root sheath ceasing before that of cortex, and the lower end of the hair shaft now becomes surrounded by keratinizing outer root sheath (see Fig. 2–32), which adds its dense keratin to form the club.[64] Wells[65] found in 1982 that hairs plucked in early telogen and put into tissue culture show outgrowth of epithelial cells from the club. What has

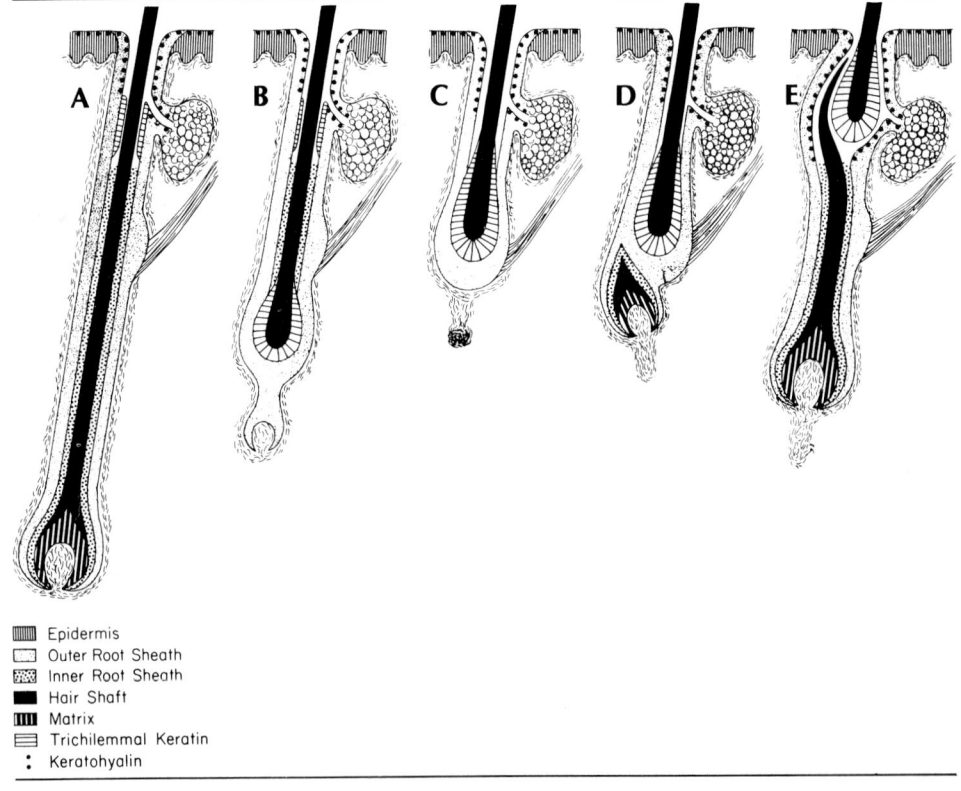

Epidermis
Outer Root Sheath
Inner Root Sheath
Hair Shaft
Matrix
Trichilemmal Keratin
Keratohyalin

Figure 2–38.
Diagram of hair cycle. **A.** Anagen. **B.** Catagen. **C.** Telogen. **D.** Early anagen. **E.** Telogen effluvium.

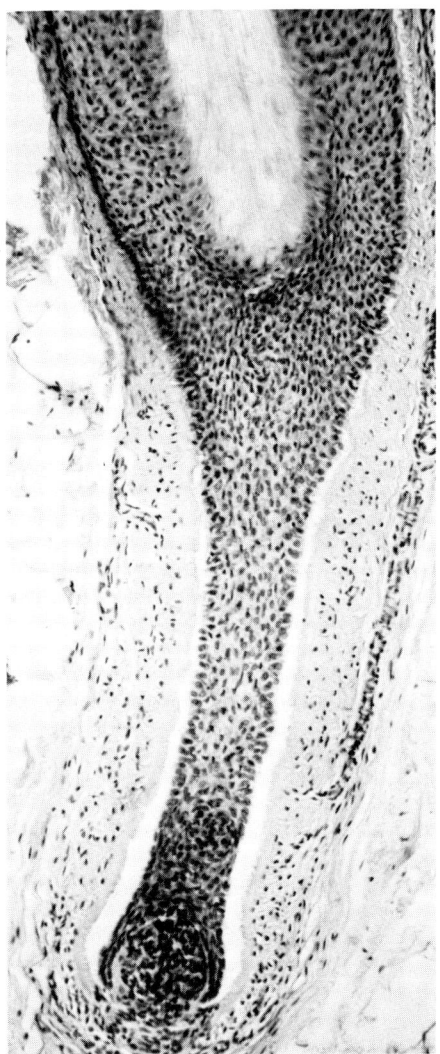

Figure 2–39.
Catagen follicle. Atrophying dermal papilla at lower end is connected with trichilemmal sac containing early club hair (at top) by epithelial hair stem, which will shorten and disappear in telogen. Fibrous root sheath (separated by artifactual cleft from epithelium) is thickened. Note darker staining nucleated trichilemmal cells beginning to lay down anchoring hair club material around the lower end of the light-staining hair shaft. H&E. X135.

been described as a brushlike spreading of keratinized hair cells actually is convergence of keratinizing outer root sheath cells into the catagen club, a picture bearing strong similarity to that seen in young trichilemmal cysts. The hair thus recedes to the level of the bulge, where it is surrounded in full telogen by a smooth contoured sac of the keratinizing outer root sheath. The fibrous cord extends downward from the lower end of this sac.

Papilla and matrix are inconspicuous during telogen, which may last from 2 to 6 months. When regrowth of hair begins, the new germ closely resembles the fetal hair germ except that it now forms at the base of the trichilemmal sac. Its axis is at an angle with the axis of the old hair, a useful sign in telling a follicle in early anagen from one in catagen. The hair matrix and papilla push downward through the channel marked by the collapsed fibrous sheath, and later the tip of the new hair protected by its inner root sheath pushes upward past the old club hair; the old club hair coexists with the new hair for a short time but eventually gets loosened from its moorings. The old hair usually falls out before the new one reaches the surface, but occasionally both hairs may be present in the follicle at the same time. This phenomenon is exaggerated in trichostasis spinulosa, where a dozen or more dead hairs may remain in the follicle. This general scheme of the hair cycle has recently been challenged by Inaba et al,[66] who found that axillary hair of the Japanese is newly formed in the region of the sebaceous duct when dermal papilla and the entire lower part of the hair follicle have been surgically removed. This phenomenon, known so far only in the vibrissae (tactile hairs) of lower mammals, needs further investigation.

ECCRINE GLAND

Contrary to apocrine glands, eccrine glands, the true sweat apparatus of man, originate directly from the epidermis, independent of hair follicles. The fetal eccrine germ first appears as a crowding of basal cells, similar to the hair germ, but it grows down straight into the dermis as a slender cord with a knobby end. It begins to coil when it reaches the subcutaneous tissue. The eccrine epithelium also grows upward through the epidermis. The epithelial cord forms a lumen in the seventh or eighth fetal month, and the entire eccrine apparatus then consists of four main portions: (1) the spiraling intraepidermal eccrine sweat duct unit (acrosyringium); (2) the straight intradermal duct, which loosely spirals and has an unpredictable course; (3) the coiled duct; and (4) the secretory portion. In skin containing relatively numerous eccrine glands, the secretory coils are found at two levels: superficial ones in the deep dermis and deep ones in the subcutaneous tissue.

The acrosyringium has two or more layers of cells that are distinctly different from the surrounding keratinocytes of the sweat duct ridge. The unit forms a spiral, which seems to have a constant length, being almost straight in acanthotic epidermis and tightly coiled in atrophic skin (Fig. 2–40). Its nonpigmented keratinized cells are exfoliated on the surface and are replenished by new cells formed in a subepidermal matrix zone,[67] in which mitoses appear in greater number (Fig. 2–41) during periods of rapid turnover, for example, after tape stripping. The lumen of the intraepidermal duct is slitlike or star shaped and coated with a PAS-positive, cuticle. Ultrastructurally there is no specific cuticle structure; numerous microvilli and vesicles are found along the luminal border. Contents of those organelles and the mucous coat of the luminal microvilli are responsible for PAS stain. As the cells move up with the epidermis, they begin to form keratohyalin and acidophilic (eosinophilic) keratin (see Fig. 2–13) at a level below the keratinizing level of the epidermis itself. The intradermal duct consists of a thin fibrous sheath, which is much less conspicuous than the fibrous hair root sheath, and two concentric layers of cuboidal epithelial cells, the outer ones of which may undergo mitosis. The lumen is covered with a PAS-positive cuticle. The epithelial cells contain much glycogen, which is apt to disappear with profuse sweating. Histochemically demonstrable enzyme activities are listed in Table 2–3.

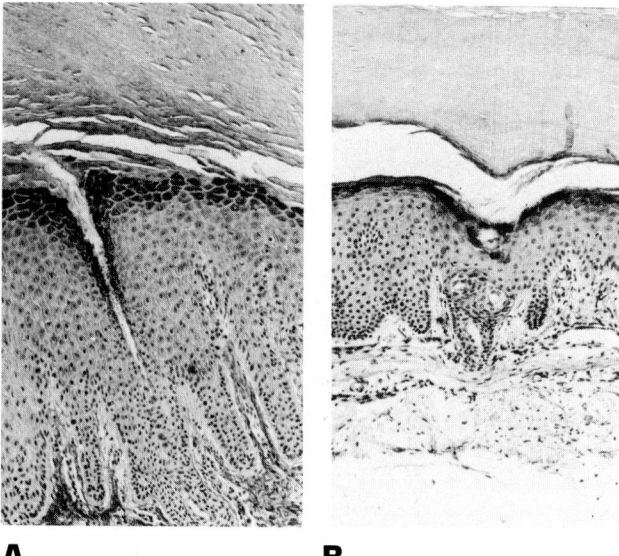

Figure 2–40.
Intraepidermal eccrine sweat duct unit (acrosyringium) in acanthotic **A.** and atrophic **B.** palmar epidermis. Respective straightening and coiling of unit suggest that it has a definite length. (From Pinkus. J Invest Dermatol 2:175, 1939.)

Figure 2–41.
Subepidermal eccrine duct 48 hours after removal of horny layer by tape stripping. Two mitoses (arrows) and several nuclei in early prophase are seen. Mitoses being extremely rare in normal ducts, this micrograph indicates that there is a matrix zone for acrosyringium that has been activated by the stripping. H&E. **A.** X180. **B.** X400.

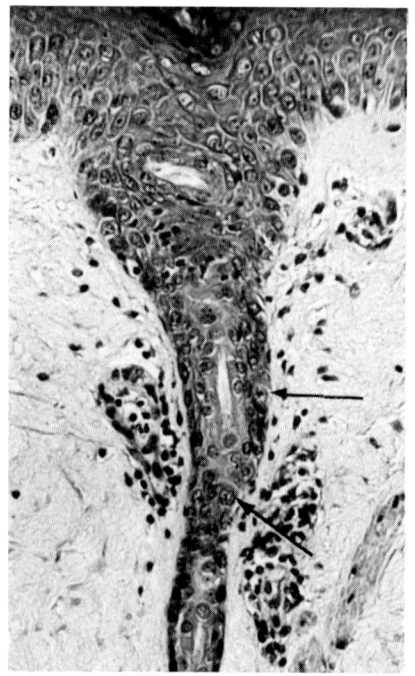
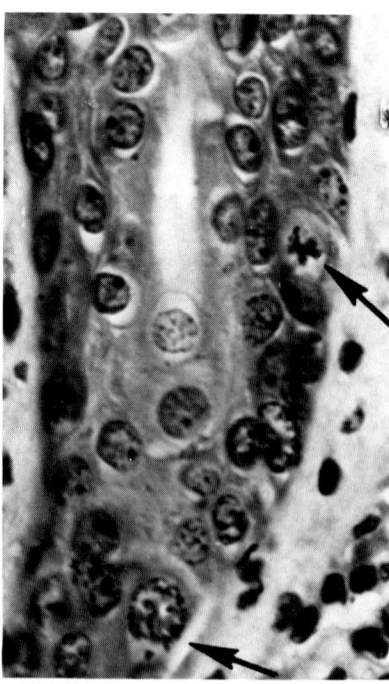

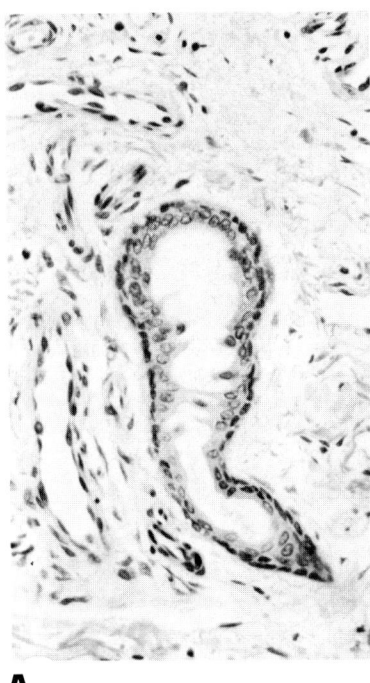 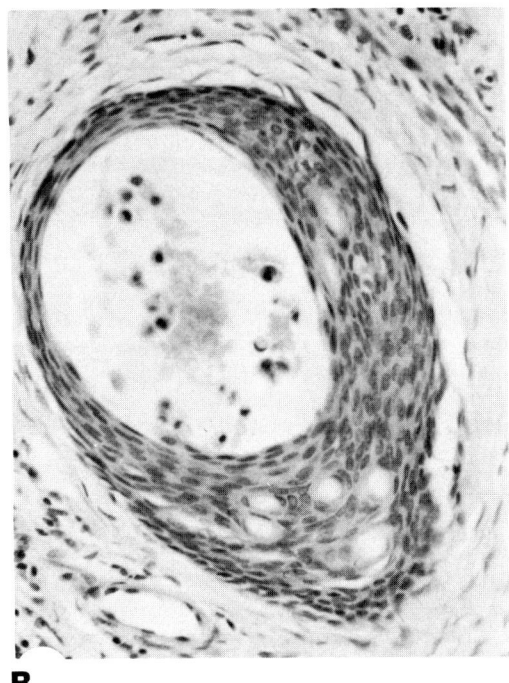

Figure 2–42.
Eccrine ducts obstructed by scar formation in dermis form small cysts with evidence of spiraling tendency. H&E. **A.** X125. **B.** X400.

The lumina of both duct and secretory part usually are smaller than one half of the total diameter of the tube, but the junction of the two portions often shows a fusiform widening, called the ampulla.[68] The secretory portion has a much less regular lining than the duct. The outer layer is composed of interrupted pavement of myoepithelial cells that differentiate from the outer layer of keratinocytes of the duct.[69] The inner layer has two components, the light and the dark cells. The light cells are located in the more basal or peripheral portion of the gland and are rich in glycogen, whereas the dark cells are located along the luminal surface and contain round mucoid granules. These granules are not visible in H&E stained sections, however, O&G stains often reveal the dark blue, coarse granules that are also acid-fast by Ziehl–Neelsen stain. S-100 protein, particularly the β subunit is strongly positive in these granules. PAS-positive granules have been described in myxedematous patients.[70] The lumen often contains PAS-positive material. The stroma of the coil consists of loose connective tissue, which may contain fat cells even when the coil is located in the dermis rather than in subcutaneous fat tissue. The stroma may be metachromatic and alcian-blue-positive and is quite vascular. Special stains for nerve such as antimyelin basic protein and neurofilament antibodies demonstrate a rich plexus of nerve endings surrounding the secretory gland.

There is a definite basement membrane zone around the secretory epithelium in which the reticular and elastic fibers form a basket impregnated with PAS-positive material.

Although the kinetics of the acrosyringeal cells and their replacement by mitotic division of dermal duct cells have been clarified by Christophers and Braun-Falco,[71] much remains to be learned about the regeneration of the eccrine apparatus. When the duct is severed experimentally in the middermis,[72] the deep stump proliferates and forms small cysts with spiraling lumen, a phenomenon also observed when ducts are obstructed by squamous cell carcinoma or other pathologic processes[73,74] (Fig. 2–42). Ductal epithelium participates in wound healing and forms new epidermis. On the other hand, when ducts are interrupted by subepidermal bullae, they often form small keratinizing cysts (sweat duct milia), which are exfoliated spontaneously. It seems possible that all sweat duct cells move upward along the basement membrane and eventually are converted into acrosyringeal cells and exfoliated. Nothing is known about regeneration of the secretory cells. Occasional mitoses may be found in sections, and epithelium of eccrine coils shows vigorous proliferative activity in tissue culture.[75]

One morphologic abnormality is occasionally encountered in the secretory portion. The cytoplasm of

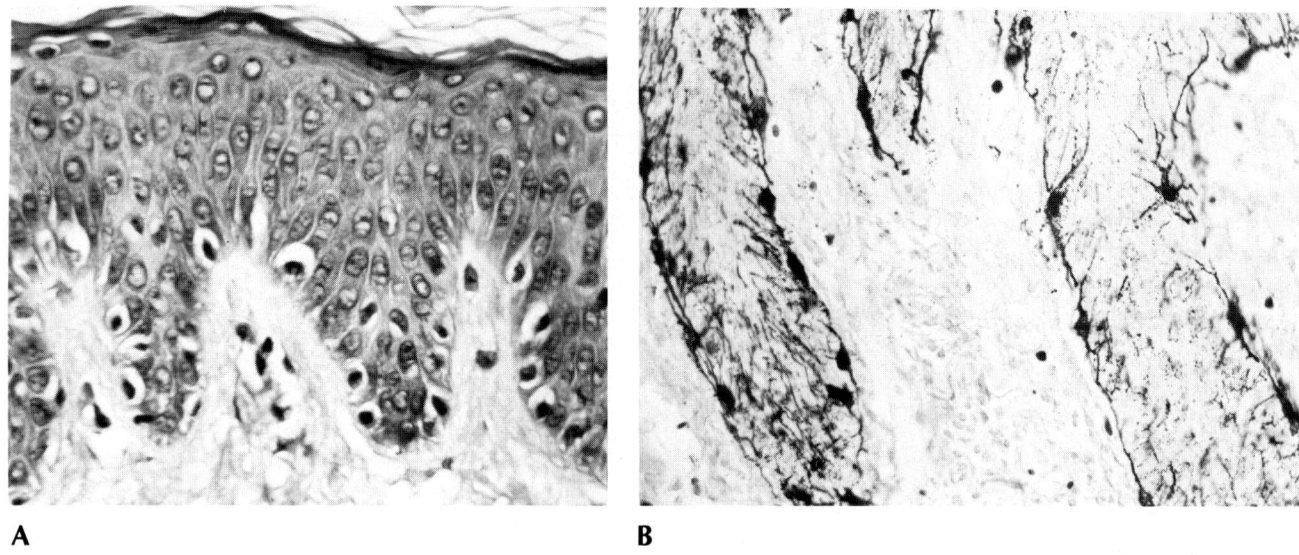

Figure 2–43.
Epidermal melanocytes. **A.** Masson's clear cells in almost nonpigmented normal epidermis. H&E. X370. **B.** Pigment block in acanthotic epidermis of eczematous dermatitis. Melanocytes are full of pigment which outlines their dendrites. Masson–Fontana silver reaction. X370.

the cells appears foamy and light staining. Acid phosphatase activity is increased,[76] but no clear association with sweat dysfunction could be established, although a single patient reported to us that his sweating was diminished. Grosshans et al[77] reported that sweat of two persons with this abnormality did not spread thinly on the skin surface and related this to the absence of the dark cells in the affected glands. A similar absence of these cells was reported in a child affected with adrenoleukodystrophy.[78]

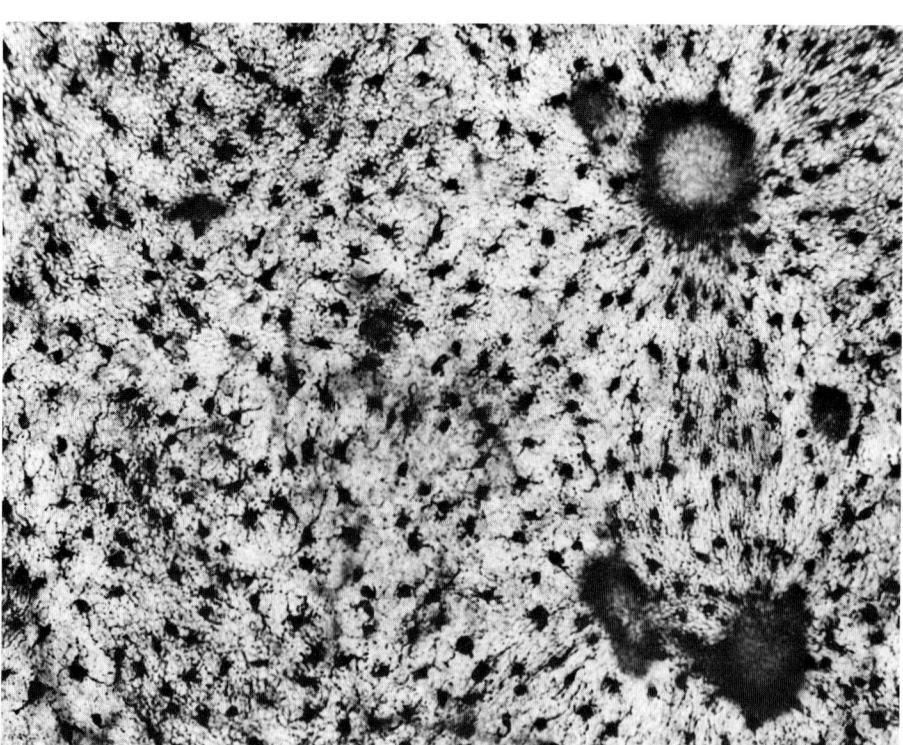

Figure 2–44.
Lower surface of an epidermal sheet separated from dermis by immersion in sodium bromide solution and stained with dopa.[81] The black rings are outlets of hair follicle and sweat ducts. The fairly even distribution of dendritic melanocytes and the faint polygonal outlines of basal keratinocytes are shown. X200 (approx).

INTRAEPIDERMAL DENDRITIC CELLS

Melanocytes

Normal epidermis contains a population of dendritic cells regularly distributed among the basal cells at the dermoepidermal junction. These cells are known as clear cells of Masson. In nonpigmented skin they are dopa-positive but pigment granules may not be seen. In pigmented skin they are Dopa-positive and contain melanin granules. They are the melanocytes (Fig. 2–43), the neuroectodermal symbionts (see Fig. 2–2) in the epidermis.

Melanocytes contribute melanin granules to the epidermal keratinocytes just as they do to keratinizing hair cells. The number of melanocytes varies from approximately 500 to 2000 per mm^2 of surface in different areas of the skin (Fig. 2–44). The number of melanocytes is, however, almost the same in all races, the difference in epidermal pigmentation being mainly one of function. In dark skinned individuals more melanin is produced more continuously by every melanocyte. In addition, highly active melanocytes produce larger melanosomes. Ultraviolet and other stimuli produce the same effects in all melanocytes,[79] but this response is very minimal in the fair-skinned individual who becomes red but never tans following sun exposure. The melanosomes transferred from the melanocyte dendrite are packaged into lysosomes of prickle cells and gradually degraded before they reach the horny layer. Melanosomes larger than approximately 0.35 μm, on the other hand, remain single and unaltered.[80] Black skin is better protected because intact melanosomes are present in the upper layers of the epidermis, whereas white and oriental skins are less protected because small melanosomes are easily digested just above the basal layer. Melanocytes are capable of phagocytosis and accumulate lipid droplets in epidermis overlying xanthomas.[81]

In normal black skin, melanocytes are not very conspicuous between the heavily pigmented basal cells unless they protrude toward the dermis. Each melanocyte seems to be associated with about 10 basal cells, with which it forms the epidermal melanin unit.[82] In dermatitis, this symbiotic relationship is easily disturbed (Fig. 2–45). Transfer of melanin into keratinocytes is blocked,[83] and the melanocytes become engorged and highly dendritic (see Fig. 2–43B). The dispersion of melanin granules in the dendrites contributes to the clinical darkening of inflamed skin in blacks, whereas in histologic sections the epidermis appears paler because the edematous keratinocytes contain less melanin.

Langerhans Cells

High-level dendritic cells (see Table 2–2) are known as Langerhans cells (Fig. 2–46). They are dopa-negative, do not contain melanin, and are usually demonstrated by gold chloride and ATPase techniques, although one can recognize them in routine sections with a fair degree of confidence. They are a separate race of nonkeratinocytes derived not from neural crest, but from the bone marrow, and they are able to undergo mitotic division in the epidermis.

Research activity has increased greatly since the role of high-level dendritic cells in primary antigen processing in contact dermatitis and in immunologic disease was recognized.[84,85] New sub-

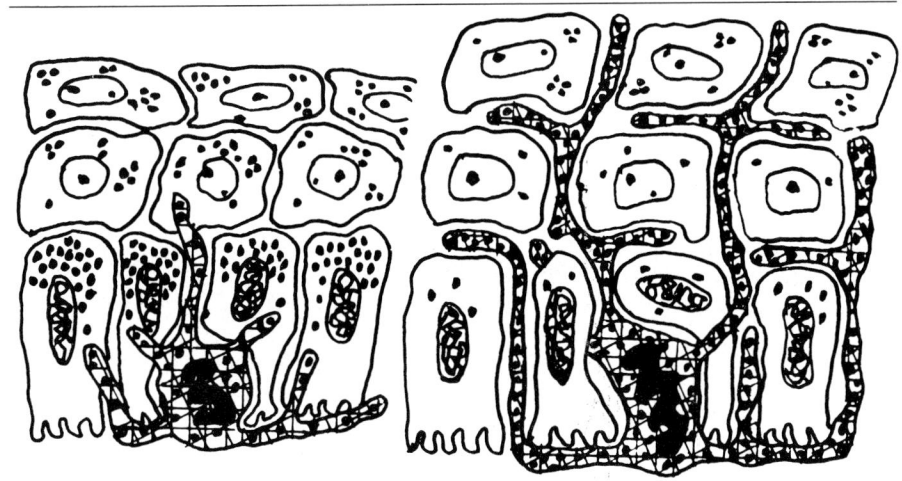

Figure 2–45.
Diagram illustrating the epidermal melanin unit (left) and its disruption in disease due to pigment block (right).

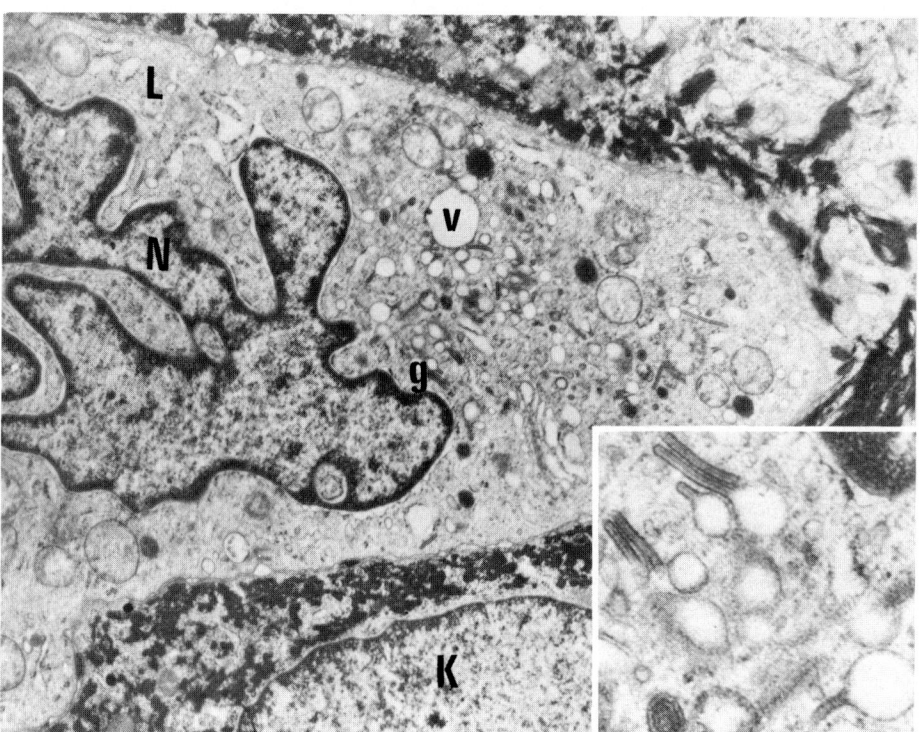

Figure 2–46.
Langerhans cell (L) between keratinocytes (K). Electron micrograph X11,200 shows the deeply indented nucleus (N). Vacuoles (V) and the Birbeck granules (g), with their tennis-racquet shape, are visible. Inset shows details of granules (Courtesy of Dr. A. P. Lupulescu.)

stances such as S-100 protein, HLA-DR, and CD1 (OKT-6)[86–88] could be stained with immunohistochemical methods but their identifying feature, besides a deeply indented nucleus, is the Langerhans cell granule (Birbeck granule), demonstrated and investigated only by electron microscopy. Langerhans cells have been found also in the dermis, in lymph nodes, and especially in the tumor cells of histiocytosis X (Chapter 25).

Merkel Cells

The Merkel cell is described in early anatomic literature as a tactile cell in connection with intraepidermal nerve endings and as possessing sparse desmosomes connecting to surrounding keratinocytes.[89] These cells appear in dermis and epidermis in the months 7 through 12 of fetal life. In recent years, they have been found by electron microscopy to contain round, dense cored granules and to occur more frequently in the haarscheibe. Merkel cells are abundant in fingertips. In fetal finger skin it is found in the mesenchyme, always accompanied by Schwann cells. Early eccrine germ contains many Merkel cells. Because they contain tonofilaments and desmosomes and may be found in the epidermis before the dermal Merkel cells are recognized, some investigators believe that they originate from the epidermis rather than from neural crest or Schwann cells. Toker[90] recognized them as the tumor cells of trabecular carcinoma, where they resemble basal cells. They are difficult to identify in routine sections unless special stains are employed such as those used for cytokeratin, neuron specific enolase, and chromogranin.[91,92]

REFERENCES

1. Montagna W, Parakkal PF: The Structure and Function of Skin, 3rd ed. New York: Academic Press, 1974
2. Pinkus H: Anatomy and embryology of the skin. In Andrade R, Gumport SL, Popkin GL, Rees TD (eds): Cancer of the Skin. Philadelphia: Saunders, 1976
3. Montagna W, Freedberg IM (eds): Cutaneous biology 1950–1975. J Invest Dermatol 67:1–230, 1976
4. Pinkus H, Tanay A: Embryologie der haut. In Jadassohn J: Handbuch der Haut- und Geschlechtskrankheiten, Ergänzungswerk, 1, 1. Berlin: Springer-Verlag, 1968
5. Holbrook KA: Human epidermal embryogenesis. Int J Dermatol 18:329, 1979
6. Flaxman BA: Cell identification in primary cell cultures from skin. In Vitro 10:112, 1974
7. Eady R: Prenatal diagnosis. Proceedings of the XVII World Congress of Dermatology, Berlin, May 1987, p 127

8. Breathnach AS: Development and differentiation of dermal cells in man. J Invest Dermatol 71:2, 1978
9. Johnson CL, Holbrook KA: Development of human embryonic and fetal dermal vasculature. J Invest Dermatol 93:105, 1989
10. Deutsch TA, Esterly NB: Elastic fibers in fetal dermis. J Invest Dermatol 65:320, 1976
11. Hashimoto K, Gross BG, Lever WF: The ultrastructure of the skin of human embryos. I. The intraepidermal eccrine sweat duct. J Invest Dermatol 45:139, 1965
12. Mishima Y, Pinkus H: Electron microscopy of keratin layer stripped human epidermis. J Invest Dermatol 50:89, 1968
13. Dale BA: Purification and characterization of a basic protein from the stratum corneum of mammalian epidermis. Biochem Biophys Acta 491:193, 1977
14. Findlay GH: Blue skin. Br J Dermatol 83:127, 1970
15. Odland GF, Holbrook K: The lamellar granules of epidermis. In Mali JWH (ed): Current Problems in Dermatology. Basel: S. Karger, 1981, p 29
16. Hashimoto K: The marginal band. A demonstration of the thickened cellular envelope of the human nail cell with the aid of Lanthan staining. Arch Dermatol 103:387, 1971
17. Baden HP, Kublis J, Phillips SB, et al: A new class of soluble basic protein precursors of the cornified envelope of mammalian epidermis. Biochem Biophys Acta 925:63, 1987
18. Hashimoto K: Cellular envelopes of keratinized cells of the human epidermis. Arch Klin Exp Dermatol 235:374, 1969
19. Plewig G, Marples RR: Regional differences of cell sizes in the human stratum corneum. J Invest Dermatol 54:13, 1970
20. Goldschmidt, H, Thew MA: Exfoliative cytology of psoriasis and other common dermatoses. Quantitative analysis of parakeratotic horny cells in 266 patients. Arch Dermatol 106:476, 1972
21. Madsen A: Diagnostic scale analysis of desquamating dermatoses. Acta Derm Venereol 52:415, 1972
22. Wright N: Cell population kinetics in human epidermis. Int J Dermatol 16:449, 1977
23. Schell H: Zur Zellkinetik der Epidermis aus biorhythmischer Sicht. Zentralbl Haut Geschl Krank 141:149, 1979 (lengthy bibliography)
24. Grove GL: Epidermal cell kinetics in psoriasis. Int J Dermatol 18:111, 1979
25. Swann MM: The control of cell division: A review. II. Cancer Res 18:1118, 1958
26. Pinkus H: The direction of growth of human epidermis. Br J Dermatol 83:556, 1970
27. Pinkus H: Die Makroskopische Anatomie der Haut. In Jadassohn J: Handbuch der Haut- und Geschlechtskrankheiten, Ergänzungswerk 1, 2. Berlin: Springer-Verlag, 1965, p 1
28. Tring FC, Murgatroyd LB: Surface microtopography of normal human skin. Arch Dermatol 109:223, 1974
29. Hodge SJ, Freeman RG: The basal lamina in skin disease. Int J Dermatol 17:261, 1978
30. Sweet RD: Orientations. Trans St Johns Hosp Dermatol Soc 57:135, 1971
31. Reed RJ, Ackerman AB: Pathology of the adventitial dermis: Anatomic observations and biologic speculations. Hum Pathol 4:207, 1973
32. Cooper JH: Histochemical observations on elastic sheath–elastic fibril system of dermis. J Invest Dermatol 52:169, 1969
33. Pinkus H, Mehregan AH, Staricco RG: Elastic globes in human skin. J Invest Dermatol 45:81, 1965
34. Hashimoto K: Normal and abnormal connective tissue of the human skin. I. Fibroblast and collagen. Int J Dermatol 17:457, 1978
35. Braverman IM, Yen A: Ultrastructure of the human dermal microcirculation. II. J Invest Dermatol 68:44, 1977
36. Mortimer PS, Cherry GW, James RI, et al: The importance of elastic fibers in skin lymphatics. Br J Dermatol 108:561–566, 1983
37. Sakai LY, Keene DR, Engvall E: Fibrillin, a new 350-KD glycoprotein, is a component of extracellular microfibrils. J Cell Biol 103:2499, 1986
38. Pierce RH, Grimmer BJ: Age and the chemical constitution of normal human dermis. J Invest Dermatol 58:347, 1972
39. Šmahel J, Charvát A: Fatty tissue in plastic surgery. Acta Chir Plast 6:223, 1964
40. Smith U, Sjostrom L, Bjorntorp P: Comparison of two methods for determining human adipose cell size. J Lipid Res 13:822, 1972
41. Whimster JW: Morbid anatomy and the skin. Trans St Johns Hosp Dermatol Soc 54:11, 1968
42. Pinkus H: Cutis punctata linearis colli. Arch Dermatol 114:625, 1978
43. Pinkus H: Embryology of hair. In Montagna W, Ellis RA (eds): The Biology of Hair Growth. New York: Academic Press, 1958, p 1
44. Holbrook KA, Odland GF: Structure of the human fetal hair canal and initial hair eruption. J Invest Dermatol 71:385, 1978
45. Kopf AW: The distribution of alkaline phosphatase in normal and pathologic human skin. Arch Dermatol 75:1, 1957
46. Madsen A: Studies on the "bulge" (Wulst) in superficial basal cell epitheliomas. Arch Dermatol 89:698, 1964
47. Straile W: Root sheath–dermal papilla relationships and the control of hair growth. In Lyne AG, Short BF (eds): Biology of the Skin and Hair Growth. Sydney: Angus & Robertson, 1965
48. Pinkus H: "Sebaceous cysts" are trichilemmal cysts. Arch Dermatol 99:544, 1969
49. Ito M, Tazawa T, Shimizu N, et al: Cell differentiation in human anagen hair and hair follicles studied with anti-hair keratin monoclonal antibodies. J Invest Dermatol 86:563, 1986
50. Knutson DD: Ultrastructural observations in acne

vulgaris: The normal sebaceous follicle and acne lesions. J Invest Dermatol 62:288, 1974
51. Duperrat B, Mascaro JM: Une tumeur bénigne développée aux dépens de l'acrotrichium ou partie intraépidermique de follicle pilaire: Porome folliculaire (acanthome folliculaire intraépidermique; acrotrichoma). Dermatologica 126:291, 1963
52. Pinkus H: Static and dynamic histology and histochemistry of hair growth. In Baccaredda-Boy A, Moretti G, Frey JR (eds): Biopathology of Pattern Alopecia. Basel: S. Karger, 1968
53. Arao T, Perkins EM JR: The interrelation of elastic tissue and human hair follicles. In Montagna W, Dobson RL (eds): Hair Growth, Oxford, New York, Pergamon Press, 1969, pp 433–440
54. Montagna W, Bell M, Strauss JJ (eds): Sebaceous glands and acne vulgaris. J Invest Dermatol 62:117, 1974
55. Plewig G, Kligman AM: Proliferative activity of the sebaceous gland of the aged. J Invest Dermatol 70:314, 1978
56. Epstein W, Kligman AM: The pathogenesis of milia and benign tumors of the skin. J Invest Dermatol 26:1, 1956
57. Hashimoto K, Ito M, Suzuki Y: "Innervation and Vasculature of Hair Follicle." In Orfanous LE, Happle R "Eds": Hair and Hair Diseases: Berlin–Heidelberg, Springer–Verlag
58. Hashimoto K, Mehregan AH, Kukira M: Tumors of Skin Appendages. Stoneham, MA, Butterworths Publishers 1987
59. Švob M: Histochemistry of sweat glands. Radovi Akad Nauka BiH 16:71, 1972
60. Hashimoto K: Ultrastructure of human apocrine glands. In Jarrett A (ed): Physiology and Pathophysiology of the Skin. London: Academic Press, 1978, p 1575
61. Perry ET: The Human Ear Canal. Springfield, Ill: Thomas, 1957
62. Pinkus F: Über Hautsinnesorgane neben dem menschlichen Haar (Haarscheiben) und ihre vergleichend-anatomische Bedeutung. Arch Mikr Anat Entwickl Gesch 65:121, 1904
63. Kawamura T, Ishibashi Y, Mori S: Haarscheibe, with special reference to its Merkel cells and perineurale Pigmenthülle. Jpn J Dermatol Ser B 81:363, 1971
64. Pinkus H: Factors in the formation of club hair. In Brown AC, Crounse RG (eds): Hair, Trace Elements, and Human Illness. New York: Praeger, 1980
65. Wells J: A simple technique for establishing cultures of epithelial cells. Br J Dermatol 107:481, 1982
66. Inaba M, Anthony J, McKinstry C: Histologic study of the regeneration of axillary hair after removal with subcutaneous tissue shaver. J Invest Dermatol 72:224, 1979
67. Christophers E, Plewig G: Formation of the acrosyringium. Arch Dermatol 107:378, 1973
68. Loewenthal LJA: The eccrine ampulla: Morphology and function. J Invest Dermatol 36:171, 1961
69. Hori K, Hashimoto K, Eto H, Dekio S: Keratin type intermediate filaments in sweat gland myoepithelial cells. J Invest Dermatol 85:453, 1985
70. Dobson RL, Abele DC: Cytologic changes in the eccrine sweat gland in hypothyroidism. J Invest Dermatol 37:457, 1961
71. Christophers E, Braun-Falco O: Zur Zellreduplikation in ekkrinen Schweissdrüsen vor and nach Stripping. Arch Klin Exp Dermatol 228:220, 1967
72. Lobitz WC Jr, Holyoke JB, Brophy D: Response of the human eccrine sweat duct to dermal injury. J Invest Dermatol 26:247, 1956
73. Santa Cruz DJ, Clausen K: Atypical sweat duct hyperplasia accompanying keratoacanthoma. Dermatologica 154:156, 1977
74. Mehregan AH: Proliferation of sweat ducts in certain diseases of the skin. Am J Dermatopathol 3:27, 1981
75. Pinkus H: Notes on structure and biological properties of human epidermis and sweat gland cells in tissue culture and in the organism. Arch Exp Zellforsch 22:47, 1938
76. Rupec M: Zur Ultrastruktur und sauren Phosphatase Aktivität in den Schweissdrüsen mit "clear reticulated cytoplasm." Arch Dermatol Res 258:193, 1977
77. Grosshans E, Juillard J, Libert JP, et al: Physiopathology of sweating response in individuals with eccrine glands of the rare reticulated clear cell type. J Invest Dermatol 74:455, 1980
78. Martin JJ, Ceuterick C, Martin L, Libert J: Skin and conjunctival biopsies in adrenoleukodystrophy. Acta Neuropathol (Berlin) 38:247, 1977
79. Toda K, Pathak MA, Parrish JA, et al: Alteration of racial differences in melanosome distribution in human epidermis after exposure to ultraviolet light. Nature (New Biol) 236:143, 1972
80. Olson RL, Gaylor J, Everett MA: Skin color, melanin, and erythema. Arch Dermatol 108:541, 1973
81. Silvers DD, Becker LE, Helwig EB: Epidermal melanocytes in eruptive xanthomas. An ultrastructural study. Arch Dermatol 107:847, 1973
82. Duchon J, Fitzpatrick TB, Seiji M: Melanin 1968: Some definitions and problems. In Kopf AW, Andrade R (eds): Year Book of Dermatology, 1967–1968. Chicago: Year Book, 1968
83. Pinkus H, Staricco RG, Kropp PJ, Fan J: The symbiosis of melanocytes and human epidermis under normal and abnormal conditions. In Gordon M (ed): Pigment Cell Biology. New York: Academic Press, 1959
84. Silberberg-Sinakin I, Baer RL, Thorbekke GJ: Langerhans cells. A review of their nature with emphasis on their immunologic functions. Prog Allergy 24:268, 1978
85. Juhlin L (ed): The Langerhans cell and contact dermatitis. Acta Derm Venereol Suppl 79:1, 1978
86. Juhlin L, Shelley WB: New staining techniques for the Langerhans cell. Acta Derm Venereol 57:289, 1977
87. Sjöberg S, Axelsson S, Falck B, et al: A new method for the visualization of the epidermal Langerhans cell

and its application on normal and allergic skin. Acta Derm Venereol Suppl 79:23, 1978
88. Miyauchi S, Hashimoto K: Epidermal Langerhans cells undergo mitosis during the early recovery phase after ultraviolet-B irradiation. J Invest Dermatol 88:703, 1987
89. Winkelmann RK, Breathnach AB: The Merkel cell. J Invest Dermatol 60:2, 1973
90. Toker C: Trabecular carcinoma of the skin. Arch Dermatol 105:107, 1972
91. Ito Y, Kawamura K, Miura T, et al: Merkel cell carcinoma. Arch Dermatol 125:1093, 1989
92. Wilson BS, Lloyd RV: Detection of chromogranin in neuroendocrine cells with monoclonal antibody. Am J Pathol 115:458, 1984

3

TECHNICAL DATA, INCLUDING PITFALLS AND ARTIFACTS

Clinical examination of skin lesions provides the dermatologist with general information upon which differential diagnosis is considered. Histopathologic examination is often needed, however, for a definitive diagnosis. Dermatopathology has developed into a medical specialty, which has an active society that meets annually and to which many American and foreign members contribute new information. In order to apply this knowledge effectively when examining biopsy sections, it is essential that submitting physicians provide detailed clinical information. This must include age and sex of the patient, shade of skin color essential for judging pigmentary change, exact site of the biopsied lesion, and a concise history and description of the dermatosis. Clinical diagnosis or a list of differential diagnoses should be given without fear of influencing the judgment of the pathologist, who is just as ready to disprove as to support the clinical diagnosis.[1]

Clinicians should be aware of the practical importance of proper selection of skin lesions for histologic examination, the estimated depth of pathology, and the steps involved in tissue preparation. They should be acquainted with factors that produce various artifacts. They should know about special stains and their requirements regarding tissue fixation or nonfixation (see Table 3–1).

SELECTION OF SITE AND LESION FOR BIOPSY

Selection of a lesion representative of a generalized eruption depends mainly on the type of lesion.[2]

In a vesiculobullous dermatitis, an early lesion (not older than 24 to 48 hours) is desirable. After this period, a significant amount of epithelial regeneration will have taken place at the floor of the blister, which may dislocate the bulla from its primary site. When only large bullous lesions are present, a punch or, preferably, an excisional biopsy specimen should be taken from the edge of a new lesion extending into the normal skin, so that sections will include the area of the initial formation of the bulla.

When the eruption is characterized by various stages of development, it is essential to select a well-formed lesion, neither too early nor too late. If the eruption shows gradual evolution of lesions, multiple biopsies of various stages are most informative. In allergic vasculitis, immunofluorescence tests for immunoglobulins and complements would be negative if one took a fresh lesion or an old one; the optimal age of the lesion for this purpose is 12 hours.

Eruptions with actively progressing borders usually assume a circular, circinate, or serpiginous shape. In these cases, an elliptical excisional biopsy

TABLE 3–1. STAINING REACTIONS OF SOME TISSUE CONSTITUENTS

Tissue Constituents	Stains	Results
Collagen	Van Gieson	Collagen, red; muscle and nerves, yellow
	Masson's trichrome	Collagen, blue; muscle, red
	Hematoxylin–eosin	Collagen, pink; nuclei, blue
Elastic fibers	Acid orcein–Giemsa	Elastic fibers, dark brown; collagen, pink; melanin, black; hemosiderin, greenish yellow; mast cell granules, deep purple
	Aldehyde fuchsin	Elastic fibers, deep purple; also sulfated AMPS (mast cell granules) and certain epithelial mucins, deep purple
Reticulum	Gomori's or Wilder's	Reticulum fibers, black; also melanin and nerves, black
Glycogen	Periodic acid–Schiff (PAS) reaction	Glycogen, magenta red; also fungous wall and certain mucopolysaccharides, red
Acid mucopolysaccharides (AMPS)	Alcian blue	AMPS, light blue
	Colloidal iron	AMPS, light blue
	Toluidine blue	AMPS, metachromatic purple
Fungi	Digested PAS	Fungous walls, red
	Grocott's methenamine silver	Fungous walls, black
Bacteria	Gram	Gram-positive bacteria, blue; gram-negative bacteria, red
	Fite	Acid-fast bacilli, red
Melanin	Masson's ammoniacal silver nitrate	Melanin, black
	Acid orcein–Giemsa	Melanin, greenish black
Iron (hemosiderin pigment)	Prussian blue and Turnbull's reactions	Tissue ferric and ferrous iron, deep blue
Calcium	Von Kossa	Calcium salts, dark brown to black
	Alizarin red	Calcium–alizarin compound, red
Amyloid	Crystal violet	Amyloid, red
	Congo red	Amyloid, red with green birefringence
	Acid orcein–Giemsa	Amyloid, light blue
	Cotton dyes (RIT)	Amyloid, orange-red

specimen including the active border of the lesion is desirable (Fig. 3–1). In atrophoderma and connective tissue abnormalities the specimen should start in normal skin, cross the active border and include part of the central portion. This procedure guarantees a comparative evaluation of the lesion against the normal connective tissue, which varies tremendously from one part of the body to another.

In the group of skin lesions characterized by areas of atrophy or sclerosis, the biopsy should also be deep enough to include the entire thickness of the skin and part of the subcutaneous fat tissue. As a second choice, one may obtain two punch biopsies, one from the inside and one from normal skin at the periphery of the lesion. These samples should be embedded side by side to provide normal and diseased area for comparative studies.

If several lesions of similar character are available, one should select a site that is above the knee for biopsy. Histologic signs of stasis vascular changes may be present below the knee even in young persons and may interfere with proper diagnosis. Psoriatic plaques or other inflammatory dermatoses over the extensor surface of elbows or knees are often complicated by lichenification. Biopsy specimens taken from other areas may be more diagnostic.

Excoriated lesions are not desirable for histologic examination (Fig. 3–2). Because of the loss of the epidermis and upper portion of the corium, an excoriated lesion is completely nondiagnostic in skin lesions involving mainly these superficial areas. This is a problem particularly in dermatitis herpetiformis, papular urticaria, and other very pruritic diseases.

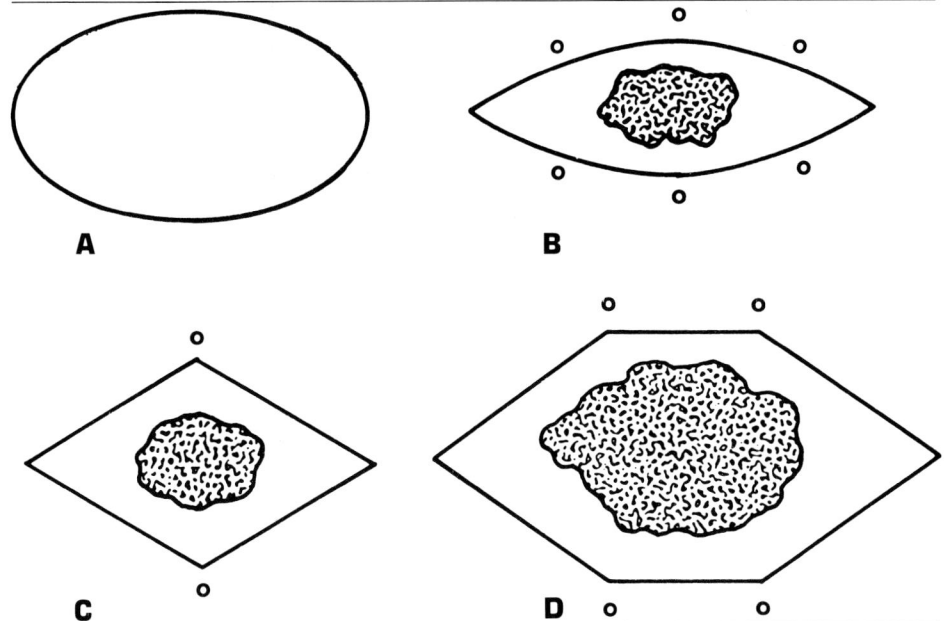

Figure 3–1.
Diagram of skin incisions. **A.** An ellipse is never the shape of a biopsy specimen. **B.** A fusiform excision is often used. It requires several interrupted sutures for adequate closure. **C.** Four straight incisions produce a diamond that can be closed with one suture. This procedure encourages the beginner to cut straight down through the entire thickness of the skin. **D.** If the lesion is large, it is outlined by two parallel incisions, which are then connected to produce a hexagon. Two interrupted sutures are usually sufficient for closure. (From Pinkus. Cutis 20:609, 1977.)

BIOPSY PROCEDURE

When a lesion has been selected for biopsy, clean the skin surface by very gentle application of an alcohol sponge, taking care not to separate any scale or crust. Local anesthesia is best obtained by infiltration under the lesion of 2 percent lidocaine solution or other suitable anesthetic. Addition of epinephrine in 1:100,000 strength greatly reduces bleeding and is rarely contraindicated. A 2- or 5-mL syringe and a No. 26 needle should be used. The injection should be made deep into the corium and subcutaneous tis-

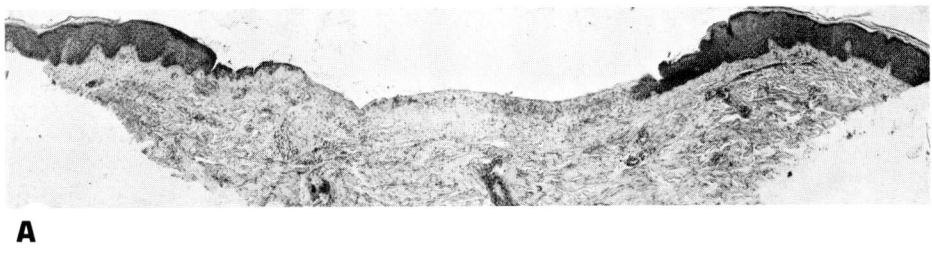

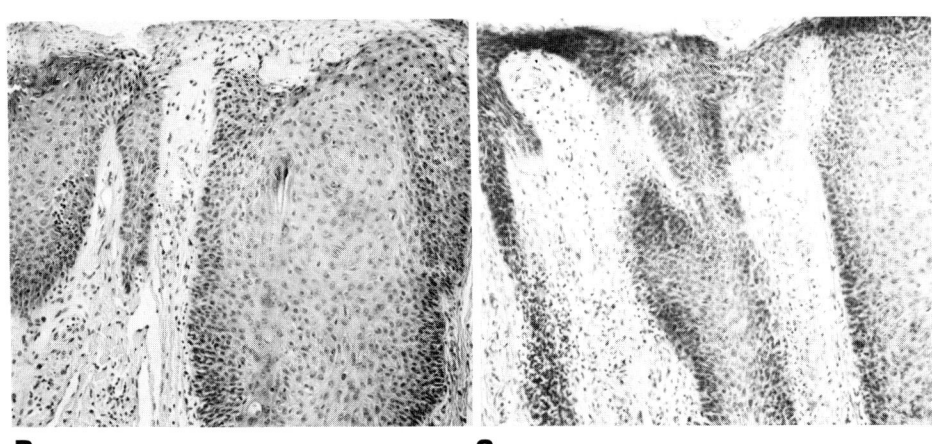

Figure 3–2.
Excoriations. **A.** Deep excoriation has removed entire epidermis. Absence of significant inflammatory infiltrate in dermis suggests that ulceration is not due to a preexistent pathologic process. H&E. X41. **B** and **C.** Hypertrophic lichen simplex chronicus with evidence of excoriation, which has removed suprapapillary plate and exposed papillary heads. H&E. X82.

sue. The Dermoject method of local anesthesia has produced artifactual changes within the epidermis and corium in the form of multiple empty vacuoles (Fig. 3–3) in the fixed tissue sections.

Punch Biopsy and Excisional Biopsy

A 3- to 4-mm punch biopsy provides an adequate amount of tissue for diagnosis of most skin lesions. The biopsy should include the entire thickness of the corium and part of the subcutaneous fat tissue. Excisional biopsy is most desirable when the tissue should be sectioned in a specific direction and is most informative in skin lesions with active borders or in atrophodermas. An excisional specimen should be immediately placed corium down on a piece of paper or cardboard to which it will adhere in order to prevent the tissue from curling. When the specimen is narrow, contraction of the dermis may produce so much overhang and curvature of the epidermis that sections show the epidermis cut at a variety of angles (see Fig. 3–15).

Various types of artifacts may be produced during the biopsy of skin lesions. Forceps pressure may deform a flat piece of skin into a seemingly pedunculated mass (Fig. 3–4). If the deep portion of a punch biopsy specimen is squeezed by forceps, the collagen bundles in the corium will show pseudosclerotic changes (Fig. 3–5) resembling scleroderma. If a toothed forceps is clamped firmly on the skin within the biopsy area, a sinuslike intrusion of epidermis into the corium may result (Fig. 3–6). This artifact usually can be recognized by its rectangular shape and because it is surrounded by compressed collagenous tissue (Fig. 3–7). A needle used for anesthesia or to pick up the specimen may cause a hole. Traumatic separation of the epidermis from the dermis (Fig. 3–8; see Fig. 3–19) may occur during biopsy, especially in skin lesions where the connection of epidermis to corium is defective, as in cases of lichen planus, porphyria, and various bullous disorders. In these cases a part of perilesional skin should be included in the biopsy.

Superficial and Deep Biopsy

Superficial skin biopsy, including the epidermis and papillary layer of the corium, is acceptable in some instances of superficial dermatoses, such as psoriasis, or certain neoplasms, such as flat warts, benign cellular nevi, or seborrheic verrucae. In most inflammatory disorders, metabolic disturbances and tumors, however, a deep biopsy including the entire thickness of the skin is necessary. An even deeper biopsy (Fig. 3–9) is essential for diagnosis of those skin diseases in which the pathologic changes reside in the lower portion of the corium and subcutaneous fat tissue. These include all types of nodular lesions of the leg and the group of panniculitides. For example, a shallow biopsy in erythema nodosum does not show the site of pathology and, therefore, is useless. Thickness of the skin in various areas should be taken into consideration. In taking a biopsy from a lesion of palm or sole, one may obtain a piece of

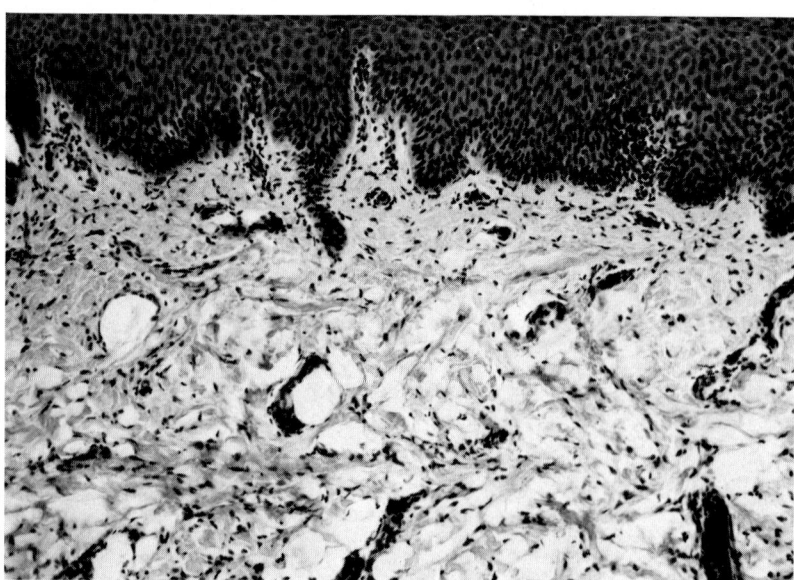

Figure 3–3.
Vacuoles in dermis resulting from Dermojet injection of anesthetic. H&E. X135. (From Mehregan and Pinkus. Arch Dermatol 94:218, 1966.)

COLOR PLATE I

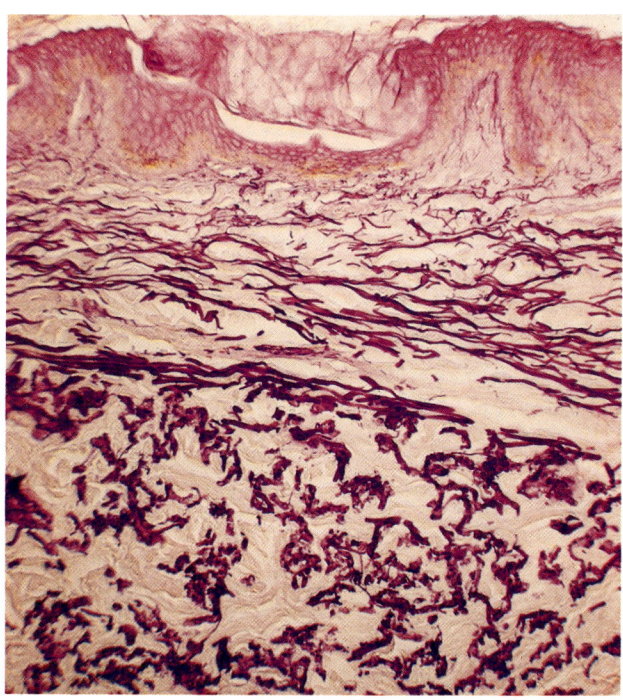

Figure 1
Pseudoxanthoma elasticum. Curled and fragmented elastic fibers in mid-dermis contrast with the normal superficial fibers. Aldehyde fuchsin × 180.

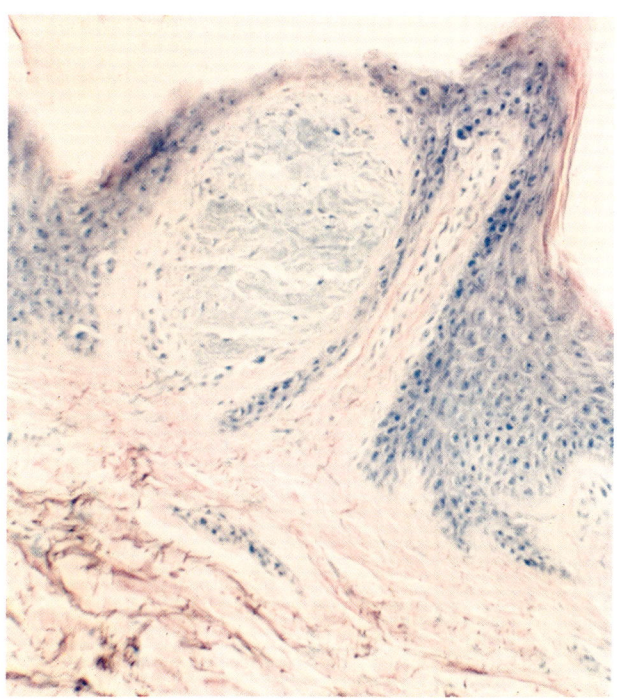

Figure 2
Lichenoid amyloidosis. The amyloid deposits stain in light grayish-blue color. Acid orcein–Giemsa × 180.

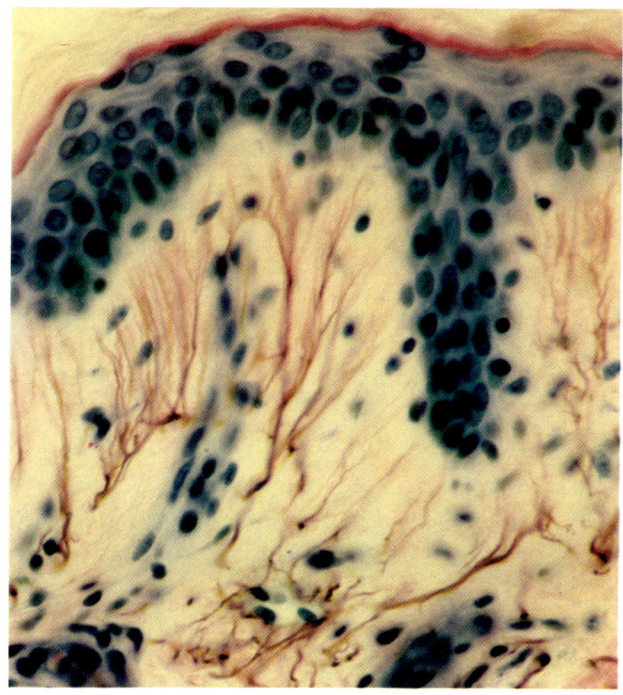

Figure 3
Normal skin. Fine network of elastic fibers in the papillary dermis. Acid orcein–Giemsa × 400.

COLOR PLATE II

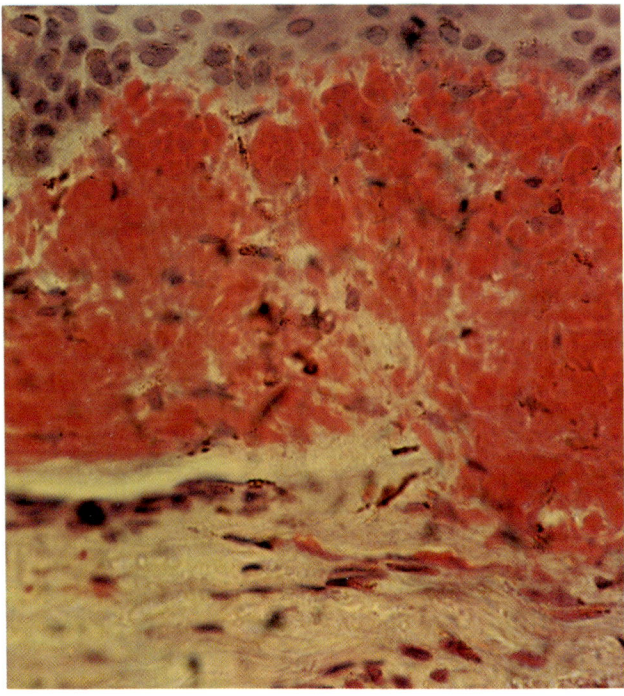

Figure 4
Macular amyloidosis. The amyloid deposits stain in a bright orange color. RIT scarlet red stain × 400.

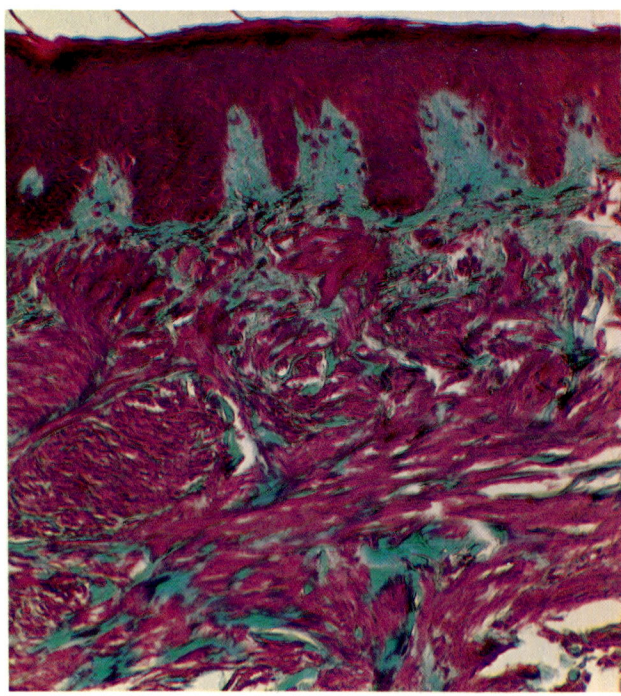

Figure 5
Leiomyoma cutis. Muscle bundles (red) are differentiated from the collagen (blue). Masson's trichrome × 135.

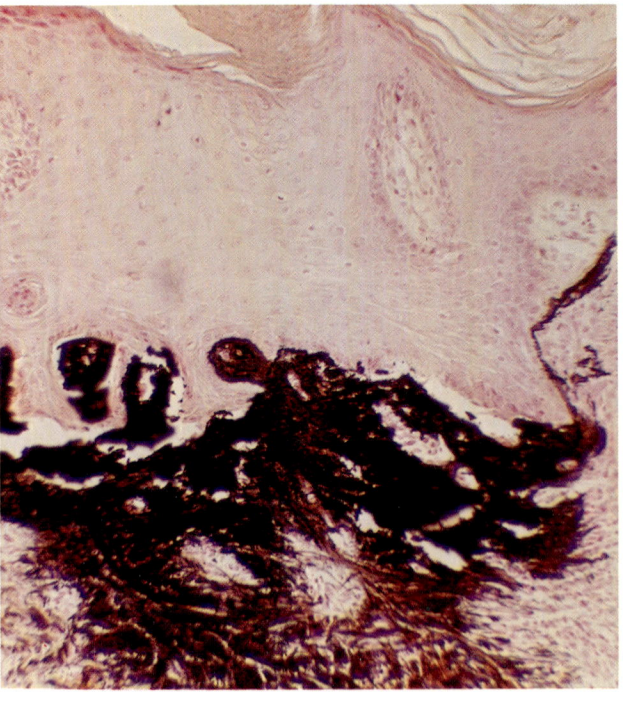

Figure 6
Calcinosis cutis. Massive calcium deposition is present below an acanthotic epidermis. Von Kossa × 135.

COLOR PLATE III

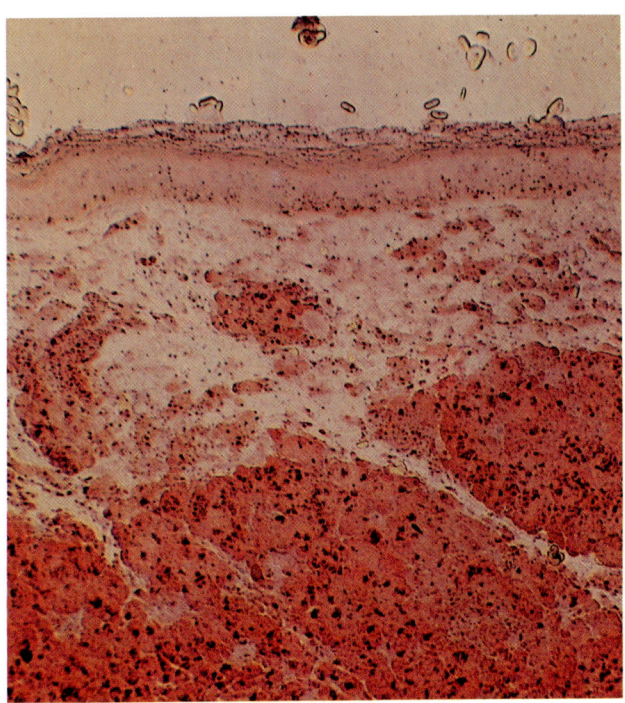

Figure 7
Xanthoma tuberosum. Masses of histiocytes contain lipid granules. Frozen section. Oil red stain × 180.

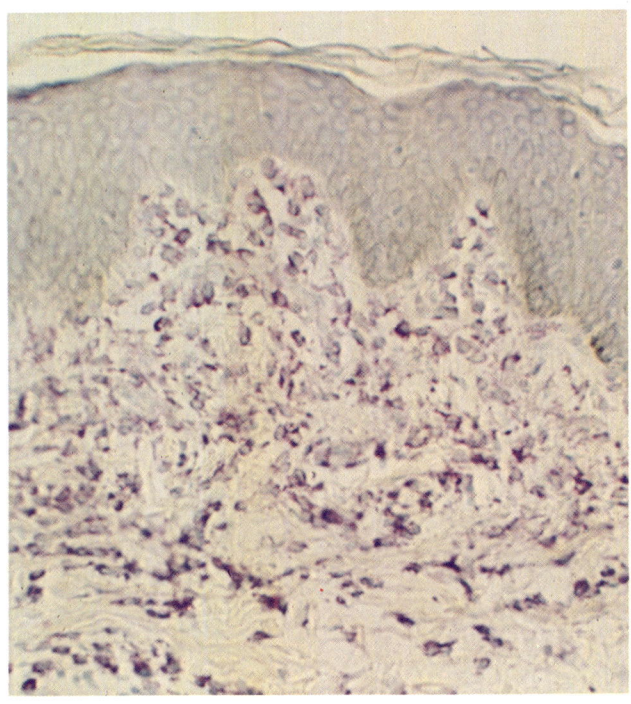

Figure 8
Cutaneous mastocytosis. Dermis shows extensive mast cell infiltrate. Toluidine blue × 200.

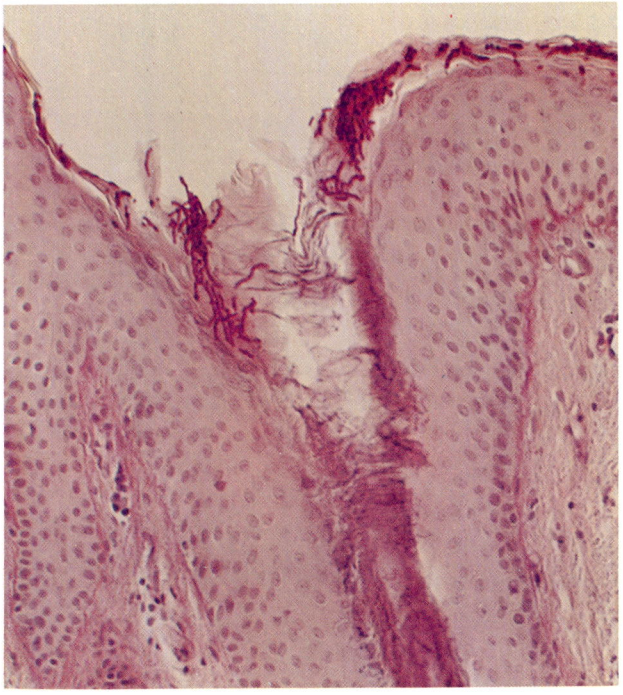

Figure 9
Superficial dermatophytosis. Fungus mycelia in the surface keratin and a hair follicle. PAS—hematoxylin × 250.

COLOR PLATE IV

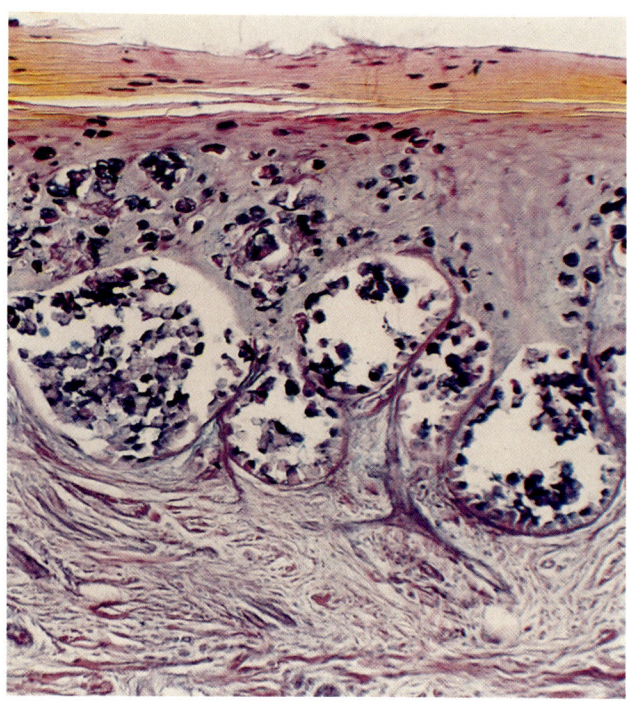

Figure 10
Extramammary Paget disease. Sialomucin in Paget cells stains with PAS and alcian blue in deep purple color. Alcian blue—PAS—picric acid × 250.

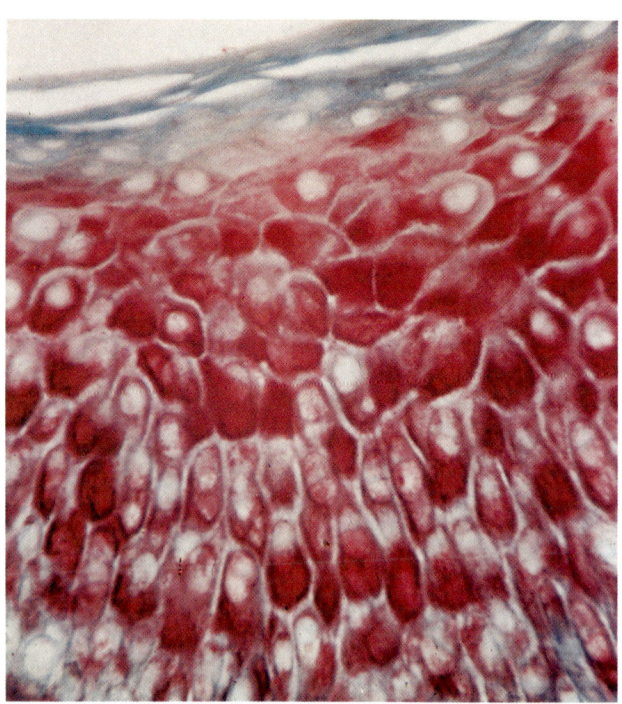

Figure 11
Chronic dermatitis. Lichenified epidermis shows cells containing glycogen granules. PAS—light green × 400.

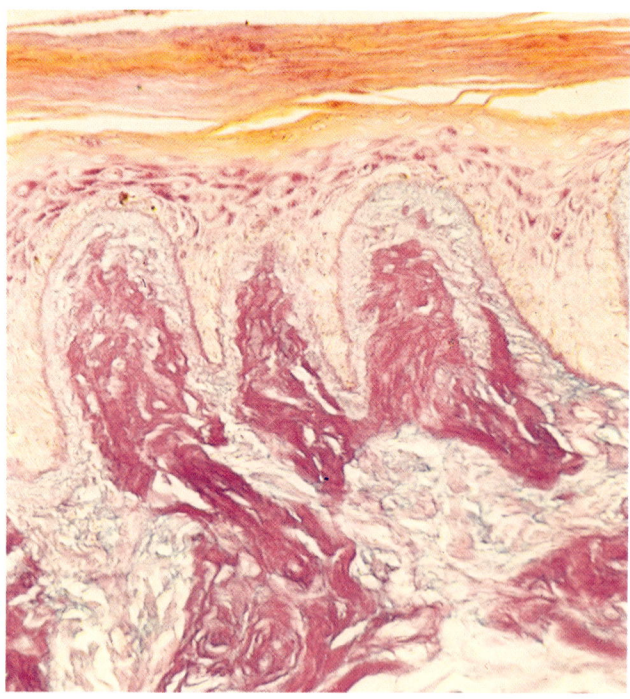

Figure 12
Erythropoietic protoporphyria. Homogeneous PAS-positive material is deposited around the superficial capillary blood vessels. Alcian blue—PAS-picric acid × 250.

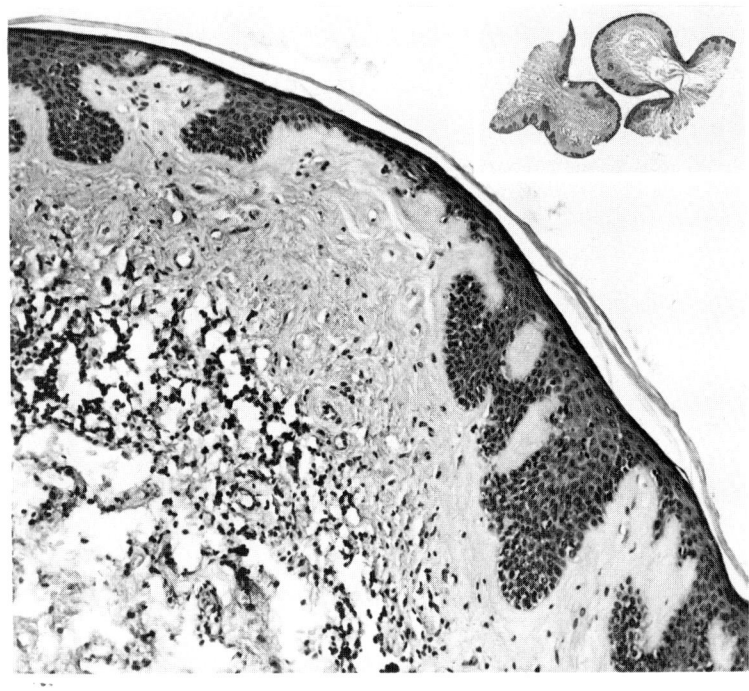

Figure 3–4.
Lesion of lichen sclerosus et atrophicus, which has been deformed into a pedunculated mass by forceps pressure. H&E. X100. Inset, H&E. X5. (From Mehregan and Pinkus. Arch Dermatol 94: 218, 1966.)

tissue that appears relatively thick and adequate and yet includes nothing more than the thick keratin of these areas.

The cutaneous punch should be pressed into the skin with a rotary motion until one feels it sink into the softer fat tissue. On withdrawal of the instrument, the plug of skin then usually pops out of the wound. It can be lifted up gently without exerting pressure, and its base can be snipped through easily with scissors. On the other hand, if the incision is made only part way through the dermis, it takes much more effort to dissect the base with scissors.

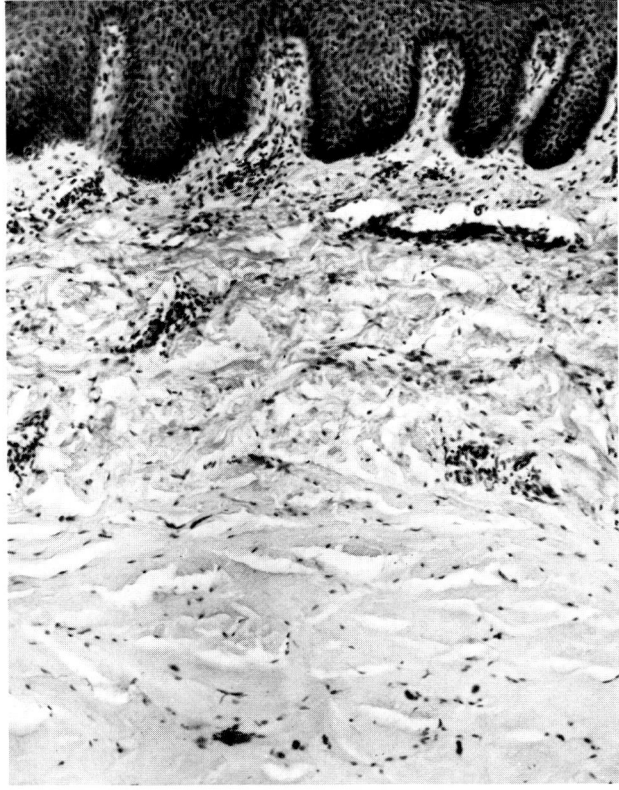

Figure 3–5.
Pseudosclerodermatous changes in deep dermis due to forceps injury. H&E. X135. (From Mehregan and Pinkus. Arch Dermatol 94:218, 1966.)

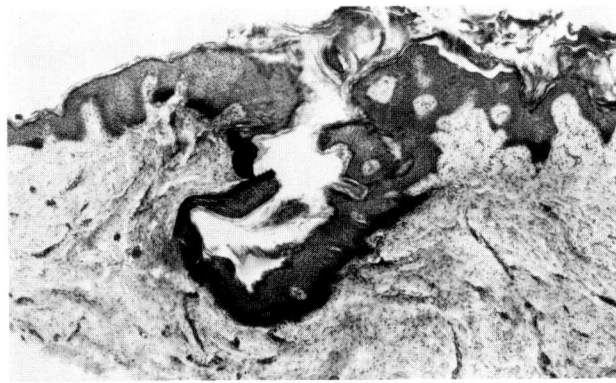

Figure 3–6.
Pseudosinus produced by toothed forceps. H&E. X75. (From Mehregan and Pinkus. Arch Dermatol 94:218, 1966.)

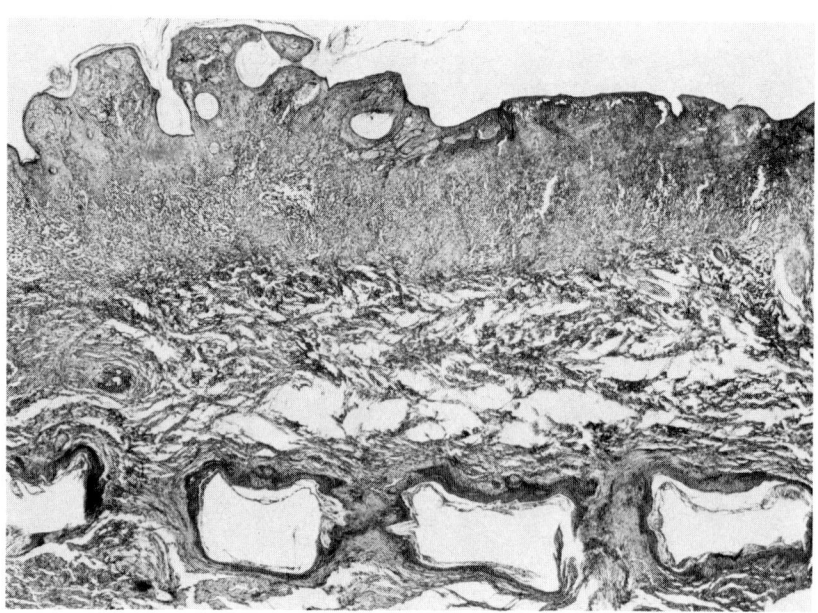

Figure 3–7.
Pseudocysts produced by toothed forceps. Note square outline and compression of epidermis and dermis around holes. H&E. X30.

Wound healing is improved by full-thickness punching if the defect is to be sutured because no tough dermal tissue remains in its base. If the site is left open a shallow biopsy heals more quickly.

If a knife is used, the blade should cut vertically through the skin into fat tissue if the wound is to be sutured (Fig. 3–10). Vertical incision also avoids the common mistake of obtaining a tissue wedge with a narrow base rather than a rectangular block. In well-anesthetized skin, a deep incision does not hurt the patient more than a shallow one and may save him the trauma of a second biopsy, which could be made necessary by an inadequate first specimen. The cosmetic result of a deep excision will be better because the wound edges can be brought together more easily by suture without undue tension. The danger of arterial bleeding is minimal, and oozing of blood can almost always be stopped by firm compression for several minutes. Today, many older patients are on anticoagulant therapy for their heart problems. It is wise to ask if your older patient is taking anticoagulant or aspirin. A 1 week drug-free period usually restores normal coagulation mechanism.

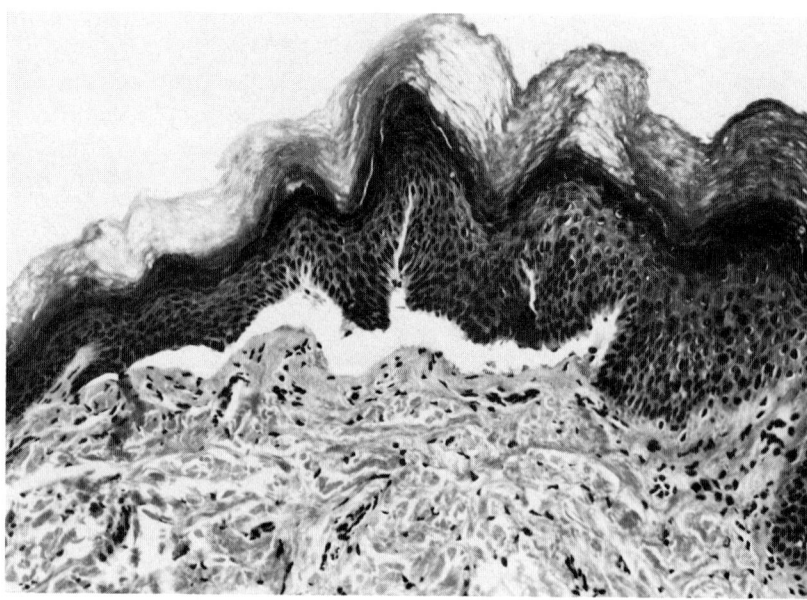

Figure 3–8.
Dermalepidermal separation due to biopsy trauma. H&E. X135. (From Mehregan and Pinkus. Arch Dermatol 94:218, 1966.)

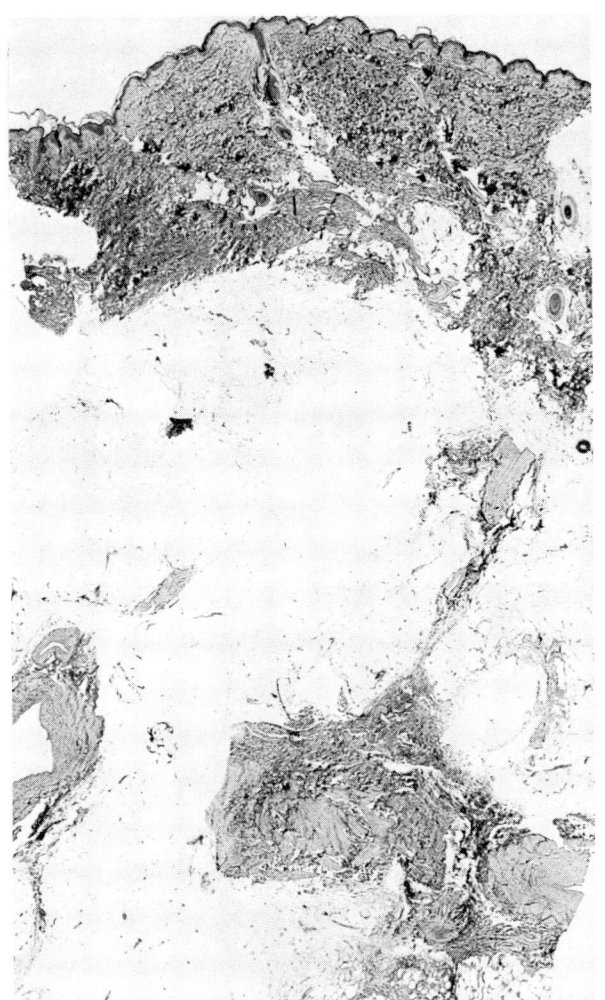

Figure 3–9.
Ideal biopsy specimen for diagnosis of cutaneous–subcutaneous lesion. Diagnosis: erythema nodosum. H&E. X9.

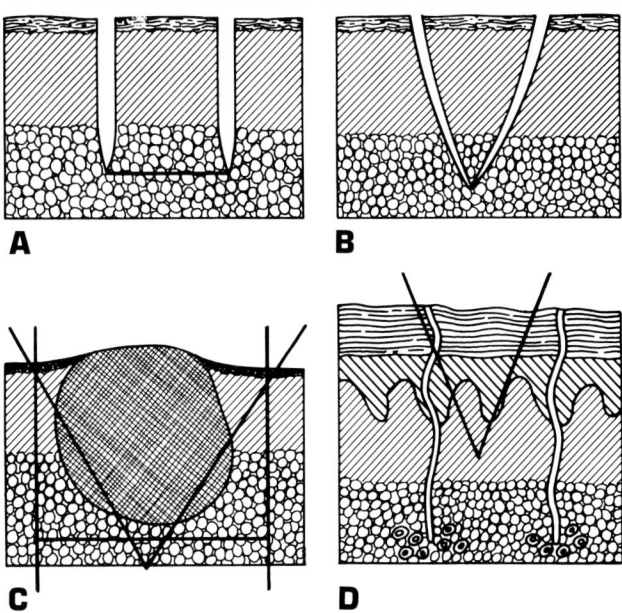

Figure 3–10.
*Diagram showing correct and incorrect incisions. **A**. Correct vertical knife incisions extending into subcutaneous fat tissue. Completion of excision by scissors is easy. **B**. Incorrect wedging of incisions produces an insufficient amount of deep tissues. **C**. The same types of incision produce complete and incomplete removal of a globular tumor. **D**. Wedge incisions in the thick skin of palms and soles often do not penetrate the dermis. (From Pinkus H. Cutis 20:609, 1977.)*

Curette Biopsy

Ordinarily, material obtained by curettage of a skin lesion is not very satisfactory for histologic examination because in such fragmented pieces, tissue orientation is difficult. If curettage is desirable for cosmetic reasons, one should attempt to obtain several large pieces of tissue early during the procedure. The material for tissue examination by curettage should be taken before the lesion is electrodesiccated. The electric current produces severe artifactual changes characterized by marked dehydration of the tissue and by elongation of cell nuclei in the direction of the current (polarization of cells) (Fig. 3–11). Tissue samples can be obtained from a nodular lesion by using a dendritic dental broach for identification of the cell infiltrate or such material as Leishman bodies.[3] Another artifact observed in curetted basal cell epitheliomas is produced by squeezing out the solid epithelial tumor masses, leaving behind empty spaces within the fibrous mesodermal stroma, which then may resemble a lymphangioma (Fig. 3–12). Similarly, whole lobes of sebaceous glands may be squeezed out of a hair follicle (Fig. 3–13). This can also occur as a natural phenomenon.[4]

FIXATION

The biopsy specimen should be placed immediately into a fixative solution. Various fixatives are available for routine purposes; 10 percent formalin or, more preferably, neutral buffered formaldehyde solutions are convenient and effective. Because the original stock solution of formalin contains only 40

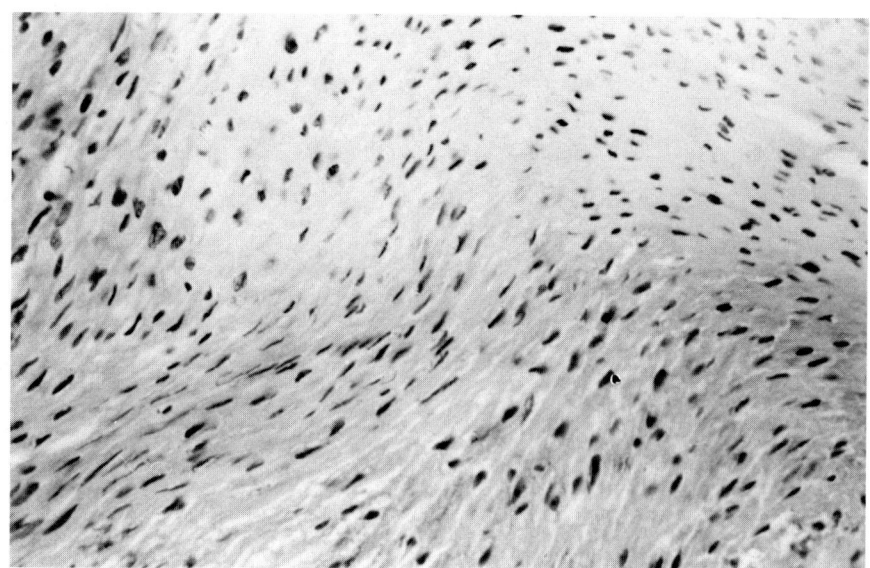

Figure 3–11.
Polarization of cell nuclei by electric current produced in a verruca vulgaris. H&E. X400.

percent formaldehyde, a 10 percent formalin solution really contains only 4 percent formaldehyde. These fixatives are prepared as follows:

10 PERCENT FORMALIN SOLUTION

Concentrated (40 percent) formaldehyde solution	100 mL
Tap water	7900 mL

NEUTRAL BUFFERED FORMALDEHYDE SOLUTION (pH 7.0)

Concentrated (40 percent) formaldehyde solution	100 mL
Tap water	900 mL
Acid sodium phosphate, monohydrate	4 g
Anhydrous disodium phosphate	6.5 g

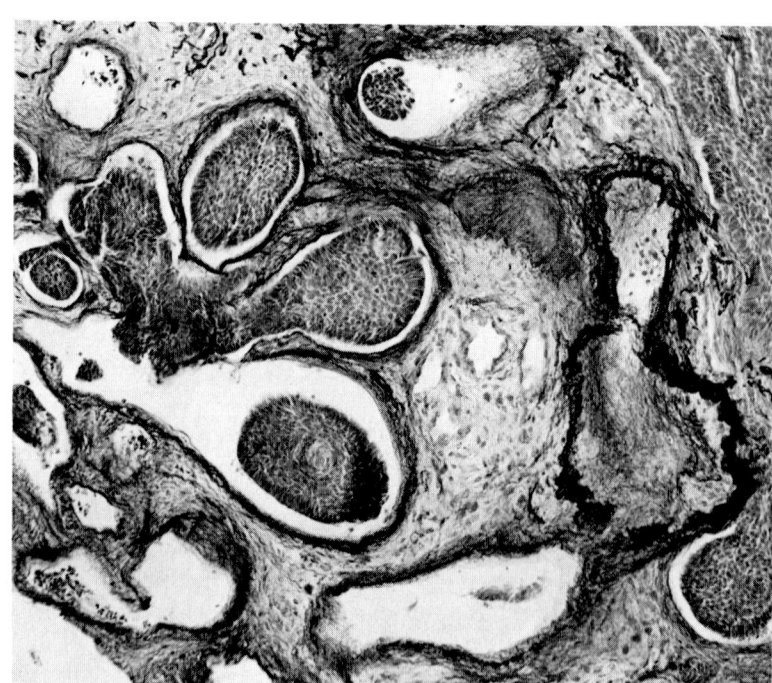

Figure 3–12.
Squeezing effect on basal cell epithelioma. Epithelial nests have been separated from their stoma, and some have been lost, causing impression of angioma. In this case, tumor stroma contains newly formed elastic fibers. O&G. X135.

Care must be taken during the winter season, especially in the northern United States. If a specimen placed in formalin fixative is deposited in an outdoor mailbox too soon, the tissue may freeze before it is completely fixed. Numerous ice crystals will form, which later become manifest (Fig. 3–14) in the tissue sections as intracellular empty vacuoles. If the process of freezing takes place slowly, larger ice crystals and intracellular vacuoles are formed, which may render the specimen completely unsuitable for interpretation. To prevent this artifact, specimens in formalin solution should be kept at room temperature for at least 6 hours before exposing them to freezing temperatures. This period allows adequate tissue fixation, and later freezing will not produce disturbing changes. Alcoholic fixatives may be substituted during the cold winter months, since they do not freeze except under extremely cold conditions. One of these (formol–alcohol) fixative is prepared as follows:

ALCOHOLIC FORMALIN
40 percent formaldehyde solution   100 mL
95 percent ethyl alcohol   900 mL

Seventy percent ethyl or isopropyl alcohol may also be used as fixatives. The alcoholic fixatives produce some shrinkage of the tissue and should not be used

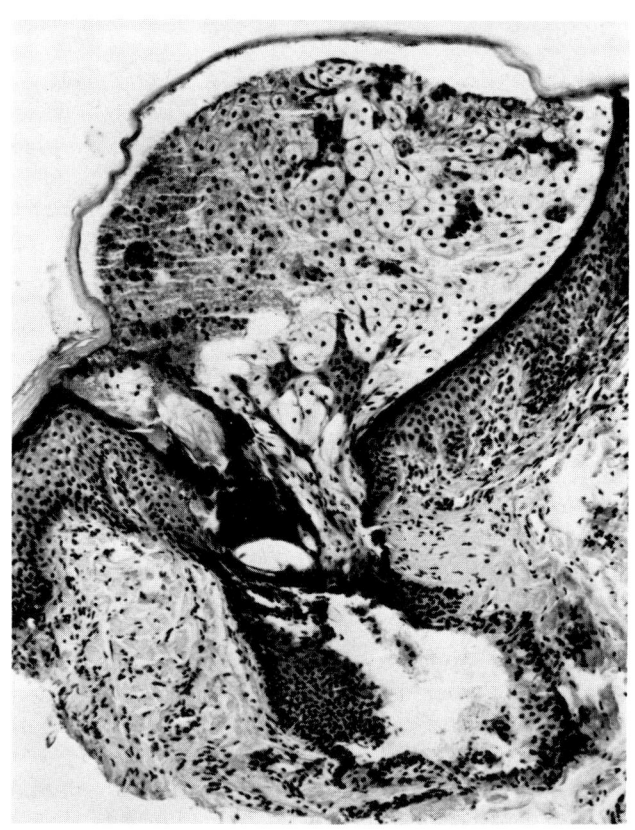

Figure 3–13.
Subcorneal displacement of sebaceous gland. H&E. X135. (From Mehregan and Pinkus. Arch Dermatol 94: 218, 1966.)

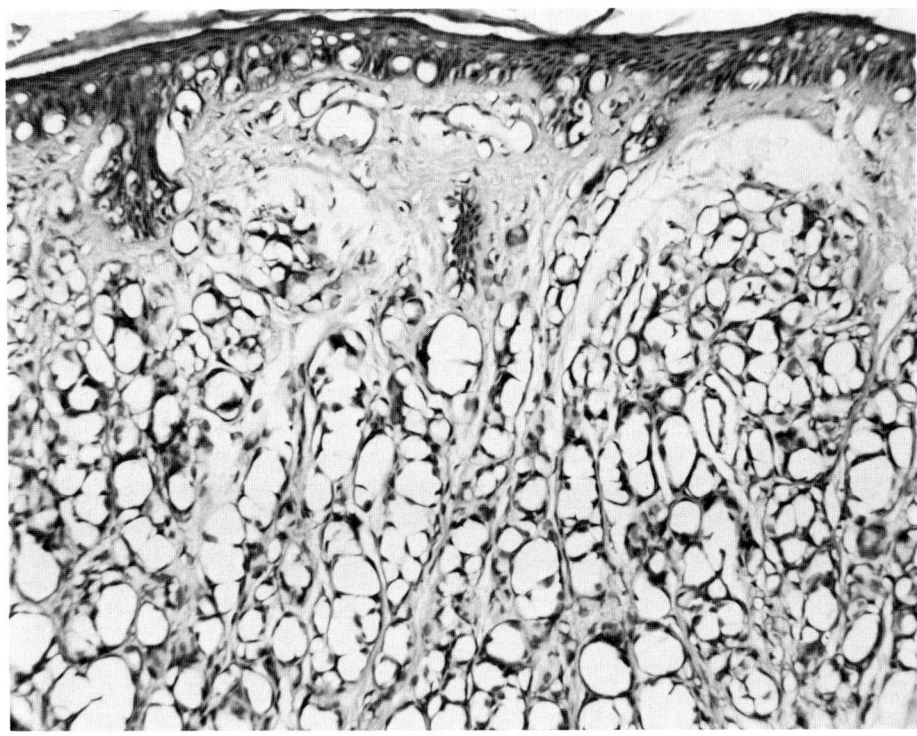

Figure 3–14.
Artifact caused by formalin fixation proceeding at freezing temperature. This section of an intradermal nevus cell nevus is almost unrecognizable because of vacuole formation in epidermal cells and nevocytes. H&E. X180.

for frozen sections for fat stain or for immunostaining for S-100 protein.

A disturbing phenomenon that occurs with the use of nonbuffered formalin is the formation of formalin pigment (acid formaldehyde hematin) by the action of acid aqueous solution of formaldehyde on blood-rich tissue.[5] It can be prevented by buffering the fixative to a pH above 6. Formalin pigment appears as dark brown microcrystalline particles, refractile under polarized light. It occurs largely within the vascular spaces among apparently intact or laked erythrocytes and also extravascularly within phagocytes.[6] The pigment may be removed from the tissue sections by either Verocay's method[7] or Kardasewitsch's method. Iron pigment deposition in tissue may occur when formalin solution is contaminated by a rusted container.

Adequate fixation time depends on the thickness of the specimen. Fixation progresses from the periphery of the tissue, with the central portion fixed last. Fixatives do not penetrate intact epidermis easily but reach it from the dermal side. Ordinarily, the amount of fixative solution should be about 20 times the volume of the specimen. Excessive amount of blood and exudate should be rinsed in normal saline because these not only dilute the solution but also interfere with the fixation.

TISSUE PROCESSING AND PREPARATION OF THE HISTOLOGIC SECTION

Every specimen received in a histopathology laboratory should be given an accession number and also identified by a short gross description. Small punch biopsies up to 4 mm usually do not require trimming. Larger punch specimens may be trimmed at one edge or divided into two pieces through the center of the specimen to provide a flat surface for embedding. Elliptical excisional specimens not wider than 4 mm also do not require trimming. Larger pieces, however, may be trimmed from one side. It is often requested of the pathologist to check an excised suspected neoplasm for completeness of the removal of the tumor. We divide such an elliptical specimen through the smaller diameter into several thin slices (step sectioning) and embed these side by side. In the sections from these pieces, one will look for evidence of tumor extension to the lateral and lower border of the specimen. If the clinical diagnosis suggests a disease in which fat stain may be necessary, one portion of the specimen may be stored in formalin solution in a cool place for frozen sections.

Dehydration

The formalin-fixed specimens pass through graded (50 percent to absolute) alcohol to become dehydrated, then through two or three changes of xylol or chloroform to become defatted and cleared, and finally through two or three changes of paraffin at a temperature of 60°C, the entire process requiring about 24 hours. A modified paraffin substance (Paraplast) is much superior to paraffin for embedding.

Embedding

Since dermatopathology has been established on morphological descriptions of skin sections that were cut perpendicular to the surface, any deviation from this standard causes problems. Figure 3–15 shows sections of pieces of normal abdominal skin embedded in the correct upright and also in incorrect tangential positions. Note the increasing degree of papillomatous appearance of the epidermis and papillary connective tissue in wrongly embedded specimens. If the specimen is embedded with the epidermal surface lying down flat, early sections will show a sheet of epidermis containing small islands representing cross sections of the connective tissue papillae. Deeper sections will contain only the corium and show the cutaneous adnexa in cross section. In such incorrrectly embedded tissue the stained section may not include superficial or deep lesions and depth measurement of melanoma becomes impossible. Embedding the skin specimens therefore requires special attention. The epidermal surface of each specimen must be identified, and then the specimen placed into a mold or a container holding the melted Paraplast in such a manner that the surface of the skin will be at a 90 degree angle to the knife when the tissue block is mounted on a microtome.

Cutting

After cooling and hardening, the Paraplast blocks are trimmed to desirable size and may be mounted on wood blocks. The specimens should be placed into the microtome in such a manner that the edge of the knife will hit the epidermis first. The epidermis, especially if thick and hyperkeratotic, represents the area of greatest resistance. If the relatively soft corium is cut first and then the knife edge meets the resistant area, artifactual separation may occur between these two parts. In addition, particles of connective tissue fibers or other intradermal material may be carried into the epidermis by the edge of the

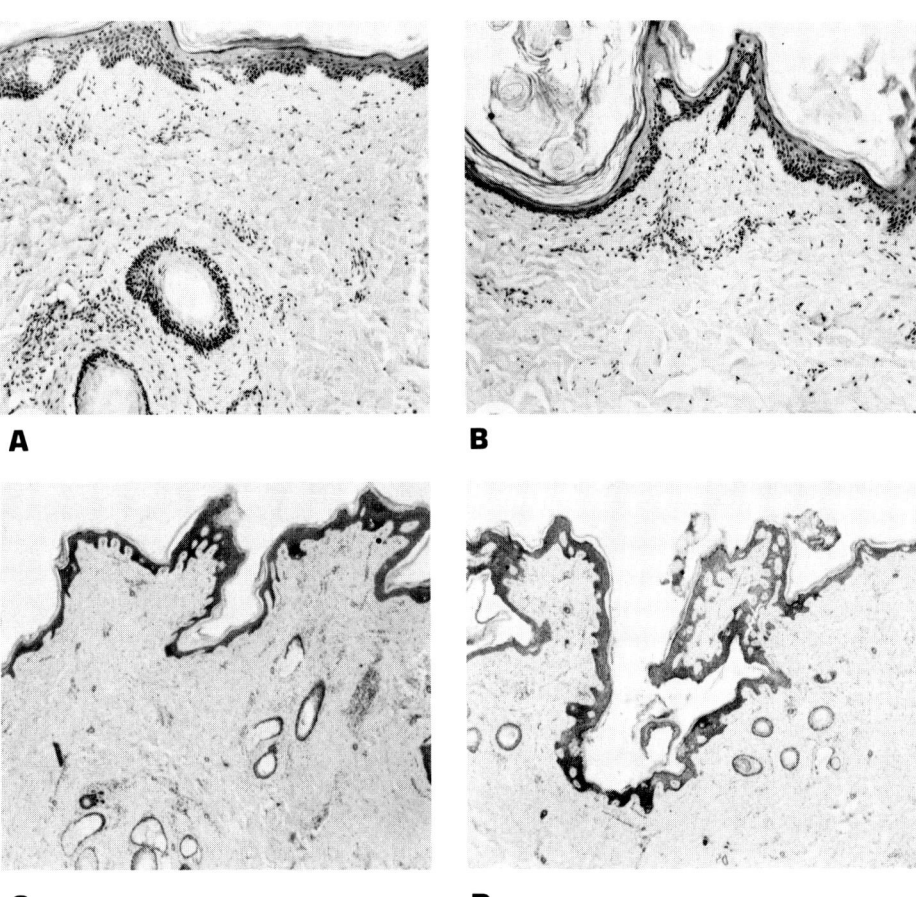

Figure 3–15.
Four pieces cut from normal skin, embedded at angles varying from vertical in **A** to 45 degrees in **D**. H&E. X60. (From Mehregan and Pinkus. Arch Dermatol 94:218, 1966.)

knife. We set the microtome at 7 μm for routine purposes because the skin is a notoriously difficult tissue to cut, and thinner sections do not give better definition of detail. The thicker sections actually provide a slightly better three-dimensional impression, which is important in the interpretation of skin structure. On the other hand, when the cytology of cells are important as in histiocytic and lymphocytic tumors, thinner sections are desirable.

In preparation of the skin sections, the result depends to a large extent on the condition of the microtome and knife. Microtomes should be cleaned at the end of the working day and lubricated regularly. The microtome knife should be carefully cleaned and sharpened by honing. Commercial knife sharpeners may be used if the knife is dull or deep nicks are present. A dull knife will cut alternating thick and thin sections. Irregularities over the cutting edge of the knife may produce linear scratch marks in tissue sections (Fig. 3–16).

Attempts should be made to cut ribbons of consecutive sections from the paraffin blocks and to mount all of them on slides (serial sections). It is desirable to prepare at least 10 to 30 consecutive sections. If histological picture is greatly deviated from clinical diagnosis, deeper cuts should be requested. Ribbons cut from paraffin sections are floated on a waterbath, cut into pieces of desirable length, and mounted on microscopic slides. The surface of the water should be cleaned after each specimen to prevent contamination (Fig. 3–17).

STAINS

Hematoxylin and eosin (H&E) is the most widely used stain in histopathology laboratories. This stain is sufficient for diagnosis of many skin diseases. It is, however, not a complete stain, since it does not demonstrate some important tissue components, such as elastic fibers or mast cells, does not differentiate between melanin and hemosiderin pigments, and only poorly shows fungal mycelia, cocci, and amyloid. To provide additional information, we use as our second routine stain the acid orcein–Giemsa (O&G) method. We find that its routine use improves our diagnostic ability in many cases and makes recut-

56 FUNDAMENTALS AND TECHNIQUES

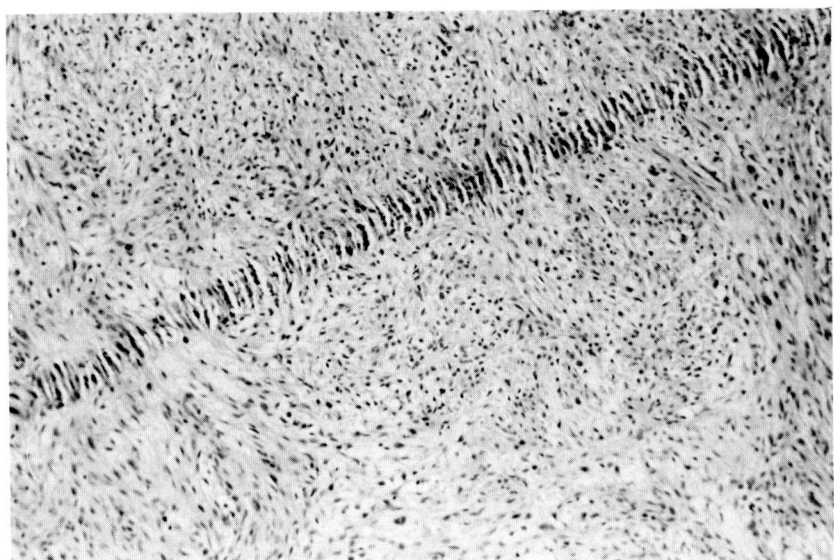

Figure 3–16.
Scratch mark produced by a nick in the knife blade. H&E. X400.

ting of blocks for special stains unnecessary in many instances. The most commonly used special stains in our laboratory are periodic acid–Schiff (PAS) stain for glycogen and with amylase digestion for fungi, and in combination with alcian blue and picric acid for glycogen and neutral and acid mucopolysaccharides[8]; and the Fite method for acid-fast bacilli. In the remainder of this chapter, hematoxylin–eosin, acid orcein–Giemsa, and periodic acid–Schiff stains are described in detail. Other stains useful in skin pathology are summarized in Table 3–1. For more information we refer you to the works of Preece,[6] Clark,[7] Bancroft and Stevens,[9] and the Manual of Histologic Staining Methods of the Armed Forces Institute of Pathology.[10]

Hematoxylin and Eosin Stain

Fixation
May be used after any fixation.

Technique
Paraffin, celloidin, or frozen sections.

Solutions

HARRIS' HEMATOXYLIN
Hematoxylin crystals	5.0	g
Alcohol, 95 percent	50.0	mL
Ammonium or potassium alum	100.0	g
Distilled water	1000.0	mL
Mercuric oxide	2.5	g

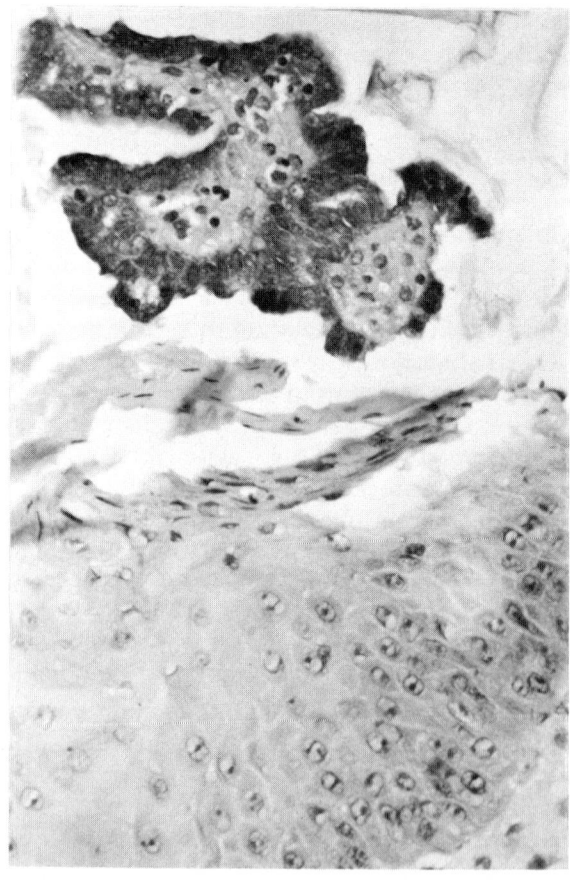

Figure 3–17.
Piece of endometrium above epidermis showing contamination from waterbath.

Dissolve the hematoxylin in the alcohol, the alum in the water with heat. Mix the two solutions. Bring the mixture to a boil as rapidly as possible and then remove from the heat and add the mercuric oxide. Reheat the solution until it becomes dark purple, about 1 minute, and promptly remove the container from the flame and plunge it into a basin of cold water. The solution is ready to use when cool.

ACID ALCOHOL
70 percent alcohol	1000.0 mL
Hydrochloric acid, concentrated	10.0 mL

ALCOHOLIC EOSIN SOLUTION
Eosin Y, water soluble	2.0 g
Distilled water	160.0 mL
Alcohol, 95 percent	640.0 mL

Dissolve eosin Y in the distilled water, then add the 95 percent alcohol. If a deeper shade is desired, add a drop of acetic acid to each 100 ml of solution.

Staining Procedure

1. Xylene, absolute alcohol, 95 percent alcohol, 70 percent alcohol, to distilled water
2. Harris' hematoxylin for 10 minutes
3. Rinse in tap water
4. Differentiate in acid alcohol—3 to 10 dips. Check the differentiation with the microscope. Nuclei should be distinct and the background very light or colorless*
5. Wash in running tap water for 10 to 20 minutes
6. Stain with eosin from 15 seconds to 2 minutes depending on the age of the eosin and the depth of counterstain desired
7. 95 percent alcohol
8. Absolute alcohol—at least two changes
9. Xylene—two changes
10. Mount in Permount or other suitable medium

Results

Nuclei—purple to blue
Cytoplasm—pink
Keratohyalin—dark purple

---

* We have replaced this step by immersing the slides in 1 percent aqueous solution of hydrochloric acid for 1 to 2 minutes. By avoiding surface tension changes between water and alcohol, the danger of sections becoming detached is minimized.

Collagen—pink
Elastic fibers—unstained
Calcium—dark purple or blue
Muscle fibers—pink

Acid Orcein and Giemsa Stain (Pinkus and Hunter)[11]

Fixation

Formalin or alcohol. Fixatives containing chromate or mercury are not suitable.

Solutions

1. Dissolve 0.2 g of Orcein Synthetic Harleco (Harleco, Inc., Philadelphia) in 100 mL 70 percent ethyl alcohol; add 0.6 ml concentrated hydrochloric acid. Solution is ready for use immediately and improves on standing. It has a long shelf life but becomes exhausted by frequent use.
2. Dilute Giemsa solution: One drop of any good Giemsa stock solution for each 20 mL of distilled water. A phosphate buffer solution adjusted to pH 7.0 may be used if distilled water is too acid.
3. A few drops of 1 percent alcoholic solution of eosin yellow are added to 95 percent alcohol for decolorization of excessively blue sections.

Staining Procedure

1. Deparaffinize sections in xylene and bring through absolute and 95 percent alcohol into 70 percent alcohol
2. Immerse in solution A for 30 minutes. This new synthetic orcein stains elastic fibers specifically and produces very little background staining. The background may be completely decolorized by short immersion of the stained sections in absolute alcohol or 0.1 percent acid alcohol. This is rarely necessary
3. Wash in running tap water for 10 minutes
4. Stain for 12 to 15 hours (preferably overnight) in solution B. Do not hurry this step. The various tissue components pick the various shades out of a very dilute solution if given enough time. One may speed up this step by having the sections stained for 1 hour in 1 percent Giemsa solution in an oven at 60C[12]
5. Wipe excess fluid off slides. Generally the sections are now stained blue. The excess blue is removed by dehydrating the sections in 95

percent alcohol to which a few drops of solution C have been added. How much eosin should be used depends on the degree of overstaining and is learned by experience. If the sections have almost the desired rose-pink color of the collagen when they come out of the Giemsa solution, omit eosin altogether in this step

6. Remove sections when the collagen of the skin begins to turn pink from blue. Finish dehydration and decolorization in two changes of absolute alcohol
7. Two changes of xylene
8. Mount in Permount or other suitable medium

Results

The nuclei should be deep blue; cytoplasm of epidermis, smooth muscle, and other cells, light blue; collagen, rose-pink; elastic fibers, dark brown to black (see Fig. 3, Color Plate I). Mast cell granules and some acid mucinous substances stain metachromatically purple,* but glandular mucin stains grayish blue, and myxedema does not stain at all. Melanin is dark green, almost black; hemosiderin, yellow-brown or light grass green. Red blood cells and eosinophilic granules are bright red; cytoplasm of plasma cells, dark blue or grayish blue. Amyloid stains a clear sky blue under ideal conditions but may be light grayish blue (see Fig. 2, Color Plate I), whereas other hyaline substances stain pink. Fibrin and fibrinoid material are greenish blue. Unna's elacin and collastin assume various shades from black to gray to blue. Trichohyalin is red; the fully keratinized inner root sheath, deep dark blue; the glassy membrane of the hair follicle, often metachromatic lavender. Keratohyalin of the epidermis usually does not stain very well, but nuclei of parakeratotic stratum corneum often stain much more distinctly than with hematoxylin. Bacteria, fungal hyphae and spores, and other microorganisms, are dark blue.

Other Elastic Fiber Stains

Other elastic fiber stains are described briefly. In Verhoeff's iodine–iron hematoxylin, elastic fibers stain in black color, as do nuclei and some other substances. Young and very thin elastic fibers (elaunin fibers) stain poorly or not at all. Weigert's resorcin fuchsin stain demonstrates the elastic fibers in black. Fullmer's orcinol new fuchsin stains elastic fibers in deep violet. Gomori's aldehyde fuchsin is listed with the acid mucopolysaccharide stains later in this chapter.

Periodic Acid–Schiff (PAS) Reaction of Hotchkiss and McManus

The PAS reaction is a fundamental stain in carbohydrate histochemistry. In this reaction, aldehyde radicals are created by mild periodic acid oxidation in the tissue sections. The free aldehyde radicals then react with Schiff reagent, forming a red to magenta color compound.

Solutions

SCHIFF'S LEUCOFUCHSIN SOLUTION

Dissolve 1.0 g basic fuchsin in 200.0 ml hot distilled water. Bring to boiling point. Cool to 50°C. Filter and add 20.0 ml normal hydrochloric acid. Cool further, and add 1.0 g anhydrous sodium bisulfite or sodium metabisulfite. Keep in the dark for 48 hours until solution becomes straw-colored. To completely decolorize, add 0.5 g activated charcoal, shake vigorously for 2 minutes, and filter. Solution should be colorless. Store in refrigerator.

To test Schiff's leucofuchsin solution, pour a few drops of Schiff's solution into 10 ml of 37 to 40 percent formaldehyde in a watch glass. If the solution turns reddish purple rapidly, it is good. If the reaction is delayed and the resultant color deep blue purple, the solution is breaking down.

0.5 PERCENT PERIODIC ACID SOLUTION

Periodic acid crystals	0.5 g
Distilled water	100.0 mL

NORMAL HYDROCHLORIC ACID SOLUTION

Hydrochloric acid, conc., sp g. 1.19	83.5 mL
Distilled water	916.5 mL

0.5 PERCENT AQUEOUS LIGHT GREEN COUNTERSTAIN

Light green	0.5 g
Distilled water	100.0 mL
(Harris' hematoxylin can also be used as counterstain)	

DIASTASE SOLUTION

Diastase of malt	1.0 g
Buffer solution	100.0 mL

---

* Substances staining purple with Giemsa solution have an affinity for the reddish azure components of the dye mixture and do not represent true metachromatic staining. The visible effect, however, is similar. It is restricted to sulfated mucin substances.

BUFFER SOLUTION
NaCl	8.0 g
Disodium phosphate	1.3 g
Sodium phosphate monobasic	0.8 g
Distilled water	1.0 liter

Staining Procedure

1. Xylene
2. Absolute alcohol
3. Alcohol, 95 percent
4. Alcohol, 70 percent
5. Rinse in distilled water
6. Periodic acid solution for 5 minutes (oxidizer)
7. Rinse in distilled water
8. Place in Schiff's leucofuchsin for 10 minutes
9. Place in running tap water for 10 minutes for pink color to develop
10. Stain in Harris' hematoxylin for 2 minutes, or light green counterstain for a few seconds. Light green is recommended for the demonstration of fungi
11. Rinse in tap water
12. Alcohol, 70 percent
13. Alcohol, 95 percent
14. Absolute alcohol, two changes
15. Xylene, two changes
16. Mount in Permount

Results

Glycogen, some mucins, reticulin, fibrin of thrombi, colloid droplets, most basement membranes, amyloid, and other elements show a positive reaction—rose to purplish red. Bacterial and fungal cell walls are deep magenta red; nuclei, blue (with hematoxylin); background, pale green (with light green).

PAS stain demonstrates glycogen and other carbohydrates in tissue sections (see Figs. 9 and 11, Color Plates III and IV*). Glycogen may be removed by the enzyme diastase in 1 percent aqueous solution. The sections are placed in the enzyme solution for a period of 30 minutes at 37°C and are then washed in distilled water. Treated sections and sections on a control slide are stained by PAS method. If the PAS-positive material present in the control sections is completely absent in the sections subjected to diastase digestion, the material is glycogen. Otherwise, it is considered a PAS-positive, diastase-

---

* Color Plate follows page 50.

resistant material. Most mucopolysaccharides except acid mucopolysaccharides (such as hyaluronic acid and chondroitin sulfate) will give positive reactions. Sialomucin and some mast cell granules are PAS-positive. Starch granules, a common contaminant of tissue sections, also are stained. PAS reaction with diastase digestion may be used for demonstration of deep or superficial fungous infections, especially in cases of sporotrichosis or where the number of organisms is small.

Alcian Blue Stain (Mowry)

In this stain,[8] a 0.1 to 1 percent solution of alcian blue 8GS in 3 percent acetic acid is used. By changing the pH values of the solution, distinction can be made[13] between sulfated and nonsulfated groups of acid mucopolysaccharides (AMPS). At pH 2.5 to 3.0, most acid mucopolysaccharides stain a blue color. But at a very low pH value (0.4), only strongly acidic groups, such as sulfated AMPS (chondroitin sulfate and heparin), will give a positive reaction. The nonsulfated AMPS and sialomucin fail to react at this low pH.

A combination of alcian blue and periodic acid–Schiff (AB–PAS) counterstained with picric acid is a very colorful and informative stain for demonstration of acid and neutral mucopolysaccharides in dermal mucinosis and alopecia mucinosa.

Colloidal Iron Stain

In Mowry's modification[8] of Hale's method, tissue sections are exposed to colloidal iron solution. The reaction is probably based on binding of colloidal iron to acidic groups. Demonstration of bound iron is made by the ferrocyanide–hydrochloric acid method. AMPS stain a blue to light green color.

Toluidine Blue Stain

Toluidine blue stain is used for demonstration of metachromasia. Metachromasia may be defined as a staining reaction in which a dye selectively stains certain tissue substances in a color that differs from the color of the dye itself. The production of metachromasia depends on the presence of free electronegative charges of certain minimal density. AMPS, nucleic acids, and other acidic groups if present in sufficient quantity will produce metachromasia (see Fig. 8, Color Plate III).[6] A 0.1 percent toluidine blue solution at pH 1.0 to 6.0 is used for demonstration of metachromasia. At pH values 3 to 6, tissue rich in hyaluronic acid will show metachromasia. At pH values 1.5 and below, only strongly acidic compounds, such as sulfated AMPS, will give metachromasia.[13]

Aldehyde Fuchsin Stain (Gomori)

Aldehyde fuchsin[14] may be used for demonstration of elastic fibers and certain groups of AMPS. The elastic fibers stain in a deep violet to purple color (see Fig. 1, Color Plate I). The same color reaction is produced by mast cell granules, sialomucin of epithelial origin, and, to a lesser degree, by chondroitin sulfate. The stain is most useful for demonstrating mucin production in cases of extramammary Paget's disease.

Enzyme Digestion

Amylase may be used for digestion of glycogen in association with PAS stain. Two other enzymes are available for investigation of AMPS. Bacterial or, more commonly, bovine testicular hyaluronidase is used for removal of hyaluronic acid from the tissue sections. Digestion is then followed by either the alcian blue or colloidal iron stain. Sialidase (neuraminidase) is used for decomposition of sialomucin in the tissue sections. Ribonuclease removes ribonucleic acid (RNA) from tissue sections.

Reticulum

The modification by either Gomori or Wilder[15] of the Bielschowsky–Maresch silver method may be used. The reticulum fibers stain in the form of delicate dark brown to black fibrils.

Amyloid

Amyloid deposits may be demonstrated by one of the following methods. Highman's crystal violet[16] will stain amyloid metachromatic in a reddish purple color. Bennhold's Congo red stain,[10] examined under polarized light, shows green birefringence. O&G stains amyloid light blue. Amyloid is also weakly PAS-positive. Three commercially used cotton dyes have been recommended for amyloid staining (Pagoda red, RIT Scarlet No. 5, RIT Cardinal Red No. 9)[17] (see Fig. 4, Color Plate II).

Lipids

Formalin calcium fixation of the specimen for a period not longer than 2 or 3 days is recommended, but routine formalin is adequate for ordinary diagnostic purposes. Frozen sections are stained by either the oil red O or Sudan black method (see Fig. 7, Color Plate III). The lipids stain deep red or greenish black, respectively. The clinician must alert the laboratory not to process the specimen through lipid solvents if a fat stain is desired.

Iron

Prussian blue and Turnbull's reaction are commonly used. Prussian blue reaction is based on the reaction of tissue ferric iron (Fe^{3+}) with potassium ferrocyanide in acid solution and formation of ferric ferrocyanide with a deep blue color in the tissue sections. Turnbull's reaction is similar. In this method, ferrous iron (Fe^{2+}) is demonstrated by reacting with potassium ferricyanide, resulting in the formation of a deep blue color. The tissue sections are best counterstained with nuclear fast red.

Melanin

Melanin pigment has a light to dark brown color in H&E stain. Exposure to a 1 to 2 percent silver nitrate solution specifically darkens melanin.[9] Fontana–Masson's ammoniacal silver nitrate technique can be used for combined demonstration of melanin and premelanin.[18] This reaction is based on the reducing capacity of the melanosome skeleton and precipitation of black silver protein compound. A similar reaction is produced by Gomori's methenamine silver stain.[19] Azure in the O&G stain causes melanin granules to appear greenish black and makes special stains unnecessary if it is used as a routine stain. Melanin pigment can be bleached out of the tissue sections by long exposure to 10 percent hydrogen peroxide or 0.5 percent potassium permanganate solution.

For demonstration of tyrosinase (dopa-oxidase), slices of rapidly frozen tissue or specimens fixed for a short time in cold formalin may be used. Special arrangements, therefore, must be made with the laboratory if the clinician desires this type of examination. The reaction takes place in two phases. In the first phase, L-tyrosine is slowly converted to L-dopa, and in the second phase, L-dopa is rapidly transformed into intermediate compounds and finally into melanin pigment.

Calcium

Two methods are commonly used for demonstration of calcium in tissue sections.

1. *Von Kossa method* (see Fig. 6, Color Plate II): It is based on the combination of silver with anions of insoluble salts, which may be phosphate, oxalate, sulfate, chloride, or sulfocyanide, and reduction to metallic silver by exposure to light.[20] In practice, it demonstrates insoluble salts of calcium.
2. *Alizarin red S:* In this method a 2 percent solution of alizarin red S adjusted to pH 4.1 to 4.3 with diluted ammonia is used. An orange-red calcium–alizarin compound is formed in 1 to 5 minutes.[20]

Silver and Other Metals

In the hematoxylin–eosin stain, silver appears as dark brown to black granules representing a silver–protein complex. Silver may be removed by placing the sections in 1 percent potassium ferricyanide in 20 percent sodium thiosulfate solution. Silver can also be demonstrated by dark-field examination of the tissue sections. Mercury[21] and gold[22] have similar properties.

Silica

Silica can be demonstrated by polarization microscopy. Polarization may be produced in any microscope by the use of two pieces of Polaroid, which is available in large sheets in photo or laboratory supply stores. One piece is introduced into the pathway of the light within or below the condenser system. Another piece may be simply placed on top of the slide. With rotation of one of these two pieces, the light field becomes darker, and double refractile crystals of silica become apparent.

Stains for Fungi

PAS stain after digestion with diastase can be used for demonstration of superficial and deep fungi (see Fig. 9, Color Plate III). Grocott stain[23] also has been widely used. In this method, the organisms stain dark brown to black. Mucicarmin has been recommended for the demonstration of *Cryptococcus neoformans*.[24]

Bacterial Stains

Most bacilli and cocci show up well in O&G-stained sections. Ziehl–Neelsen's carbolfuchsin and methylene blue stain is used for demonstration of acid-fast bacteria in smears or tissue sections. Acid-fast bacilli and ceroid stain red. Cell nuclei are blue, and mast cell granules take a blue-violet color. Certain granules in sweat glands and keratinized hair and inner root sheath (Chapter 2) also are apt to retain the red color. Hansen's bacilli need special precautions and are best demonstrated by the Fite method.[25]

Gram stain can be used on smears or tissue sections. Gram-positive bacteria stain blue-black, and gram-negative organisms stain red.

PREPARATION OF TZANCK SMEAR AND TISSUE IMPRINTS

Tzanck smears are useful procedures for the rapid diagnosis of herpes simplex and less frequently for pemphigus vulgaris. Smears should be taken from an early vesiculobullous lesion that shows no sign of secondary infection. The top of the bulla is opened up by the tip of a surgical blade. The contents of the bulla and material obtained by gentle scraping of the floor of the bulla are collected by the edge of the blade and spread evenly over a glass slide. The preparation may be air dried or fixed by dipping four or five times into 95 percent ethyl alcohol. The slide is stained with a few drops of stock Giemsa solution for 2 or 3 minutes or by Paragon multiple stain for frozen sections.[26] Tissue imprints may be prepared by touching the punch biopsy specimen to a clean, dry glass slide in multiple spots. The slides are air dried and stained with either Giemsa or Wright stain.[27] They are then rinsed in distilled water, air dried, and cover-slipped for examination under high, dry power of the microscope or, if necessary, under oil immersion.

FOREIGN BODIES

Various foreign materials may be observed in the examination of tissue sections. Some of these may have been introduced into the skin at various times before biopsy and may have produced a variety of tissue reactions.[28] Others appear during tissue processing. Silica and other substances producing granulomatous reactions are discussed in Chapter 21. Wood and other plant material are highly birefringent and can be thus identified. Pencil lead, other forms of carbon, and other substances such as cinnabar, are encountered in accidental or purposeful tattoos (Chapter 28). Silver and other metals were mentioned earlier. Suture material may have been

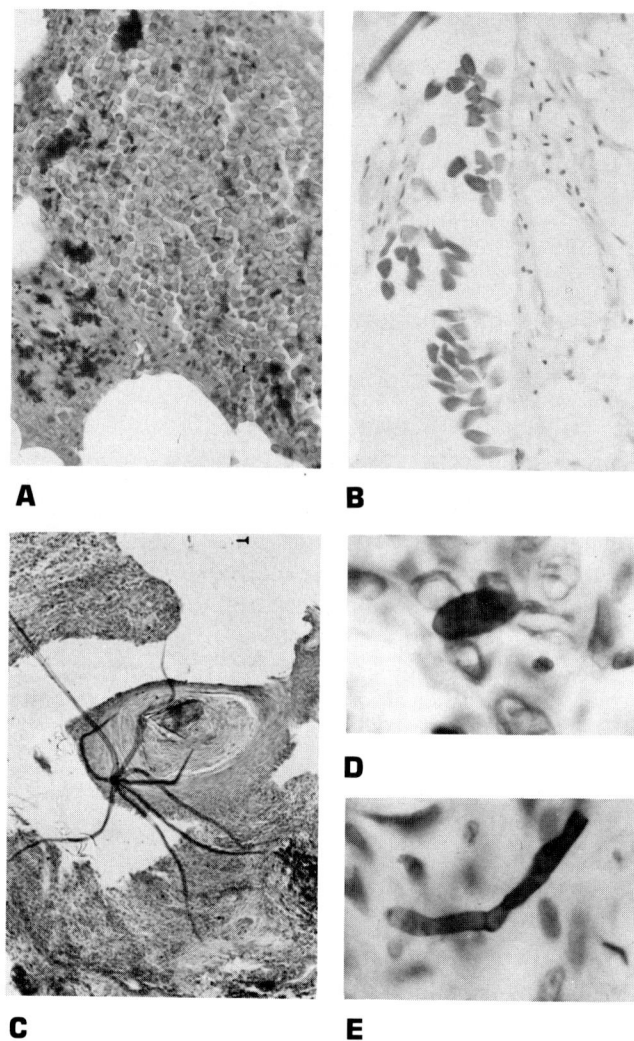

Figure 3–18.
Foreign bodies encountered in tissue sections. **A.** Formalin pigment in hemorrhagic tissue. H&E. X280. **B.** Suture material, probably nylon thread. H&E. X180. **C.** Plant hair contaminant. O&G. X60. (From Pinkus. Arch Dermatol 100:96, 1969.) **D.** Alternaria spore. H&E. X400. **E.** Fungous mycelium. H&E. X400.

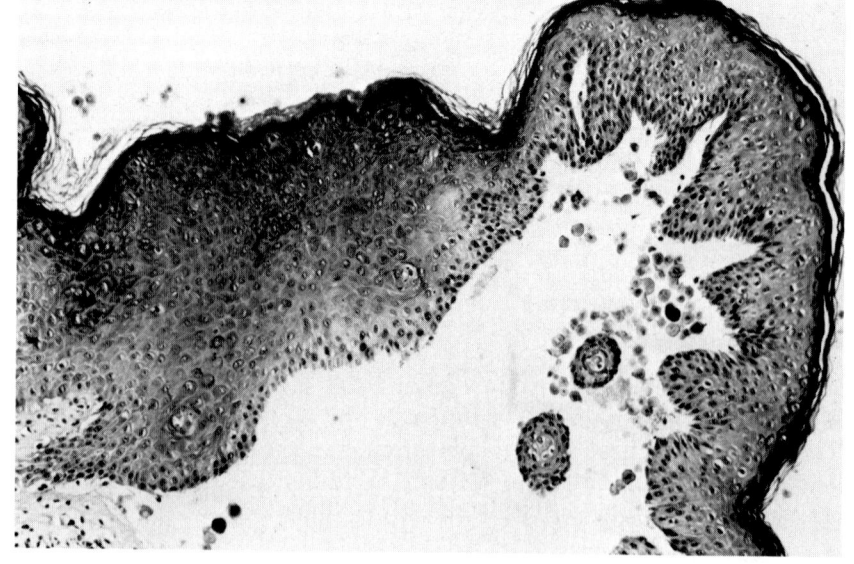

Figure 3–19.
Starch granules in artificial cleft between epidermis and dermis. Artifact is indicated by emptiness of space except for dislodged hair follicles and foreign bodies. The latter are identified as starch by size, roundish or polygonal shape, and dark center that represents air bubble. They could be further identified by positive reaction to PAS. H&E. X135.

left in the tissue from previous surgery or may have been placed by the surgeon with the purpose of tissue orientation. Formalin pigment, previously mentioned in this chapter, may form as a result of formalin fixation of blood-rich tissues. Starch granules, plant hairs,[29] alternaria spores, fungus hyphae, and pollen are ordinary tissue contaminants (Figs. 3–18 and 3–19).

ARTIFACTS

In addition to being aware of the artifacts that may result from the biopsy procedure and tissue processing, the dermatopathologist must be cognizant of tissue alterations that arise in vivo but are not classifiable as dermatoses in the usual sense of the word. One of these, excoriation, was illustrated at the beginning of this chapter. There are other physical and medicamentous influences that may produce characteristic changes. Suction[30] may induce paranuclear vacuoles and later, dermoepidermal separation. Friction[31] leads to rupture of cell membranes following intercellular edema. Electric current produces severe deformity of cells (see Fig. 3–11). Sunburn leads to the formation of characteristic pyknotic cells in the epidermis.[32] Freezing was shown many years ago to induce multinucleated epidermal giant cells. The chemical action of podophyllin in the treatment of warts causes characteristic clumped mitoses (see Fig. 32–10), and systemic administration of methotrexate and hydroxyurea has been shown to produce peculiar pyknotic prickle cells with eosinophilic cytoplasm in psoriatic epidermis.[33] The application of cantharidin leads to acantholysis, and this list of artifacts could be greatly expanded. The pathologist should suspect that any unusual and bizarre changes in epidermis and dermis may be due to accidental or intentional artifact. Being able to identify some specific alterations will make pathologists very useful to the clinician in obscure cases.

REFERENCES

1. Pinkus H: Skin biopsy: A field of interaction between clinician and pathologist. Cutis 20:609, 1977
2. Mehregan AH, Pinkus H: Artifacts in dermal histopathology. Arch Dermatol 94:218, 1966
3. Griffiths WAD, Dutz W: Repeated tissue sampling with a dental broach. Br J Dermatol 93:43, 1975
4. Weigand DA: Transfollicular extrusion of sebaceous glands: Natural phenomenon or artifact? A case report. J Cutan Pathol 3:239, 1976
5. Ackerman AB, Penneys NS: Formalin pigment in skin. Arch Dermatol 102:318, 1970
6. Preece A: A Manual for Histologic Technicians, 3rd ed. Boston: Little, Brown, 1972
7. Clark G: Staining Procedures. 4th edition. Baltimore: Williams and Wilkins 1981
8. Mowry RW: The special value of methods that color both acidic and vicinal hydroxyl groups in the histochemical study of mucins, with revised directions for the colloidal iron stain, the use of alcian blue G8X and their combinations with the periodic acid–Schiff reaction. Ann NY Acad Sci 106:402, 1963
9. Bancroft JD, Stevens A: Theory and Practice of Histological Techniques. New York: Churchill Livingstone, 1977
10. Luna LG: Manual of Histologic Staining Methods of the Armed Forces Institute of Pathology, 3rd ed. New York: McGraw-Hill, 1968
11. Pinkus H, Hunter R: Simplified acid orcein and Giemsa technique for routine staining of skin sections. Arch Dermatol 82:699, 1960
12. Krobock E, Rahbari H, Mehregan AH: Acid orcein and Giemsa stain. Modification of a valuable stain for dermatologic specimens. J Cutan Pathol 5:37, 1978
13. Johnson WC, Johnson FB, Helwig EB: Effect of varying the pH on reactions for acid mucopolysaccharides. J Histochem Cytochem 10:684, 1962
14. Gomori G: Aldehyde fuchsin: A new stain for elastic tissue. Am J Clin Pathol 20:665, 1950
15. Wilder HC: An improved technique for silver impregnation of reticulum fibers. Am J Pathol 11:817, 1935
16. Highman B: Improved methods for demonstrating amyloid in paraffin sections. Arch Dermatol 41:559, 1946
17. Yanagihara M, Mehregan AH, Mehregan, DR: Staining of amyloid with cotton dyes. Arch Dermatol 120:1184–1185, 1984
18. Mishima Y: New technique for comprehensive demonstration of melanin, premelanin, and tyrosinase sites: Combined dopa-premelanin reaction. J Invest Dermatol 34:355, 1960
19. Gomori G: Chemical character of the enterochromaffin cells. Arch Pathol 45:48, 1948
20. McGee-Russell SM: Histochemical methods for calcium. J Histochem Cytochem 6:22, 1958
21. Burge KM, Winkelmann RK: Mercury pigmentation: An electron microscopic study. Arch Dermatol 102:51, 1970
22. Cox AJ: Gold in the dermis following gold therapy for rheumatoid arthritis. Arch Dermatol 108:655, 1973
23. Grocott RG: A stain for fungi in tissue sections and smears. Using Gomori's methenamine–silver nitrate technic. Am J Clin Pathol 25:975, 1955
24. Lopez JF, Lebron RF: *Cryptococcus neoformans:* Their identification in body fluids and cultures by mucicarmin stain (Mayer). Bol Assoc Med PR 64:203, 1972
25. Fite GL, Cambre PJ, Turner MH: Procedure for demonstrating lepra bacilli in paraffin sections. Arch Pathol 43:624, 1947

26. Barr RJ: Cutaneous cytology. Int J Dermatol 17:552, 1978
27. King DT, Sun NCJ: Touch preparation in diagnosis of skin disorders. Arch Dermatol 115:1034, 1979
28. Mehregan AH, Faghri B: Implantation dermatoses. Acta Derm Venereol 54:61, 1974
29. Pinkus H: Stellate plant hair contaminant in the laboratory. Arch Dermatol 100:96, 1969
30. Hunter JAA, McVittie E, Comaish JS: Light and electron microscopic studies of physical injuries to the skin. I. Suction. Br J Dermatol 90:481, 1974
31. Hunter JAA, McVittie E, Comaish JS: Light and electron microscopic studies of physical injuries to the skin. II. Friction. Br J Dermatol 90:491, 1974
32. Daniels F Jr, Brophy D, Lobitz WC Jr: Histochemical responses of human skin following ultraviolet irradiation. J Invest Dermatol 37:351, 1961
33. Smith C, Gelfant S: Effects of methotrexate and hydroxyurea on psoriatic epidermis. Arch Dermatol 110:70, 1974

4
IMMUNOPATHOLOGY OF THE SKIN

Besides special stains for various components of cells and tissues such as PAS or acid orcein–Giemsa, immunopathologic techniques have become indispensable procedures in the diagnosis of inflammatory skin diseases and cutaneous neoplasms. Some immunologic patterns are disease specific. Others are of value only when combined with the clinical information and other laboratory findings. Four major routine immunofluorescence methods are applied.

DIRECT IMMUNOFLUORESCENCE

This method is used for in situ demonstration or direct detection of various substances in the tissue and cells. If the specific antibody is present for a suspected substance in the lesion, a 4–6 μm fresh frozen section is cut and incubated with the antibody, which is conjugated with a fluorescent dye such as fluorescein isothiocyanate or rhodamin. If the suspected substance (antigen) is present, the antigen–antibody reaction takes place and the sites of antigen are identified by the presence of fluorescence under a fluorescence microscope. This method is simple and specific because in the skin only elastic fibers and lipid granules of eccrine secretory coil are autofluorescent. The disadvantage of this method is a high cost of fluorescence microscope.

A 4-mm punch biopsy specimen may be taken and divided into two parts. One part is processed for paraffin embedding and routine stains. The other part is put aside for immunofluorescence study. If a cryostat is available, 4- to 6- μm sections of the tissue are made immediately, placed on a glass slide, and transported to the laboratory. If the laboratory is located within driving distance, the sections may be stored in a freezer and transported in dry ice within 1 week. If there is neither cryostat nor laboratory in the institution, the biopsied specimen should be wrapped in normal saline-soaked gauze, placed in a Petri dish, and stored in freezer compartment of refrigerator. It should be transported in dry ice within a week. If Michel's solution[1] is available, the specimen could be shipped in this solution to a commercial laboratory within 1 week.

Frozen sections cut in a cryostat are placed on a glass slide that has been coated with an adherent agent such as poly-L-lysine. This is necessary because these sections undergo several incubations and washings. Air-dried sections on a glass slide are incubated with fluorescein-conjugated antihuman immunoglobulins such as IgG, IgA, IgM, anticomplement C_3, and antifibrinogen. After 30 minutes incubation in a moist chamber and subsequent rinse in phosphate buffered saline, the sections are covered with glycerine jelly with 1 percent paraphenylenediamine, which preserves fluorescence. The sections incubated with antihuman IgG, IgM, and complement C_3 antibodies show an apple green flu-

TABLE 4–1. IMMUNOHISTOCHEMICAL STAINING PATTERN FOR FORMALIN FIXED, PARAFFIN EMBEDDED TISSUES

	Keratinocytes	Melanocytes	Fibroblast–Histiocyte
	BCE, Seb K, AK Bowen, SCC	Nevi, Melanoma	Atypical fibroxanthoma or fibrous histiocytoma Non-X histiocytic tumors

Antikeratin
  DAKO: antikeratin
  ENZO: MA 903
         MA 904
  DAKOPATTS: Prekeratin
	All (+)	All (−)	All (−)

Antimelanoma ENZO HMB 45	All (−)	All (+), except spindle cell melanoma	All (−)
ENZO MEL 5	All (−)	Melanosome (+)	All (−)
Antifibrohistiocyte Vimentin	Some (+)	Some (+)	All (+)
α-Chymotrypsin α-Trypsin	All (−)	All (−)	All (+)
Lysozyme	All (−)	All (−)	All (+)
S-100 antibody	All (−)	All (+)	Some (+)

BCE = basal cell epithelioma, Seb K = seborrheic keratosis, SCC = squamous cell carcinoma.

orescence in dermoepidermal junction or basement membrane zone under properly set filters in a fluorescence microscope.

Modification of Direct Immunofluorescence

Direct demonstration of substances is not limited to immunoglobulins and C_3. These are frequently studied substances and fluorescein conjugates are commercially available. For less frequently studied materials such as keratin, vimentin, surface antigens of lymphocyte subset etc., fluorescein-conjugated antibodies are not commercially available. In this case the indirect method should be used. First, one must know in what animals these antibodies were produced and what class of immunoglobulins they are. If they were produced in a mouse and are IgG class immunoglobulins, the section is first incubated with that antibody, and after a rinse with buffered saline, reincubated with antimouse IgG conjugated with fluorescein, which is commercially available. For example, if a nodular lesion is removed from the face of an elderly individual and histologically shows massive spindle cell proliferation, the possibilities of spindle cell malignant melanoma or malignant fibrous histiocytoma may be considered. The decision depends on demonstration of melanoma-associated antigens or vimentin for fibroblasts (Table 4–1). Frozen sections are cut and incubated with the antimelanoma antibody of IgG class made in the mouse or with antivimentin of IgG class, also made in the mouse. These antibodies are not conjugated with fluorescein and, therefore, the sections are rinsed and reincubated with antimouse IgG* conjugated with fluorescein. IgG became fluorescent in the section that was incubated with antimelanoma antibody but no fluorescence is seen in the section that was incubated first with antivimentin; therefore the diagnosis of spindle cell melanoma was established.

INDIRECT IMMUNOFLUORESCENCE

This test is used to determine if the patient has circulating autoantibodies in his peripheral blood. Nonheparinized blood is allowed to clot in a test tube and the separated serum is stored in the freezer until use. Normal human or animal skin or mucous membranes are obtained, sectioned at 4–6 μm, and adhered to a glass slide. The sections are incubated with patient's serum for 30 minutes in a moist chamber. If auto-antibody against nuclear DNA, for example, is present in the serum, it combines with the

---

* If antimouse IgG is produced in a horse, the sections should be ideally incubated with normal horse serum to plug all nonspecific sites that might bind with normal horse immunoglobulins. This step is usually omitted in routine testing.

nucleus of epidermal keratinocytes and those of connective tissue cells during this incubation. The sections are rinsed with phosphate buffered saline and reincubated with antihuman IgG, IgM, or IgA, depending on suspected autoantibody class. These antihuman immunoglobulins are conjugated with fluorescein and the binding sites (nuclei in this case) become fluorescent under fluorescence microscopy.

For example, if a patient is suffering from oral blisters and ulcerations, the possibility of pemphigus vulgaris may be considered. A biopsy specimen should be taken that includes part of the blister and the surrounding normal area. The diagnosis of pemphigus vulgaris is confirmed if direct immunofluorescence is positive in the intercellular spaces of the epidermis with antihuman IgG and C_3 (Table 4–2).

Before the therapy is implemented, however, we may like to know the serum titer of his antiintercellular antibodies. Peripheral blood is drawn and the serum is separated. Since the autoantibodies are directed toward the intercellular substance, the epithelial tissue rich in this substance should be selected. Normal human foreskin may be utilized that has been sectioned to 4–6 μm in a cryostat. After being put on a glass slide the section is first incubated with the patient's own serum without dilution. After a brief rinse, the sections are reincubated with antihuman IgG conjugated with fluorescein; a strong intercellular fluorescence is observed. The serum is serially diluted up to 240 times and the test repeated. If intercellular fluorescence is observed up to 120 dilutions, the titer is reported as 120.

The term "indirect immunofluorescence" is also used if direct fluorescein conjugate is not available even when the lesional biopsy tissue is used as test substrate (see Modified Immunofluorescence).

TABLE 4–2. DIRECT AND INDIRECT IMMUNOFLUORESCENCE TEST: INDICATIONS AND PATTERNS

Disease	Direct	Indirect	Biopsy Site
Pemphigus			
vulgaris	Intercellular IgG, (G_1, G_4), C_3	Intercellular IgG, C_3	Perilesional
vegetans	Intercellular IgG, C_3	Intercellular IgA, C_3	Lesional or perilesional
foliaceus	Intercellular, sometimes only upper epidermis IgG, (G_1, G_4), C_3	Sometimes intercellular IgG	Perilesional
Pemphigoid			
bullous	Linear BMZ IgG, (G_1, G_4), C_3	Linear BMZ IgG, (G_1, G_4), C_3; (may be −)	Perilesional
gestationis	Linear BMZ IgG_1	Linear BMZ with full term placenta as substrate IgG_1, C_3	Perilesional
		Herpes gestationis factor is IgG_1, which combines C_3	Perilesional
cicatricial	Linear BMZ IgG, IgM, IgA, C_3	Linear BMZ (mostly −) IgG	
Dermatitis herpetiformis	Granular in dermal papillae IgA, IgG, IgM, fibrin	Negative or rarely IgA in BMZ	Perilesional or normal skin
Linear IgA dermatosis	Linear BMZ IgA	Frequently positive	Perilesional
Lupus			
discoid	Granular or linear IgG, IgM, C_3	Negative	Non-treated, several weeks old lesion
subacute (SCLE)	Granular IgG, IgM, C_3	Ro/SSA, La/SSB	Non-treated, several weeks old lesion
systemic	Linear IgG, IgG, C_3 fibrinogen	ANA > 1:160	Lesional Lupus band test: normal sun-exposed skin
bullous	Linear BMZ IgG, IgA	Linear BMZ IgG, IgA; (may be −)	
Epidermolysis bullosa acquisita	Linear sub-basement membrane (25–50%) IgG, IgA, IgM, C_3	Linear sub-basement membrane (variable) IgG	Perilesional

IMMUNOPEROXIDASE AND OTHER IMMUNOHISTOCHEMICAL METHODS

Preservation of stained tissue sections using immunofluorescence is difficult because the tissue is not fixed and fluorescein degrades rapidly. If peroxidase-conjugated antibodies were used instead of fluorescein conjugates and the reaction sites are identified by various histochemical staining of peroxidase such as the diaminobenzidine reaction, which produces brown-black insoluble pigment, the specimens can be stored semipermanently. Then a regular microscope, instead of an expensive fluorescence microscope, is sufficient and universally available. If the specimen is fixed with periodic acid lysine paraformaldehyde (PLP) before the peroxidase procedure, it could be processed for electron microscopy after light microscopic observation because the peroxidase–diaminobenzidine complex is electron dense. The sensitivity of the peroxidase method has been enhanced greatly by the recent development of the avidin–biotin complex (ABC) method. It utilizes the affinity between avidin and biotin. In the direct method the sections are incubated with biotinylated antibody (primary antibody) and after a brief rinse are reincubated with avidin. In this reaction several biotin binding sites of avidin are used but others are still available. After a brief rinse, biotinylated peroxidase is added, which binds to these available biotin binding sites (Fig. 4–1). A premixed avidin and biotinylated peroxidase may be used. The color reaction of peroxidase makes the reaction site of the primary antibody visible.

A disadvantage of the peroxidase method in dermatopathology is the presence of granulocyte and erythrocyte peroxidase in inflammatory lesions. Preincubation of the tissue sections with 0.3–1.0 percent hydrogen peroxidase in 80 percent methanol will exhaust these cellular peroxidases.

In pigmented cells such as melanocytes or macrophages (melanophages), the brown-black color of the peroxidase—diaminobenzidine reaction product is confused with melanin pigments. In such cases chromogens other than diaminobenzidine should be used. Examples are chloronaphthol (blue) and aminoethylcarbazole (red).

Application of Direct and Indirect Immunofluorescence and Immunoperoxidase Methods

Any disease in which a deposition of immunoglobulin or other substances in specific sites or patterns is

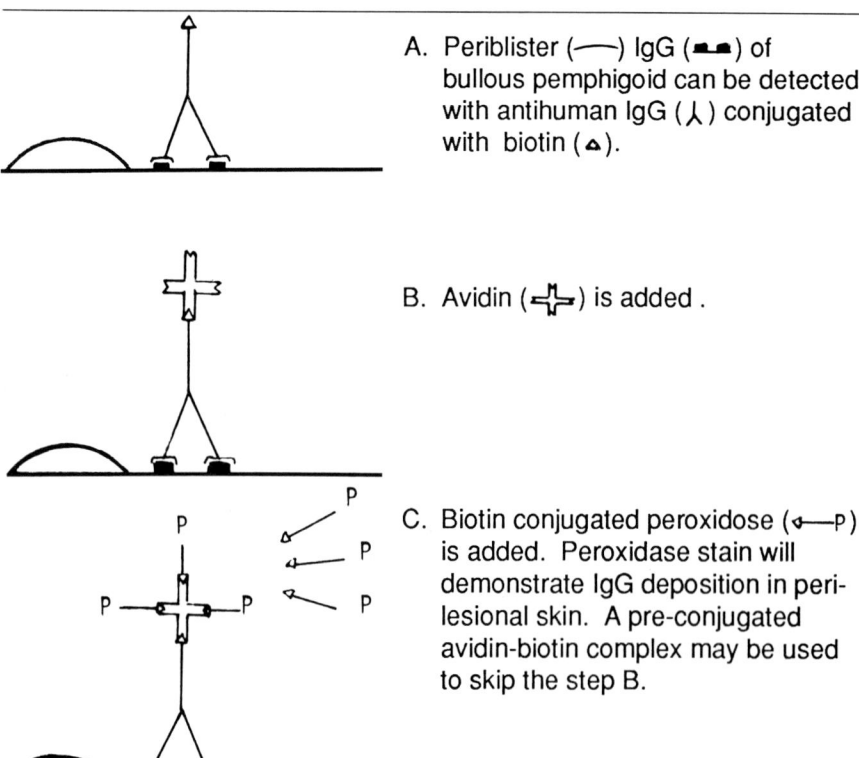

Figure 4–1. Direct avidin–biotin immunoperoxidase technique.

A. Periblister (——) IgG (■■) of bullous pemphigoid can be detected with antihuman IgG (⅄) conjugated with biotin (▲).

B. Avidin (⇦) is added.

C. Biotin conjugated peroxidose (◆——P) is added. Peroxidase stain will demonstrate IgG deposition in perilesional skin. A pre-conjugated avidin-biotin complex may be used to skip the step B.

diagnostic could be diagnosed by these methods. The diseases in which the direct test is frequently performed are listed in Table 4–2 with the specific sites and pattern of deposition of substances. Indirect test is used for the diseases in which circulating autoantibodies in the peripheral blood are diagnostic or titer of such autoantibodies is important to estimate the disease progression or effect of therapy. It is also used when the direct conjugate is not commercially available. The diseases in which indirect tests are indicated are also listed in Table 4–2.

MONOCLONAL ANTIBODY TECHNIQUE

Monoclonal antibodies are produced mostly in mice by repeated injection of purified or semipurified immunogen. If the serum of the immunized mouse is found to contain the desired antibody, the spleen lymphocytes (B cells) are isolated and hybridized with mouse myeloma cells.

Hybridized cells that are tested to produce the desired antibody are selected and propagated into continuous cell lines in culture (hybridoma). This hybridization with self-propagating myeloma cells guarantees a permanent supply of the identical quality of monoclonal antibody derived from the B cell. Supernatants of such culture media or ascites produced in other mice into which the cultured hybridoma was injected intraperitoneally contain the desired monoclonal antibody. Since each spleen B cell produces antibodies against a limited number of molecules (e.g., 10–15 amino acid sequence) each hybridized cell produces antibody against very specific antigenic determinant or epitope. Isolation of desired hybridized cells by repeated dilution (limiting dilution) or manual picking enables us to establish the desired cell lines.

The advantages of monoclonal antibody over conventional antisera (polyclonal antibodies) are as follows:

1. It can be produced in a large quantity in culture.
2. The production is permanent (as long as the cloned cell line lives) and the product is always uniform in its specificity. This allows longitudinal, long-term studies and comparative studies between several laboratories.
3. A high specificity avoids nonspecific background staining due to contamination of unwanted antibodies as encountered in immune sera. For example, polyclonal antikeratin antibodies produced by immunization of rabbit or mouse with epidermal homogenate stain the whole epidermis. Monoclonal antibody specific for 50 Kd keratin (EKH4, AEl, etc.) stains mostly the basal cells.
4. Antigen that cannot be isolated easily for immunization may be selectively recognized by spleen B cells out of a relatively crude mixture of antigens, and thus monoclonal antibodies can be produced.

The disadvantage of monoclonal antibodies is mainly their inability to stain formalin-fixed, paraffin-embedded specimens. In conventional immune sera or polyclonal cocktail antibodies recognize several antigenic sites, whereas monoclonal antibody reacts with only one determinant and if it is damaged during fixation and embedding, the reaction does not occur. The cell membrane antigens such as CD antigens of lymphocytes are more delicate and vulnerable than cytoplasmic ones such as keratin and S-100 proteins.

Applications of various monoclonal antibodies in diagnostic dermatopathology are summarized in Tables 4–1 and 4–3.

DIAGNOSIS OF INFLAMMATORY DISEASES OF THE SKIN

Pemphigus Vulgaris

A high incidence of this disease occurs among Mediterranean races, particularly in Jews. It is also seen in Orientals and other races. Oral mucous membrane erosion may be the initial manifestation. As the disease progresses, face, neck and friction areas of the trunk are gradually involved. Large flaccid bullae are formed and soon break down, leaving areas of superficial ulceration.

Immunofluorescence

Direct immunofluorescence of immunoperoxidase test on perilesional skin shows IgG (mainly G_1) and complement C_3 deposition in the intercellular spaces of the epidermis (Fig. 4–2). The substance with which IgG and C_3 combine seems to be the desmosomal proteins with a molecular weight of 130 Kd.[2] Desmoglein I protein of 150 Kd binds pemphigus vulgaris antibody as well as pemphigus foliaceus antibodies.[2] This test is almost always positive in untreated perilesional skin. Indirect immunofluorescence using normal human skin or animal esophagus as substrate is also positive, except during very

TABLE 4–3. IMMUNOSTAINING REACTIVE PATTERNS

Antibody	Reactive Cells	Conditions
S-100	Melanocyte, Schwann cell, Langerhans cell, histiocyte	Melanoma, neurogenic tumor, histiocytosis-X Histiocytic tumors
HMB-45	Melanocytic and nevocytic cell	Melanoma, nevus; MEL 5, only pigmented lesions
MEL 5	MEL 5 stains melanosome	
Neuron-specific enolase (NSE)	Neurogenic cells Merkel cells	Neurogenic tumors and conditions Merkel cell carcinoma
α_1-Antitrypsin, α_1-Antichymotrypsin (α_1-ACT), Lysozyme	Histiocyte/phagocyte	Histiocytic tumors, granulomatous conditions
Carcinoembryonic antigen (CEA)	Sweat gland cells, breast gland cells, GI tract cells	Tumors of these cells, Paget's cell
MA-902 904 MAK-6 AEI-3 DAKO antikeratin	Keratin-containing cells	Tumors of epidermal and appendage origins, e.g., squamous cell carcinoma
Vimentin	Connective tissue cells	Fibroblastic and histiocytic tumors
Desmin	Muscle cells	Leiomyomas, rhabdomyosarcomas
EMA (epithelial membrane antigen)	Glandular and ductal epithelium, mesodermal cells	Adenocarcinomas Connective tissue tumors Eccrine, apocrine, and sebaceous glands, Paget's cell
Factor VIII-related antigen (Factor VIII RA)	Blood vessels	Angiomas, angiosarcomas
B-15	Blood vessels	Vascular tumors
Type IV collagen	Basement membrane	Vascular tumors
Leukocyte common antigen	Lymphocyte, myelogenous leukemia cells	Lymphoma, leukemia
Myelin basic proteins	Nerves	Neural tumors
Cytokeratin CAM 5.2 synaptophysin	Merkel cell	Merkel cell carcinomas
Papilloma virus common antigen	Papilloma virus	All types of verruca and condyloma

early stages of the diseases, with variable titers usually reflecting disease activities. False positive reactions are seen in the sera from various diseases such as thymic diseases (hyperplasia, thymoma, myasthenia gravis), epidermal infections (*T. rubrum* infection) or necrosis (toxic epidermal necrolysis, various bullous disorders, burn), and drug eruptions (penicillin-induced morbilliform eruption, penicillamine). In these conditions, the epidermal keratinocytes are sufficiently destroyed or modified and intercellular antigens seem to be released into blood circulation to elicit autoantibody formation. Thymus is antigenically similar to the epidermis. False negative tests may result from very low titer after corticosteroid therapy (remission), very high titer (prozone), or interference with other antibodies such as ANA. Some patient's autoantibody is species specific and does not combine with animal intercellular substances; neonatal foreskin obtained by circumcision is probably the best substrate. Calcium may be added to the incubation media because it enhances the sensitivity of the substrate and, thus, the rate of detection of serum autoantibody.

Pemphigus Vegetans

Mucous membranes of mouth and genitalia are invariably involved. The presentation is often beefy red denudation covered with verrucous crusts. In the Hallopeau type, vegetative reaction is prominent (pyodermite végétante), particularly in the groin, axilla, lips, and toes, while in the Neumann type, vegetation is milder and it is often converted to pemphigus vulgaris.

Immunofluorescence

Direct test is always positive with anti-IgG and C_3. Indirect test is inconsistent.

Pemphigus Erythematosus (Senear–Usher Syndrome)

Mainly face and neck areas are involved with erythematous, scaly plaques which may easily be

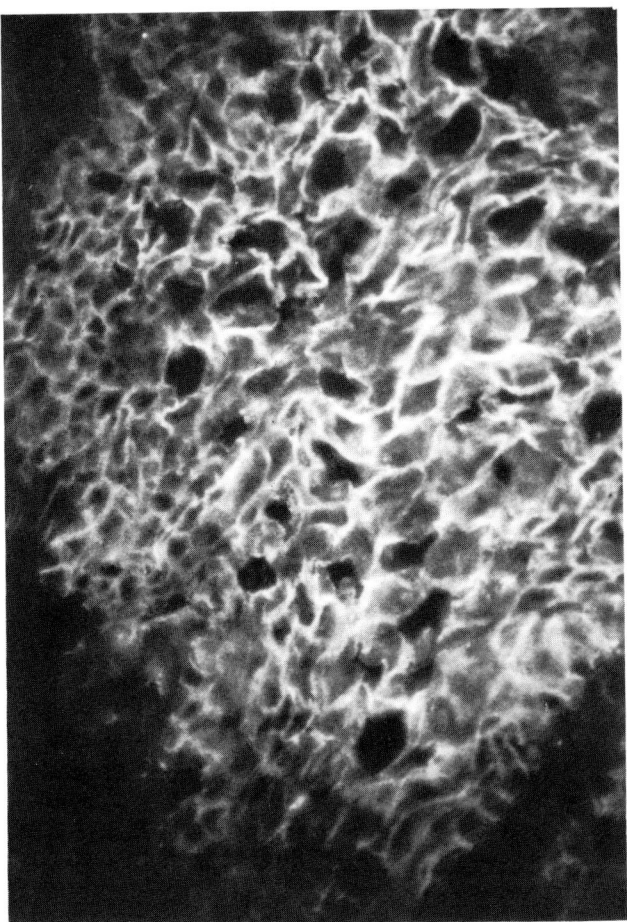

Figure 4–2.
Pemphigus vulgaris. Note the fishnet pattern of intercellular IgG deposits in the epidermis.

mistaken for seborrheic dermatitis, polymorphous light eruption or lupus erythematosus.

Immunohistology
Direct test demonstrates intercellular deposition of IgG and C_3, either in entire epidermis or more concentrated toward upper layers. In addition, IgG and C_3 deposits are seen in basement membrane zone (BMZ) in linear or granular patterns. BMZ deposition of immunoglobulins is also found in the uninvolved skin of patient (positive lupus band test) (Fig. 4–3), particularly if sun-exposed normal skin is tested. Association with true lupus erythematosus may occur with positive ANA.

Pemphigus Foliaceus

Relatively small bullae or vesicles are initially formed but are very fragile because of their superficial location. In advanced cases the clinical picture resembles exfoliative dermatitis.

Sometimes large, leafy scales are dry; however, when peeled, the underlying skin is wet or oozing if not denuded.

Immunofluorescence
The subcorneal blister so much resembles the blister of impetigo and subcorneal pustular dermatosis that the demonstration of intercellular immunofluorescence is important. Bacterial culture may not be a reliable criterion to separate impetigo from pemphigus foliaceus because secondary infection is always present in the latter. Direct test shows IgG and often C_3 deposition in the intercellular spaces of the whole layers of the epidermis. Desmoglein I, the glue substance of desmosome, seems to be the antigenic site.[2] A subset of pemphigus foliaceus may give a positive test limited to the upper layers of the epidermis corresponding to the actual sites of acantholysis. Indirect test is inconsistent. Direct test is always negative in impetigo and subcorneal pustular dermatosis.

Bullous Pemphigoid

This disease was separated from pemphigus by Lever in 1953[3] based on the histology of nonacantholysis. The formation of large bullae is similar to pemphigus but there are several different features in clinical observation. (1) There is no racial predilection. (2) An older age group (>60) is affected. (3) Blisters do not spread after breakage. (4) Erythema or urticaria-like induration often develops first and blisters form within it or a chain of vesicles festoon along its periphery. (5) The disease process is usually self-limiting.

Immunofluorescence
Direct test shows a linear deposition of IgG (G_4, G_1) and C_3 along the BMZ of periblister skin (Fig. 4–4). In the blister area the immunofluorescence or immunoperoxidase stain is split and occurs on the roof and the floor of the blister. In severe cases in which autoantibody is present in peripheral blood in a high titer, normal appearing skin also shows IgG deposition. Indirect test shows the identical BMZ binding of IgG of patient's serum autoantibody if normal human skin or mucous membrane is used as substrate, however, if the substrate is treated with 1.0 M saline and partially separated at the dermoepidermal junction through the lamina lucida, the autoantibody reacts only on the roof, that is, the basilar surface of the basal cells. The most likely antigen present on

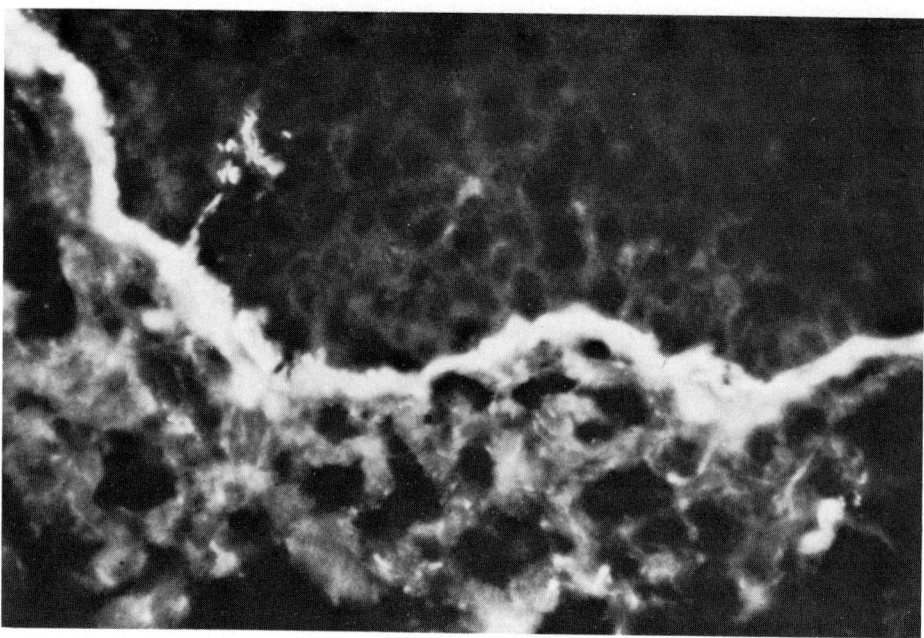

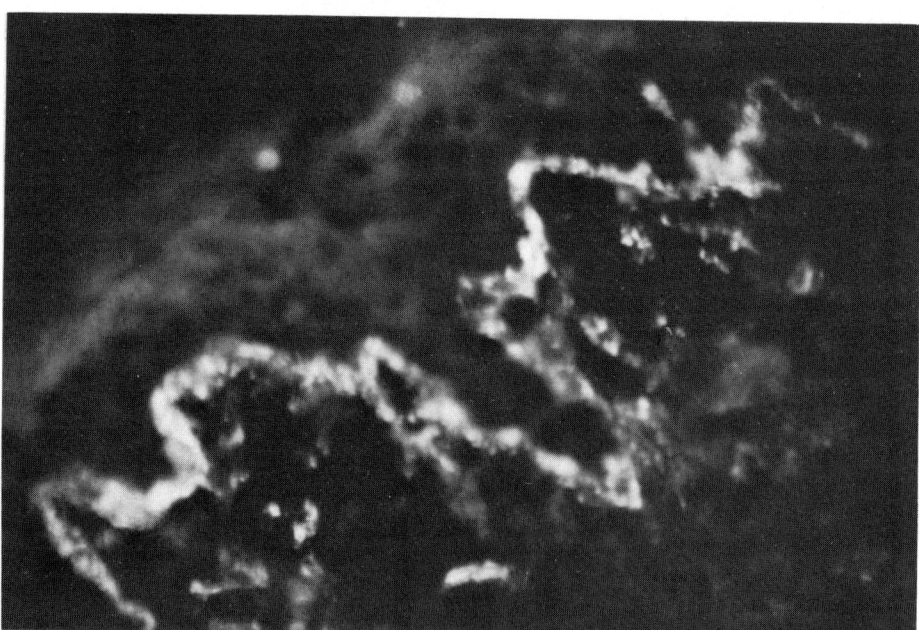

Figure 4–3.
Lupus band. Note IgM deposition along the dermal–epidermal junction in a solid pattern **(A)** and in a granular pattern **(B)**.

the basilar surface of the basal keratinocytes is hemidesmosome (see below).

Immunoelectron Microscopy

The search for bullous pemphigoid antigen to which the patient's autoantibodies bind has been long and controversial. By immunoelectron microscopic technique, at least three patterns of antibody localization are recognized[5]: (1) hemidesmosomes of basal cell, (2) lamina lucida, and (3) basal lamina. The reaction products are absent beneath the melanocytes, which lack hemidesmosomes. This observation and the most frequent localization of immunoreactants on the hemidesmosome–tonofilament complex when the keratinocyte cell membrane is rendered leaky[6] suggest that hemidesmosomes of the epidermis are the major target antigen of bullous pemphigoid autoantibodies.[7] It has been suggested that target molecules could be heterogeneous. Within or on the surface of keratinocytes, several glycoproteins could serve as binding targets of different autoantibodies from different patients.[6] It has

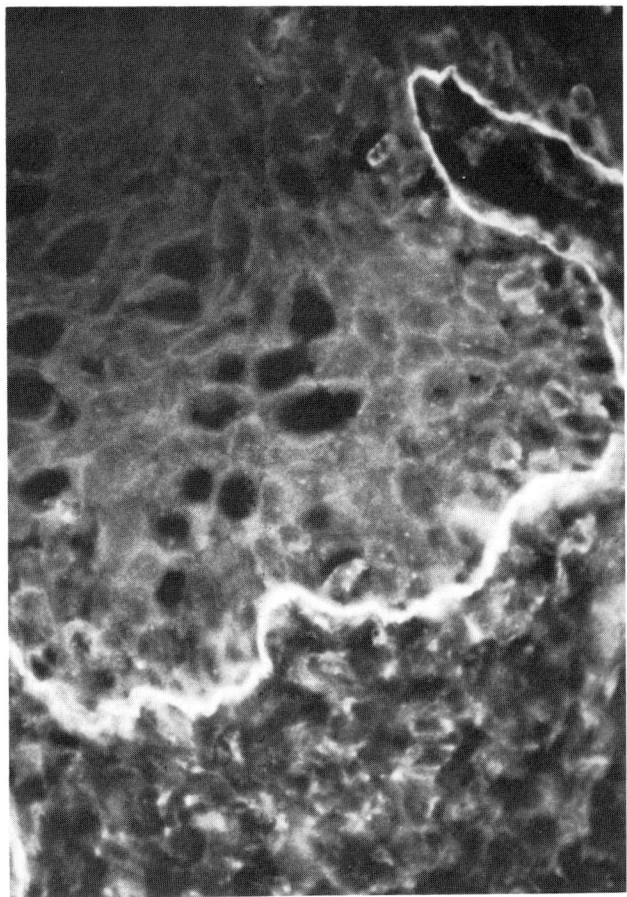

Figure 4-4.
Bullous pemphigoid. Note linear (tubular) deposition of IgG along the basement membrane zone.

also been suggested that some patients' autoantibodies recognize more than one antigen, that is, 200–240 Kd and 100-116 Kd glycoproteins of the BMZ.[8,9]

Recently cDNA of 230 Kd antigen was cloned and the antigenic protein (fusion proteins) was produced in E coli phages (42). If such antigenic fusion proteins become available for other autoimmune bullous diseases, immunoprecipitation or ELISA methods will soon replace indirect immunofluorescence which is less quantitative and more expensive.

It is not known if antigens on keratinocytes including the hemidesmosome–tonofilament complex elicit autoantibody production, although it is conceivable that keratinocyte cell membrane-associated glycoproteins are sufficiently modified in aged skin to become antigenically foreign. It is also possible that a truly antigenic substance is present elsewhere and the autoantibodies against it cross-react with the keratinocyte components. No matter what the source of the antigen, the autoantibodies produced against it come to the skin but can neither cross the basal lamina freely nor penetrate the basal cell membrane to attach to the hemidesmosome–tonofilament complex. The antibodies stay around the BMZ and the antigen–antibody complex activates the complement system, which in turn chemoattracts leukocytes, particularly eosinophils.[10] Pericapillary mast cells may release eosinophilic chemotactic factor. At any rate, degranulation of eosinophils and neutrophils releases proteolytic enzymes that damage the BMZ[11] and contribute to the accumulation of tissue fluid and blister formation.

Cicatricial Pemphigoid (Occular or Benign Mucous Membrane Pemphigoid)

Mucous membranes of mouth, genitalia, and conjunctivae of middle-aged individuals are affected with repeated blister formation and erosion, leading to scar formation. Erosions may extend to the larynx and esophagus. Conjunctival scarring may eventually lead to synechiae, symblepharon, and blindness. Skin lesions may be seen most frequently in the scalp and face, in combination with mucosal lesions or independently. In the Brunsting–Perry type, recurrent blistering occurs on a limited patch of scalp and neck without mucosal lesions.

Immunofluorescence

In a direct test a linear deposition of IgG, IgA, and complement C_3 are found in the BMZ in most cases[12] (Fig. 4–5). Only rarely can low-titer circulating autoantibodies against BMZ be detected by indirect test.[12] Immunoelectron microscopy shows depositions of these immunoreactant in lamina densa, lamina lucida, and occasionally in anchoring fibril area. The target molecules (antigenic substance) of the immunoglobulins are 230–240 Kd and 180 Kd proteins of BMZ;[12] the major epidermolysis acquisita antigen (240 Kd) is not recognized by patient's serum. Cicatricial pemphigoid is, therefore, considered as a variant of bullous pemphigoid. Unlike bullous pemphigoid, these antigens are expressed also on the lamina lucida and deeper part of BMZ; this may explain the scarring course of the disease.[12]

Herpes Gestationis

Clinical presentation is similar to those of bullous pemphigoid except that it occurs during pregnancy and, therefore, affects a younger female population. The abdomen, particularly the periumbilical region is the predilection site but inner thighs, palms, and soles are also affected.

Immunofluorescence

Basement membrane zone (BMZ) staining is seen in both direct (perilesional) and indirect tests. IgG_1,

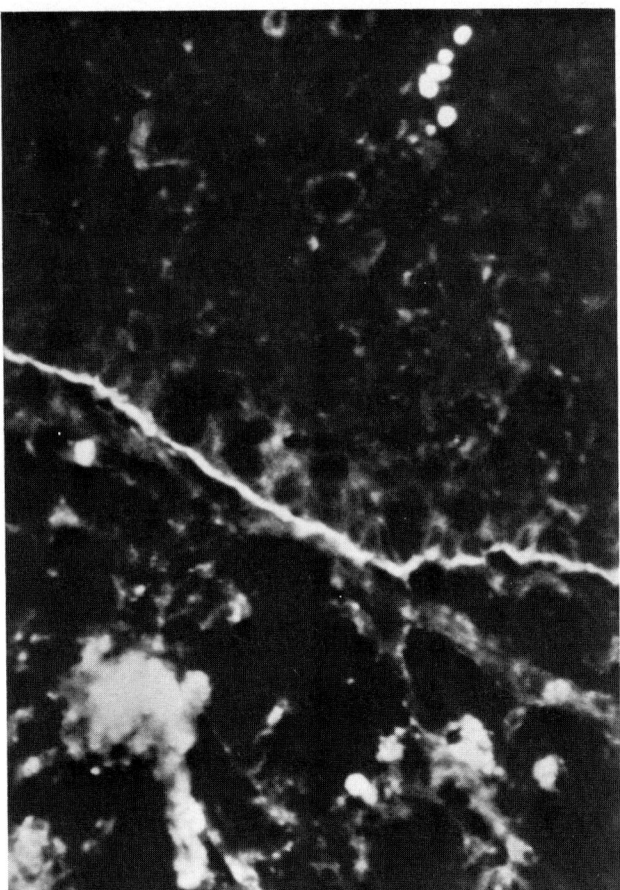

Figure 4-5.
Cicatricial pemphigoid. Note linear IgG deposition along the mucosal basement membrane zone.

which fixes complement, activated through the classical pathway, is the dominant immunoglobulin in the lesion as well as in patient sera.[4] This explains why a dense deposition of C_3 is always seen in the lesion in direct test. In indirect test a special procedure was used to detect the complement-fixing factor or "herpes gestationis factor" of patient's serum. Sections of normal skin as substrate are incubated with patient serum, fresh human serum as the source of complement, and fluorescein-labeled antihuman C_3. If one uses monoclonal anti-IgG$_1$ in both direct and indirect test and C_3 simultaneously, this will eliminate the test for herpes gestationis factor. Amniotic epithelium of patient's placenta shows BMZ depositions of IgG_1.[4] The newborn baby may have transient blisters with the same histological and immunohistological findings.

Epidermolysis Bullosa Acquisita

This condition, first named by Kablitz[13] in 1904 as a subset of epidermolysis bullosa, is now considered to be a different entity from the hereditary disorders grouped together under the name of epidermolysis bullosa. Rather, it is an immunologic disorder in which the patient develops autoantibodies against type-VII collagen present in anchoring fibrils and lower parts of the lamina densa.[9] Clinically, the disease is not congenital or hereditary; it usually begins after 50 with pruritic vesicle and blister formation often on traumatized skin and leaves atrophic scars.

Subepidermal blisters are found. The BMZ is hazy because connective tissue in the papillary dermis is degenerated. PAS stain may delineate basement membrane on the roof of the blister or split between the floor and the roof of the blister. Cellular infiltration is adjacent to the basement membrane and consists of neutrophils and some monocytes. Eosinophils, in contrast to bullous pemphigoid, are not predominant.

Immunofluorescence

The direct test is most frequently positive in linear homogeneous fashion for IgG, C_3, and fibrinogen and less frequently for IgA and IgM.[14-17] The presence of more than two classes of immunoglobulin is more frequent in this disease than in bullous pemphigoid.[4] Circulating autoantibodies are demonstrable in less than 20 percent of patients.[5] By immunoelectron microscopy, the immunoglobulin depositions were localized in the sublamina densa region to the lower part of lumina densa.[15,18] The dermal end of anchoring fibrils, but not the banded central portion, and lower part of lamina densa were labeled with patient sera which bind specifically with the carboxyl terminal of type-VII collagen by immunoblotting.[8] Therefore, it is very likely that one of the antigens of epidermolysis bullosa acquisita is related to anchoring fibrils. Indirect immunofluorescence may be able to separate this entity from bullous pemphigoid by using a substrate skin that was treated with 1 M NaCl for 72 hrs at 4°C and then the epidermis is gently removed.[12] In epidermolysis bullosa acquisita the patient's autoantibodies bind to the lamina densa left on the surface of the dermal piece and do not label the peeled epidermis. In bullous pemphigoid the dermal side is negative and the basal surface of peeled epidermis is positive.

By direct immunoelectron microscopy Fine et al[17] showed that the early separation takes place in the lamina lucida, whereas the immunoglobulin deposition in the lesion or perilesion is in the sublamina densa anchoring fibrils. This discrepancy is explained by the presence of leukocytes, chemoattracted by bound immunoreactants directly underneath the cleavage; that is, proteolytic enzymes derived from leukocyte degranulation attack the weakest structural unit, in this case the lamina lucida.[17] A similar situation exists in dermatitis herpetiformis.

Dermatitis Herpetiformis

This is usually a life-long disease affecting young as well as older individuals. Very pruritic, grouped vesicles (like herpes simplex) and rarely large bullae are surrounded with erythema. The predilection sites are broad areas of frequent friction such as extensor surface of extremities, particularly elbows and knees, buttocks, and shoulders.

Immunofluorescence

IgA deposition in dermal papillae in disrupted, granular aggregations is diagnostic (Fig. 4–6). In some cases, fibrillar deposition of IgA on bundles of microfibrils is seen. Fibrin deposition is not specific for this disease but is frequently detected. Complement C_3, IgG, IgM, and properdin may be present. Circulating IgA class autoantibodies are found in about 2 percent of patients.[19] It is likely that IgA is produced in the jejunum in response to gluten and transported to the skin to fix with some unknown papillary dermis components. This immune complex stimulates an alternative (properdin) pathway; chemotactic complements are produced; neutrophils and eosinophils are attracted to papillary dermis; and degranulation causes initial tissue damage leading to blister formation.

Adult Linear IgA Bullous Dermatosis

Patients are usually female aged between 20 and 70 years.[11] Polymorphous vesiculobullous eruptions occur on the trunk and extremities. Mucous membrane involvement is frequent.

Immunofluorescence

Direct test demonstrates linear IgA deposition along the dermoepidermal junction. As in dermatitis herpetiformis this deposition is also observed in the normal skin of the patient. Circulating IgA class autoantibodies against linear BMZ antigen has also been reported.[20,21] By immunoelectron microscopy the IgA deposition was detected in the lamina lucida, sublamina densa, or both. It is suggested that the difference of sites of immunoreactant deposition explains various clinical features of this group of diseases.

Benign Chronic Bullous Dermatosis of Childhood

Benign chronic bullous dermatosis of childhood, or juvenile linear IgA dermatosis, shares with the adult type a linear IgA deposition at dermoepidermal junction but clinical presentations are different. Children up to age 10 years are affected with annular or serpiginous erythematous plaques with the peripheral rim of vesicles/blisters.

Immunofluorescence

Same as adult linear IgA dermatosis. The presence of circulating anti-BMZ autoantibodies of IgA class is frequent but in low titers.

Discoid Lupus Erythematosus (DLE)

Discoid lesions are predominantly found in the sun-exposed areas such as face, malar prominences, nose,

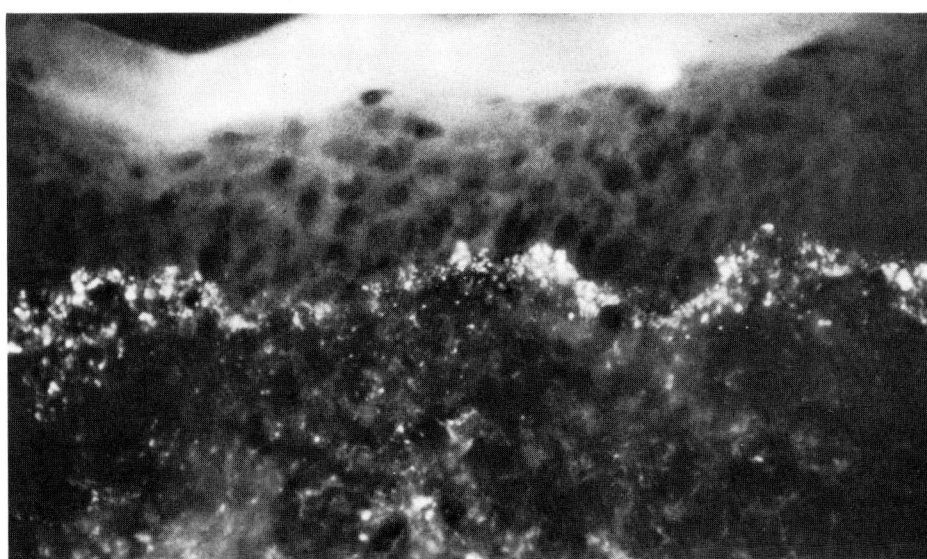

Figure 4–6.
Dermatitis herpetiformis. Note granular IgA deposits in the tips of dermal papillae. (From Korkij and Soltani. Seminars in Dermatol, 3:22, 1984.)

and forehead. These together form the "butterfly" lesion.

Immunoglobulins (IgG, IgM, IgA, IgE) and complement ($C1_q$, C_3, C_4, C_5) are commonly found along the thickened basement membrane of the lesion as uneven granular depositions.[22–24] The granular deposit of immunoglobulins and complement is seen only in the lesional skin in DLE, whereas it is also observed in the normal-appearing skin in SLE.[22] Many cytoid bodies derived from degenerated basal cells (hydropic degeneration) of the epidermis and hair follicles are scattered in papillary and reticular dermis. They absorb various immunoglobulins, particularly large molecules of IgM.

Systemic Lupus Erythematosus (SLE)

Systemic involvement is seen in kidney, heart, central nervous system, pleura, pericardium, hematopoietic organs, and joints.[25] Cutaneous lesions are present in about 20 percent of SLE patients at the onset of the disease[26] and no skin lesions develop throughout the course in about 20 percent.[27]

Granular deposition of immunoglobulins and complement is found along the dermoepidermal junction as in DLE. In SLE, however, normal-appearing skin also shows similar deposition; this phenomenon called a positive "lupus band test" is found in 60 percent of SLE patients and, if positive, can differentiate SLE from DLE.[23] The positive lupus band test in sun-protected normal skin such as buttocks may suggest a severe prognosis of the patient with diffuse renal disease. Using electron microscopy these immunoglobulins and complement components are found on fine collagen fibers beneath the lamina densa.[28] Patients with a positive lupus band test may have a poorer prognosis than those with a negative lupus band test.[29] Immunoglobulins (IgG, IgM, IgA), complement, and fibrin are often found not only on the dermal blood vessels but also diffusely between collagen bundles, justifying the designation as a collagen vascular disease.

Patient's blood serum contains antinuclear antibodies (ANA) (Fig. 4–7) and their immunofluorescence patterns are significant. ANA titers of 1:160 or higher are generally considered to be significant,[30] particularly if the reaction patterns are homogeneous (DNA, DNP, histone) or particularly peripheral (double stranded or native DNA).[31] Other patterns such as speckled or nucleolar are also found in systemic sclerosis.[31] Smith (Sm) antibody is relatively infrequent (25 percent) but is said to be very specific for SLE and indicative of renal involvement.[32,33] Antinuclear ribonucleoprotein (anti-nRNP) antibodies or antibodies against extractable nuclear antigen are diagnostic for mixed connective tissue disease (MCTD).[34]

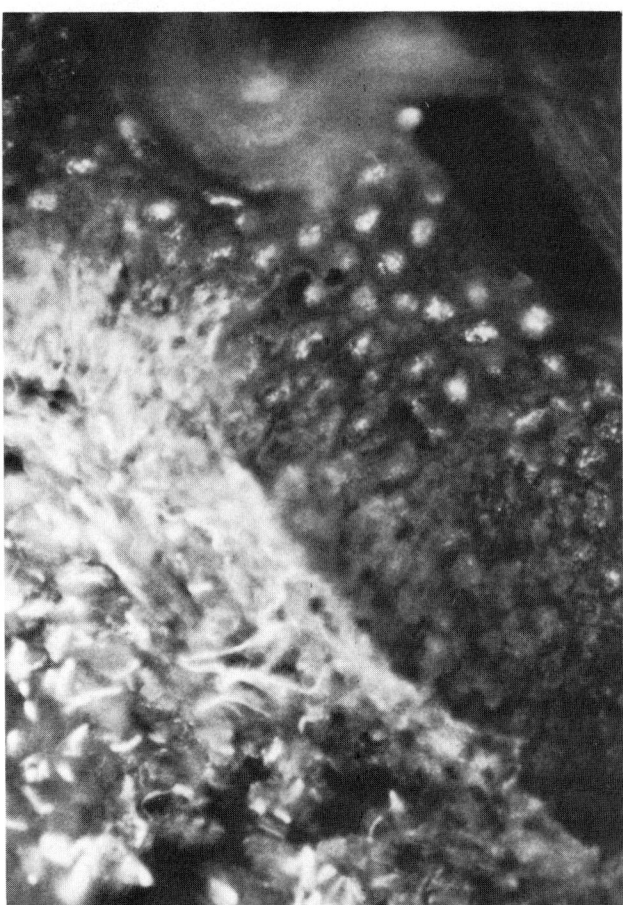

Figure 4–7.
Speckled epidermal nuclear fluorescence. Note in vivo IgG deposits in the epidermal cell nuclei.

Subacute Cutaneous Lupus Erythematosus (SCLE)

This subgroup is characterized by a severe photosensitivity manifesting as annular, polycyclic, or psoriasiform lesions. Involvement of internal organs is mild or totally absent. Recently the close relationship of patients with SCLE and Sjögren's syndrome and a mother of a neonatal lupus erythematosus (NLE) infant was established; SSA (Ro) and SSB (La) were the common denominators.[35] Further, HLA-B8, DR3, DQw2, and DRW52 phenotypes are commonly found among these three groups of patients. NLE has been known to cause severe photosensitivity. Ultraviolet B (290–320 nm) can induce the keratinocyte membrane expression of SSA, SSB, and ENA[36]; it is postulated that sun sensitivity of SCLE and NLE may be caused by the binding of antibodies to these easily accessible antigens and basal cell vacuolization is caused by the antibody–antigen–complement reaction and its chemotactic attraction of cytotoxic lymphocytes. Since SSA (Ro) antigen is not a nuclear component but a cytoplasmic glycoprotein, ANA is negative. SCLE is, therefore, often misdiagnosed by testing only for ANA.

Mixed Connective Tissue Disease (MCTD)

Overlap syndrome between scleroderma, myositis, and lupus has been known for many years. The discovery of serum autoantibody against saline-extractable nuclear antigen among this group of patients[34] established a new entity, now called MCTD. Cardinal clinical symptoms are Raynaud's phenomenon, sclerodactyly, sausage-like swelling of fingers, and myopathy including esophageal hypomotility. The LE like pictures are found in about half of the patients and are usually subacute, nonscarring lesions.[37] The absence of DNA antibody may explain a good prognosis without renal involvement. Patient's serum contains autoantibody against saline-extractable nuclear antigen that can be digested with ribonuclease, however, the epidermal keratinocytes of patient's normal skin show nuclear deposition of IgG in speckled pattern.

Scleroderma

Antinuclear antibodies are demonstrated in patient's sera in both morphea and systemic sclerosis, particularly if HEp-2 cells (human epithelial papilloma cells) are used as substrate.[38] The common fluorescence patterns are speckled and nucleolar. In acrosclerosis, anticentromere antibodies, which are also the markers of CREST syndrome, are demonstrated. Since anticentromere antibodies are absent in systemic sclerosis[39] and CREST syndrome carries a good prognosis, these antibodies are considered to indicate a good prognosis.[40] On the other hand, if SC-170, which is most frequently found in systemic sclerosis, is absent in acrosclerosis patients who have positive anticentromere antibodies, it may signify a poor prognosis. Direct immunofluorescence of the lesional and normal skin of systemic sclerosis may be positive with nucleolar IgG staining of the epidermal keratinocytes if patient's serum contains a high titer of antinucleolar antibodies.[41]

REFERENCES

1. Michel B, Milnery, David K: Preservation of tissue-fixed immunoglobulins in skin biopsies of patients with lupus erythematosus and bullous diseases. Preliminary report. J Invest Dermatol 59:449, 1972
2. Hashimoto T, Ogawa MM, Konohana A, Nishikawa T: Detection of pemphigus vulgaris and pemphigus foliaceus antigens by immunoblot analysis using different antigen sources. J Invest Dermatol 94:327–331, 1990
3. Lever WF. Pemphigus. Medicine 32:1–123, 1953
4. Kelly SE, Cerio R, Bhogal BS, Black MM: The distribution of IgG subclasses in pemphigoid gestationis: PG factor is an IgG1 autoantibody. J Invest Dermatol 92:695–698, 1989
5. Labib RS, Anhalt GJ, Patel HP, et al: Molecular heterogeneity of the bullous pemphigoid antigens as detected by immunoblotting. J Immunol 136:1231–1235, 1986
6. Yamane Y, Kitajima Y, Yaoita H: Characterization of bullous pemphigoid antigen synthesized by cultured human squamous cell carcinoma cells. J Invest Dermatol 93:220–223, 1989
7. Mutasim DF, Takahashi Y, Labib RS, et al: A pool of bullous pemphigoid antigen(s) is intracellular and associated with the basal cell cytoskeleton-hemidesmosome complex. J Invest Dermatol 84:37, 1985
8. Meyer LJ, Taylor TB, Kadunce DP, Zone JJ: Two groups of bullous pemphigoid antigens are identified by affinity-purified antibodies. J Invest Dermatol 94: 611–616, 1990
9. Tanaka T, Korman NJ, Shimizu H, et al: Production of rabbit antibodies against carboxy-terminal epitopes encoded by bullous pemphigoid cDNA. J Invest Dermatol 94:617–623, 1990
10. Gammon WR, Lewis DM, Carlo JR, et al: Pemphigoid antibody mediated attachment of peripheral blood leucocytes at the dermal-epidermal junction of human skin. J Invest Dermatol 75:334, 1980
11. Naito K, Morioka S, Ogawa H. The pathogenic mechanism of blister formation in bullous pemphigoid. J Invest Dermatol 79:303, 1982
12. Bernard P, Prost C, Lecerf V, et al: Studies of cicatricial pemphigoid autoantibodies using direct immunoelectron microscopy and immunoblot analysis. J Invest Dermatol 94:630–635, 1990
13. Kablitz R. Ein Beitrag zur Frage der epidermolysis bullosa traumatica (hereditaria et acquisita). Rostock Med Diss Rostock April 20, 1904
14. Wilson BD, Birnkrant AF, Beutner EH, Maige JC. Epidermolysis bullosa acquisita: A clinical disorder of varied etiologies. J Am Acad Dermatol 3:280, 1980
15. Ueki H, Yaoita H: A Colour Atlas of Dermato-Immunohistocytology. London:Wolfe Medical Publications, 1989
16. Gammon WR, Briggaman RA, Inman AO III, et al:

Differentiating anti-lamina lucida and anti-sublamina densa anti-BMZ antibodies by indirect immunofluorescence on 1.0 M sodium chloride-separated skin. J Invest Dermatol 82:139–144, 1984
17. Fine J-D, Tyring S, Gammon WR: The presence of intralamina lucida blister formation in epidermolysis bullosa acquisita: possible role of leukocytes. J Invest Dermatol 92:27–32, 1989
18. Shimizu H, McDonald JN, Gunner DB, et al: Epidermolysis bullosa acquisita antigen and C-terminal of type VII collagen have common immuno-localization on anchoring fibrils and lamina densa of basement membrane. (Abstract) 92:518, 1989
19. Yaoita H, Katz SI: Circulating IgA anti-basement membrane zone antibodies in dermatitis herpetiformis. J Invest Dermatol 69:558, 1977
20. Chorzelski TP, Jablonska SJ, Beutner EH, et al: Linear IgA bullous dermatosis. In: Beutner EH, Chorzelski TP Bean SF (eds): Immunopathology of the Skin. 2nd ed. New York: John Wiley and Sons, 1979, pp 315–323
21. Pehamberger H, Konrad K, Holubar K: Circulating IgA anti-basement membrane antibodies in linear dermatitis herpetiformis Duhring. IF and immuno-electron studies. J Invest Dermatol 59:490, 1977
22. Burnham TK, et al: The application of fluorescent antibody technique to the investigation of lupus erythematosus and various dermatoses. J Invest Dermatol 41:451, 1963
23. Cormane RH: 'Bound' globulin in the skin of patient with chronic discoid lupus erythematosus. Lancet 1:534, 1964
24. Tuffanelli DL, Epstein JH: Discoid lupus erythematosus. In: Dubois EL (ed): Lupus Erythematosus, 2nd ed. Los Angeles: University of Southern California Press, 1974, p 225
25. Wechsler HL: Editorial: Lupus Erythematosus. A clinician's coign of vantage. Arch Dermatol 119:877–882, 1983
26. Provost TT: Commentary: Neonatal Lupus Erythematosus. Arch Dermatol 119:619–622, 1983
27. Estes D, Christian CL: The natural history of systemic lupus erythematosus by prospective analysis. Medicine (Baltimore) 50:85–95, 1971
28. Ueki H, Wolff HH, Braun-Falco O: Cutaneous localization of human-globulins in lupus erythematosus. An electron microscopical study using the peroxidase-labelled antibody technique. Arch Dermatol Res 248:297–314, 1974
29. Davis BM, Gilliam AN: Prognostic significance of subepidermal immune deposits in uninvolved skin of patients with systemic lupus erythematosus: 10-year longitudinal study. J Invest Dermatol 83:242, 1984
30. Nisengard RJ, Jablonska S, Chorzelski T, et al: Diagnosis of systemic lupus erythematosus. Importance of antinuclear antibody titers and peripheral staining patterns. Arch Dermatol 111:1298–1300, 1975
31. Burnham TK: Antinuclear antibodies. Arch Dermatol 114:1343–1344, 1978
32. Michelson S: Systemischer Lupus erythematodes, die Bedeutung immunologischer Tests. Z Hautkr 61:667–670, 1986
33. Beaufils M, Kouki F, Mignon F, et al: Clinical significance of anti-Sm antibodies in systemic lupus erythematosus. Am J Med 74:201–205, 1983
34. Sharp GC, Anderson PC: Current concepts in the classification of connective tissue diseases. Overlap syndromes and mixed connective tissue disease (MCTD). J Am Acad Dermatol 2:269–279, 1980
35. Alexander EL, McNicholl J, Watson RM, et al: The immunogenetic relationship between anti-Ro (SS-a)/La(SS-B) antibody positive Sjögren's/Lupus erythematosus overlap syndrome and the neonatal lupus syndrome. J Invest Dermatol 93:751–756, 1989
36. Furukawa F, Kashihara-Sawami M, Lyons MB, Norris DA: Binding of antibodies to the extractable nuclear antigens SS-A/Ro and SS-B/La is induced on the surface of human keratinocytes by ultraviolet light (UVL): Implications for the pathogenesis of photosensitive cutaneous lupus. J Invest Dermatol 94:77–85, 1990
37. Prystowsky SD, Gilliam JN: Discoid lupus erythematosus as part of a larger disease spectrum. Arch Dermatol 111:1448–1452, 1975
38. Balanga V, Medsger TA Jr, Reichlin M: Antinuclear and anti-single-stranded DNA antibodies in morphea and generalized morphea. Arch Dermatol 123:350–353, 1987
39. Jarzabek-Chorzelska M, Blasczyk M, Jablonska S, et al: Scl 70 antibody, a specific marker of systemic sclerosis. Br J Dermatol 115:393–401, 1986
40. Chorzelski TP, Jablonska S, Beutner EH, et al: Anti-centromere antibody. Br J Dermatol 113:381–398, 1985
41. Prystowsky SD, Gilliam JN, Tuffanelli D: Epidermal nucleolar IgG deposition in clinically normal skin. Arch Dermatol 114:536–538, 1971

5
GENERAL PATHOLOGY: TERMINOLOGY

Many phenomena encountered in dermatohistopathology are unique to the skin and are best described in specific terms not often used in general pathology. Exact definition and application of these terms aid greatly in precise description and communication.

Similarly, it is advisable to follow a systematic pattern in the description of skin sections. Every normal constituent of the skin should be mentioned in order to show that it has not been overlooked. It is convenient to start at the surface and work down toward the subcutaneous layer, but a few modifications are recommended. If a section represents a tumor, of either the epidermis or the dermis, this is best stated at the outset. A good description of a skin section should make it possible for the reader to visualize the pathologic change, and the statement that we are dealing with a tumor and where it is located is very helpful in this respect. Also, if the principal abnormal feature is located deep in the dermis or subcutis, it is wise to mention this right away, before proceeding with the routine detailed description.

Another modification that we recommend is to begin with the living major portion of the epidermis. Start with the rete malpighi or prickle cell layer, then trace these cells in their natural course through the granular into the horny layer. This is followed, if necessary, by details concerning the condition of the basal layer and junction. Papillary and subpapillary portions of the dermis are described next, then the reticular portion (middermis and deep dermis), and finally the subcutaneous fat tissue, if the submitting physician was circumspect enough to include it in his biopsy. Absence of the deeper layers should be recorded, as they often contain invaluable clues to the diagnosis, which in their absence may remain unclear. The outlined scheme will be followed in this chapter, and photomicrographs of various skin diseases will be used to illustrate and name the phenomena of cutaneous general pathology.

There are several reasons for our recommendations. Unless we can be content with the short statement, "The epidermis shows no significant changes," we have to keep in mind that all pathobiologic alterations of the epidermis start in its living portion. All changes in the horny layer (with the exception of external trauma) are initiated in the prickle cell layer. The basal layer, on the other hand, less frequently shows tangible pathology, and if it does, this is best discussed in terms of its two principal functions: as a rgenerative layer and as a part of the epidermodermal interface.

Another reason is the fact that the true baseline in the structural organization of the skin is the superficial dermis at the base of the papillae, as shown so vividly in Figure 2–11 and mentioned in Chapter 2. The normal epidermis resembles a moldable cover over the dermis and fills all the spaces between the papillae. In pathologic biology, if the papillae become edematous or hypertrophic, they elevate the epidermis above them, and the rete ridges become exaggerated. When the epidermis becomes hyperplastic, it also thickens toward the outside of the body. If its ridges grow high and large, the spaces between them are filled by the accommodating papillae, and the suprapapillary plate is pushed up. With very few exceptions (see lichen simplex chronicus in Chapter 7 and pseudoepitheliomatous proliferation in Chapter 35), there is no downgrowth of rete ridges, and this often misused descriptive term should be applied with the utmost caution.

EPIDERMIS

General Configuration

The epidermis may be thicker or thinner than normal. Figure 5–1A shows a case of chronic eczematous dermatitis. The epidermis is thicker than normal and contains a larger number of prickle cells. It exhibits acanthosis (akanthos, Greek for spine or prickle), which is defined as epidermal "hyperplasia," through overabundance of prickle cells. Figure 5–1B, in contrast, shows a thick epidermis consisting of relatively few and very large prickle cells. This state is best called epidermal "hypertrophy" (sometimes called pseudoacanthosis). A rough estimate of the number of prickle cells can be obtained by counting the number of nuclei along a vertical line between basal layer and granular (or parakeratotic) layers. Normally, four to seven nuclei are present, depending on whether one chooses the area above a papilla or that in a rete ridge. In Figure 5–1A, 10 to 12 nuclei are found in a vertical row in a ridge, four to five above the papilla. In Figure 5–1B, the range is four to seven, indicating that there is no overproduction (hyperplasia) of cells. Epidermal "atrophy" and "hypoplasia" are shown in Figure 5–2. The number and vertical diameter of cells are diminished, and, at the same time, rete ridges are short or absent. Note that hyperplasia, hypertrophy, hypoplasia, and atrophy are judged by the number and size of the prickle cells. The basal layer by definition is always single, as pointed out in Chapter 2. The condition of its cells must be described separately and is discussed later.

The condition of the rete ridges and the suprapapillary plate (that part of the epidermis above a line connecting the tips of the papillae) should be noted separately. The latter can be thick or thin. The ridges may be absent, short, long, thin, thick, clubbed, or pointed. They may be even or uneven in length and width. A word of caution is necessary. Because we ordinarily examine thin vertical sections, rete ridges may be cut at any angle. Cross sections look like pegs, but tangential and oblique sections may look like very broad blocks. It is only by comparing size and shape of ridges in a long section, or better, in serial sections, that one can get an

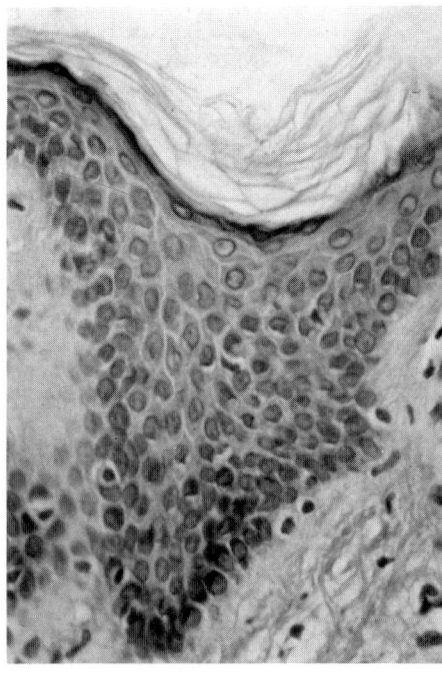 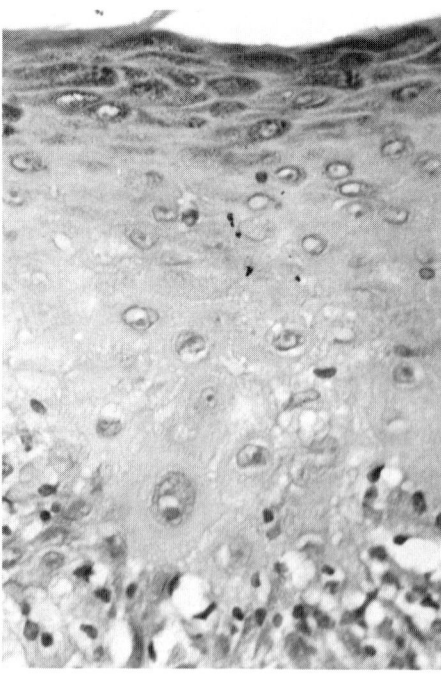

Figure 5–1.
Hyperplasia and hypertrophy of epidermis. **A.** Mildly acanthotic epidermis of chronic lichenification. **B.** Hypertrophic epidermis of lichen planus. Compare number and size of keratinocytes in these photos taken at identical magnification. H&E. X352.

A   B

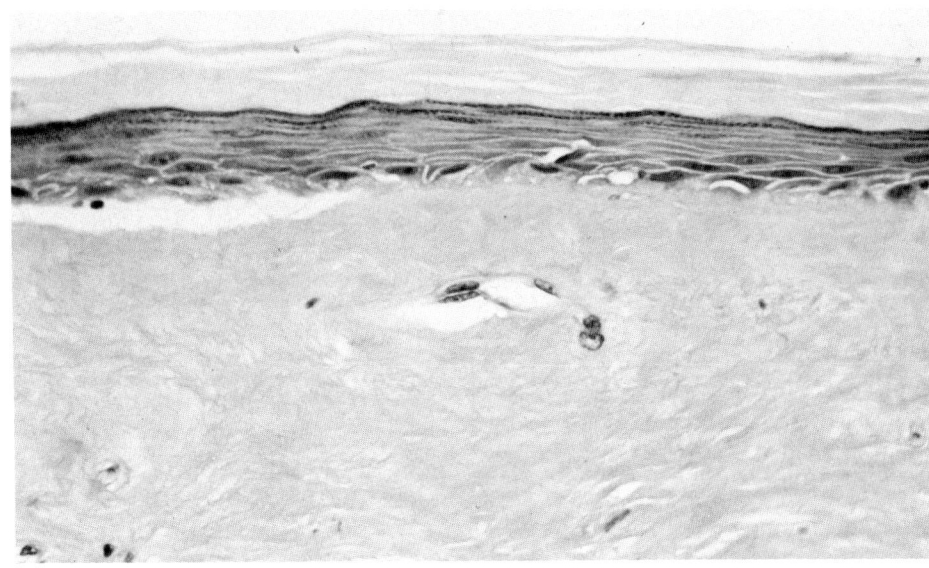

Figure 5-2.
Epidermal atrophy in lichen sclerosus et atrophicus. H&E. X370.

approximate estimate of their true configuration in any biopsy specimen. For this purpose the split skin preparations are highly instructive (Fig. 5–3). The tendency to describe any acanthotic epidermis as "psoriasiform" is regrettable.

Special Features in the Prickle Cell Layer

Prickle cells may be smaller than normal (atrophic) but more commonly are larger, either through hypertrophy or intracellular edema. The size of the nucleus in nonneoplastic disease varies within narrow limits. It has been well shown that every prickle cell nucleus contains approximately the same amount of chromatin (diploid). Therefore, a smaller nucleus will stain darker than a larger one. The size of the cell body varies considerably, and whether this is due to hypertrophy or edema is difficult to judge in routine sections. The depth of staining is a poor indicator. Prickle cells of acanthotic epidermis may contain much glycogen (Fig.

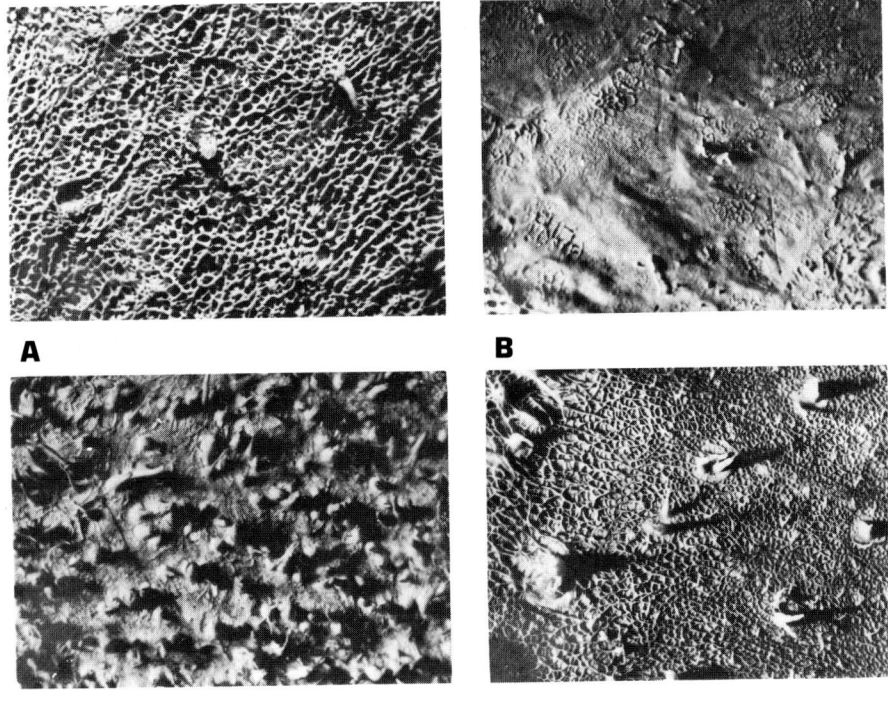

Figure 5-3.
Lower surface of epidermis in various skin diseases. Specimens prepared by Oberste–Lehn according to Horstmann's method and photographed in oblique incident light. The projecting peglike structures are the stumps of hair roots and sweat ducts. **A.** Psoriasis. Note even pattern of accentuated rete ridges. **B.** Lichen planus. Note atrophy of ridges. **C.** Chronic discoid lupus erythematosus. Large number of small facial hair follicles, distended by keratinous plugs. **D.** Lichen simplex chronicus at left, normal skin at right. Gradually increasing hyperplasia of rete ridges becoming excessive in left upper corner. (From Pinkus. Arch Dermatol 82:681, 1960.)

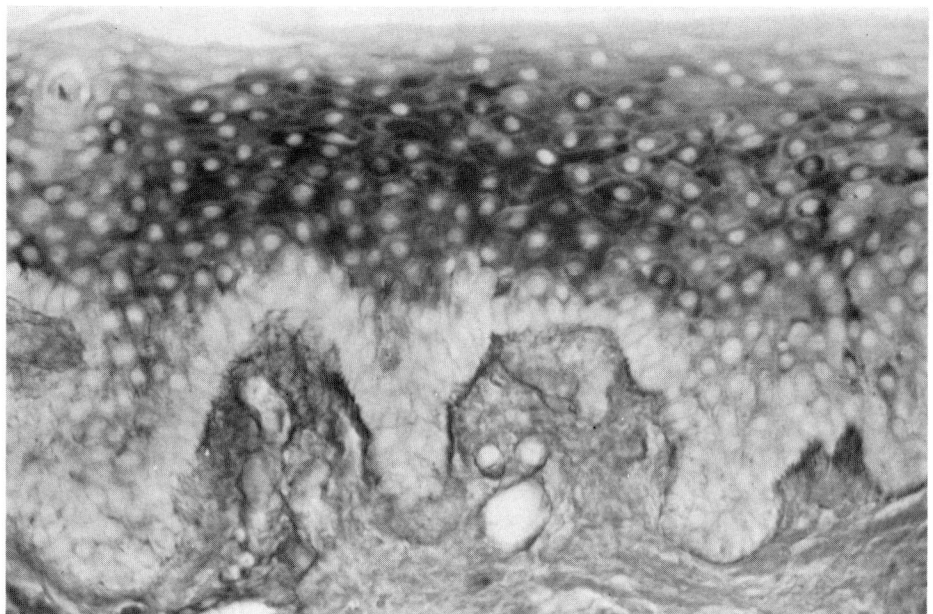

Figure 5–4.
Glycogen (dark because PAS-positive) in canthotic epidermis. Note absence of glycogen in basal cells and in keratinizing layers. PAS–light green. X285.

5–4) and, therefore, may appear pale in H&E and other stains without being edematous. A high degree of intracellular edema usually is indicated by a perinuclear or paranuclear empty space due to retraction of the nucleus from the tonofibril-containing peripheral cytoplasm during routine fixation (Fig. 5–5).

More important for diagnostic purposes are the presence, quantity, and distribution of intercellular edema. This widens the intercellular spaces and accentuates the intercellular bridges (see Figs. 2–5 and 7–4). The relationship of intercellular bridges, desmosomes, and tonofibrils was discussed in Chapter 2. It should be noted in the description whether edema is diffuse or focal. A pronounced degree of intercellular edema is called "spongiosis" because it makes an epidermal section resemble a sponge (Fig. 5–6). Once the overstretched intercellular bridges rupture, vesiculation is initiated. Intraepidermal vesicles of this type are referred to as spongiotic vesicles.

Vesiculation plays an important part in clinical diagnosis, and the pathologist is often called upon to decide the type and location of the vesicle. A classification and differentiation of vesiculating processes is given in Chapter 11. Here we point out that vesicles and bullae can arise at any level within and just below the epidermis. They may be *subcorneal* (above the granular layer, see Fig. 11–22), *intragranular* (see Fig. 11–21), *intraepidermal* (see Fig. 11–17), and *subepidermal*. Subepidermal vesicles can result from separation at the dermoepidermal

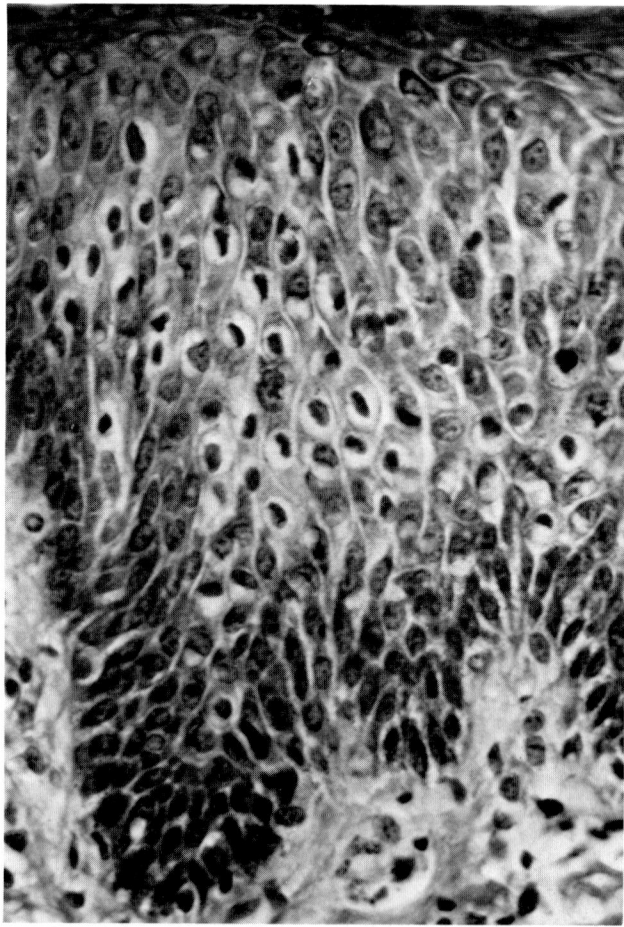

Figure 5–5.
Intracellular edema producing perinuclear halos. H&E. X465.

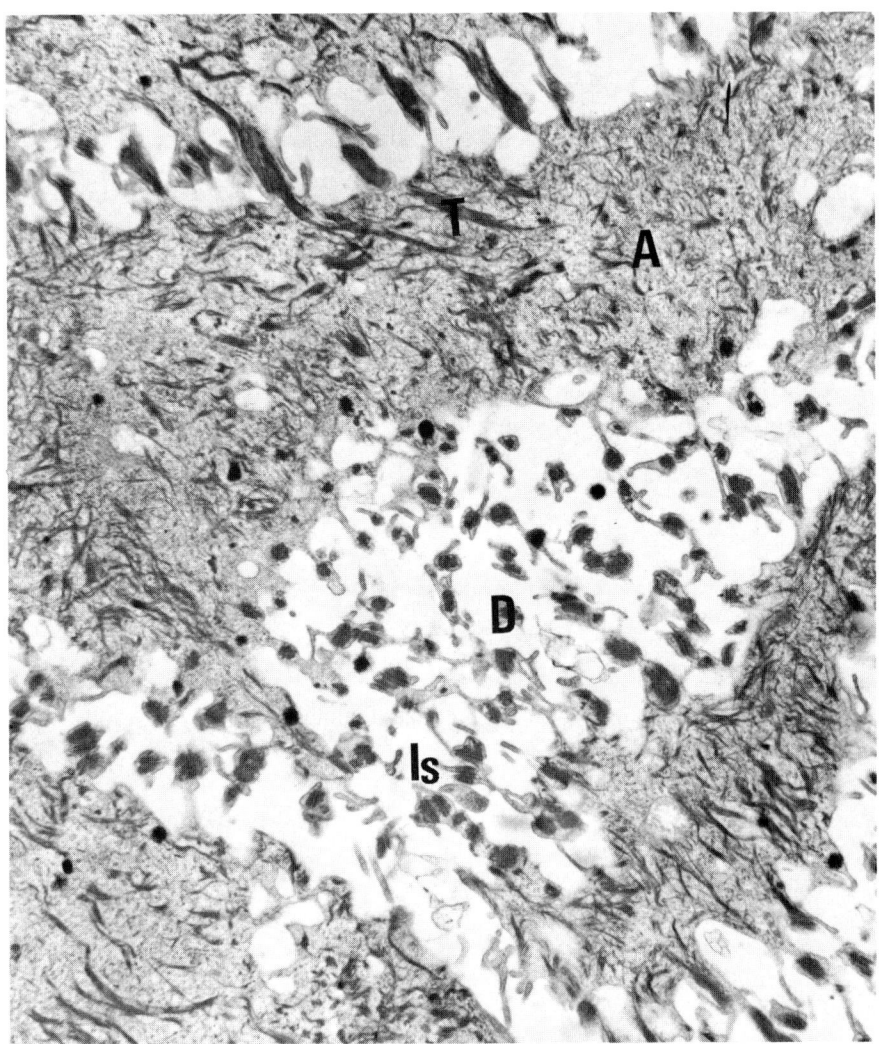

Figure 5–6.
Spongiosis. Intercellular edema more severe than in Figure 2–6. Intercellular space (Is) filled with partly broken intercellular bridges (D) and microvilli. Tonofilaments (T) in cytoplasm (A) extend to intercellular bridges. Electron micrograph. X8000. (Courtesy of Dr. A. P. Lupulescu.)

junction (see Fig. 11–8), sometimes in association with basal cell degeneration (see Fig. 9–3), or they may be "intradermal bullae" resulting from bullous edema of the papillae (see Fig. 10–4).

Intraepidermal vesicles and bullae may result from spongiosis through rupture of stretched intercellular bridges or from acantholysis (dissolution and disappearance of intercellular connections, see Fig. 11–1) or from necrosis and disappearance of entire cells. The latter is the mechanism of reticulating degeneration, which is particularly common in viral diseases (see Fig. 12–1). Empty spaces within or below the epidermis that do not contain recognizable fluid and may be due to retraction of separated elements during fixation are referred to as "clefts" (e.g., Fig. 29–1 in Darier's disease, also lichen planus). Flat, flaccid vesicles resulting from acantholysis are called "lacunae" (e.g., in Hailey–Hailey's disease, Fig. 29–6). Unique processes are the edema and rupture of hypertrophic granular cells (see Figs. 30–3 and 30–4), leading to the bullae of epidermolytic hyperkeratosis (bullous form of ichthyosiform erythroderma), and the basal cell disintegration of epidermolysis bullosa.

Not only tissue fluid but formed elements of various types may be present within the epidermis. Inflammatory cells, including neutrophilic and eosinophilic polymorphonuclear leukocytes as well as lymphocytes, easily enter through temporary breaks (see Fig. 8–7) in the basement membrane (exocytosis). They may migrate singly in the intercellular spaces or may accumulate in vesicles. Accumulations of polymorphonuclear cells between the damaged cells of the suprapapillary plate of psoriasiform tissue reactions (see Fig. 8–12) are known as "spongiform pustules" (Kogoj). Groups of pyknotic

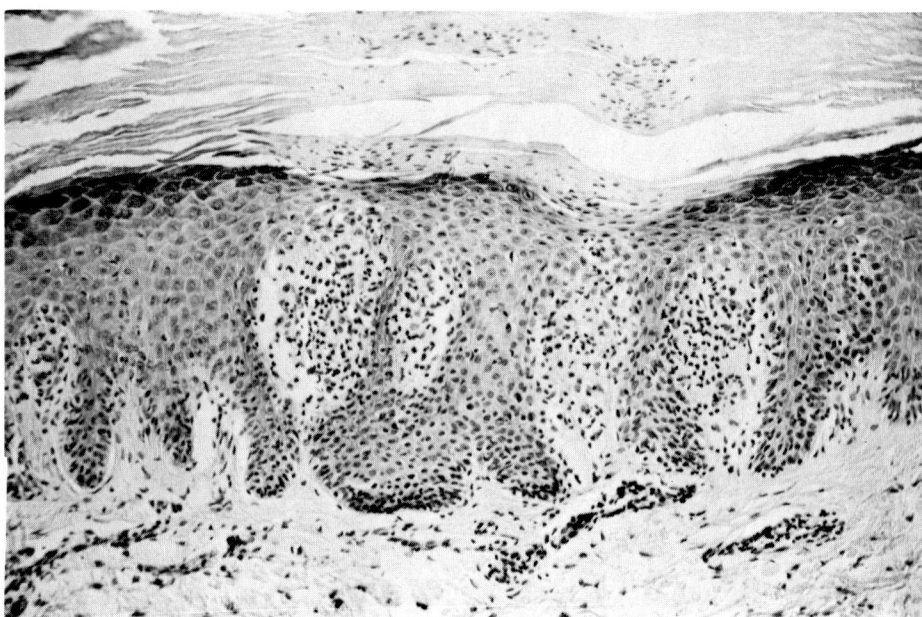

Figure 5–7.
Psoriasiform lesion showing association of parakeratosis and loss of granular layer with heads of papillae. H&E. X135.

leukocytes found in the keratinizing layers are known as Munro microabscesses (see Fig. 8–3). Other cells, such as mast cells, but particularly reticuloendothelial and lymphomatous cells, invade the epidermis. This is an important diagnostic feature in histiocytosis X (monocytes and Langerhans cells, see Fig. 25–1) and in mycosis fungoides (atypical mononuclear cells, Pautrier abscesses, see Fig. 45–6). Red blood cells also get into the epidermis, as do fragments of elastic and collagenous fibers and clumps of amyloid. These and other nonmotile elements are gradually pushed outward with the stream of keratinocytes and are eliminated on the surface (transepidermal elimination).[1,2] Transepidermal elimination should, however, be kept separate from transepidermal perforation, which is a much more massive process.

Stratum Granulosum and Stratum Corneum

Vertical sections of normal epidermis usually show one or two rows of granular (keratohyalin) cells except on the acral parts of the extremities, where this layer is thicker. Multiple layers of granular cells are described as "hypergranulosis." Reduction ("hypogranulosis") or absence of granular layer is abnormal and should always be mentioned in description.

Hypergranulosis and absence of granular layer may be found together in one section, in alternating or focal distribution. Because it may be of diagnostic significance, the state of the granular layer in topical relation to rete ridges or papillae should be mentioned. In Figure 5–7, for example, the granular layer is absent from the suprapapillary portions, whereas it is thickened in the interpapillary stretches.

The horny layer (stratum corneum) varies considerably in width and compactness in different parts of the normal skin (see Fig. 2–1).[3] It is, therefore, very important to know exactly from which locality a biopsy specimen has been obtained. "Hyperkeratosis" means increased thickness of the horny layer. It may be *orthokeratotic* (consisting of morphologically normal cells without nuclei) or *parakeratotic* (containing pyknotic nuclei). Hyperkeratosis may be relative in comparison to the atrophic or hypoplastic prickle cell layer, or it may be absolute, and often it is both. The normal horny layer often is described as having a basketweave appearance because our routine sections stain mainly the cell walls, whereas the body of the cell appears empty. This state is exaggerated in some diseases, for example, verruca plana. In other sections (see Fig. 9–1), the horny layer looks compact or compressed, similar to that of palms and soles. A compressed horny layer may be relatively thin and yet represent hyperkeratosis. In other conditions (e.g., psoriasis), we encounter a lamellated stratum corneum, composed of alternating layers of orthokeratosis and parakeratosis (see Fig. 8–8).

Scale and Crust

Hyperkeratosis usually corresponds to the clinical aspect of scaliness, especially if it is parakeratotic or lamellated. One can often judge the clinical characteristics in the sections. The large lamellar scales of psoriasis tend to separate in histologic sections; the fine branny scale of seborrheic dermatitis appears as moundlike foci (see Fig. 8–2). The thin, disclike scale of pityriasis lichenoides chronica can be recognized and is a help in diagnosis (see Fig. 13–4).

If tissue fluid (serum) is mixed with horny material, usually of parakeratotic type, a scale–crust results (Fig. 5–8). The inspissated and dried-up serum appears in the sections as amorphous material that is eosinophilic and usually PAS-positive. The term "colloid keratosis"[14] has been applied to conditions in which large blobs of dense PAS-positive material are found in the hyperplastic horny layer (see Fig. 47–20).

An essential part of the examination of the horny layer is a search for microorganisms, such as fungi and bacteria, which may solve an otherwise puzzling histopathologic picture. Hyphae and spores are sometimes visible in H&E sections and are easily recognized in O&G sections (see Fig. 13–1A), although it must be admitted that the PAS procedure furnishes a much more dramatic demonstration (see Figs. 13–1B and 13–3). Bacteria also are stained by the Giemsa solution. Scabies mites (see Fig. 13–13) and various foreign particles that may or may not have significance may be found in the stratum corneum. It is worthwhile to examine red and white blood cells that adhere to the skin surface. They may give a clue to sickling or other erythrocyte abnormalities and to leukemia, even if the small vessels in the skin do not contain blood.

Disturbances in the Basal Layer

It must be said at the outset that nothing has caused more confusion in dermatopathology than the indiscriminate application of the designation "basal cell" to any epithelial cell that has a relatively small dark nucleus and scant cytoplasm (Chapter 2). The concept of basal cell carcinoma as a tumor of basal cells and opposed to spinous or squamous cell carcinoma as a tumor composed of prickle cells has had repercussions extending into other fields of pathology and has injected dualistic concepts into biologic and embryologic investigations. Fortunately, the electron microscopists have reconfirmed classic concepts and have securely established the unity of all keratinocytes. Basal cells, prickle cells, and keratinized cells are the same strain of cell at different ages. The germinal basal cell is eternally young. It does not produce progeny but splits into two cells equal to itself. That one of these daughters usually goes on to maturation and death may be explained by its becoming separated from immaturity-preserving contact with the dermis.

The numerous applications of the term basal cell and suggested substitutes are listed in Table 2–2. In most instances, substitution of "basaloid cell" is acceptable and self-explanatory. It has become abundantly clear that similarity in H&E-stained paraffin sections does not mean morphologic or functional or biologic identity of small, dark-staining epithelial cells.

The term "basal cell" is then reserved for cells in the *basal layer* of the epidermis or at the periphery of adnexal structures. Cells that are in contact with subserving mesoderm, in most circumstances, are also the only type of cell undergoing mitotic division. If mitotic activity is greatly increased, for example, in psoriasis, however, two to three strata of the epidermis may contain mitoses[5] and form the *germinal layer* (stratum germinativum) of the hy-

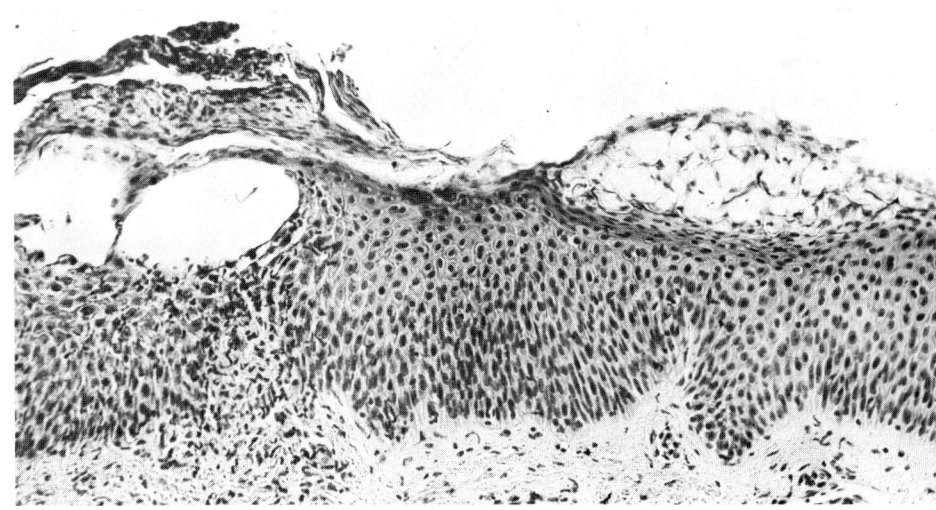

Figure 5–8.
Two types of parakeratotic crust in cases of seborrheic dermatitis. At left, dense parakeratotic lamellae are mixed with pyknotic leukocytic nuclei. At right, coagulated serum is caught between cells and produces a spongy appearance. H&E. X126. (From Sutton. Diseases of the Skin, 11th ed. 1956. Courtesy of Dr. R. L. Sutton, Jr. Contributed by H. Pinkus.)

perplastic epidermis. The cells of these layers may be relatively small and immature; they are basaloid cells.

Basal cells of normal or abnormal epidermis may be flat (Fig. 5–2), cuboidal, or columnar (Figs. 5–4 and 5–8). In most instances, it suffices to state that the layer is intact. In some diseases, basal cells are said to undergo liquefaction degeneration (see Fig. 9–5) or hyalinization (see Fig. 9–4). An organized basal layer may be absent for short or longer stretches of the epidermis, and cells having the morphologic appearance of prickle cells border on the dense inflammatory infiltrate present in all these cases. Usually, this phenomenon is associated with subepidermal cleft formation (see lichen planus, lupus erythematosus). The peripheral cells of squamous cell carcinoma usually have little morphologic resemblance to basal cells.

Melanocytes

The basal layer normally contains a complement of melanocytes. Their number being fairly constant for any given area, an unusual scarcity or abundance may have pathologic significance. Individual sections may show great variations, however, and judgment must be based on examination of a series of sections. One also has to remember that nonpigmented basal melanocytes are indistinguishable by light microscopy from similarly situated Langerhans cells.

Melanin in granular form is normally present in basal cells, except in very light skin. It is also found (see Fig. 2–13) in prickle cells and horny cells of more darkly pigmented skins. The decision whether absence or presence of melanin has pathologic significance depends on clinical information, which is essential. Many skins under a variety of chronic inflammatory conditions present pigment block (see Fig. 2–45). The keratinocytes seem unable to accept melanin from the melanocytes, which become engorged with pigment (see Figs. 2–43 and 2–44) and highly dendritic. The epidermal melanin unit becomes dissociated. Failure of pigment transfer on a congenital basis was found to be the cause of universal dyschromatosis in two Bantu.[6] Other disturbances of melanization are discussed in the corresponding chapters, especially Chapter 31.

Dyskeratosis, Dysplasia, Anaplasia

These terms need special discussion because their significance has changed over the years, and they are often loosely applied. Without going into historical details, it may be said that *dyskeratosis* has a very specific meaning and is practically synonymous with individual cell keratinization. In certain diseases, for example, Darier's (see Fig. 29–1) and Bowen's (see Fig. 35–12) individual cells become separated from their neighbors through acantholysis. They may proceed to keratinize as round isolated bodies (corps ronds, grains) (Fig. 5–9). Some authors distinguish between *benign* and *malignant* dyskeratosis. Thus, Darier's disease is said to be characterized by benign dyskeratosis and Bowen's

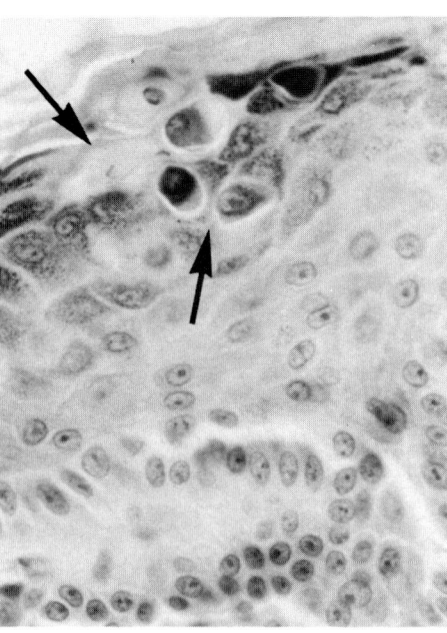
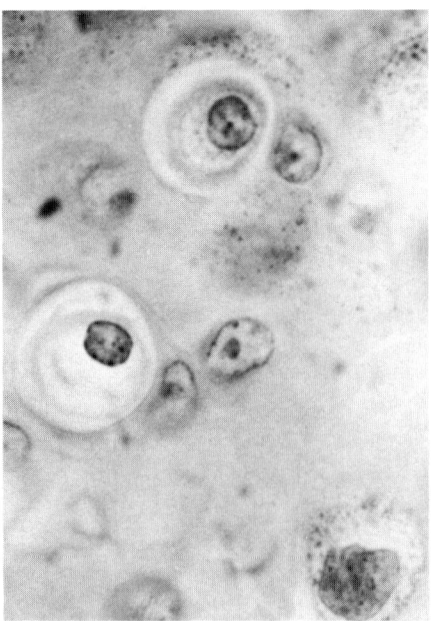

Figure 5–9.
Darier's disease. **A.** Suprabasal cleft as sign of acantholysis. Dyskeratotic cells near granular layer. Corps ronds have a nucleus within a cytoplasm, which is separated from surrounding cells by a cleft (lower arrow). Grain is a keratinized body with remnant of a nucleus (upper arrow). H&E. X600. **B.** Several corps ronds, one (lower right) with keratohyaline granules. H&E. X800.

A   **B**

disease by the malignant counterpart. Any cell on its way toward keratinization, however, has no malignant potentialities, and diagnosis of benign or malignant in these diseases is based on other criteria.

Cytologic characteristics, which stigmatize Bowen's dermatosis as carcinoma in situ, usually are called "anaplasia." This term was introduced to convey the concept that cancer results from a reversion of normal adult cells to embryonic cells. It is obvious that the significance of the word has been changed completely in present usage. There is no similarity between the highly atypical, uneven, and often hyperchromatic cells of Bowen's disease and the well-organized, though immature cells of the embryo. In the skin at least, it is preferable to substitute "dysplasia" for anaplasia as a descriptive term. More details are given in Chapter 35 on precanceroses. A certain degree of uneven size and irregular arrangement of basal and prickle cells may exist without diagnostic significance, especially in atrophic epidermis or in instances of heavy exocytosis. Considerable experience is needed to differentiate such changes from true neoplastic dysplasia, and multiple sections should be examined in doubtful cases. Inasmuch as carcinoma in situ of the skin is not a highly dangerous condition, it is better to err on the conservative side and to ask for rebiopsy at a later date, should the clinical lesion persist. Multinucleated epidermal giant cells (Fig. 5–10) are encountered occasionally without diagnostic implications and may be present in dysplastic conditions, especially Bowen's disease, in viral infections (see Fig. 5–15D), in chronic and lichenified dermatitis, and as a result of freezing.

Cell Death

Epidermal cells normally die through the intricate maturation process of keratinization. The most common deviation from this process is "parakeratosis," usually encountered in inflammation, in which no keratohyalin is formed and the nuclei persist as flat, stainable disks. Several other forms of cell death were mentioned in the preceding paragraphs or will be discussed under specific diseases (reticulating and ballooning degeneration in viral diseases, acantholytic degeneration in pemphigus, epidermolytic hyperkeratosis, basal cell disappearance in epidermolysis bullosa, and lichenoid tissue reactions). Cell-sized hyaline bodies in lichen planus and other diseases are known as "Civatte bodies" (see Fig. 9–6), and peculiar pyknotic prickle cells have been described after ultraviolet irradiation, in graft-vs.-

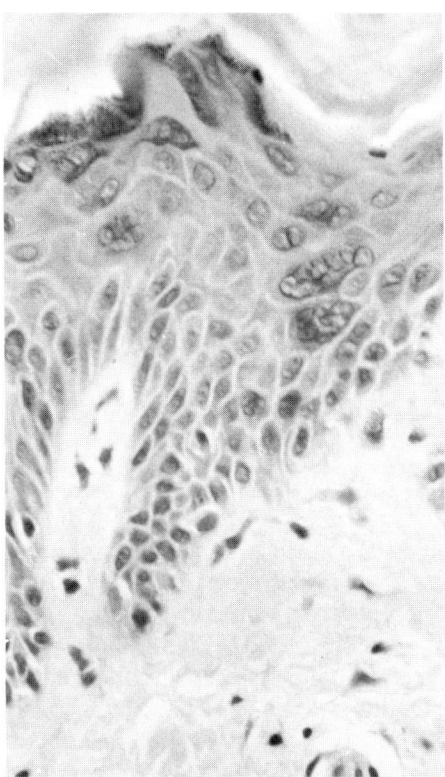
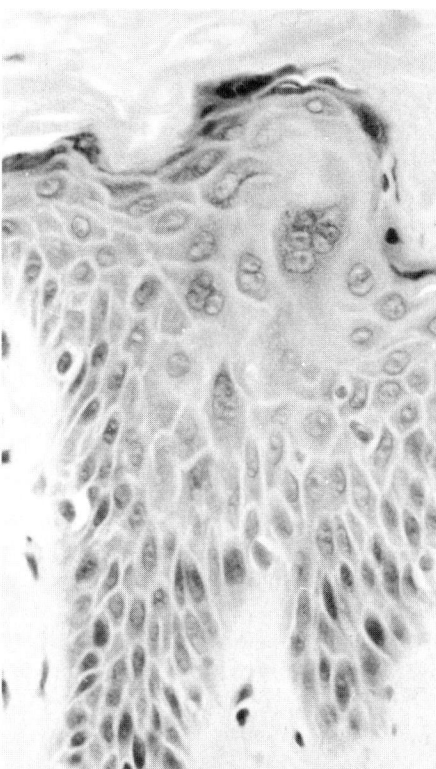

A **B**

Figure 5–10.
Multinucleated giant cells in epidermis have no diagnostic significance in many cases. These examples were found in lichenified dermatitis. H&E. X600.

host reaction, and following podophyllin treatment of condyloma acuminatum. Other types of tissue cells, especially in neoplasms but also in embryologic development (e.g., hair germ), undergo a peculiar type of pyknosis and fragmentation to which the botanical term "apoptosis" has been applied,[7] intimating the concept of programmed cell destruction as a countermeasure to mitotic cell multiplication.[8]

Transepithelial Elimination

Under a variety of circumstances, nonepidermal elements enter the epidermis from the dermis and are eliminated to the outside (Fig. 5–11). This process of transepithelial elimination was discussed in detail by Mehregan.[1] Four subdivisions may be made.

(1) The entry of motile cells, such as neutrophils or treponemas, may be called transmigration.

(2) The entry of nonmotile cells, such as erythrocytes, or of nonirritating particles, such as amyloid or carbon, through a break in the basement membrane leads to their being surrounded by epithelial cells and gradually being moved outward with the stream of keratinocytes until they are incorporated in the horny layer and exfoliated. If the particles are small, no definite disturbance of epidermal architecture will occur.

(3) Another type of transepithelial elimination involves larger blocks of material, which may be a foreign body, such as calcium, or may be a devitalized portion of the dermis, such as collagen or elastic fibers or a mass of necrotic tissue, more or less infiltrated with inflammatory cells. These materials press against the epidermis from below and cause damage. Damage may vary from precocious keratinization forming a shell around the foreign body to definite epidermal necrosis and superficial ulceration. Ulceration secondarily induces epidermal repair and hyperplasia and leads to eventual elimination and healing. Smaller defects of this type appear as intraepidermal channels, as in perforating elastosis or collagenosis, but larger defects, as found in perforating granuloma annulare or chondrodermatitis nodularis, merge with the processes of ulceration (see Fig. 23–5), in which considerable portions of epidermis are sloughed off. Where the borderline should be drawn is a matter of definition.

(4) The last type of transepithelial elimination involves hair follicles, as in perforating folliculitis. Here the follicular epithelium surrounds a mass of necrotized and inflamed dermis and incorporates it into the follicular lumen. This bolus formation is followed by slow elimination to the surface. A similar process was also described for the necrobiotic material of granuloma annulare.[2]

DERMIS

Basement Membrane

The junction or interface between epithelial and mesodermal structures is discussed in Chapter 2. In routine sections stained with either H&E or O&G, the only plainly visible basement membrane is the vitreous membrane of the hair follicle (see Figs. 2–27, 2–28, and 2–29). The PAS procedure, on the other hand, shows red lines at the lower border of the epidermis (see Fig. 2–15), around the periphery of hair follicles and sweat glands, and also around capillary blood vessels. It should be kept in mind that other substances also take the stain.

The PAS-positive subepidermal basement membrane may be thickened or reduplicated in lupus erythematosus and other dermatoses and then becomes visible in H&E sections as a hyaline eosinophilic band. The region of the basement membrane has assumed great significance in immunofluorescent studies because autoantibodies, immune complexes, and other substances may be bound here. In many inflammatory dermatoses, such as psoriasis, close observation will show small breaks in the basement membrane (see Fig. 8–7). Every time a leukocyte crosses from dermis into epidermis, the basement membrane is pierced. Breaks in the basement membrane do not enable epidermal basal cells to invade the dermis; examination of the membrane, however, does have significance in tumor pathology. Benign epithelial tumors and basal cell epitheliomas usually have PAS-positive membranes. Squamous cell carcinomas usually have none, and basement membrane disappears when a precancerous keratosis becomes invasive.

Pars Papillaris

In descriptive histopathology, papillae and subpapillary layer should be mentioned separately. Papillae can be absent, short, long, narrow, wide, club-shaped, edematous, or even branching. If they are sufficiently long to elevate the covering (suprapapillary) portion of the epidermis above the general level of the skin surface, the term "papillomatosis" is appropriate. A tumor consisting of such elongated and possibly branching papillae and other epidermal cover is called a "cutaneous papilloma." A cel-

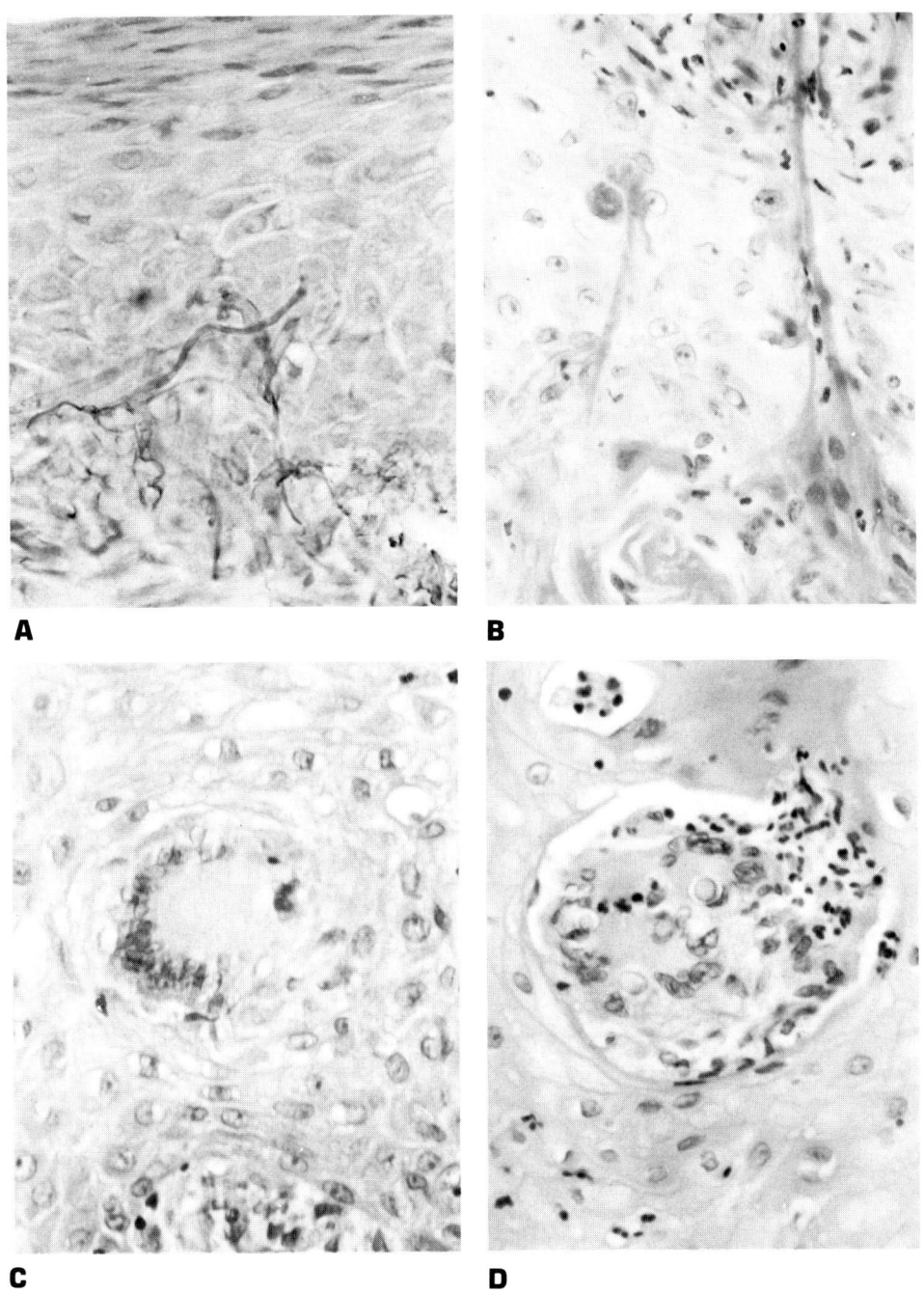

Figure 5-11.
Transepidermal elimination. **A.** *Elastic fibers in epidermis. O&G. X600.* **B.** *Vertical collagenous fibers in epidermis in a case of perforating collagenosis. H&E. X600.* **C.** *Langhans multinucleated giant cell incorporated in epidermis in a case of sarcoidosis. Epithelioid cell infiltrate visible below the epidermis. H&E. X600.* **D.** *Intraepidermal abscess containing blastomyces in a case of North American blastomycosis. H&E. X600. Note attempted keratinization of surrounding keratinocytes in* **C** *and* **D.**

lular nevus or other specific tumor may have papillomatous configuration.

The condition of the intrapapillary capillaries should be mentioned separately, when indicated. They may be tortuous, engorged, or hyalinized or may form tufts. Foreign substances, such as hyalin, amyloid, or melanin, may be present in the papillae.

The subpapillary layer, including the subpapillary precapillary and postcapillary vessels, should then be described. It may be diffusely edematous or show perivascular edema. The latter may be obvious as an empty space around vessels, or if cellular infiltrate is present, it is evident in the spacing or separation of the cells in an empty-appearing area. This feature differentiates the lymphocytic infiltrate of lupus erythematosus from the closely packed lymphocytic mass of leukemia. Blood vessels may show thin or swollen endothelia, may be wide open, engorged, or ectatic. Their walls may be hyalinized or thickened through apposition of outer cell layers.

The usually thin collagen fibrils of the subpapillary layer may be sclerosed, homogeneous, or, on the contrary, separated by edema. Macrophages containing either melanin (melanophages, Fig. 5–12) or hemosiderin are found not infrequently. If the presence of melanophages is associated with absence of epidermal pigment, the term "incontinentia pigmenti" may be used.

Red blood cells are fairly commonly seen outside vessels in biopsies of a variety of inflammatory dermatoses, especially in punch biopsy specimens. Extravasation may be the result of surgical trauma, especially when vascular walls are weakened by inflammation. Only if erythrocytes are found in various stages of disintegration and possibly associated with hemosiderin is one justified in considering a preexisting purpuric condition. Presence of red cells within the epidermis also justifies that assumption. A few small round cells (lymphocytes) and an occasional neutrophilic or eosinophilic leukocyte are of no pathologic significance. Any appreciable number should be evaluated. Neutrophils have a short life span, and their nuclei begin to become pyknotic or disintegrate into nuclear dust after a few days in the tissue (leukocytoclasia). In other cases, nuclear dust may be the result of breakdown of lymphocytes or other cells. Mast cells occur normally but are difficult to identify in H&E sections, whereas O&G sections show them clearly. To judge pathologic increase requires considerable experience. Presence of mast cells in the stroma of benign or malignant epithelial tumors or nevus cell nevi has no diagnostic significance.

Pars Reticularis

The major portion of the dermis, constituted by relatively coarse collagen bundles, thick elastic fibers, and a small number of fibrocytes, is much less frequently involved in cutaneous disease than is the pars papillaris. As a rule, none of the common inflammatory dermatoses, such as eczematous dermatitis, psoriasis, or lichen planus, affect the pars reticularis with more than an extension of lymphocytic infiltrate around smaller vessels. If significant inflammatory infiltrate is present, it may be associated with hair follicles and sweat glands, or it may be diffuse. Its distribution and composition must be noted because the pars reticularis is the common seat of *granulomatous inflammation*. In addition to polymorphonuclear leukocytes, eosinophils, and lymphocytes, we commonly encounter plasma cells and histiocytes in all their various disguises.

Lymphocytes

The term "lymphocyte" has been used rather indiscriminately for many years to identify a small cell

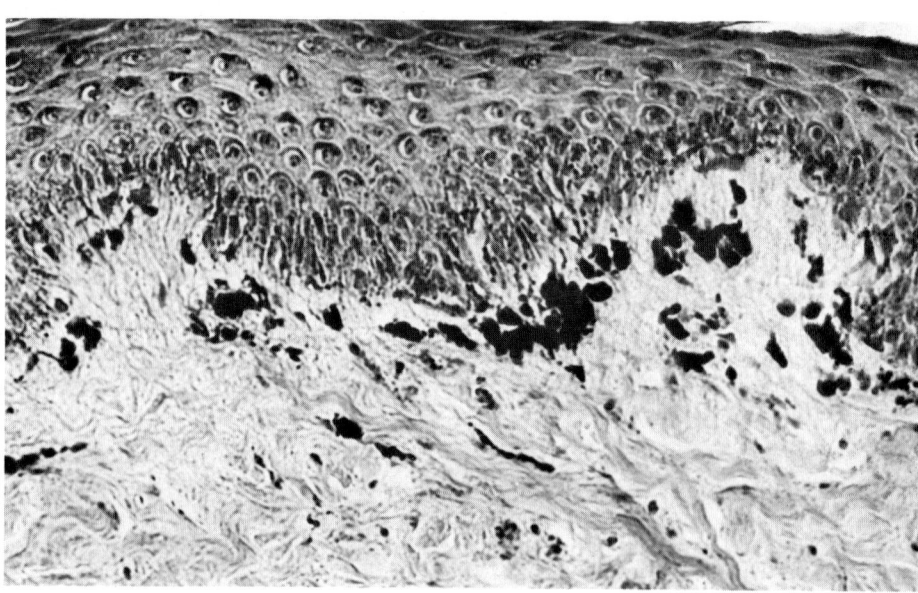

Figure 5–12.
Melanophages (macrophages containing clumped melanin) in a case of postinflammatory pigmentation. H&E. X180. (From Sutton. Diseases of the Skin, 11th ed, 1956. Courtesy of Dr. R. L. Sutton, Jr. Contributed by H. Pinkus.)

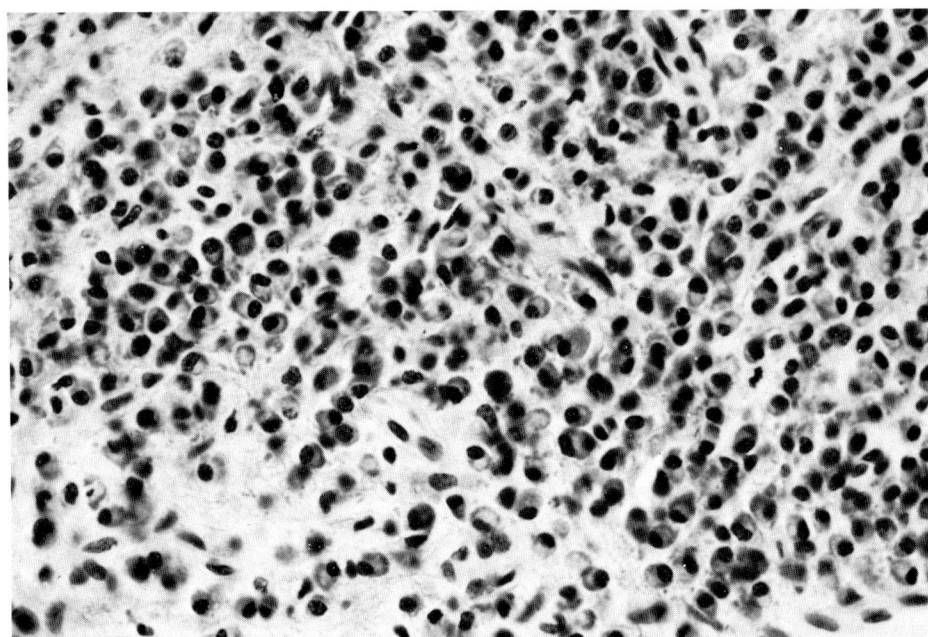

Figure 5–13.
Plasma cells in cutaneous plasma-cytoma. H&E. X800.

with a roundish dark nucleus. One has to realize, however, that any cell, whether fibroblast, histiocyte, or smooth muscle cell, when cut exactly across, may resemble a lymphocyte. Second, pathologists can identify lymphocytes with fair ease if they see a small cell in a lymph node. Identification of such cells in the skin is much more difficult, as new techniques have proved. It is fortunate that enzyme cytochemical and immunologic methods are now available to tell apart not only lymphocytes from monocytes, but T lymphocytes from B lymphocytes in properly prepared sections of a variety of skin diseases.[9,10] The term T lymphocyte refers to a cell that has been modified in the thymus gland and is concerned with cell-to-cell interactions. B lymphocytes are cells that secrete antibodies and other substances (under the influence, in birds, of the bursa fabricii) and are important in immunologic processes. Methods for identification of T and B cells and their subsets are now commercially available for routine application.[11,12]

Plasma Cells

Plasma cells (Figs. 5–13, 21–8, and 45–2) are derived from B lymphocytes and secrete immunoglobulins. They are identified by their larger nucleus, possessing coarse chromatin particles and sitting eccentrically in a round or ovoid cell body. The latter is basophilic and is apt to retain hematoxylin unless the sections are thoroughly decolorized. The cytoplasm stains prominently dark blue or grayish blue in O&G sections but does not exhibit granularity or metachromasia, in distinction from mast cells. Usually, there is a lighter staining paranuclear zone. Plasma cells undergoing a peculiar type of hyalinization are known as "Russell bodies" (Fig. 5–14).

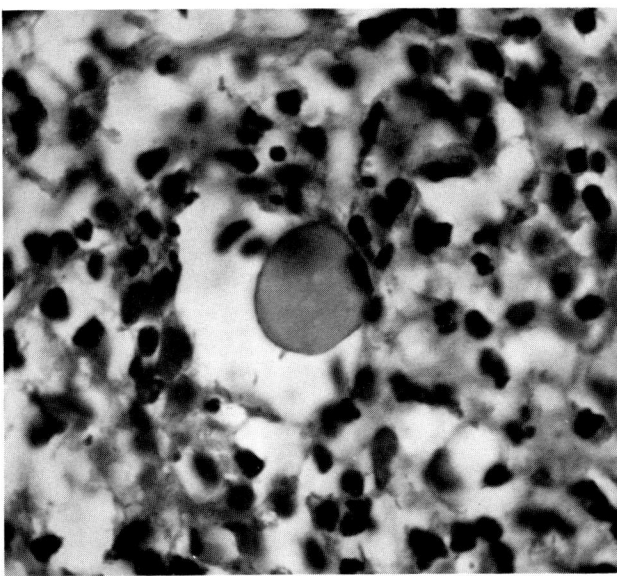

Figure 5–14.
Russell body in rhinoscleroma, a granulomatous disease characterized by mixed infiltrate containing many plasma cells. H&E. X800.

Histiocytes and Multinucleated Giant Cells

Histiocytes were considered members of Aschoff's reticuloendothelial system, generally benign cells, and the precursors of macrophages. Modern hematologists have chosen to replace the name "reticulum cell" with "histiocyte" and to point out that many malignant lymphomas are histiocytic rather than reticulum cell sarcomas. Early precursor cells are monoblasts in the bone marrow, which develop into monocytes in the blood and into mature tissue macrophages (another synonym for histiocytes) and into Langerhans cells.[13] In the quiescent state, skin histiocytes are difficult to differentiate from fibroblasts, although their nuclei may be slightly larger, and they have more cytoplasm. It is appropriate to say "fixed-tissue-type cell," if one cannot identify a cell as either a fibroblast or a histiocyte. When histiocytes contain phagocytized substances, we call them by specific names, such as "melanophages" or "lipophages." The latter are usually called foam cells. Cells containing no visible inclusions in H&E sections may be shown to harbor acid-fast bacilli by special stain. These and other microorganisms are discussed in the chapters on granulomatous inflammation. If histiocytes with large homogeneous cell bodies aggregate closely without intervening connective tissue fibers, they are described as "epithelioid cells," a term that can be used only in the plu-

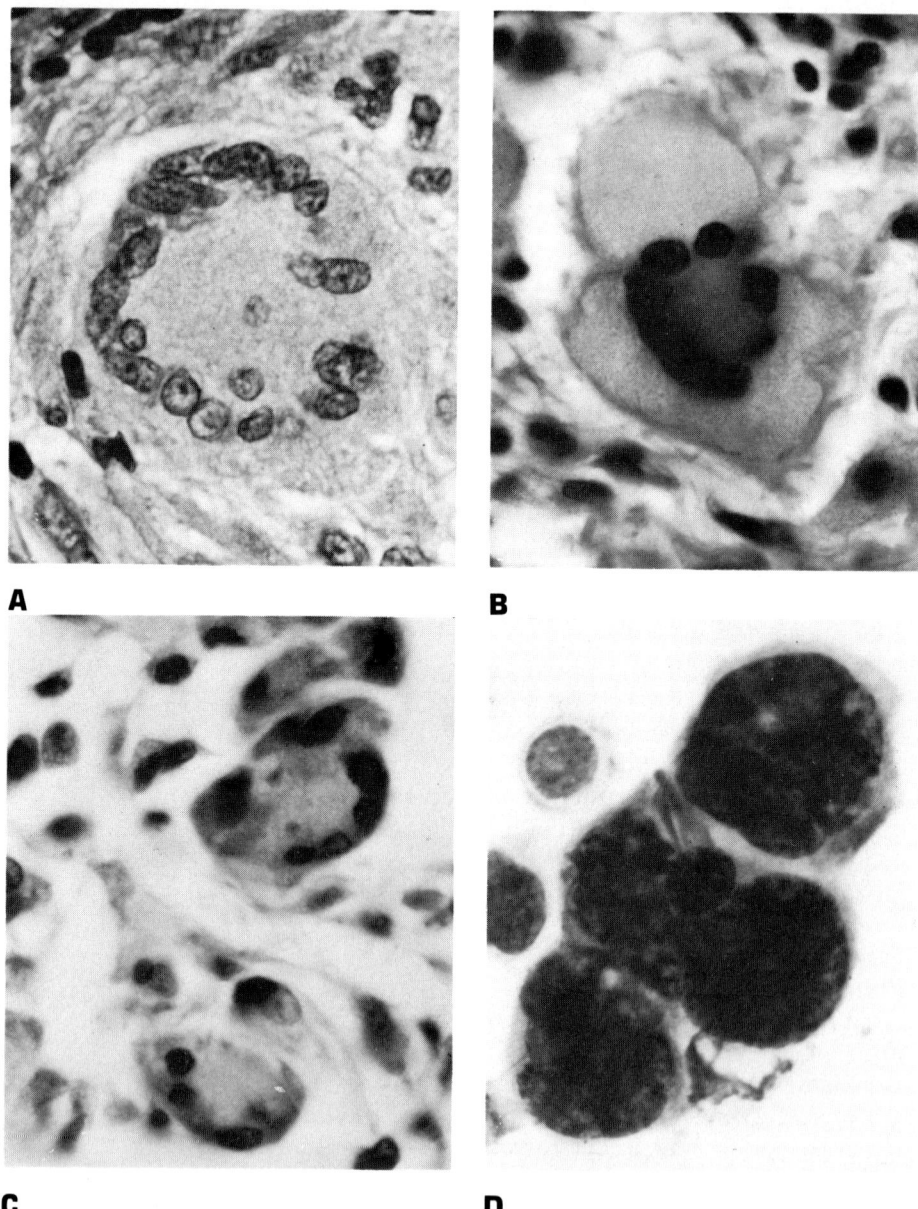

Figure 5–15.
Multinucleated giant cells. **A.** Langhans type. **B.** Touton type. **C.** Foreign body type. **D.** Epidermal cells in Tzanck smear of zoster. **A, B, C.** H&E. X800. **D.** Giemsa. X800.

ral form. Nodular aggregates of epithelioid cells often are called "tubercles" regardless of etiology.

Multinucleated large histiocytes, which probably originate through fusion of several cells more often than from repeated nuclear division, are known as "multinucleated giant cells," a term that should be used in its entirety because there also are mononuclear giant cells of different significance. Multinucleated giant cells may be of *Langhans type* (Fig. 5–15A, nuclei form a horseshoe), of *foreign body type* (Fig. 5–15C, nuclei in irregular clusters), or of *Touton type* (Fig. 5–15B, nuclei form a circle between central and peripheral portions of the cytoplasm, which usually is foamy). Although these variants are most commonly associated with specific disorders, the association is by no means absolute. Some multinucleated giant cells contain peculiar asteroid bodies (Fig. 5–16), which are not pathognomonic for any specific disease. Fragments of elastic fibers and a variety of crystalline and amorphous foreign substances may be enclosed in multinucleated histiocytes.

Tumor Cells

Various types of tumor cells may occur in the dermis singly or in groups, cords, nests, or masses. They should be described according to their characteristics. The term "sheets of tumor cells" should be avoided because it describes only the two-dimensional appearance of a mass of cells in a thin section.

Noncellular Components

In order to recognize and evaluate structural abnormalities of the noncellular components of the dermis, the student should carefully examine their normal appearance in the many biopsy specimens that exhibit no significant alterations. It is not easy to determine edema or sclerosis unless one is thoroughly familiar with normal variation and is aware also of the technical fallacies mentioned in Chapter 3. Any marked degree of edema, especially *myxedema* and *lymphedema*, will not only widen interfascicular spaces but split the collagen bundles into thinner ones or into fibers. The tissue will stain diffusely blue in O&G sections if myxedema is present. Alcian blue will reveal blue-staining fine fibrils.

In the evaluation of elastic fibers, their three-dimensional distribution in the skin must be kept in mind. Short pieces with sharp edges mean that a fiber has been cut transversely (Fig. 5–17) by the microtome knife. Fragmentation of elastic fibers is

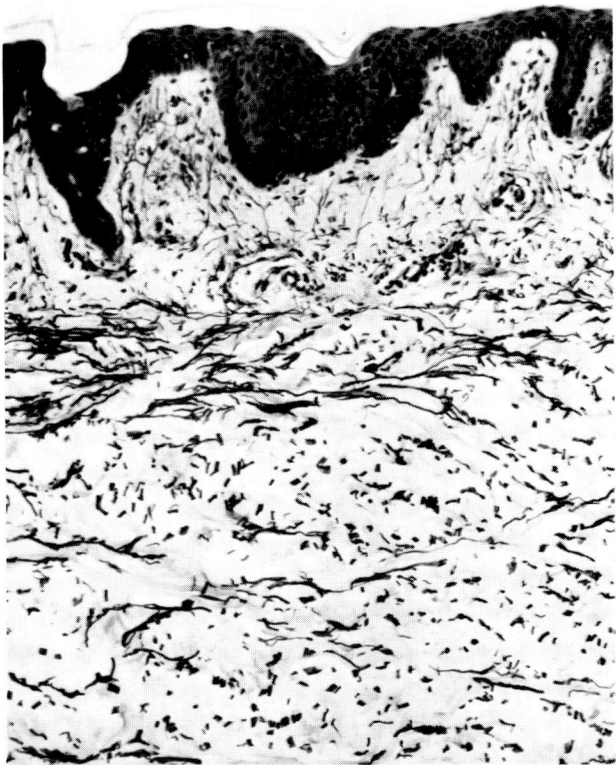

Figure 5–17.
Pseudofragmentation of elastic fibers. These are normal elastic fibers cut by microtome knife into fragments of different length owing to their three-dimensional orientation in tissue. Note the difference in thickness and arrangement between the fibers of pars reticularis and pars papillaris (see Fig. 2–18). O&G. X135.

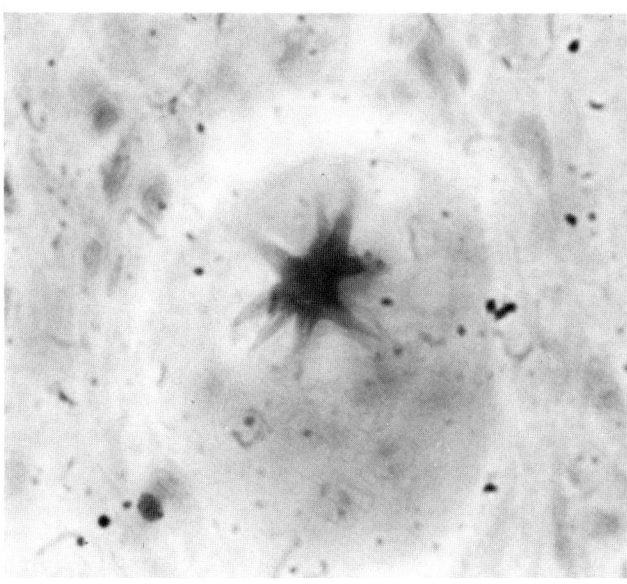

Figure 5–16.
Crystalline asteroid body in multinucleated giant cell (nuclei are out of focus). O&G. X1000.

very difficult to prove because they weave in and out of the thin section, and the rounded end of a truly fragmented fiber is a rare sight. Roughness, unevenness along their length, and curling are encountered occasionally and may be significant. The characteristic change of pseudoxanthoma elasticum is best compared to a heap of "raveled wool thread," as Zola Cooper used to say. Dissolution into short pieces and granules is found in rare cases of *elastolysis* (see Fig. 27–3). The most frequent pathologic change of elastic fibers is their complete absence in localized areas. Inasmuch as elastic fibers are not easily formed anew, their absence often indicates past inflammatory, and especially granulomatous, processes. If new fibers are formed, they usually remain much thinner and are apt to form parallel strands (e.g., striae, see Fig. 27–14) or an irregular meshwork (old lesions of lupus erythematosus). Elastic fibers give valuable diagnostic clues in many cases and should be examined routinely (see O&G stain in Chapter 3).

Pathologic changes of blood vessels and nerves are similar to those of other organs. Alterations of hair follicles, sweat glands, and subcutaneous fat tissue are discussed in their respective chapters. In cases of purpura, erythrocytes may be ingested and decomposed in epidermal cells. This phenomenon helps in the identification of purpuric lesions.[14]

REFERENCES

1. Mehregan AH: Transepithelial elimination. In Mali JWH (ed): Current Problems in Dermatology. Basel: S. Krager, 1970, Vol 3, pp 124–147
2. Woo TY, Rasmussen JE: Disorders of transepidermal elimination. Int J Dermatol 24:267, 1985
3. Anderson RL, Cassidy JM: Variations in physical dimensions and chemical composition of human stratum corneum. J Invest Dermatol 61:30, 1973
4. Alkiewicz J, Lebioda J, Rokita Z: Über Kolloidkeratose. Dermatol Monatsschr 158:329, 1972
5. Van Scott EJ, Ekel TM: Kinetics of hyperplasia in psoriasis. Arch Dermatol 88:373, 1963
6. Findlay GH, Whiting DA: Universal dyschromatosis. Br J Dermatol 85 (Suppl 7):66, 1971
7. Grubauer G, Romani N, Kofler H, et al: Apoptotic keratin bodies as autoantigen casing the production of IgM-anti-keratin intermediate filament autoantibodies. J Invest Dermatol 87:466, 1986
8. Wyllie AH, Kerr JFR, Currie AR: Cell death: The significance of apoptosis. Int Rev Cytol 68:251, 1980
9. Burg G, Braun-Falco O: Cutaneous non-Hodgkin lymphoma: Re-evaluation of histology using enzyme cytochemical and immunologic studies. Int J Dermatol 17:496, 1978
10. Souteyraud P, Thivolet J, Alaria A, et al: Étude immunocytologique des lymphomas cutanés malins. Essai de classification. Dermatologica 157:269, 1978
11. Jaworsky C, Murphy GF: Special techniques in dermatology. Arch Dermatol 125:963, 1989
12. Murphy GF, Bhan AK, Harrist TJ, Mihm MC Jr: In situ identification of T6-positive cells in normal human dermis by immunoelectron microscopy. Br J Dermatol 108:423–431, 1983
13. Lesser A: The mononuclear phagocytic system: a review. Human Pathol 14:108, 1983
14. Boiron G, Surleve-Bageille JE, Tamisier JM, Guiliet G: Phagocytosis of erythrocytes by keratinocytes in human and animal epidermis. Dermatologica 115:158–167, 1982

6

SYSTEMATICS OF HISTOPATHOLOGIC INTERPRETATION

In the preceding chapter, a systematic course of description of a skin section was outlined. In order to make a diagnosis from this morphologic analysis, one should also follow a systematic course of mental analysis. Some diagnoses are so obvious that a short glance through the low-power lens is sufficient. However, one should never be satisfied with a snap diagnosis because closer examination may show features that modify or reverse the first impression. It is human nature that a first opinion gives a bias to the mind, and the beginner is apt to search out features favorable to his opinion and to overlook unfavorable ones. It is therefore highly recommended, after arriving at a diagnosis, that two searching questions be asked: What else could it be? What speaks against my diagnosis? One should act as the devil's advocate to one's own interpretation. Moreover, the dermatopathologist has no right to make a diagnosis of nonspecific dermatitis or inflammation. Every biopsy specimen is a sample of some specific process, but the visible changes may be noncharacteristic and may not permit a diagnosis. Similarly, if one is dealing with granulomatous inflammation, the expression *of undetermined etiology* should be used instead of "nonspecific."

TECHNIQUE

For an ideal interpretation, there are two prerequisites. The section should include all of the skin and some of the subcutaneous tissue, and it should be large enough to show all spaced skin structures, such as hair complexes and sweat glands. Even then, one should examine multiple, and preferably serial, sections in order to be sure that the features of the first section are characteristic of the entire biopsy specimen. With the commonly encountered 4-mm punch, examination of at least 30 serial sections is highly desirable. Only a few of these may include a follicle or a sweat gland or may show the most characteristic alterations, especially the center of the clinical lesion. A 2-mm punch (never an ideal specimen) should be sectioned practically from end to end, and of a 6-mm punch or larger excisional biopsy enough sections should be prepared to insure a representative sample. This can be made easier by dividing the specimen as outlined in Chapter 3.

One should always look at the slide first with the naked eye to see how large the sections are and whether there are perhaps sections of several tissue fragments. The next step must be scanning of the sections under low power. Beginners should be instructed that they may go to high power if their attention is attracted by a detail that they cannot identify with the scanning lens but that they should quickly revert to the low magnification until they have scanned all the sections on the slide, preferably all the slides available, and certainly all the stains.

CATEGORIZING

Once we have satisfied ourselves that we have seen everything the clinician was good enough to provide, it is best to decide first into which of the major categories of disease the lesion belongs, then to subcategorize until a specific diagnosis is decided upon.

Thus, we try to decide first whether the section represents a tumor or an inflammatory process or neither and whether the epidermis or the dermis is involved mainly. Sometimes, this decision cannot be made immediately, or it may have to be reversed later, but in most cases it is fairly easy and permits one to concentrate on only one major portion of the pathologic field. Tumors and certain metabolic or degenerative diseases then are categorized according to rules given in later chapters.

Inflammatory lesions often can be assigned without too much difficulty to one of two subgroups. Involvement of only the papillary part of the dermis speaks for nongranulomatous processes, whereas granulomatous inflammation practically always involves also the pars reticularis. Exceptions, such as lupus erythematosus, a nongranulomatous disease involving most of the dermis, and lichen nitidus, a granuloma involving papillae only, are recognized just because of their exceptional features. It is always much easier to ascertain the seat of an inflammatory or neoplastic process by looking for the differential characteristics of superficial and deep elastic fibers in O&G sections. This is one of the most valuable features of the routine use of this stain. Specific instances will be found in several chapters.

A special point for consideration is the involvement of hair follicles in inflammatory disease. Not infrequently, examination of the first section and even of several sections presents a puzzling picture until a subsequent section reveals a follicle in the center of the lesion. The same is true, though much less frequently, for sweat glands. Involvement of larger blood vessels, on the other hand, is sometimes overlooked because their structure may be so altered as to be almost unrecognizable (see Fig. 16–4A) in H&E sections. Here, O&G stain (see Fig. 16–4B) not only is apt to show remnants of the elastic coat but also usually permits identification of vein or artery by the specific arrangement of the fibers.

Lesions that are neither inflammatory nor neoplastic but consist of specific alteration of connective tissue fibers or deposits of unusual substances, such as mucin and amyloid, require a high level of suspicion in many cases. Here again, except in the case of calcification, the O&G stain usually is more revealing than the H&E, but special procedures may be called for.

Anybody who teaches students and residents will have the experience that the diagnosis of epithelial tumors is easiest, with that of mesodermal tumors and specific granulomatous lesions next in line. The greatest difficulty is encountered in the field of simple inflammation, and this, unfortunately, includes the greatest number of all skin lesions encountered in clinical practice and roughly one third of the specimens submitted for histologic diagnosis. Even the expert often is stumped and frequently can do no better than to favor one diagnosis over one or several others. If it seems impossible to arrrive at a positive diagnosis, it is often helpful to use the negative approach and to rule out all the dermatoses one feels could not be represented by the specimen. By doing so one can often narrow the diagnosis down to a reasonable choice or even to a single possibility. In this connection, it must be stressed that in the interpretation of tissue reactions, and even of tumors, we are laying down rules, not laws. In the chapters that follow, the words "usually," "often," and "rarely" are found only too frequently, and we assure the reader that we eliminated them in many places in order not to appear too indecisive. The beginner may be led astray by putting too much stress on a conspicuous but insignificant feature; the pundit may know so many exceptions that his willingness to make a definite diagnosis sags. It is the task of the successful diagnostician to thread his way between the two extremes.

CLINICOPATHOLOGIC COORDINATION

Because a simple report of subacute or chronic dermatitis is of no value to the practicing skin specialist, the dermatopathologist must be familiar with clinical dermatology as well, and he must insist on the clinician's cooperation in submitting sufficient information and a list of differential diagnoses. Practitioners who believe that the pathologist should arrive at a diagnosis objectively and not be influenced by clinical data or opinions should realize that the pathologist cannot give the best service to either physician or patient unless he knows the entire story. We gently remind the clinician that we are just as happy to disprove his diagnosis as to support it.

Clinical information should include the physi-

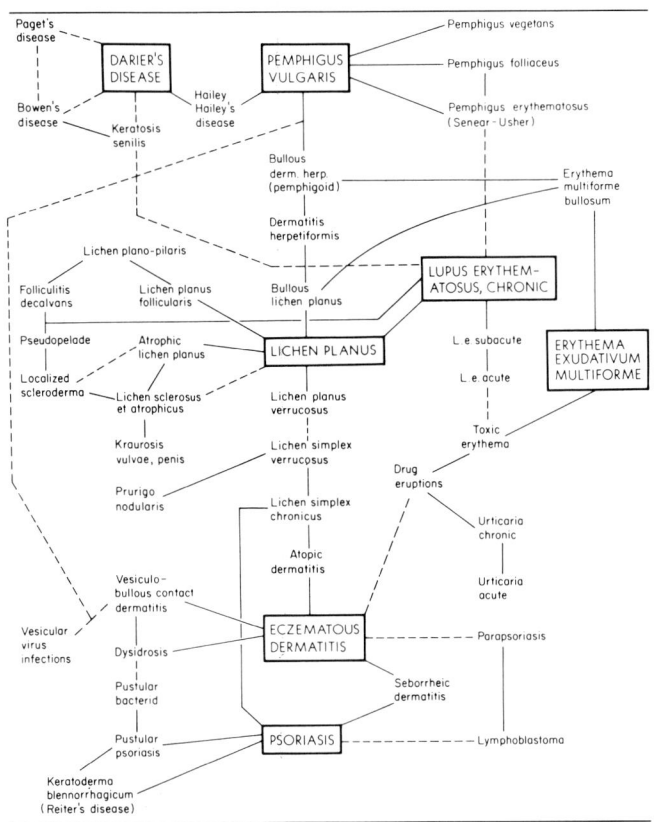

Figure 6–1.
Diagrammatic representation of histomorphologic similarities of tissue reaction and resulting differential diagnostic considerations in inflammatory skin diseases.

cian's and the patient's name for identification. Sex and age are essential in judging the general characteristics of the skin specimen and sometimes are helpful in diagnostic deliberations. The question of color or shade of skin is not discriminatory when a cutaneous biopsy must be examined. Details, such as blond, brunet, olive, Oriental, light or dark black, and Native American, are much more helpful than white, Caucasian, colored, or black in judging whether the amount of pigment in the section is normal or abnormal for the individual. The exact anatomic site of biopsy is highly important in view of the great topical differences encountered in the skin. A simple sketch is helpful.

A concise clinical history is of inestimable value for the pathologist in throwing out completely inapplicable diagnoses or explaining unusual features. The same is even more true of a clinical description of the eruption. Finally, there should be a clinical diagnosis or a list of differential diagnoses. By comparing the clinician's list with his own, the pathologist may be able to rule out certain diagnoses, to favor others, and perhaps to come up with a single one that fits clinical and pathologic data alike. Cooperation between clinician and pathologist is more important in the field of skin disease than in almost any other field if the patient is to derive the greatest benefit from the biopsy.

Figure 6–1 should help students in their differential diagnostic deliberations. It lists the most common types of tissue reaction as centers of gravity or foci of crystallization, for example, eczematous dermatitis and psoriasis. Other diagnoses are arranged in between according to the degree of morphologic similarity in tissue sections. Nosologic relations are not necessarily implied. Solid lines indicate common differential problems, dashed lines uncommon ones. Although the diagram may seem confusing at first, we hope its study will help the student to be aware of diagnostic possibilities. One example is the morphologic row from eczematous dermatitis to lichen planus. Chronic dermatitis with lichenification resembles lichen simplex chronicus, and this, in turn, resembles hypertrophic lichen planus.

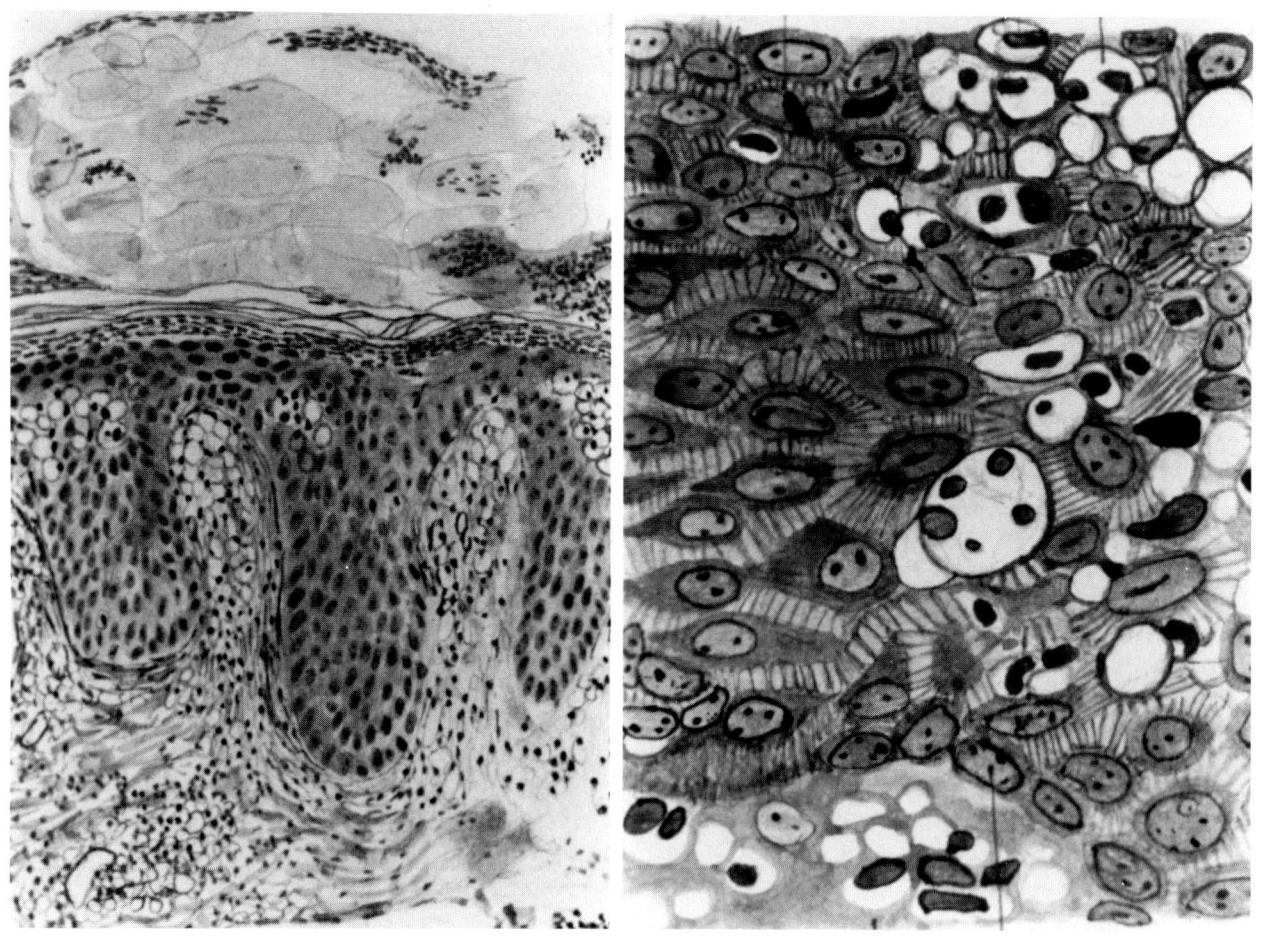

Seborrheic dermatitis (*left*). Spongiosis and Exocytosis (*right*).

SECTION 11

SUPERFICIAL INFLAMMATORY PROCESSES

The terms *superficial* and *inflammatory* are used here in a very wide sense. We include lesions that histologically have their seat predominantly in the pars papillaris of the dermis, with or without involvement of the epidermis, and that are not neoplastic or obviously granulomatous.[1] Inasmuch as the word *dermatitis* means inflammation of skin, we do not use it as a specific diagnostic term but always add a modifying adjective, such as *eczematous* or *seborrheic*. We exclude from this section lesions in which the pathognomonic disturbance is alteration of the noncellular components of the dermis or deposition of metabolic products, such as amyloid or calcium.

We deal, therefore, with the most common dermatoses, such as eczematous dermatitis, psoriasis, lichen planus, drug eruptions, and the so-called papulosquamous lesions. Many of these are caused by known external or internal agents to which the skin reacts. In others, the cause is unknown, but we can conceive of them as reactions to injury, as will be pointed out in the individual discussions. Reaction to injury is the most basic definition of inflammation and gives us the courage to include all these dermatoses under one heading. Reaction to injury is also the common denominator under which we can try to analyze the colorful variety of lesions that we encounter in this group. The concept of reaction to injury explains why the skin may respond to a great variety of agents with identical or similar alterations. Great as its repertoire is, the skin has a limited number of expressions. Erythema exudativum multiforme may be the response to a dozen or more different agents and contact-type eczematous dermatitis to thousands of sensitizing externa.

The histopathologist, therefore, deals with the expression of tissue reaction, and in each individual biopsy section we deal with one fixed moment of the reaction, one that the clinician chooses more or less judiciously from several or many lesions in various stages of development. Our ability to diagnose a disease from the tissue reaction depends on interpretation and is influenced by our knowledge of clinical dermatology, our concept of the disease in question, and our individual experience with the limits of variability of the disease.[2] The pathologist and the submitting clinician must be aware that the report rendered includes interpretation. In our laboratory we sum up our findings, not under the heading of "microscopic diagnosis" but as "conclusions," and we are not ashamed if occasionally we have to revise our conclusions on the basis of follow-up information.

The following chapters, then, will bear such headings as "eczematous reactions," "psoriasiform reactions," and "Lichenoid reaction" rather than the names of individual diseases.

REFERENCES

1. Ackerman AB: Histologic Diagnosis of Inflammatory Skin Diseases. Philadelphia: Lea & Febiger, 1987
2. McKee PH: Pathology of the Skin with Clinical Correlations. Philadelphia: JB Lippincott, 1989

7

ECZEMATOUS TISSUE REACTIONS

Eczematous tissue reactions include lesions encountered in all types of contact dermatitis, in atopic dermatitis, lichen simplex chronicus, and dyshidrosiform dermatitis. Exfoliative dermatitis and prurigo are considered. Seborrheic dermatitis, asteatotic dermatitis, and the related nummular eczema are discussed in the differential diagnosis of psoriasiform tissue reactions (Chapter 8). Stasis dermatitis is considered under the heading of vasculitides (Chapter 15) and photosensitivity reactions in the differential diagnosis of lupus erythematosus (Chapter 14). Eczematous tissue reactions are also encountered in some of the papulosquamous diseases discussed in Chapter 13.

"Eczema" is an old word that has been used in the clinic with so many meanings that it has become practically meaningless.[1] *Eczematous tissue reaction*, however, has a well-defined connotation: It is the epidermal reaction to injurious agents encountered typically in contact dermatitis due to sensitization. The dermal reaction is secondary and rather noncharacteristic, except that it involves the blood vessels of the superficial plexus, as do many other dermatoses. The typical epidermal change involves four principal features: intercellular edema (spongiosis), acanthosis, parakeratosis, and exocytosis, all present in a focal, spotty distribution. From these changes are derived others, such as vesiculation and lichenification.[2] Synonyms for eczematous dermatitis are spongiotic dermatitis and spongiotic dermoepidermitis.[3]

CONTACT DERMATITIS

Primary Irritant Type

Contact dermatitis is commonly divided into *primary irritant* or *sensitization dermatitis*.[4] When a primary irritant is not strong enough to cause necrosis, it is apt to produce more damage to superficial living cells than to deeper structures. The reaction to the injury will consist of exudation of fluid and polymorphonuclear cells from the blood capillaries into the epidermis, which becomes edematous and may show cell degeneration. Figure 7–1 illustrates the site of a patch test 48 hours after application of a primary irritant. Horny and granular layers show no or minor morphologic alterations because cell bodies and intercellular connections are quite rigid in these strata. The upper strata of prickle cells are separated by spongiotic edema (edema that widens intercellular spaces and lengthens intercellular bridges so that they resemble the fibers crossing the spaces in a sponge) and inflammatory cells, with the production of an intraepidermal vesicle resulting from breakage of intercellular bridges.

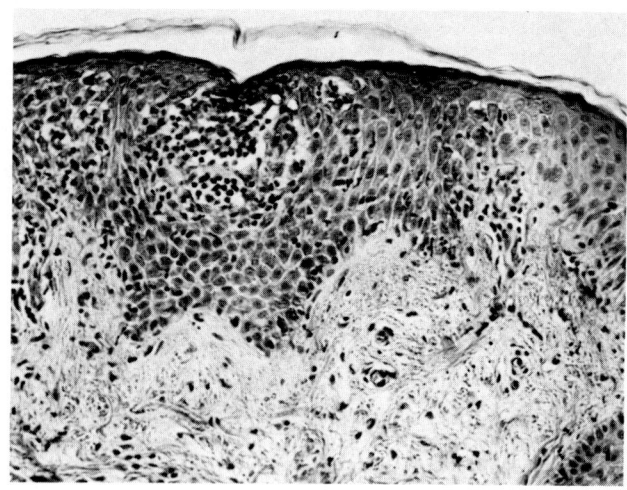

Figure 7-1.
Primary irritant type of contact dermatitis. Patch test with sodium lauryl sulfate after 48 hours. H&E. X135.

There is a degree of acanthosis, suggesting that mitotic proliferation has started to replace the damaged upper layers.

There are apparently no significant differences between the induced allergic contact dermatitis and the primary irritant contact dermatitis in sequences of cellular events or responding cell types. Both show apposition of Langerhans cells to lymphocytes in the epidermis and a predominantly T-lymphocyte infiltrate.[5]

Epidermal Regeneration

In primary irritant dermatitis, the outpouring of fluid and scavenger cells is due to the presence of chemically damaged epithelium, but the basic repair mechanism of the epidermis is similar when we remove the horny layer by tape stripping,[6] thus exposing the prickle cells to dehydration. In this case, edema and exudate remain minimal, and the regenerative sequence is more clearly seen (Fig. 7–2). One-half hour after stripping, the uppermost cells look parakeratotic as they begin to dry out. Most of the prickle cells later are involved in this process, whereas the basal cells become very large.

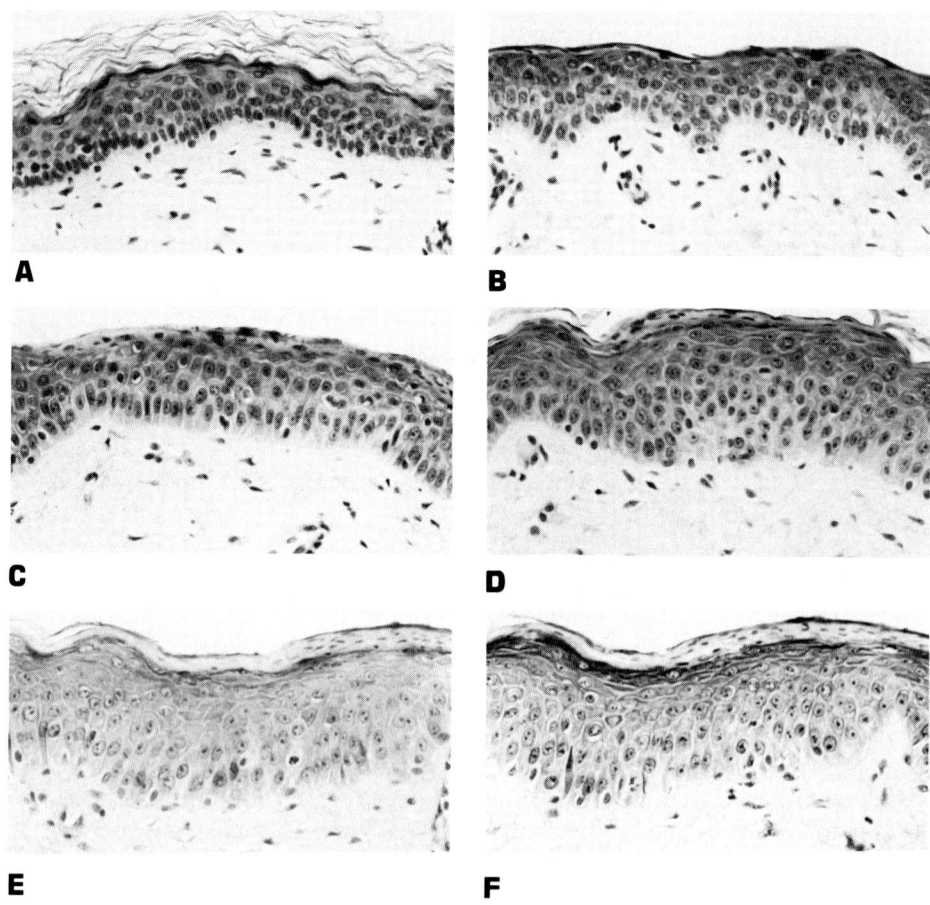

Figure 7-2.
Epidermal response to tape stripping. **A.** Control. **B.** After 12 hours. **C.** After 24 hours. **D.** After 36 hours. **E** and **F.** After 48 hours. H&E. X205.

Their edematous appearance is due to accumulation of glycogen. After 36 to 48 hours, a great burst of mitotic activity develops in the basal layer and replaces, within a few days, the cells lost through stripping and dehydration. A new and usually hyperplastic granular layer is formed, followed by maturation of a new horny layer. Most of the original epidermis is exfoliated as a parakeratotic scale.

Pictures of this type are occasionally encountered in biopsy sections and can be interpreted as accelerated epidermal regeneration if one is familiar with them. In contact dermatitis and other inflammations, the picture is variously modified, but the basic process persists. Old and damaged material is eliminated toward the surface and is replaced, often in excess, by mitotic division of germinal cells at the base of the epidermis. Awareness of this process makes it possible to interpret fixed sections in terms of temporal sequence.

Sensitization Dermatitis

If contact dermatitis is due to a substance to which the skin was sensitized previously, the picture (Fig. 7–3) may be slightly different from the primary irritant type. The epidermal Langerhans cells recognize and bind contact allergens and carry them to lymph nodes.[7-9] On subsequent exposure to the allergen, sensitized lymphocytes enter the epidermis from below and cause the eczematous reaction. Therefore, edema and cell damage are found early in the lower prickle cell layers. The upper layers are involved by extension and because the damaged cells are carried quickly toward the outside. Simultaneously, the epidermis will react with excessive regeneration, resulting in acanthosis and accentuation of rete ridges. Unless the damaging contact is a fleeting one, new cells will sustain damage, and the process of edema spongiosis, and vesiculation will be found in different stages of development and varying degrees of severity throughout the epidermis.

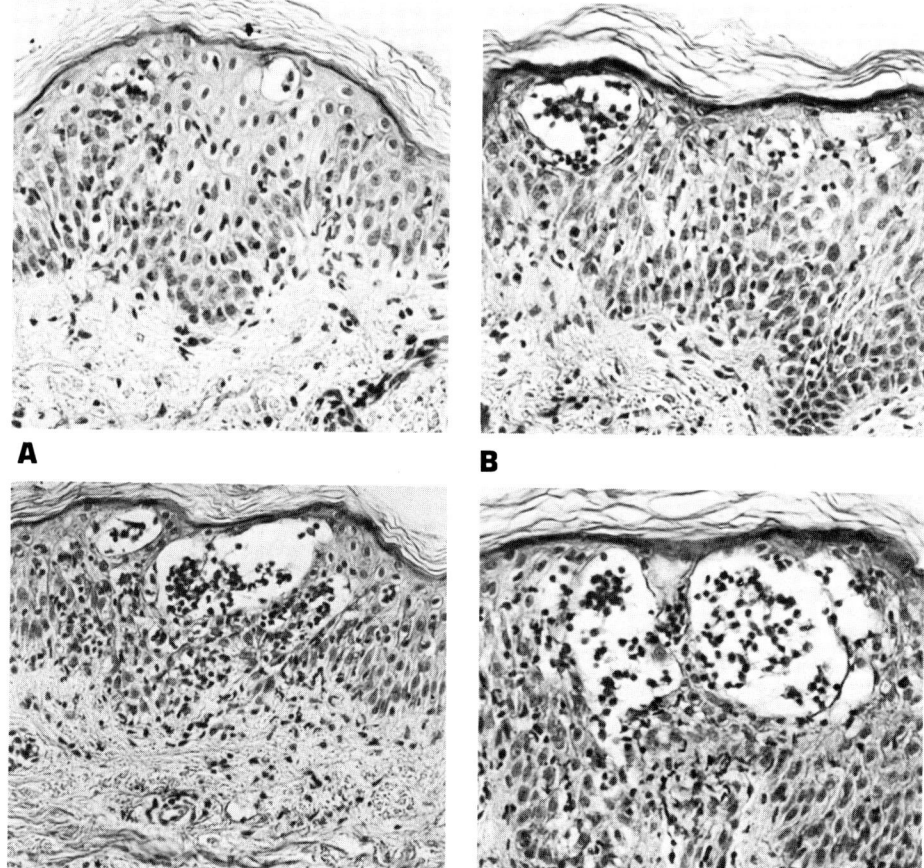

Figure 7–3.
Sensitization-type contact dermatitis. Figures represent several fields from a 48-hour patch test reaction to 5 percent nickel sulfate solution. Compare with Figure 7–8, showing dermal sensitivity reaction to nickel sulfate in another patient. Some vesicles contain mainly degenerating epithelial cells. Such pictures should not be confused with Pautrier abscesses of mycosis fungoides (see Fig. 45–5B). H&E. X128.

The cardinal epidermal features of sensitization-type contact dermatitis are (1) edema, which is mainly intercellular and may lead to spongiosis and vesiculation; (2) acanthosis; (3) parakeratosis; and (4) exocytosis, including T lymphocytes and polymorphonuclear cells (Fig. 7–4). A highly important fifth feature is the focal, spotty character of all these changes, in horizontal and vertical direction. As one scans a section from end to end, one encounters relatively normal portions interspersed with areas of spongiosis and intraepidermal vesiculation. Different ages of such changes can be inferred from their vertical distribution. Dermal changes are edema and cellular infiltrate in papillae and subpapillary layer. T lymphocytes predominate; eosinophils may be few or fairly numerous; neutrophils are absent except inside dilated blood vessels. Closer examination reveals degranulation of mast cells and basophils as an essential early change.[10]

Acute Contact Dermatitis

Figure 7–5 illustrates a case of acute contact dermatitis caused by a drawing ointment applied to the skin near the knee 4 days previously. The onset of dermatitis within 24 hours and the character of the response are evidence of previous sensitization. The focal distribution of the cardinal features is well shown. It is interesting to note that the original thick horny layer of the knee is present intact above the inflamed epidermis. This fact provides objective evidence that the dermatitis can be only a few days old. The malpighian layer is about 10 times thicker than normal, not only through edema and vesiculation but through an actual increase in the number of cells. It is truly acanthotic, and mitotic division of basal cells could be demonstrated in the sections but is not illustrated in the photomicrograph. The vesicles in the higher layers are smaller and contain dense basophilic material. This indicates that they are beginning to dry up and are older and have moved up from deeper layers. In contrast to the impressive epidermal changes, those of the dermis are mild and noncharacteristic.

The combination of the four cardinal features varies with duration and severity of the dermatitis. The fifth feature, spottiness, is always evident. In a mild case of acute dermatitis, there may be vesiculation and relatively little acanthosis, as illustrated in Figure 7–6. In more prolonged cases, acanthosis becomes more prominent, but the epidermis may not be as thick because there is less edema. After the first few days, any trace of the normal stratum corneum is lost, and the surface is covered by parakeratotic scale–crust. The granular layer disappears quickly but may return just as quickly in subsiding areas. This feature adds to the impression of spottiness. Because focal conditions may change repeatedly, parakeratosis may be underlaid by a new granular layer, and orthokeratotic lamellae may alternate with parakeratotic material.

Interesting modifications are introduced when the dermatitis is due to spicules that have mechanically irritating as well as sensitizing properties.

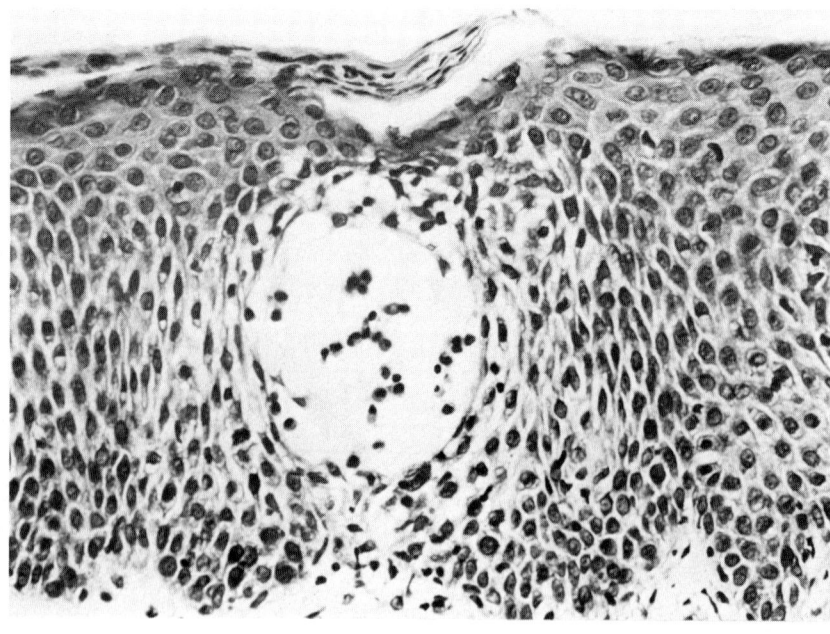

Figure 7–4.
Acute sensitization-type contact dermatitis shows spongiotic vesicle and early parakeratosis. H&E. X250.

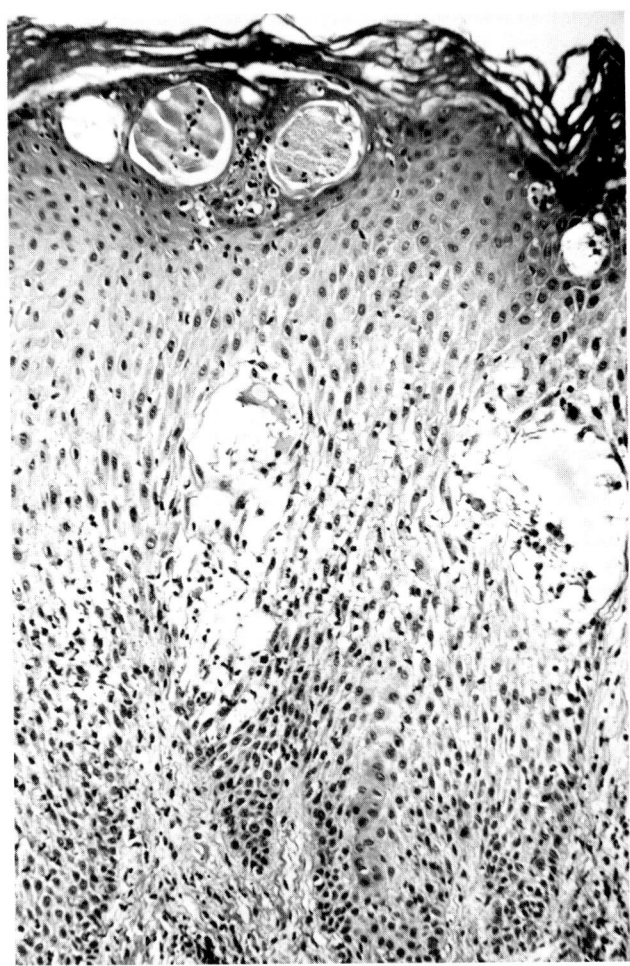

Figure 7–5.
Acute sensitization-type contact dermatitis 4 days after application of a drawing ointment to skin near knee. H&E. X135.

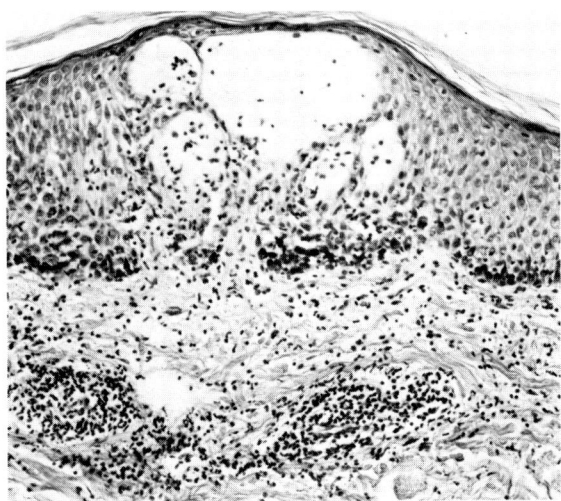

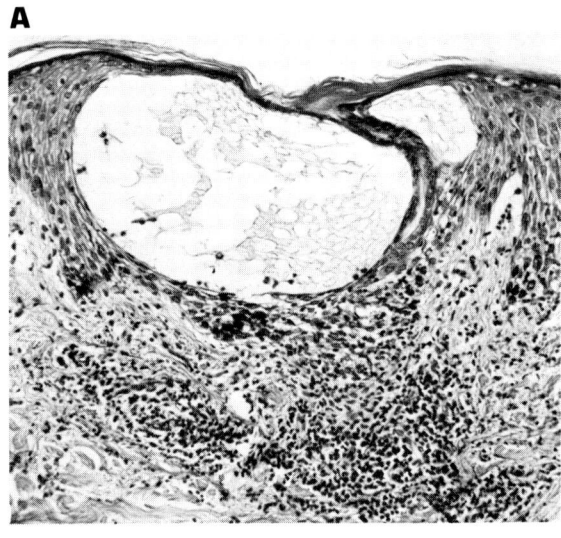

Figure 7–6.
A. Acute vesicular contact dermatitis without much acanthosis. **B.** Note sweat duct winding its way between vesicles. H&E. X185.

Mineral wool,[11] fiberglass, possibly coated with epoxy resins,[12] and the hairs of caterpillars containing a sensitizing substance[13] are examples. Both the epidermal damage and the dermal response may be modified.

Chronic Contact Dermatitis

In chronic contact dermatitis (Fig. 7–7), vesiculation often is completely absent, and evidence of intercellular edema may be scant. Even parakeratosis and loss of granular layer may be minor. Acanthosis is the outstanding feature. The picture then is that of lichenification and merges with that of lichenification originating from other causes. Minor differences are discussed under atopic dermatitis, lichen simplex circumscriptus, and psoriasis.

Histologic examination makes it evident that the clinical thickening and stiffness of the skin in lichenification are due mainly to acanthosis and hyperkeratosis. The characteristic coarse folds are due to the uneven size and shape of rete ridges and a degree of papillomatosis. Inflammatory infiltrate may be minor and restricted to the periphery of small subpapillary vessels. The latter usually show no appreciable thickening of their walls, a feature often found in lichenified atopic dermatitis and circumscribed lichen simplex.

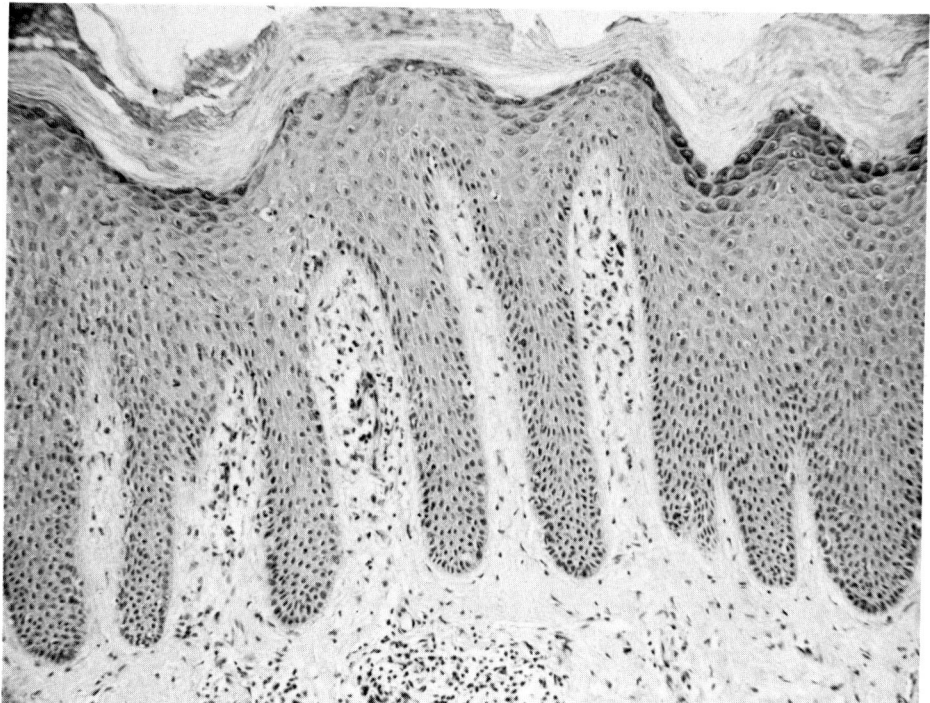

Figure 7–7.
Lichenified chronic contact dermatitis. Rete ridges even and long as in psoriasis, but suprapapillary thick and without Munro abscesses. Granular layer almost intact, partly thickened. Only minor indication of intercellular edema in left half of picture. Some parakeratosis indicates earlier loss of granular layer. No excess mitotic activity. Mild inflammatory infiltrate in papilla and subpapillary layer. No exocytosis. H&E. X135.

The histologic features of contact dermatitis are best studied in biopsy specimens obtained from clear-cut cases. In everyday diagnostic work, they may not be so convincing because the picture may have been modified by topical applications, by scratching, or by systemic steroid treatment. Combination of atopic dermatitis with acute medicamentous contact dermatitis, or chronic contact dermatitis lichenified by scratching may puzzle the most astute observer. An outstanding example is diaper dermatitis.[14]

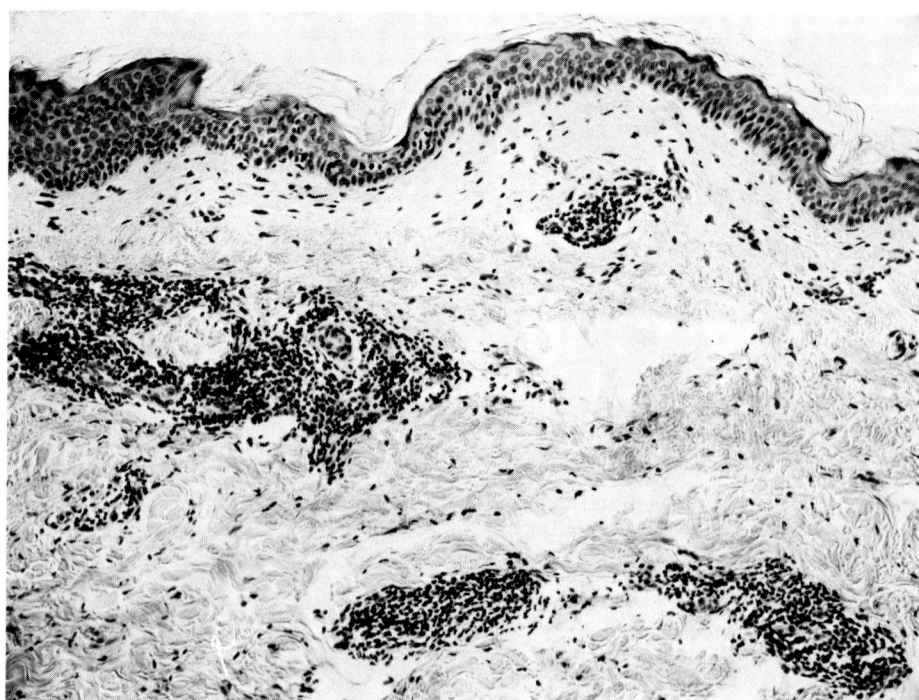

Figure 7–8.
Dermal contact sensitivity reaction. Patch test with nickel sulfate after 48 hours in a nickel-sensitive patient. Compare with Figure 7–3, which represents epidermal response to nickel sulfate in another patient. H&E. X135.

One should remember that histologic pictures closely resembling the eczematous tissue reaction can be caused by infectious organisms, ranging from diphtheria bacilli[15] to dermatophytes (Chapter 13), if they remain in the surface layers of the skin. Unrelated papulosquamous eruptions, especially pityriasis rosea, and seborrheic dermatitis also may mimic eczematous dermatitis.

Dermal Contact Sensitivity Reaction

The situation becomes even more complicated by the introduction of the concept of the dermal type of contact sensitivity reaction. These cases[16,17] are often caused by nickel or neomycin but possibly by many other substances. The clinical picture may imitate atopic dermatitis. Histologically (Fig. 7–8), epidermal changes may be minor[18] and, if present, are restricted to acanthosis with some parakeratosis. Infiltrate in the dermis is prominent, usually perivascular, often nodular, and frequently not restricted to the pars papillaris. There usually is a mixture of lymphocytes, plasma cells, and eosinophils. Fixed-tissue-type cells or larger mononuclear round cells may contribute aspects of a granulomatous, or even lymphomatous, infiltrate. This impression is enhanced by immigration of mononuclear cells into the epidermis. The dermal type of contact sensitivity reaction can be a stumbling block to clinician and pathologist alike. It should always be considered in the differential diagnosis of chronic itching dermatoses, in which the suspicion of mycosis fungoides arises.[19] Chronic photosensitivity dermatitis also may produce the picture of dermal contact sensitivity reaction (see actinic reticuloid in Chapter 45).

DYSHIDROSIFORM DERMATITIS

The term "dyshidrosiform" is chosen because there is no histologic involvement of sweat ducts in the lesions usually diagnosed as dyshidrosis or pompholyx by clinicians. Pathologic changes of sweat ducts are readily demonstrable in miliaria (Chapter 20), but the sweat ducts thread their way between the vesicles of dyshidrosiform dermatitis. This type of tissue reaction (Fig. 7–9) is simple vesicular eczematous dermatitis modified by the terrain of thick epidermis covered by a thick, horny layer.[20] Spongiotic vesicles forming in the normally bulky rete of palms and soles have room to grow and are prevented from rupturing by the physiologic hyperkeratosis of these regions. Differential diagnosis of other vesiculopustular lesions of palms and soles is discussed in Chapter 8 (see Fig. 8–13).

ATOPIC DERMATITIS

Pure atopic dermatitis (Fig. 7–10) (the effects of scratching are practically always evident), either in infants or older children, rarely presents vesicles or even much intercellular edema but has acanthosis, parakeratosis, and some exocytosis. Acanthosis usually is quite even, the epidermal cells are relatively small, and mitoses are significantly increased[21] and

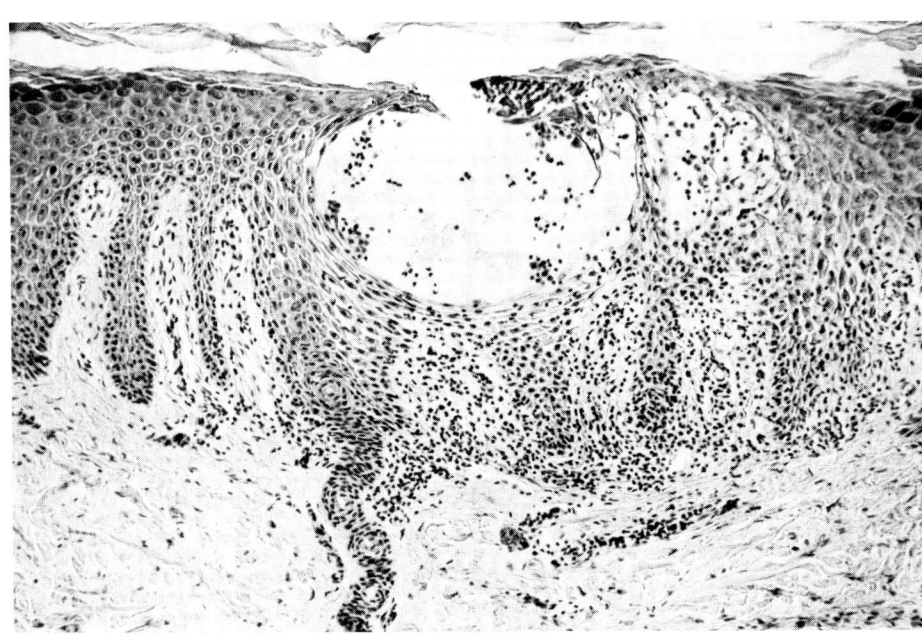

Figure 7–9.
Dyshidrosiform type of eczematous dermatitis. This specimen was obtained from acral skin with relatively thin horny layer. Note sweat duct not involved in vesiculation. H&E. X135.

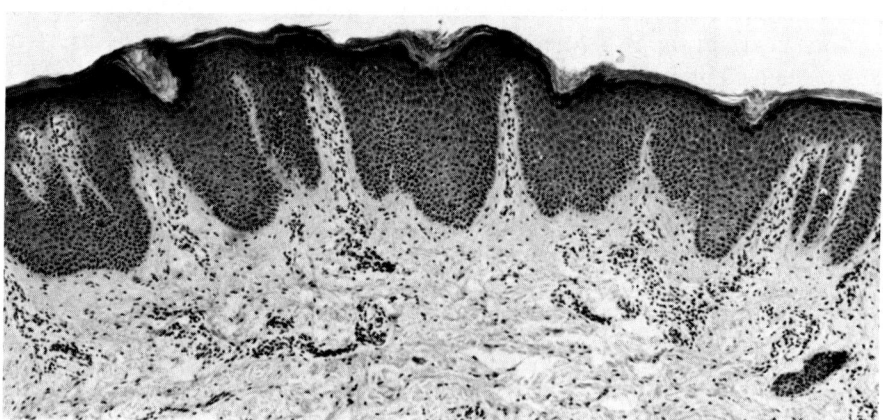

Figure 7–10.
Atopic dermatitis (flexural eczema) in a child, which did not present clinical evidence of excoriation or irritation. Note relatively small size of prickle cells in the absence of intracellular and intercellular edema. Uneven ridges and thick suprapapillary plate differ from psoriasis. H&E. X90. (From Pinkus. Ann Allergy 12:671, 1954.)

are present in suprabasal layers. In older people the picture resembles that of chronic lichenification. One outstanding feature of atopic skin is a peculiar prominence of the walls of small subpapillary vessels.[22] It is due to endothelial thickening and apposition of a few peripheral cells—nothing very definite but recognizable if one pays attention to it. It is an expression of the factor of vascular reaction. The quantity of inflammatory infiltrate varies according to the activity of the process at the time of biopsy. The cells are lymphocytes and histiocytes; eosinophils may or may not be present, and mast cells are increased in number.

Atopic dermatitis, because of its chronicity, often leads to a loss of superficial elastic fibers and later to some increase of collagen and to fibrosis. An elastic fiber stain, therefore, is helpful. The rather characteristic histologic features of excoriation (see Fig. 3–2) are frequently present in all types of eczematous tissue reaction, but especially in atopic dermatitis and lichenification; one must learn to recognize them.

Individuals with chronic atopic dermatitis often have ichthyotic dry skin especially in winter season. Dry skin areas may show low grade eczematous changes, abnormal keratinization resembling ichthyosis vulgaris and atrophy of sebaceous glands.[23,24]

INFANTILE ACROPUSTULOSIS

Recurrent crops of 1–2 mm pruritic vesiculopustules occur over the palms and soles most often male

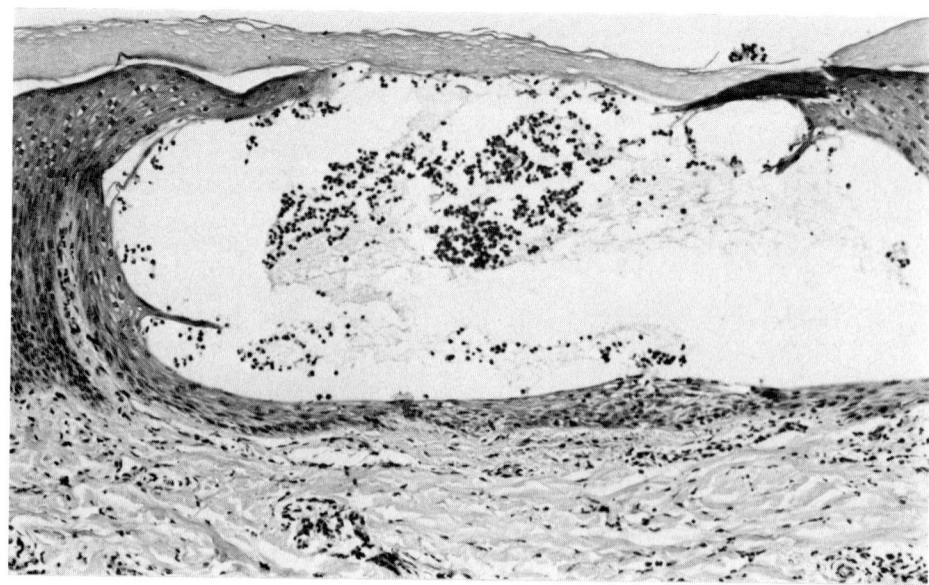

Figure 7–11.
Infantile acropustulosis. An intraepidermal pustule containing polymorphonuclear cells. H&E. X125.

Asian and black infants between 2 and 18 months of age. Disease disappears within 2 or 3 years (Fig. 7–11). Histologically superficial intraepidermal pustules are presently filled with neutrophils or eosinophils.[24–29]

ERYTHEMA TOXICUM NEONATORUM

Erythema toxicum neonatorum occurs within the first 2 weeks of life and lasts only 2 or 3 days. Yellow papules, 1 to 3 mm in size, and pustules are seen over an erythematous base (Fig. 7–12). Histologically, subcorneal pustules are located at the orifices of the pilosebaceous structures and are filled with eosinophils.[30]

ACROKERATOSIS PARANEOPLASTICA

Scaly dermatitic lesions involving the extremities, ears, and bridge of the nose, occurring in association with malignancies of the laryngopharyngeal region, are known as acrokeratosis paraneoplastica or Bazex syndrome.[31,32] Histologically, the cutaneous lesions show irregular epidermal acanthosis with spotty spongiotic edema and parakeratosis. The superficial dermal capillary blood vessels may show fibrinoid deposition and are surrounded with lymphocytes and eosinophils.[33]

EXFOLIATIVE DERMATITIS

Exfoliative dermatitis is a clinical term applied to generalized involvement of the skin with erythema,

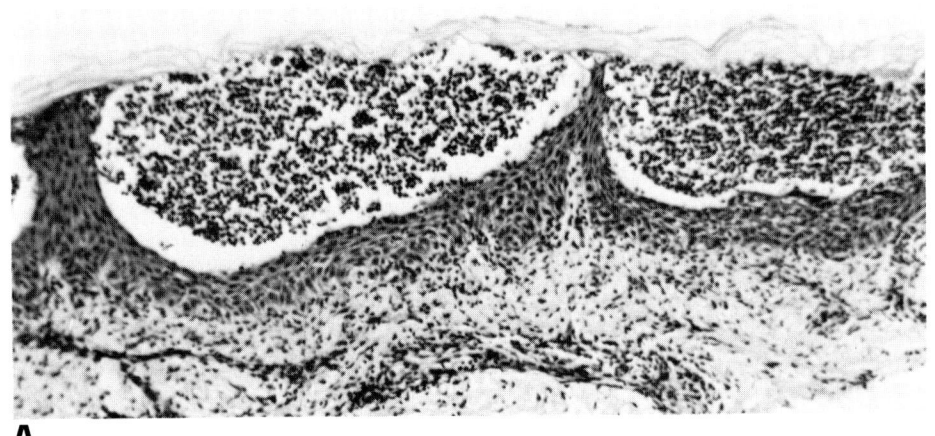

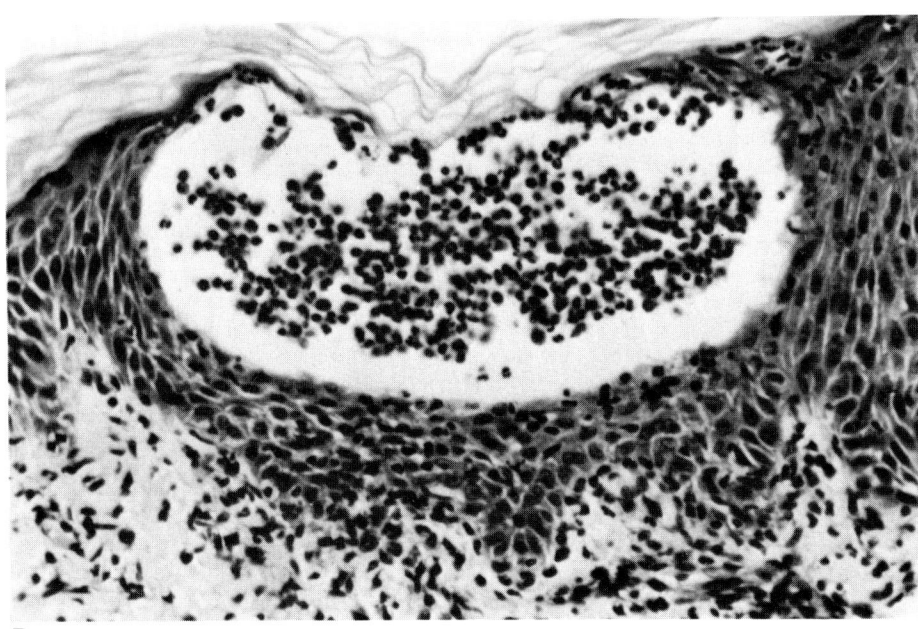

Figure 7–12.
Erythema toxicum neonatorum. Multiple subcorneal pustules filled with eosinophils. **A.** H&E. X125. **B.** H&E. X400.

swelling, and diffuse copious scaling. The presence of exfoliating scales differentiates this dermatosis from certain forms of universal erythroderma, although the two terms are sometimes used interchangeably. The histopathologist must try to determine whether the clinical picture has developed as the most severe manifestation of eczematous dermatitis, psoriasis, or drug sensitivity reaction or whether it represents cutaneous lymphoma. Rarer disorders, such as pityriasis rubra pilaris and ichthyosiform erythroderma, also may come into differential diagnosis. It is usually not too difficult to come to a conclusion on the basis of careful histologic examination if the differential features mentioned in this and the other pertinent chapters are taken into consideration.

PRURIGO

Prurigo is an old dermatologic term attached to various diseases by different authors. Prurigo Besnier is a synonym for atopic dermatitis. Prurigo ferox and prurigo hiemalis are obsolete; the latter probably is synonymous with asteatotic dermatitis. Prurigo nodularis is discussed later in this chapter. That leaves prurigo simplex, a clinical diagnosis made in patients who have ill-defined and very pruritic papular lesions with a great deal of excoriation.[34]

Grouping prurigo has a chronic course characterized by appearance of inflammatory papules within a fairly well-defined plaque over the trunk and extremities.[35] The clinical course is different in prurigo pigmentosa in which acute eruption disappears within a week leaving areas of reticulated pigmentation.[36] The histopathologist usually is requested to rule out dermatitis herpetiformis, eczematous dermatitis, and papular urticaria. The epidermal changes are minimal or absent unless the lesion is excoriated. The perivascular infiltrate is often coat-sleeve type and consists of lymphocytes and eosinophils.

LICHEN SIMPLEX CHRONICUS

Contact dermatitis as well as atopic dermatitis may lead to lichenification. Being concerned with tissue reactions, we need not discuss the controversial subject of neurodermatitis beyond stating that chronic itching leads to chronic scratching and rubbing and that the histologic picture reflects the effects. The purest example of this type of tissue reaction is represented by solid plaques of circumscribed lichen simplex chronicus (Fig. 7–13) as they are found in the ulnar and tibial regions and the nape of the neck. Its chief components are epidermal hyperplasia, fibrosis of superficial dermis, and thickening of the walls of small blood vessels. Inflammatory infiltrate usually is minor and may be absent.

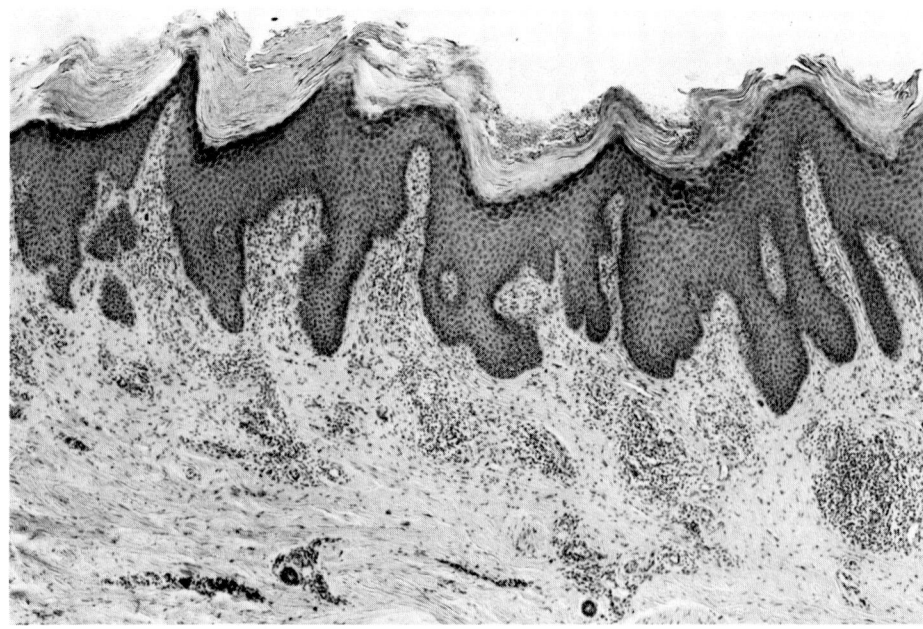

Figure 7–13.
Lichen simplex chronicus circumscriptus. Note mild papillomatosis, uneven rete ridges, and papillae, hypergranulosis, and hyperkeratosis with only small foci of parakeratosis. Dermal infiltrate concentrated around small blood vessels, the lumina and walls of which are recognizable at this relatively low magnification. H&E. X75.

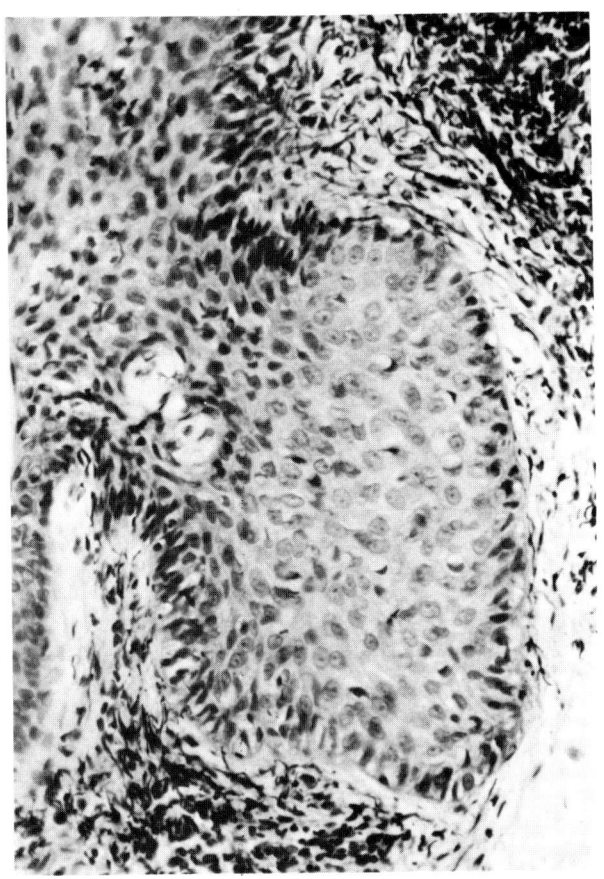

Figure 7–14.
Chronic alarm reaction of sebaceous gland, which is transformed into a solid epithelial mass with only a few lipidized cells near the junction with the hair follicle. Heavy inflammatory infiltrate. H&E. X220. (From Mehregan. J Am Acad Dermatol 1:56, 1979.)

Epidermal hyperplasia of the type to be described now should not be called psoriasiform. It must, in fact, be distinguished from psoriasiform reactions as described in the next chapter. It is characterized by acanthosis, hypergranulosis, and orthokeratotic hyperkeratosis and may be considered the attainment of a new level of homeostasis in the chronically stimulated epidermis. In experiments with tritium-labeled thymidine, Marks and Wells[37] found that the labeling index measuring cells in the DNA-synthesizing phase is at least as high as in psoriasis but that the life span of cells, measured by their transit time through the stratum spinosum, is much longer. They explain this, in part, by the greater mass of the epidermis and, in part, by the fact that some of the labeled cells in the higher strata probably are Langerhans cells and not keratinocytes. The suprapapillary plate in lichen simplex is indeed thick in contrast to psoriasis, and the rete ridges are long and massive but uneven in size (Figs. 5–3 and 7–13). The epidermal surface often shows minor degrees of papillomatosis due to elongation of dermal papillae. Ordinarily, edema, hypogranulosis, and parakeratosis are absent. Their focal presence signifies activity of the underlying eczematous process or response to acute injury by excoriation or infection. In all these respects the lichenified epidermis is quite distinct from psoriatic epidermis, with its evenly long rete ridges, thin suprapapillary plate, and elongated papillae with dilated capillaries. Papillae and subpapillary layers contain vessels that appear rigid and thick walled through apposition of cells and fibers. The pars papillaris may show generalized fibrosis and loss of elastic fibers as the result of many bouts of inflammatory and mechanical injury and repair. Sebaceous glands may be transformed into solid epidermoid plugs (chronic alarm reaction, Chapter 2) (Figs. 7–14 and 7–15), and this feature often adds to the faulty impression of pseudoepitheliomatous downgrowth of epidermis.[38]

PICKER'S NODULE AND PRURIGO NODULARIS

All histologic features of chronic and lichenified dermatitis are exaggerated in lesions diagnosed as giant lichenification and Picker's nodule[39] (Fig. 7–16). In *Prurigo nodularis* multiple lesions often involve the upper and lower extremities. Histologic findings include marked epidermal thickening with or without follicular involvement,[40] superficial dermal fibrosis, and a low grade inflammatory cell infiltrate. Hyperplasia of the cutaneous nerve bundles may or may not be present.[41,42]

Figure 7–15.
Alarm reaction of hair follicles and sebaceous glands in lichen simplex chronicus. Reduction in size, premature and displaced keratinization of hair, absence of lipidization of glands, and extrusion of parts of follicular contents. Relatively mild inflammatory infiltrate and partial devitalization of epidermis point to effects of excoriation. H&E. X125. (From Mehregan. J Am Acad Dermatol 1:56, 1979.)

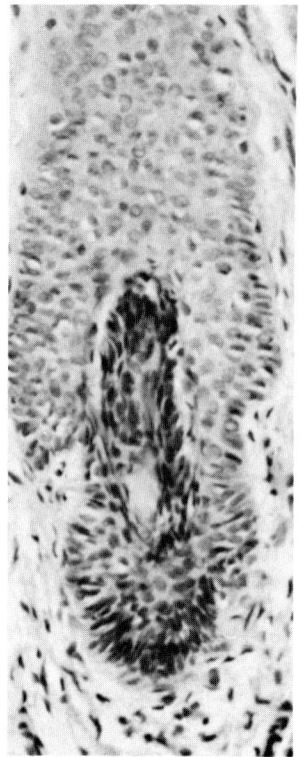
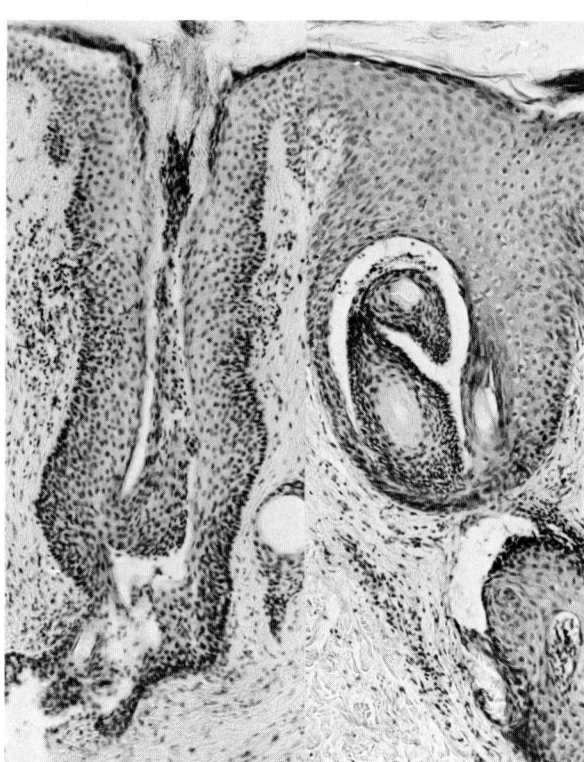

Figure 7–16.
Hypertrophic lichen simplex chronicus (Picker's nodule). Some of the massive epithelial structures are rete ridges, others are hyperplastic walls of hair follicles and possibly sweat ducts. Note fibrosis and vascularity of stroma. H&E. X41. (From Mehregan. Dermatol Digest 4:55, 1965.)

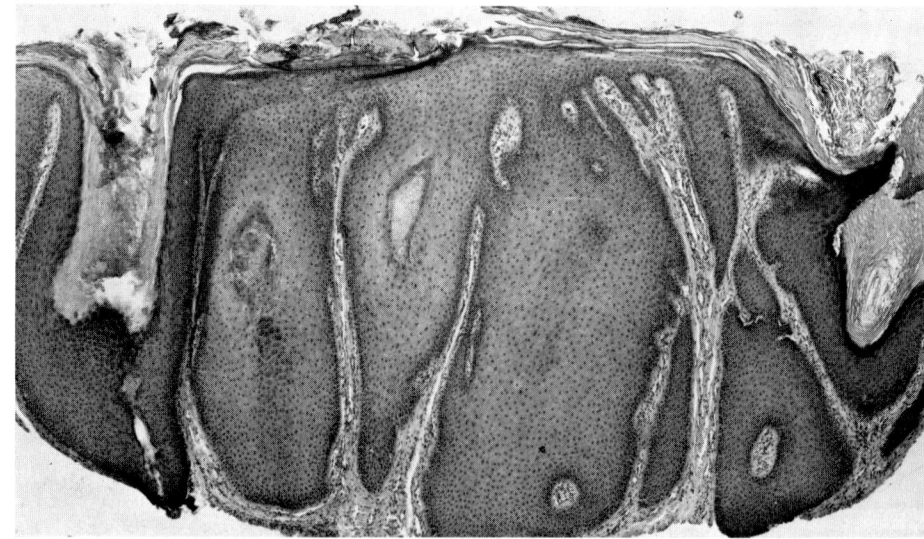

REFERENCES

1. Ackerman AB, Ragaz A: A plea to expurge the word "eczema" from the lexicon of dermatology and dermatopathology. Am J Dermatopathol 4:315, 1982
2. Jones RB: The histogenesis of eczema. Clin Exp Dermatol 8:213, 1983
3. Hornstein OP: Definition and classification of eczemas. A pertinent challenge to dermatologists. J Dermatol (Tokyo) 13:81, 1986
4. Fisher AA: Contact Dermatitis. Philadelphia: Lea & Febiger, 1986
5. Willis CM, Young E, Brandon DR, Wilkinson JD: Immunopathological and ultrastructural findings in hu-

man allergic and irritant contact dermatitis. Br J Dermatol 115:305, 1986
6. Pinkus H: Examination of the epidermis by the strip method, II. Biometric data on regeneration of the human epidermis. J Invest Dermatol 19:431, 1952
7. Cormane RM, Husz S, Hammerlinck FF: Immunoglobulin and complement-bearing lymphocytes in eczema. Br J Dermatol 88:307, 1973
8. Silberberg-Sinakin I, Thorbecke SJ, Baer RL, et al: Antigen-bearing Langerhans cells in skin, dermal lymphatics, and in lymph nodes. Cell Immunol 25: 137, 1976
9. Shelley WB, Juhlin L: Selective uptake of contact allergens by the Langerhans cell. Arch Dermatol 113: 187, 1977
10. Dvorak HF, Mihm MC, Dvorak AM: Morphology of delayed-type hypersensitivity reactions in man. J Invest Dermatol 67:391, 1976
11. Björnberg A, Löwhagen G-B: Patch testing with mineral wool (Rockwool). Acta Derm Venerol 57:257, 1977
12. Cuypers JMC, Hoedemaeker PJ, Nater JP, DeJong MGM: The histopathology of fiberglass dermatitis in relation to von Hebra's concept of eczema. Contact Dermatol 1:88, 1975
13. DeJong MCMJ, Hoedemaeker PJ, Jongeblood WF, Nater JP: Investigative studies of the dermatitis caused by the larva of the brown-tail moth (*Euproctis chrysorrhaea* Linn). II. Histopathology of skin lesions and scanning electron microscopy of their causative setae. Arch Dermatol Res 255:177, 1976
14. Montes LF: The histopathology of diaper dermatitis. J Cutan Pathol 5:1, 1978
15. Lamy M, Novak F, Duboscq MF, et al: La chenille processionnaire de chene (Thaunetopoea processionea L.) et l'homme: Appareil urticant et mode d'action. Ann Dermatol Venereol 115:1023, 1988
16. Epstein S: Epidermal and dermal reactions in a case of sensitivity to nickel. J Invest Dermatol 38:37, 1962
17. Epstein S: Contact dermatitis due to nickel and chromate. Observations on dermal delayed (tuberculintype) sensitivity. Arch Dermatol 73:236, 1956
18. Rudner EJ, Hudson P, Mehregan AH: Sensibilidad por contacto dermico: Evaluación clinica y dermatopatologica. Arch Argent Dermatol 22:69, 1972
19. Gomez Orbaneja J, Iglesias Diaz L, Sanchez Lozano JL, Conde Salozar L: Lymphomatoid contact dermatitis. A syndrome produced by epicutaneous hypersensitivity with clinical features and a histopathologic picture similar to that of mycosis fungoides. Contact Dermatol 2:139, 1976
20. Castelain P-Y: Les dysidroses. Ann Dermatol Venereol 114:579, 1987
21. Kaplan AP, Buckley RH, Mathews KP: Allergic skin disorders. JAMA 258:2900, 1987
22. Mihm MC Jr, Soter NA, Dvorak HF, Austen KF: The structure of normal skin and the morphology of atopic eczema. J Invest Dermatol 67:305, 1976
23. Uehara M, Miyauchi H: The morphologic characteristics of dry skin in atopic dermatitis. Arch Dermatol 120:1186, 1984
24. Uehara M: Clinical and histological features of dry skin in atopic dermatitis. Acta Derm Venereol Suppl 114:82, 1985
25. Sturman SW: Infantile acropustolosis. Semin Dermatol 3:50, 1984
26. Laudren A, Chevrant-Breton J, Lancien G: Acropustulose infantile: Un Cas. Ann Dermat./Venereol 112: 251, 1985
27. Newton JA, Salisbury J, Marsden A, McGibbon DH: Acropustulosis of infancy. Br J Dermatol 115:735, 1986
28. Vignon-Pennamen MD, Wallach D: Infantile acropustulosis. A clinicopathologic study of six cases. Arch Dermatol 112:1155, 1986
29. Jorda E, Moragon M, Verdeguer JM, et al: A propos d'un cas d'acropustulose infantile avec immunofluorescence direct positive. Ann Dermatol Venereol 115: 39, 1988
30. Freeman RG, Spiller R, Knox JM: Histopathology of erythema toxicum neonatorum. Arch Dermatol 82: 586, 1960
31. Jacobsen FK, Abildtrup N, Laursen SO, et al: Àcrokeratosis paraneoplastica (Bazex syndrome). Arch Dermatol 120:502, 1984
32. Obasi OE, Garg SK: Bazex paraneoplastic acrokeratosis in prostate carcinoma. Br J Dermatol 117:647, 1987
33. Wishart JM: Bazex paraneoplastic acrokeratosis: a case report and response to Tigason. Br J Dermatol 115:595, 1986
34. Kocsard E: The problem of prurigo. Australas J Dermatol 6:156, 1962
35. Ofuji S, Ogino A: Grouping prurigo. J Dermatol (Tokyo) 15:60, 1988
36. Nagashima M: Prurigo pigmentosa-clinical observations of our 14 cases. J Dermatol (Tokyo) 5:61, 1977
37. Marks R, Wells GC: Lichen simplex. Morphodynamic correlates. Br J Dermatol 88:249, 1973
38. Mehregan AH: Alarm reaction of pilosebaceous apparatus. J Am Acad Dermatol 1:55, 1979
39. Mehregan AH: Picker's nodule. Dermatol Digest 4:55, 1965
40. Miyauchi H, Uehara M: Follicular occurrence of prurigo nodularis. J Cutan Pathol 15:208, 1988
41. Doyle JA, Connolly SM, Hunziker N, Winkelmann RK: Prurigo nodularis: A reappraisal of the clinical and histologic features. J Cutan Pathol 6:392, 1979
42. Lindley RP, Payne CME R: Neural hyperplasia is not a diagnostic prerequisite in nodular prurigo. A controlled morphometric microscopic study of 26 biopsy specimens. J Cutan Pathol 16:14, 1989

8
PSORIASIFORM TISSUE REACTIONS

Under the heading of psoriasiform tissue reaction we consider the dermatoses listed inside the oval of Figure 8–1. Those listed outside the oval are discussed in other chapters. The two principal features uniting psoriasiform tissue reactions are suprapapillary exudate and focal parakeratosis related to it. The exudate may consist of fluid, leukocytes, or a mixture of both. Of great importance is its intermittent character, which is expressed[1,2] in the easily remembered term, "the squirting papilla." All modifications of intensity and character of the exudate and frequency of the discharges may be encountered, and their varying combinations produce different pictures that make the histologic diagnosis of the individual diseases (Table 8–1).

The focal parakeratosis is the expression of damage to suprapapillary cells and acts as a stimulant to mitosis in the deep epidermal germinative strata. Just as complete removal of superficial cells stimulates mitosis and leads to temporary hyperregeneration of the epidermis, so does intermittently repeated injury by suprapapillary exudate and the resulting parakeratosis. If the stimulus is mild, not much acanthosis will follow. If it is severe, the highest degrees of psoriasiform epidermis will be the result. Figure 8–10 illustrates the vicious cycle, in which acanthosis is a most dramatic but secondary result of cyclic suprapapillary exudate. More will be said about this concept of the disease process in the discussion of psoriasis, but Table 8–1 shows that psoriasiform acanthosis is only one feature of the psoriasiform tissue reaction, and not a very constant one.

There is no claim that the dermatoses discussed in this chapter are necessarily related. The squirting papilla and its products are biologic–morphologic features and may be due to a variety of causes.

SEBORRHEIC DERMATITIS

The simplest form of this tissue reaction is seen in seborrheic dermatitis, especially in Unna's *petaloid* form, so frequently encountered in the presternal area of hairy-chested men. Sections of this lesion (Fig. 8–2) show the epidermis mildly to moderately acanthotic, with somewhat uneven development of ridges and papillae. There is perivascular infiltrate in the subpapillary layer and, on the surface, focal parakeratosis, which often takes the shape of tapering *mounds* and may contain a few pyknotic leukocytes. It is only when one examines serial sections that one becomes aware of the constant association of the parakeratotic areas with the suprapapillary thin portions of the epidermis. Papilla and overlying rete may not look particularly abnormal below a well-developed mound because in these areas one sees the last, exfoliating stage of a tiny inflammatory focus. One has to look closely to find the earlier stages, which are reconstructed in the series shown in Figure 8–3. The very earliest stage of the cycle is a highly edematous papilla with engorged capillaries; the epidermis appears unaltered. In the next stage, fluid and a few polymorphonuclear cells enter the suprapapillary plate and cause some intercellular edema. This is followed by loss of granular layer and formation of parakeratotic cells between which the fluid and granulocytes are trapped. Meanwhile, the papillary edema has subsided, and the papilla may become quite inconspicuous. Edema of the suprapapillary plate at first produces a flat mound, which then increases in height by the accumulation of parakeratotic cells and the products of the squirting papilla. Still later, normal horny cells are produced, and the granular layer is reconstituted. The parakeratotic mound now becomes a lenticular focus in the stratum corneum and is eliminated onto the surface.

Individual papillae squirt and subside at different times in seborrheic dermatitis and thus produce focal mounds. Their number, size, and degree of admixture of inflammatory products vary greatly with the intensity of the dermatitis. The described petaloid form is intermediate, being chronic but relatively mild. In acute seborrheic dermatitis, larger parakeratotic crusts may form, the epidermis may become quite acanthotic and spongiotic, and there may be formation of small spongiotic vesicles in the edematous suprapapillary plate (see Fig. 5–8). In the follicular form, spongiosis and abscess formation also involve the upper hair follicle and give rise to the characteristic, tiny, pointed pustules of the clinical picture (Fig. 8–4). In other cases of seborrheic dermatitis, the rete ridges may become long and the suprapapillary plate so thin that the tips of the papillae are covered only by parakeratotic material. This picture, which is usually associated with much

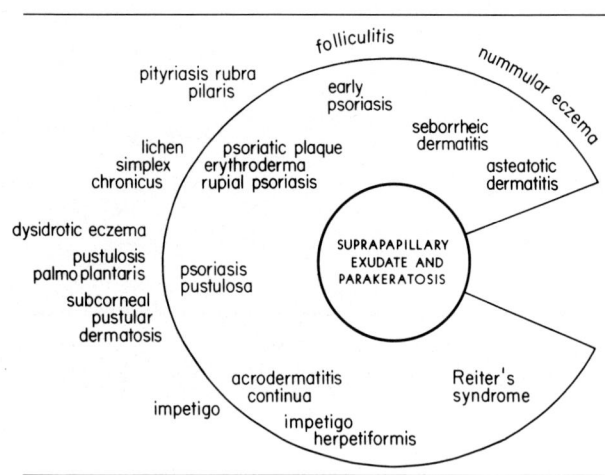

Figure 8–1.
Psoriasiform tissue reactions. Diagrammatic guide to differential diagnosis.

epidermal and dermal edema and inflammatory infiltrate, merges by degrees into that of "nummular eczema."[3]

On the other hand, a fresh lesion of seborrheic dermatitis, impressive clinically by its swollen appearance, may be very disappointing under the microscope, where vascular engorgement and dermal edema have been lost in the paraffin-embedded sections. Sometimes one has to look for a few early parakeratotic mounds and a few emigrating leukocytes in order to make a diagnosis. It is a good rule to think of seborrheic dermatitis whenever the clinician describes a florid lesion and the microscopist sees practically normal skin.

The role of Pityrosporum in pathogenesis of seborrheic dermatitis is not yet fully understood.[4] An increase in the incidence of seborrheic dermatitis

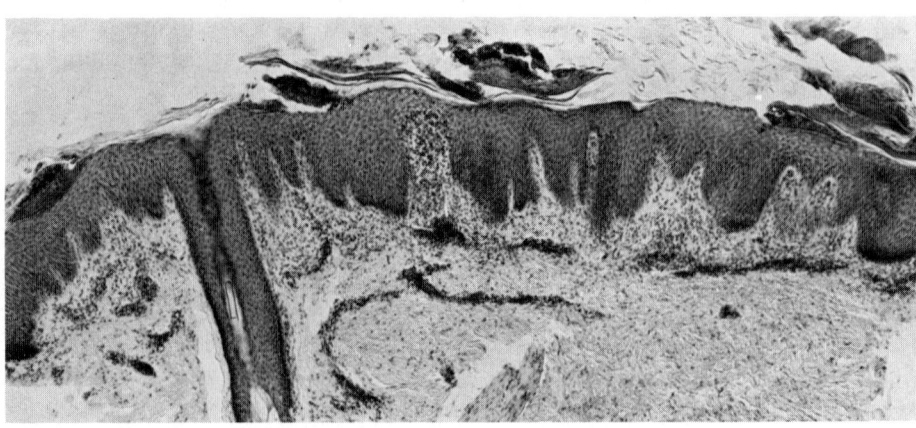

Figure 8–2.
Seborrheic dermatitis. H&E. X60.

TABLE 8–1. DIFFERENTIAL DIAGNOSTIC FEATURES IN THE GROUP OF PSORIASIFORM TISSUE REACTIONS

Diagnostic Feature	Asteatotic Dermatitis	Seborrheic Dermatitis (Simple)	Early Psoriasis	Fully Developed Psoriasis	Rupial Psoriasis	True Pustular Psoriasis of Palms	Acrodermatitis Continua	Impetigo Herpetiformis, Ps. Pustulosa	Keratoderma Blennorrhagicum, Reiter's Disease
Suprapapillary exudate	Scattered	Scattered	Magnified	Grouped and repeated	Exaggerated	Obscured	Exaggerated	Obscured	Massed
Spongiform pustule	Very rare	Very rare	Yes	Rare	Yes	At borders	Well developed	At borders	Massive
Munro abscess	Rare, tiny	Rare, tiny	Well developed, large	Yes	Many, large	No	No	No	Many
Macropustule	No	Rare	Rare	No	No	Typical	Typical	Typical	Early
Parakeratosis	Focal, scattered	Focal, scattered	Yes	Focal, aggregated, repeated	Aggregated, repeated	Minor	Yes	Yes	Massive, layered
Serous exudate	Focal, scattered	Focal, scattered	Mild	Minor	Pronounced	Much	Much	Much	Varying
Leukocytic exudate	Hardly any	Hardly any	Focal, pronounced	Focal, minor	Pronounced	Massive	Massive	Massive	Focal, varying
Acanthosis	Minor	Some	Yes	Pronounced	Exaggerated papillomatous	Rete compressed	Moderate or compressed	Moderate	Pronounced
Edema of papillary heads	Focal, scattered	Focal, scattered	Yes	Yes	Pronounced	No	Focal	Focal	Focal
Inflammatory infiltrate	Scattered	Little	Some	Some	Moderate	Moderate	Moderate	Moderate	Considerable
Eczematous spongiosis	Occasionally	Occasionally	No	No	No	No	No	No	No
Acantholysis	No	No	No	No	No	No	No	Occasionally	No

From Pinkus. Australas J Dermatol 18:31, 1965.

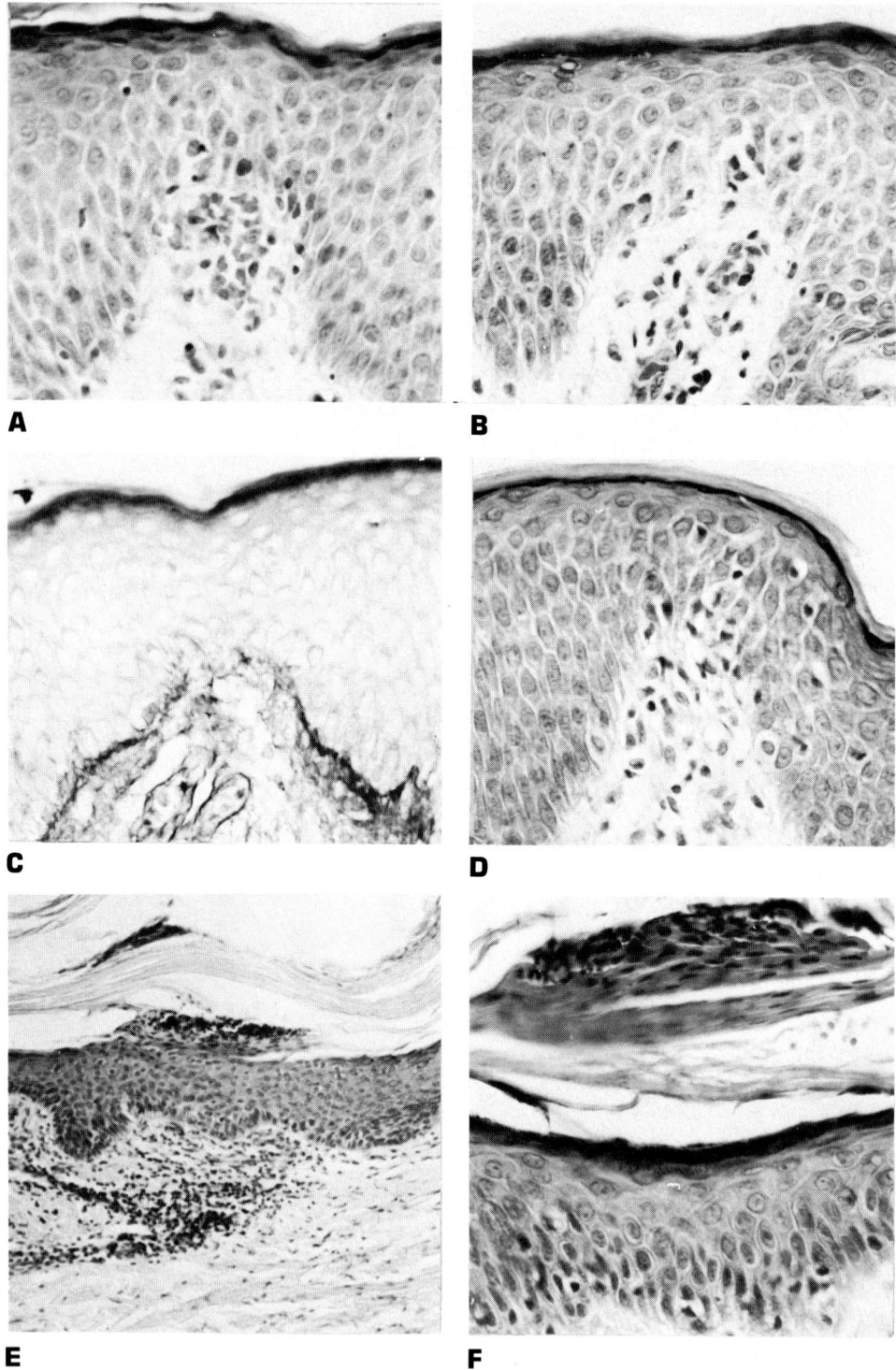

Figure 8–3.
Cycle of suprapapillary exudate in seborrheic dermatitis. **A, B,** and **D.** Early stages before parakeratosis develops. H&E. X400. **C.** Temporary break in basement membrane. Alcian blue–PAS. X400. **E.** Later stage in which a parakeratotic mound includes polymorphonuclear leukocytes, whereas papilla has become inconspicuous. Lenticular parakeratotic inclusion in horny layer is end product of a previous squirt. H&E. X135. **F.** Details of microabscess in a parakeratotic mound that has been lifted up by normal horny material underlaid by a granular layer. H&E. X400.

has been reported in patients with Parkinson's disease or acquired immunodeficiency syndrome.[5-7] Another study suggests close association between infantile seborrheic dermatitis and atopic disease.[8]

Perioral Dermatitis

A recalcitrant, erythematous, scaly, and papular eruption, originally described as light-sensitive seborrheid,[9] has become an increasingly vexing problem to dermatologists.[10,11] Biopsies are done in order to rule out rosacea, lupus erythematosus, and seborrheic dermatitis. The histologic changes[12] are not pathognomonic (Fig. 8–4) and resemble eczematous dermatitis with parakeratotic scaling and spongiotic edema in epidermis and follicular epithelium, the latter causing a resemblance to follicular seborrheic dermatitis. Scattered dermal infiltrate consists of lymphocytes, some histiocytes, and occasional plasma cells.

Similar eruptions may occur following long-term application of fluorinated corticosteroids in periocular distribution. Histologic findings in "periocular dermatitis" consist of a chronic granulomatous reaction in relation with the pilosebaceous structures.[13]

ASTEATOTIC DERMATITIS

The differential diagnosis of seborrheic dermatitis may have to include pemphigus erythematosus in rare instances, but a common source of error is the close resemblance of the microscopic picture of asteatotic dermatitis (winter eczema). The latter usually has less acanthosis, but all other features are quite similar, and asteatotic (xerotic) dermatitis also may merge histologically and clinically into the picture of nummular eczema in aggravated cases (Fig. 8–5). The presence or absence of well-formed sebaceous glands is helpful in differential diagnosis but requires examination of multiple sections in order to judge the size of glands fairly.

PSORIASIS

Classic

Typical lesions of psoriasis (Fig. 8–6) are characterized by a high degree of acanthosis of the rete ridges, which are evenly long and alternate in the section with long edematous and often club-shaped papillae. The suprapapillary plate is thin, and the surface is covered by a lamellated scale in which orthokeratotic and parakeratotic areas alternate. Papillary capillaries appear rigid and tortuous, and there is a rather small amount of perivascular lymphocytic infiltrate in the subpapillary layer. The presence of small accumulations of pyknotic neutrophilic leukocytes in the horny layer (*Munro abscesses*[14]) completes the picture. This generalized description is quite adequate for the diagnosis of typical cases but

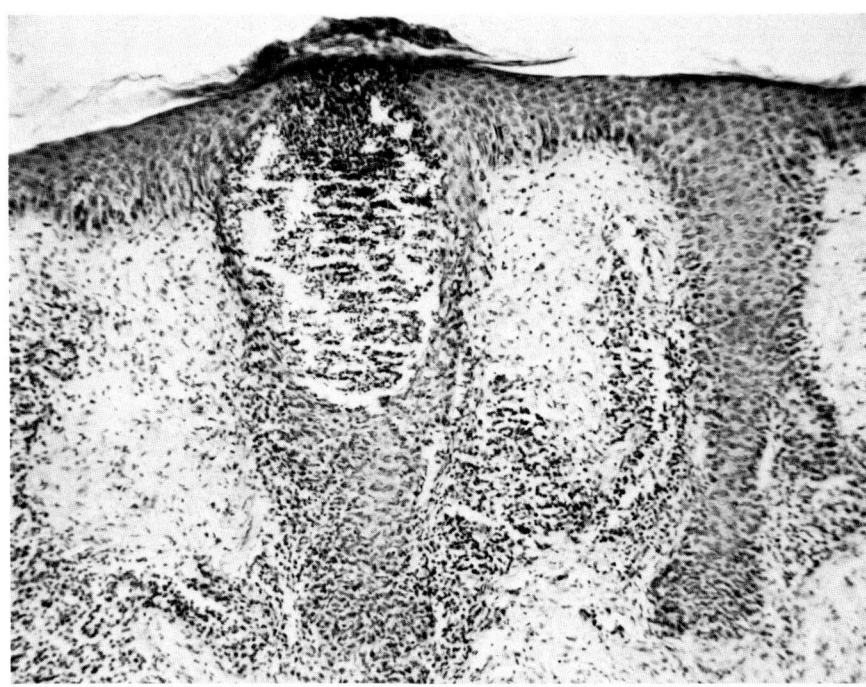

Figure 8–4.
Perioral dermatitis. Heavy involvement of upper portion of hair follicle and admixture of polymorphonuclear leukocytes to the generally lymphocytic infiltrate make the picture similar to the follicular type of seborrheic dermatitis. H&E. X135.

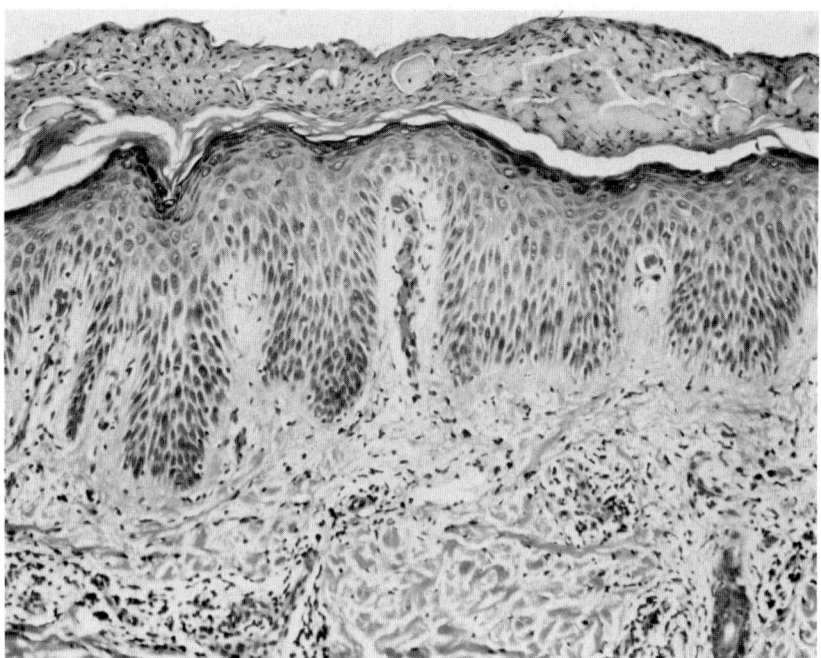

Figure 8–5.
Asteatotic dermatitis. Note the generally eczematous character of the changes in this specimen, which obviously was obtained at a moment when a much more exudative phase had been replaced by normalizing processes expressed in acanthosis and hypergranulosis. Highly edematous papilla with prominent vessel below relatively thin suprapapillary plate and eddies in the parakeratotic scale—crust are reminders of the cyclic character of the acute process. Minimal perivascular infiltrate also speaks against a true eczematous dermatitis. H&E. X135.

says nothing about the pathobiology of the psoriatic process, nor is it helpful in atypical cases or in the numerous variants of psoriasis.

Examination of sections for evidence of squirting papillae is revealing in both respects. It is easy to find a cycle of events very similar to that in seborrheic dermatitis, except that the amount of serum discharged from the tip of a papilla is usually smaller and the number of leukocytes larger. Lymphocytes and neutrophils often migrate individually through breaks in the basement membrane (Fig. 8–7A) into the suprapapillary plate (Fig. 8–7B), then aggregate in the parakeratotic mound, where we call them a "microabscess" (Fig. 8–8). The rhythmic discharges from one papilla seem to last a little longer, and they repeat themselves at shorter intervals so that one may find two or several cycles, one above the other in different stages of development. Moreover, numerous papillae squirt in close vicinity.

These phenomena seem to explain most of the features of psoriasis. The papillae, and especially their tips remain in a state of edema and engorgement of capillaries. Polymorphonuclear leukocytes are often visible in the vascular lumen, but rarely in the dermis and practically never in the rete ridges, which are solid without much evidence of edema

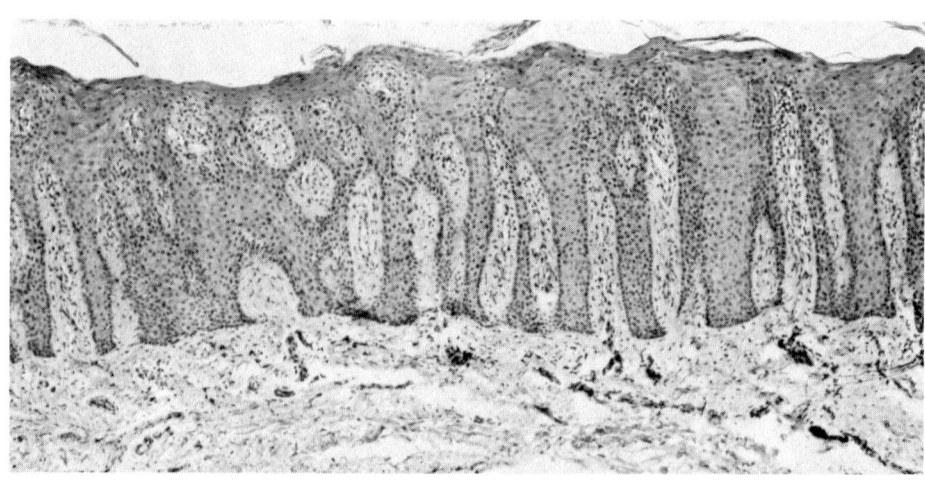

Figure 8–6.
Psoriasis, plaque. Only fragments of the scale are present because the lamellated psoriatic stratum corneum easily disintegrates during histologic processing. Although some papillae are shown full length, others are cut obliquely and only the upper or the lower portions appear in the section. H&E. X70.

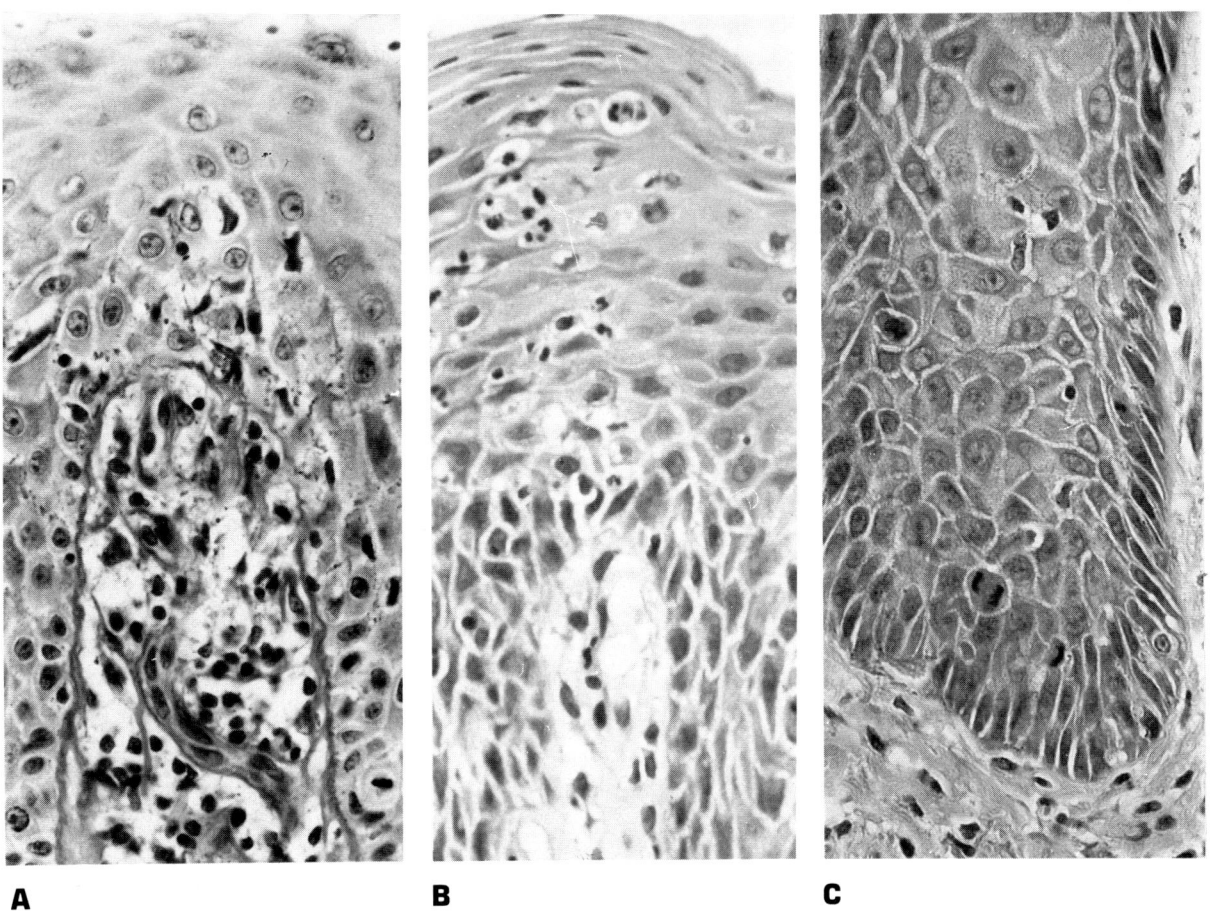

Figure 8–7.
Details of psoriatic epidermis. **A.** Shows telangiectasia, papillary edema, and disruption of PAS-positive basement membrane within the suprapapillary area. **B.** Migration of individual leukocytes from tip of papilla into and through suprapapillary plate associated with loss of granular layer and parakeratosis. **C.** Lower part of long rete ridge stains darker (no edema) and shows several mitoses, indicating division of epidermis into a vigorously proliferating lower portion and a damaged and rapidly exfoliating upper portion. H&E. X400.

(Fig. 8–7C). Instead, leukocytes are found between the living cells of the suprapapillary plate above papillary tips (Fig. 8–9) and between the parakeratotic cells of mounds and lenticular inclusions within the horny layer, which thus becomes lamellar. If one follows one lamella sideways through the length of the section, one sees it swell up (Fig. 8–8) into a lentil-shaped mass of parakeratotic cells, farther on subside and continue as an orthokeratotic thin lamella for a stretch, then become parakeratotic again. The trapping of air between the lamellae contributes to the silvery aspect of the clinical lesion. The inflammatory process varies in intensity from spot to spot and from time to time. Most important, it is always associated with heads of papillae. These events are obscured in the center of very active chronic plaques of psoriasis because of the rapid succession of squirts from many papillae. Intelligent and careful examination is needed to recognize them. Manifest clinical psoriasis is a rhythmic, repeated pathologic event, not a continuous one.

Much research of the last several years has focused on the earliest events in the development of the psoriatic lesion. The results can be separated into those that call psoriasis a primarily epidermal disease with dermal alterations as secondary byproducts, and others that stress underlying changes in the dermis and especially in blood vessels, which precede and cause the visible epidermal alterations.[15,16] Staricco[17] noted in 1980 that tape

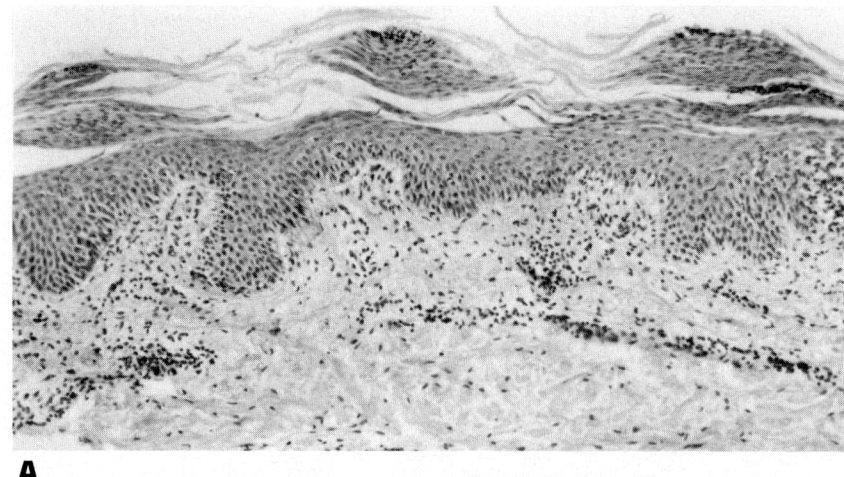
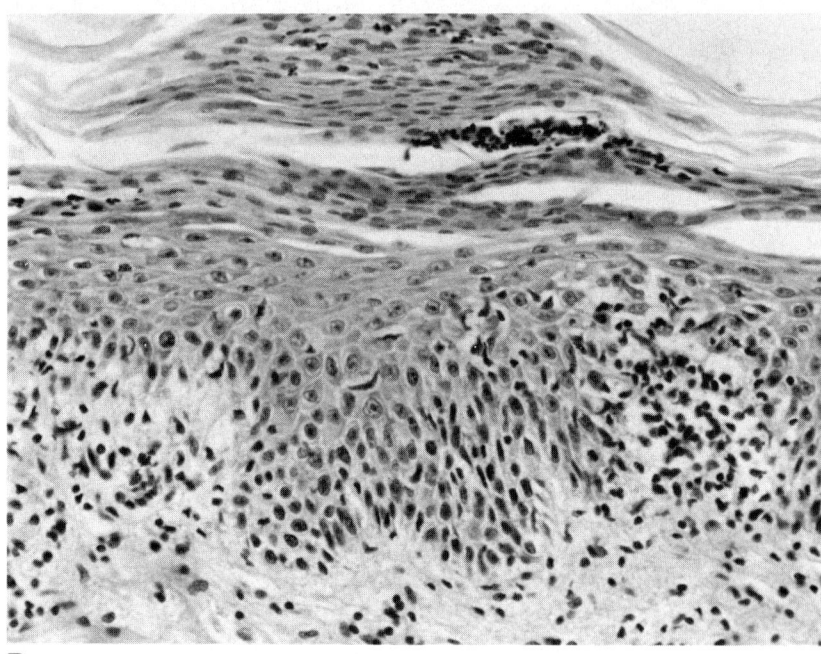

Figure 8–8.
Acute guttate psoriasis. Layered scale consists of thin orthokeratotic lamellae and lenticular parakeratotic mounds harboring microabscesses. H&E. **A**, X125, **B**, X400.

stripping of normal forearm skin induces petechiae after 9 strips in psoriatic subjects against 19 strips in normal people or patients with other skin diseases. The petechial threshold is lowered in normal skin of psoriatics. Jablonska et al.[18] found that tape stripping produces prepinpoint papules, developing into typical psoriatic lesions in a high percentage of psoriatics. One may postulate that the constantly repeated inflammatory insult to the suprapapillary epithelial cells forces the undamaged rete ridges to become hyperplastic and to speed up mitotic division (Fig. 8–7C) in an effort to replace the prematurely lost suprapapillary portion. Either hypothesis will explain the data that mitoses are about 10 times as common in psoriasis as in normal epidermis and occur not only in the basal layer but in two to three rows of basaloid germinal cells,[19,20] and that turnover of the epidermal population is correspondingly speeded up. Similar conditions have been found in control studies of atopic dermatitis and lichen simplex chronicus. It is not possible at this time to prove which phenomenon is primary, but as a mental aid in diagnosis, the thought is helpful that mitotic speedup is secondary to epithelial damage, which is secondary to papillary squirting (Fig. 8–10). Investigations of early and later manifestations of psoriasis have led several authors[21] to the tentative conclusion that psoriatic epidermal hyperplasia may develop in association with antecedent and persisting vascular events in the dermis.

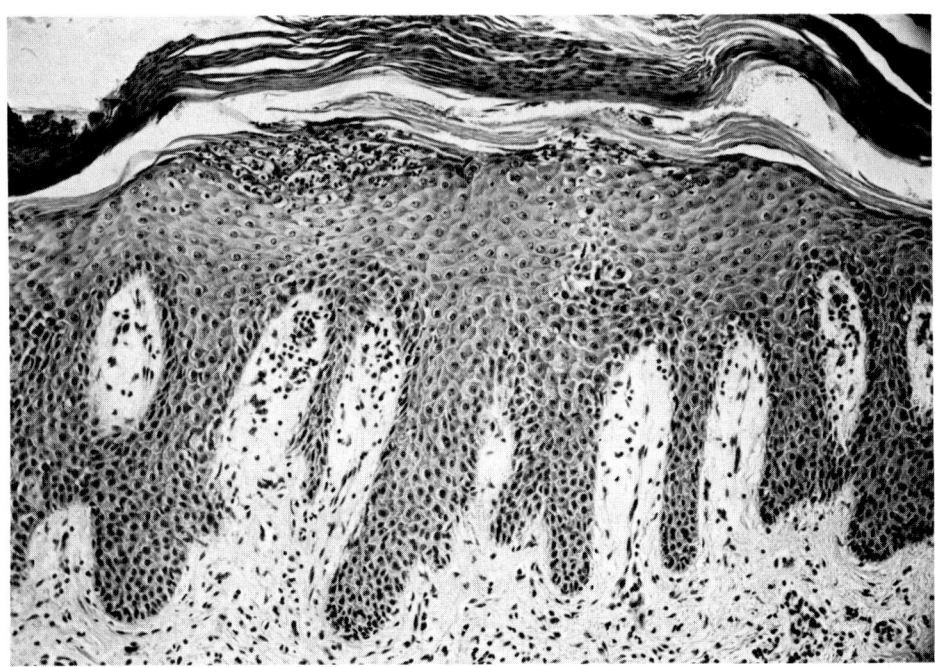

Figure 8–9.
Psoriasis with spongiform pustule. Suprapapillary plate appears thick in section because head of squirting papilla is not encountered in section. Stream of leukocytes in right half of picture indicates that a papillary head would be encountered in one of subsequent serial sections. H&E. X135.

Ultrastructural changes include microvascular dilatation, bridged fenestrations and gaps in endothelium, edematous areas in the cytoplasm of endothelial cells, pericytes and myocytes, basement membrane thickening, and cell extravasation, indicating increased vascular permeability.[22]

Variants

Most of the variants of psoriasis can be understood as variations of the interlocking sequence of events illustrated in Figure 8–10. If papillary exudate and subsequent acanthosis are reduced in quantity, we encounter the picture of *seborrheic psoriasis* or may have difficulty in making a decision between psoriasis and seborrheic dermatitis. The latter is more likely if rete ridges are uneven and if spongiotic edema is evident. Psoriasis is practically ruled out if spongiosis affects the ridges.

We come closer to the features of *pustular psoriasis* when the amount of exocytosis increases. This is often seen in cases of acute psoriatic flare-up, when each new lesion clinically appears as a tiny pustule, then spreads into a scaly erythematous papule. Histologically (Fig. 8–11), we see an aggregate of discharging papillae capped by a huge parakeratotic mound. At this stage, the suprapapillary plate is paradoxically thickened, due mainly to edema. Such cases simply represent an exaggeration of the exudative process of typical psoriasis. However, the picture is not too different in cases of generalized

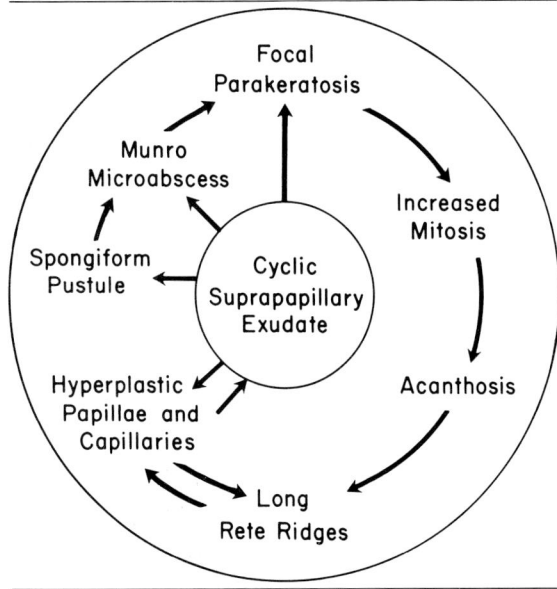

Figure 8–10.
Diagram illustrating the hypothesis that cyclic suprapapillary exudate is the main driving force of the established psoriatic process (regardless of possibility that some abnormality in the epidermis may initiate the exudate). According to this view, damage to superficial epidermal layers secondarily induces regenerative mitotic activity in the rete ridges and other histologic changes. (Adapted from Pinkus. Arch Dermatol 107:840, 1973.)

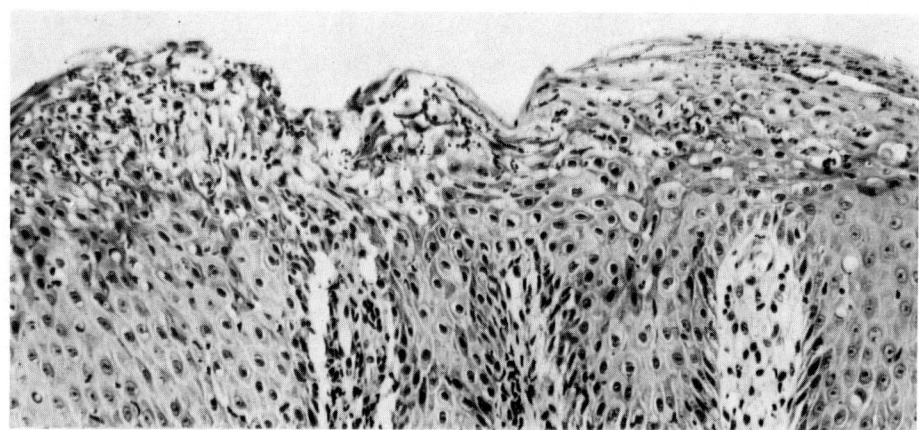

Figure 8–11.
Very early, clinically pustular lesion in an acute burst of psoriasis. While suprapapillary plate is relatively thick, most of keratinocytes are damaged and are in the process of being converted into parakeratotic elements. H&E. X280. (From Sutton. Diseases of the Skin, 11th ed, 1956. Courtesy of Dr. R. L. Sutton, Jr. Contributed by H. Pinkus.)

pustular psoriasis of the von Zumbusch type, except that the acanthotic response of the epidermis is much reduced. Microabscesses become macroabscesses (Fig. 8–12), and their precursor state among the still living epidermal cells represents Kogoj's spongiform pustule (see Fig. 8–9).[23]

The spongiform pustule is the hallmark of Hallopeau's acrodermatitis continua. Personal experience convinces us as clinicians that this dermatosis is a variant of psoriasis.

Impetigo Herpetiformis

Almost indistinguishable from generalized pustular psoriasis, either clinically or histologically, is a rare disease called "impetigo herpetiformis." Originally described as a severe affection of pregnant women, it has also been found in nonpregnant women and in men. It is related to hypoparathyroidism,[24,25] and cases exhibiting no disturbance of calcium–phosphorus metabolism probably should be labeled pustular psoriasis.[26,27] Histologically, there is a tendency to dissociation in the upper epidermal layers affected with spongiform pustulation, and some rounded acantholytic cells are found in the macropustule (Chapter 11). In this respect, impetigo herpetiformis resembles the subcorneal pustular dermatosis of Sneddon and Wilkinson.

Psoriasis of Palms and Soles: Pustulosis Palmaris et Plantaris

Another special case is pustular psoriasis of palms and soles. Here, the concept of suprapapillary ex-

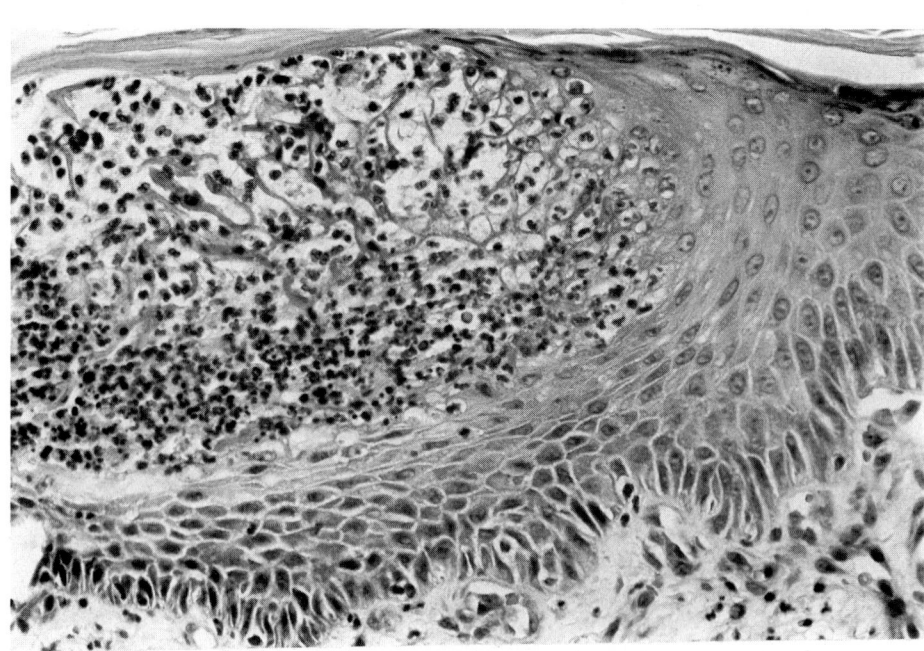

Figure 8–12.
Pustular psoriasis of von Zumbusch type. Note spongiform pustulation in the shoulder of this early lesion characterized by massive leukocytic exudate and minimal acanthosis (mitotic activity). H&E. X180.

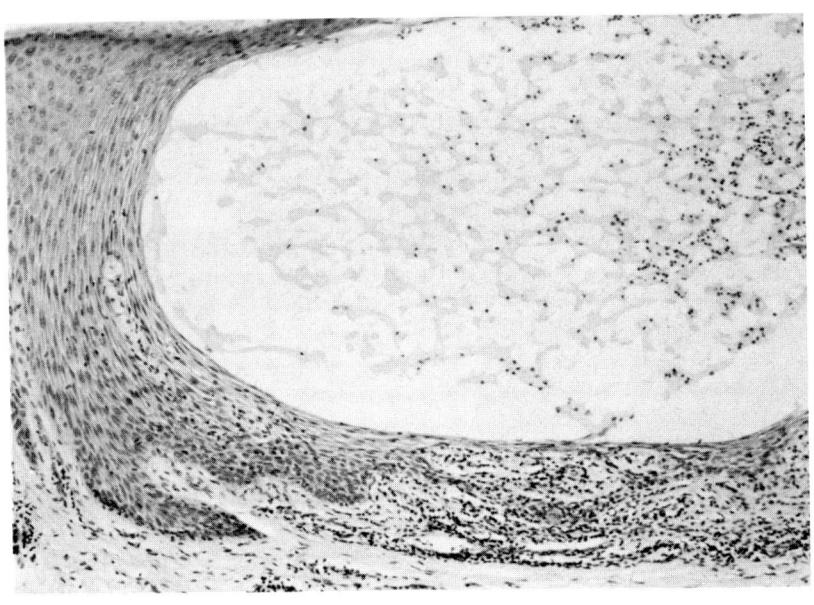

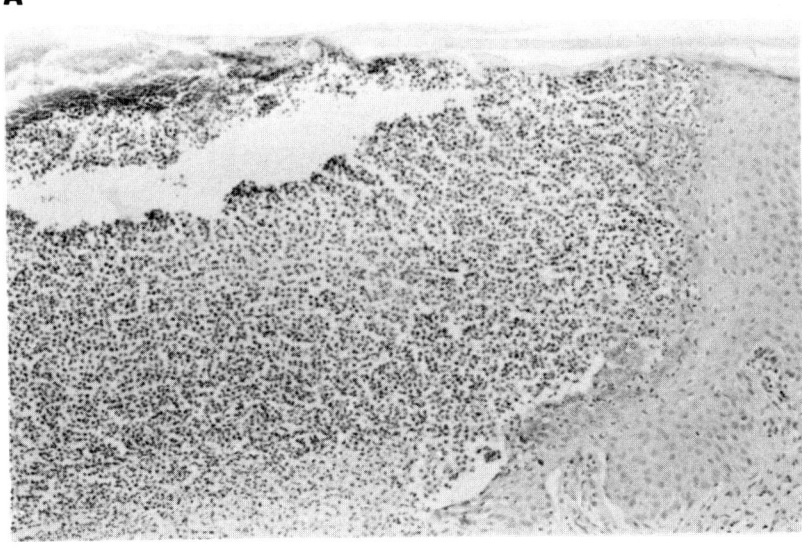

Figure 8-13.
Comparison of pustulosis palmaris et plantaris and true pustular psoriasis at low power. **A.** The vesicopustule probably began intraepidermally and compressed keratinocytes all around it without evidence of spongiosis or spongiform pustulation visible in **B**. **B.** Pustular psoriasis shows a picture identical with Figure 8–12 taken from a lesion of generalized pustular psoriasis. H&E. X125.

udation helps in the differential diagnosis from pustulosis palmaris et plantaris and dyshidrosiform eczematous dermatitis. The vesicle of the latter (see Fig. 7–9) is derived from spongiotic intraepidermal edema, and the roof of the blister contains living epidermal cells unless the entire rete is destroyed. The former two (Fig. 8–13) begin in the superficial epidermal layers and soon become subcorneal. The entire rete malpighi is compressed in the bottom of the blister. True pustular psoriasis has at least some evidence of the spongiform pustule in the shoulders of the lesion (Fig. 8–14) or in the septa between adjoining cavities. This sign is absent in pustulosis palmaris et plantaris, which is a rare condition synonymous with Andrews' pustular bacterid and not related to psoriasis.[28,29]

There is yet another relatively rare type of volar psoriasis. The clinical picture resembles a dry eczematous eruption and is biopsied for differentiation from occupational chronic hand dermatitis. In this type, suprapapillary exudate and all accompanying changes are reduced to a minimum. The naturally thick epidermis shows little acanthosis, and the thick horny layer contains only a few scattered lenticular foci of parakeratotic cells and pyknotic leukocytes. Capillaries may be wide, but subepidermal inflammation is almost absent.

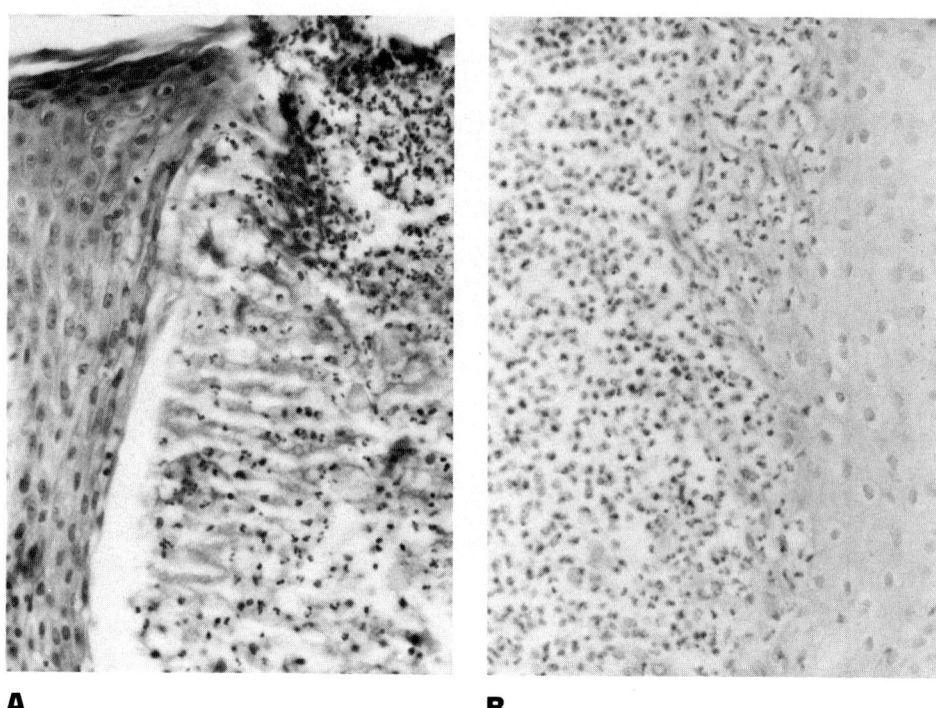

Figure 8-14.
Higher magnification of the shoulders of pustules in previous illustration shows the absence **(A)** and presence **(B)** of spongiform pustulation in pustulosis palmaris et plantaris **(A)** and pustular psoriasis **(B)** of palm. H&E. X250.

Psoriatic Erythroderma

The psoriatic eruption may progress to universal erythroderma or exfoliative dermatitis. The clinical picture is indistinguishable from other forms of erythroderma, especially in malignant lymphoma (Chapter 45). Histologically, however, the picture is that of classic psoriasis with acanthosis, parakeratosis, and Munro abscesses, and there is relatively little cellular infiltrate in the upper dermis.

Psoriasis of Oral Mucosa

The question of psoriasis of the oral mucosa and its possible relationship to geographic tongue are discussed in Chapter 46.

REITER'S DISEASE

The last member of the family of psoriasiform reactions (see Fig. 8-1) is the keratotic or crusted lesion of Reiter's disease (Keratoderma blennorrhagicum).

Figure 8-15 shows a typical but relatively small lesion from the palm. The old thick horny layer has been lifted up by a truncated cone of parakeratotic crust, which actually represents a huge mound including dozens of microabscesses and parakeratotic lenticles. The suprapapillary layer is thick because it is highly edematous. If we look for details, we find typical squirting papillae, similar to those of any of

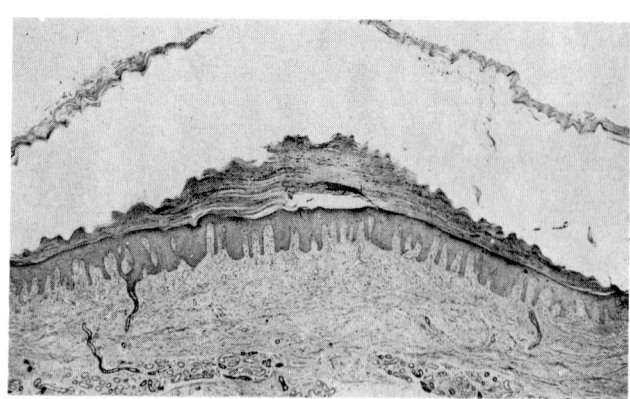

Figure 8-15.
Small and relatively dry lesion of Reiter's disease. H&E. X30.

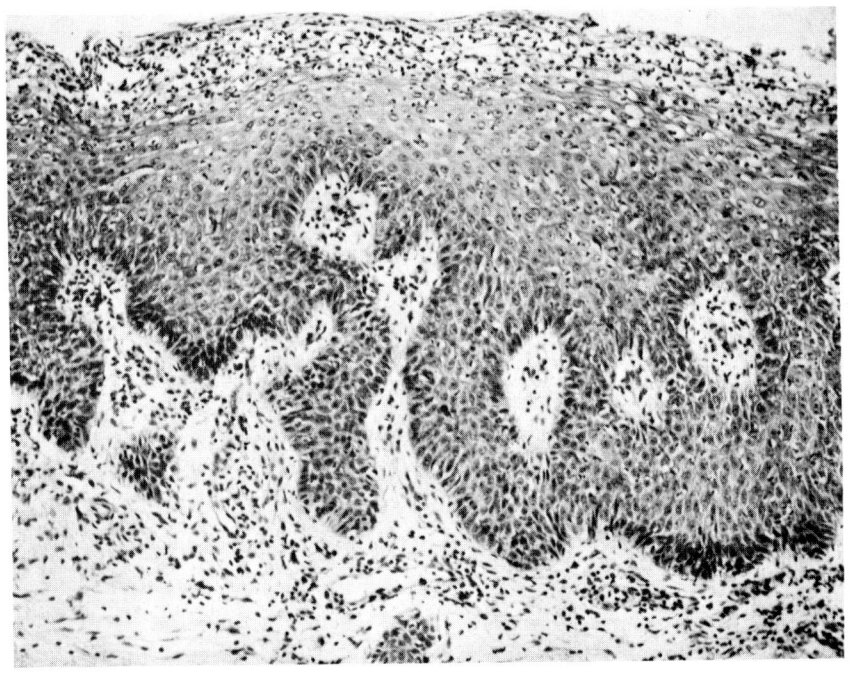

Figure 8–16.
More exudative form of Reiter's disease. Transmigration of leukocytes from papillae to disintegrating stratum corneum. H&E. X135.

the other entities (Fig. 8–16). The difference is quantitative. There is also much edema and inflammatory infiltrate in papillae and the subpapillary layer. In very acute cases, the exudate may almost destroy the suprapapillary plate and may lead to vesiculation under the crust. Lesions of the Reiter syndrome on the glans penis are known as "balanitis circinata." They closely resemble psoriatic plaques of this area both clinically and histologically. Differential diagnosis must be based on the evaluation of the entire case history.[30–32] Reiter's syndrome is another condition reported as occurring in patients with the acquired immunodeficiency syndrome.[33]

NUMMULAR ECZEMA

Just as the clinical picture of nummular eczema often develops in an asteatotic or seborrheic soil, so do the histopathologic features suggest an exacerbation of asteatotic and seborrheic dermatitis (Fig. 8–17), with the addition of eczematous features. Edema and

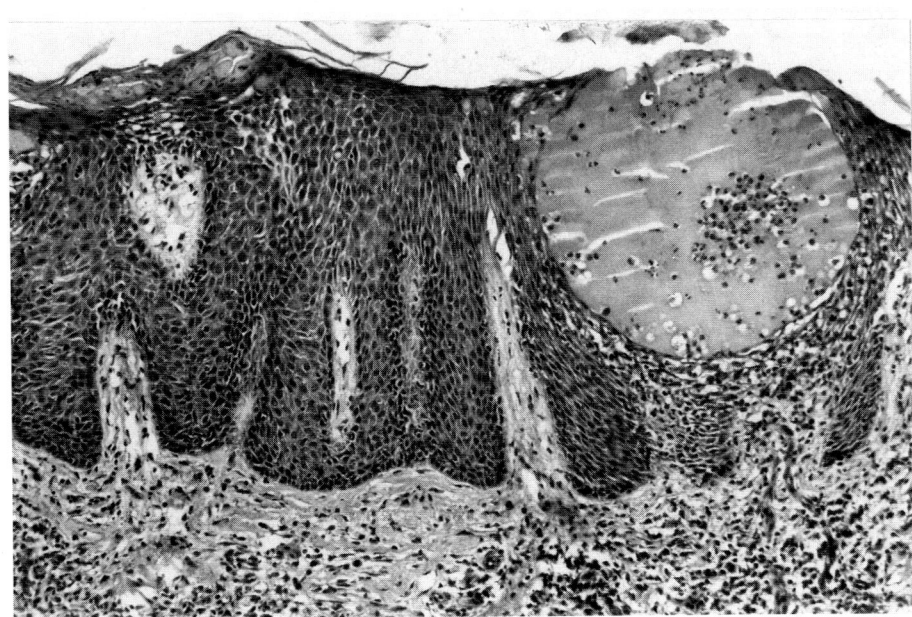

Figure 8–17.
Nummular eczema combines eczematous and psoriasiform features. H&E. X135.

leukocytic exudate dominate the picture. Evenly or unevenly sized rete ridges are riddled by spongiosis and exocytosis. The suprapapillary plate may be completely disrupted so that edematous papillary heads are exposed, and the surface is covered by parakeratotic crust containing pyknotic granulocytes and dried serum. Bacterial colonies occasionally are seen in the crust and support the clinical impression of an infectious factor in this disease.[34] Cellular infiltrate consisting of small round cells and granulocytes in the edematous pars papillaris complete the picture, which combines features of the eczematous and psoriasiform tissue reactions.

SULZBERGER–GARBE DISEASE

Nine cases of a distinctive, exudative, discoid, and lichenoid chronic dermatosis were described by Sulzberger and Garbe in 1937. The disease is peculiarly localized in its distribution, being predominantly encountered among middle-aged Jewish males in the New York area. In a review,[35] Sulzberger differentiates it from a great variety of other dematoses, the most important ones being mycosis fungoides and nummular eczema. We, therefore, discuss it at this point. The epidermal changes resemble those of nummular eczema but are rarely seen unaltered due to the severe pruritus. The arterioles and capillaries of the upper dermis are dilated and have thickened walls. The infiltrate consists of small round cells, fixed tissue type cells, polymorphs, and numerous plasma cells. The latter are found close to vascular walls and are the most characteristic feature except in early lesions. The true pathogenetic relations of this disease are unknown.[36] Fortunately, it responds well to corticosteroids.

REFERENCES

1. Pinkus H, Mehregan AH: The primary histologic lesion of sehorrheic dermatitis and psoriasis. J Invest Dermatol 46:109, 1966
2. Chowaniec O, Jablonska S, Beutner EH, et al: Earliest clinical and histological changes in psoriasis. Dermatologica 163:42, 1981
3. Metz J, Metz G: Ultrastruktur der Epidermis bei seborrhoischem Ekzem. Arch Dermatol Forsch 252:285, 1975
4. Grosshans E, Bressieux A: L'eczema seborrheique (la pityrosporose). Ann Dermatol Venereol 115:79, 1988
5. Eisenstat BA, Wormser BP: Seborrheic dermatitis and butterfly rash in AIDS. N Engl J Med 311:189, 1984
6. Mathes BM, Douglass MC: Seborrheic dermatitis in patients with acquired immunodeficiency syndrome. J Am Acad Dermatol 13:947, 1985
7. Soeprono FF, Schinella RA, Cockerell CJ, Comite SL: Seborrheic-like dermatitis of acquired immunodeficiency syndrome. J Am Acad Dermatol 14:242, 1986
8. Podmore P, Burrows D, Eedy DJ, Stanford CF: Seborroeic eczema—A disease entity or a clinical variant of atopic eczema? Br J Dermatol 115:341, 1986
9. Frumess GM, Lewis HM: Light sensitive seborrheic dermatitis. Arch Dermatol 75:245, 1957
10. Wilkinson DS, Kirton V, Wilkinson JD: Perioral dermatitis: A 12 year review. Br J Dermatol 101:245, 1979
11. Wilkinson D: What is perioral dermatitis? Int J Dermatol 20:485, 1981
12. Marks R, Black MM: Perioral dermatitis. A histopathologic study of 26 cases. Br J Dermatol 84:242, 1971
13. Fisher AA: Periocular dermatitis akin to the perioral variety. J Am Acad Dermatol 15:642, 1986
14. Munro WJ: Note sur l'histopathologie du psoriasis. Ann Dermatol Syphiligr 9:961, 1898
15. Van Scott EJ, Flaxman BA: Lesion kinetics in psoriasis; tissue, cellular, and subcellular compartments. Acta Derm Venereol Suppl 73:75, 1973
16. Braun-Falco O: The initial psoriatic lesion. In Farber EM, Cox AJ (eds): Psoriasis, Proceedings of the Second International Symposium of Stanford Univ, 1976. New York: Yorke Medical Books, 1976
17. Staricco RG: Altered capillary response to tape stripping in psoriasis and some other dermatoses: Petechial threshold test. Dermatologica 160:315, 1980
18. Jablonska S, Chowaniec O, Beutner EH, et al: Stripping of the stratum corneum in patients with psoriasis. Production of pre-pinpoint papules and psoriatic lesions. Arch Dermatol 118:652, 1982
19. Weinstein GD, Frost P: Abnormal cell proliferation in psoriasis. J Invest Dermatol 50:254, 1968
20. Farber EM, Nall L, Strefling A: Psoriasis: A disease of the total skin. J Am Acad Dermatol 12:150, 1985
21. Braverman IM, Yen A: Ultrastructure of the capillary loops in the dermal papillae of psoriasis. J Invest Dermatol 68:53, 1977
22. Mordovtseu VN, Albanova VI: Morphology of skin microvasculature in psoriasis. Am J Dermatopathol 11:33, 1989
23. Colomb B, LaBatie J-P: La pustule spongiforme de Kogoj. Apports de le microscope electronique. Ann Dermatol Venereol 104:707, 1977
24. Moynihan GD, Ruppe JP Jr: Impetigo herpetiformis and hypoparathyroidism. Arch Dermatol 121:1330, 1985
25. Oumeinish OY, Farraj SE, Bataineh AS: Some aspects of impetigo herpetiformis. Arch Dermatol 118:103, 1982

26. Osterling RJ, Nobrega RE, DuBoeuff JA, Van der Mear JB: Impetigo herpetiformis or generalized pustular psoriasis. Arch Dermatol 114:1527, 1978
27. Lotem M, Katzenelson V, Rotem A, et al: Impetigo herpetiformis: A variant of pustular psoriasis or a separate entity. J Am Acad Dermatol 20:338, 1989
28. Uehara M, Ofuji S: The morphogenesis of pustulosis palmaris et plantaris. Arch Dermatol 109:518, 1974
29. Pierard J, Kint A: La pustulose palmo-plantaire chronique et recidivante. Etude histologique. Ann Dermatol Venereol 105:681, 1978
30. Perry HO, Mayne JG: Psoriasis and Reiter's syndrome. Arch Dermatol 92:129, 1965
31. Sehgal VN, Koranne RV, Basunatary RK, et al: Reiter's disease. J Dermatol Tokyo 9:145, 1982
32. Sehgal VN, Jain MK, Srivastava G, Saha MM: Reiter's disease. A radiological assessment of joints. J Dermatol Tokyo 15:535, 1988
33. Winchester R, Bernstein DH, Fischer HD, et al: The co-occurrence of Reiter's syndrome and acquired immunodeficiency. Ann Intern Med 106:19, 1987
34. Röckl H: Untersuchungen zur Klinik und Pathogenese des mikrobiellen Ekzems. Hautarzt 7:70, 1956
35. Sulzberger MB: Distinctive exudative discoid and lichenoid chronic dermatosis (Sulzberger and Garbe) reexamined—1978. Br J Dermatol 100:13, 1979
36. Rongioletti F, Corbella L, Rebora A: Exudative discoid and lichenoid chronic dermatosis (Sulzberger–Garbe). A fictional disease? Int J Dermatol 28:40, 1989

9
LICHENOID AND POIKILODERMATOUS TISSUE REACTIONS

The botanic term "lichen" signifying dry, scurfy forms of lower plant life, has been applied to dry scaly skin disease in such expressions as pityriasis lichenoides or lichenification. The prototype, however, of a lichen of the skin is *lichen planus* (lichen ruber planus). When we call a clinical eruption "lichenoid," we usually mean it resembles lichen planus. Similarly, there is a histologic reaction that is typically expressed in the papule and plaque of lichen planus. Clinically atrophic, hypertrophic, and bullous forms of the disease have histologic features easily recognized as variants of this reaction. The lichenoid tissue reaction, however, is also found in nosologically unrelated dermatoses, such as lichen nitidus, certain types of lupus erythematosus, and some solar keratoses.[1-3] Some of its features are encountered in lichenoid drug eruptions and in erythema dyschromicum perstans. Furthermore, it blends with the tissue reactions characterizing the various types of poikiloderma, a term applied to any clinical picture that combines the four features of telangiectasia, hyperpigmentation, depigmentation, and atrophy in a mottled distribution. Lichen planuslike tissue reactions have also been described in the graft-vs-host reaction. We are thus dealing in this chapter with a heterogeneous assembly of clinical dermatoses, all of which may enter differential diagnosis in the examination of a biopsy specimen.[4] Clinicopathologic correlation is even more essential in this field than in the areas covered in previous chapters, and determination of the correct diagnosis can be a difficult, stimulating and, in the end, gratifying process.

LICHEN PLANUS

The basic histobiologic feature of lichen planus is basal layer damage. Just as we used the suprapapillary exudate to explain most of the other features of psoriasis, so can we derive most of the histologic details of lichen planus by considering that damage to the germinal layer must be reflected in the epidermis and must lead to inflammatory reaction in the subepidermal zone.

Histology

The classic histologic features of lichen planus (Fig. 9–1) include hyperkeratosis, hypergranulosis, and hypertrophy of the rete, liquefaction or colloid degeneration of basal cells, and a bandlike subepidermal lymphocytic infiltrate that invades the lower layers of the epidermis. Focal separation of epidermis and dermis (*Max Joseph spaces*) may occur (Fig. 9–2). Sawtooth-shaped rete ridges and deposition of melanin in dermal macrophages complete the picture (Fig. 9–3).

132 SUPERFICIAL INFLAMMATORY PROCESSES

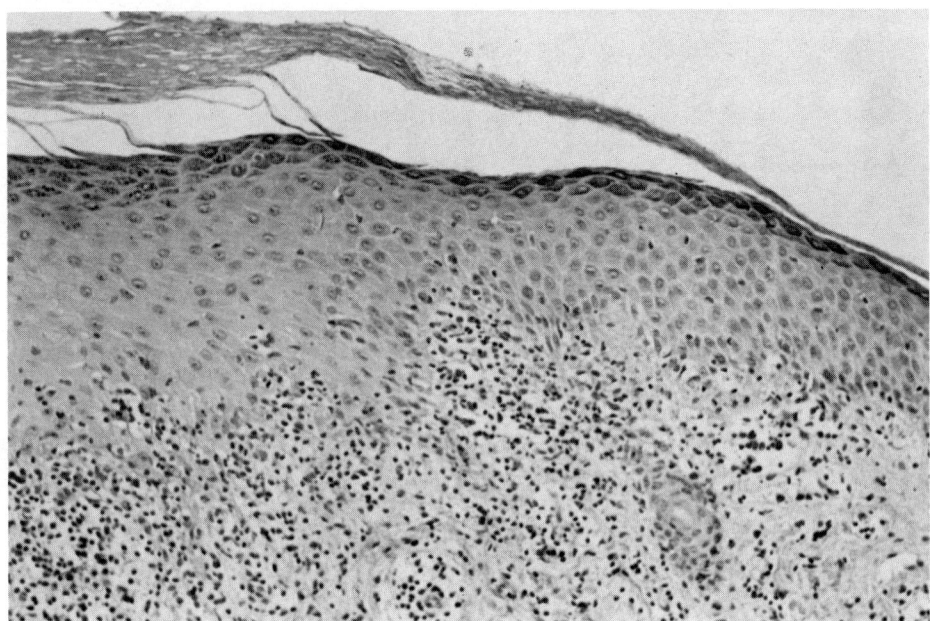

Figure 9–1.
Lichen planus, edge of plaque.
H&E. X135.

Damage to the basal layer in lichen planus is manifested in several ways. Normal, regularly aligned, cuboid, or columnar basal cells are rarely seen. The lowest cells of the epidermis often look more like prickle cells. Their arrangement is disturbed by the presence of lymphocytes between them. Peculiar round or oval acidophilic bodies about the size of a basal cell may be present in scant or large numbers within or just below the epidermis (*Civatte bodies*, apoptotic cells, Fig. 9–4).[5] Occasionally, the impression is gained that most of rete ridge has been transformed into these colloid bodies, leaving only a pointed sawtooth. Melanocytes are more or less absent or seem degenerating. Melanin granules evidently have been discharged from the damaged basal layer and have been engulfed by macrophages in the subepidermal zone. The darker the skin is normally, the more conspicuous is this feature.

Mitotic figures are rarely seen under the light

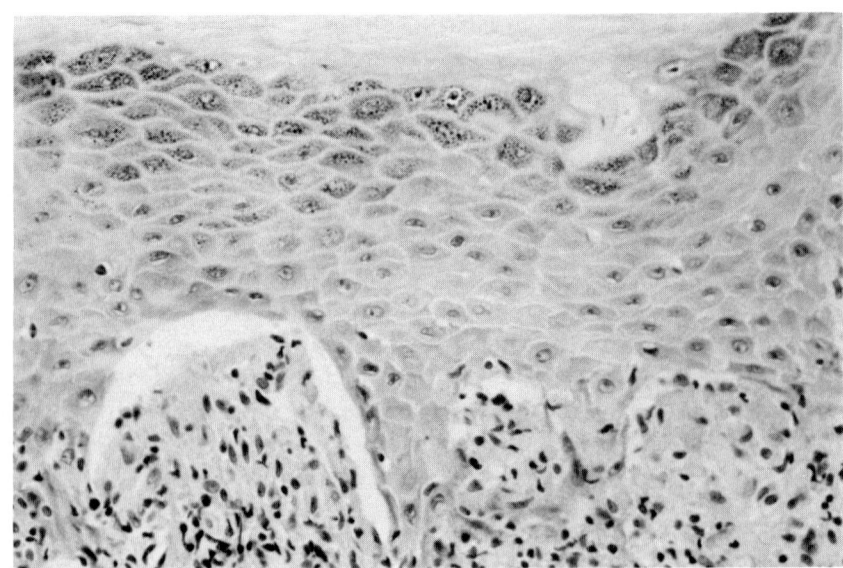

Figure 9–2.
Lichen planus. Focal separation between epidermis and dermis due to loss of basal cells (Max Joseph space). Keratohyalin develops halfway through epidermis. Some hyalinized (Civatte) bodies in place of basal cells in right half of picture between inflammatory cells. H&E. X600.

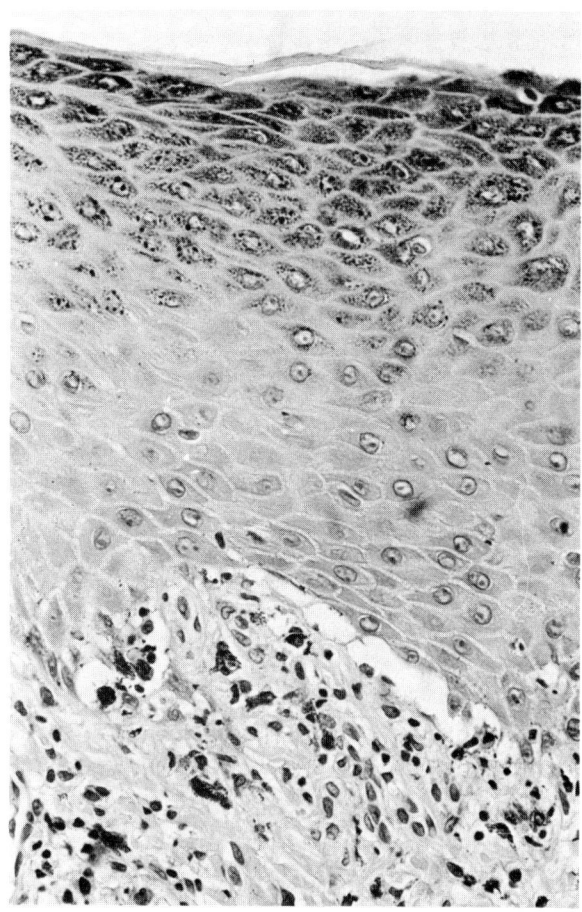

Figure 9–3.
Lichen planus. Max Joseph space, thick stratum granulosum, and loss of pigment granules into the dermis, where some are taken up by macrophages. H&E. X600.

phy (pseudoacanthosis) rather than with hyperplasia (acanthosis).

Close inspection and the use of special stains reveal features that set the dermal infiltrate of lichen planus (Fig. 9–5) apart from the plain inflammatory infiltrate of most other superficial dermatoses. Although T lymphocytes[9] predominate, plasma cells may be present. Fixed-tissue-type cells are always increased in number, most of them being histiocytes and some containing phagocytized melanin. Others are endothelial cells, with the number of capillaries definitely increased. Elastic fiber stain shows two important facts: the infiltrate is always restricted to the papillary layer, and the superficial fine elastic fibers usually are destroyed. There are, thus, certain aspects of a granulomatous infiltrate, and it is not too rare to find an occasional multinucleated giant cell. These features also may be explained as a reaction to the damaged basal layer. The cascade of histobiologic events resulting from basal cell damage is illustrated diagrammatically in Figure 9–6.

Clinicohistologic Correlation

It is rewarding to correlate the clinical signs of lichen planus plaque with the histologic ones. Although lichen planus often is counted among the papulosquamous dermatoses, it usually does not have an exfoliating scale but has an adherent horny layer, which is removed with difficulty. This phenomenon is explained by facts already mentioned. The keratohyaline layer is generally preserved. The whitish *Wickham's striae* are expressed in the varying thickness of the granular layer. Keratohyaline granules reflect and diffuse light (Chapter 2), and their accumulation makes the skin look white. They also influence the transmission of the color of blood, causing a bluish tint. This and the deposition of melanin below the epidermis produce the violaceous hue of the disease. Vascularity of the infiltrate and damage to the basal layer are responsible for a diagnostic procedure well known in France: methodic scraping of a lesion, which will produce the Auspitz phenomenon of capillary bleeding in psoriasis, instead produces subepidermal hemorrhage in lichen planus (Brocq phenomenon[1]). Scraping is also quite painful to the patient, and the paradox that lichen planus patients usually do not have excoriations in spite of intense pruritus is explained by the pain produced by scratching skin, the free nerve endings of which are in the very layer that is affected by the inflammatory process.

Lichen planus of the mouth and other mucous

microscope in lichen planus, but treatment with tritiated thymidine has shown a greatly increased labeling index,[6] and electron microscopic observations have revealed excessive mitotic activity.[7] The reason for this discrepancy is not clear. It seems likely that many of the labeled cells do not achieve mitosis. The epidermis responds as it always does when mitosis is suppressed: the cells get larger, and the proportion of maturing cells increases.[8]

There is a reciprocal relationship between mitotic activity and length of epidermal cell life. In psoriasis, high mitotic rate and short life span are associated; in lichen planus, low mitotic rate leads to long retention of cells in a cohesive granular and horny layer. The epidermis may be thick, but actual count reveals that the number of nucleated cells is not much increased. We are dealing with hypertro-

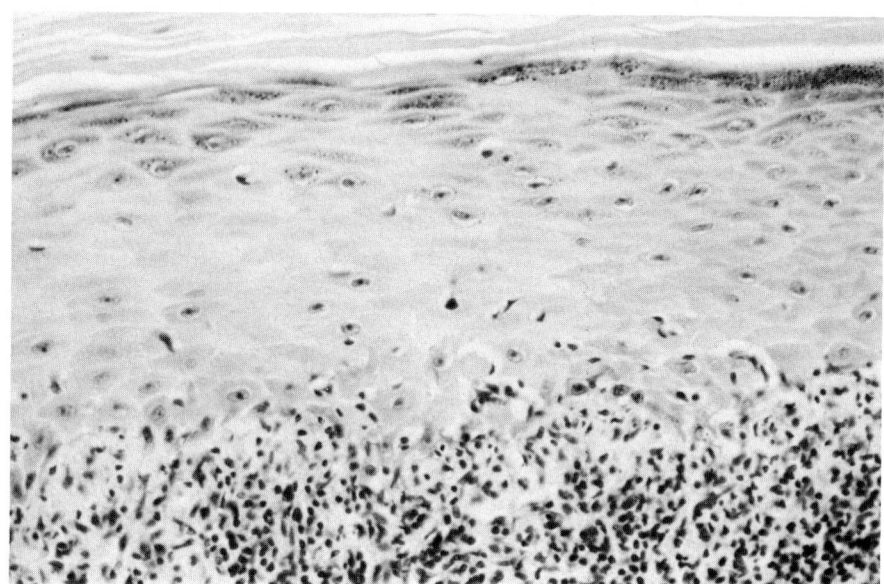

Figure 9–4.
Lichen planus. Typical invasion of lower epidermis by lymphocytes, with dissociation of basal layer and formation of Civatte bodies (see Fig. 5–1B). H&E. X600.

membranes are discussed in Chapter 46 and nail involvement is discussed in Chapter 47.

Atrophic, Verrucous, and Follicular Lesions

One or the other of the specific histologic features of lichen planus becomes modified in its clinical variants. Atrophic (Fig. 9–7) and annular forms usually show typical lichen planus features in the periphery, sometimes only for the width of one or two rete ridges. Centrally, the lymphocytic infiltrate is washed out, leaving behind the skeleton of capillary vessels, fixed tissue cells, and macrophages below the now plainly atrophic epidermis. The absence of elastic

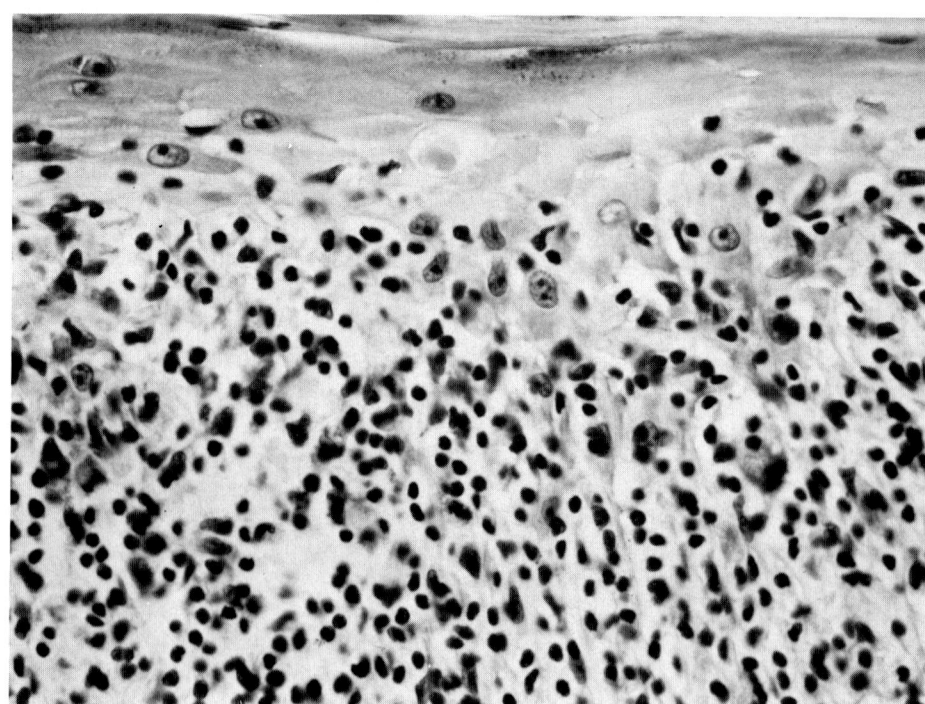

Figure 9–5.
Infiltrate of lichen planus. Note obliteration of lower epidermal contour. H&E. X465.

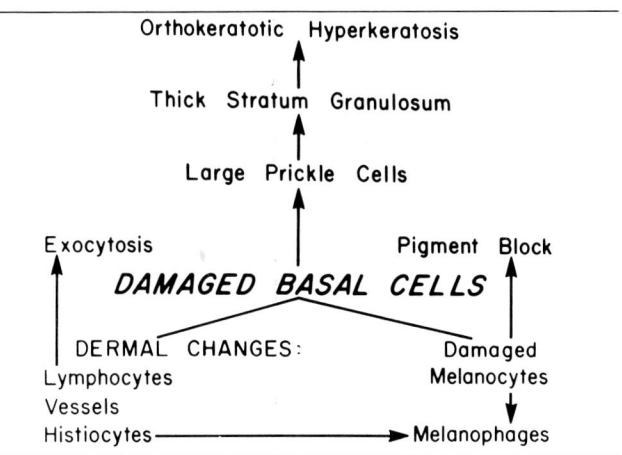

Figure 9–6.
Cascade of histobiologic events associated with epidermal basal cell damage. (Adapted from Pinkus. Arch Dermatol 107:840, 1973.)

fibers in this zone is evident in O&G sections and adds to the clinical impression of atrophy. In hypertrophic (Fig. 9–8) and verrucous cases, on the other hand, the epidermis seems to overcompensate the damage, and the rete ridges, sweat ducts, and follicular sheaths become truly acanthotic, although preserving their composition of large hypertrophic prickle cells. The infiltrate tends to hug the lower circumference of the ridges, whereas the suprapapillary portions of the epidermis may appear quite normal, with a good columnar basal layer. This discrepancy is accentuated in follicular lichen planus (Fig. 9–9), in which the infiltrate hugs the damaged layer of the follicular sheaths.[10] The hair root usually atrophies completely, and the entire follicle is converted into a cup-shaped bag filled with a keratin plug. It is characteristic for lichen planus that the keratin plug is ovoid and often wider below the surface (see Fig. 14–5), in contrast to the conical or tack-shaped plug of lupus erythematosus. The Graham–Little syndrome of scarring alopecia of the scalp seems to be closely related to, if not identical with, lichen planopilaris.[11]

Bullous Lesions

The rare bullous form of lichen planus has found a variety of interpretations. There is little doubt that in older times overtreatment with arsenic could provoke inflammatory edema and that the preformed cleft at the junction led to a bullous exacerbation.[12] There is, however, always a question whether lichen planus pemphigoides, in which bullae arise on normal skin and is associated with papular lichen planus, represents an association of lichen planus and bullous pemphigoid. Direct and indirect immunofluorescent studies may confirm coexistence of the two diseases.[13–15]

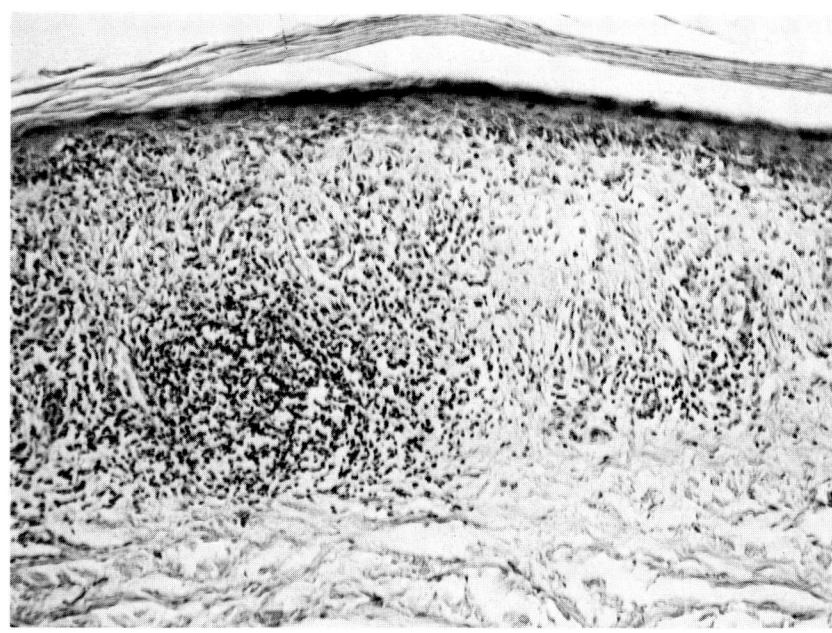

Figure 9–7.
Atrophic lichen planus. The active border is at left. Toward the center of the lesion at the right, lymphocytic infiltrate becomes sparse, but basal cell damage persists. H&E. X135.

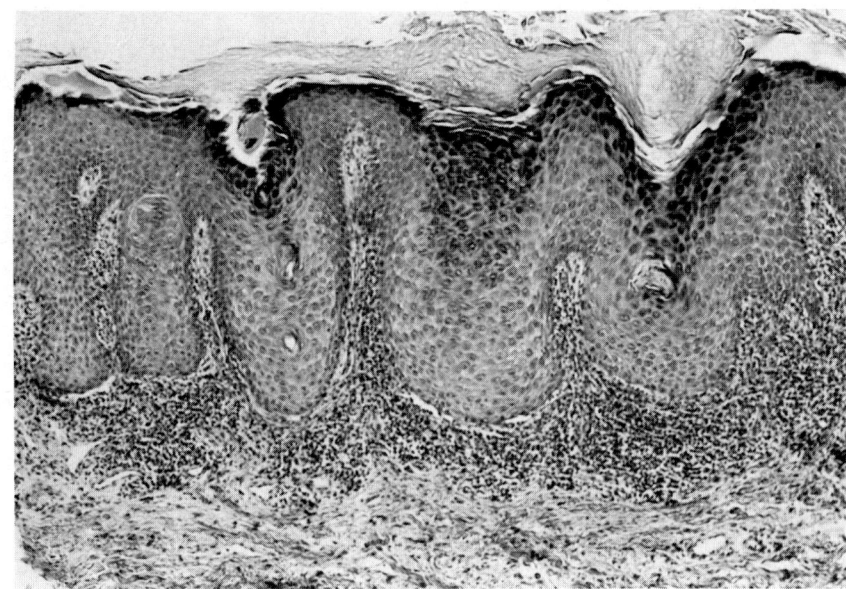

Figure 9–8.
Hypertrophic lichen planus. The infiltrate hugs the lower circumference of rete ridges, and the tips of papillae are normal. Note difference in size of epidermal cells.

Pigmented Lichen Planus, Lichen Pigmentosus, and Erythema Dyschromicum Perstans

Healing lichen planus often leaves behind a slightly atrophic, hyperpigmented skin. The pigment is melanin deposited in macrophages and resembles that found in other instances of postinflammatory pigmentation. The pigmentation may persist for many months, even in cases in which the inflammatory phase was minimal (lichen invisible pigmenté of Gougerot).[16,17] The histologic diagnosis may be approached by looking for occasional foci of basal cell

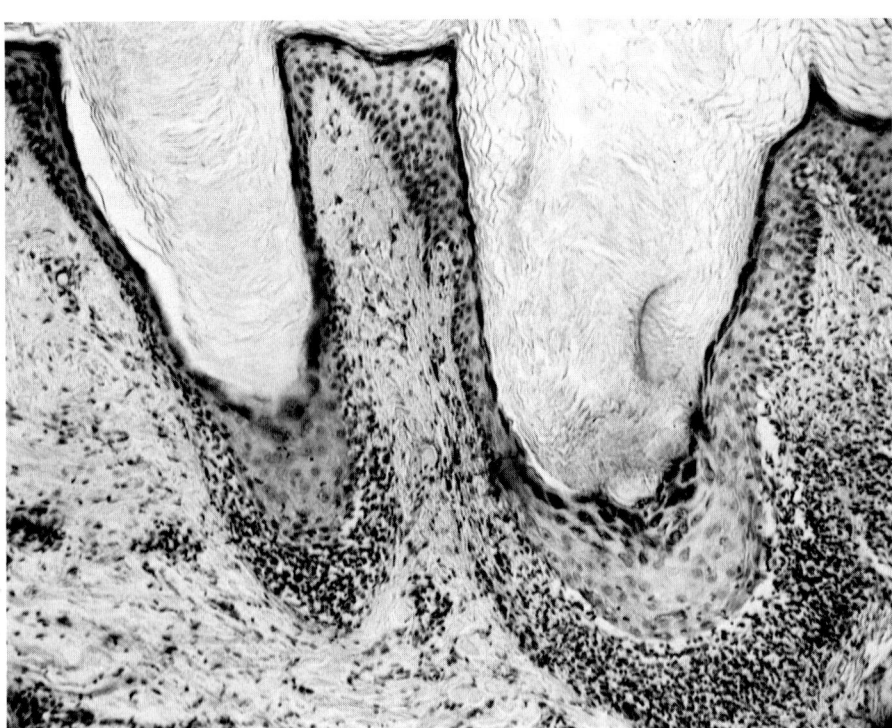

Figure 9–9.
Lichen planopilaris. Note almost normal condition of interfollicular epidermis and rounded horny plugs in cupshaped follicles. H&E. X135.

damage, loss of superficial elastic fibers, and increased vascularity.

Clinical and histologic features of healing lichen planus are simulated by two other dermatoses, *lichen pigmentosus*, as described in Japan[18] and India,[19] and *erythema dyschromicum perstans*,[20] originally identified in South America as dermatosis cenicienta.[21,22] Erythema dyschromicum perstans (Fig. 9–10) was also observed later in the United States[23] and other countries[24–26] in the form of long-standing macular pigmentation preceded clinically by a mild erythematous and scaly phase and exhibiting histologically occasional foci of basal cell damage, with associated epidermal consequences, mild round cell infiltrate, and pronounced macrophage pigmentation. We suspect,[1] on the basis of our biopsy material, that this dermatosis may be the response to some unidentified environmental noxious agent. It may occur also in light-skinned people,[27] where histologic diagnosis may become difficult because there is much less deposition of melanin in macrophages.

LICHEN PLANUS ACTINICUS

Lichen planus actinicus or tropicus (lichenoid melanodermatitis) occurs in subtropical countries.[28–30] Macular and hyperpigmented plaques appear over the light-exposed skin areas, such as face, neck, upper chest, and extremities. Circular lesions may give a false impression of central atrophy. Typical lichen planus papules may be present over the extremities

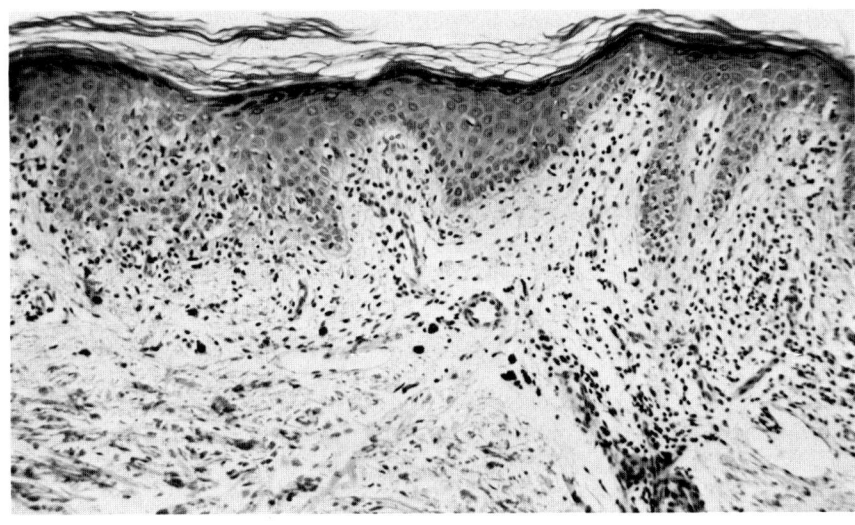

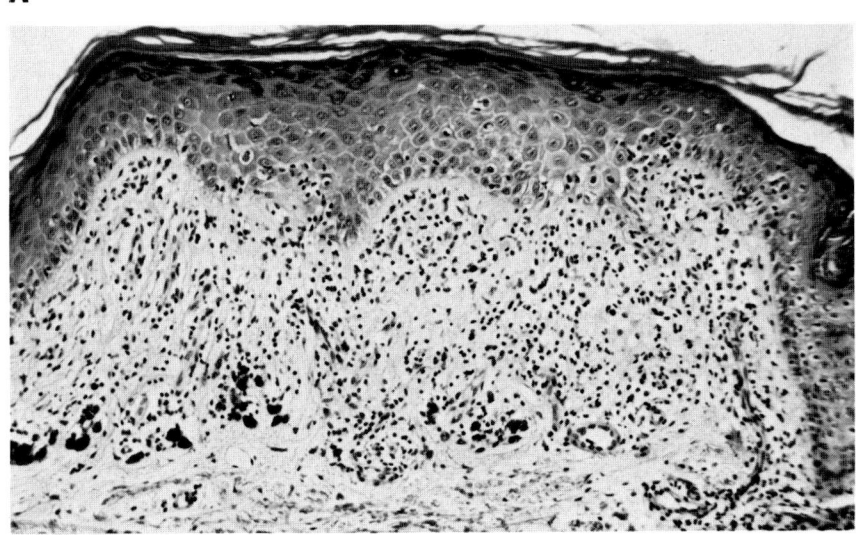

Figure 9–10.
Erythema dyschromicum perstans, as seen in a Native American. **A.** An early lesion showing poikilodermatous changes of focal basal cell degeneration in relation to spotty inflammatory infiltrate and ectasia of blood and lymph capillaries. **B.** An older stage resembling atrophying lichen planus except for the relatively thick epidermis. Note melanophages at lower border of fading infiltrate. H&E. X180.

(Fig. 9–11). Histologic findings are indistinguishable from the classic lichen planus.[31]

SOLITARY LICHEN PLANUSLIKE KERATOSIS

Another condition that occurs predominantly over the light-exposed areas of face, arms, and presternal regions is known as solitary lichen planuslike keratosis (lichenoid benign keratosis).[32] Histologically, there is marked resemblance to lichen planus with a few minor exceptions (Fig. 9–12). These include spotty parakeratosis, the presence of plasma cells and eosinophils in the superficial dermal infiltrate, and lentigo senilis-type epidermal changes at the periphery of the lesion.[33,34]

GRAFT-VS-HOST DISEASE

Graft-vs-host disease is a frequent complication of allogeneic bone marrow transplantation.[35] Erythematous maculopapular eruption shows predilection for head, neck, upper thorax, hands, and feet (Fig. 9–13). Histologic findings include vacuolar degeneration of basal cells, individual epidermal cell necrosis, superficial dermal infiltrate of T lymphocytes, and lymphoid cell exocytosis with individual or several lymphocytes associated with the necrotic keratinocytes (satellite cell necrosis).[36–38] Lip biopsy including the underlying mucous glands show similar changes.[39]

POIKILODERMA

We agree with others[40,41] that poikiloderma atrophicans vasculare is not a nosologic entity and that we should relate poikilodermatous manifestations to the underlying diseases, which include mycosis fungoides or its precursors, parapsoriasis of the plaque, lichenoid and retiform varieties, and, dermatomyositis and lupus erythematosus. In addition, poikiloderma of Civatte, the related Riehl's melanosis (melanodermatitis toxica), congenital poikiloderma of Thomson,[42] dyskeratosis congenita,[43] and two familial forms, hereditary sclerosing poikiloderma[44] and acrokeratotic poikiloderma, share certain clinical and histologic features. Pinta (Chapter 20) may have to be considered. The clinical differential diagnosis includes chronic x-ray dermatitis (Chapter 15) and erythromelanosis follicularis colli (Chapter 30). The distinctive histologic marker of all forms of this group is focal basal cell damage, so-called liquefaction degeneration, with the cascade of events that we found in the lichenoid tissue reaction, only in milder form, and spotty distribution corresponding to the clinical mottling. There is variable epidermal thickness from slight hyperplasia to definite atrophy. Epidermal pigmentation is focal, and there is macrophage pigmentation (Fig. 9–14). Spotty te-

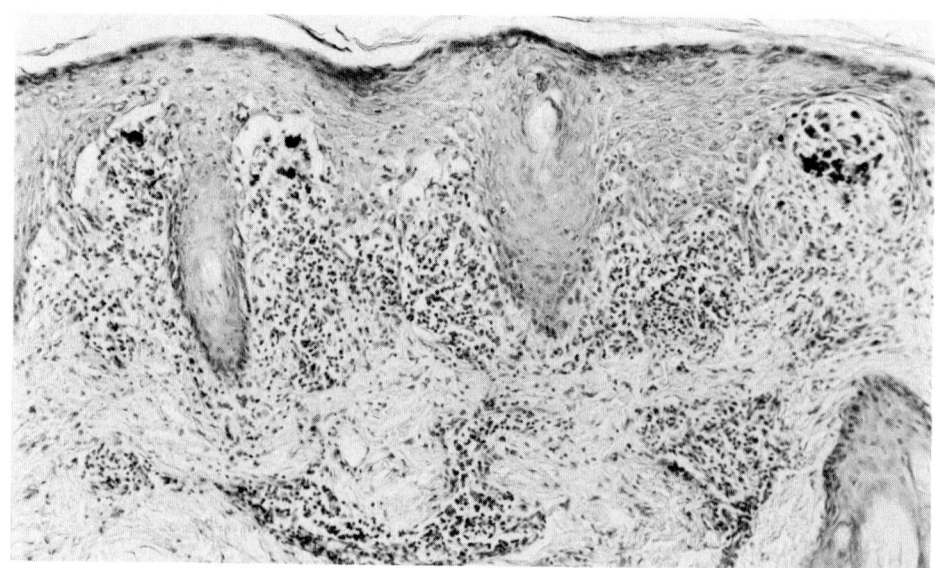

Figure 9–11.
Lichen planus actinicus. Facial plaque shows histologic changes indistinguishable from the classic lichen planus. H&E. X125.

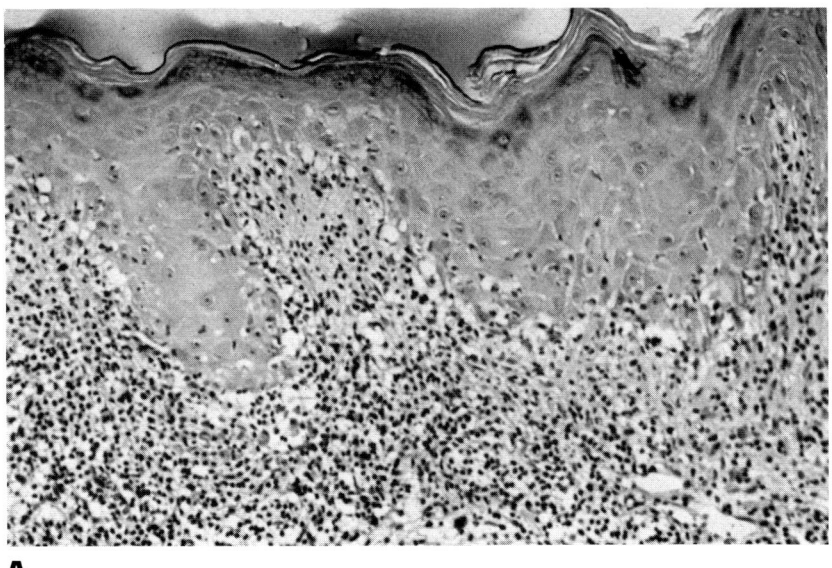

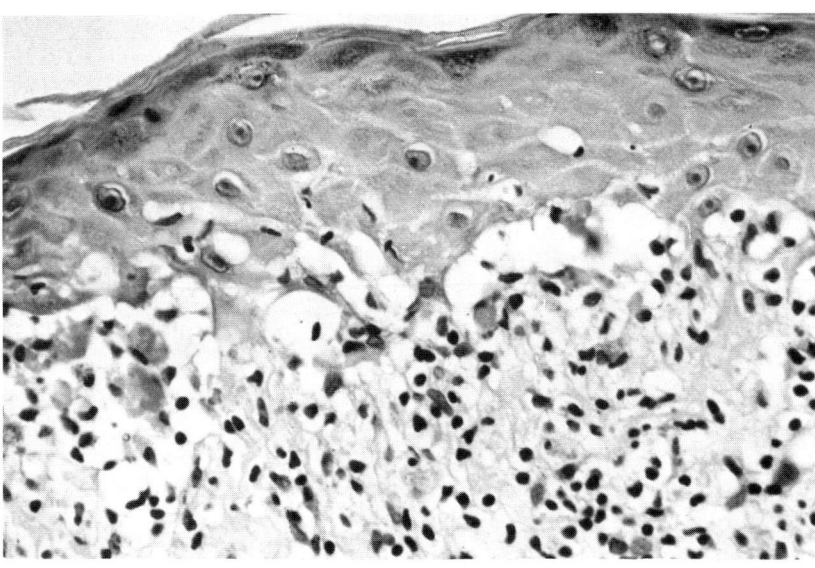

Figure 9–12.
Solitary lichen planuslike keratosis. **A.** Lichenoid tissue reaction with epidermal thickening, liquefaction degeneration of basal cells, and lymphocytic infiltrate. H&E. X180. **B.** Severe liquefaction degeneration of basal cells with formation of Civatte bodies. H&E. X225.

langiectasia and loss of superficial elastic fibers complete the picture of the poikilodermatous tissue reaction, to which the underlying dermatoses add their distinctive features. Thus, the appearances illustrated in Figures 5–12, 9–10A, 14–2, and 14–4 should evoke the thought that one is dealing with poikiloderma.

KERATOSIS LICHENOIDES CHRONICA

The condition originally described by Kaposi as *lichen ruber verrucosus et reticularis* occurs as purplish papulonodular lesions in a linear fashion over the extremities.[45,46] Scaly facial eruption, mucosal involvement, and nail changes are often present. Histologically (Fig. 9–15), epidermal acanthosis with hypergranulosis, hyperkeratosis, and liquefaction degeneration of basal cells resemble those of lichen planus. Dermal infiltrate, however, is both bandlike and perivascular and contains a number of plasma cells.[47]

LICHEN NITIDUS

The supposed nosologic relation of lichen nitidus to lichen planus is based on the fact that a very early

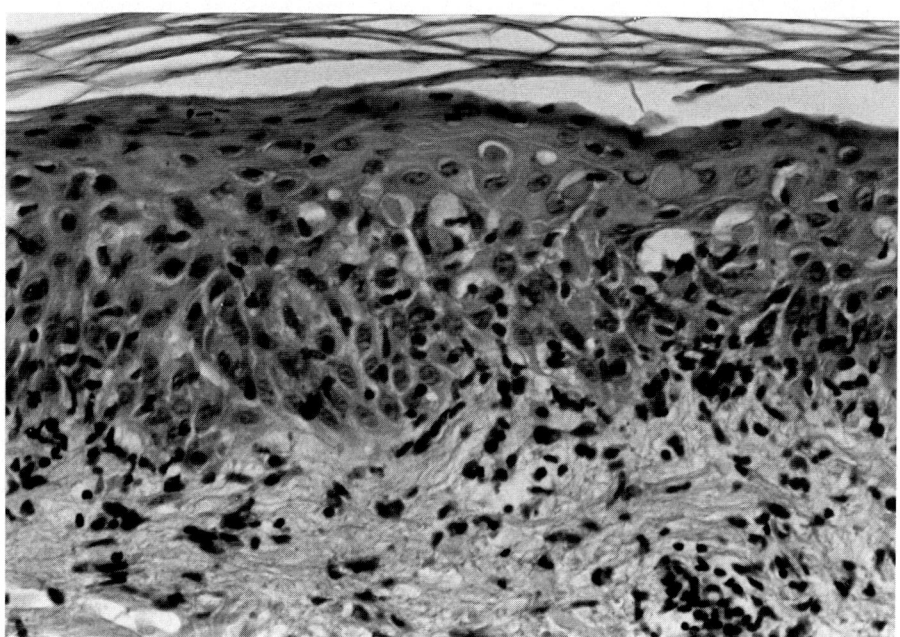

Figure 9–13.
Graft-vs-host disease shows disruption of the dermoepidermal interface with inflammatory infiltrate and scattered necrotic keratinocytes. H&E. X225.

lichen planus papule may indeed be almost indistinguishable from a lichen nitidus papule under the microscope. The lichen planus papule invariably grows and becomes confluent with others, however, to form a plaque, whereas the lichen nitidus lesion never exceeds a certain small size, and the papules retain their individuality even if closely grouped, linear, or in generalized variety.[48,49] In addition, the typical lichen nitidus papule (Fig. 9–16) has a central parakeratotic cap, often associated with a slight clinical depression of the epidermis. This feature is exaggerated in palmar lesions[50] and has considerable diagnostic significance because it is practically never found in lichen planus. The common denominator of both dermatoses appears to be damage to basal cells and melanocytes. The dermal reaction in

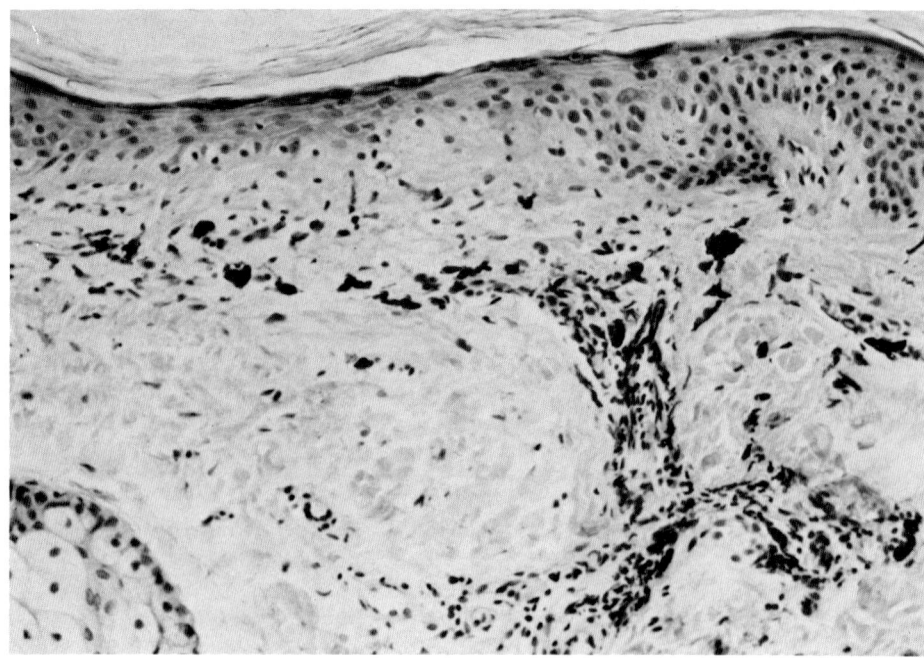

Figure 9–14.
Poikiloderma atrophicans vasculare. H&E. X285.

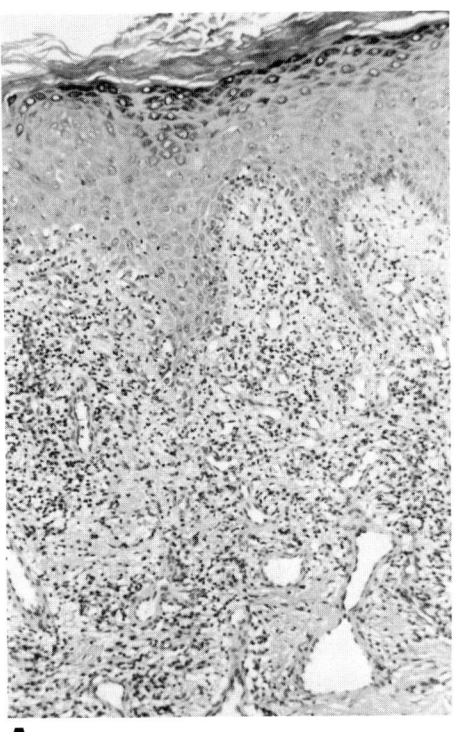 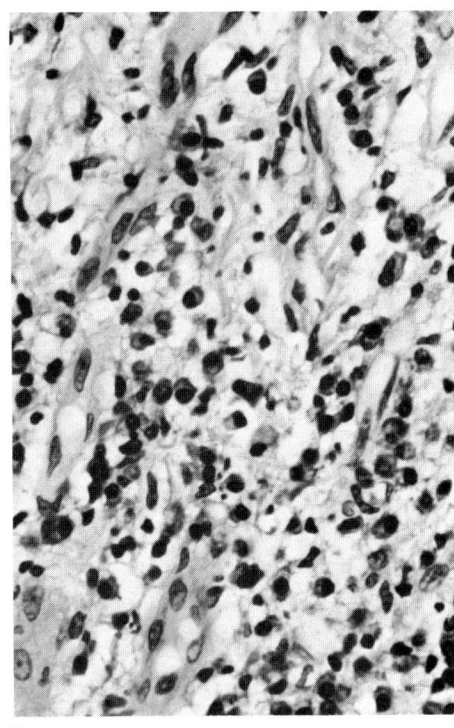

Figure 9–15.
Keratosis lichenoides chronica. **A.** Picture resembles lichen planus, but the infiltrate is not so dense. **B.** Mixed infiltrate includes many plasma cells. H&E. **A,** X125. **B,** X600.

lichen nitidus is definitely granulomatous. Often, especially in pigmented skin, it contains one or more multinucleated giant cells full of melanin. The granulomatous infiltrate is limited to a single dilated dermal papilla. In contrast to lichen planus, there are no deposits of γ-globulin.[51] The almost globular little granuloma resembles a ball pressed against the epidermis from below. The epidermis is thin, completely free of pigment, and lacks a basal layer. In the diagnostic examination for lichen nitidus, it is essential to have serial sections.

LICHENOID DRUG ERUPTIONS AND OTHER LICHENOID LESIONS

The clinical impression of a lichenoid drug eruption is often reflected histologically in hyperkeratosis of the epidermis and spotty damage to basal cells (Fig. 9–17). However, the inflammatory infiltrate usually is perivascular and lymphocytic or is mixed with a few eosinophils and does not have the specific localization and composition of lichen planus. Parakeratosis often is present, whereas it is a rare feature in lichen planus.[52,53] There are many variations of clinical manifestations and histologic findings.

A startling dermatosis was seen toward the end of World War II in men who had taken chloroquin hydrochloride (Aralen) for prolonged periods. The histologic picture of this atypical lichenoid dermatitis[54] was variable, with epidermal acanthosis and atrophy, and, in many cases, led to permanent dermal atrophy and to atrophy of sweat ducts and anhidrosis.

Lichenoid drug eruption that occurs following oral intake of antihypertensive medications (methyldopa-chlorothiazide) may show epidermotropic multinucleated giant cells.[55] Psoriasiform lesions showing the histologic picture of lichen planus have been seen after practolol intake.[56] These cases are mentioned here as a reminder that the field of lichenoid tissue reactions probably is not exhausted by the dermatoses discussed in this chapter.

Other dermatoses carrying the name of lichen have quite different histologic features. Lichen simplex is discussed under the eczematous reactions (Chapter 7), lichen sclerosus et atrophicus is dealt with in the chapter on scleroderma (Chapter 26), and lichen striatus is discussed under the papulosquamous eruptions, where pityriasis lichenoides also is found (Chapter 13). Still other lichens are listed in the index. It must be mentioned here that the histologic differential diagnosis between lichen

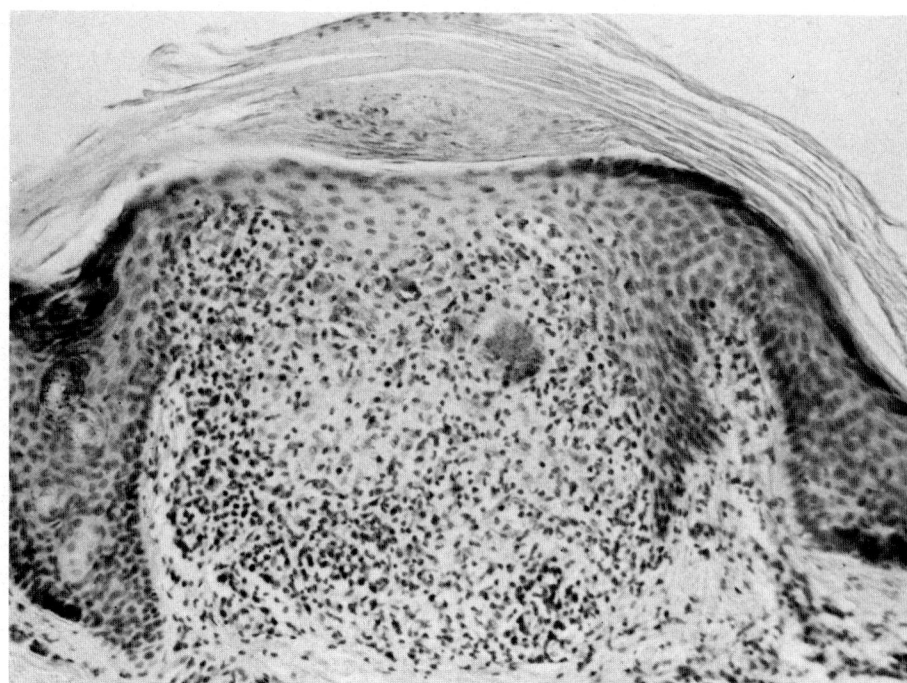

Figure 9–16.
Lichen nitidus papule in characteristic (but not universal) location close to a sweat duct. Note absence of granular layer and parakeratosis. The infiltrate appears granulomatous and contains a multinucleated giant cell. Pictures of this type suggested relationship to tuberculosis to earlier observers, a concept that is now forgotten. H&E. X180.

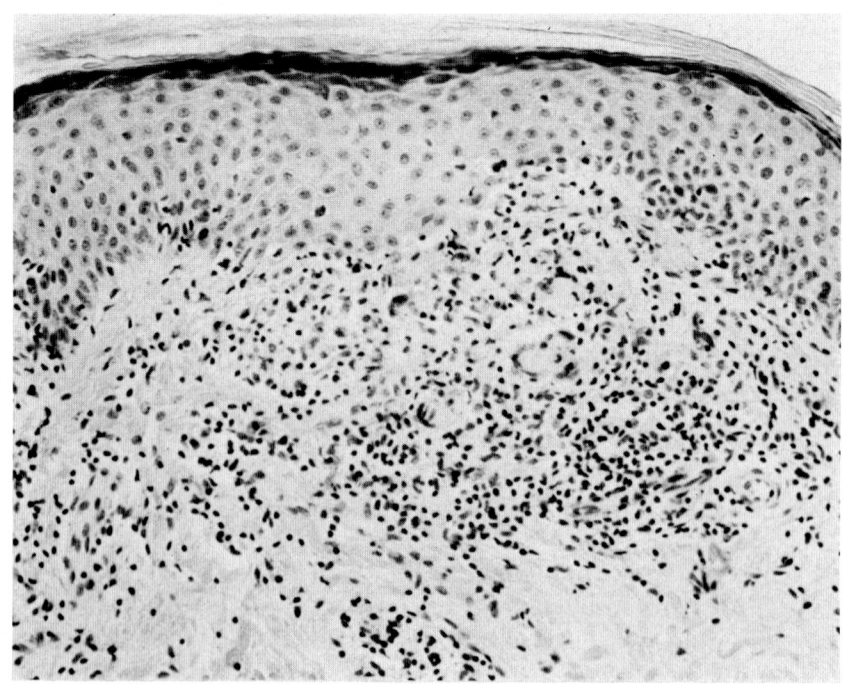

Figure 9–17.
Lichenoid eruption due to gold injections. H&E. X150.

planus and lupus erythematosus in extrafacial localization may be extremely difficult (Chapter 14) and that a lichen planuslike histologic picture may be encountered in syphilis.

REFERENCES

1. Pinkus H: Lichenoid tissue reactions. A speculative review of the clinical spectrum of epidermal basal cell damage with special reference to erythema dyschromicum perstans. Arch Dermatol 107:840, 1973
2. Comisa C: Lichen planus and related condition. In Callen JP et al (eds): Advances in Dermatology. Chicago: Year Book Med Pub, 1987, Vol. 2, 47
3. Fergus G, Winkelmann RK, Muller SA: Lichenoid dermatitis: A clinicopathologic and immunopathologic review of sixty-two cases. J Am Acad Dermatol 21:284, 1989
4. Bleicher PA, Dover JS, Arndt KA: Lichenoid dermatoses and related disorders. II. Lichen nitidus, lichen sclerosus et atrophicus, benign lichenoid keratoses, lichen aureus, pityriasis lichenoides, and keratosis lichenoides chronica. J Am Acad Dermatol 22:671, 1990
5. Ebner H, Gebhart W: Light and electron microscopic differentiation of amyloid and colloid or hyaline bodies. Br J Dermatol 92:637, 1975
6. Ebner H, Gebhart W: Epidermal changes in lichen planus. J Cutan Pathol 3:167, 1976
7. Ebner H, Gebhart W, Lassman H, Jurecka W: The epidermal cell proliferation in lichen planus. Acta Derm Venereol 57:133, 1977
8. Bullough WS: The control of epidermal thickness. Br J Dermatol 87:187, 1972
9. Bjorke JR, Krogh HK: Identification of mononuclear cells in situ in skin lesions of lichen planus. Br J Dermatol 98:605, 1978
10. Matta M, Kibbi A-G, Khattar J, et al: Lichen planopilaris: A clinicopathologic study. J Am Acad Dermatol 22:594, 1990
11. Bernardi D, Caroti A, Torregrossa F: Sindrome di Graham-Little-Piccardi-Lasseur: A proposito di due casi clinici. Chron Dermatol 17:373, 1986
12. Juliusberg F: Lichen ruber and pityriasis rubra pilaris. In Jadassohn J (ed): Handbuch der Haut- und Geschlechtskrankheiten. Berlin: Springer Verlag, 1931, Vol. 7, Part 2, p 36
13. Okochi H, Nashiro K, Tsuchida T, et al: Lichen planus pemphigoides: Case report and results of immunofluorescence and immunoelectron microscopic study. J Am Acad Dermatol 22:626, 1990
14. Mora RG, Nesbitt LT Jr, Brantley JB: Lichen planus pemphigoides: Clinical and immunofluorescent findings in four cases. J Am Acad Dermatol 8:331, 1983
15. Comisa C, Neff JC, Rossana C, Barrett JL: Bullous lichen planus: Diagnosis by direct immunofluorescence and treatment with Dapsone. J Am Acad Dermatol 14:464, 1986
16. Bologa EI, Luncan Malene G, Stroe A: Considerations cliniques, histopathologiques et histochimiques sur le lichen-plan pigmentaire d'emblée. Arch Belg Dermatol, 28:85, 1972
17. Grupper C, Buisson J, Durepaire R, et al: Lichen plan invisible de Gougerot. Bull Soc Fr Derm Syphiligr 78:598, 1972
18. Shima T: Supplementative study on lichen pigmentosus. Jpn J Dermatol Ser B 66:353, 1956
19. Bhutani LK, Bedi TR, Pandhi RK, et al: Lichen planus pigmentosus. Dermatologica 149:43, 1974
20. Convit J, Kerdel-Vegas F, Rodriguez G: Erythema dyschromicum perstans. A hitherto undescribed skin disease. J Invest Dermatol 36:457, 1961
21. Ramirez CO: Dermatosis cenicienta. Dermatología Méx 7:232, 1963
22. Navarro Jimenez BR, Sanchez Navarro LM: Dermatosis cenicienta (erithema dyschromicum perstans): Estudio prospectivo de 23 pacientes. Med Cutanea Ibero Lat Am. 16:407, 1988
23. Knox JM, Dodge BG, Freeman RG: Erythema dyschromicum perstans. Arch Dermatol 97:262, 1968
24. Holst R, Mobacken H: Erythema dyschromicum perstans (ashy dermatosis). Acta Derm Venereol 54:69, 1974
25. Phay KL, Goh CL: Erythema dyschromicum perstans/ashy dermatosis. A report of eight cases from Singapore. J Dermatol Tokyo 14:502, 1987
26. Miyagawa S, Komatsu M, Okuchi T, et al: Erythema dyschromicum perstans. Immunopathologic studies. J Am Acad Dermatol 20:882, 1989
27. Byrne DA, Berger RS: Erythema dyschromicum perstans: A report of two cases in fair-skinned patients. Acta Derm Venereol 54:65, 1974
28. El–Zawahri M: Lichen planus tropicus. Derm Int 4:92, 1965
29. Verhagen ARHB, Koten JW: Lichenoid melanodermatitis. A clinicopathological study of 51 Kenyan patients with so-called tropical lichen planus. Br J Dermatol 101:651, 1979
30. Zahaf A, Fraitag S, Sevestre H, et al: Le lichen plan actinique: Sept observations tunisiennes. Nouv Dermatol 8:317, 1989
31. Salman SM, Kibbi A-G, Zaynoun S: Actinic lichen planus. A clinicopathologic study of 16 patients. J Am Acad Dermatol 20:226, 1989
32. Berger TG, Graham JH, Goette DK: Lichenoid benign keratosis. J Am Acad Dermatol 11:635, 1984
33. Mehregan AH: Lentigo senilis and its evolutions. J Invest Dermatol 65:428, 1975
34. Barranco VP: Multiple benign lichenoid keratoses simulating photodermatoses: Evolution from senile lentigines and their spontaneous regression. J Am Acad Dermatol 13:201, 1985
35. Del Forno C, Sloane JP, Sanderson KV, et al: The histologic diagnosis of cutaneous graft versus host disease: Relationship of skin changes to marrow purg-

ing and other clinical variables. Histopathology 11: 145, 1987
36. Lever R, Turbitt M, Mackie R, et al: A prospective study of the histological changes in the skin in patients receiving bone marrow transplantation. Br J Dermatol 114:161, 1986
37. Elliott CJ, Sloane JP, Sanderson KV, et al: The histological diagnosis of cutaneous graft versus host disease: Relationship of skin changes to marrow purging and other clinical variables. Histopathology 11: 145, 1987
38. Hood AF, Vogelsang GB, Black LP, et al: Acute graft-vs-host disease. Development following autologous and syngeneic bone marrow transplantation. Arch Dermatol 123:745, 1987
39. Nakhleh RE, Miller W, Snover DC: Significance of mucosal vs salivary gland changes in lip biopsies in the diagnosis of chronic graft-vs-host disease. Arch Pathol Lab Med 113:932, 1989
40. Lever WF, Schaumbaerg-Lever G: Histopathology of the Skin. 6th ed. Philadelphia: J. B. Lippincott Co, 1983
41. Demis JD: Clinical Dermatology. Philadelphia: J. B. Lippincott Co, 1988
42. Wozniak KD, Böhm W: Zum Problem der Poikilodermia congenita Thomson. Z Hautkr 47:625, 1972
43. Nazzaro P, Argentieri R, Bassetti F, et al: Dyskératose congénitale de Zinsser–Cole–Engman, deux cas. Bull Soc Fr Derm Syphiligr 79:242, 1972
44. Greer KE, Weary PE, Nagy R, Robinow M: Hereditary sclerosing poikiloderma. Int J Dermatol 17:316, 1978
45. Mehregan AH, Heath LE, Pinkus H: Lichen ruber moniliformis and lichen ruber verrucosus et reticularis of Kaposi. J Cutan Pathol 11:1, 1984
46. Elnékavé FL, Kuffer R, Erner J et al: Kératose lichénoïde striée (KLS). Ann Dermatol Venereol 113: 959, 1986
47. Fraitag S, Oberlin P, Bourgault I, et al: Keratose lichenoide striae. Ann Dermatol Venereol 116:900, 1989
48. Prigent F, Cavalier-Balloy B, Lemarchand-Venencie F, Civatte J: Lichen nitidus lineaire. Ann Dermatol Venereol 116:814, 1989
49. Ocampo J, Torne R: Generalized lichen nitidus. Report of two cases treated with Astemizol. Int J Dermatol 28:49, 1989
50. Weiss RM, Cohen AD: Lichen nitidus of the palms and soles. Arch Dermatol 104:538, 1971
51. Waisman M, Dundon BC, Michel NB: Immunofluorescent studies in lichen nitidus. Arch Dermatol 107:200, 1973
52. Penneys NS, Ackerman AB, Gottlieb NL: Gold dermatitis: A clinical and histopathological study. Arch Dermatol 109:372, 1974
53. Van den Haute V, Antoine JL, Lachapelle JM: Histopathological discriminant criteria between lichenoid drug eruption and idiopathic lichen planus: Retrospective study on selected samples. Dermatologica 179:10, 1989
54. Alden HS, Frank LJ: Atypical lichenoid dermatitis. A drug eruption due to quinacrine hydrochloride (Atabrine). Arch Dermatol 56:13, 1947
55. Gonzales JG, Marcus MD, Santa Cruz DJ: Giant cell lichenoid dermatitis. J Am Acad Dermatol 15:87, 1986
56. Cochran RET, Thomson J, Fleming K, McQueen A: The psoriasiform eruption induced by practolol. J Cutan Pathol 2:314, 1975

10

TOXIC, ALLERGIC, AND MULTIFORM ERYTHEMAS

In clinical dermatology, the word "erythema" is attached as a diagnostic term to several manifestations, some of which are characterized only by redness, whereas others exhibit more or less pronounced swelling and induration and, in some cases, blistering. None of them, however, have scales or other evidence of primary epidermal disease. Correspondingly, in this chapter, emphasis shifts from the epidermis to the dermis, although the epidermis may show highly diagnostic alterations. Figure 10–1 illustrates morphologic rather than nosologic relations. It is grouped around a vascular reaction that includes endothelial swelling and evidence of increased vascular permeability in the form of edema and cellular exudate. The latter, as it is common in the skin, consists mainly of lymphocytes. Usually, there are at least a few eosinophils. Neutrophils may be absent or present; they predominate in Sweet syndrome. Changes of this type may be found without epidermal changes in acute and chronic urticaria and in eruptions due to drugs.

If there is morphologic evidence of leukocytoclasia, granulomatous infiltration of vessel walls, or vascular necrosis, we deal with a true vasculitis, and these phenomena are discussed in Chapter 15. This chapter is devoted mainly to urticaria and to a type of tissue reaction that finds its most complete expression in idiopathic erythema exudativum multiforme. In addition, the role of eosinophils in skin disease is considered.

URTICARIA

The wheal of *acute urticaria*, in keeping with its fleeting clinical course, is characterized mainly by dermal edema, which is difficult to recognize in paraffin sections, and by some endothelial swelling of small vessels of the superficial plexus and a few lymphocytes and eosinophils around them.[1] Somewhat more chronic lesions show predominantly lymphocytic infiltrate (Fig. 10–2). Neutrophils are present within and around the superficial capillaries in cholinergic urticaria.[2,3] In dermographism the perivascular infiltrate is largely lymphocytic.[4]

Lichen Urticatus

The tense and quickly excoriated superficial vesicle of so-called "papular urticaria," also known as "lichen urticatus," and in Europe by the picturesque and noncommittal name "strophulus," is a tissue reaction most commonly seen in young children as an allergic reaction to insect bites.[5,6] Inasmuch as the characteristic middermal reaction of ordinary insect bites (see following discussion) is absent, it would seem likely that one or few bites provoke a crop of urticated lesions as an allergic reaction in previously affected sites. Histologically, pronounced perivascular infiltrate and edema of the dermis are associated with a spongiotic epidermal vesicle

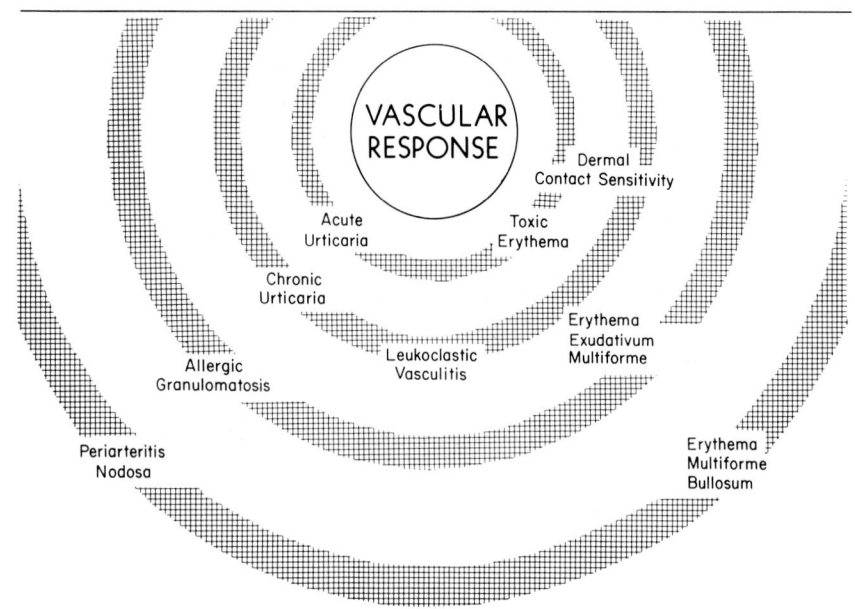

Figure 10–1.
Diagram of morphologic relations of various entities involving vascular response and vasculitis, used as a guide in differential diagnosis.

containing eosinophils in lesions that have not been excoriated. The resulting protruding papule is almost conical and strictly limited to the reacting focus (Fig. 10–3). The experimental implantation of rickettsiae in Rocky Mountain spotted fever and other manifestations of rickettsial diseases, as well as some minor viral exanthems, produces a similar reaction.

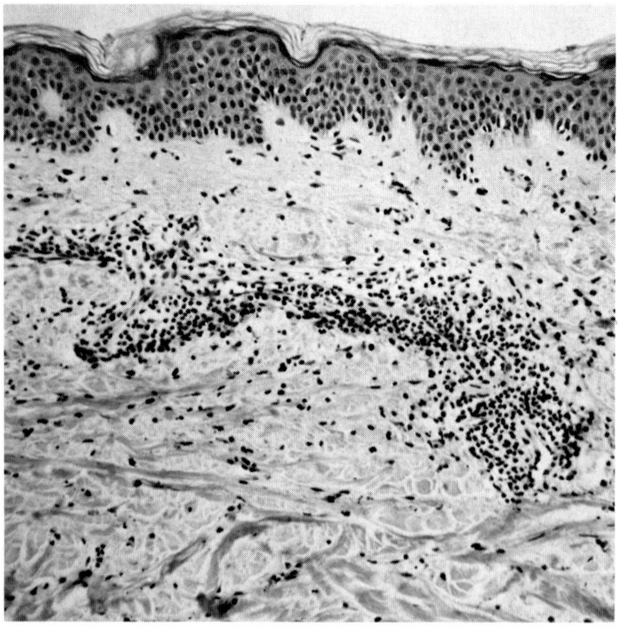

Insect Bites

The histologic hallmark of real insect (mosquito, flea) bites is a middermal center of reaction, which corresponds to the site of deposition of the toxin and may vary from plain edema to tissue necrosis surrounded by heavy perivascular infiltrate including round cells, fragmenting polymorphs, and often eosinophils.[5,6]

The epidermal changes may be minimal or may range from formation of a central spongiotic vesicle to frank epidermal necrosis. Continued epidermal and dermal necrosis at the site of tick bite can produce an eschar. Two fatal cases were reported by Walker et al.[7]

ERYTHEMA EXUDATIVUM MULTIFORME

We are dealing here with the typical Hebra type of erythema multiforme, which has sudden onset and spontaneously involutes within a few weeks.[8]

Figure 10–4 is a low-power view in which the three zones of the clinical *iris lesion* can be identified: peripheral erythema, intermediate swelling, and central bulla with epidermal necrosis. It is noteworthy that in erythema multiforme, in contrast to

Figure 10–2.
Chronic urticaria, representing purest type of reversible inflammatory vascular response of superficial plexus. H&E. X135.

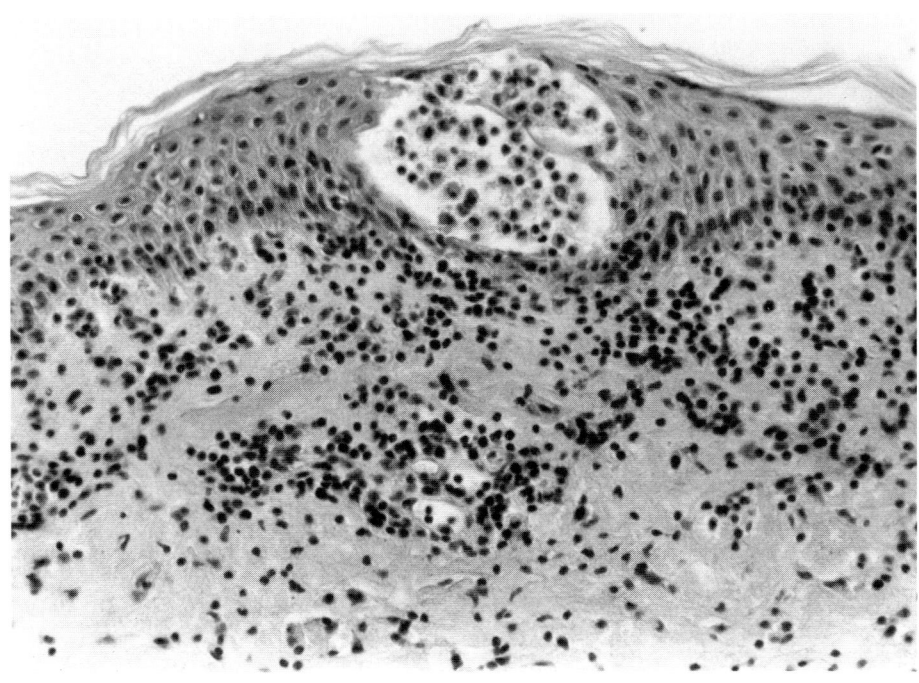

Figure 10–3.
Lichen urticatus. H&E. X185.

the punctiform changes scattered through the lesion of eczematous dermatitis and psoriasis, we are dealing with a zonal arrangement. This has to be kept in mind in the examination of a section, which preferably should come from a radial biopsy specimen, including all zones.

The earliest changes in the advancing rim of the lesion are inflammatory infiltrate around small subpapillary vessels. The infiltrate consists predominantly of T lymphocytes of helper and suppressor types and include occasional eosinophils.[9] The inflammatory changes may also affect the pars reticularis. Toward the center, as dermal edema increases, the epidermis also becomes affected by intercellular edema. This stretches all the cells vertical to the skin surface because the stream of exudate is stopped at the granular layer, which, together with the horny layer, remains unaltered.

This purely passive edema (Fig. 10–5) of the epidermis is highly characteristic. It does not lead to spongiosis and intraepidermal vesiculation. In other cases, many keratinocytes become pyknotic and even necrotic (Fig. 10–6), but there is barely any evidence of epidermal proliferation or parakeratosis.

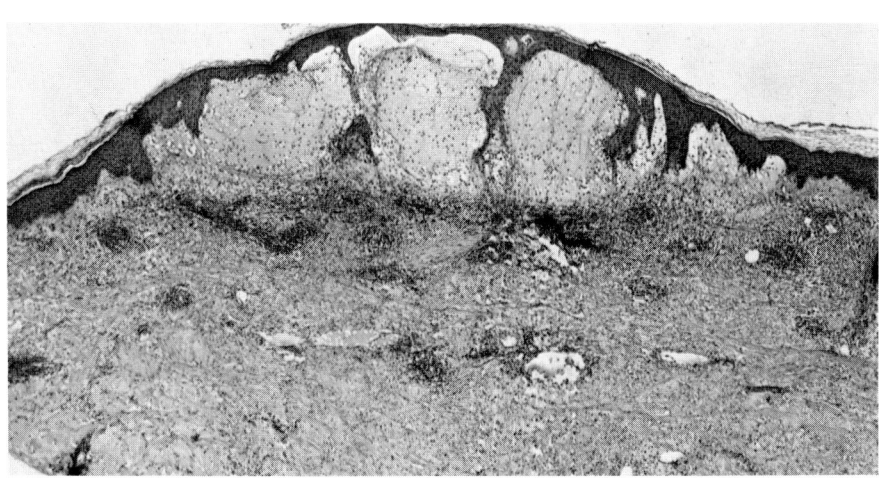

Figure 10–4.
Erythema exudativum multiforme exhibiting three concentric regions—vasodilatation (erythema), inflammatory edema, and central subepidermal vesiculation. In later stages, the center of the bulla collapses and dries, producing the clinical target lesion. H&E. X75.

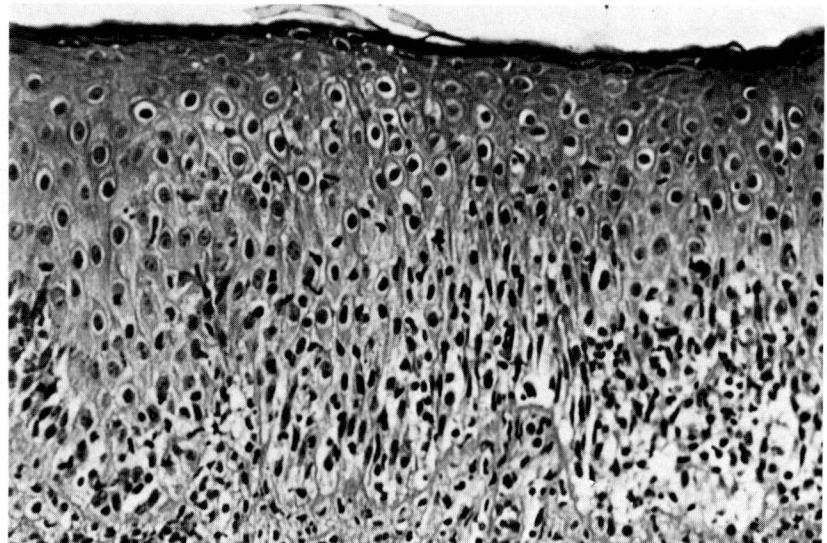

Figure 10–5.
Characteristic epidermal edema of erythema multiforme. All cells are elongated vertical to skin surface, nuclei are pyknotic, and there is intracellular and intercellular edema. Granular layer is present, and horny layer, if preserved, would be orthokeratotic. H&E. X180. (From Pinkus. Ann Allergy 12:67, 1954.)

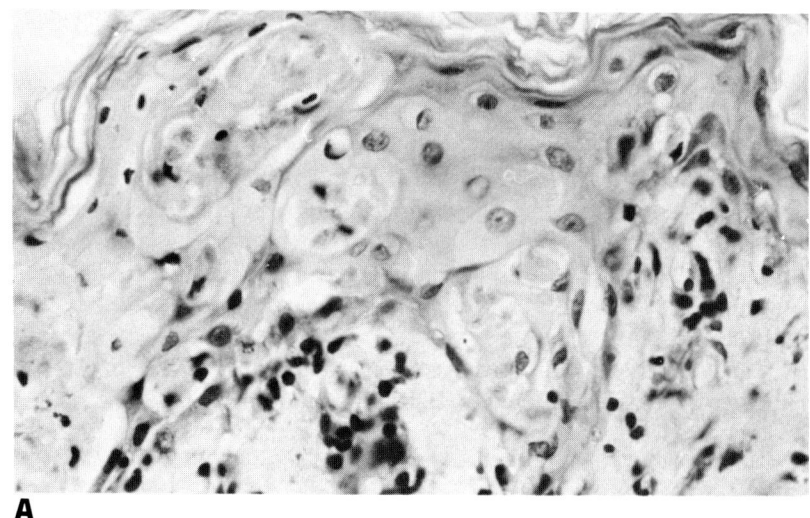

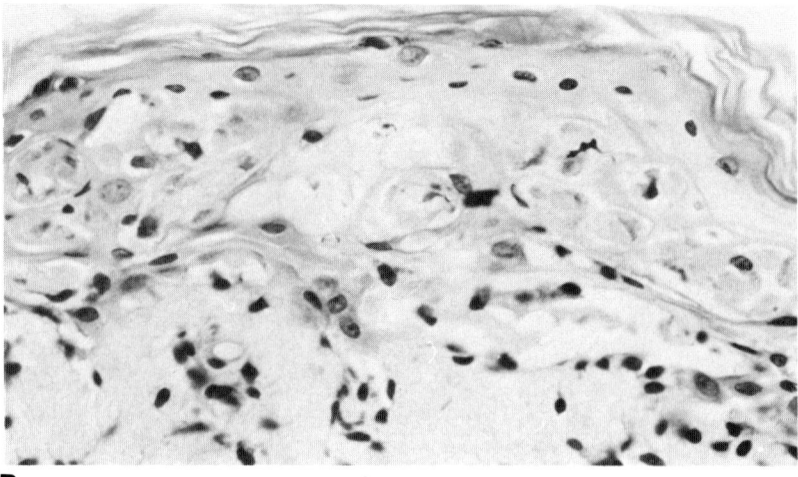

Figure 10–6.
Epidermal cell necrosis in erythema multiforme. In these cases, infiltrate in the dermis may be sparse, and the histologic picture may be similar to that of toxic epidermal necrolysis (Chap. 11). This has been called the "epidermal type" of erythema multiforme. H&E. X400.

Centrally, in the full-blown lesion, bullous edema of the papillae leads to separation between epidermis and dermis. A subepidermal bulla is formed (see Table 11–1), the roof of which consists of the entire epidermis in a state of degeneration or necrosis. Shreds of connective tissue fibers often remain attached to the lower epidermal surface. At the same time, the entire thickness of the dermis may become involved with pronounced inflammatory infiltrate, edema, and even hemorrhage. As the lesion extends, the acuteness of the process subsides in the center, the bulla collapses, and the damaged epidermis is eliminated as a necrotic or hemorrhagic crust.

The tissue reaction is similar, whether we are dealing with an idiopathic or postherpetic case of *erythema exudativum multiforme,* with a bullous drug eruption, or with a lesion secondary to systemic infection. Variations may occur in the number of eosinophils or in the severity of the inflammation. Deposition of immune complexes along the dermoepidermal junction and in the wall of small superficial vessels has been found.[10] Eosinophils may be very numerous, raising the suspicion of bullous disease (Chapter 11). Early and not very severe lesions of paravaccinia (Chapter 12) may exhibit features very similar to acute erythema multiforme in the prebullous phase. It must be understood that the bulla is the final and most severe manifestation of erythema exudativum multiforme, that not every lesion proceeds to this stage, and that a biopsy specimen of an early papule may not show a bulla. It is in these cases that epidermal edema of the type illustrated in Figure 10–5 is especially helpful in diagnosis.

Involvement of the dermoepidermal interface with individual necrotized keratinocytes, vacuolar alteration of basal cells (Fig. 10–6), and sparse lymphohistiocytic infiltrate has been emphasized as the earliest manifestation.[11,12] Others have divided erythema multiforme into dermal and epidermal types.[13] There are, no doubt, iris lesions in which inflammatory cellular infiltrate is practically absent, whereas the epidermis undergoes acute necrosis and separates from the dermis. The picture then is almost indistinguishable from the adult form of toxic epidermal necrolysis (Chapter 11).

The skin eruption in toxic shock syndrome may resemble erythema multiforme. Eosinophilic necrosis of epidermal cells is observed in association with dermal vascular changes characterized by endothelial swelling and an infiltrate of lymphocytes, histiocytes, and plasma cells.[14]

TOXIC ERYTHEMA

When a biopsy section shows superficial perivascular inflammatory changes without any appreciable epidermal involvement and without evidence of vasculitis, we prefer to label it toxic erythema as a generic morphologic diagnosis. In this group are cases of chronic urticaria (see Fig. 10–2), erythema marginatum,[15] drug eruptions (Fig. 10–7) of morbilliform, plaque, or other papular types, papular eruptions of pregnancy (Chapter 11), and the various forms of erythema perstans.[16] Histologic differentiation within this group is extremely difficult and must remain tentative, subject to clinical evaluation.

Erythema Annulare Centrifugum

Many cases of erythema annulare centrifugum (Fig. 10–8) may be identified with some confidence because the infiltrate is unusually heavy, shows coat-sleeve-type arrangement, and extends into the deeper parts of the dermis. The infiltrate may resemble Jessner's lymphocytic infiltration, or it may include a few larger mononuclear cells and require differentiation from lymphocytic-type lymphoma. Cases have been seen in infants of mothers who had lupus erythematosus.[17]

Erythema Chronicum Migrans

Erythema chronicum migrans (Lyme disease[18]) has been known in Europe for many years, but recently cases have cropped up in America. It is known to follow tick bite and can also be transferred by inoculation of involved skin. The name "Lyme disease" refers to a small Connecticut town in which many early observed patients lived. It was found that the majority of skin lesions contain spirochetes and are successfully treated with antibiotics such as penicillin, erythromycin, or ceftriaxone.[19,20]

Histologically, a superficial and deep perivascular dermal infiltrate is present, consisting mainly of lymphocytes. Eosinophils are observed in the center of the lesion. Erosion of the lower border of the epidermis and extravasation of erythrocytes may be present. Spirochetes are demonstrated by the Warthin–Starry silver stain in superficial dermis and at the dermoepidermal junction.[21]

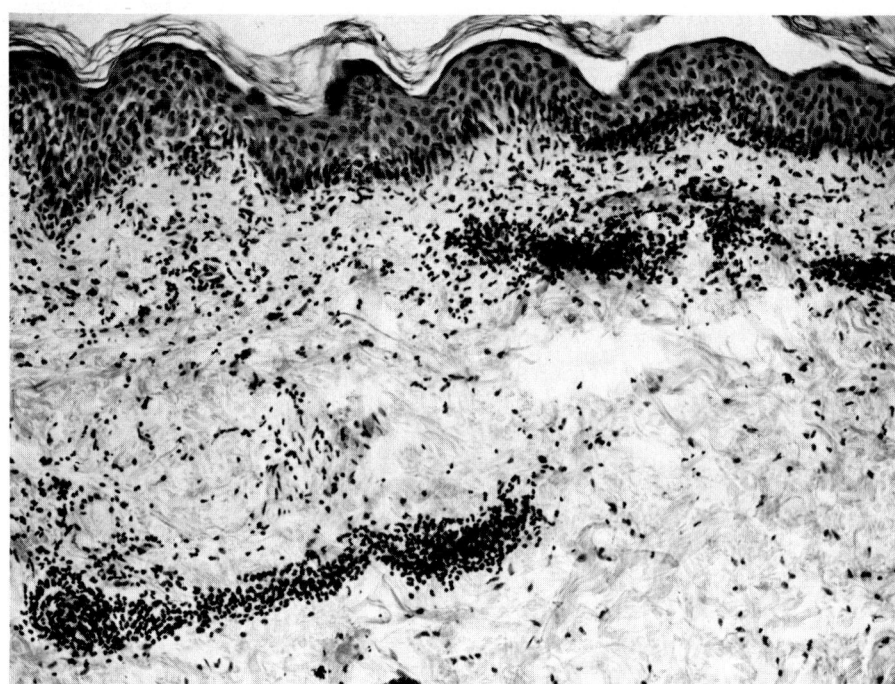

Figure 10-7.
Toxic erythema type of drug eruption. Although there is some exocytosis and mild intercellular edema in the lower epidermal layers, there is no significant epidermal reaction as in eczematous dermatitis. H&E. X135.

Erythema Gyratum Repens

The name "erythema gyratum repens" was given by Gammel[14] to an extraordinary figurate, scaling erythema that moved from day to day and disappeared after removal of a carcinoma of the breast. Approximately 83 percent of reported cases had an associated internal malignancy including lung cancer, uterine, cervical and breast carcinoma, and neoplasms of stomach, bladder, and prostate.[22]

The eruption is remarkable clinically because of its slow movement, configuration, and evidence of a scale on the subsiding border. Histologic examination has not been helpful in explaining this configuration. Mild parakeratosis is reported, in addition to variable superficial dermal infiltrate.[23] Holt and Davies[24] reported an absence of T lymphocytes and coarse granular deposits of IgG and C3 at the basement membrane. The necrolytic migratory erythema associated with carcinoma of the pancreas is discussed in Chapter 11.

Differential Diagnosis

Differential diagnosis of all forms of toxic erythema includes cases of vasculitis of the small dermal vessels (Chapter 15), papules of secondary syphilis (Chapter 21), the pigmented purpuric eruptions and some other papulosquamous dermatoses (Chapter 13), and dermal contact sensitivity reaction (Chapter 7), which itself may resemble eruptions due to photosensitivity. It is obvious that definite conclusions are extremely difficult in this field and that the histologic diagnosis of toxic erythema should be made by exclusion if no signs of more specific alterations of either epidermis, vessels, or other constituents of the dermis can be recognized. When we have settled on the diagnosis "toxic erythema," we often add "compatible with drug eruption" in order to stimulate the clinician to make a thorough search, not only for medicaments but also for the possible role of food additives and other ingested chemicals, which are not classified as drugs.

ACUTE FEBRILE NEUTROPHILIC DERMATOSIS

Dermatosis described by Sweet in 1964 is now generally accepted as a distinctive clinicopathologic entity.[25,26] Sweet syndrome is characterized by the appearance of multiple raised tender erythematous plaques or vesiculopustular lesions with superficial ulceration in a patient with fever and neutrophilia. It occurs in association with acute myelogenous leukemia or solid malignant tumors of ovary, testicle, prostate, rectum, inflammatory bowel disease, or upper respiratory infection.[27,32] Histologically, (Fig. 10-9), there is extensive dermal involvement, with

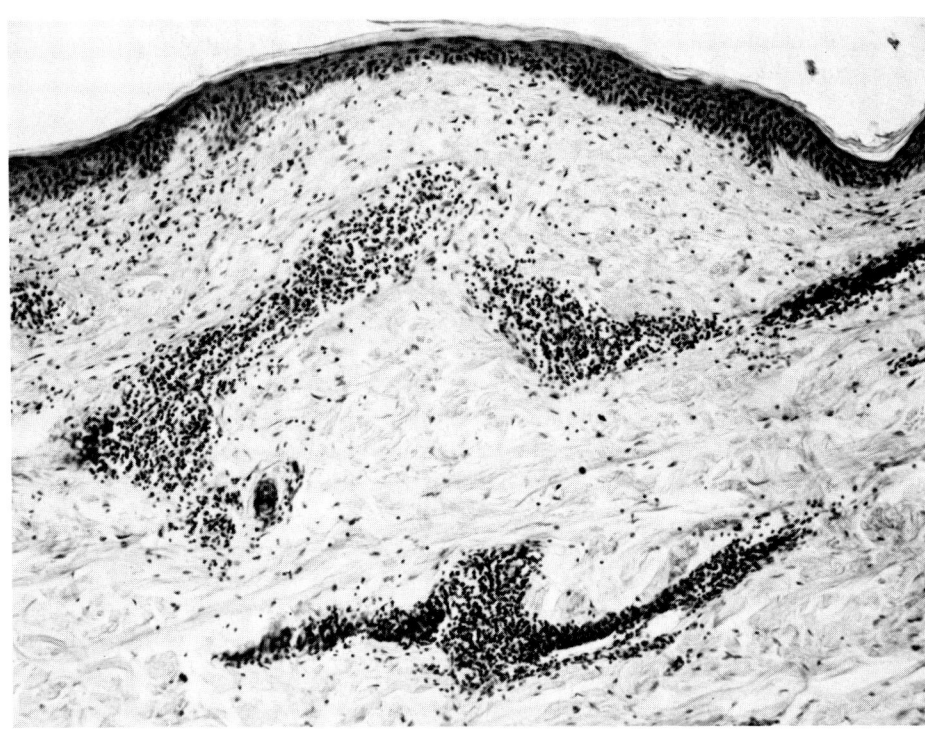

Figure 10–8.
Erythema annulare centrifugum. Infiltrate involves the deep vascular plexus. No significant epidermal changes. H&E. X135.

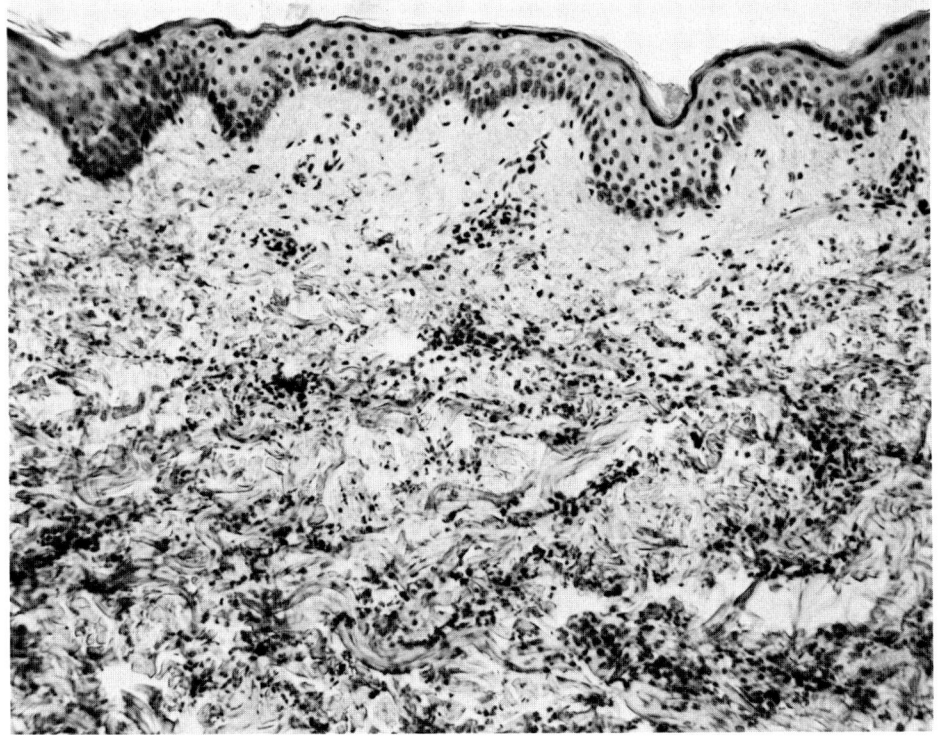

Figure 10–9.
Acute febrile neutrophilic dermatosis (Sweet). Most of the cells of the infiltrate have polymorphic nuclei. H&E. X225.

edema and heavy exudate of polymorphonuclear neutrophilic leukocytes with some nuclear dust formation.

CELLULITIS AND ERYSIPELAS

The histologic picture of Sweet syndrome may be observed in acute cellulitis and erysipelas. Extensive edema, basophilic staining of dermal connective tissue, and diffuse infiltrate of polymorphonuclear neutrophils are present. Demonstration of gram-positive cocci will confirm the diagnosis.[33] A similar picture has been reported in the erysipelas-like skin lesions of familial Mediterranean fever.[33]

EOSINOPHILIC CELLULITIS

The initial skin lesion of eosinophilic cellulitis (Wells syndrome) may be a single erythematous plaque that will extend over 1 or 2 days to cover a major portion of an extremity.[34-36] Edematous swollen plaques may be covered with superficial blisters resembling an acute cellulitis.[37] The affected area remains cool. There is no response to antibiotics. The lesions have a protracted course with recurrences occurring for several years.[38] General health of the patient is good. Peripheral eosinophilia is present in one half of the patients. In a few cases the clinical appearance suggests a tick bite reaction.[39] Histologic findings in an early lesion is characterized by diffuse edema and extensive infiltration of eosinophils involving the entire thickness of dermis and the fat tissue.[40] Later on, histiocytes appear around basophilic collagen bundles encrusted with free eosinophilic granules forming flame figures (Fig. 10–10).[41]

HYPEREOSINOPHILIC SYNDROME

The presence of eosinophils in many of the lesions discussed in this chapter makes it advisable to discuss eosinophilia in context, especially since the introduction of the hypereosinophilic syndrome and its various manifestations into the literature.[28] The occurrence of an increased eosinophil count in the peripheral blood triggers a search for allergic reactions, for intestinal parasites, and for dermatitis herpetiformis by the classically trained physician. The finding of eosinophils in tissue sections should stimulate suspicion of entities other than those mentioned in this chapter. It is known that intraepidermal vesicles in the newborn often carry eosinophils. Urticaria pigmentosa develops eosinophilia after stroking. Eosinophilic spongiosis may be found in pemphigus. In granulomatous inflammation, eosinophils take on special significance. Kimura's disease or angiolymphoid hyperplasia with eosinophilia comes to mind. Scabies and tick bites often are rich in eosinophils. Thus, eosinophils in blood or tissues are a warning signal that should be carefully evaluated and correlated with other pathologic and clinical signs.

The hypereosinophilic syndrome is diagnosed when all other possibilities are eliminated and in the presence of eosinophil counts of over 1.5×10^9 (hypereosinophilia).[42,43] The skin manifestations are associated with signs of multiple internal organ involvements and range from urticarial eruption to maculopapular plaques involving trunk and extremities.[44,45] Histologically, there is endothelial thickening of dermal vessels and infiltration of eosinophils.

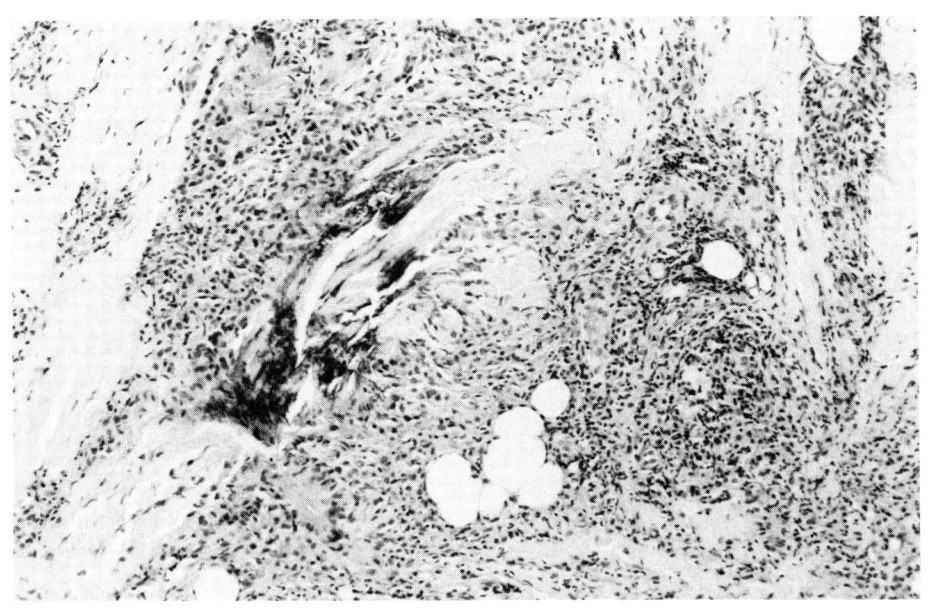

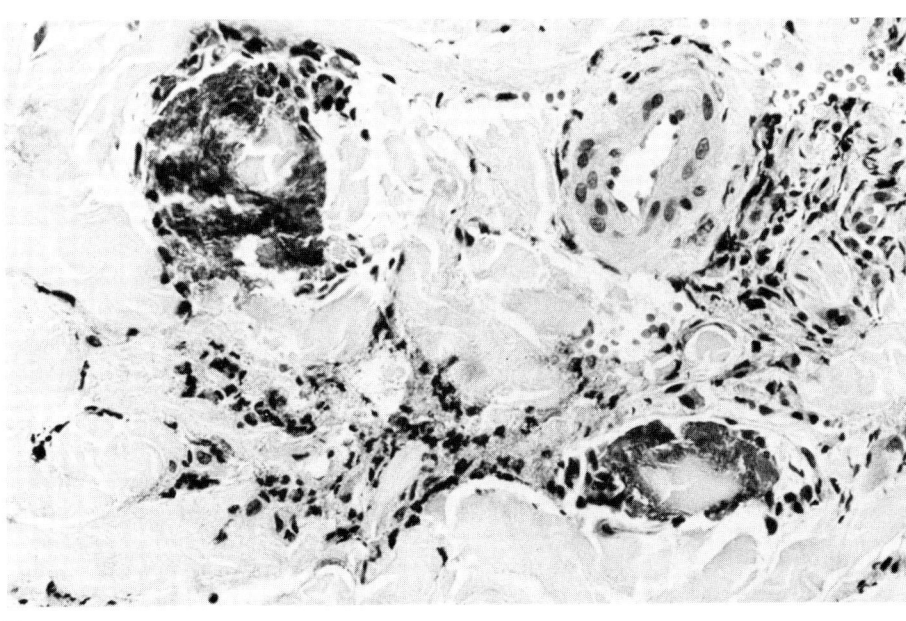

Figure 10–10.
Eosinophilic cellulitis (Wells) shows extensive dermal infiltrate of histiocytes and eosinophils. Flame figures consist of collagen bundles encrusted with free eosinophilic granules. H&E. **A,** X225, **B,** X400. (Courtesy of Dr. J. B. Stern.)

REFERENCES

1. Boonk WJ, Nieboer C, Huijgens PC: Pathogenetic studies in chronic urticaria. Failure to demonstrate vasculitis, complement activation and fibrinolysis. Dermatologica 173:264, 1986
2. Peters MS, Winkelmann RK: Neutrophilic urticaria. Br J Dermatol 113:25, 1985
3. Hirschmann JV, Lawlor F, English JSC, et al: Cholinergic urticaria. A clinical and histologic study. Arch Dermatol 123:462, 1987
4. Winkelmann RK: The histology and immunopathology of dermographism. J Cutan Pathol 12:486, 1985
5. Shaffer F, Jacobson C, Beerman H: Histopathologic correlation of lesions of papular urticaria and positive skin test reactions to insect antigens. Arch Dermatol 70:437, 1954
6. Bazex A, Bazex J, Broussy F, Balas D: Étude anatomopathologique optique et ultra-structurale des papules de prurigo strophulus en phase de début. Bull Soc Fr Derm Syphilgr 82:369, 1975
7. Walker DH, Gay RM, Valdes-Depena M: The occurrence of eschars in Rocky Mountain spotted fever. J Am Assoc Dermatol 4:571, 1981
8. Goldberg GN: Erythema multiforme. Controversies and recent advances. In Callen JP, et al (eds): Advances in Dermatology. Chicago: Year Book Medical Publishers, 1987, Vol 2, p 73
9. Zaim MT, Giorno RC, Golitz LE et al: An immunopathological study of herpes associated erythema multiforme. J Cutan Pathol 14:257, 1987
10. Howland WW, Golitz LE, Weston WL, Huff JC: Erythema multiforme: Clinical, histopathologic, and immunologic study. J Am Acad Dermatol 10:438, 1984
11. Ackerman AB, Penneys NS, Clark WH: Erythema multiforme exudativum: Distinctive pathological process. Br J Dermatol 84:554, 1971
12. Reed RJ: Erythema multiforme. A clinical syndrome and a histologic complex. Am J Dermatopathol 7:143, 1985
13. Orfanos CE, Schaumburg-Lever G, Lever WF: Dermal and epidermal types of erythema multiforme. Arch Dermatol 109:682, 1974
14. Vuzevski VD, Van Joost Th, Wagenvoort JHT, Michiels Dey JJ: Cutaneous pathology in toxic shock syndrome. Int J Dermatol 28:94, 1989
15. Brauner GJ, Mihm MC Jr, Des Groseilliers JP: Erythema marginatum in streptococcal endocarditis without rheumatic heart disease. Cutis 12:206, 1973
16. Ellis F, Friedman AA: Erythema annulare centrifugum (Darier's). Arch Dermatol 70:496, 1954
17. Hammar H, Rönnerfält L: Annular erythemas in infants associated with autoimmune disorders in their mothers. Dermatologica 154:115, 1977
18. Krafchik B: Lyme disease. Int J Dermatol 28:71, 1989
19. Berger BW, Clemmensen OJ, Ackerman AB: Lyme disease is a spirochetosis. A review of the disease and evidence for its cause. Am J Dermatopathol 5:111, 1983
20. Dattwyler RJ, Halperin JJ, Volkman BJ: Treatment of late Lyme borreliosis-randomized comparison of ceftriaxone and penicillin. Lancet 1:1191, 1988
21. Waldo ED, Sidhn SS: The spirochete in erythema chronicum migrans. Demonstration by light and electron microscopy. Am J Dermatopathol 5:125, 1983
22. Appell ML, Ward WQ, Tyring SK: Erythema gyratum repens, a cutaneous marker of malignancy. Cancer 62:548, 1988
23. Levy-Klotz B, Janier M, Cavalier-Balloy B, et al: Erythema gyratum repens. Ann Dermatol Venereol 114:1428, 1987
24. Holt PJA, Davies MG: Erythema gyratum repens—An immunologically mediated dermatosis? Br J Dermatol 96:343, 1977
25. Sweet RD: An acute febrile neutrophilic dermatosis. Br J Dermatol 76:349, 1964
26. Jordaan FH: Acute febrile neutrophilic dermatosis. A histopathological study of 37 patients and a review of the literature. Am J Dermatopathol 11:99, 1989
27. Gisser SD: Acute febrile neutrophilic dermatosis (Sweet's Syndrome) in a patient with hairy-cell leukemia. Am J Dermatopathol 5:283, 1983
28. Cooper PH, Innes DJ Jr, Greer KE: Acute febrile neutrophilic dermatosis (Sweet's syndrome) and myeloproliferative disorders. Cancer 51:518, 1983
29. Hazen PG, Kark EC, Davis BR, et al: Acute febrile neutrophilic dermatosis in children. Arch Dermatol 119:998, 1983
30. Elsner P, Hartmann AA, Lechner W: Sweet's syndrome associated with Yersinia enterocolitica infection. Dermatologica 173:85, 1986
31. Cohen PR, Kurzrock R: Sweet's syndrome and malignancy. Am J Med 82:1220, 1987
32. Kemmett D, Hunter JAA: Sweet's syndrome: A clinicopathologic review of twenty-nine cases. J Am Acad Dermatol 23:503, 1990
33. Azizi E, Fisher BK: Cutaneous manifestations of familial Mediterranean fever. Arch Dermatol 112:364, 1976
34. Wells GC, Smith NP: Eosinophilic cellulitis. Br J Dermatol 100:101, 1979
35. Fisher GB, Greer KE, Cooper PH: Eosinophilic cellulitis (Wells' syndrome). Int J Dermatol 24:101, 1985
36. Aberer W, Konrad K, Wolff K: Wells' syndrome is a distinctive disease entity and not a histologic diagnosis. J Am Acad Dermatol 18:105, 1988
37. Correia S, Garcia E, Silva L: Sindroma de Wells infantil. Med Cutanea Ibero Lat Am. 16:221, 1988
38. Dijkstra JWE, Bergfeld WF, Steck WD, Tuthill RJ: Eosinophilic cellulitis associated with urticaria. A report of two cases. J Am Acad Dermatol 14:32, 1986
39. Schorr WF, Tauscheck L, Dickson KB, Melski JW: Eosinophilic cellulitis (Wells' syndrome): Histologic and clinical features in arthropod bite reactions. J Am Acad Dermatol 11:1043, 1984
40. Ferrier MC, Janin-Mercier A, Souteyrand P, et al: Eosinophilic cellulitis (Wells' syndrome): Ultrastruc-

tural study of a case with circulating immune complexes. Dermatologica 176:299, 1988
41. Stern JB, Sobel HJ, Rotchford JP: Wells' syndrome: Is there collagen damage in the flame figures? J Cutan Pathol 11:501, 1984
42. Spry CJF: The hypereosinophilic syndrome: Clinical features, laboratory findings and treatment. Allergy 37:539, 1982
43. Van den Hoogenband HM: Skin lesions as the first manifestation of the hypereosinophilic syndrome. Clin Exp Dermatol 7:267, 1982
44. Elnekave FL, Calvo F, Erner J, et al: Manifestations cutanees d'un syndrome hypereosinophile. Ann Dermatol Venereol 113:961, 1986
45. Prost C, Schnitzler L, Perroud AM, et al: Syndrome hypereosinophilique: Etude ultrastructurale des manifestations cutanees. Ann Dermatol Venereol 110:761, 1983

11

VESICULAR AND BULLOUS DISEASES

The skin can produce vesicles and bullae from many different causes, by many different mechanisms, and in all the different layers from the stratum corneum of the epidermis to the stratum papillare of the dermis. The various possibilities are listed in Table 11-1.

Some types of blistering were discussed under eczematous, psoriasiform, lichenoid, and erythematous tissue reactions. Others are taken up in Chapters 12, 29, 30, and 46. In this chapter, we deal mainly with the histopathologic features of pemphigus vulgaris, bullous pemphigoid, dermatitis herpetiformis, their variants, and some other disorders in which the formation of vesicles or bullae is the outstanding characteristic.

Epidermal cells, when isolated from their neighbors, quickly acquire smooth contours, and desmosomes disappear. We now know that desmosomes split in acantholytic disease, whereas the joint remains temporarily intact and cells become motile as a result of breaks in the plasma membrane in certain types of injury, such as tape stripping, and perhaps in other dermatoses. Moreover, serum of pemphigus patients contains antibodies directed against complexes that contain polypeptides found in adhering junctions,[1] although these are not present in other diseases, such as subcorneal pustular dermatosis, in which acantholytic cells may occur. The presence of antibasement-membrane antibody in patients with bullous pemphigoid correlates well with the light microscopic impression of a clean separation at this level and adds a welcome tool to the differential diagnosis of erythema multiforme and dermatitis herpetiformis in which such antibodies have not been found. Finding and identifying deposits of immunoglobulins and factors of complement at the basement membrane have become helpful procedures. These are covered extensively in Chapter 4.

ACANTHOLYTIC DISORDERS

Although acantholysis is also a basic feature in Hailey–Hailey's and Darier's diseases, these are discussed in Chapter 29 as inborn errors of epidermal metabolism, and we concentrate here on pemphigus vulgaris and its relatives. Of these, pemphigus vegetans is the closest kin, and pemphigus foliaceus and pemphigus erythematosus, owing to the higher level at which acantholysis occurs, seem to form a separate group histologically as well as clinically. Acrodermatitis enteropathica is mentioned in differential diagnosis.

Pemphigus Vulgaris

Vesiculation in pemphigus is intraepidermal and usually suprabasal.[1] In contrast to the spongiotic edema of eczematous dermatitis, which eventually

TABLE 11-1. VESICULOBULLOUS ERUPTIONS

Diagnosis	Level of Separation	Characteristics of Epidermis	Histomechanism	Prevalent Inflammatory Cells
Eczematous dermatitis	Prickle layer	Spongiosis	Intercellular edema	Lymphocytes and PMNs
Impetigo	Subcorneal	Mild edema	Exocytosis	PMNs
Subcorneal pustular dermatosis	Subcorneal	Acantholysis, minimal	Exocytosis	PMNs
Pustulosis palmaris et plantaris	Subcorneal	Compressed below bulla	Exocytosis and transmalpighian exudate	PMNs and lymphocytes
Psoriasiform eruptions	Suprapapillary	Spongiform pustule, microabscess	Squirting papilla	PMNs in epidermis, lymphocytes in dermis
Impetigo herpetiformis	Suprapapillary	Spongiform pustule, microabscess	Suprapapillary exudate and acantholysis	PMNs, lymphocytes
Benign familial pemphigus	Suprabasal	Intraepidermal lacunae and budding ridges	Acantholysis	Lymphocytes
Pemphigus vulgaris	Suprabasal	Intraepidermal bulla	Acantholysis	Lymphocytes, some eosinophils
Pemphigus vegetans	Suprabasal, extending into hair follicles	Vegetating hyperplasia, clefts	Acantholysis	Lymphocytes, plasma cells, eosinophils
Pemphigus foliaceus	Subgranular or intragranular	Intraepidermal clefts	Acantholysis	Lymphocytes, some eosinophils
Acrodermatitis enteropathica	Suprabasal or higher	Acanthosis, partial necrosis, parakeratosis	Derangement of lipid metabolism, zinc deficiency	Mixed
Pemphigoid, bullous	Subepidermal	Complete and viable	Junctional separation	Lymphocytes, eosinophils, PMNs
Pemphigoid, cicatricial	Subepidermal	Viable	Junctional separation	Granulation tissue
Dermatitis herpetiformis	Subepidermal	Complete and viable or basal cell necrosis	Papillary necrosis, junctional separation	PMNs, lymphocytes, eosinophils
Chronic bullous dermatosis of childhood	Subepidermal	Viable	Junctional separation	Mixed
Herpes gestationis	Intradermal	Necrosis of basal cells	Papillary edema, HG factor	Mixed, eosinophils
Erythema multiforme	Intradermal	Primary or secondary necrosis	Bullous papillary edema, focal malpighian necrosis	PMNs, lymphocytes
Toxic epidermal necrolysis (TEN), infantile	Intraepidermal	Necrosis of upper half	Staphylococcal toxin	Minimal
TEN, adult type	Subepidermal	Complete necrosis	Drug sensitivity or unknown	Minimal
Porphyria cutanea tarda	Subepidermal	Complete and viable	Junctional separation with persistent papillae	Minimal
Epidermolysis bullosa simplex	Subepidermal	Viable above basal layer	Basal cell edema and necrosis	Mild
Epidermolysis dystrophica	Intradermal	Viable	Absence of anchoring fibrils	Variable
Glucagonoma syndrome	Upper epidermal layers	Acanthotic, parakeratotic	Degeneration of upper prickle cells	Polymorphs, mixed
Intranuclear viruses	Prickle layer	Necrotizing, multinucleated giant cells	Reticulating and ballooning degeneration	Mild to severe, lymphocytes, PMNs
Cytoplasmic viruses	Prickle layer	Degenerating	Cellular edema and death	Lymphocytes, PMNs
Bullous incontinentia pigmenti	Prickle layer	Often acanthotic	Toxic?	Eosinophils
Epidermolytic hyperkeratosis	Granular layer	Hyperplastic	Granular cell rupture	Absent
Burn blisters	Subepidermal	Necrotic	Death of epidermis and dermis	Inconspicuous

leads to the rupture of intercellular bridges, and also in contrast to the reticulating degeneration of infected epidermal cells in viral diseases, the bulla of pemphigus results from primary acantholytic separation between keratinocytes above the basal layer. The early stage can be seen under the light microscope as a cleft between basal layer and lower prickle cells and between the latter (Fig. 11–1). Most patients with pemphigus vulgaris demonstrate IgG autoantibodies directed against an antigen located on the surface of keratinocytes.[2] Electron microscopic observations suggest that the intercellular cement is affected and that desmosomes split before they disappear. Fluid accumulates in the clefts thus created, and the acantholytic cells lie in the bulla like grains of sand. They show peculiar degenerative processes (Fig. 11–2), expressed in a washed-out appearance of the nucleus and a basophilic outer rim of the cytoplasm. Inflammatory infiltrate of moderate amount is usually present in the upper dermis. It is made up of lymphocytes[3] with variable, but usually small, numbers of eosinophils.

The roof of the bulla consists of the fairly intact upper layers of the epidermis, the base of the isolated basal layer, often presenting the appearance of a row of tombstones (Figs. 11–3 and 46–4), still adherent to the dermis. It is important to biopsy early blisters, preferably not older than 24 hours, because later lesions may show too much degeneration of the roof and disintegration of the base or, on the other hand, beginning reepithelization. It is the acantholytic prickle cells and the residual basal cells that are obtained by the Tzanck procedure and are seen in the stained smear (see Fig. 11–2 inset).

Pemphigus Vegetans

Acantholysis in pemphigus vegetans usually is suprabasal as in pemphigus vulgaris but becomes very extensive and often descends deep into hair follicles. Simultaneously, the epidermis becomes thickened and papillomatous, and a heavy inflammatory infiltrate develops, characterized by a high percentage of plasma cells in addition to lymphocytes and often by eosinophils that may form intraepithelial microabscesses.[4] Bullae often are not formed, and the histologic picture (Fig. 11–3) reflects the mushy vegetations seen clinically.

Pemphigus Foliaceus, Pemphigus Erythematosus

The acantholytic cleft usually forms in higher strata, often in the granular layer (Fig. 11–4), in pemphigus foliaceus and the closely related pemphigus erythematosus. Thus, there is no coherent roof to form a bulla, the amount of exudate is usually less, and a greater thickness of viable epidermis is preserved to protect the dermis (Fig. 11–5). If the acantholytic process repeats itself at short intervals, the multiple foliations of this type of pemphigus result. Antibodies reacting with the higher epidermal layers were demonstrated in the sera of patients.[5,6]

Fogo Selvagem

The endemic Brazilian pemphigus (fogo selvagem) has been called identical with pemphigus foliaceus[7] or has been attributed to a virus. Histologic studies

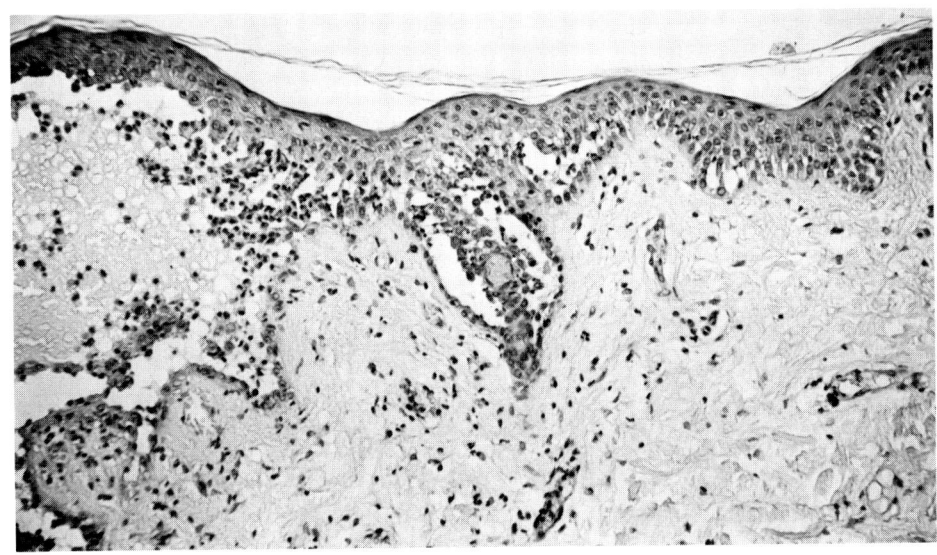

Figure 11–1.
Pemphigus vulgaris, edge of bulla. Note acantholysis extending along a sweat duct. H&E. X135.

160 SUPERFICIAL INFLAMMATORY PROCESSES

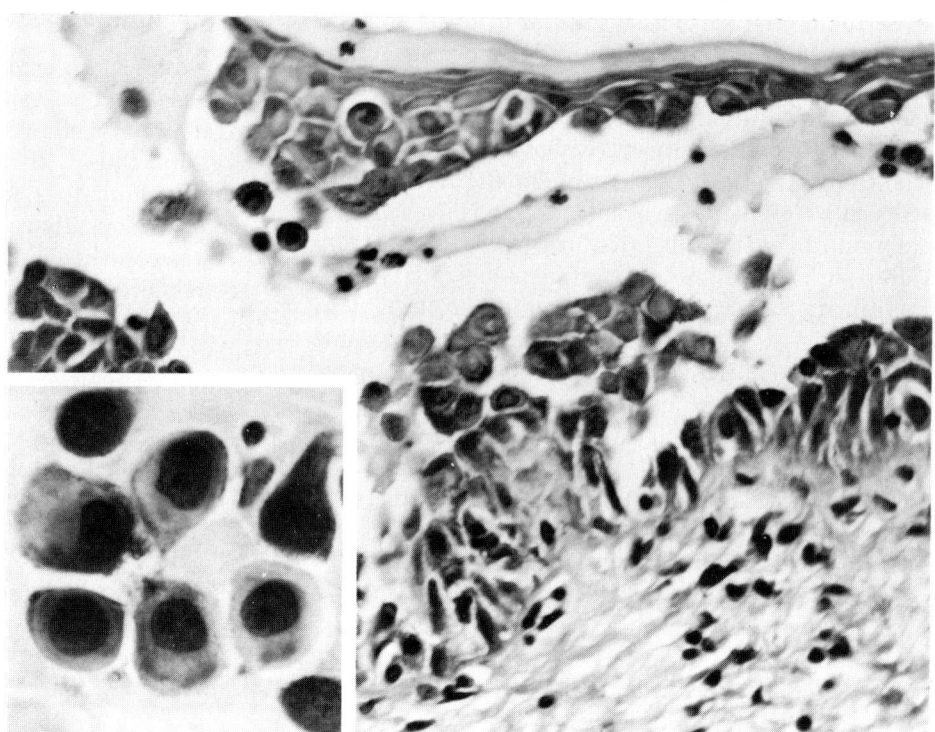

Figure 11–2.
Acantholytic cells in pemphigus vulgaris, in section. H&E. X465. Inset shows Tzanck smear. Wright stain. X800.

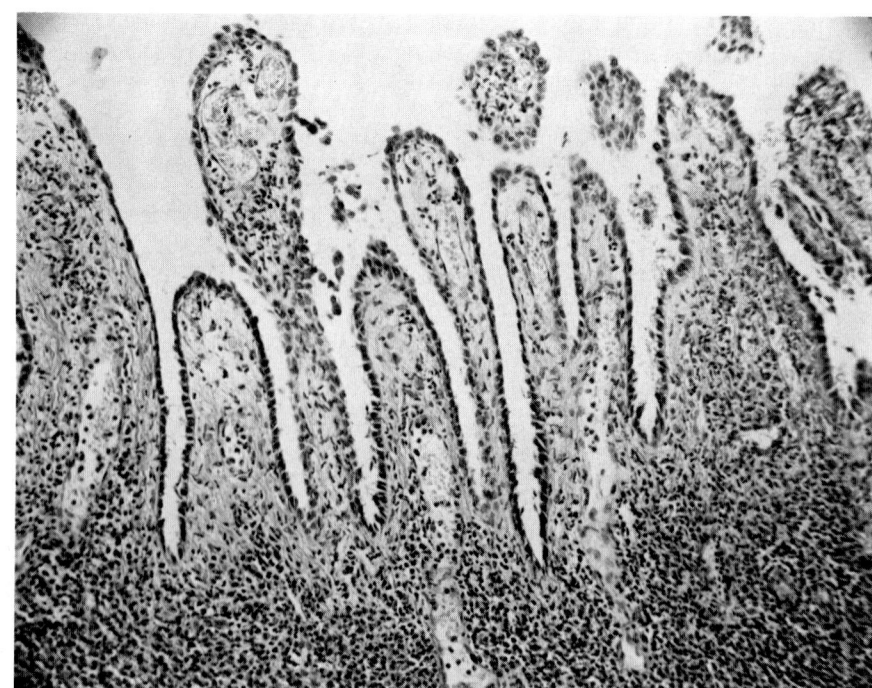

Figure 11–3.
Pemphigus vegetans. Upper layers of papillomatous epidermis are completely lost; some acantholytic cells are preserved. Basal layer shows tombstone pattern. Dense infiltrate of round and plasma cells in dermis. H&E. X135.

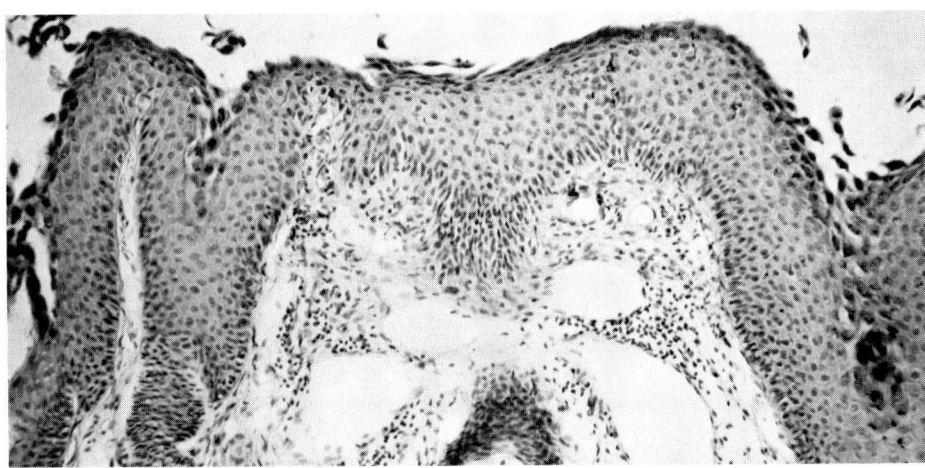

Figure 11–4.
Pemphigus foliaceus with acantholytic dissociation of granular layer. H&E. X135.

show no significant differences, but electron microscopic examination of one case showed evidence of dyskeratosis and the presence of viruslike particles.

Eosinophilic Spongiosis

Emmerson and Wilson-Jones[8] reported in 1968 that the skin of patients who later developed pemphigus could present a picture of spongiosis with eosinophils in early stages. This has been confirmed by others,[9,10] and it explains the existence of mixed cases of dermatitis herpetiformis and pemphigus. The existence of this—to the dermatopathologist—very disturbing feature (Fig. 11–6) must be kept in mind. Cases have been reported[11] in which eosinophilic spongiosis was not associated with pemphigus.

Differential Diagnosis

Differentiating features of pemphigus and other dermatoses that may form vesicles, bullae, or pustules are listed in Table 11–1. The most difficult problem in the group of acantholytic lesions is posed by the benign familial pemphigus (Hailey–Hailey's disease). One of the best distinctions is the good preservation of acantholytic cells in that eruption (see Fig. 29–6) against the features of cell degeneration in pemphigus vulgaris and vegetans. Individual cell keratini-

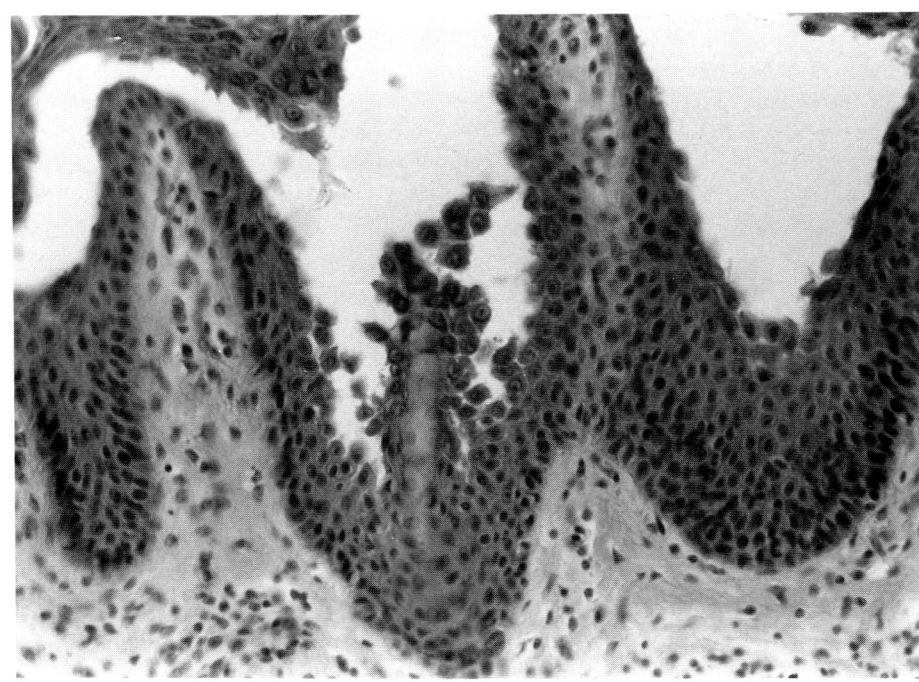

Figure 11–5.
Pemphigus erythematosus. Acantholysis occur high within the granular layer of the epidermis. H&E. X250.

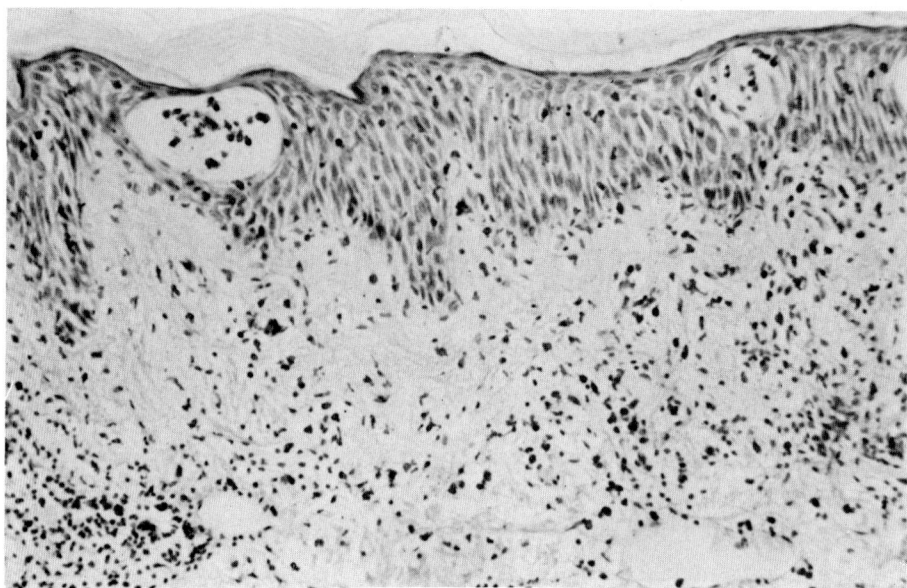

Figure 11–6.
Eosinophilic spongiotic pemphigus. Note absence of acantholysis and presence of eosinophils (large dark-appearing cells) in infiltrate. H&E. X225.

zation distinguishes Darier's disease (see Table 29–1). In mild forms of pemphigus erythematosus, the epidermal change may resemble the parakeratotic mounds and scale–crusts of seborrheic dermatitis just as the clinical picture does. The presence of acantholytic granular cells should make the diagnosis.

The use of D-penicillamine has been followed by eruptions indistinguishable from pemphigus vulgaris or other forms.[12]

Acrodermatitis Enteropathica

A disease in which acantholysis and intraepidermal vesicle formation are found on the basis of deranged lipid metabolism in zinc deficiency is acrodermatitis enteropathica. Acantholysis and the presence of dyskeratotic cells were described quite a few years ago, but electron microscopy has recently revealed[13] severe cytoplasmic disorganization with formation of multiple lipid vacuoles in basal cells and prickle cells. Large portions of the upper epidermis can become necrotic.[14] In addition to acantholysis,[15] there is acanthosis and parakeratosis of variable degree associated with considerable mixed dermal infiltrate (Fig. 11–7). *Candida* has been found in many cases as a secondary invader.

BULLOUS PEMPHIGOID

In contrast to pemphigus vulgaris and its variants, pemphigoid has a subepidermal bulla that seems to be due to a clean split between epidermis and dermis (Fig. 11–8A) similar to the separation one can obtain by the action of enzymes or acids or salts that act on the basement membrane region.[16–18] The entire epidermis forms the roof of the bulla and shows no degenerative changes (Fig. 11–8B) in early lesions. If the epidermis is pigmented, the lowest layer can be seen to consist of the pigmented and somewhat flattened intact basal cells.[19] The denuded papillary layer forms the base of the bulla. Although papillae may still be recognized in very early lesions, they flatten out under the pressure of the fluid contents of the bulla. Inflammatory infiltrate varies greatly from case to case, as does the number of eosinophils that are mixed with lymphocytes and neutrophilic leukocytes. It is obvious that scraping of the blister base in the Tzanck procedure will not procure any epithelial cells. Only inflammatory and red cells will be seen. After only 24 hours, however, reepithelization of the base may begin from the edges and from hair follicles and sweat ducts. Smears from older bullae then may show modulated epithelial cells (Chapter 2), hard to differentiate from acantholytic cells. Most patients with bullous pemphigoid demonstrate circulating autoantibodies reactive with an antigen located in the lamina lucida region of the basement membrane zone.[20]

CICATRICIAL PEMPHIGOID

Although the pemphigoid lesions of mucous membranes are discussed in Chapter 46, cicatricial pem-

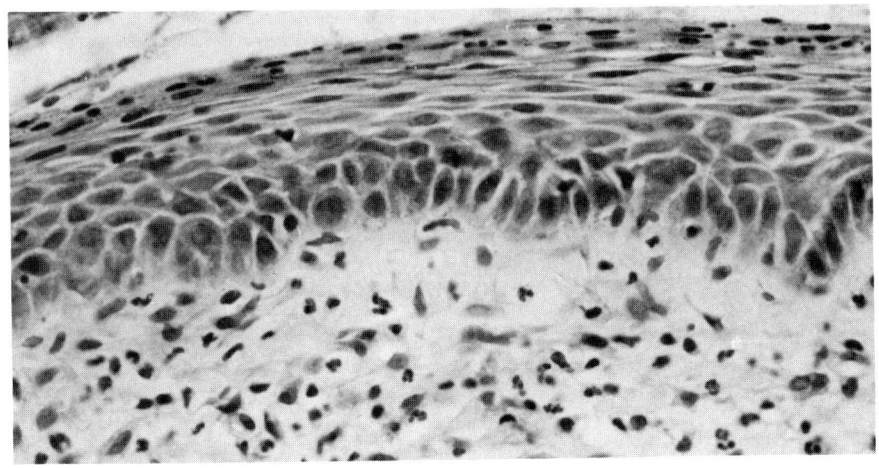
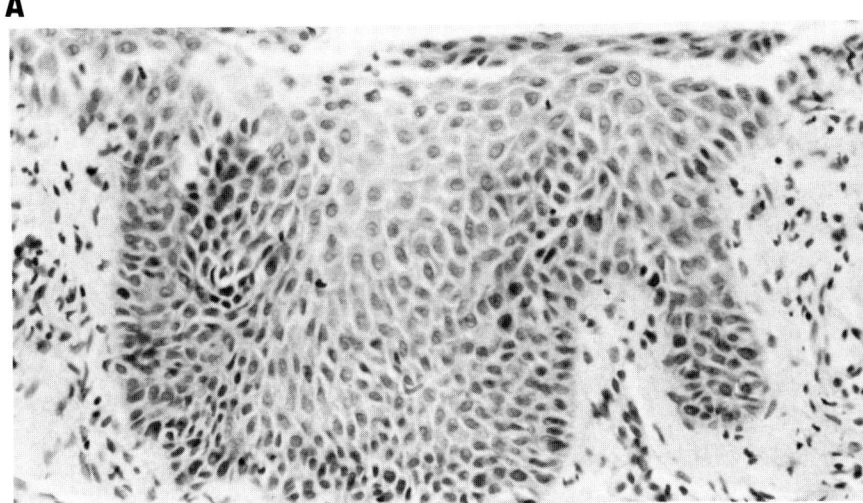

Figure 11–7.
Acrodermatitis enteropathica.
A. Epidermis rather thin with large uneven basal cells, lack of stratum granulosum, and some exocytosis. This picture may represent epidermal regeneration (Chap. 5). Moderate inflammatory infiltrate in dermis.
B. Epidermal hyperplasia with acantholytic cleft formation above basal cells and upper prickle cell layer. H&E. X400.

phigoid may show generalized or localized skin manifestations. The localized variety (Brunsting–Perry type) may occur predominantly over the extremities or may show involvement of face, neck or scalp resulting in scarring alopecia.[21,22] The subepidermal separation may extend along the hair follicles and is associated with increased vascularity and fibrosis (Fig. 11–9). There are immunoglobulin deposits at the junction.[23]

DERMATITIS HERPETIFORMIS

Duhring's disease (Fig. 11–10) probably has the most variable picture of all the bullous dermatoses. Vesicles and bullae of greatly varying size are encountered. Although separation is subepidermal in principle, the growing vesicle may dissect between epidermal layers (tension bulla). Eosinophilia, although often pronounced, is not as constant as classic descriptions suggest. The most diagnostic feature of dermatitis herpetiformis is present before the vesicle develops, giving a clue to its histogenesis. This feature is a small accumulation of neutrophilic and occasional eosinophilic leukocytes in the tips of individual papillae, which often have a basophilic tinge. The papillary tissue seems to disintegrate, and the epidermis becomes separated. Confluence of several such foci leads to the formation of vesicles. Electron microscopic study of classic lesions with granular IgA deposits beneath the epidermis and gluten-sensitive enteropathy show that the initial changes leading to blister formation are neutrophilic invasion above the basal lamina and subsequent degeneration of the basal cells.[24]

Immunofluorescence shows constant deposition of IgA at the dermoepidermal junction,[25] sometimes

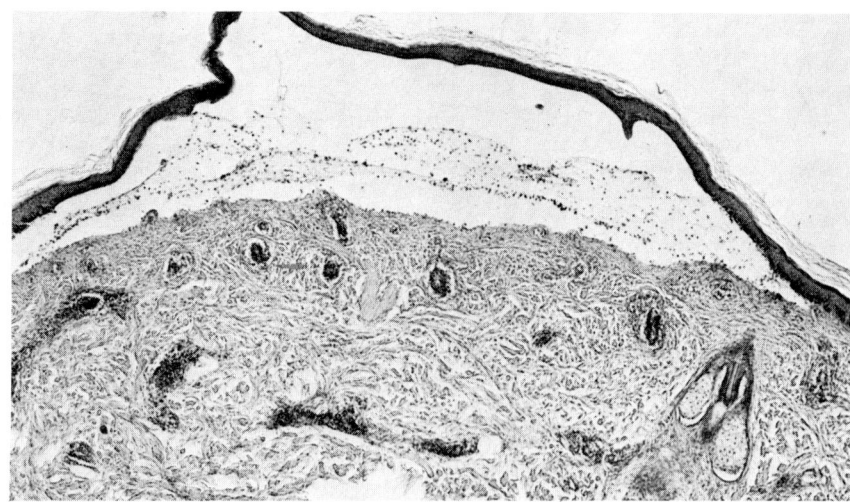

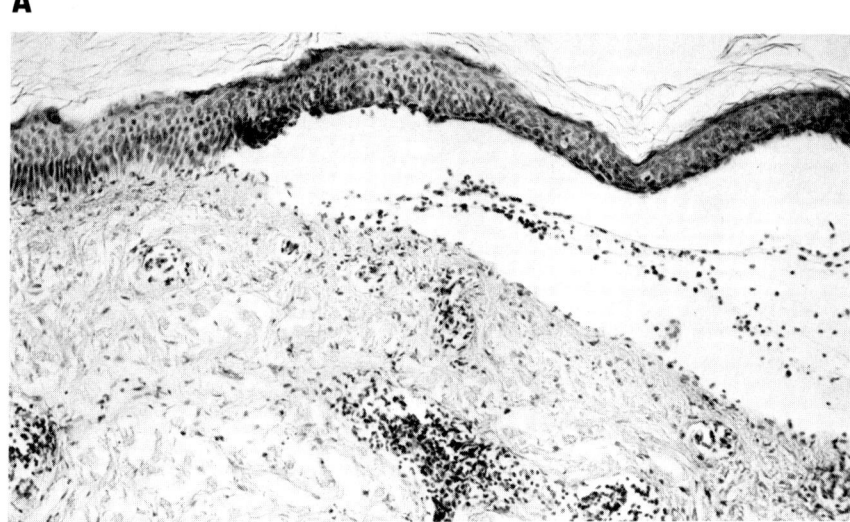

Figure 11–8.
Bullous pemphigoid. **A.** Entire bulla. H&E. X75. **B.** Edge of bulla to show clean separation between viable epidermis and intact dermis with flattening of papillae and rete ridges. The bulla contains a mixture of inflammatory cells but no epidermal cells. H&E. X135.

accompanied by other immunoglobulins or components of serum. IgA is deposited in granular form in 85–95 percent and in linear pattern in 10–15 percent of the cases.[26,27]

CHRONIC BULLOUS DERMATOSIS OF CHILDHOOD

Chronic bullous eruptions are rare in children. Although some are probably dermatitis herpetiformis, others show clinical features and immunologic findings that are different from those of dermatitis herpetiformis or bullous pemphigoid.[28–30] This group of subepidermal blistering disease are now recognized as chronic bullous dermatosis of childhood.[31] Blisters appear over the lower face, neck, lower abdomen, and diaper areas. Histologically, blisters are formed by separation of the epidermis from dermis. A mixed-type inflammatory cell infiltrate of lymphocytes and eosinophils is present in the upper dermis (Fig. 11–11). Papillary microabscesses are absent. All affected patients show continuous linear band of IgA at the dermoepidermal junction.[32]

DERMATOSES OF PREGNANCY

Two diseases, *impetigo herpetiformis* and *herpes gestationis,* have long been known to be related to pregnancy and to endanger the life of the mother or the

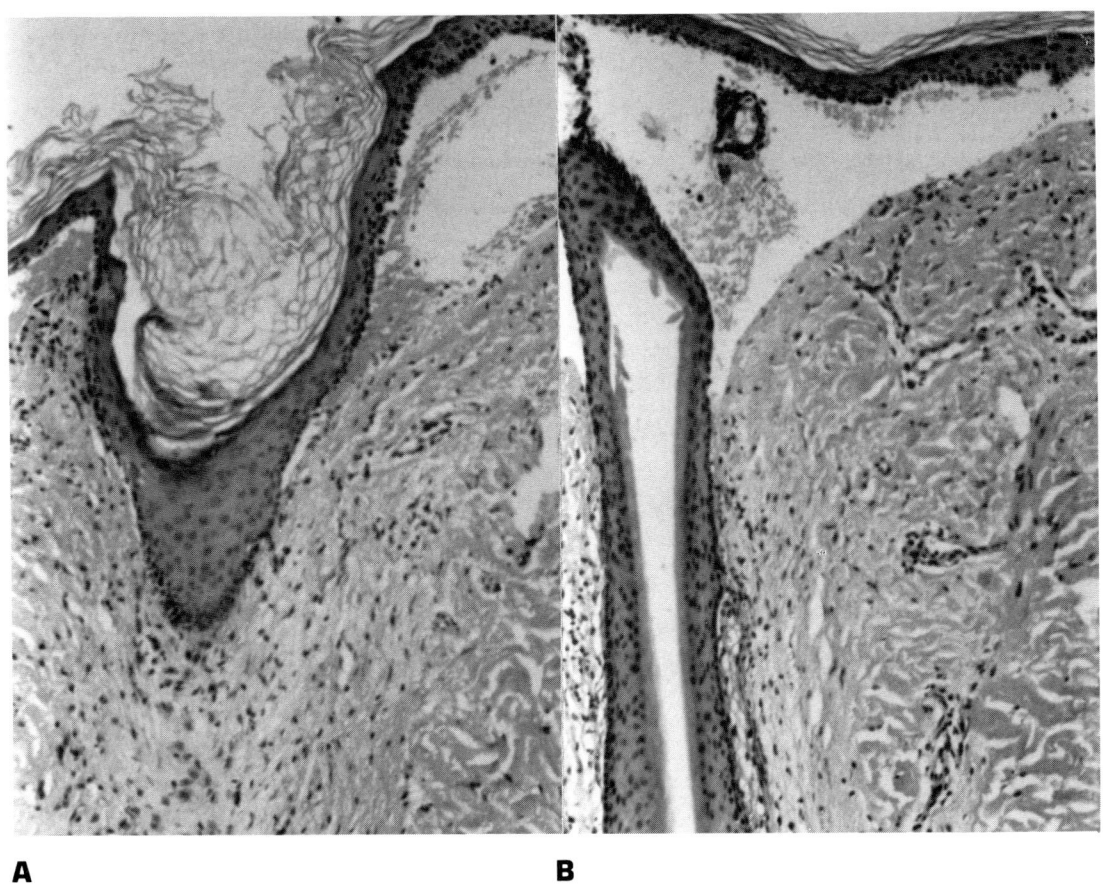

Figure 11–9.
Localized bullous pemphigoid (Brunsting–Perry type). **A** and **B** show subepidermal blisters extending around the hair follicles. Perifollicular fibrosis is leading to scarring alopecia. H&E. X125.

fetus. Recently, two nonbullous disorders, *papular dermatitis of pregnancy*[33] and *autoimmune progesterone dermatitis of pregnancy*,[34] have been added. The last named case was exceptional, as the eruption was not pruritic and was characterized by intense eosinophilic infiltrate.

Spangler et al.[33] did not give a histopathologic description of their cases. In our own experience,[35] pruritic papules of pregnancy are characterized by lymphohistiocytic infiltrates around the small vessels of the superficial dermis, with some extension around deeper vessels. There is an admixture of polymorphs and eosinophils. The epidermis shows some parakeratosis and crust formation as the result of excoriation, but there is no evidence of subepidermal or intraepidermal bulla. The changes are those of toxic erythema.[36]

Impetigo herpetiformis resembles generalized pustular psoriasis so closely in its clinical and histologic features that their identity has been postulated. Presence of acantholytic cells in the zone of spongiform pustulation and disturbances in calcium–phosphorus metabolism in impetigo herpetiformis seem to remain distinguishing features.

Vesicular pruritic eruptions in pregnancy (herpes gestationis) (Fig. 11–12) vary greatly in severity. In the last decade, there have been several publications that clarify the histopathologic picture and pathogenesis. The sera of most patients contain a specific complement-fixing factor—herpes gestationis factor (HGF)—that binds to immunoglobulins and complement deposited in linear fashion along the basement membrane.[37] The histologic picture[38,39] shows a mixed inflammatory cell infiltrate containing eosinophils around the vessels of the superficial and deep plexus and pronounced dermal papillary edema, leading to subepidermal and intraepidermal vesiculation with necrosis of basal cells, which may resemble Civatte bodies of lichen planus. Eosinophils may be found in spongiotic foci in the epidermis. This picture is sufficiently different from erythema multiforme, dermatitis herpeti-

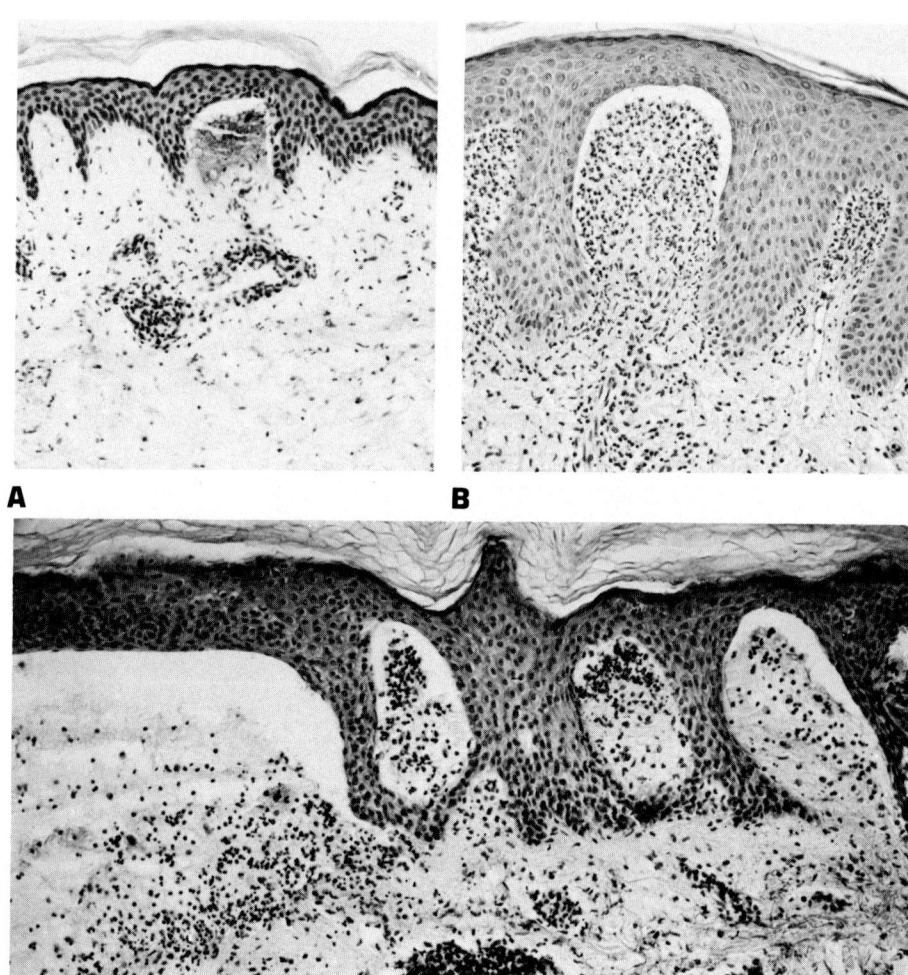

Figure 11–10.
Dermatitis herpetiformis. **A.** Basophilic papillary necrosis. H&E. X90. **B.** Neutrophilic and eosinophilic leukocytes in papilla and early epidermal separation. H&E. X135. **C.** Confluence of primary vesicles to form the subepidermal bulla. H&E. X135.

formis, and bullous pemphigoid to establish herpes gestationis as a disease entity, in association with the characteristic immunofluorescent findings.

TOXIC EPIDERMAL NECROLYSIS

Lyell syndrome,[40] which is clinically characterized by large areas of epidermis becoming detached so that they slide over their base, similar to the appearance of scalded skin[41] but without the formation of fluid-filled bullae, seems to become separated into two histologically and pathogenetically distinct groups. In many of the adult cases, a medicamentous cause can be established, the entire thickness of the epidermis becomes necrotic, and the separation is subepidermal (Fig. 11–13B). These features relate this type of case histologically to certain forms of erythema exudativum multiforme. Most of the cases in infants and a few in adults[42] are caused by staphylococcal toxin and show necrosis of the upper epidermal layers only. The epidermal changes occur in the absence of significant dermal inflammatory cell infiltrate (Fig. 11–13A). These cases seem identical to Ritter's disease (dermatitis exfoliativa neonatorum).

PORPHYRIA CUTANEA TARDA

The bulla of porphyria cutanea tarda is subepidermal (Fig. 11–14)[43] and characterized by two features: almost complete absence of inflammatory infiltrate and persistence of the papillae, which stick up into the blister. It seems possible that the latter feature is due mainly to the tougher weave of the

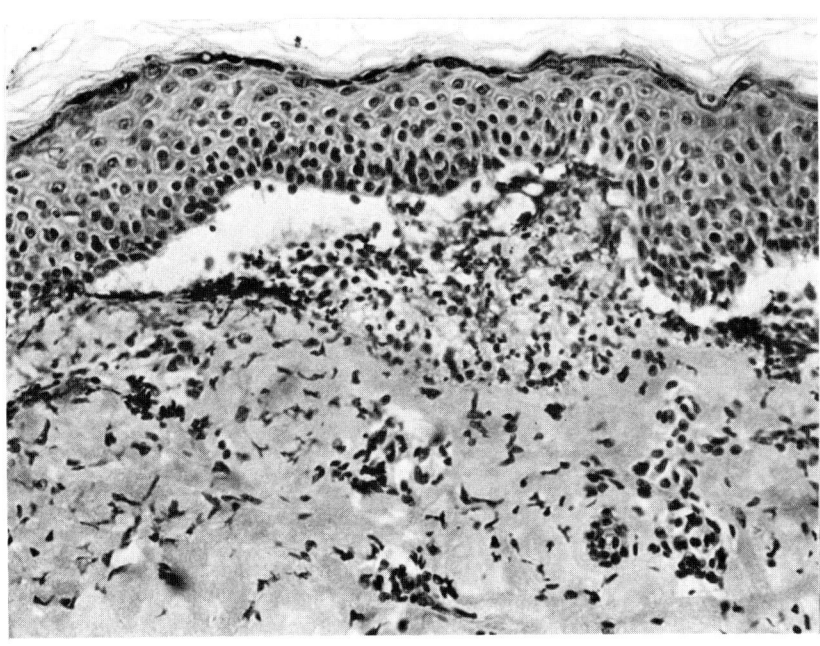

Figure 11–11.
Chronic bullous dermatosis of childhood. An early subepidermal blister contains a number of neutrophils and eosinophils. H&E. X250.

acral skin, where these blisters occur. O&G stain usually shows a heavy elastic fiber support in the papillae. Deposition of PAS-positive, diastase-resistant material, and immunoglobulins around superficial blood vessels has been pointed out as characteristic of all porphyric skin lesions.[44] Porphyria like but reversible changes have been observed after photosensitization due to tetracycline.[45]

Other forms of cutaneous porphyria are discussed in Chapters 14 and 28.

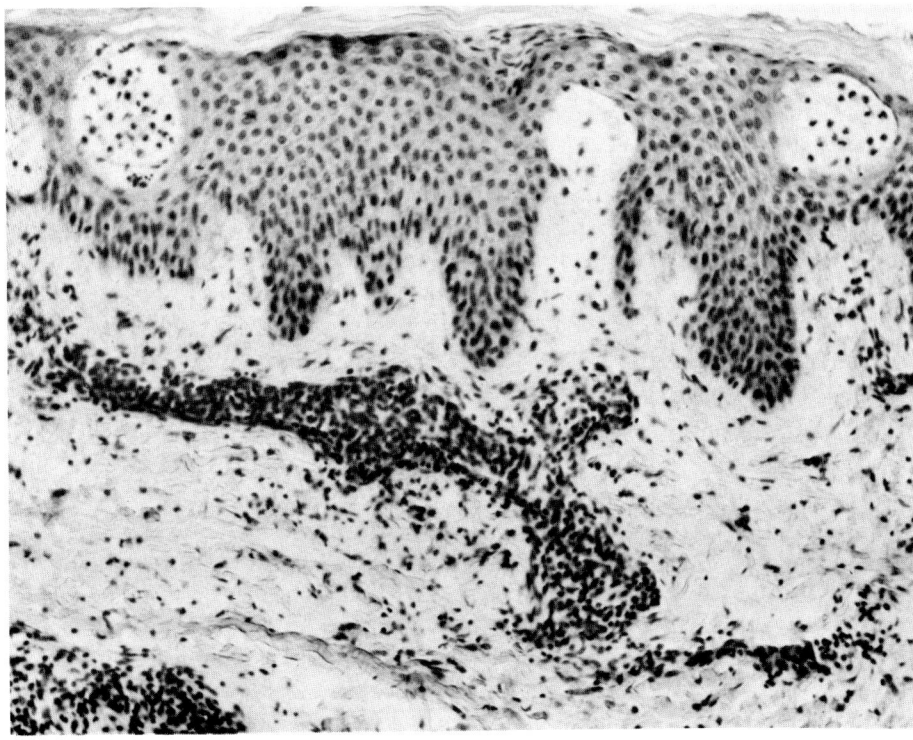

Figure 11–12.
Herpes gestationis. In this case, there is subepidermal and intraepidermal vesiculation, moderate acanthosis with focal loss of granular layer and parakeratosis, and considerable perivascular infiltrate consisting mainly of lymphocytes and some eosinophils. H&E. X180.

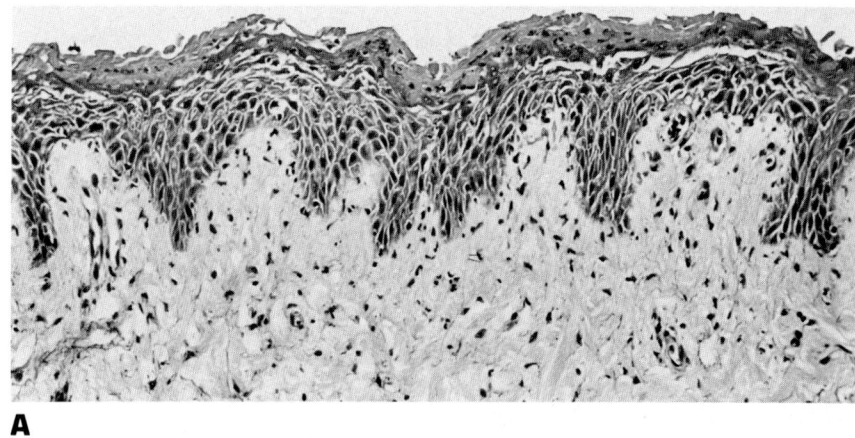

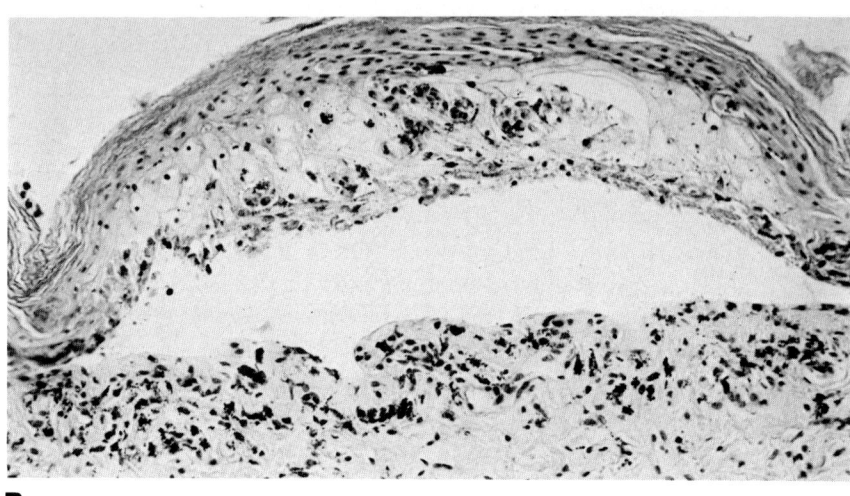

Figure 11–13.
Toxic epidermal necrolysis (Lyell). **A.** Represents a case in which only upper epidermal layers become necrotic, while lower layers exhibit peculiar intercellular edema and cell shrinkage, often seen as an effect of bacterial toxins. **B.** Complete epidermal necrosis (compare with Fig. 10–6). Note relative absence of inflammatory infiltrate in both cases. H&E. X185.

EPIDERMOLYSIS BULLOSA

"Epidermolysis bullosa" (EB) is a misnomer for this group of diseases except for epidermolysis bullosa simplex in which lysis of the epidermis truly occurs. In all other forms of this disease, separation occurs either at the dermoepidermal junction or in the dermis.[46,47] The term "mechanobullous diseases" better represents the major clinical features of these diseases. In familial cases, fetal biopsy by fetoscopy between 18 and 24 weeks would provide vital information.[48,49] Biopsy should be taken from a fresh blister in an affected newborn because secondary degenerative and regenerative changes in an old lesion make such specimen useless for electron microscopic examination. The biopsy should include the edge of the blister and the surrounding normal skin; an elliptical excision with a sharp knife is recommended. Ideally, a new blister should be induced by a rotary action of a new flat-topped pencil eraser on intact skin. However, induction of the blister may take a long time and in some cases of EB of feet and hands it does not occur. Fig. 2–17 illustrates relevant ultrastructure.

Epidermolysis Bullosa Simplex

This variety shows typical basal cell degeneration; the level of cleavage is therefore through the basal layer of the epidermis (Fig. 11–15). All forms are dominantly inherited and clinical severity is mild, often nothing but a nuisance or an inconvenience for the patient.[50] Scarring is minimal. In generalized EB simplex the superficial blisters are seen in early infancy and widely scattered.[51] Symptoms flare up in hot weather. In localized form (i.e., EB of feet and hands) of Weber and Cockayne[52,53] the onset is dur-

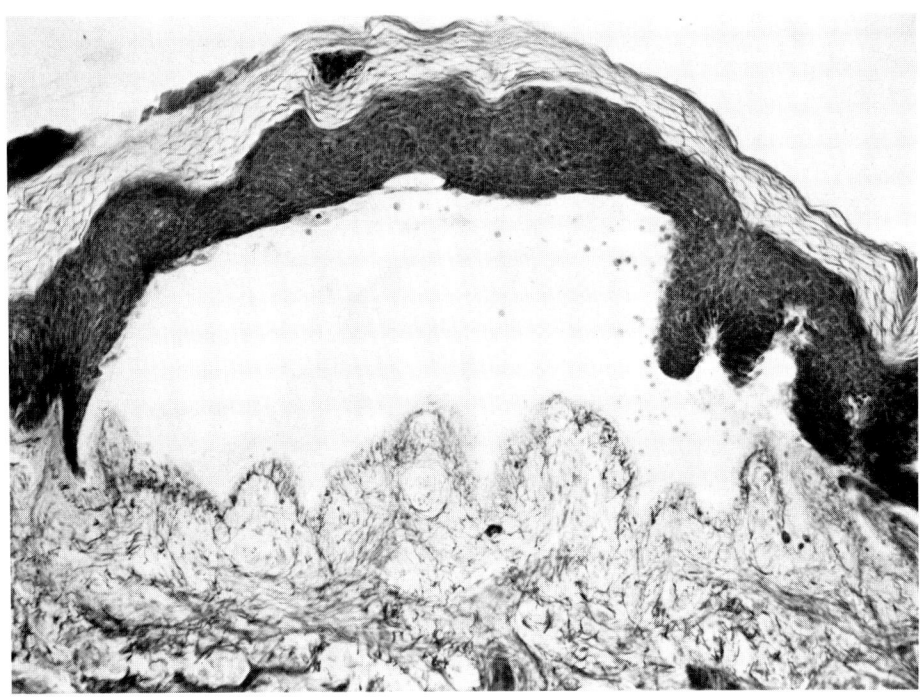

Figure 11–14.
Porphyria cutanea tarda. Separation of viable epidermis from almost reactionless dermis with preservation of papillae and elastic fibers. O&G. X135.

ing childhood and first noticed in friction areas such as heels, toes, and hands. Warm weather may also aggravate this variety. In EB herpetiformis of Dowling–Meara type, grouped vesicles occur at birth. Generalized large blisters may occur and fatality in early infancy has been reported.[54] Because of the intraepidermal separation, PAS-positive basement membrane is found along the blister floor (Fig. 11–16). Lamina densa and its associated antigens are also found at the bottom of the blister (Table 11–2). Electron microscopy shows rupture and degeneration of tonofilaments in the basal keratinocytes (Fig. 11–17). In EB herpetiformis, tonofilament aggregations and subse-

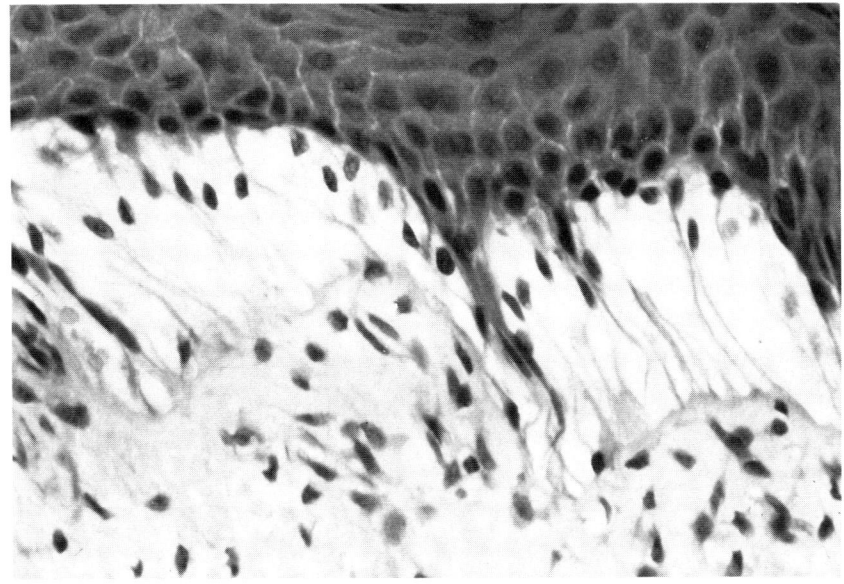

Figure 11–15.
Epidermolysis bullosa simplex. An early lesion shows degeneration of basal cells and beginning dermoepidermal separation. H&E. X400.

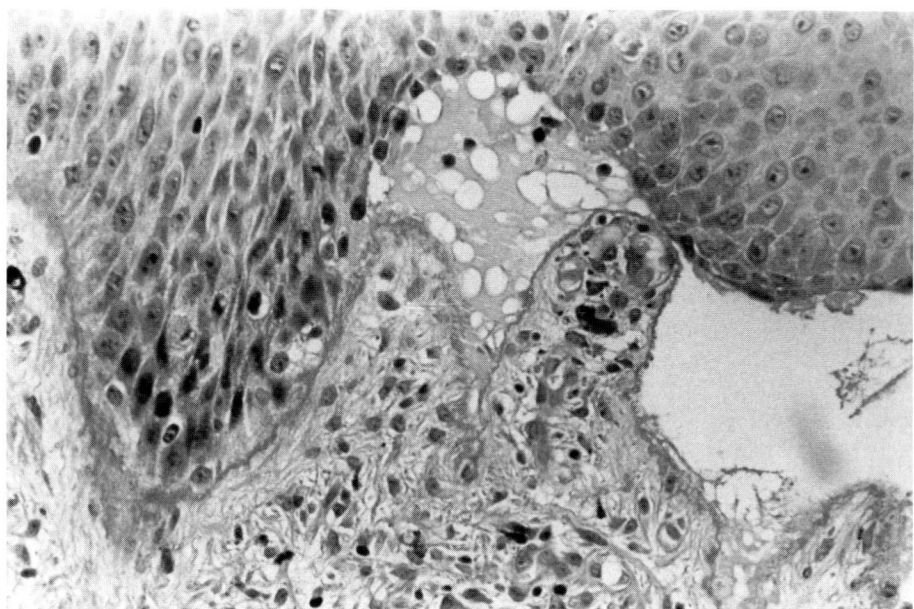

Figure 11–16.
Epidermolysis bullosa simplex shows a clean subepidermal blister. Note the PAS-positive basement membrane at the floor of the blister. PAS–H. X250.

quent degenerations are seen in the basal keratinocytes (Fig. 11–18).

Epidermolysis Bullosa Letalis

This entity is also called junctional EB because the level of the cleavage is at the dermoepidermal junction or through the lamina lucida. "Junctional EB" may be a better designation because one of this group, generalized atrophic benign type, is not lethal. The more common Herlitz type is invariably lethal early in infancy. In this type subepithelial separation is also found in the upper gastrointestinal tract, respiratory mucosa, and urinary tract.[55,56] Atresia of the duodenum may result in early death of the infant.[57] The PAS-positive basement membrane stays on the floor of the blister as do other markers of the basement membrane zone (Table 11–2). In particular the hemidesmosome–anchoring filament marker 19 DEJ-1 is always negative (Fig. 11–19).[58] Using electron microscopy one can see the severance through the lamina lucida, that is, between the lamina densa (basal lamina) and the basal cells. Hemidesmosomes are reduced or absent and anchoring filaments are torn. No damage is seen in either lamina densa or basal cells. Dermal collagen and anchoring fibrils are intact. Relevant fine structures are illustrated in Fig. 2–17.

Epidermolysis Bullous Dystrophica

In the *generalized recessive* type, severe erosions and ulcers may occur not only in the skin, oral mucosa, esophagus, and nails but may result in formation of

TABLE 11–2. ANTIBODIES AND ULTRASTRUCTURAL CHANGES USEFUL FOR EB CLASSIFICATION

Subtypes	Antibodies[a]	Location of Bulla ultrastructural changes
Simplex	All antibodies (+)	Epidermis
Junctional	GB3, AA3 ↓ 19 DEJ-1 (−)	Lamina lucida Hemidesmosome ↓
Dominant dystrophic	KF-1 ↓ AF-1, AF-2 normal	Below lamina densa Anchoring fibril (type VII) collagen ↓ Collagenase ↑ Collagenolysis (mild)
Recessive dystrophic	KF-1 (−), AF-1 (−) AF-2 (−), LH7:2 (−)	Below lamina densa Anchoring fibril ↓ ↓ Collagenase ↑ ↑ Collagenolysis (severe)
Transient dermolysis of the newborn	Type VII collagen (−) at D-E junction but (+) in basal cell inclusions	Below lamina densa Absence of anchoring fibrils in blistered areas Collagenolysis (moderate)

[a] Lamina lucida antibodies: GB3, AA3, 19-DEJ-1; lamina densa antibodies: KF-1, LH7:2; anchoring fibril-associated antibodies: AF-1, AF-2.
(J-D Fine et al, Arch Dermatol 125:520, 1989.)

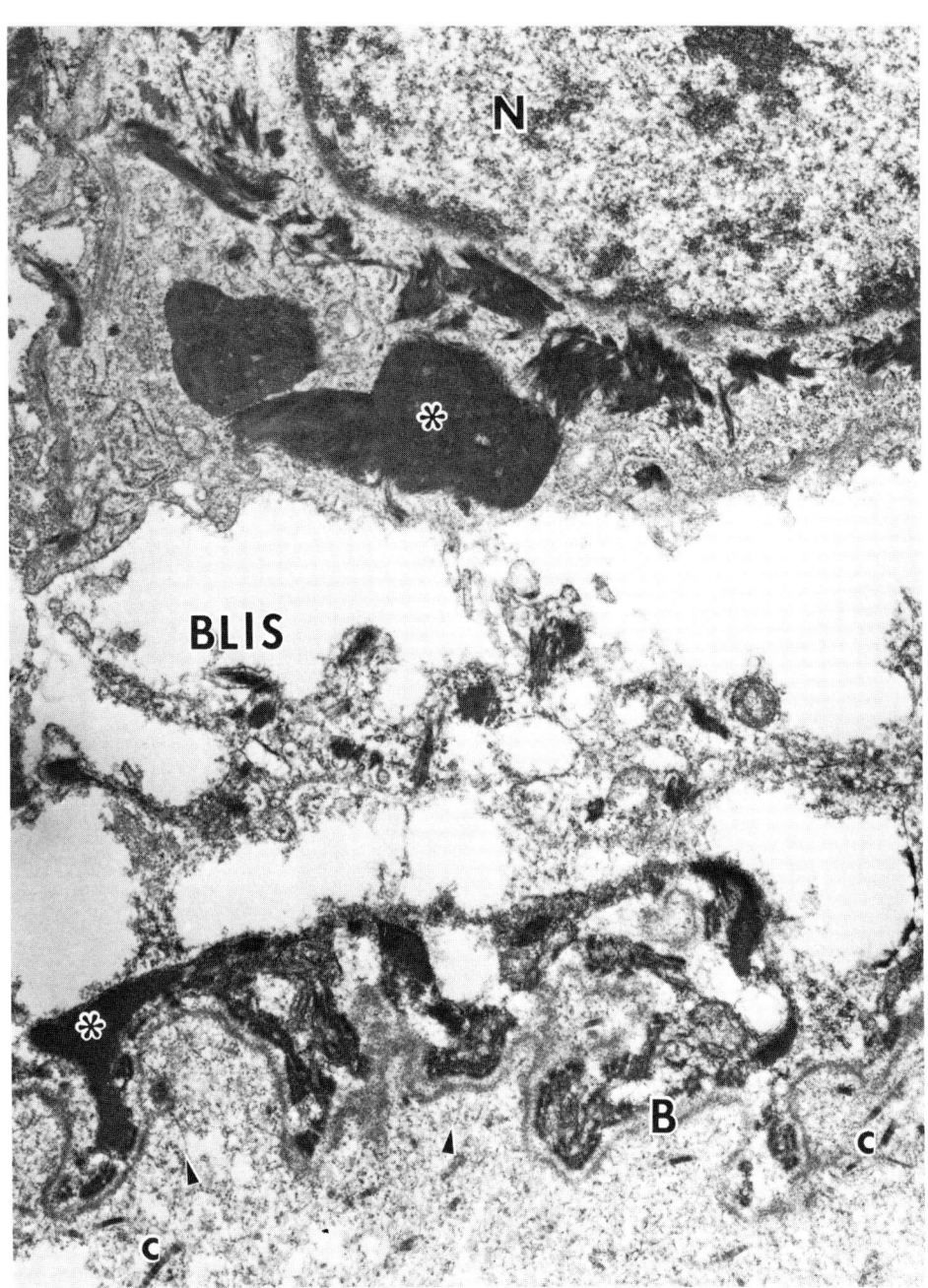

Figure 11–17.
Epidermolysis bullosa simplex. The intraepidermal blister (BLIS) shows on both sides aggregates of clumped tonofilaments (*). At the top is part of an epidermal cell nucleus (N). Below is basement membrane (B), anchoring fibrils (arrows) and collagen bundles (C). Original ×21,000. (Courtesy of Dr. K. Hashimoto.)

hypertrophic scars and esophageal stenosis.[59,60] Chronic lesions may become complicated with development of squamous cell carcinoma and metastasis.[61] Survival rate is less than in dominant type. In *localized recessive* type, symptoms are less severe and prognosis is better than in generalized type. In *inversa* type the blisters are mainly limited to the trunk instead of extremities and symptoms are milder than other types. In *dominant variant* type, clinical symptoms are much milder and scarring and keloid formation are tolerable. In both forms the separation takes place through the sublamina densa zone. In *recessive* type collagenolysis is so severe that PAS-positive basement membrane is obscured and papillary dermis appears chewed up. In *dominant* type, PAS-positive basement membrane zone is often preserved in early blisters and can be seen on the roof of the blister. Other basement membrane antigens are also on the roof of the blister if preserved (Table 11–2). Anchoring fibril antigens (type VII collagen) is absent even in the unaffected skin (Fig. 11–20).[62] Electron microscopy

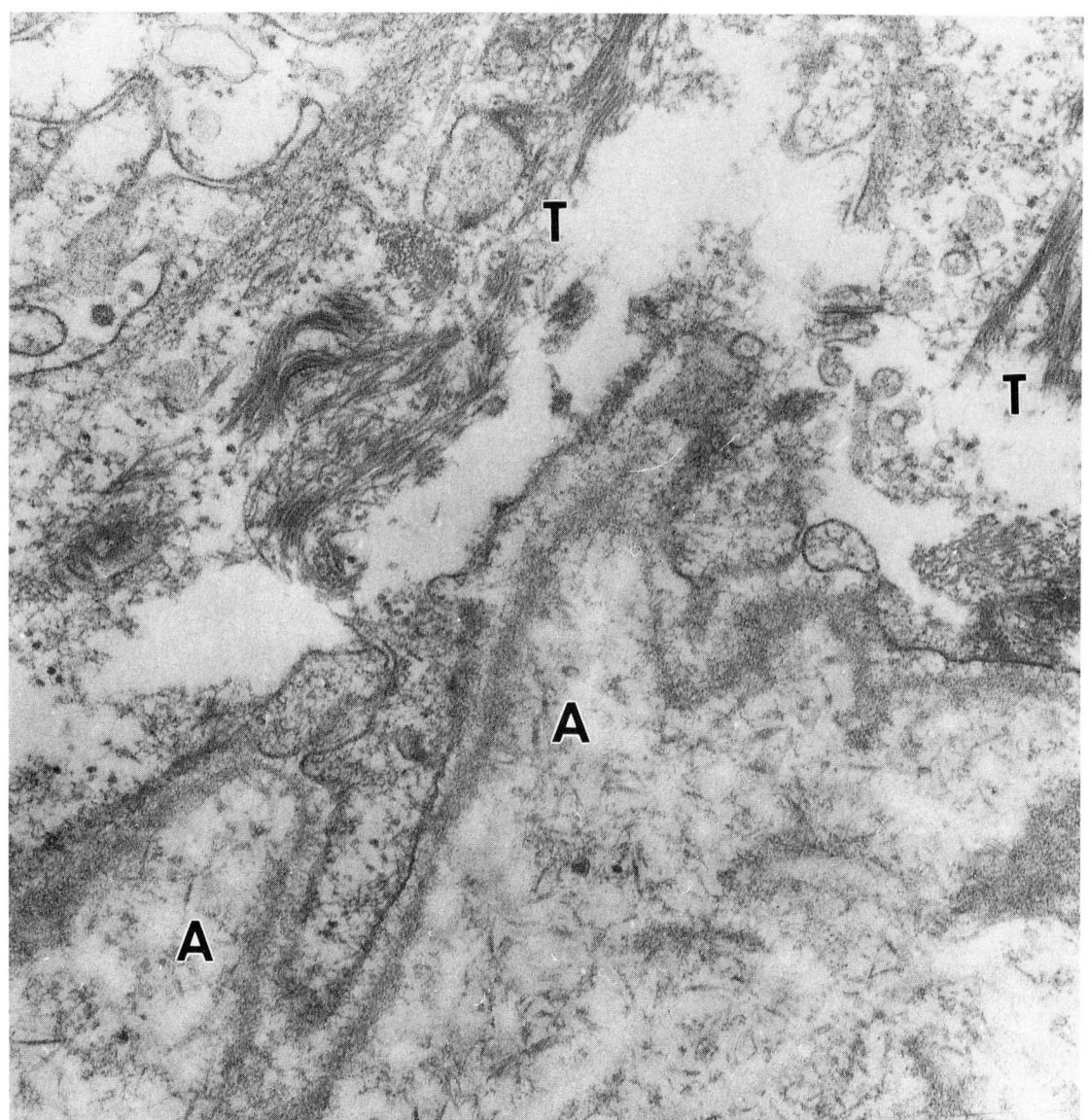

Figure 11–18.
Epidermolysis bullosa simplex. Electron microscopy shows disruption of tonofibrils.
(T). Anchoring fibrils (A) are intact. X60,000.

reveals a severe collagenolysis in papillary dermis and absence or greatly diminished number of anchoring fibrils. In generalized recessive type, the severest variety, anchoring fibrils are often diminished or absent in the nonblistered, nonscarred skin[63] (Fig. 11–20). In localized and dominant types structurally normal anchoring fibrils can be detected in the lesion. Collagenolysis is most prominent in generalized recessive type and the least in dominant type.

Transient Bullous Dermolysis of the Newborn (Hashimoto et al)

This new entity is the most recent subtype of mechanobullous disorders.[64,65] The infant is born with blisters or develops them shortly after birth. The fact that the babies delivered by Cesarian section had normal skin suggests that the severe friction through the birth canal or against bed sheets is required for the induction of blisters. Interestingly,

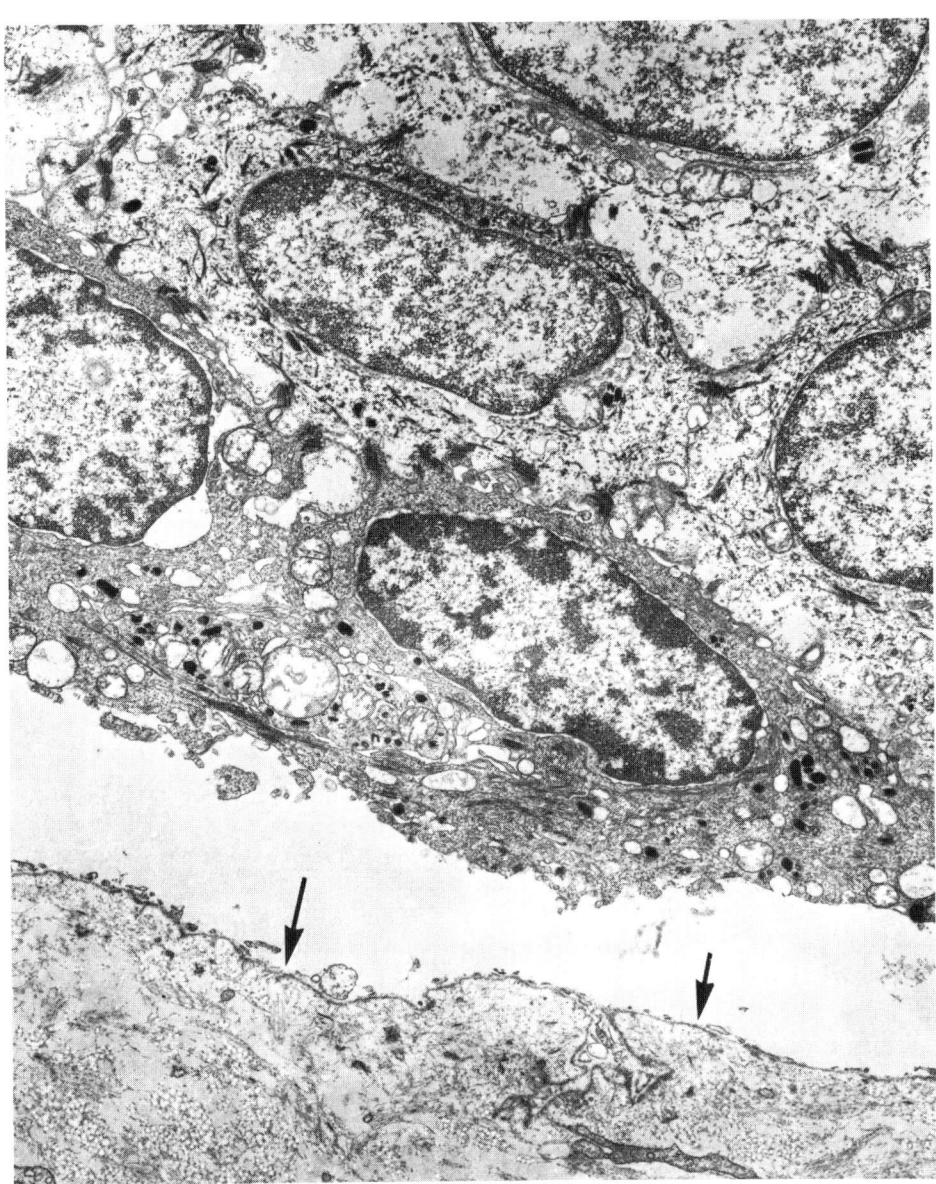

Figure 11–19.
Epidermolysis bullosa letalis.
Separation occurs above the
basal lamina (arrows).
X12,000. (Courtesy of Dr.
K. Hashimoto.)

all blisters cease to develop within a few weeks to several months.[64–66] A slight atrophic scar and milia are the only sequelae. Some cases show dominant genetic background.[16] Histologically the lesional epidermal basal cells contain PAS-positive inclusions and vacuoles. The vacuoles and large cavities are best visualized in plastic embedded specimens. Under electron microscopy, basal cell inclusions are resolved into stellate or dot-like electron-dense materials in which filament bundles with periodicity similar to that of anchoring fibrils are seen.[65] Recent studies[66,67] demonstrated the presence of type-VII collagen (anchoring fibril) antigens in these vesicles and the absence of the same antigen in dermoepidermal junction of the lesion. It is postulated, therefore, that in this disease the discharge mechanism of type-VII collagen, which is known to be produced by the epidermal keratinocyte,[68] is disturbed and anchoring-fibril-like filament bundles are crystallized within the basal cell; the lack of sufficient anchoring fibrils causes the separation of the epidermis. Many cases of so-called Bart's syndrome[69] and congenital self-healing (transient) mechanobullous dermatosis[70] probably belong to this variety.

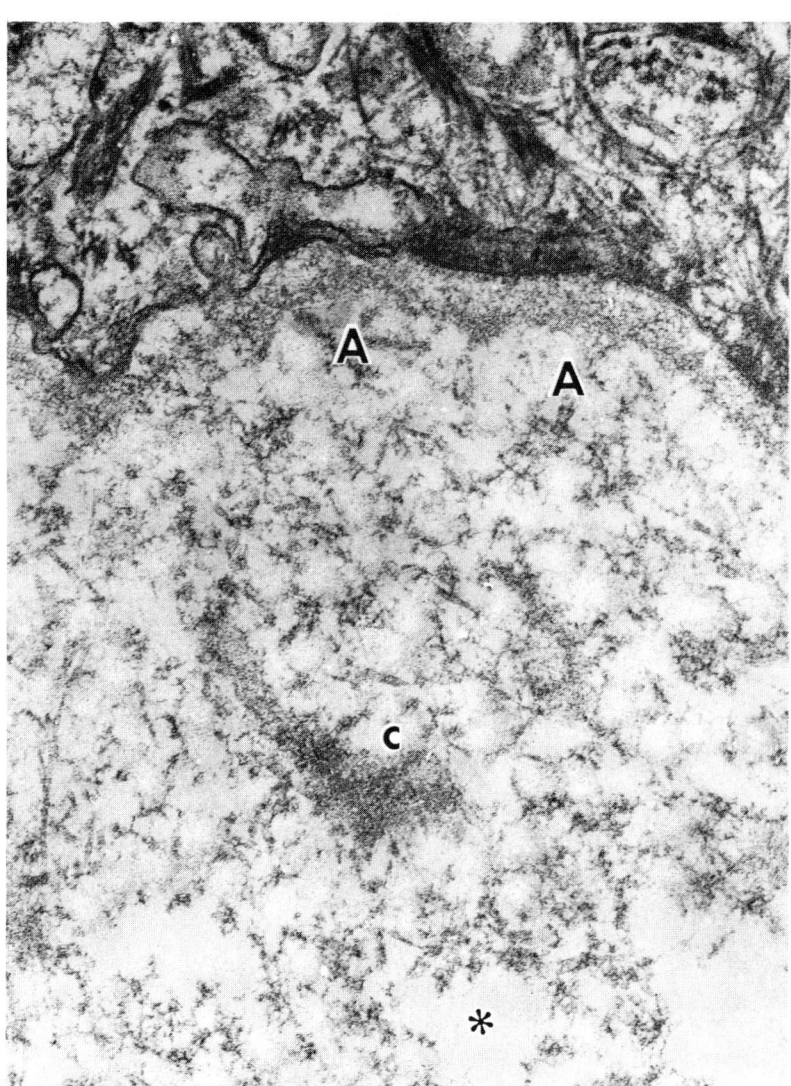

Figure 11–20.
Epidermolysis bullosa dystrophica shows damaged anchoring fibrils (A). Collagen fibers (C) are few and poorly stained. Early cavity formation (*) below the basal lamina. Original X90,000. (Courtesy of Dr. K. Hashimoto.)

IMPETIGO AND SUBCORNEAL PUSTULAR DERMATOSIS

The most superficial type, the subcorneal separation, manifests itself usually as a pustule or purulent bulla. The commonest, but rarely biopsied, disease in this group is *impetigo contagiosa* (Fig. 11–21), which may form true subcorneal bullae in infants, whereas in older children and adults one usually sees only crusts on denuded surfaces. It is important to keep bullous impetigo in mind in the differential diagnosis of subcorneal pustular dermatosis (Fig. 11–22) because their histologic pictures are almost indistinguishable.

In both dermatoses we find polymorphonuclear leukocytes migrating through the epidermis and accumulating between granular and horny layers, often without too much disturbance of epidermal architecture.[71] Inflammatory infiltrate in the dermis varies and may be minimal. A few acantholytic cells may be found in the blister of Sneddon–Wilkinson's disease, but larger numbers raise a question of pemphigus foliaceus. Association with monoclonal (IgA) gammopathy has been reported.[72] A patient identified in a publication as having subcorneal pustular dermatosis was found to have Von Zumbusch-type psoriasis.[73] Similar observations have raised the question as to whether subcorneal pustular dermatosis exists as a distinctive entity.[74]

Pustular and crusted clinical lesions are encountered in association with many other dermatoses, especially pruritic ones. We use the term "impetiginization" in cases that are clearly due to superinfection by scratching. Histologically, the pic-

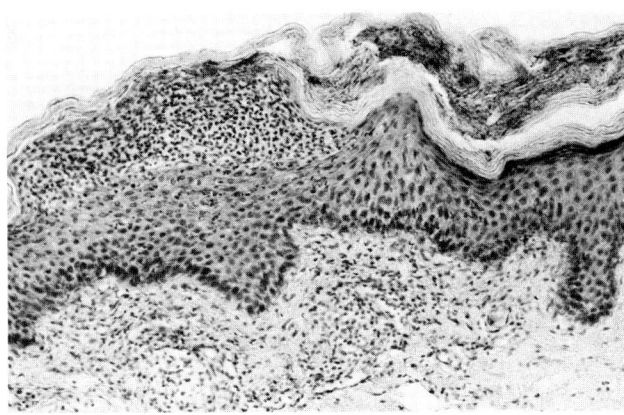

Figure 11–21.
Bullous impetigo contagiosa. Transmigration of leukocytes through epidermis and abscess formation below the elevated horny layer at left. At right, pyknotic leukocytes between old and newly formed horny layer. Stratum granulosum absent under fresh lesion, reconstituted under old one. H&E. X250.

ture may be confusing in the absence of clinical information. Presence of colonies of cocci, often already evident in H&E sections and identifiable by O&G or Gram stain, in the superficial pustules and crusts of any inflammatory dermatosis gives a lead to a diagnosis of impetiginization. In other cases, pyodermatous lesions indistinguishable from ordinary impetigo are manifestations of immune deficiency syndromes, such as the Wiscott–Aldrich syndrome[75] and granulomatous disease of childhood.[76] Table 11–3 gives a survey of dermatoses associated with polymorphonuclear leukocytes.[77]

NECROLYTIC MIGRATORY ERYTHEMA

During the past decade a distinctive dermatosis has been recognized as a paraneoplastic manifestation of islet cell carcinoma of the pancreas, especially glucagonoma. These migrating erythematous lesions had been observed occasionally since 1948, but histologic examination brought out specific changes that were observed in 1973 as necrolytic migratory erythema.[78,79] The disease causes blisters that are intraepidermal, situated in the higher prickle cell layer, and associated with transformation of epithelial cells into flat or ballooning elements without keratohyalin.[80] Occasionally, truly acantholytic cells have been observed.[81] Acanthosis varies. Inflammatory infiltrate in the dermis is mild. Polymorphonuclear cells accumulate in the bulla. The differential diagnosis includes acrodermatitis enteropathica and the various bullous dermatoses.

OTHER BULLOUS LESIONS

Bullous eruptions resembling bullous pemphigoid have been reported in association with internal malignant disease. Inasmuch as bullous pemphigoid is

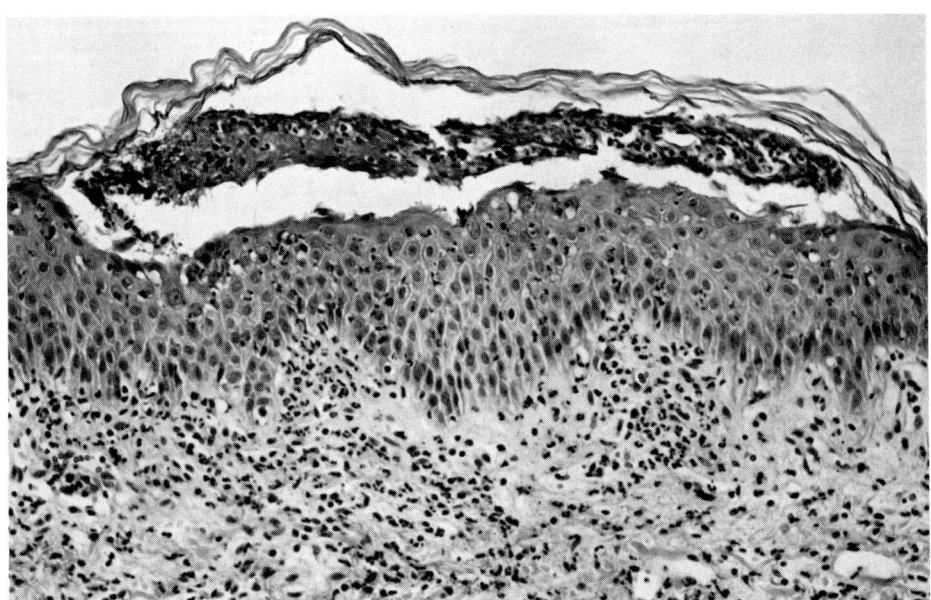

Figure 11–22.
Subcorneal pustular dermatosis. H&E. X185.

TABLE 11–3. DERMATOSES REGULARLY ASSOCIATED WITH POLYMORPHONUCLEAR LEUKOCYTES

Location of PMNs	Mechanics or Distribution	Disease Entities
Subcorneal	Superficial infection or injury	Impetigo, yeast or fungal infections, chemical injury (nickel, turpentine)
	Unknown cause	Psoriasiform tissue reactions, subcorneal pustular dermatosis
	Secondary	Pustulosis palmaris et plantaris, transepidermal elimination of products of deeper inflammation
Intraepidermal		Psoriasiform tissue reaction, nummular eczema, pustulosis palmaris et plantaris, some viral infections, halogen eruptions, deep fungal infections
Dermal	Adnexal	Staphylococcal infections, acne vulgaris, rosacea, halogen eruptions
	Diffuse	Cellulitis and erysipelas, neutrophilic febrile dermatosis, anthrax, DNA autosensitivity, some bullous diseases
	Vascular	Leukocytoclastic vasculitis, periarteritis nodosa, erythema elevatum diutinum
	Granulomatous	Erythema nodosum (early), all mixed cell granulomas, granuloma faciale, mycosis fungoides

Modified from Wilkinson.[77]

a disease of the older age group in which cancer is more common, and some bullous eruptions that wax and wane with the ups and downs of the cancer have atypical features, it is advisable to reserve judgment until more of these rare cases have been investigated by modern methods. It may well be that the association of true bullous pemphigoid with malignancy is coincidental[82] and that bullous eruptions of different character[83] are indeed related to cancer. Association of subepidermal bullae with carbon monoxide or barbiturate poisoning (Fig. 11–23), phototoxic bullae from frusemide medication[84] or psoralens, and bullae in diabetes mellitus[85–87] and a variety of neurologic disorders[88] are being recorded

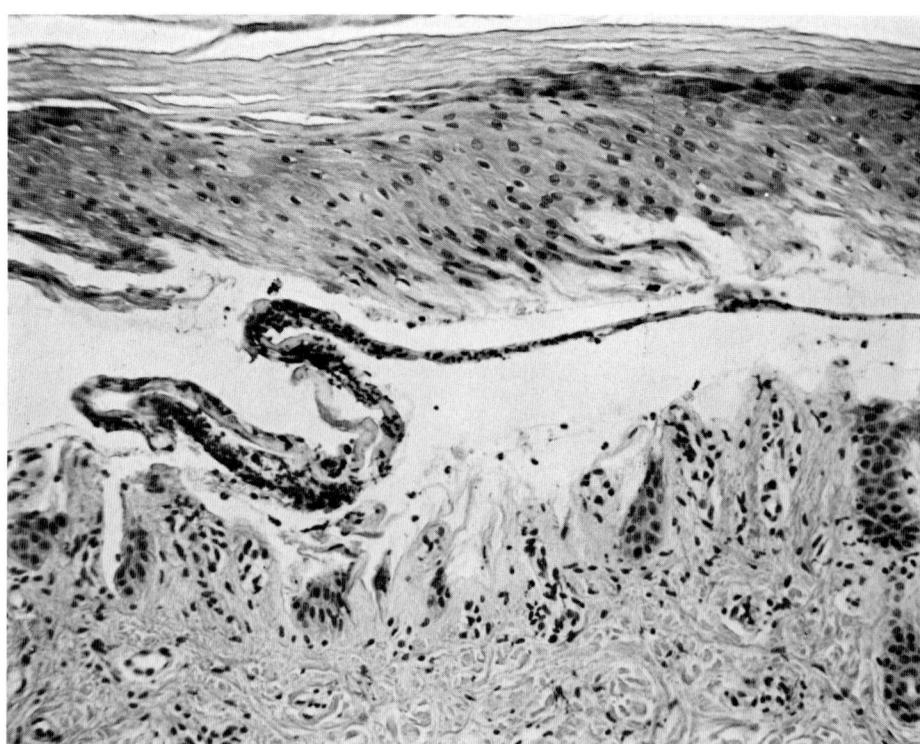

Figure 11–23.
Bulla associated with barbiturate coma. Epidermal cells deformed and pyknotic. Papillary connective tissue frayed. Tips of some rete ridges adhere to dermis. Pyknotic polymorphonuclear leukocytes and fibrin in the bulla. The entire aspect suggests separation due to shearing forces. H&E. X180.

more and more frequently. One should not forget bullae due to burns and friction. All these are subepidermal and may be associated with epidermal damage. These lesions evidently are not related to the disease, bullous pemphigoid.

MUCOUS MEMBRANE LESIONS

The oral manifestations of the bullous diseases and the mucous membrane pemphigoid are discussed in Chapter 46.

REFERENCES

1. Stanley JR: Pemphigus. Skin failure mediated by autoantibodies. JAMA 264:1714, 1990
2. Korman N: Pemphigus. J Am Acad Dermatol 18:1219, 1988
3. Nestor MS, Cochran AJ, Razzaque Ahmed A: Mononuclear cell infiltrates in bullous disease. J Invest Dermatol 88:172, 1987
4. LeRoy D, Lebrun J, Maillard V, et al: Pemphigus végétant à type clinique de dermatite pustuleuse chronique de Hallopeau. Ann Dermatol Venereol 109:549, 1982
5. Bystryn J-C: Pemphigus foliaceus. Subcorneal intercellular antibodies of unique specificity. Arch Dermatol 110:857, 1974
6. Jones SK, Schwab HP, Norris DA: Childhood pemphigus foliaceus: Case report and review of the literature. Pediatr Dermatol 3:459, 1986
7. Guimaraes Proenca N, Rivitti E: Antiepithelial antibodies in Brazilian pemphigus foliaceus. Int J Dermatol 16:799, 1977
8. Emmerson RW, Wilson-Jones E: Eosinophilic spongiosis in pemphigus. A report of an unusual histological change in pemphigus. Arch Dermatol 97:252, 1968
9. Knight AG, Black MM, Delaney TJ: Eosinophilic spongiosis. A clinical histological and immunofluorescent correlation. Clin Exp Dermatol 1:141, 1976
10. Degos R, Civatte J, Belaïch S, Bonvalet D: Spongiose à éosinophiles. A propos de deux cas. Bull Soc Fr Dermatol 83:14, 1976
11. Kennedy C, Hodge L, Sanderson KV: Eosinophilic spongiosis: A localized bullous dermatosis unassociated with pemphigus. Clin Exp Dermatol 3:117, 1978
12. Enjolras O, Sedel D, Leibowitch M, Escande J-P: Pemphigus induits. Ann Dermatol Venereol 114:25, 1987
13. Ginsburg R, Robertson A Jr, Michel B: Acrodermatitis enteropathica. Abnormalities of fat metabolism and integumental ultrastructures in infants. Arch Dermatol 112:653, 1976
14. Brazin SA, Johnson WT, Abramson LJ: The acrodermatitis enteropathica-like syndrome. Arch Dermatol 115:597, 1979
15. Juljulian HH, Kurban AK: Acantholysis: A feature of acrodermatitis enteropathica. Arch Dermatol 108:105, 1971
16. Hadi SM, Barnetson R St C, Gawkrodger DJ et al: Clinical, histological and immunological studies in 50 patients with bullous pemphigoid. Dermatologica 176:6, 1988
17. Liu H-H H, Su DWP, Rogers RS: Clinical variants of pemphigoid. Int J Dermatol 25:17, 1986
18. Castanet J, LaCour J-P, Ortonne J-P: Forms cliniques atypiques de pemphigoid bulleuses. Ann Dermatol Venereol 117:73, 1990
19. Ookusa Y, Takata K, Nagashima M, Hirano H: Bullous pemphigoid—A scanning electron microscopic study. Dermatologica 172:6, 1986
20. Korman N: Bullous pemphigoid. J Am Acad Dermatol 16:907, 1987
21. Salomon RJ, Briggaman RA, Wernikoff SY, Kayne AL: Localized bullous pemphigoid. A mimic of acute contact dermatitis. Arch Dermatol 123:389, 1987
22. Leenutaphong V, von Kries R, Plewig G: Localized cicatricial pemphigoid (Brunsting-Perry): Electron microscopic study. J Am Acad Dermatol 21:1089, 1989
23. Sugihara K, Dekio S, Tohgi K, Jidoi J: Localized pemphigoid: A case report showing in situ deposition as well as presence in serum of IgG and IgA antibasement membrane zone antibodies. J Dermatol Tokyo 14:73, 1987
24. Horiguchi Y, Danno K, Toda K et al: Ultrastructural sites of blister formation in dermatitis herpetiformis: Report of a case and retrospective electron microscopy using routine histologic preparations. J Dermatol Tokyo 14:462, 1987
25. Katz SI, Strober W: The pathogenesis of dermatitis herpetiformis. J Invest Dermatol 70:63, 1978
26. Hall RP: The pathogenesis of dermatitis herpetiformis: Recent advances. J Am Acad Dermatol 16:1129, 1987
27. Combemale P, Prost C: Maladie a IgA lineaire de l'adulte. Revue de la literature. Ann Dermatol Venereol 114:1605, 1987
28. Smith SB, Harrist TJ, Murphy GF, et al: Linear IgA bullous dermatosis V dermatitis herpetiformis. Quantitative measurements of dermoepidermal alterations. Arch Dermatol 120:324, 1984
29. Pothupitiya GM, Wojnarowska F, Bhogal BS, Black MM: Distribution of the antigen in adult linear IgA disease and chronic bullous dermatosis of childhood suggests that it is a single and unique antigen. Br J Dermatol 118:175, 1988
30. Wojnarowski F, Marsden RA, Bhogal B, Black MM: Chronic bullous disease of childhood, childhood cicatricial pemphigoid, and linear IgA disease of adults. J Am Acad Dermatol 19:792, 1988
31. Roberts LJ, Sontheimer RD: Chronic bullous dermatosis of childhood: Immunopathologic studies. Pediatr Dermatol 4:6, 1987

32. Akahoshi Y, Kanda G, Anan S, Yoshida H: Dermoepidermal blister formation by linear IgA dermatosis sera in normal human skin in organ culture. J Dermatol Tokyo 14:352, 1987
33. Spangler AS, Reddy W, Bardanil WA, et al: Papular dermatitis of pregnancy. A new clinical entity? JAMA 181:577, 1962
34. Bierman SM: Autoimmune progesterone dermatitis of pregnancy. Arch Dermatol 107:896, 1973
35. Rahbari H: Pruritic papules of pregnancy. J Cutan Pathol 5:347, 1978
36. Winton GB, Lewis CW: Dermatoses of pregnancy. J Am Acad Dermatol 6:977, 1982
37. Carruthers JA: Herpes gestationis: A reappraisal. Clin Exp Dermatol 3:199, 1978
38. Hertz KC, Katz SI, Maize J, Ackerman AB: Herpes gestationis. A clinicopathologic study. Arch Dermatol 112:1543, 1976
39. Harrington CI, Bleehen SS: Herpes gestationis: Immunopathological and ultrastructural studies. Br J Dermatol 100:389, 1979
40. Lyell A: Toxic epidermal necrolysis (the scalded skin syndrome). A re-appraisal. Br J Dermatol 100:67, 1979
41. Sturman SW, Malkinson FD: Staphylococcal scalded skin syndrome in an adult and a child. Arch Dermatol 112:1275, 1976
42. Roujeau J-C, Guillaume J-C, Fabre J-P, et al: Toxic epidermal necrolysis (Lyell syndrome): Incidence and drug etiology in France, 1981–1985. Arch Dermatol 126:37, 1990
43. Cormane RH, Szabò E, Hoo TT: Histopathology of the skin in acquired and hereditary porphyria cutanea tarda. Br J Dermatol 85:531, 1972
44. Epstein JH, Tuffanelli DL, Epstein WL: Cutaneous changes in the porphyrias; a microscopic study. Arch Dermatol 107:689, 1973
45. Epstein JH, Tuffanelli DL, Seibert JS, Epstein WL: Porphyria-like cutaneous changes induced by tetracycline hydrochloride photosensitization. Arch Dermatol 112:661, 1976
46. Fine J-D: Epidermolysis bullosa. Clinical aspects, pathology, and recent advances in research. Int J Dermatol 25:143, 1986
47. Pearson RW: Clinicopathologic types of epidermolysis bullosa and their nondermatological complications. Arch Dermatol 124:718, 1988
48. Eady RAJ: Prenatal diagnosis. In Orfanos CE, Stadler R, Gollnick H (eds): Dermatology in Five Continents: Proceedings of the XVII World Congress of Dermatology Berlin, May 24–29, 1987, Springer-Verlag: Berlin, p 127
49. Blanchet-Bardon C, Dumez Y, Nazzaro V, et al: Le diagnostic antenatal des epidetmolyses bulleuses hereditaires. Ann Dermatol Venereol 114:525, 1987
50. Haber RM, Hanna W, Ramsay CA, Boxall LBH: Hereditary epidermolysis bullosa. J Am Acad Dermatol 13:252, 1985
51. Lowe LB: Hereditary epidermolysis bullosa. Arch Dermatol 95:587, 1967
52. Anton-Lamprecht I, Schnyder UW: Epidermolysis bullosa Dowling-Meara. Dermatologica 164:221, 1982
53. Haneke E, Anton-Lamprecht I: Ultrastructure of blister formation in epidermolysis bullosa hereditaria. V. Epidermolysis bullosa simplex localisata type Weber-Cockayne. J Invest Dermatol 78:219, 1982
54. Buchbinder LH, Lucky AW, Ballard E et al: Severe infantile epidermolysis bullosa simplex. Dowling-Meara type. Arch Dermatol 122:190, 1986
55. Pearson W: The mechanobullous diseases. In: Fitzpatrick TB, Arndt KA, Clark WH Jr, et al (eds): Dermatology in General Medicine. New York: McGraw-Hill 1971, p 621
56. Schachner L, Lazarus GS, Dembitzer H: Epidermolysis bullosa hereditaria letalis. Br J Dermatol 96:51, 1977
57. Chung-Ho C, Perrin EV, Bove KE: Pyloric atresia associated with epidermolysis bullosa: Special reference to pathogenesis. Pediatr Pathol 1:449, 1983
58. Fine J-D, Horiguchi Y, Couchman JR: 19-DEJ-1, A hemidesmosome-anchoring filament complex-associated monoclonal antibody: Definition of a new skin basement membrane antigenic defect in junctional and dystrophic epidermolysis bullosa. Arch Dermatol 125:520, 1989
59. Pearson RW, Paller AS: Dermolytic (dystrophic) epidermolysis bullosa inversa. Arch Dermatol 124:544, 1988
60. Bergenholtz A, Olsson O: Die Epidermolysis bullosa hereditaria dystrophic mit Oesophagusveranderungen. Arch Klin Exp Dermatol 271:518, 1963
61. Reed WB, College J Jr, Francis MJO et al: Epidermolysis bullosa dystrophica with epidermal neoplasms. Arch Dermatol 110:894, 1974
62. Bruckner-Tuberman L, Ruegger S, Odermatt B, et al: Lack of type VII collagen in unaffected skin of patients with severe recessive dystrophic epidermolysis bullosa. Dermatologica 176:57, 1988
63. Tidman MJ, Eady RAJ: Evaluation of anchoring fibrils and other components of the dermal–epidermal junction in dystrophic epidermolysis bullosa by a quantitative ultrastructural technique. J Invest Dermatol 84:374, 1985
64. Hashimoto K, Matsumoto M, Iacobelli D: Transient bullous dermolysis of the newborn. Arch Dermatol 121:1429, 1985
65. Hashimoto K, Burk JD, Bale GF, Eto H, et al: Transient bullous dermolysis of the newborn: Two additional cases. J Am Acad Dermatol 21:708, 1989
66. Fine J-D, Horiguchi Y, Stein DH et al: Intraepidermal type VII collagen. J Am Acad Dermatol 22:188, 1990
67. Smith LT, Sybert VP: Intra-epidermal retention of type VII collagen in a patient with recessive dystrophic epidermolysis bullosa. J Invest Dermatol 94:261, 1990
68. Regauer S, Seiler GR, Compton CC: Epidermal origin

of cutaneous anchoring fibrils. Clin Res 38:613A, 1990
69. Bart BJ, Gorlin RJ, Anderson VE, et al: Congenital localized absence of skin and associated abnormalities resembling epidermolysis bullosa. Arch Dermatol 93:296, 1966
70. Fisher GB Jr, Greer KE, Cooper PH: Congenital self-healing (transient) mechanobullous dermatosis. Arch Dermatol 124:240, 1988
71. Sneddon IH: Subcorneal pustular dermatosis. Int J Dermatol 16:640, 1977
72. Kasha EE, Epinette WW: Subcorneal pustular dermatosis (Sneddon–Wilkinson disease) in association with a monoclonal IgA gammopathy: A report and review of the literature. J Am Acad Dermatol 19:854, 1988
73. Beck AL, Kipping HL, Crissey JT: Subcorneal pustular dermatosis. Arch Dermatol 83:627, 1961
74. Chimenti S, Ackerman AB: Is subcorneal pustular dermatosis of Sneddon and Wilkinson an entity sui generis? Am J Dermatopathol 3:363, 1981
75. Scher PK: Wiskott–Aldrich syndrome. Cutis 12:566, 1973
76. Bass LJ, Voorhees JJ, Dubin HV, et al: Chronic granulomatous disease of childhood. Superficial pyoderma as a major dermatologic manifestation. Arch Dermatol 106:68, 1972
77. Wilkinson DS: Pustular dermatoses. Br J Dermatol 81 (Suppl 3):38, 1969
78. Wilkinson DS: Necrolytic migratory erythema with carcinoma of the pancreas. Trans St Johns Hosp Dermatol Soc 59:244, 1973
79. Verbov J: Necrolytic migratory erythema associated with an islet cell tumour of the pancreas. Dermatologica 163:189, 1981
80. Kahan RS, Perez-Figaredo RA, Neimanis A: Necrolytic migratory erythema. Distinctive dermatosis of the glucagonoma syndrome. Arch Dermatol 113:792, 1977
81. Swenson KH, Amon RB, Hanifin JM: The glucagonoma syndrome. A distinctive cutaneous marker of systemic disease. Arch Dermatol 114:224, 1978
82. Paslin DA: Bullous pemphigoid and hypernephroma. A critical review of the association of bullous pemphigoid and malignancy. Cutis 12:554, 1973
83. Skog J: Cutaneous manifestations associated with internal malignant tumors with particular reference to vesicular and bullous lesions. Acta Derm Venereol 44:117, 1964
84. Burry JN, Lawrence JR: Phototoxic blisters from high frusemide dosage. Br J Dermatol 94:495, 1976
85. Bernstein JE, Medenica M, Soltani K, Criem SF: Bullous eruption of diabetes mellitus. Arch Dermatol 115:324, 1979
86. Toonstra J: Bullosis diabeticorum. Report of a case with a review of the literature. J Am Acad Dermatol 13:799, 1985
87. Mazer JM, Belaich S: Bullous idiopathique des diabetiques. Ann Dermatol Venereol 114:593, 1987
88. Arndt KA, Mihm MC, Parrish JA: Bullae: a cutaneous sign of a variety of neurologic diseases. J Invest Dermatol 60:312, 1973

12

INFLAMMATORY VIRUS DISEASES

Long-known human diseases characterized by an inflammatory reaction of the skin to viruses are the varicella-herpes group, variola-vaccinia, paravaccinia, ecthyma contagiosum, as well as rubella, rubeola, and related exanthems. To these have been added "minor" virus rashes caused by Coxsackie and other recently identified agents. The Gianotti–Crosti syndrome also seems to be caused by a virus. Various skin lesions associated with acquired human immunodeficiency virus (HIV) infection are listed in Table 12–1 for convenience. Specific lesions are discussed in related chapters. Other viruses that cause primarily epithelial proliferation are covered in Chapter 32.

INTRANUCLEAR VIRUSES

Herpes simplex, zoster, and *varicella* have in common not only the intranuclear localization of the virus but also the specific epidermal reaction described as reticulating and ballooning degeneration[1] (Fig. 12–1). Infection and death of individual cells lead to defects in the malpighian layer, which are quickly filled with fluid and produce vesicles of netlike appearance.[2,3] This process can be best observed in early or mild lesions or in the borders of larger ones in which the center forms a vesicle characterized by almost complete disintegration of the living parts of the epidermis (Fig. 12–2). In the vesicle are edematous cells and cell groups floating like balloons. Multinucleated epithelial cells are common.

These often huge elements, whether mononucleated or multinucleated are the characteristic feature in Tzanck smears (see Fig. 5–15D). In well-stained preparations, especially with O&G stain, one sees eosinophilic inclusion bodies in some or many nuclei. In H&E sections, the nucleus more commonly has a pale ground-glass appearance with a thin hematoxylin-stained rim (Fig. 12–1).

The vesicle thus is intraepidermal, but the individual features depend very much on the age of the lesion and the acuteness of the process. Herpes simplex is apt to produce the most severe destruction accompanied by heavy dermal infiltrate. The infiltrate consists predominantly of lymphocytes.

Varicella (Fig. 12–3) usually has relatively mild and superficial inflammation,[4] whereas the infiltrate of vesicular zoster is intermediate in amount and extends deep into the subcutaneous tissue, often involving nerve trunks. In hemorrhagic and necrotizing cases of zoster, tissue changes will be, of course, correspondingly severe. In herpes simplex, viral colonization of outer root sheath is not uncommon, and typical cytologic changes may be found more easily there than in

TABLE 12–1. CUTANEOUS MANIFESTATIONS OF ACQUIRED IMMUNODEFICIENCY SYNDROME

1. Inflammatory dermatoses
   Severe seborrheic dermatitis, eosinophilic pustular folliculitis, severe cystic acne, granuloma annulare-like lesions, acrodermatitis enteropathica.
2. Common infections
   Superficial dermatophytosis, tinea pedis, onychomycosis, herpes simplex, herpes zoster, palmoplantar warts, perianal condylomas, molluscum contagiosum, mucocutaneous candidiasis, oral hairy leukoplakia, pseudomonas infection, scabies.
3. Uncommon infections
   Mycobacterial infections, cryptococcosis, histoplasmosis, nocardiosis, fusarium infection, aspergillosis, bacillary epithelioid angiomatosis.
4. Malignant neoplasms
   Kaposi's sarcoma, lymphoma, basal cell epithelioma, squamous cell carcinoma.

(From Cockerell CJ: Cutaneous manifestations of HIV infection other than Kaposi's sarcoma: Clinical and histologic aspects. J Am Acad Dermatol 22:1260, 1990.)

the destroyed epidermis. Superinfection of inflamed skin, especially in atopic dermatitis, with herpes simplex virus is known as "Kaposi's varicelliform eruption" or "eczema herpeticum,"[5] which can be differentiated by Tzanck smear from the clinically similar "eczema vaccinatum."

The demonstration of virus-infected large nuclei in genital ulcers proves herpes simplex even in the simultaneous presence of chancroid (see Fig. 17–2). On the other hand, one must not forget that large and sometimes multinucleated cells may be found in the epidermis for a variety of nonspecific reasons (see Fig. 5–10).

VARIOLA AND VACCINIA

Smallpox is said to have been eradicated, but *vaccinia* is to be considered in the differential diagnosis of vesicular dermatoses because it may be spread by contamination, as in eczema vaccinatum. The mechanism of vesiculation in these two diseases consists of reticulating and ballooning degeneration of prickle cells. The process in vaccinia is slower and starts in the upper layers, with formation of multiloculated vesicles, while edema and inflammatory infiltrate of the dermis may be already well devel-

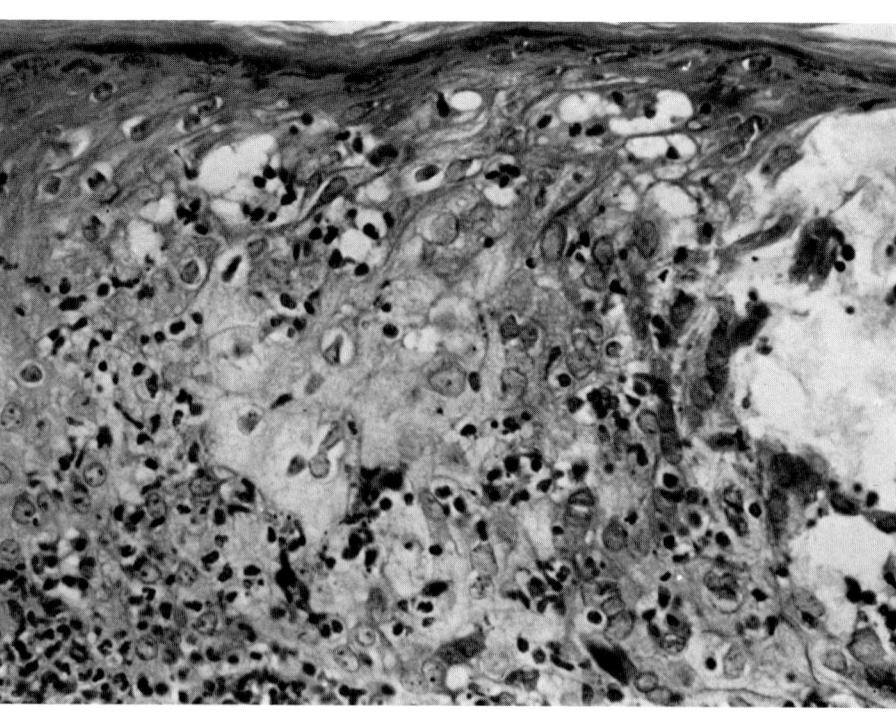

Figure 12–1.
Edge of herpes zoster vesicle showing ground-glass appearance of nuclei due to intranuclear inclusions, reticulating degeneration due to complete disappearance of individual cells, and ballooning degeneration with formation of multinucleated giant cells. H&E. X370. (From Sutton. Diseases of the Skin, 11th ed, 1956. Courtesy of Dr. R. L. Sutton, Jr. Contributed by H. Pinkus.)

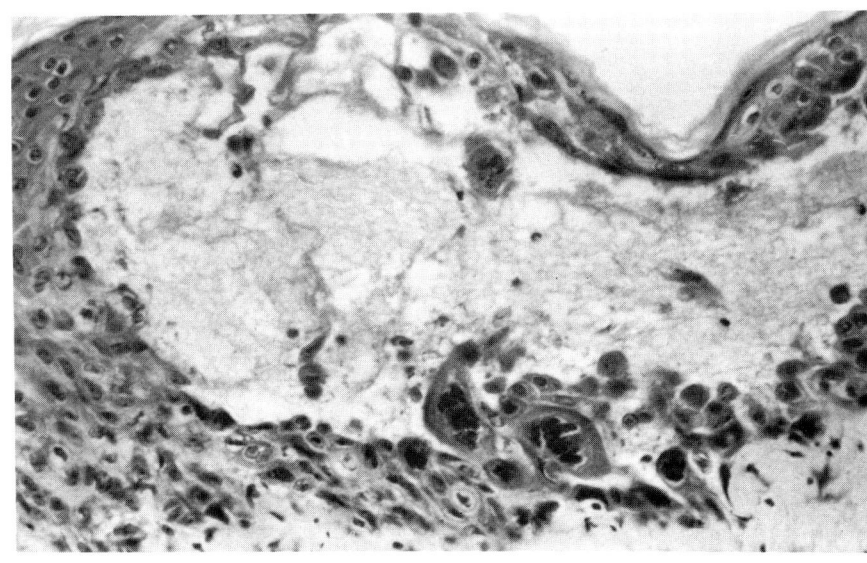

Figure 12–2.
Herpes simplex. Reticulating degeneration and formation of multinucleated epithelial giant cells within an intraepidermal blister. H&E. X250.

oped. Inclusion bodies, if present, are intracytoplasmic (Guarneri bodies).

PARAVACCINIA AND ECTHYMA CONTAGIOSUM

The so-called "milker's nodule" (Fig. 12–4) owes its hard consistency (stone pox) to a combination of epidermal acanthosis high degree of edema, and much cellular infiltrate.[6] Early stages may resemble erythema multiforme with beginning bullous edema of papillae (Fig. 12–5), but the epidermis does not necrotize but shows vacuolization of the higher prickle cell layers and fingerlike elongation of rete ridges. The vacuolated cells contain eosinophilic inclusion bodies in cytoplasm and nucleus. Inflammatory infiltrate (Fig. 12–4) consists of a mixture of polymorphs, lymphocytes, and plasma cells. Most of the infiltrate remains fairly superficial. Virus has been cultured in bovine fetal kidney and resembles that of sheep pox.

"Sheep pox" or orf (Fig. 12–6) exhibits ballooning and reticular degeneration of the epidermis in the early stage and may produce pseudoepithelioma-

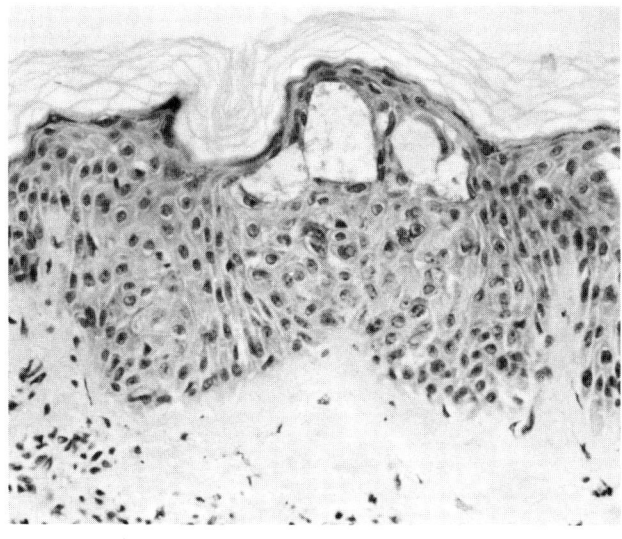

Figure 12–3.
Varicella. Relatively mild derangement of epidermis with several small vesicles due to reticulating degeneration of keratinocytes. Horny layer intact, mild inflammatory infiltrate in dermis. H&E. X250.

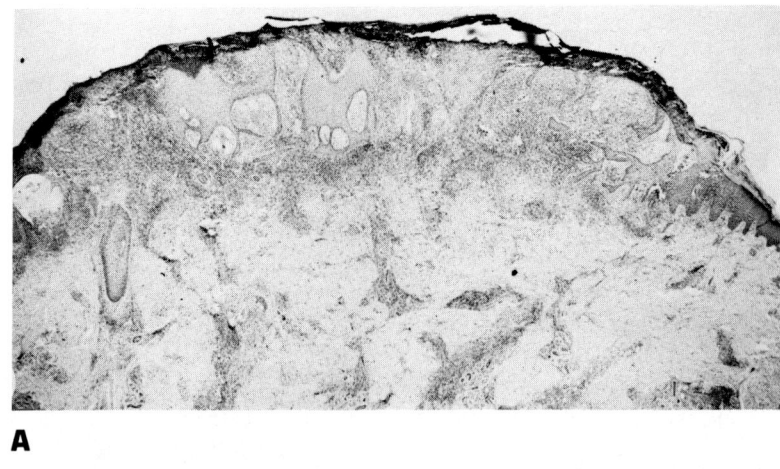
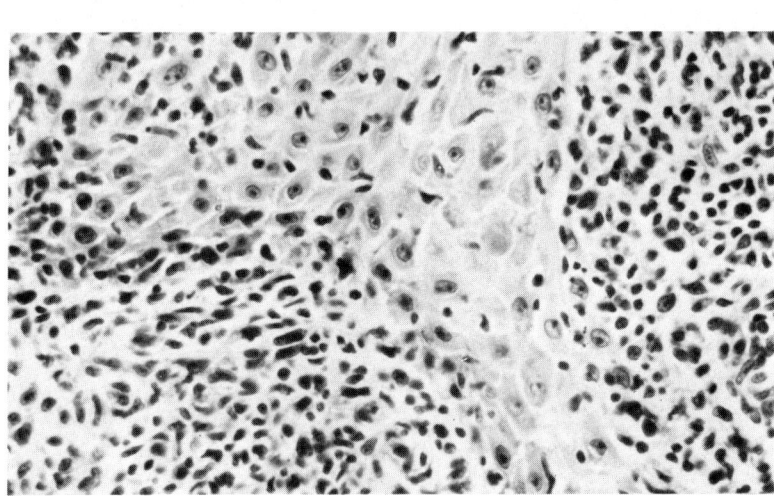

Figure 12–4.
A. Milker's nodule (paravaccinia). Note resemblance to erythema exudativum multiforme at low power. H&E. X14. **B.** Acanthosis and mixed, almost granulomatous infiltrate at high power. H&E. X280.

tous proliferation later.[7,8] The dermis is highly vascular and edematous and contains severe inflammatory infiltrate of mixed character. Eosinophilic inclusion bodies may be demonstrable in the cytoplasm of inflammatory cells (Fig. 12–7). The virus of ecthyma contagiosum is a DNA-containing poxvirus.

MEASLES AND GERMAN MEASLES

The histologic picture of *rubeola* and *rubella* is more or less that of a toxic erythema. Multinucleated epidermal cells may be found in true measles,[9] but the pathognomonic mesenchymal cells with numerous nuclei are usually present only in lymphoid tissues. A morbilliform exanthem having histologic features of periarteritis nodosa develops in cases of Kawasaki's disease (Chapter 15).

COXSACKIE AND ECHO VIRUSES

Exanthems have been described due to various newly identified viruses. Figure 12–8 illustrates a case and shows an intraepidermal vesicle with some degeneration of prickle cells, localized dermal edema and hemorrhage, and some perivascular round cell infiltrate. The histologic picture of all these diseases is of diagnostic value only in coordination with the clinical features and possibly corroborative laboratory evidence of rising antibody titers. The most common clinical differential diagnosis is with drug exanthems, and these rarely produce intraepidermal vesicles or multinucleated giant cells. Lichen urticatus (Chapter 10) and possibly pityriasis rosea (Fig. 12–9) may enter histologic differential diagnosis.

A special case is hand-foot-and-mouth disease, caused by a Coxsackie virus.[10] Histologically, this

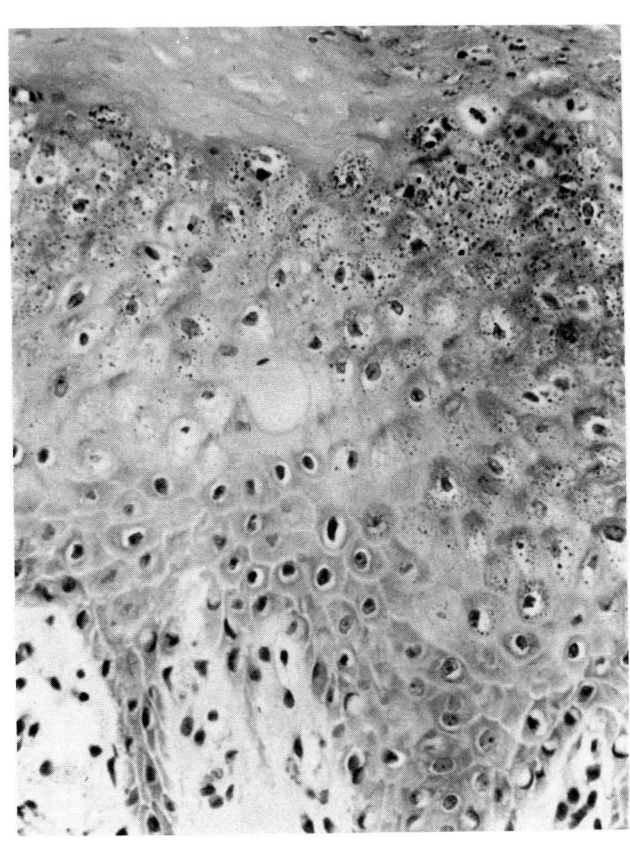

Figure 12–5.
Milker's nodule showing marked vacuolization of prickle cells high in the epidermis. H&E. X225.

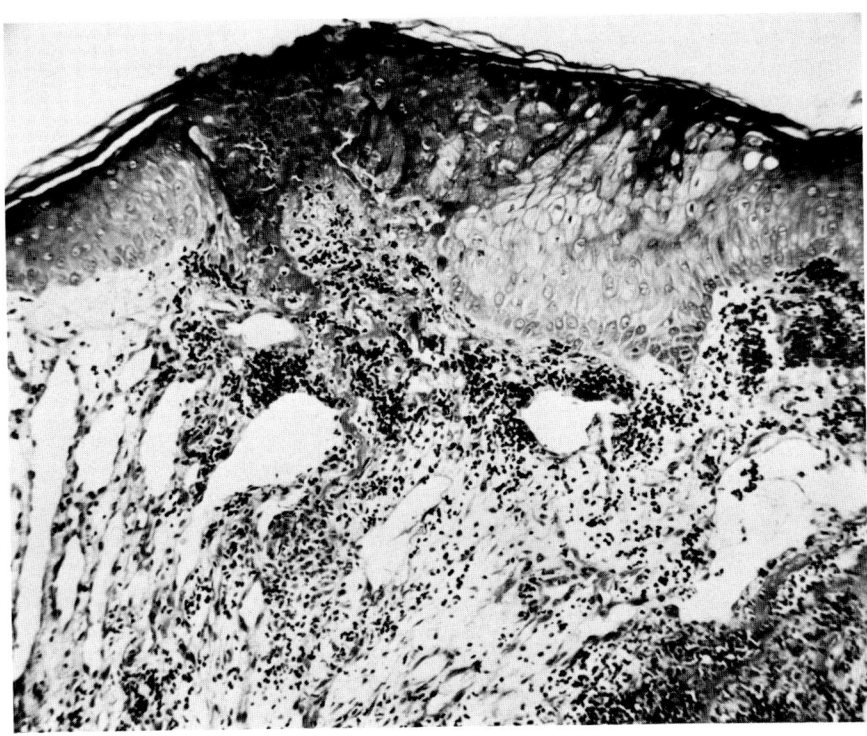

Figure 12–6.
Ecthyma contagiosum (orf). Epidermis is in part necrotic and shows beginning proliferative changes. Edema, telangiectasia, and inflammatory infiltrate in dermis. H&E. X135.

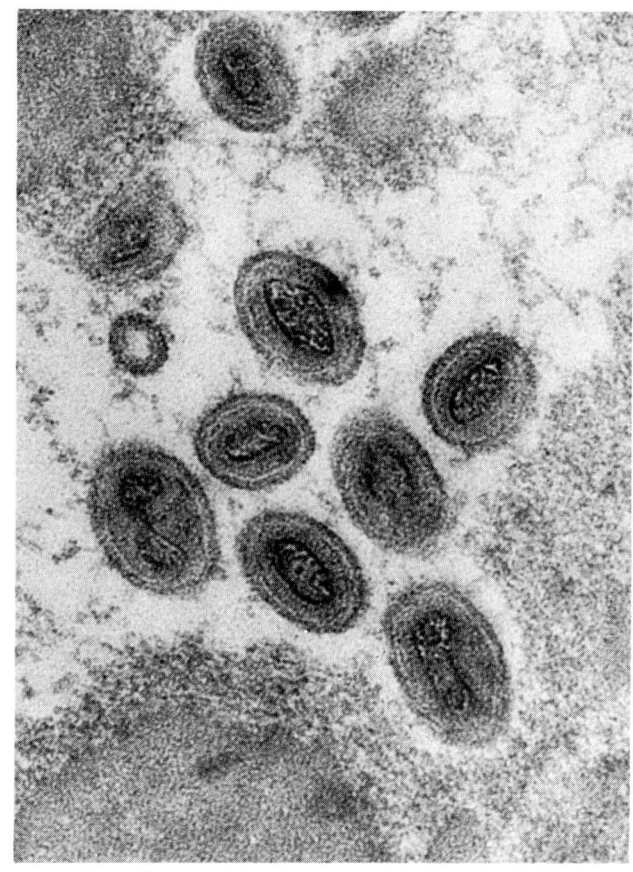

Figure 12–7.
Ecthyma contagiosum (orf). Electron micrograph of intracytoplasmic elongated virus particles. X116,000. (Courtesy of Drs. A. Eng and K. Soltani.)

also shows ballooning and reticulating degeneration of the epidermis with neutrophils and mononuclear cells in the vesicles. The dermis shows a mixed cellular infiltrate.

Skin lesions associated with spotted fever group of Rickettsioses appear on the third day of illness in the form of petechial maculopapules in 50 percent of cases. A predominantly T-lymphocyte and histiocyte infiltrate is present around dermal capillaries. Polymorphs are absent.[11]

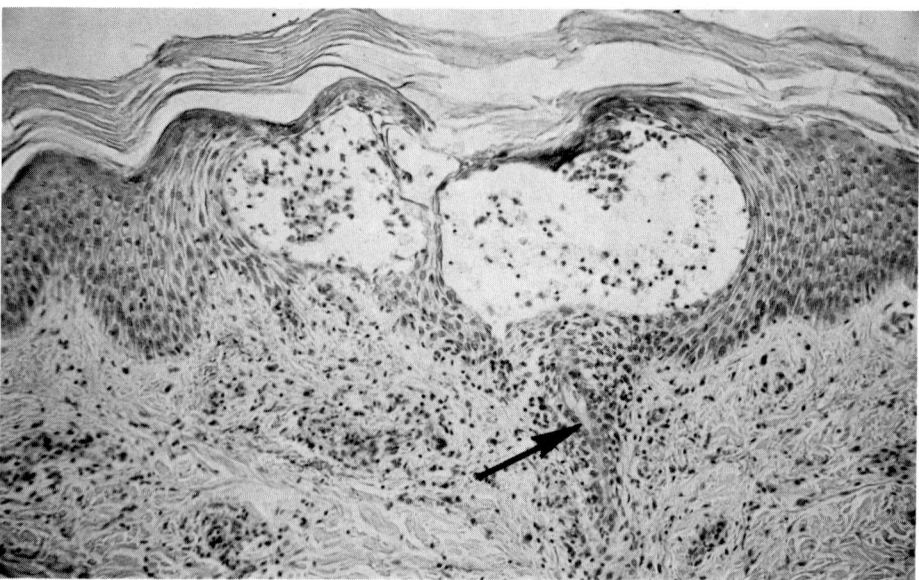

Figure 12–8.
Viral exanthem, suspected to be caused by echo virus. H&E. X135. Note sweat duct (arrow) near center of lesion.

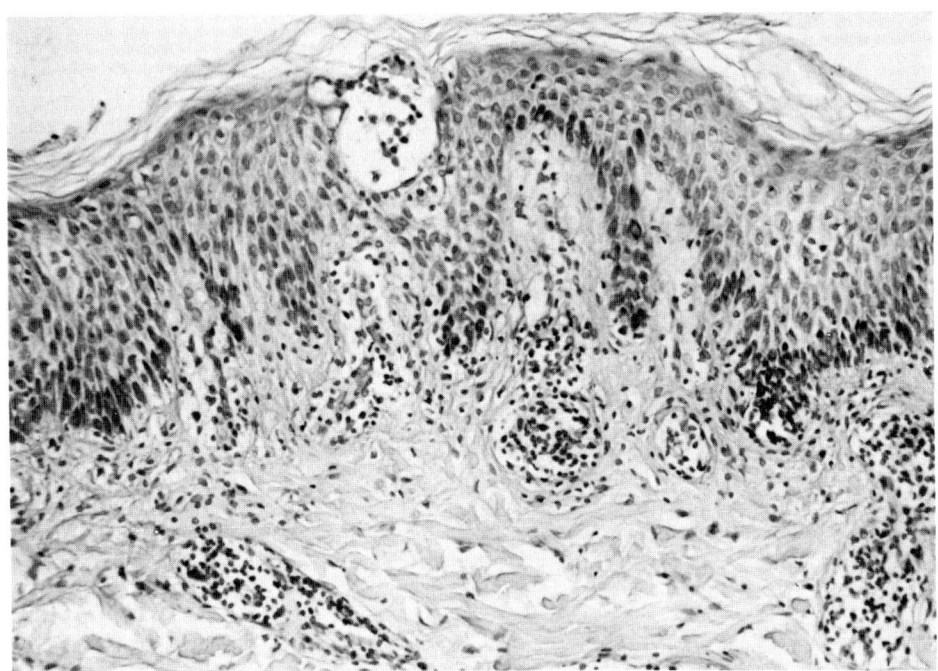

Figure 12–9.
Pityriasis rosea showing characteristic solitary intraepidermal vesicle at point of greatest activity. There are two other foci of less severe spongiotic edema, and the epidermis in the left side of the picture shows the earliest stage of parakeratosis, which farther into the lesion (not shown in the photo) will replace the normal horny layer and lead to scale formation. H&E. X180.

GIANOTTI–CROSTI SYNDROME

A large body of literature has accumulated concerning *papular acrodermatitis of childhood,* first described in 1955,[12] which has been recognized as the skin manifestation of infection with hepatitis B virus. A peculiar feature of the disease is that it has been extensively reported from Europe,[13] and there is one report of an epidemic occurrence in Japan,[14] but there are only a few reports from the United States.[15–18] The reasons for this low incidence in this country of an apparently striking febrile disease in children is unclear. The histologic picture is said to consist of some acanthosis, spongiosis, and parakeratosis of the epidermis and a mixed lymphohistiocytic infiltrate of the upper dermis with Pautrier-like monocytic accumulations in the epidermis. Therefore, the picture is, at best, compatible with the clinical diagnosis but not diagnostic.

PITYRIASIS ROSEA

If one examines a dozen or more typical cases of active pityriasis rosea by taking complete cross sections of small lesions or radial slices extending from normal skin into the center of large ones, one arrives at a fairly consistent concept of the histologic changes.

A well-oriented section of a typical lesion is characterized by definite zonal arrangement.[19,20] Farthest out, under still normal epidermis, there is mild to moderate edema of the pars papillaris, engorgement of widened subpapillary vessels, and moderate perivascular infiltrate of T lymphocytes predominantly of helper–inducer subset.[21,22] These changes increase toward the center of the lesion, and now the epidermis becomes slightly thickened, more through edema than actual acanthosis. At the height of the inflammatory process, there is usually one, sometimes two, small intraepidermal vesicle (Fig. 12–9) of spongiotic type, accompanied by some exocytosis of mononuclear cells.

Adjacent to the vesicle, parakeratosis and loss of granular layer are found for a relatively short distance. As edema and inflammatory infiltrate subside toward the center of the plaque, the parakeratotic scale moves upward and is replaced by normal keratinization in the clearing center. The scale thus has a free end at the central side of the lesion corresponding to the collarette effect of the clinical lesion. There is nothing very specific about any of these alterations. It is only their combination and arrangement that determines the diagnosis. The changes resemble eczematous dermatitis, and contact dermatitis, tinea, and drug eruptions, especially gold dermatitis, may produce similar pictures. Perhaps the most impressive feature is the almost regular presence of an intraepidermal vesicle in a clinically dry dermatosis. The long-standing suspicion of virus origin of the disease has been emphasized by the description of viruslike particles in the herald patch of pityriasis rosea.[23] In other studies, elevated titers of antibodies against *Borrelia burgdorferi* has been reported.[24]

REFERENCES

1. Demis JD: Clinical Dermatology, Section 14. Philadelphia: J. B. Lippincott Co. 1988
2. Jarratt M: Herpes simplex infection. Arch Dermatol 119:99, 1983
3. Huff JC, Krueger GG, Overall JC, et al: The histopathological evolution of recurrent herpes simplex labialis. J Am Acad Dermatol 5:550, 1981
4. McSorley J, Shapiro L, Brownstein MH, et al: Herpes simplex and varicella zoster: Comparative histopathology of 77 cases. Int J Dermatol 13:69, 1974
5. Bork K, Brauninger W: Increasing incidence of eczema herpeticum: Analysis of seventy-five cases. J Am Acad Dermatol 19:1024, 1988
6. Sanchez RL, Herbert A, Lucia H, Swendo J: Orf. Arch Pathol Lab Med 109:166, 1985
7. Shelley WB, Shelley ED: Farmyardpox: Parapox virus infection in man. Br J Dermatol 108:725, 1983
8. Mendez B, Burnett JW: Orf. Cutis 44:286, 1989
9. Ackerman AB, Suringa DWR: Multinucleate epidermal cells in measles. Arch Dermatol 103:180, 1971
10. Kimura A, Abe A, Nakao T: Light and electron microscopic study of skin lesions of patients with hand, foot, and mouth disease. Tohoku J Exp Med 122:237, 1977
11. Walker DH: Rickettsioses of the spotted fever group around the world. J Dermatol Tokyo 16:169, 1989
12. Gianotti F: Papular acrodermatitis of childhood and other papulo-vesicular acro-located syndromes. Br J Dermatol 100:49, 1979
13. Taieb A, Plantin P, Du Pasquier P, et al: Gianotti–Crosti syndrome: A study of 26 cases. Br J Dermatol 115:49, 1986
14. Ishimaru Y, Ishimaru H, Toda G, et al: An epidemic of infantile papular acrodermatitis (Gianotti's disease) in Japan associated with hepatitis B surface antigen subtype ayw. Lancet 1:707, 1976
15. Rubenstein D, Esterly NB, Fretzin O: The Gianotti–Crosti syndrome. Pediatrics 61:433, 1978
16. Castellano A, Schweitzer R, Tong MJ, Omata M: Papular acrodermatitis of childhood and hepatitis B infection. Arch Dermatol 114:1530, 1978
17. San Joaquin VH, Ward KE, Marks MI: Gianotti disease in a child and acute hepatitis B in mother. JAMA 246:2191, 1981
18. Lee S, Kim KY, Hahn CS, et al: Gianotti–Crosti syndrome associated with hepatitis B surface antigen (subtype adr). J Am Acad Dermatol 12:629, 1985
19. Panizzon R, Bloch PH: Histopathology of pityriasis rosea Gilbert. Qualitative and quantitative light-microscopic study of 62 biopsies of 40 patients. Dermatologica 165:551, 1982
20. Aiba S, Tagami H: Immunohistologic studies in pityriasis rosea. Evidence for cellular immune reaction in the lesional epidermis. Arch Dermatol 121:761, 1985
21. Parsons JM: Pityriasis rosea update: 1986. J Am Acad Dermatol 15:159, 1986
22. Fox BJ, Odom RB: Papulosquamous diseases: A review. J Am Acad Dermatol 12:597, 1985
23. Aoshima T, Komura J, Ofuji S: Virus-like particles in the herald patch of pityriasis rosea. Dermatologica 162:64, 1981
24. Kuske B, Schmidli J, Hunziker T: Antibodies against *Borrelia burgdorferi* in patients with pityriasis rosea (PR). Dermatologica 177:255, 1988

13

MISCELLANEOUS PAPULOSQUAMOUS ERUPTIONS

In this chapter a number of superficial skin diseases that cannot be easily fitted into one of the patterns discussed in previous chapters are brought together. Rather than trying to classify them as specific types, we prefer to distinguish them by their particular characteristics.

Because papulosquamous disorders often have confusing or indistinct clinical features, they constitute a considerable percentage of specimens in a dermatopathologic laboratory. Some answers are easy: Psoriasis and lichen planus may be confused clinically but are at diametric ends of the histologic spectrum. Other differentiations may be difficult because the diseases belong to the same group of tissue reaction, for instance, seborrheic dermatitis and psoriasis.

The dermatoses to be discussed here are superficial fungous infections, various forms of parapsoriasis, the pigmented purpuric eruptions, lichen striatus, and scabies. We thus include considerably more territory than is covered by the classic clinical group. Seborrheic dermatitis, psoriasis, lichen planus, and other possible candidates were discussed in previous chapters. Secondary syphilis is considered together with other forms of the disease in Section IV.

SUPERFICIAL FUNGOUS INFECTIONS

Histologic examination of skin changes caused by dermatophytes in the widest sense illustrates three biologic phenomena. (1) Microorganisms do not have to invade living tissue in order to cause inflammation and immune reactions.[1–3] (2) The number of demonstrable organisms is inversely related to the degree of inflammatory reaction. (3) Fungal elements found in tissue sections are not necessarily the cause of the dermatosis but may be secondary parasites or even innocent bystanders. The dermatophytes, with the occasional exception of *Trichophyton rubrum* and *Candida,* live only in the dead horny layers of epidermis, hair, or nail. The inverse relation of number of organisms to inflammatory tissue reaction is described under the individual diseases, and we shall encounter a related principle in the chapters on granulomatous inflammation. *Candida* is the outstanding example of an opportunistic organism that may or may not be the principal cause of the dermatosis in which it is encountered. Hyphae and spores of nonpathogenic molds also may be seen in tissue sections and may be mistaken morphologically for dermatophytes. An exhaustive review of the dermal pathology of superficial fungous infection is available.[4]

Noninflammatory Lesions

Among the tineas, *tinea versicolor* occupies a singular place, histologically as well as clinically. There is almost complete absence of edema or inflammatory infiltrate. The epidermis also is practically normal, although it may be slightly thickened. Characteristic filaments and grouped spores usually can be seen within the horny layer in H&E sections. Minor histologic variations occur in different clinical manifestations. Horny layer is thickened and contains numerous organisms in hyperpigmented lesions (Fig. 13–1). Light microscopic impression of pigment block, lessened epidermal pigmentation, and melanocytic damage has been confirmed by electron microscopy of hypopigmented areas.[5,6]

Two rare conditions that share the features of large numbers of microorganisms and absence of inflammation with tinea versicolor are *tinea nigra palmaris*,[7] due to *Cladiosporum* species, and *pitted keratolysis,* from which *Streptomyces* and the organism of erythrasma have been cultured (see Chapter 34). The more typical clinical forms of erythrasma may also be mentioned here, although the causative microbe has been reclassified as *Corynebacterium minutissimum*. This organism is so small that it can be recognized only by oil immersion examination, and even then identification in thin tissue sections is hazardous. Skin scrapings stained with methylene blue or tape strippings[8] of the horny layer are advisable. The second technique is also the easiest way to demonstrate the tinea versicolor organism.

Tinea Superficialis

Other superficial fungous infections usually are due to *Trichophyton* species and often are the *tinea circinata* type.[9] They present a more or less eczematous reaction, but the picture frequently is somewhat bizarre, with very spotty spongiosis, acanthosis, and parakeratosis punctuated by occasional intraepider-

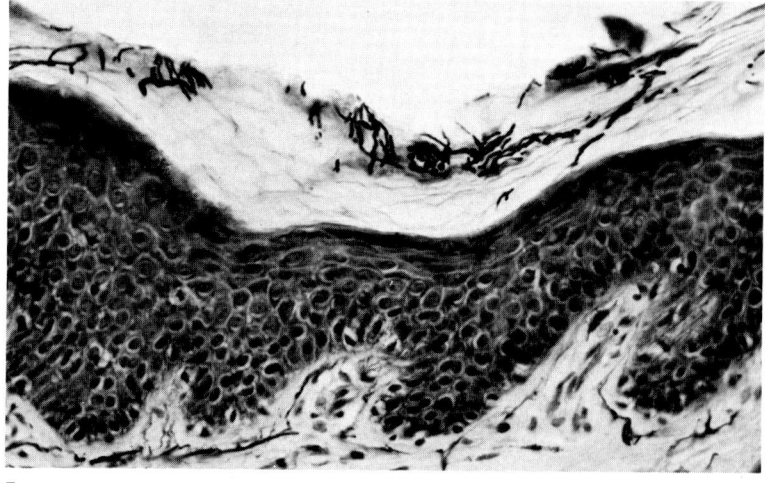

A

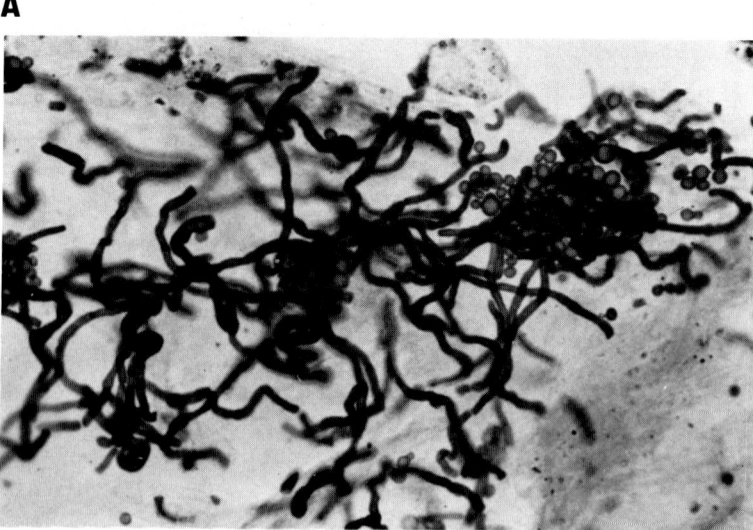

B

Figure 13–1.
Tinea versicolor. **A.** Demonstration of fungi in horny layer. O&G. X180. **B.** Fungi in a scale stained by PAS. X460.

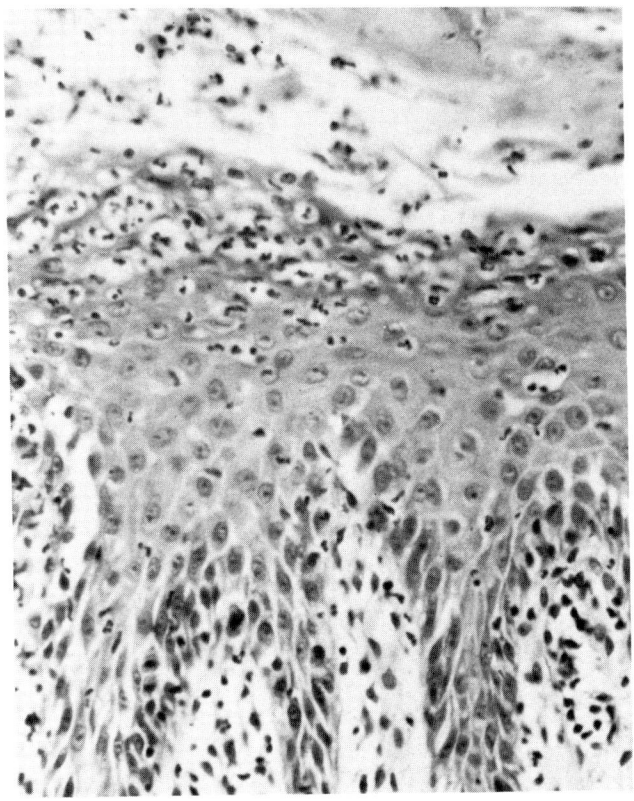

Figure 13–2.
Inflammatory dermatophytosis. Psoriasiform tissue reaction with spongiform pustule formation, mycelia in the keratin layer. H&E. Original X250.

mal vesiculation. Another tissue reaction is characterized by foci of spongiform edema and exocytosis with formation of subcorneal microabscesses resembling pustular psoriasis (Fig. 13–2).[10] Histologic findings are prominent at the active border of the lesions. Dermal infiltrate consists mainly of T lymphocytes of helper and suppressor subsets.[11]

It is important to keep in mind that mycelia are found only in the horny layer and often only in a short stretch peripheral to the inflammatory zone. Mycelia cannot be expected above the area of heaviest inflammation. Although thin paraffin sections are far from ideal objects in the search for dermatophytes, it happens occasionally that the histopathologist finds dermatophytes (Fig. 13–3) when the clinician either did not think of the diagnosis or was unsuccessful in the search. It is also well to remember that mycelia may be absent from the surface layer but present in the follicular ostium, especially in intertriginous areas and in tinea faciei.[12] O&G sections usually are satisfactory for finding dermatophytes, but PAS stain should be done for confirmation.

Inflammatory vesiculobullous eruption on the feet, especially between the toes, may be secondary to dermatophytes or erythrasma.[13] Mycelia may or may not be present in the surface scale of the lesion. Other lesions due to dermatophytes and *Candida* are discussed in Chapters 18, 46, and 47.

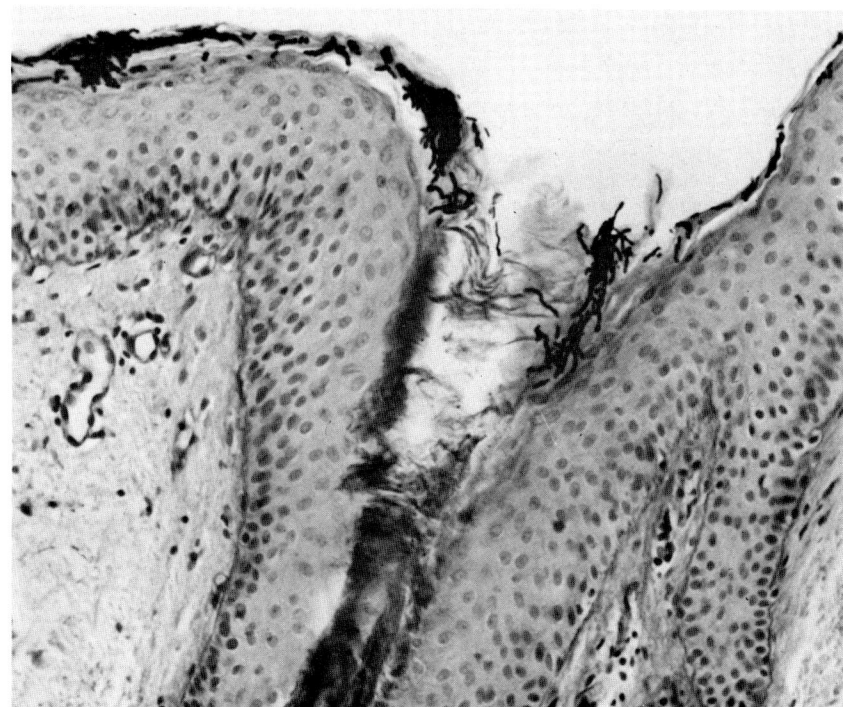

Figure 13–3.
Tinea faciei showing mycelia in the horny layer of the epidermis and the follicular infundibulum. Mild reactive changes of epidermis and dermis. PAS–hematoxylin. X225.

PARAPSORIASIS

On both clinical and histologic grounds, we prefer to separate the guttate forms of Brocq's parapsoriasis under the name of pityriasis lichenoides from those with larger or ill-defined lesions (parapsoriasis en plaques). We also believe that pityriasis lichenoides should be subdivided into chronic, subacute, and acute (and possibly varioliform) types, and the acute form is not to be set up as a separate entity.

Pityriasis Lichenoides

Among the most striking features of the guttate lesions under the microscope (Fig. 13–4A) are their sharp definition and their constant size, which hardly ever exceeds the limits of a widefield eyepiece under low power (total magnification ×40). This latter feature is one good clue. Another is the character of the scale in the fully developed chronic and subacute lesion, with some modification in the acute form. The scale is flat (Fig. 13–4B), and although it shows parakeratotic inclusions and even occasional microabscesses, it is not split into lamellae as is the psoriatic scale. It either adheres to the underlying epidermis or separates as a whole, a feature typical also in clinical examination. In the acute forms, the scale often is converted into a crust and may contain serum, leukocytes, and red cells (Fig. 13–5). The third outstanding feature is the peculiar, passive behavior of the epidermis.[14] Although it may be slightly thickened in the chronic type, it rarely gives the appearance of active regenerative or reactive inflammatory changes. It just seems to sit there suffering the invasion by inflammatory cells. That these are predominantly lymphocytic is another important difference from psoriasis. The subpapillary dermis exhibits variable degrees of edema and perivascular infiltrate of T lymphocytes, relatively mild in the chronic form and becoming increasingly

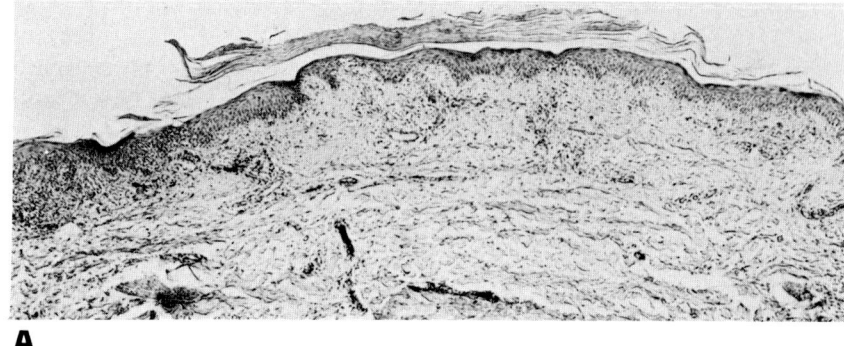

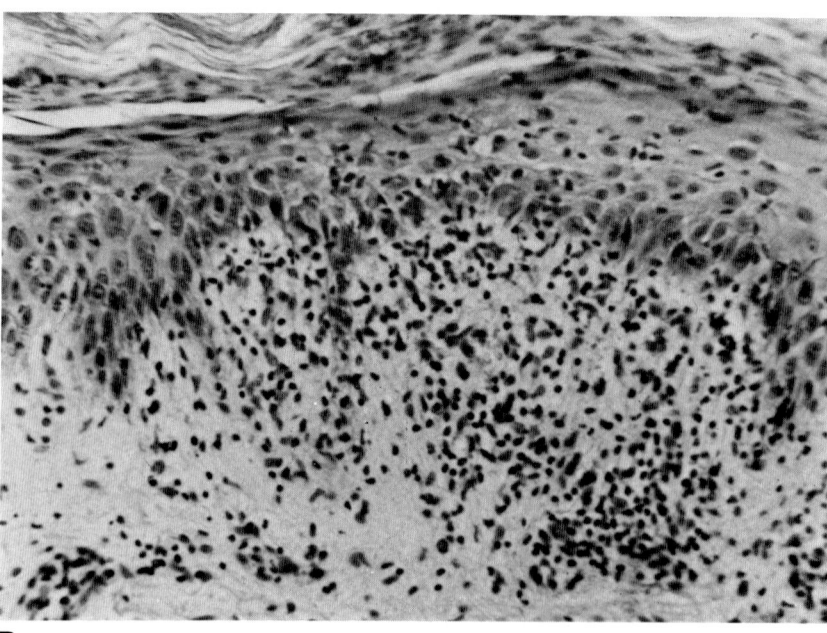

Figure 13–4.
Pityriasis lichenoides chronica. **A.** Typical size and appearance at low magnification. H&E. X45. **B.** Disk-like parakeratotic scale with suggested microabscesses, epidermal invasion by round cells, and perivascular infiltrate. Epidermis is more acanthotic than usual. H&E. X135.

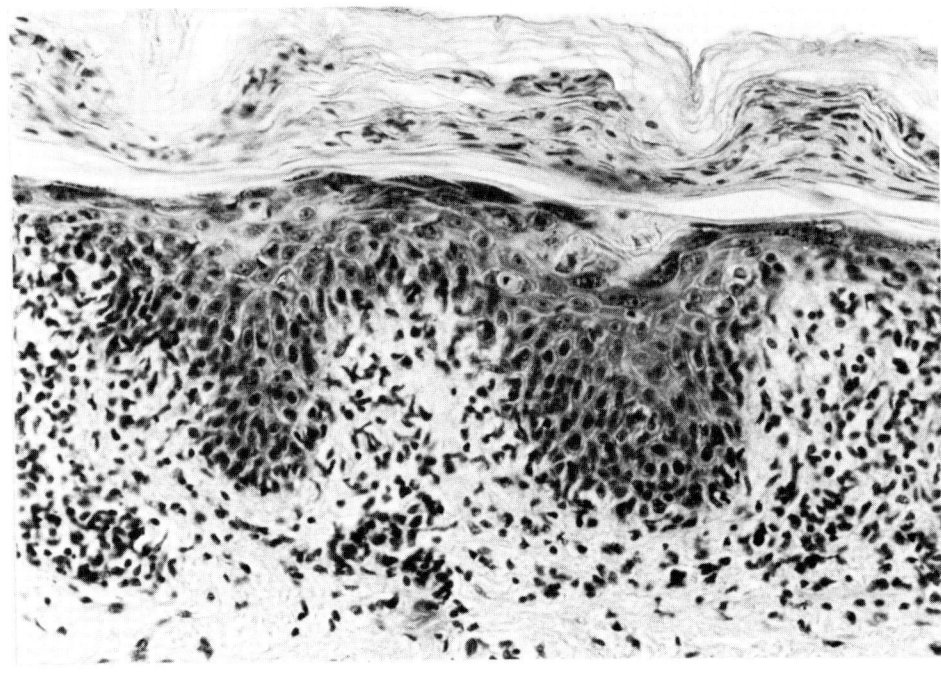

Figure 13–5.
Pityriasis lichenoides chronica. The epidermis is diffusely infiltrated by lymphocytes. The granular layer is replaced by a layer of parakeratotic crust. H&E. X250.

severe in the subacute (Fig. 13–6) and acute (Fig. 13–7) types. Black and Marks[15] find many histiocytes and no evidence of vascular disease. Wood et al,[16] in their survey of immunohistologic findings, have confirmed our long-held opinion that the varioliform type is probably a variant of the more chronic form (Juliusberg's disease). It is our impression that the name "Mucha–Habermann disease" has been applied too liberally to cases that show occasional crusted lesions and that it might be more properly reserved for more hyperacute and severely necrotic cases.[17] There are many intermediate cases

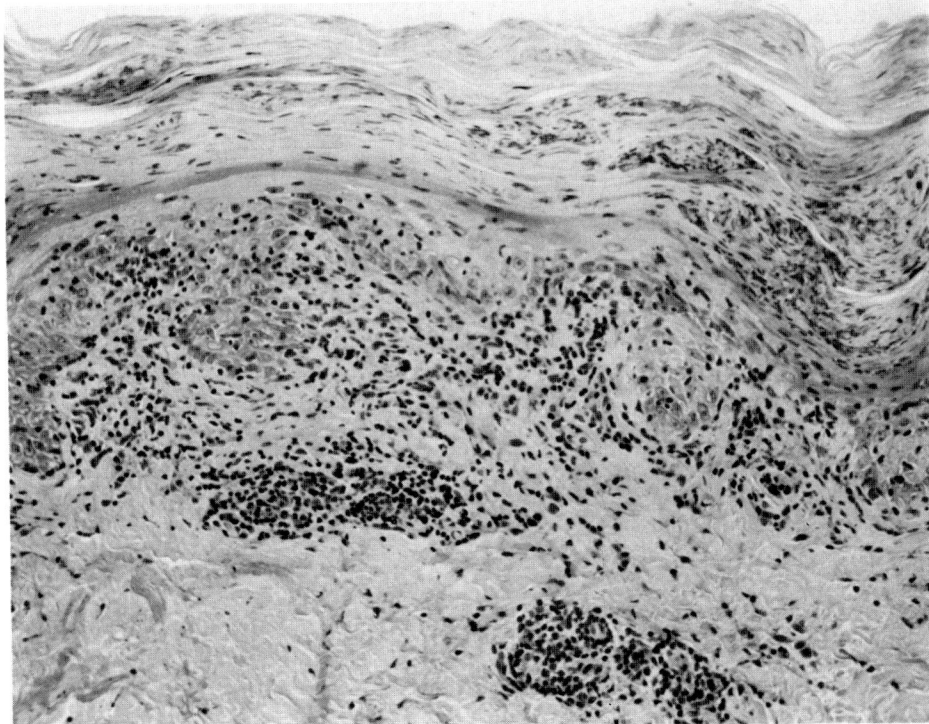

Figure 13–6.
Pityriasis lichenoides subacuta. Fading of epidermal nuclei, exocytosis of small round cells, layered parakeratotic scale with microabscesses. Dermal infiltrate somewhat heavier than in chronic form. Papules of this type may be found associated with more chronic and with more acute lesions in the same patient. H&E. X180.

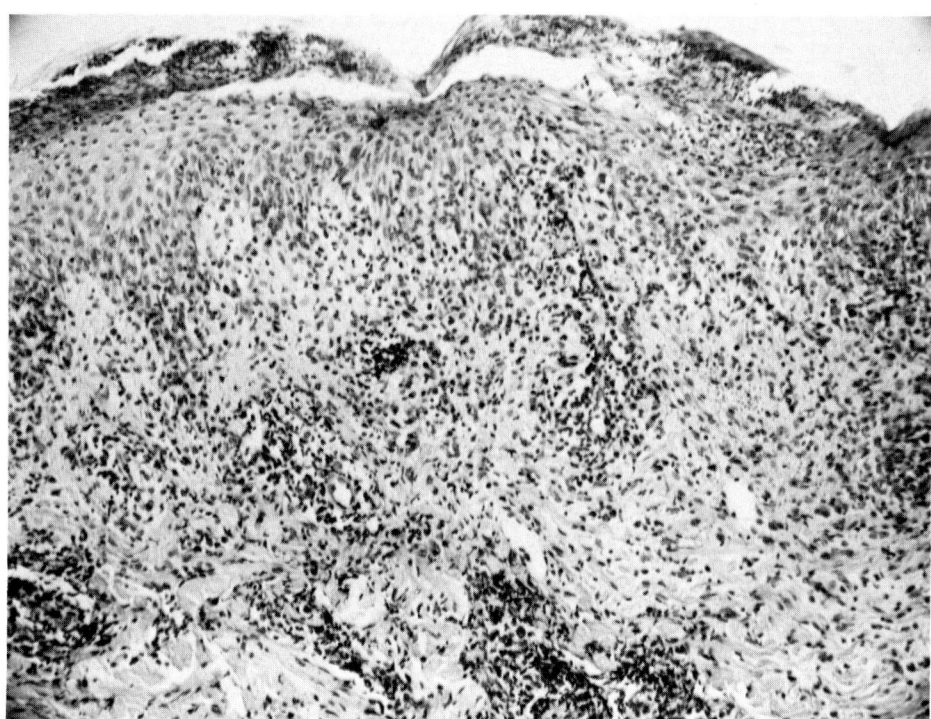

Figure 13–7.
Pityriasis lichenoides et varioliformis acuta. Fairly early lesion of moderate intensity. Beginning breakdown of epidermis. Infiltrate consists of mononuclear cells. H&E. X135.

in which the severity of the tissue reaction depends a lot on the individual lesion and the stage in which it was taken for biopsy. In really severe lesions, the entire epidermis and part of the pars papillaris undergo necrosis, and there is hemorrhage associated with much edema and inflammatory infiltrate. A papulonecrotic lesion is produced that has very little in common with the histologic picture of variola.

Thus, the various forms of pityriasis lichenoides are characterized by their typical size, by relatively minor though characteristic, epidermal participation, and by histiocytic and small round cell infiltrate, which has a peculiar tendency to invade the epidermis. There is no evidence of vasculitis. These latter features tie the histologic picture of pityriasis lichenoides to the other forms of parapsoriasis. For a discussion of lymphoma-like lesions (lymphomatoid papulosis) see Chapter 45.

Parapsoriasis en Plaques

It becomes more increasingly obvious[18,19] that parapsoriasis en plaques should be divided into two forms with decidedly different prognosis and recognizable clinical and histologic differences. One type, which has been called "digitate dermatosis" and "chronic superficial dermatitis" and which we prefer to call small-plaque parapsoriasis, has no serious significance, whereas large-plaque parapsoriasis sooner or later progresses toward mycosis fungoides, sometimes through the intermediate state of poikiloderma.[20] Histologic differences may not be striking in early lesions but become more pronounced as the large-plaque type progresses.[21,22]

Just as the plaques of parapsoriasis are barely palpable clinically, so may the histologic features be very mild. A practically normal epidermis (Fig. 13–8) has an almost normal horny layer with occasional foci of parakeratosis. A few round cells may have migrated into the epidermis, most often singly, only occasionally simulating an eczematous vesicle or a Pautrier abscess (Fig. 13–9A). The subepidermal infiltrate also is mild, somewhat diffuse and accentuated around subpapillary vessels. It presents one feature characteristic of all types of parapsoriasis: the admixture of a fair proportion of fixed-tissue-type cells to small round cells. This phase of parapsoriasis en plaques, therefore, has features that suggest a mild and benign proliferative process of lymphoreticular cells rather than an inflammatory disease. The small-plaque variant remains in this state indefinitely. The large type, if biopsied at intervals, will show a row of progressively heavier alterations. These do not concern the epidermis, although it may be somewhat acanthotic and may have more parakeratosis and even an occasional microves-

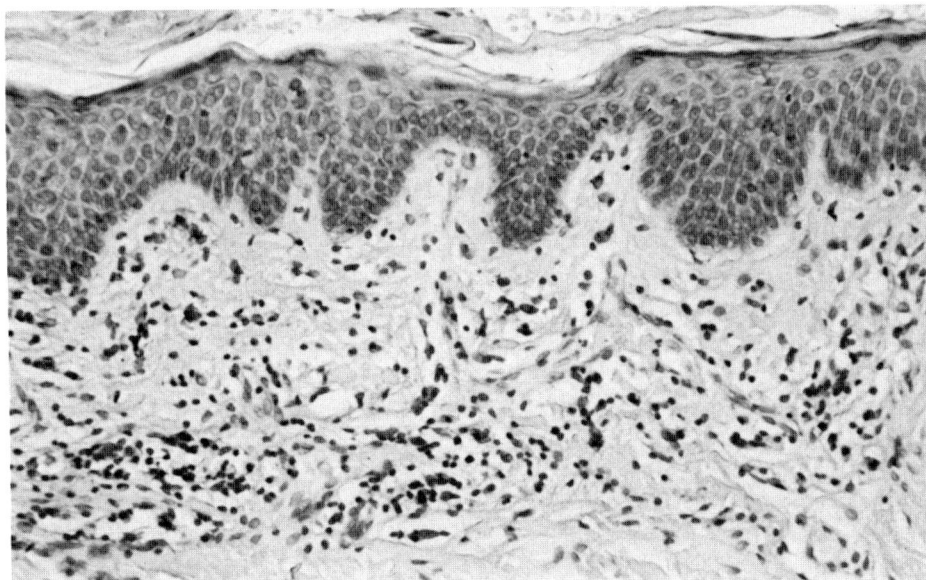

Figure 13–8.
Small-plaque form of parapsoriasis. Almost normal epidermis with minimal parakeratosis. Moderate diffuse infiltrate consisting of small round cells and fixed-tissue-type cells. No sign of the poikilodermatous tissue reaction. The picture is characterized more by the absence of specific features of other diseases than by any outstanding hallmarks of its own. H&E. X225.

icle. It is the infiltrate that increases in severity and tendency to epidermal invasion (Fig. 13–9B). Its composition of small round cells and fixed-tissue-type cells remains unchanged (Fig. 13–10). Careful search may reveal an occasional very large and dark-staining nucleus. Eosinophils and plasma cells are rare occurrences. The question that so often prompts biopsy in these cases—Is it still parapsoriasis en plaques, or is it changing into mycosis fungoides?—should be answered with great reserve. Actually, the turning point is more sharply defined by the clinical observation of increase in thickness of skin lesions

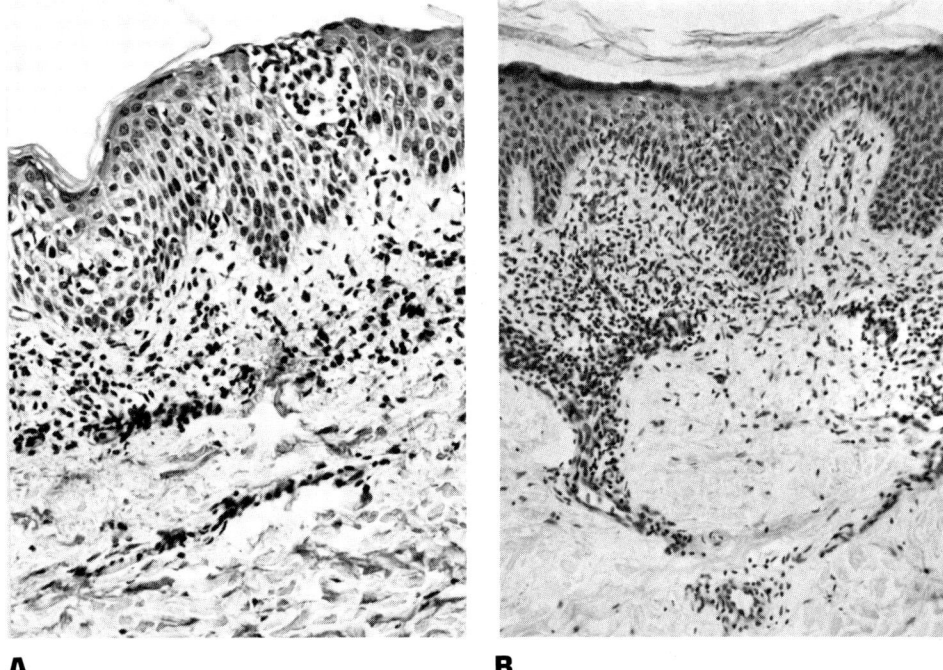

A   **B**

Figure 13–9.
Parapsoriasis en plaques. **A.** Intraepidermal vesicle combining features of eczematous reaction (see Fig. 7–3) and Pautrier abscess (see Fig. 45–5B) in a lesion exhibiting mild infiltrate and no acanthosis. **B.** Less epidermal invasion in a case with considerable acanthosis and fairly heavy infiltrate. H&E. X135.

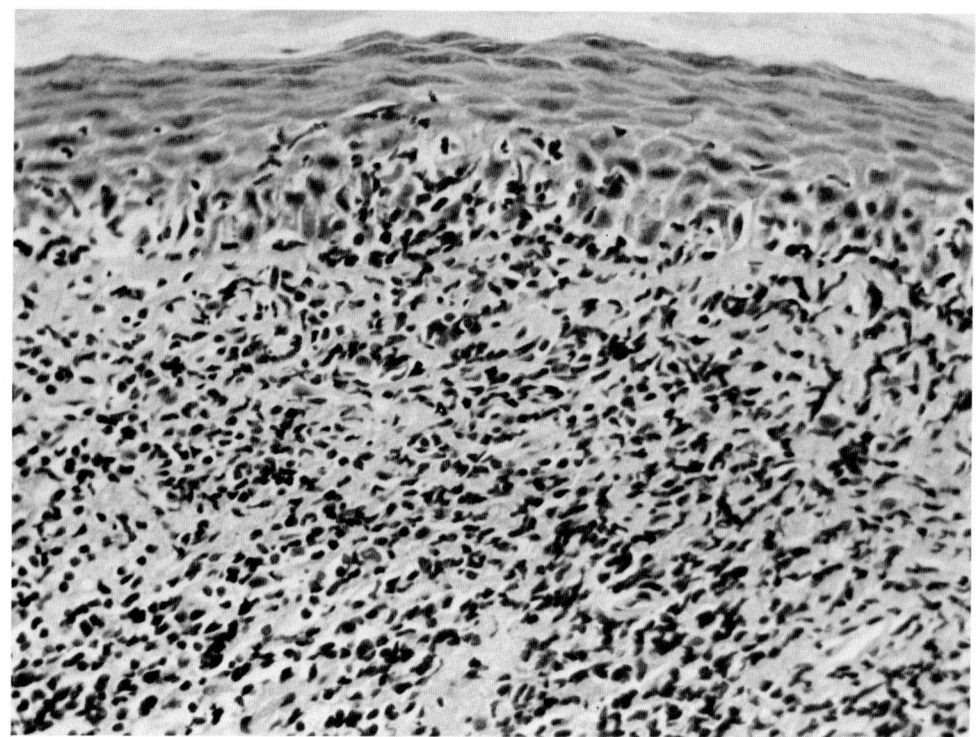

Figure 13–10.
Premycotic phase of large-plaque type of parapsoriasis. More diffuse and polymorphous infiltrate with strong tendency to invade the lower layers of the atrophic epidermis in a clinically poikilodermatous lesion. H&E. X375.

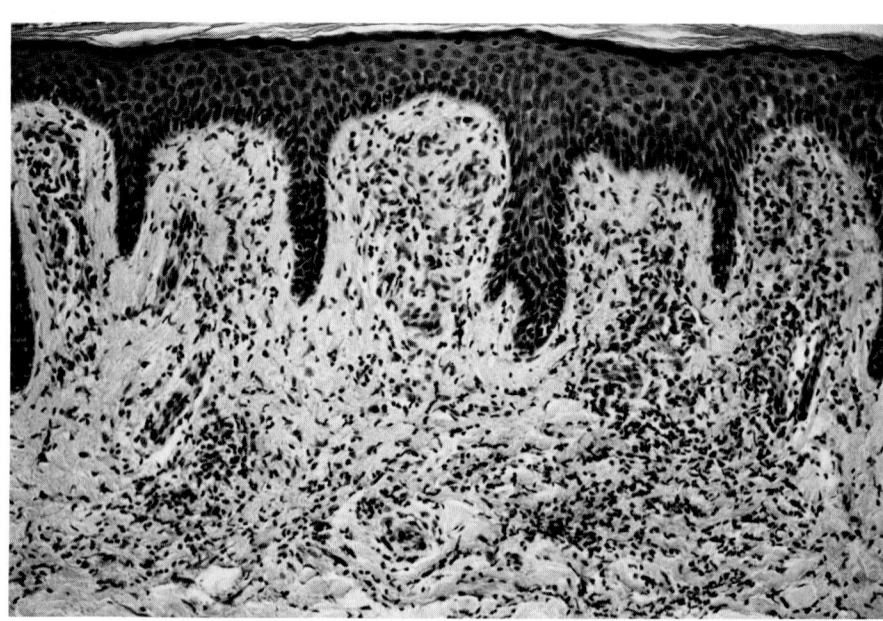

Figure 13–11.
Pigmented purpuric eruption of Schamberg–Majocchi type. H&E. X135.

and developing pruritus. Histologic indications include a much heavier dermal infiltrate containing cells with hyperchromatic and hyperconvoluted nuclei and more prominent microabscess formation.

Parapsoriasis Lichenoides and Poikiloderma

The histologic features of the rare *lichenoid* and *retiform* types of parapsoriasis are similar to parapsoriasis en plaques and may evoke from them, but often tend toward those of poikiloderma, into which the clinical features also merge. Indeed, parapsoriasis is one of the three diseases that can cause the clinicopathologic symptom complex of poikiloderma atrophicans vasculare. Dermatomyositis and lupus erythematosus are the other two. The poikilodermatous lesions show epidermal atrophy with preservation of granular and horny layer, spotty liquefaction degeneration of basal cells, and a bandlike, superficial dermal infiltrate of lymphocytes, histiocytes, and macrophages with melanin pigment granules.[23]

PIGMENTED PURPURIC ERUPTIONS

There seems to be little doubt that Schamberg's and Majocchi's diseases are variants of the same process. Gougerot–Blum's lichenoid purpuric eruption and lichen aureus have somewhat distinctive features. Hutchinson's angioma serpiginosum has been separated[24] as a noninflammatory, purely angiomatous, and very rare entity (Chapter 43).

Schamberg–Majocchi Eruption

The first low-power impression (Fig. 13–11) in a case of Schamberg–Majocchi eruption is that of a peculiarly ragged infiltrate, which is neither diffuse nor strictly perivascular, is widespread in the subpapillary layer but not dense, and is somewhat focal without forming definite papules. The infiltrate is predominantly lymphocytic. The epidermis usually is not much changed, except for focal invasion by inflammatory cells, which may cause some edema and parakeratosis. Closer inspection reveals ectatic small vessels with swollen endothelia, and in favorable sections, one may recognize the hyaline degeneration of vessel walls that is the hallmark of these affections. Hemorrhage by diapedesis, decomposed red cells, and hemosiderin deposits complete the picture.

In routine diagnostic work, the two principal clinical features of purpura and pigmentation are of little help. Extravasation of red blood cells is common in skin sections due to surgical trauma, especially in punch biopsy. It is only if disintegrating red cells are recognized that one can diagnose in vivo hemorrhage. Hemosiderin is peculiarly difficult to see in H&E sections, when only small amounts are present. Usually, the clinician will submit a fresh lesion in which the gradual process of conversion of hemoglobin in hemosiderin has barely begun. O&G sections are not helpful either. While they show erythrocytes more clearly, they leave hemosiderin unstained and often obscure in contrast to melanin. Specific stain for iron, therefore, is required if blood pigment has to be demonstrated. This is rarely necessary, however, because other histologic features are sufficiently characteristic.

Gougerot–Blum Eruption

Gougerot–Blum eruption usually shows a considerably heavier infiltrate, some epidermal acanthosis, and considerably more invasion by inflammatory cells associated with edema and parakeratosis. Inasmuch as this disease usually forms more persistent plaques, the amount of hemosiderin also is apt to be greater.

Lichen Aureus (Purpuricus)

An often linear (zosteriform) eruption on legs or trunk of young adults has been described under the striking name of "lichen aureus," although the clinical color is more often the red-brown color of hemosiderosis (lichen purpuricus). The cause is unknown, and the course is protracted as in all the pigmented purpuric eruptions.[25] The histologic features are similar to those seen in Schamberg–Majocchi's eruption. The bandlike lymphocytic infiltrate is heavier and there are larger numbers of macrophages containing hemosiderin granules. The presence of Langerhans cells has been demonstrated by electron microscopy.[26] The infiltrate is often separated from the epidermis by edematous papillae, and there is no evidence of epidermal invasion.[27]

Differential Diagnosis

The differential diagnosis of all pigmented purpuric eruptions, if found on the legs below the knees, must include stasis dermatitis (Chapter 15) and drug eruptions. Any medicamentous dermatitis that produces a maculopapular exanthem on other

198 SUPERFICIAL INFLAMMATORY PROCESSES

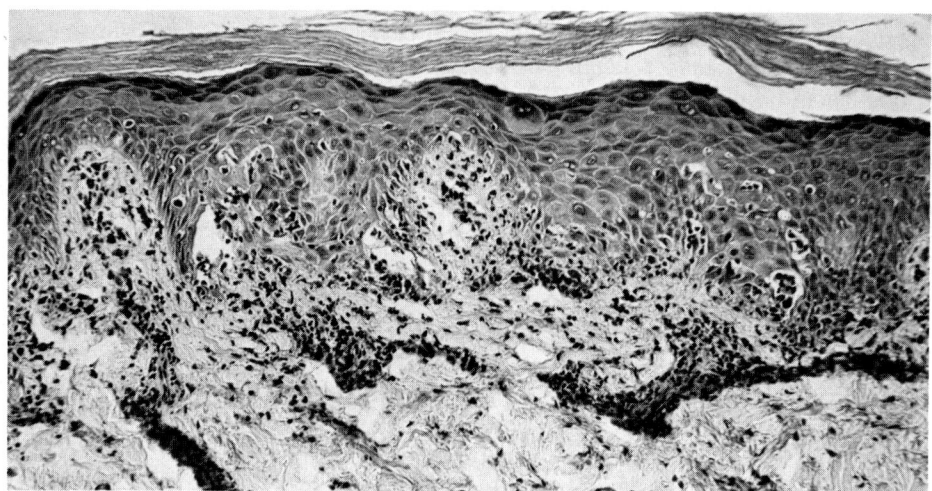

Figure 13–12.
Lichen striatus. Note individual cell keratinization and heavy perivascular infiltrate extending below superficial plexus. H&E. X135.

parts of the body is apt to become purpuric on the lower legs and to produce pictures barely distinguishable from Schamberg–Majocchi's disorder. Tufting of capillaries in the papillary layer without evidence of hyalinization of the walls speaks for stasis. Active microvasculitis speaks for a drug-induced lesion.[28]

LICHEN STRIATUS

The most typical feature of lichen striatus, its linearity, cannot be appreciated under the microscope.[29] There are, however, certain fairly characteristic histologic features (Fig. 13–12) that can make one suspect the diagnosis even without clinical information. There is some similarity to the pigmented purpuric eruptions in the ragged appearance of the infiltrate. Closer inspection, however, shows that one can delineate fairly well-defined papules and there is an unusually heavy lymphocytic infiltrate around selected subpapillary vessels and their extensions into the middermis. Within the papule, the infiltrate invades the epidermis almost as heavily as in lichen planus but is accentuated in some papillae, whereas others may

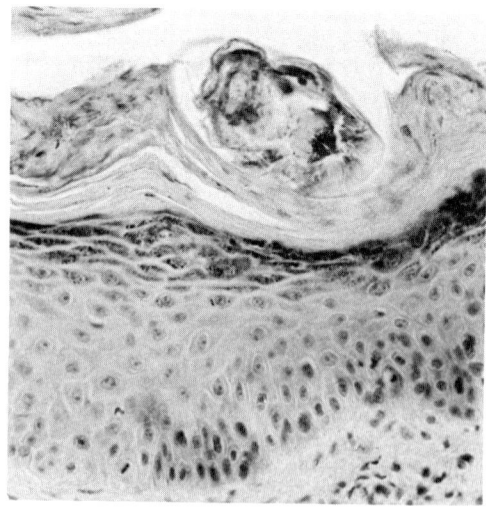
A

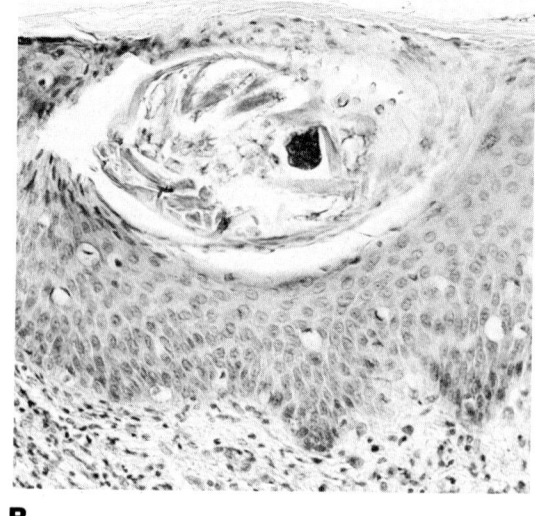
B

Figure 13–13.
Scabies. **A.** Cross sections of female acari in parakeratotic horny layer of a papule. Mild epidermal and considerable dermal inflammatory reaction. Note spines on abdomen of mite in **B.** H&E. X185.

be almost free, in contrast to the continuous band of lichen planus infiltrate.[30] The epidermis correspondingly varies in thickness and degree of edema. In later stages,[31] the basal cells degenerate and microvesicles result. The desmosomes retract,[32] and individual necrotic epidermal cells with homogeneous and eosinophilic cytoplasm are present in about half of the cases.[33]

SCABIES

The histologic diagnosis of scabies is usually unsatisfactory but sometimes gratifying. Submission of a biopsy specimen means that the clinical diagnosis has been missed. Otherwise, the patient would have been treated with or without demonstration of the acarus (Fig. 13–13B) in a fresh horny-layer preparation. The papulosquamous and often excoriated lesions on the skin of an infested individual usually do not contain the mite; it is mainly found in the characteristic linear burrows.[34] The histologic findings combine the features of an eczematous tissue reaction with foci of spongiotic edema and exocytosis covered by moundlike masses of parakeratotic crust together with a pronounced perivascular inflammatory cell infiltrate in which the eosinophils predominate.[35] Occasionally, however, an unexpected, peculiar body (Fig. 13–13A) is discovered in a circumscribed thickening of the parakeratotic horny layer and can be identified as a sectioned acarus. In even rarer instances, the histopathologist may discover large numbers of mites in the greatly thickened horny layer of a clinically verrucous lesion from a case of Norwegian scabies (Fig. 13–14).[36-38] Persistent nodular lesions occur in connection with scabies, as with other arthropods (Chapter 45), and should always be thought of in unclear nodular lesions. The nodular lesions show variable degrees of epidermal thickening and a rather heavy perivascular dermal infiltrate of lymphocytes, histiocytes, plasma cells, and eosinophils. No mites are found in these cases.[39]

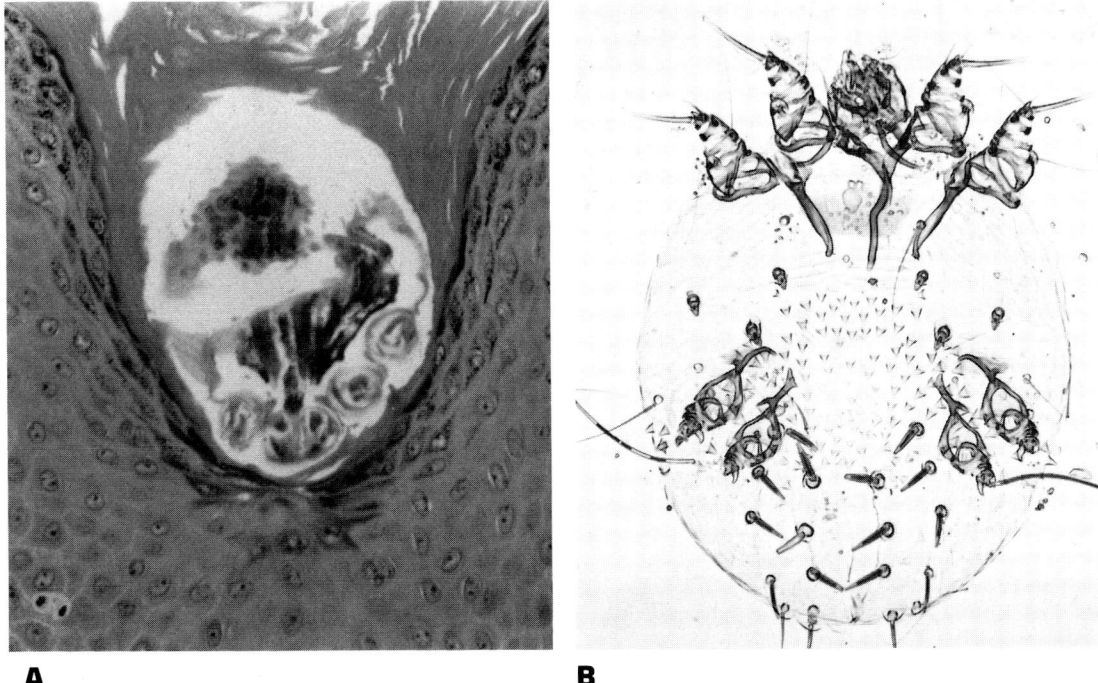

Figure 13–14.
Scabies. **A.** Sectioned mites in the acanthotic epidermis of Norwegian scabies. H&E. X180. **B.** Female acarus in native preparation obtained from a burrow. Unstained in water. X400.

REFERENCES

1. Svegaard E: Immunologic investigations of dermatophytes and dermatophytosis. Semin Dermatol 4:201, 1985
2. Jones HE: Cell-mediated immunity in the immunopathogenesis of dermatophytosis. Acta Derm Venereol (Suppl) 121:73, 1986
3. Tagami H, Kudoh K, Takematsu H: Inflammation and immunity in dermatophytosis. Dermatologica 179 (Suppl 1):1, 1989
4. Graham JH, Barroso-Tobila C: Dermal pathology of superficial fungus infections. In Baker RD (ed): The Pathologic Anatomy of Mycoses. Handbuch der speziellen pathologischen Anatomie und Histologie. Berlin, New York: Springer-Verlag, 1971, vol 3, pt 5
5. Karaoui R, Bou-Resli M, Al-Zaid NS, Mousa A: Tinea versicolor: Ultrastructural studies on hypopigmented and hyperpigmented skin. Dermatologica 162:69, 1981
6. Galadari I: Histologic and ultrastructural investigation of pigmentary changes in pityriasis versicolor. Thesis from MD degree in Dermatology. Univ. of Cairo. 1988
7. Sayegh-Carreno R, Abramovits-Ackerman W, Giron GP: Therapy of tinea nigra plantaris. Int J Dermatol 28:46, 1989
8. Marks R, Ramnarain ND, Bhogal B, et al: The erythrasma microorganism in situ: Studies using the skin surface biopsy technique. J Clin Pathol 25:799, 1972
9. Jacobs PH: Dermatophytes that infect animals and humans. Cutis 42:330, 1988
10. Kakutani H, Takahashi S: Experimental chronic dermatophytosis in human skin grafted to nude mouse: Inoculation of trichophytons and histopathologic evaluation. J Dermatol Tokyo 15:230, 1988
11. Sugiura H, Uehara M, Watanabe S: An analysis of infiltrating cells in human ringworm. Acta Derm Venereol 67:166, 1987
12. Alteras I, Sandbank M, David M, Segal R: 15-year survey of tinea faciei in the adult. Dermatologica 177:65, 1988
13. Grigorin D, Delacrétaz J: La forme vesiculo-bulleuse de l'érythrasma interdigito-plantaire. Dermatologica 152, 1, 1976
14. Marks R, Black MM: The epidermal component of pityriasis lichenoides. Br J Dermatol 87:106, 1972
15. Black MM, Marks R: The inflammatory reaction in pityriasis lichenoides. Br J Dermatol 87:533, 1972
16. Wood GS, Strickler JG, Abel EA, et al: Immunohistology of pityriasis lichenoides et varioliformis acuta and pityriasis lichenoides chronica. Evidence for their interrelationship with lymphomatoid papulosis. J Am Acad Dermatol 16:559, 1987
17. Longley J, Demar L, Feinstein RP, et al: Clinical and histologic features of pityriasis lichenoides et varioliformis acuta in children. Arch Dermatol 123:1335, 1987
18. Samman PD: The natural history of parapsoriasis en plaques (chronic superficial dermatitis) and prereticulotic poikiloderma. Br J Dermatol 87:405, 1972
19. Hu CH, Winkelmann RK: Digitate dermatosis. A new look at symmetrical, small plaque parapsoriasis. Arch Dermatol 107:65, 1973
20. Lindae ML, Abel EA, Hoppe RT, Wood GS: Poikilodermatous mycosis fungoides and atrophic large-plaque parapsoriasis exhibit similar abnormalities of T-cell antigen expression. Arch Dermatol 124:366, 1988
21. Bonvalet D, Colan-Gohm K, Belaich S, et al: Les différentes formes du parapsoriasis en plaques. A propos de 90 cas. Ann Derm Venereol 104:18, 1977
22. Lambert WE, Everett MA: The nosology of parapsoriasis. J Am Acad Dermatol 5:373, 1981
23. Altman J: Parapsoriasis: A histopathologic review and classification. Semin Dermatol 3:14, 1984
24. Barker LP, Sachs PM: Angioma Serpiginosum. Arch Dermatol 92:613, 1965
25. Price ML, Wilson Jones E, Calnan CD, Macdonald DM: Lichen aureus: A localized persistent form of pigmented purpuric dermatitis. Br J Dermatol 112:307, 1985
26. Geiger J-M, Grosshans E, Brauch-Wolff Y, Fabre M: Ultrastructure du lichen aureus. Ann Dermatol Venereol 113:1123, 1986
27. Del Forno C, Caresana G, Baldanza T, et al: Lichen aureus. Chron Dermatol 20:381, 1989
28. Nishioka K, Katayama I, Masuzawa M, et al: Drug-induced chronic pigmented purpura. J Dermatol Tokyo 16:220, 1989
29. Toda K-I, Okamoto H, Horio T: Lichen striatus. Int J Dermatol 25:584, 1986
30. Baran R, Dupre A, Lauret P, Puissant A: Le lichen striatus onychodystrophique. A propos de 4 cas avec revue de la literature (4 cas). Ann Dermatol Venereol 106:885, 1979
31. Stewart WM, Lauret P, Pietrini P, Thomine E: "Lichen striatus." Critères histologiques (à propos de 5 cas). Ann Derm Venereol 104:132, 1977
32. Charles R, Johnson BL, Robinson TA: Lichen striatus. A clinical, histologic and electron microscopic study of an unusual case. J Cutan Pathol 1:265, 1974
33. Staricco RG: Lichen striatus. Arch Dermatol 79:311, 1959
34. Van Neste DJJ: Human scabies in prospective. Int J Dermatol 27:10, 1988
35. Hejazi N, Mehregan AH: Scabies. Histological study of inflammatory lesions. Arch Dermatol 111:37, 1975
36. Suzumiya J, Sumiyoshi A, Kuroki Y, et al: Crusted (Norwegian) scabies with adult T-cell leukemia. Arch Dermatol 121:903, 1985
37. Suzumiya J, Sumiyoshi A, Kuroki Y, Inoue S: Crusted (Norwegian) scabies with adult T-cell leukemia. Arch Dermatol 121:903, 1985

38. Jucowics P, Ramon ME, Don PC, et al: Norwegian scabies in an infant with acquired immunodeficiency syndrome. Arch Dermatol 125:1670, 1989

39. Fernandez F, Torres A, Ackerman AB: Pathologic findings in human scabies. Arch Dermatol 113:320, 1977

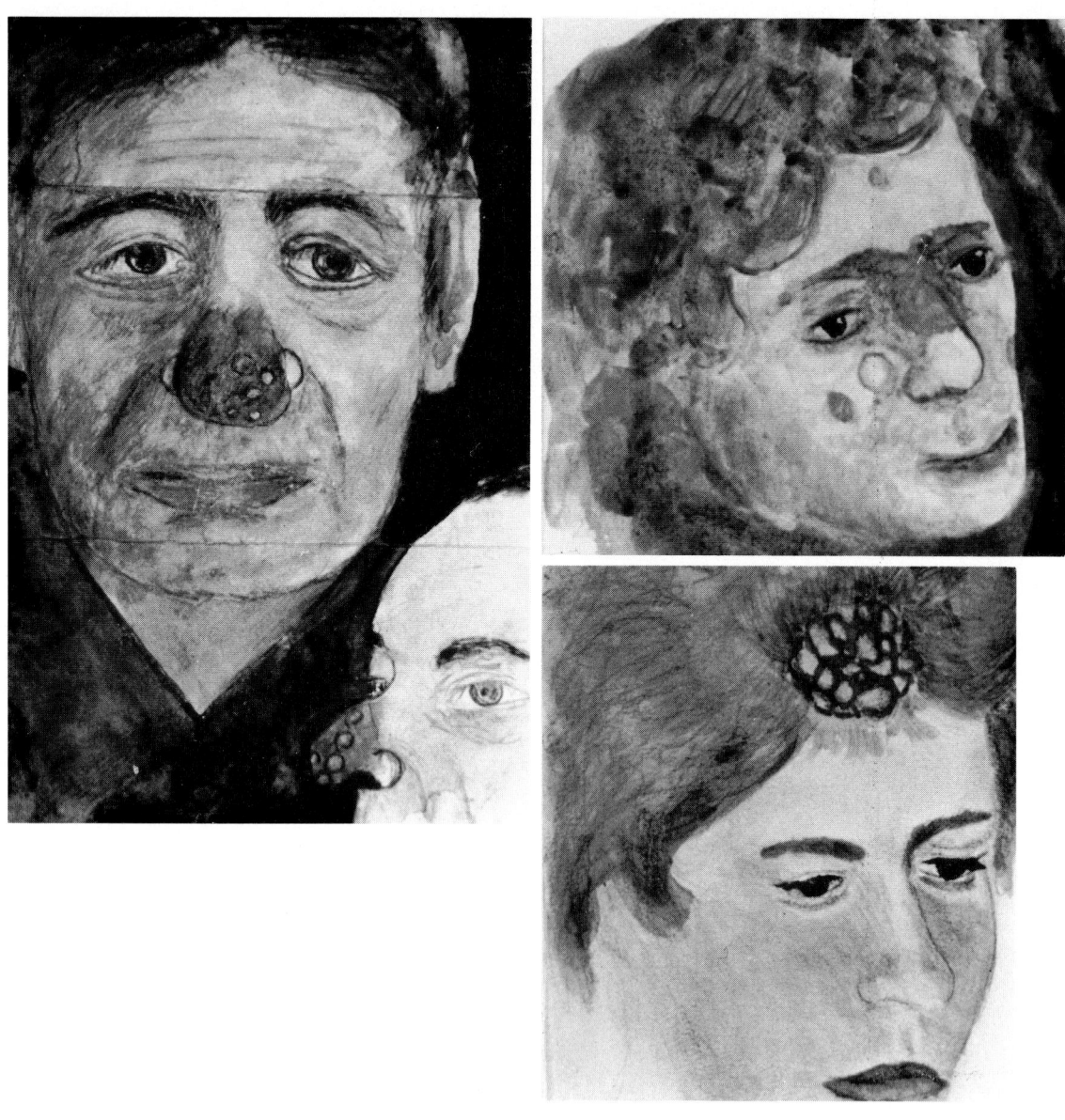

Portraits of patients from charts; acne rosacea (*upper left*), chronic discoid lupus erythematosus (*upper right*), and organoid nevus of scalp (*lower right*).

SECTION III

DEEP INFLAMMATORY PROCESSES

All dermatoses discussed so far involve predominantly the epidermis and the pars papillaris of the dermis. If low-power inspection reveals abnormal aggregates of cells mainly in the pars reticularis or the subcutaneous fat tissue, we can immediately rule out the superficial inflammatory dermatoses. The next step is to ascertain the nature of the abnormally present cells. Epithelial and mesodermal tumor cells, with the exception of some undifferentiated metastatic carcinomas, are easily recognized. Lymphomatous infiltrates are more difficult to identify, but we shall leave this point for Chapter 45. If the infiltrate consists of a mixture of cells, one should look particularly for any appreciable number of histiocytes and macrophages and put the lesion into the category of granulomatous inflammation, whether or not they are present in the form of epithelioid nodules (Section IV). The following chapters, then, deal with deep inflammatory infiltrates composed of small round cells (lymphocytes) mainly. Polymorphonuclear leukocytes and plasma cells may also be present.

Classification within the group is made according to the particular structures with which the infiltrate is associated. Thus, we can separate out vasculitides in which sizable blood vessels are affected, inflammation of fat lobes (panniculitis) or interlobar septa, and lesions associated with hair follicles or sweat glands. Finally, there are some dermatoses in which only small vessels seem to serve as the centers of inflammation. The outstanding example of this type is lupus erythematosus.

14

LUPUS ERYTHEMATOSUS AND RELATED CONDITIONS

HISTOLOGY OF LUPUS ERYTHEMATOSUS

Testimony to the close biologic interactions between mesoderm and epithelium, the diagnostic features of all manifestations of cutaneous lupus erythematosus involve changes in the dermis, in the epidermis, and in the pilosebaceous follicles. The changes are qualitatively similar but are combined in varying quantity. Inasmuch as the clinical criteria of discoid and systemic cannot be recognized under the microscope, it seems best to list the histologic forms of the disease as chronic, subacute, and acute (Figs. 14–1, 14–2, 14–3, and, 14–4).[1-3]

For diagnostic and differential purposes, it is then recommended to look for triads of alteration in epidermis and hair follicles and for five features in the dermis. If all or most are present, a diagnosis can be made with considerable assurance, but one has to keep in mind the biologic limitations of some of the criteria. For instance, one cannot expect keratotic plugging of follicles if all the hair roots have been destroyed by the disease. The diagnostic criteria are listed in Table 14–1. Important diagnostic features have been added by immunofluorescent findings[4-6] (Chapter 4).

Special Features

It may seem strange that epithelial changes play such an important part in the diagnosis of a connective tissue disease. One may resolve this paradox by considering the close interaction between mesoderm and ectoderm. It is also paradoxical that fibrinoid and vascular changes, which play such a prominent part in lupus erythematosus of internal organs, are barely worth looking for in routinely stained sections of skin. One should further realize that many of the diagnostic changes develop slowly. It is generally best to biopsy a well-established lesion of at least several weeks' duration.

The epidermal changes (Fig. 14–3) have much similarity to those of lichen planus and, for the same reason, damage to basal cells. This is apt to be more spotty in lupus erythematosus (Fig. 14–2) and restricted to the areas where lymphocytic infiltrate touches the epidermis. Sawtooth appearance of rete ridges is hardly ever seen, and hyaline bodies are extremely rare. Atrophy of the malpighian layer (Fig. 14–4) may be extreme in subacute and acute cases and makes a striking contrast to the thick horny layer, which usually rests on a well-developed or even thickened granular layer. Occasional spots of parakeratosis may be found in the circinate or psoriasiform lesions of the subacute variety.[7,8]

Some cases of chronic discoid lupus erythematosus, clinically of the verrucous type, show marked acanthosis alternating with atrophic stretches of epidermis. Close inspection of H&E-stained sections may reveal changes of the basement membrane, which are more obvious with the PAS procedure.

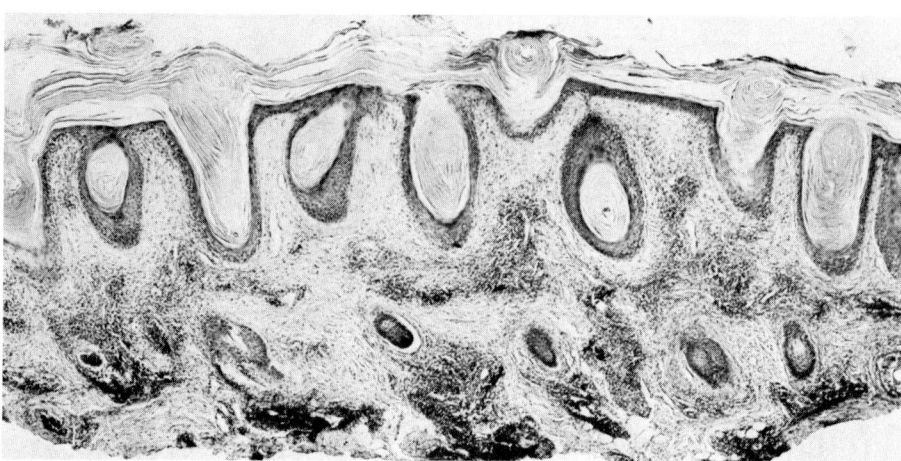

Figure 14–1.
Chronic lupus erythematosus of beard. Section shows all typical features except that follicular plugs are less conical than usual. Note orthokeratotic hyperkeratosis and epidermal and sebaceous atrophy. Edema and telangiectasia are more pronounced in the superficial dermis; perivascular lymphocytic infiltrate in the deeper layers. H&E. X60.

The membrane is of uneven width but more commonly thickened and even reduplicated. In other areas, it may appear frayed or lost.

The earliest follicular change is sebaceous atrophy. Even this takes some weeks to develop, however, and usually affects the small superficial glands of the vellus follicles of the face first, while the large, deep-seated glands of the sebaceous follicles may remain of fair size for some time. Therefore, sebaceous atrophy is usually of less diagnostic value in subacute and acute lesions. The keratotic plug also develops gradually but may be quite pronounced in acute cases where general epithelial atrophy is severe. It need not be present in every follicle. Basal layer damage of follicular sheath is seen particularly well on strong scalp hairs associated with a hugging lymphocytic infiltrate similar to that of lichen planopilaris. It is an empiric rule that the plug in lupus erythematosus often is conical, whereas that of follicular lichen planus is rounded and sits in a cup-shaped or even bottle-shaped follicle (Fig. 14–5). Eventually the pilosebaceous structures may disappear completely, leaving behind remnants of fibrous sheath and the hair muscle. In these late stages, one must not expect keratotic plugs histologically or carpet-tack scale clinically.

The most prominent dermal sign is the pure lymphocytic infiltrate (Fig. 14–1) that is apt to be

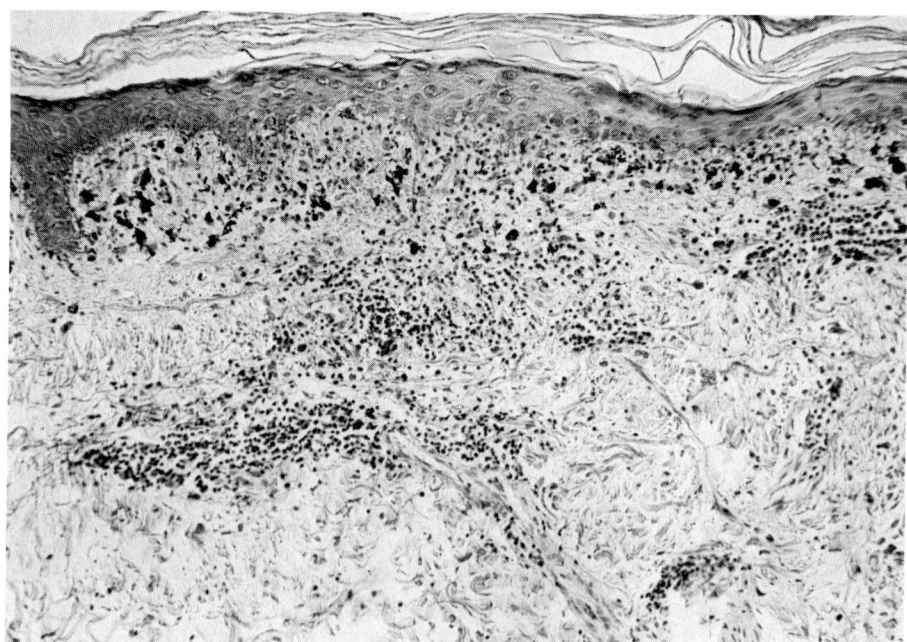

Figure 14–2.
Subacute lupus erythematosus. Note numerous pigmented macrophages below nonpigmented atrophic epidermis (symptomatic incontinentia pigmenti). H&E. X135.

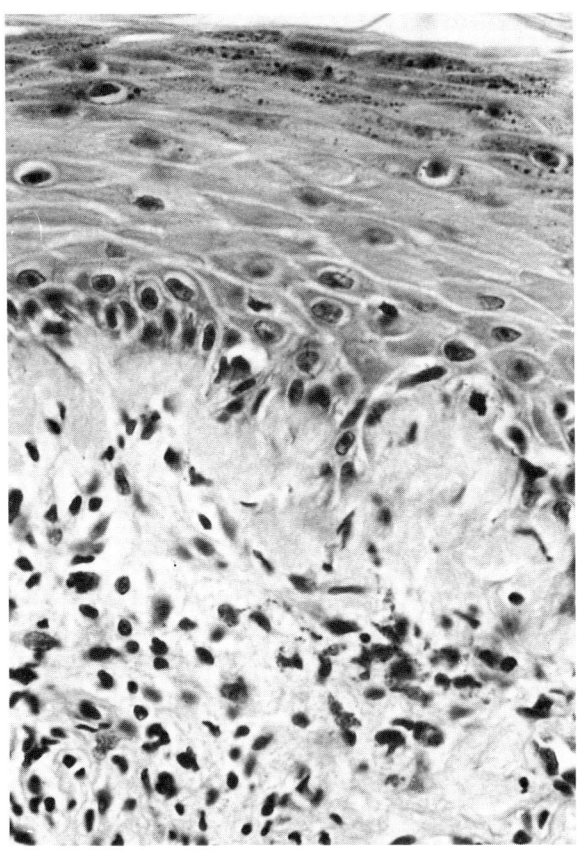

Figure 14–3.
Subacute lupus erythematosus shows liquefaction degeneration of basal cells and hyalin bodies. H&E. X400.

present in all layers of the dermis, but most regularly in the middle third. It is arranged around small vessels and, therefore, is mainly found in the vicinity of hair follicles. It is heavy and nodular in chronic cases but differs from the massive infiltrate of a lymphocytic lymphoma by the fact that all cells are neatly spaced rather than packed close. This is a sign of the edema that is present at the same time. The infiltrate is mainly T lymphocytes. The population of helper/inducer and suppressor/cytotoxic cells, however, vary in the acute (systemic) and the chronic discoid lesions.[9] A few plasma cells, even an occasional eosinophil, are permissible, but a heavier admixture of these cell types raises doubts. They are more commonly present in the polymorphous light eruptions. The infiltrate practically always approaches the epidermis in a few places and is associated with basal cell degeneration. One may have to scan a number of sections to find this feature, but its complete absence favors "Jessner's lymphocytic infiltration." The infiltrate is in reciprocal relation to the amount of edema as one goes from chronic to subacute and acute lesions. It may be entirely absent in very acute cases, which show only a generally red skin clinically. This produces the peculiar picture illustrated in Figure 14–4. A specific stain would reveal considerable amounts of dermal hyaluronic acid in this type of case. Edema is noticeable in various ways: by spacing of the lymphocytes, splitting of collagen bundles, and a peculiarly empty look

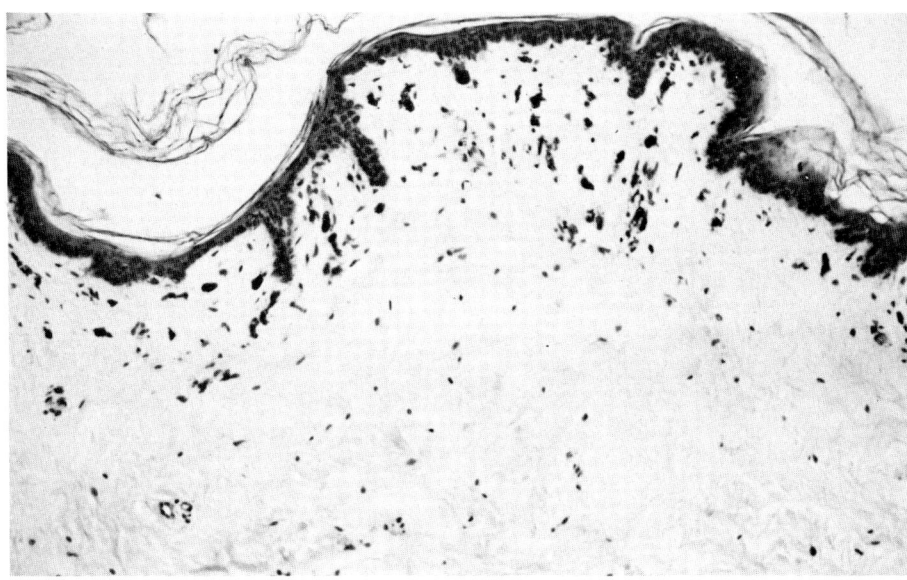

Figure 14–4.
Acute lupus erythematosus. Atrophic epidermis with relative hyperkeratosis. Papillary layer highly edematous. Practically no inflammatory infiltrate. Numerous melanophages appear in skin of this black patient. H&E. X180.

TABLE 14-1. DIAGNOSTIC FEATURES OF LUPUS ERYTHEMATOSUS

Epidermis
Hyperkeratosis and hypergranulosis
Atrophy (rarely hyperplasia) of the malpighian layer
Focal liquefaction necrosis of the basal layer

Pilary Complex
Conical keratotic plugs
Sebaceous atrophy
Pilar atrophy

Dermis
Lymphocytic infiltrate with focal invasion of epidermis and follicular sheath
Edema
Telangiectasia
Subepidermal macrophage pigmentation
Focal destruction of elastic fibers

of the subpapillary zone (Fig. 14–1). Edema usually is associated with telangiectasia, not only of blood vessels but also of lymph vessels. Since the latter are rarely recognized in normal skin or other dermatoses, the presence of open spaces lined only by occasional endothelial cells is a good clue for lupus erythematosus.

As in lichen planus, the damaged basal layer releases melanin granules, which are taken up by macrophages. This sign (Figs. 14–2 and 14–4) is apt to be minimal in very fair skin and is striking in brown skin. It has no diagnostic value in itself because it is also present in fixed drug eruptions, Riehl's melanosis, lichen planus, and various other dermatoses, but its presence should make one suspicious.

The fifth dermal feature, spotty absence of elastic fibers, is of considerable diagnostic value in chronic cases. It is due to the fact that elastic fibers are easily destroyed by chronic inflammatory infiltrate and not easily formed anew. Chronic lesions of lupus erythematosus, therefore, will reveal loss of preexisting elastic fibers in areas previously involved by infiltrate. This feature persists long after the lesion has become quiescent and all infiltrate has disappeared. In some cases, especially in young patients, new elastic fibers may be formed, but these are thin and abnormally arranged. Areas of elastic fiber destruction may look quite normal in H&E sections but are conspicuous with O&G stain. The feature may be present in Jessner's lymphocytic infiltration but is rarely seen in polymorphous light eruption.

Variants

In the *hypertrophic* or *verrucous* form of chronic lupus erythematosus, epidermal atrophy may be replaced by considerable acanthosis.[10-12] Clinically

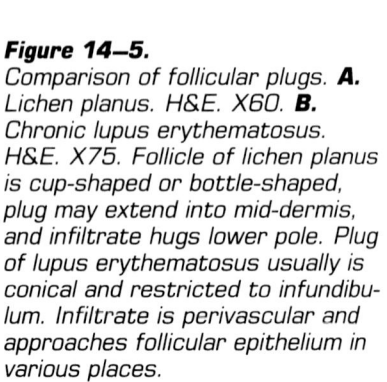

Figure 14–5.
Comparison of follicular plugs. **A.** Lichen planus. H&E. X60. **B.** Chronic lupus erythematosus. H&E. X75. Follicle of lichen planus is cup-shaped or bottle-shaped, plug may extend into mid-dermis, and infiltrate hugs lower pole. Plug of lupus erythematosus usually is conical and restricted to infundibulum. Infiltrate is perivascular and approaches follicular epithelium in various places.

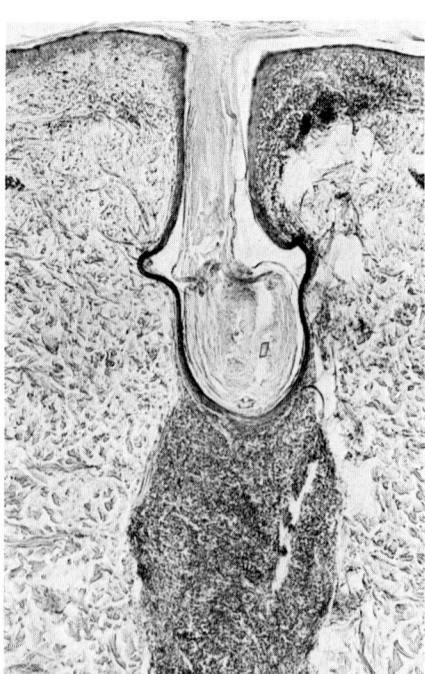
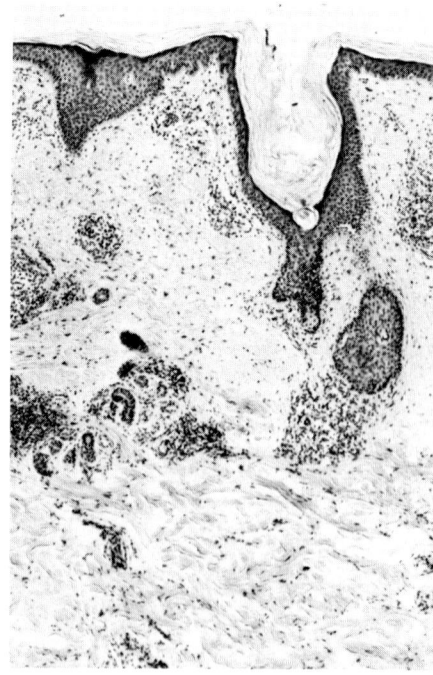

A B

the lesions may resemble hypertrophic lichen planus or multiple keratoacanthomas. Histologically, however, all other diagnostic features such as spotty liquefaction degeneration of basal cells, dermal edema, telangiectasia, perivascular lymphocytic infiltrate, and atrophy of the pilosebaceous structures are present.

"Bullous systemic lupus erythematosus" shows a subepidermal blister associated with infiltration of neutrophils resembling dermatitis herpetiformis.[13,14] The eruption may be localized to the face or generalized. Final diagnosis is made by demonstration of basement membrane zone antibodies.

"Lupus erythematosus profundus (lupus panniculitis)" appears as subcutaneous nodules in any locations.[15,16] In 20 percent of the cases the subcutaneous nodules are associated with the chronic discoid lupus erythematosus-type changes within the overlying epidermis. Poikiloderma-like changes are observed on the surface in another 20 percent of the lesions. Dermis shows edema, mucin deposition, and hyaline sclerosis at the level of sweat glands (Fig. 14–6 and 14–7). The infiltrate involving the subcutaneous fat tissue is predominantly lymphocytic. Small and large blood vessels are involved with endothelial cell hyperplasia, edema, and occlusion and are surrounded by hyalinized collagenous tissue. Lymphoid follicles are present in half of the cases.

"Lupus erythematosus of the scalp" is to be differentiated from other forms of scarring alopecia (Chapter 19) by the extrafollicular changes in the epidermis and around blood vessels, where lymphocytic infiltrate and loss of elastic fibers should be looked for. Flat plaques of lupus erythematosus on the body and extremities, where hair follicles are few, may be extremely hard to tell from lichen planus. The distribution of the infiltrate—exclusively superficial in lichen planus, extending deeper around vessels in lupus erythematosus—is the best clue.

The syndrome of mixed connective tissue disease may present cutaneous lesions of discoid or systemic lupus erythematosus in a high percentage of cases.[11] There is no histologic differentiation except by immunofluorescence. Cutaneous changes of lupus anticoagulant consist of lividoid or pyoderma gangrenosum like changes of the extremities or generalized necrotic skin lesions. Histologically extensive thrombosis of small dermal blood vessels occur in the absence of vasculitis.[17–19]

"Lupus erythematosus of the oral mucosa" cannot be differentiated from lichen planus with any degree of assurance (Chapter 46).[20]

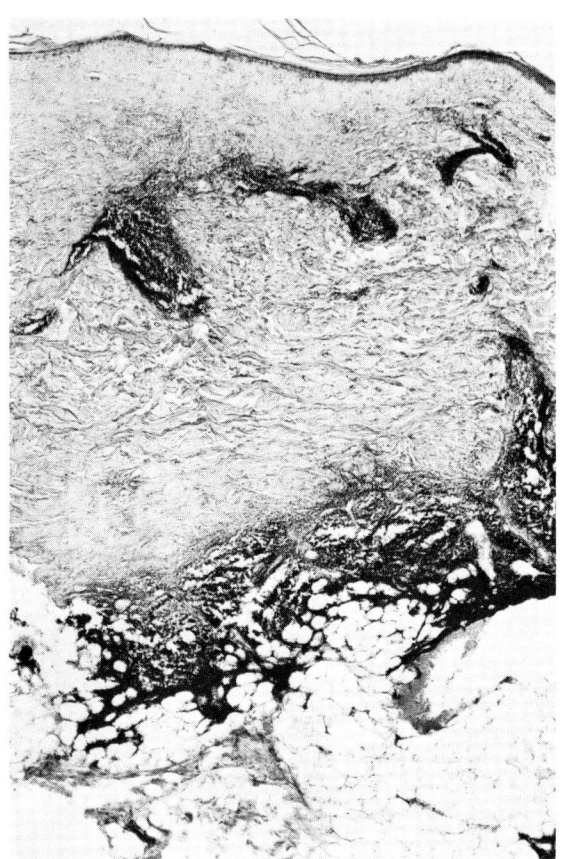

Figure 14–6.
Lupus erythematosus profundus. Diagnosis must be based on clinicopathologic correlation. H&E. X30.

JESSNER'S LYMPHOCYTIC INFILTRATION

In spite of the noncharacteristic name and the abortive way[21] in which the disease was announced to the world, Jessner's distinguishing his lymphocytic infiltration (Fig. 14–8) from lupus erythematosus was a highly welcome event. Jessner's lymphocytic infiltration[22] is an entity worth differentiating from discoid lupus erythematosus because it has a much better prognosis. The principal histologic deviations are the absence of epidermal involvement and of follicular plugging. Some sebaceous atrophy and loss of elastic fibers may be present. The infiltrate is mainly T lymphocytes. It has been demonstrated that the population of Leu-8 positive cells is four times higher in Jessner's disease than in chronic discoid lupus erythematosus.[23] Edema and telangiectasia usually are not pronounced. On the other hand, Jessner's disease can be differentiated from lymphocytoma by the fact that its lymphocytic infiltrate has an inflammatory perivascular character even though it

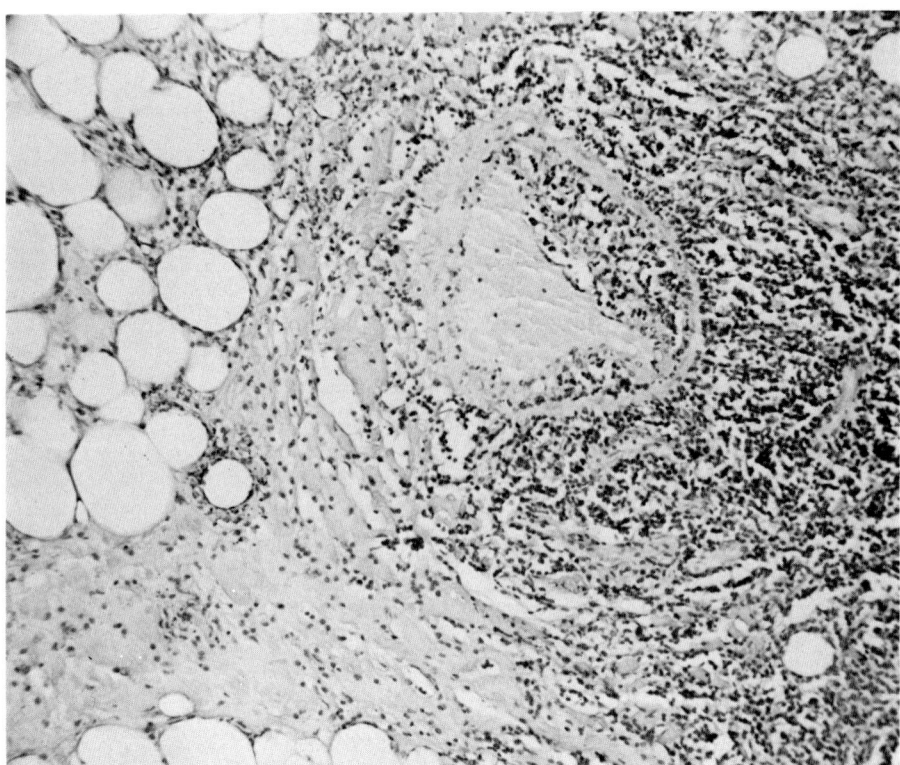

Figure 14–7.
Panniculitis of lupus erythematosus profundus. Lymphocytic infiltrate disrupts the structural integrity of a large vein (phlebitis) and extends between fat cells. H&E. X135.

may be nodular and dense in some cases.[24] Histiocytes and lymphoid structures are not present. We therefore exclude it from the group of benign cutaneous lymphoplasias.

PHOTOSENSITIVITY REACTIONS

One of the more perplexing diagnostic problems is the field of inflammatory tissue reactions related to light sensitivity. Not only are many lesions of lupus erythematosus aggravated or triggered by light, but eruptions caused by actinic exposure have multiplied in recent years owing to the photosensitizing propensities of numerous internal medications and external additives to soaps, bleaches, and cosmetics. Essentially, we are dealing with three classes of photodermatitis.[25-26] *Phototoxic* eruption occurs in all individuals exposed to sufficient doses of the phototoxic agents and resembles an exaggerated sunburn.[27] Histologically, necrosis of individual or small groups of epidermal cells is present with foci of vesicle formation (Fig. 14–9).

Polymorphous light eruption (PLE) is the most common form of photodermatitis. Etiology is unknown. The clinical manifestations include papular eruption, papular urticaria like lesions, plaque type, erythema multiforme, and vesiculobullous dermatitis (Fig. 14–10). The common histologic feature is perivascular infiltrate of T lymphocytes involving the upper and mid-dermis.[28,29] Subepidermal edema, vacuolar degeneration of basal cells, and spongiotic edema are present in various severity. There is no atrophy of the pilosebaceous structures or loss of elastic fibers. In the plaque type, the infiltrate tends to be lichenoid, in bandlike distribution involving the lower surface of the epidermis.[30] Erythema multiforme-like lesions show extensive subepidermal edema leading to blister formation and epidermal necrosis. The vesiculobullous variety shows both subepidermal edema and spongiotic vesicle formation.[31]

Photoallergic (photocontact) dermatitis is based on cell-mediated hypersensitivity and includes benign summer light eruption and the persistent light reaction. It appears within a few hours or days following light exposure as an acute dermatitis indistinguishable from an eczematous contact dermatitis.[32,33] Histologically, there are areas of spongiotic edema and exocytosis with intraepidermal vesicle formation. The perivascular dermal infiltrate is predominantly T lymphocytes. Persistent light reactors show plaques of chronic dermatitis with histologic

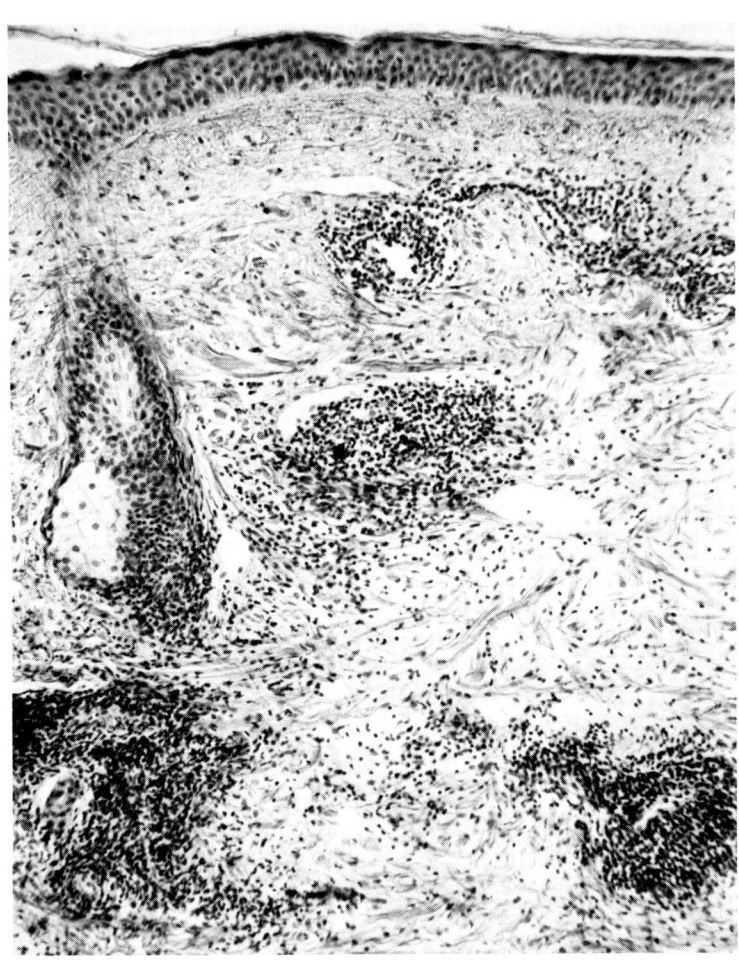

Figure 14–8.
Jessner's lymphocytic infiltration. Although epidermis is not affected by infiltrate, this does invade follicular sheath, an exceptional feature. There is, however, no sebaceous atrophy or follicular plugging. H&E. X135.

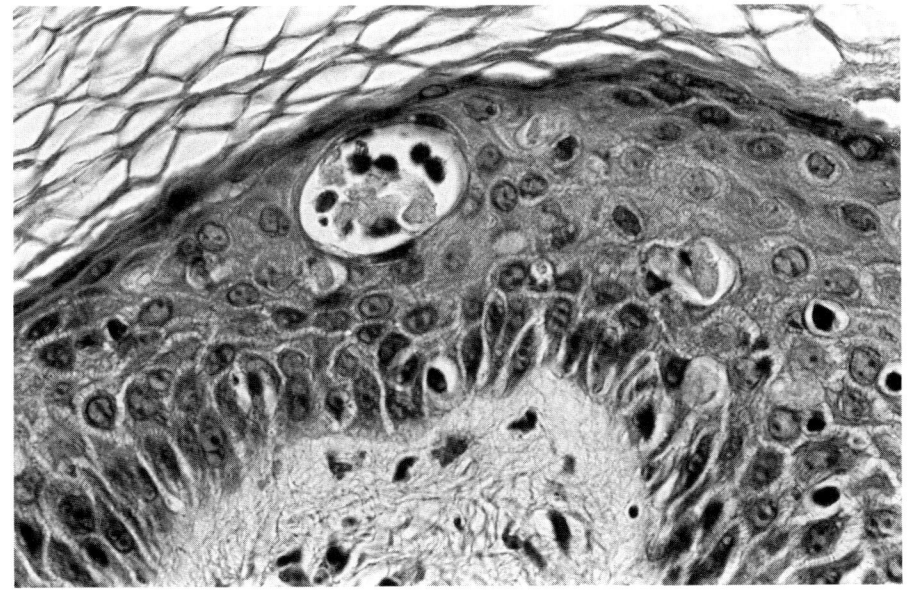

Figure 14–9.
Phototoxic light eruption shows necrotic keratinocytes and an intraepidermal vesicle. H&E. X400.

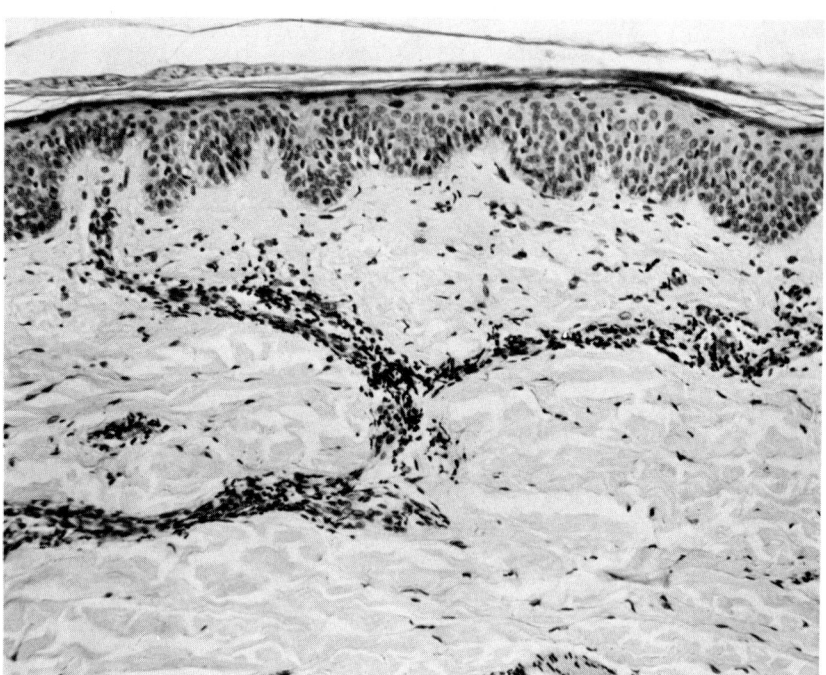

Figure 14–10.
Light sensitivity reaction. Photo patch test 5 days after application of 3 MED to sensitized skin. A thin layer of parakeratosis between two orthokeratotic layers remains as evidence that the epidermis has undergone an acute inflammatory phase (in this case, a sunburn reaction) and has recovered, now exhibiting mild acanthosis and a rather thick granular layer. The dermal infiltrate is similar to that of dermal contact sensitivity reaction (see Fig. 7–8) and of drug eruption (see Fig. 10–7), with which it also shares a tendency to invasion of the epidermis. H&E. X135.

features of dermal contact sensitivity. Minimal epidermal changes are associated with a rather heavy perivascular dermal infiltrate of lymphocytes, histiocytes, plasma cells, and a few eosinophils. The presence of occasional large mononuclear cells within the rather heavy and mixed dermal infiltrate may suggest cutaneous lymphoma (actinic reticuloid).[34–36]

Hydroa vacciniforme is a rare form of chronic photodermatitis occurring in childhood with vesicular lesions over the light-exposed areas healing with formation of varioliform scars.[37,38] Histologically, intraepidermal vesicles are formed by reticular degeneration and necrosis of the epidermal cells with underlying perivascular lymphocytic infiltrate.

Pellagra

A different mechanism of light sensitivity causes the cutaneous manifestations of pellagra and of Hartnup's disease, which have the common denominator of nicotinamide deficiency. In the acute dermatitic stage, there is chronic inflammatory infiltrate, and predominantly subepidermal bullae may form. Later, epidermal hyperkeratosis, parakeratosis, and hyperpigmentation are seen, followed by epidermal atrophy. The dermis often shows the elastic changes

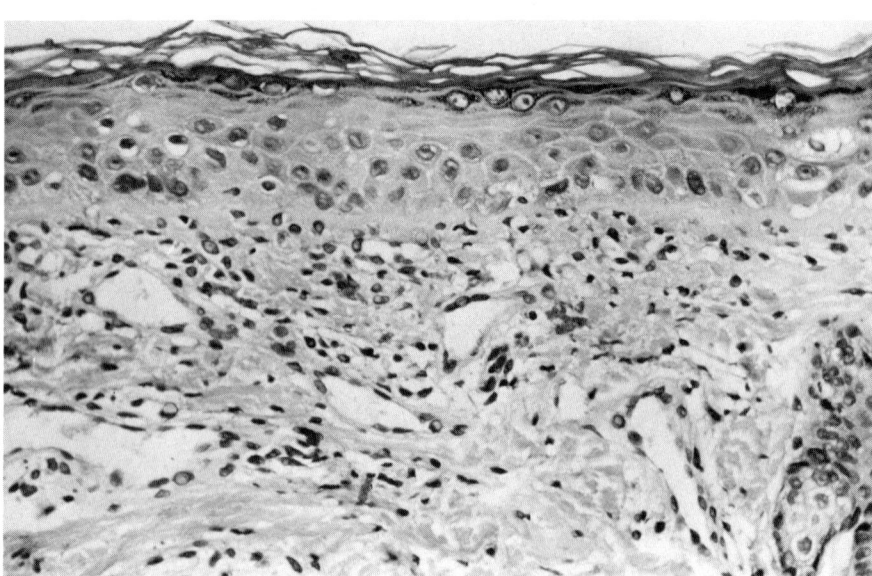

Figure 14–11.
Dermatomyositis. Poikilodermatous eruption shows mild epidermal atrophy, telangiectasia, and scattered inflammatory cells. H&E. X250.

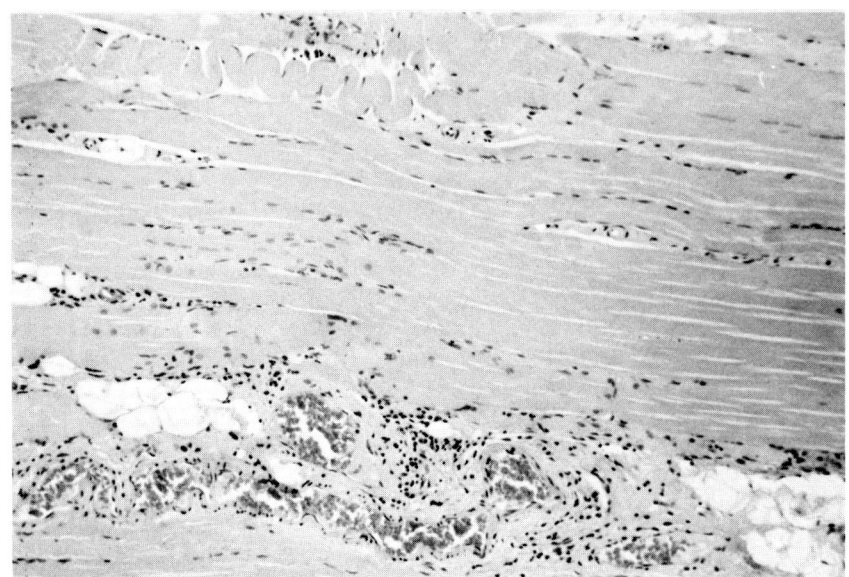

Figure 14–12.
Myositis of dermatomyositis. Lymphocytic infiltrate of interstitial connective tissue (containing some fat cells). Severe atrophy of skeletal muscle fibers showing long stretches without nuclei. H&E. X250.

of chronic actinic influence and may exhibit hyalinization of collagen in the deeper layers.[39] Tissue changes are confirmatory of a clinical diagnosis rather than diagnostic.

DERMATOMYOSITIS

It seems convenient to discuss the skin manifestations of dermatomyositis at this point because they cause diagnostic difficulties with systemic lupus erythematosus. Cutaneous lesions in dermatomyositis may be present more than a year before the onset of muscle weakness.[40] The skin changes include violaceous or heliotrope periorbital edema, periungual telangiectasia, poikilodermatous eruption, photodermatitis, and Guttron's papules. Many of these manifestations are as noncharacteristic histologically as they are clinically. The trained eye, however, looks for evidence of edema, especially around small vessels, and a fairly mild perivascular infiltrate in which plasma cells and an occasional eosinophil join the small round cells (Fig. 14–11). Definite diagnosis is rarely possible in the absence of striated muscle pathology (Fig. 14–12). Occasionally, degenerative changes have been observed in smooth muscle. Hyaluronic acid is surprisingly plentiful in the edematous skin, a feature shared with systemic lupus.[41]

Diagnosis becomes easier when poikilodermatous features are present. Here again, it is easier to differentiate dermatomyositis from a simple dermatitis than from a poikilodermatous form of lupus erythematosus (Fig. 14–13). The latter is apt to have a heavier and purely lymphocytic infiltrate in the subacute form and much more extensive damage to the basal layer and epidermal atrophy in the acute type.

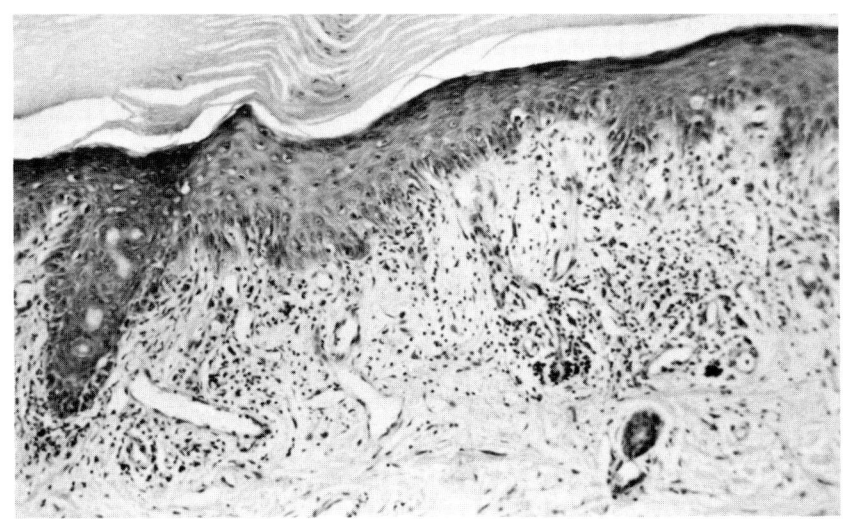

Figure 14–13.
Poikilodermatous form of lupus erythematosus. Skin of finger. Telangiectasia, lymphocytic infiltrate, and basal cell damage causing epidermal atrophy are features fitting lupus erythematosus as well as poikilodermatous dermatomyositis. H&E. X250.

REFERENCES

1. Moschella SL: Dermatologic overview of lupus erythematosus and its subsets. J Dermatol (Tokyo) 16:417, 1989
2. Bangert JL, Freeman RG, Sontheimer RD, Gilliam JN: Subacute cutaneous lupus erythematosus and discoid lupus erythematosus. Comparative histopathologic findings. Arch Dermatol 120:332, 1984
3. Jerdan MS, Hood AF, Moore WG, Callen JP: Histopathologic comparison of the subsets of lupus erythematosus. Arch Dermatol 126:52, 1990
4. Nieboer C: The reliability of immunofluorescence and histopathology in the diagnosis of discoid lupus erythematosus and lichen planus. Br J Dermatol 116:189, 1987
5. Johansson-Stephansson E, Koskimies S, Partanen J, Kariniemi AL: Subacute cutaneous lupus erythematosus. Genetic markers and clinical and immunological findings in patients. Arch Dermatol 125:791, 1989
6. Williams REA, Mackie RM, O'Keefe R, Thomson W: The contribution of direct immunofluorescence to the diagnosis of lupus erythematosus. J Cutan Pathol 16:122, 1989
7. Herrero C, Bielsa I, Font J, et al: Subacute cutaneous lupus erythematosus: Clinicopathologic findings in thirteen cases. J Am Acad Dermatol 19:1057, 1988
8. Mooney E, Wade TR: Subacute cutaneous lupus erythematosus in Iceland. Int J Dermatol 28:104, 1989
9. Kohchiyama A, Oka D, Ueki H: T-cell subsets in lesions of systemic and discoid lupus erythematosus. J Cutan Pathol 12:493, 1985
10. Spann CR, Callen JP, Klein JB, Kulick KB: Clinical, serologic, and immunogenetic studies in patients with chronic cutaneous (discoid) lupus erythematosus who have verrucous and/or hypertrophic skin lesions. J Rheumatol 15:256, 1988
11. Eskreis BD, Eng AM, Furey NL: Surgical excision of trauma-induced verrucous lupus erythematosus. J Dermatol Surg Oncol 14:1296, 1988
12. Rubenstein DJ, Huntley AC: Keratotic lupus erythematosus: Treatment with isotretinoin. J Am Acad Dermatol 14:910, 1986
13. Fleming MG, Bergfeld WF, Tomecki KJ, et al: Bullous systemic lupus erythematosus. Int J Dermatol 28:321, 1989
14. Rappersberger K, Tschachler E, Tani M, Wolff K: Bullous disease in systemic lupus erythematosus. J Am Acad Dermatol 21:745, 1989
15. Sanchez NP, Peters MS, Winkelmann RK: The histopathology of lupus erythematosus panniculitis. J Am Acad Dermatol 5:673, 1981
16. Winkelmann RK: Panniculitis in connective tissue disease. Arch Dermatol 119:336, 1983
17. Alegre VA, Winkelmann RK: Histopathologic and immunofluorescence study of skin lesions associated with circulating lupus anticoagulant. J Am Acad Dermatol 19:117, 1988
18. Grob JJ, Bonerandi JJ: Cutaneous manifestations associated with the presence of the lupus anticoagulant. A report of two cases and a review of the literature. J Am Acad Dermatol 15:211, 1986
19. Frances C, Tribout B, Boisnic S, et al: Cutaneous necrosis associated with the lupus anticoagulant. Dermatologica 178:194, 1989
20. Van Joost TH, Stolz E, Van Der Sluis JJ, et al: Oral lupus erythematosus: Markers of immunologic injury. J Cutan Pathol 12:500, 1985
21. Jessner M: Lymphocytic infiltration of the skin. Arch Dermatol 68:447, 1953
22. Toonstra J, Wildschut A, Boer J, et al: Jessner's lymphocytic infiltration of the skin. A clinical study of 100 patients. Arch Dermatol 125:1525, 1989
23. Ashworth J, Turbitt M, Mackie RA: A comparison of the dermal lymphoid infiltrate in discoid lupus erythematosus and Jessner's lymphocytic infiltrate of the skin using the monoclonal antibody Leu-8. J Cutan Pathol 14:198, 1987
24. Cerio R, Oliver GF, Wilson Jones E, Winkelmann RK: The heterogeneity of Jessner's lymphocytic infiltration of the skin. Immunohistochemical studies suggesting one form of perivascular lymphocytoma. J Am Acad Dermatol 23:63, 1990
25. Lim HW, Baer RL, Gange RW: Photodermatoses. J Am Acad Dermatol 17:293, 1987
26. Taylor CR, Stern RS, Leyden JJ, Gilchrest BA: Photoaging/photodamage and photoprotection. J Am Acad Dermatol 22:1, 1990
27. Toback AC, Anders JE: Phototoxicity from systemic agents. Dermatol Clin 4:223, 1986
28. Hölzle E, Plewig G, Von Kries R, Lehmann P: Polymorphous light eruption. J Invest Dermatol 88(March Suppl):32, 1987
29. Lecha M, Marti R, Mascaro JM: Erupcion polimorfa luminica. Estudio del infiltrado con anticuerpos monoclonales. Med Cutan Iber Lat Am 16:451, 1988
30. Wolf R, Dorfman B, Krakowski A: Quinidine-induced lichenoid and eczematous photodermatitis. Dermatologica 174:285, 1987
31. Hood AF, Elpern DJ, Morison WL: Histopathologic findings in papulovesicular light eruption. J Cutan Pathol 13:13, 1986
32. Wojnarowska F, Calnan CD: Contact and photocontact allergy to musk ambrette. Br J Dermatol 114:667, 1986
33. Bonvalet D, Baddoura R, Jeanmougin M: Interet de l'etude histologique du phototest dan les photodermatoses. Ann Dermatol Venereol 113:1205, 1986
34. Kaidbey KH, Messenger JL: The clinical spectrum of the persistent light reactor. Arch Dermatol 120:1441, 1984
35. Vandermaesen J, Roelandts R, Degreef H: Light on the persistent light reaction-photosensitivity dermatitis-actinic reticuloid syndrome. J Am Acad Dermatol 15:685, 1986
36. Lim HW, Buchness MR, Ashinoff R, Soter NA: Chronic actinic dermatitis. Study of the spectrum of

chronic photosensitivity in 12 patients. Arch Dermatol 126:317, 1990
37. Eramo LR, Garden JM, Esterly NB: Hydroa vacciniforme. Diagnosis by repetitive ultraviolet-A phototesting. Arch Dermatol 122:1310, 1986
38. Sonnex TS, Hawk JLM: Hydroa vacciniforme: A review of ten cases. Br J Dermatol 118:101, 1988
39. Moore RA, Spies TD, Cooper ZK: Histopathology of the skin in pellagra. Arch Dermatol 46:100, 1942
40. Rockerbie NR, Woo Ty, Callen JP, Giustina T: Cutaneous changes of dermatomyositis precede muscle weakness. J Am Acad Dermatol 20:629, 1989
41. Nesbitt LT Jr: Cutaneous immunofluorescence in dermatomyositis. Int J Dermatol 19:270, 1980

15

DERMAL VASCULITIDES AND OTHER VASCULAR DISORDERS

All inflammatory processes involve blood vessels. True inflammation depends on the presence of blood vessels. The terms *vasculitis* or *angiitis* therefore should not be used loosely for those inflammatory changes that we have considered up to now, all of which exhibit reversible endothelial swelling, perivascular edema, and perivascular cell infiltrates. Vasculitis means inflammation of the vascular wall. In order to diagnose vasculitis, we need evidence of organic damage to the wall in the form of necrosis, hyalinization,[1] fibrinoid change, or granulomatous involvement. The fact that a vascular wall is occupied by many polymorphonuclear leukocytes is not necessarily evidence of vasculitis: All inflammatory leukocytes go from the bloodstream into the tissue, and they must migrate through the walls of the vessels. It is much easier to diagnose vasculitis if there is a vascular wall substantial enough for us to recognize damage in routine sections. Many cutaneous vessels do not fulfill this requirement, and the question of presence or absence of vasculitis remains in doubt. Of the diseases discussed so far, only the pigmented purpuric eruptions are apt to show vasculitic changes in the form of hyalinization of the walls of very small vessels. Vascular damage is difficult to demonstrate in cutaneous lupus erythematosus. In later chapters on granulomatous inflammation, vasculitis is encountered more often.

In this chapter, the first tissue reaction discussed is leukocytoclastic vasculitis,[2] the more severe expressions of which merge with cutaneous forms of polyarteritis nodosa and other types of necrotizing vasculitis (Table 15–1). Embolic and thrombotic phenomena are discussed next. Other types of vascular disease that do not fit conveniently into other chapters are given attention. The so-called lymphocytic vasculitis of pityriasis lichenoides acuta and of certain drug eruptions comes so close to a heavy perivascular infiltrate that we prefer not to single it out as an entity.

NECROTIZING ANGIITIS

Leukocytoclastic Vasculitis

The outstanding histologic features of leukocytoclastic vasculitis (Fig. 15–1) include involvement of dermal blood vessels with endothelial swelling, neutrophilic invasion of the blood vessel wall, fragmentation of the leukocytic nuclei (nuclear dust), fibrinoid deposition (Fig. 15–2), and extravasation of erythrocytes.[3-7] A relatively mild form of this tissue reaction involving small blood vessels occurs in the clinical forms of palpable purpura, urticarial vasculitis, and Schönlein–Henoch purpura.[8-14] More severe involvement of larger and deeper blood vessels merge into necrotizing vasculitis and periarteritis nodosa.[15] The eruption may be limited to the skin or

TABLE 15–1. CLASSIFICATION OF NECROTIZING VASCULITIS

Small vessels: Leukocytoclastic vasculitis
   Schölein–Henoch's purpura
   Palpable purpura
   Urticarial vasculitis
   Erythema elevatum diutinum
   Diseases of the connective tissue
   Drug-induced reactions
   Pustular vasculitis in Behcet disease and in bowel-associated dermatosis-arthritis syndrome
Large vessels
   Periarteritis nodosa
   Wegener's granulomatosis
   Churg–Strauss syndrome
   Lymphomatoid granulomatosis
   Temporal arteritis

other organ systems may be involved, particularly the joints, kidneys, and gastrointestinal tract. Immune complex pathogenesis is most likely in which a variety of antigens such as bacteria, viruses, drugs, or chemicals are involved.

Pustular vasculitis is another variant seen predominantly in cutaneous lesions of Behcet disease,[16] in bowel-associated dermatosis–arthritis syndrome,[17] skin eruption of gonococcemia, and chronic meningococcemia.[18,19] Dermal vascular changes are not as severe as in leukocytoclastic vasculitis. Fibrinoid deposition and extravasation of erythrocytes are not prominent, but the neutrophilic cell infiltrate is very heavy and resembles that seen in Sweet syndrome.[20]

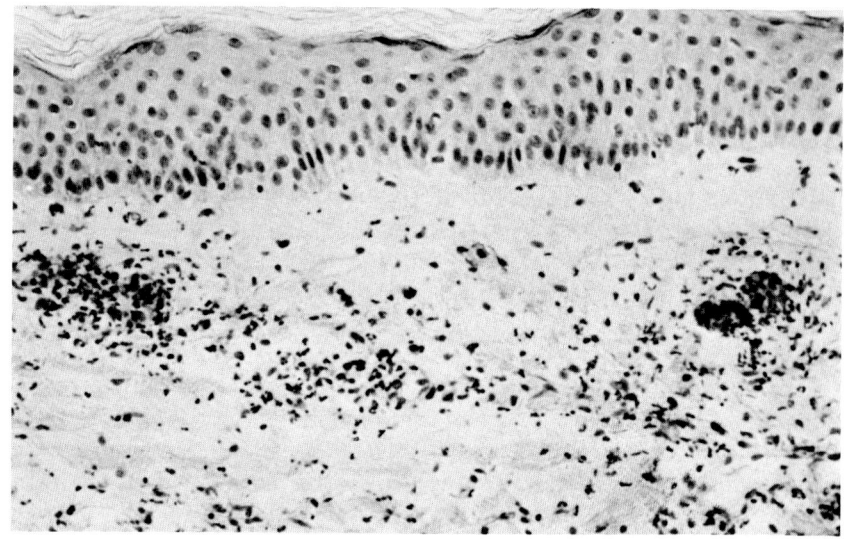

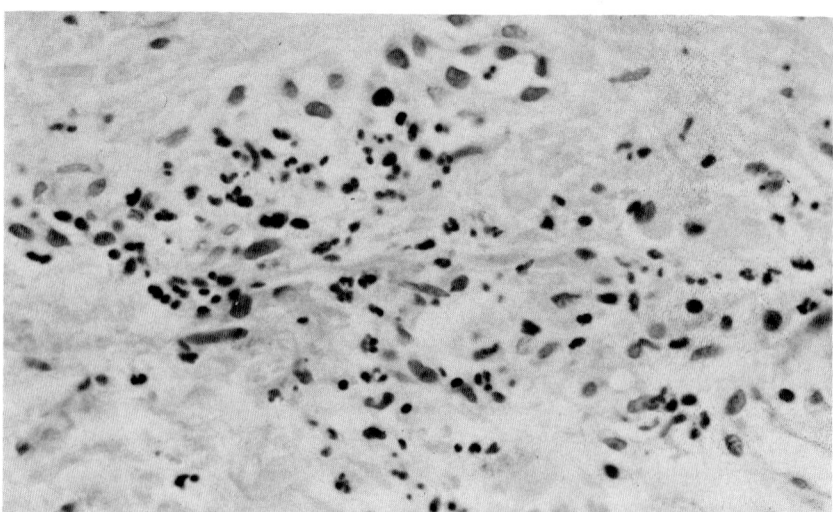

Figure 15–1.
Leukocytoclastic vasculitis. Vessels of the subpapillary plexus are involved. Polymorphonuclear leukocytes break down, leaving nuclear dust. **A.** H&E. X225. **B.** H&E. X465.

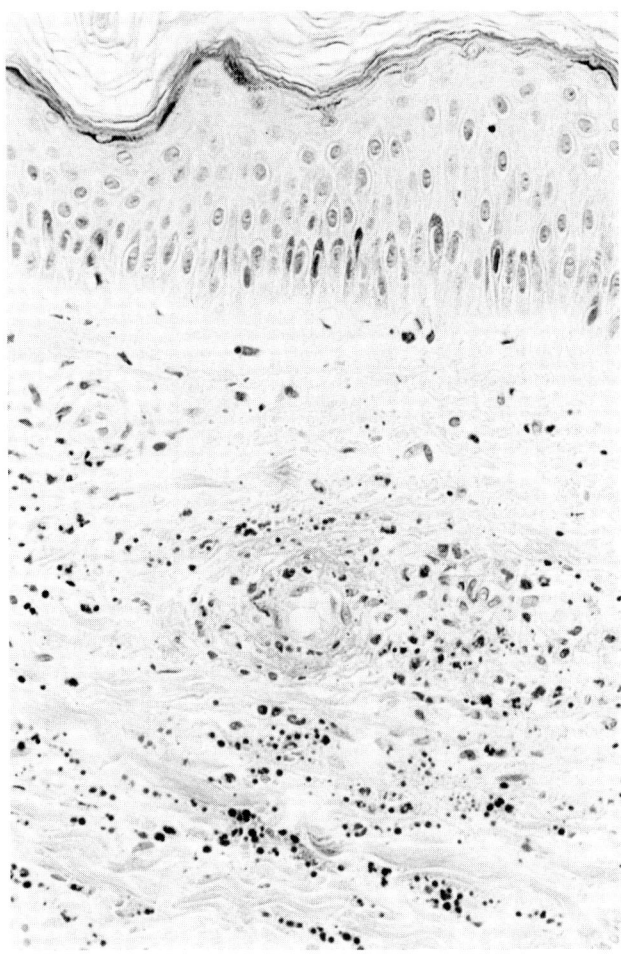

Figure 15–2.
Leukocytoclastic vasculitis. Superficial vessels show endothelial swelling and deposition of fibrinoid material and nuclear dust. H&E. X250.

Periarteritis (Polyarteritis) Nodosa

Polyarteritis nodosa (Fig. 15–3) usually involves somewhat larger and deeper vessels that have sizable walls.[21] Surprisingly, this fact may not help in the diagnosis when H&E sections are examined. The structure of the vessel may be altered so much that it is hard to recognize. O&G sections are very helpful because the subintimal elastic ring of arteries and the elastic coats of veins are usually well preserved. The histologic hallmark of polyarteritis nodosa is necrosis of all or part of the vascular wall. This occurs early and is accompanied by neutrophilic and eosinophilic infiltrate. It is followed by more chronic inflammation, often by thrombosis, and sometimes by rupture and hemorrhage and eventual

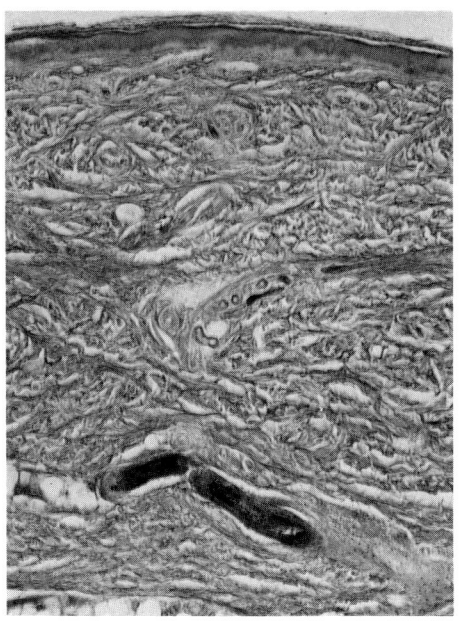

A

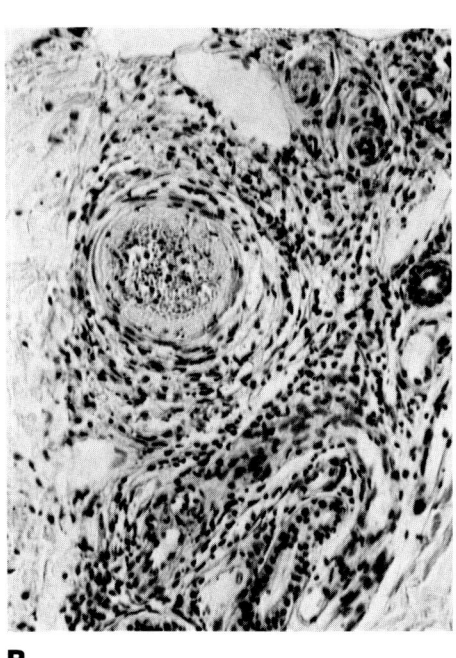

B

Figure 15–3.
Segmental arteritis in case of clinical livedo racemosa (livedo reticularis). All layers of wall of a deep, medium-sized vessel are involved. **A.** O&G. X70. **B.** H&E. X225.

replacement by scar tissue. The picture in individual sections, therefore, depends on the stage of the disease, but evidence of destruction of the vessel wall and presence of eosinophils are requirements for diagnosis. The vascular involvement may be limited to the skin or associated with the systemic manifestations.[22]

Other Forms

Other forms of necrotizing vasculitis with strongly granulomatous tissue reaction have been described. *Wegener's granulomatosis*,[23,24] *allergic granulomatous angiitis* (Churg–Strauss syndrome), and *lymphomatoid granulomatosis*[25,26] often have cutaneous and multisystem involvement. In Churg–Strauss syndrome patients have asthma, pulmonary infiltration, and peripheral eosinophilia. Histologic sections show involvement of small- and medium-sized blood vessels and areas of necrosis and destruction of collagen bundles with deposition of fibrinoid and eosinophilic material and Charcot–Leyden crystals surrounded by infiltration of eosinophils, macrophages, and multinucleated giant cells in palisaded arrangement. Churg–Strauss-type of granulomatous vasculitis may be observed in the cutaneous lesions of patients with Takayasu's arteritis.[27] Another special form of granulomatous vasculitis occurring subsequent to excessive solar exposure is temporal arteritis (Fig. 15–4).[28,29]

KAWASAKI'S DISEASE

An infantile acute febrile *mucocutaneous lymph node syndrome* described in Japan and later in Hawaii and the continental United States[30] seems to be related to cutaneous polyarteritis nodosa. Children affected are usually younger than 5 years of age and develop a polymorphous scarlatiniform, morbilliform, or erythema multiformelike exanthem, which is followed by general exfoliation beginning at the edge of the fingernails and toenails. In 1 or 2 percent of cases, death has resulted from cardiac failure, and the cutaneous lesions have features of polyarteritis nodosa histologically. All attempts to find a toxic or infectious agent have failed.[31]

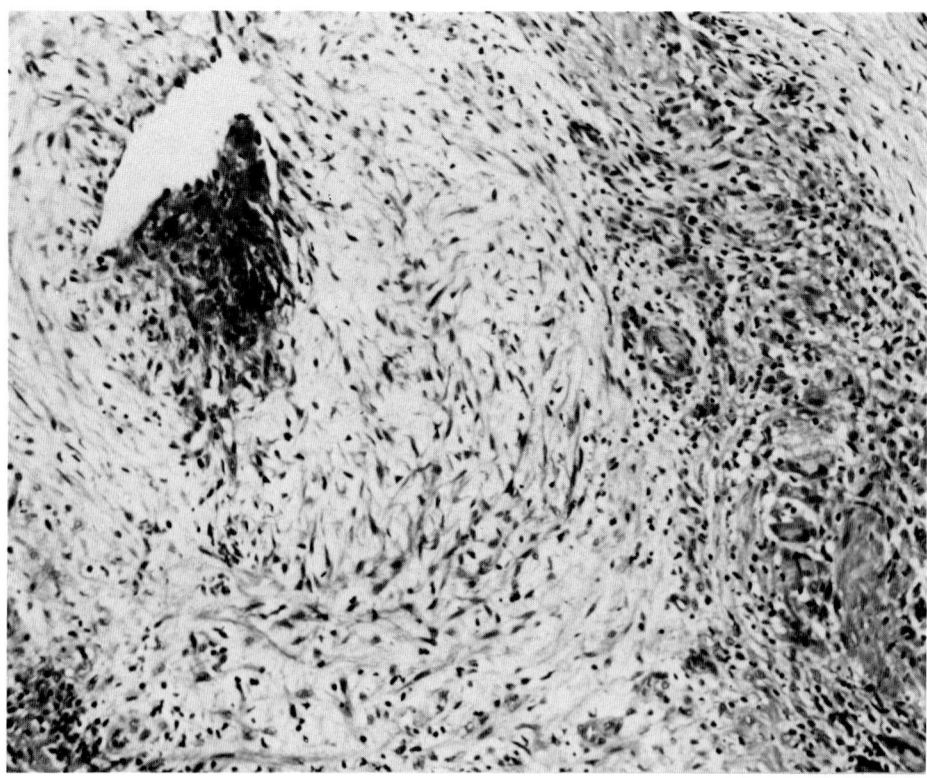

Figure 15–4.
Temporal arteritis. A branch of the temporal artery is partly occluded by subendothelial proliferation, and its wall is affected by granulomatous infiltrate, including multinucleated giant cells. H&E. X135.

EMBOLISM, THROMBOSIS, AND INFARCTION

Embolism

Other forms of vasculitis are due to, or at least are associated with, embolism or thrombosis. To the first type belong skin lesions in certain cases of chronic sepsis. Cutaneous eruption associated with gonococcemia and meningococcemia has already been mentioned under pustular vasculitis. Fat embolisms in small cutaneous vessels and resulting purpura are encountered after fracture of long bones.[32] Embolism of tubercle bacilli in the small vessels may cause *miliary tuberculosis* of the skin and is the supposed origin of *lichen scrofulosorum* and *papulonecrotic tuberculids* (Chapter 21).

Thrombosis

Thrombotic phenomena often involve larger vessels and produce several different manifestations. The most impressive one histologically is *thromboangiitis obliterans*,[33] in which a large artery or vein at the subcutaneous border is occluded by an organizing thrombus, and the wall is frayed and occupied by chronic inflammatory infiltrate. This disorder, together with polyarteritis nodosa, must be taken into consideration in the differential diagnosis of deep nodose lesions (Chapter 16).

Two special cases are *Mondor's disease* and *nonvenereal sclerosing lymphangiitis* of the penis. Mondor's disease, whether spontaneous or induced by trauma, involves superficial veins of the anterior thorax with a thrombophlebitis that goes through the classic three stages: (1) formation of an intraluminal thrombus, (2) organization of the thrombus with fibroblasts, and (3) recanalization.[34,35] The same is true for the somewhat frightening firm cord in the postcoronal area of the penis, which has usually been interpreted as lymphangiitis but probably also is a phlebitis that dissolves spontaneously.[36,37]

Livedo

A peculiar clinical manifestation is livedo reticularis or racemosa,[38] which must be differentiated from the purely functional cutis marmorata seen mainly in children. The cause of the chronic and permanent types of livedo is subtotal occlusion of larger vessels deep in the dermis or subcutaneous tissue (Fig. 15–5). A rare form of tissue reaction is livedoid vasculitis characterized by involvement of small- and medium-sized blood vessels with intimal thickening, endothelial proliferation, and hyalin degeneration of vascular walls with minimal perivascular inflammatory cell infiltrate.[39] Involvement of superficial dermal blood vessels with livedoid vasculitis occurs in patients with cryoglubulinemia and other forms of dysproteinemic purpura with ulceration. Livedoid vasculitis is also observed in the early stage of atrophie blanche and in patients with systemic lupus erythematosus.[40,41]

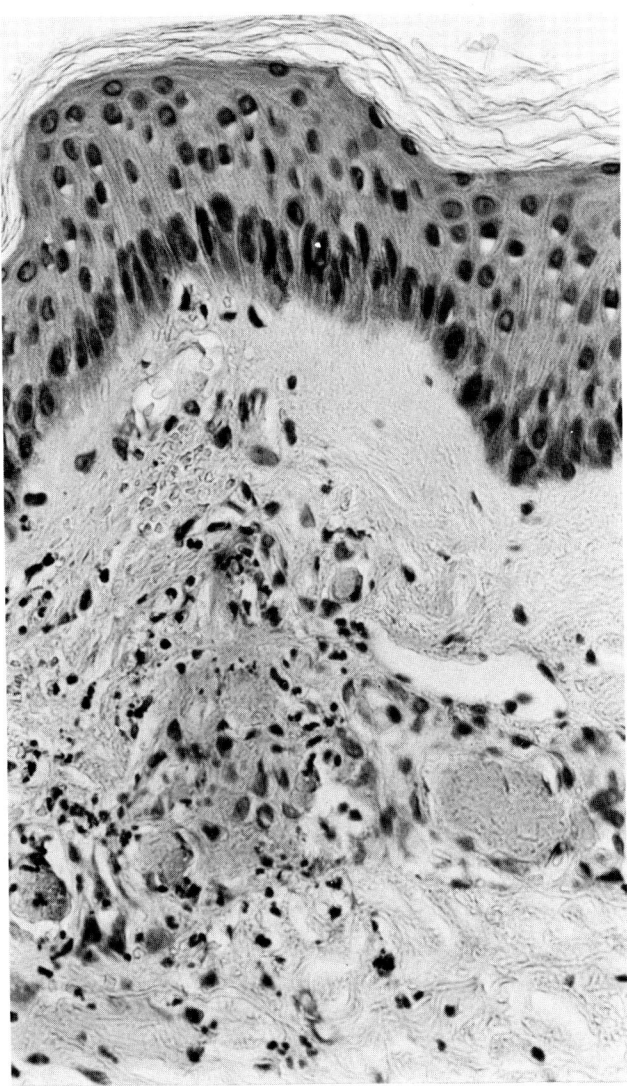

Figure 15–5.
Superficial vascular occlusion with fibrinoid deposition of livedoid vasculitis. H&E. X250.

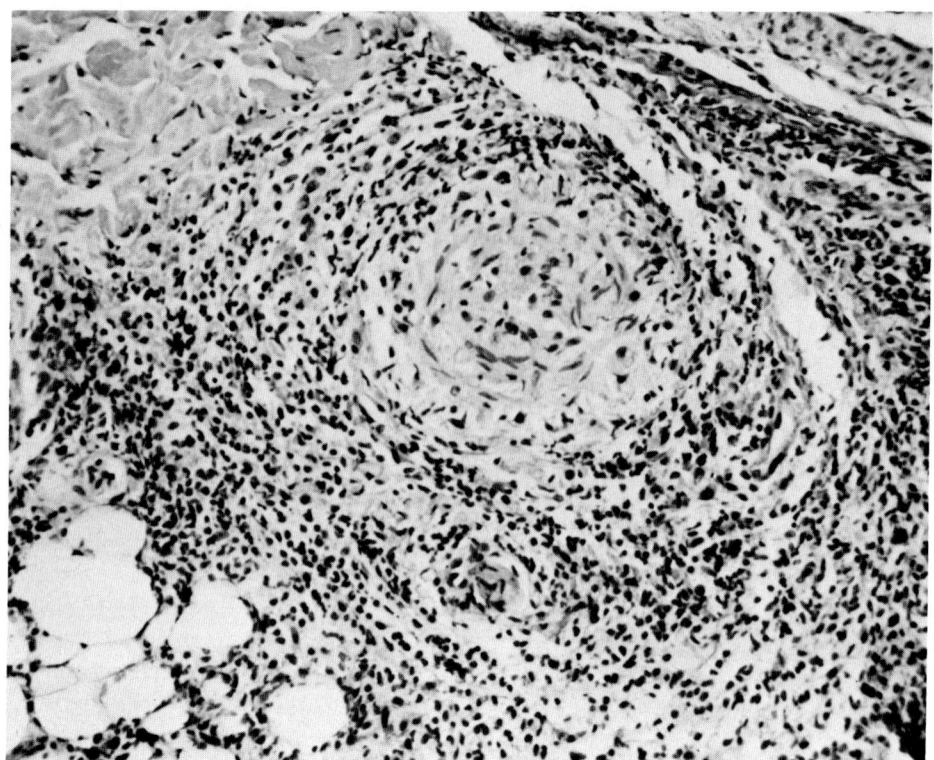

Figure 15–6.
Acute pernio. Thrombotic occlusion of a small vessel at deep cutaneous border. Structure of wall obliterated by subacute inflammatory infiltrate, which also extends into surrounding tissue. H&E. X225.

Acute and chronic *pernio*, on the other hand (Fig. 15–6), exhibits obliteration of deeper dermal vessels by intimal proliferation and, at times, adherent thrombi. There is associated mixed inflammatory infiltrate of varying degree.[42]

Infarction

Purpuric and necrotic lesions of various types and subcutaneous hematomas may be manifestations of disseminated intravascular coagulation.[43] Similar necrotic lesions may occur following administration of coumarin or intravenous heparin therapy.[44–46] Skin biopsy may lead to early diagnosis and shows extensive vascular involvement with fibrin thrombi located centrally in the lumen and with no significant perivascular inflammatory cell reaction (Fig. 15–7).

Another disease that fulfills the clinical and histologic criteria of anemic infarct is *malignant atrophic papulosis* of Degos, characterized by appearance of many scattered sunken porcelain-white skin lesions.[47–49] The epidermis is atrophic. The dermis shows a conical zone of sclerotic connective tissue at the lower tip of which is an occluded blood vessel (Fig. 15–8). Inflammatory cell reaction is minimal.[50–52]

CHRONIC X-RAY DERMATITIS

Another not uncommon dermatosis in which severe vascular damage plays a role in addition to damage affecting all other constituents of the skin is chronic x-ray dermatitis (Fig. 15–9). Epidermal changes include hypertrophy or atrophy and spotty pigmentation and may progress to dysplasia and neoplasia.[53] The epidermis, however, does not exhibit the focal basal cell liquefaction of poikilodermas to which the clinical picture has great similarity. All layers of the dermis show severe sclerosis, uneven distribution and clumping of elastic fibers, and obliteration of large vessels with some new formation of ectatic, thin-walled vessels. A peculiar and almost pathognomonic feature is the presence of giant fibroblasts (Fig. 15–9B) similar to those seen in poorly growing tissue cultures. They seem to compensate for their inability to multiply by hypertrophy of nucleus and cytoplasm.

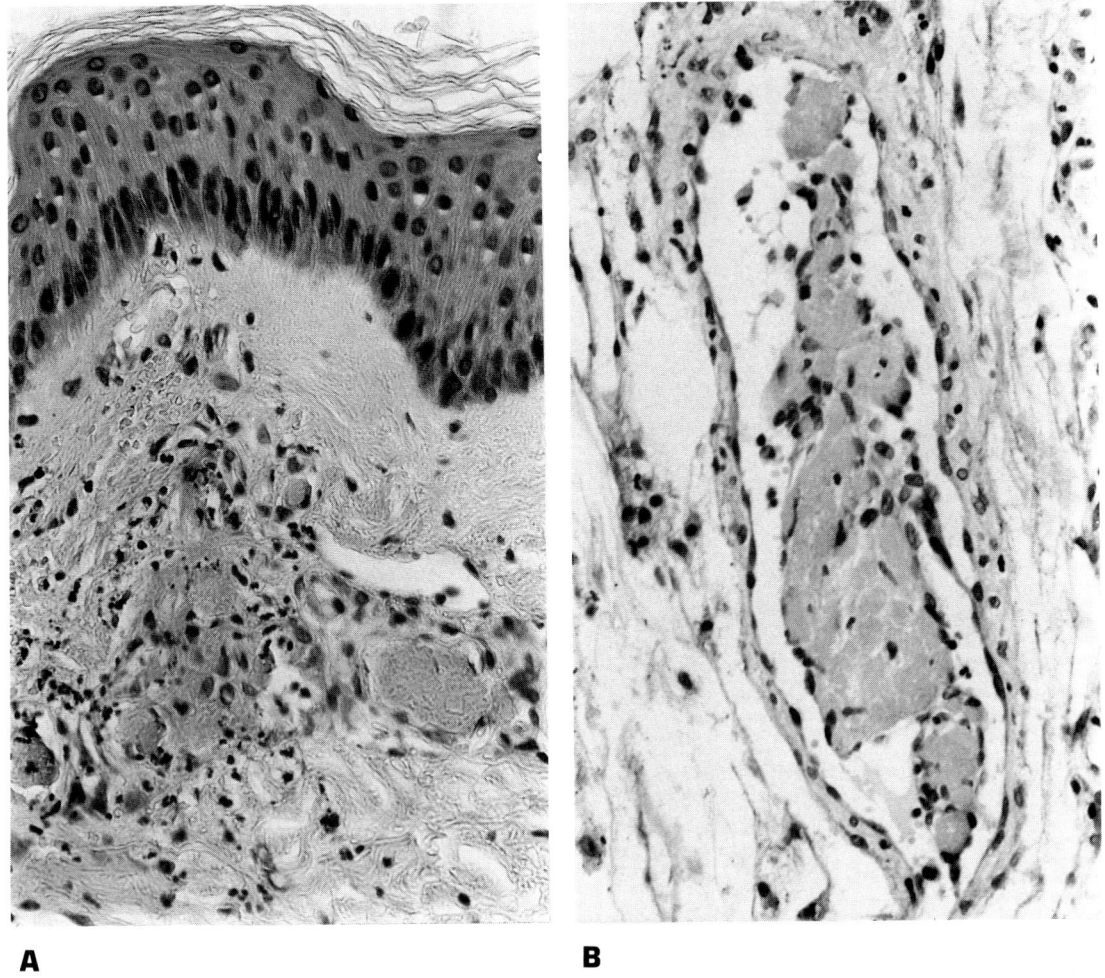

Figure 15–7.
Coumarin necrosis. **A.** and **B.** Extensive dermal vascular involvement with fibrin thrombi. H&E. X225.

ERYTHEMA ELEVATUM DIUTINUM

An unusual type of leukocytoclastic vasculitis is encountered in erythema elevatum diutinum (Fig. 15–10). The disease[54] is characterized by the paradox that the cellular infiltrate consists almost entirely of neutrophils and eosinophils in spite of the chronic course.[55] The substance called "toxic hyalin" by Weidman is similar to fibrinoid in its staining reactions. It occupies a zone broader than the actual vessel wall and is seen as a coarse trabeculation of the connective tissue, similar to that found in granuloma faciale (Fig. 15–11). Older lesions show increase in vascularity and dermal fibrosis.[56] The histologic differential diagnosis includes Sweet syndrome, in which the peculiar perivascular changes are absent, and granuloma faciale, in which many histiocytes are present as proof of a granulomatous response.

GRANULOMA FACIALE

Granuloma faciale derives its name from the fact that it occurs almost exclusively on the face[57,58] although a few disseminated cases have been recorded. Once considered a member of the group of eosinophilic granulomas, this peculiarly indolent disease has highly characteristic histologic features (Fig.

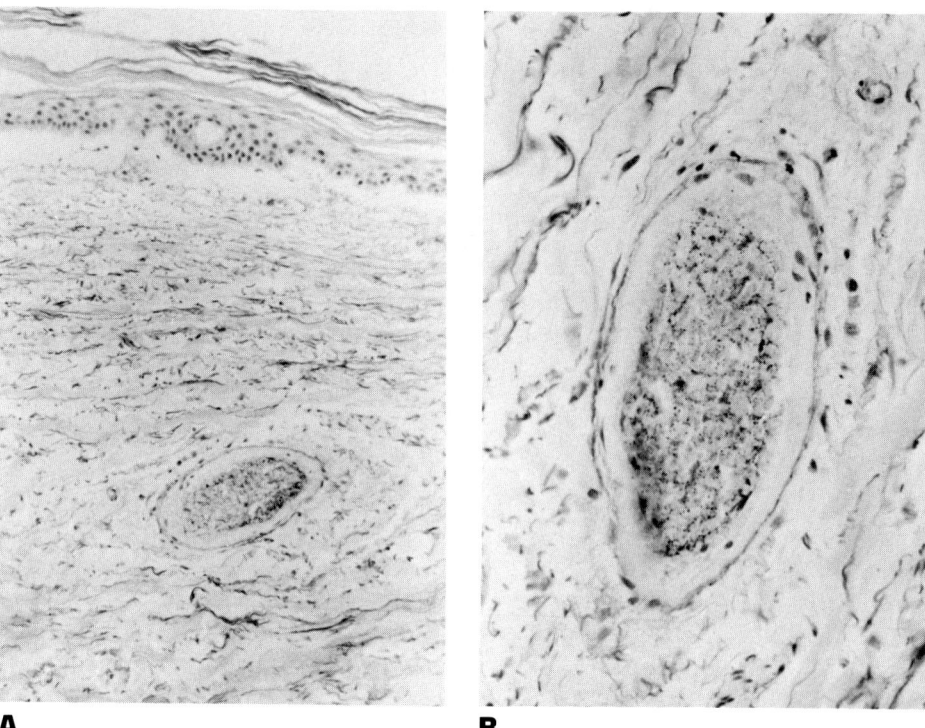

Figure 15—8.
Degos' disease. Infarction and necrosis of a medium-sized artery in deep dermis without inflammation. Elastica interna of artery well shown. O&G. **A.** X125. **B.** X400.

15–11B), the most prominent of which is presence of neutrophilic leukocytes in a clinically chronic affection. Eosinophilic leukocytes are also usually present, sometimes in large numbers, but are not absolutely necessary for diagnosis. Other features are the presence of histiocytes, lymphocytes, and plasma cells, a peculiar trabeculation of connective tissue (fibrinoid?) around thin-walled wide vessels, often associated with leukocytoclasia, and a free subepidermal zone (grenz zone).[59,60] Multinucleated giant cells are rare, a few foam cells may occur, but phagocytosis of hemosiderin and melanin is more common. The epidermis usually shows no particular changes, and ulceration is most uncommon. Hair follicles and sweat glands slowly undergo atrophy. The granulomatous infiltrate may extend into the subcutaneous tissue.

The picture thus combines prominent granulomatous inflammation with leukocytoclastic vasculitis, a unique experience. There is some similarity to the Arthus phenomenon.[61] Granuloma faciale differs from erythema elevatum diutinum, in which there may be considerable fibrosis but rarely much histiocyte or plasma cell reaction.

STASIS DERMATITIS

Finally, we have to discuss common cutaneous changes of the lower extremities that are often called stasis dermatitis in the widest sense. It was recommended in Chapter 3 to avoid biopsy of lesions below the knee, if there is a choice. Even relatively young persons without obviously diseased skin may exhibit dilatation, tortuosity, and tufting of capillaries and thickening of the walls of deeper vessels as early signs of stasis. These changes lead to excessive fragility of capillary walls and diapedesis of red cells with advanced age, and it is a common experience that a generalized maculopapular drug eruption will become purpuric below the knees and heal with residual hemosiderin pigmentation. Vascular changes of this type, mild round cell infiltrate, and a moderate quantity of hemosiderin in dermal macrophages should be discounted in the diagnosis of other dermatoses if the specimen was obtained from the lower extremities. More definite vascular alterations are needed for a diagnosis of pigmented purpuric eruption. Heavier deposits of hemosiderin that extend

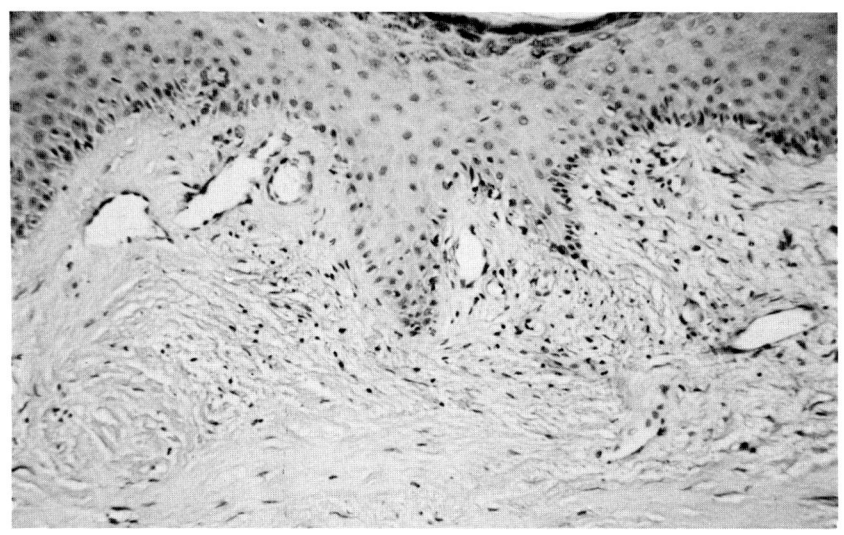

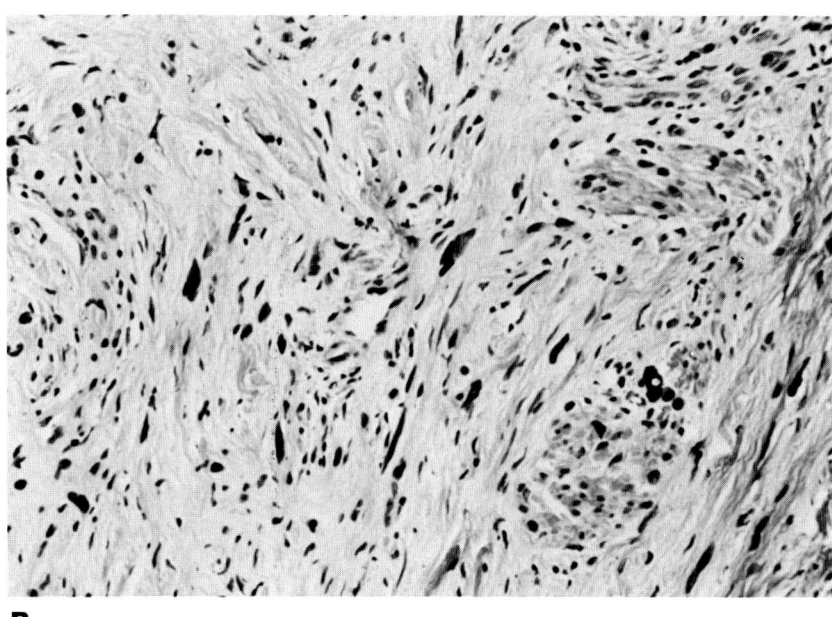

Figure 15–9.
Chronic x-ray damage. **A.** The epidermis is somewhat hypertrophic and hyperplastic, and the dermis shows paucity of cells in the sclerotic pars reticularis and telangiectasia and distortion of collagen fibers in the pars papillaris. H&E. X135. **B.** Higher magnification shows damaged smooth muscle bundles in right half of picture, nuclei of giant fibroblasts in center, and unevenly sized collagen bundles in left half. H&E. X375.

into the deeper layers together with pericapillary fibrin deposition are often associated with venous insufficiency.[62] Variable degrees of dermal fibrosis, loss of elastic fibers, and atrophy of epidermis and adnexal structures (hair muscles, however, usually survive and actually increase in size) are additional nonspecific changes in leg skin that may be quite disturbing in the interpretation of biopsy specimens.

In cases that show clinical evidence of stasis dermatitis, one should, of course, expect evidence of subacute or chronic eczematous tissue reaction in addition to the changes just described (Fig. 5–12). In a special variant extensive proliferation of endothelial-lined blood vessels occurs in a broad zone below the epidermis associated with heavy accumulation of hemosiderotic macrophages producing nodules and infiltrated plaques resembling Kaposi's

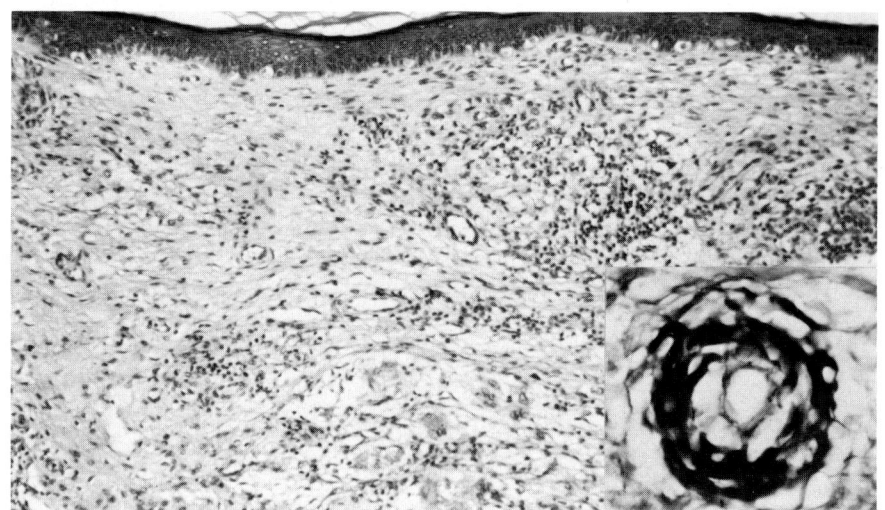

Figure 15–10.
Erythema elevatum diutinum. Several of the involved vessels are surrounded by hyaline material. H&E. X135. Inset shows trabeculation of PAS-positive material surrounding a small vessel. Alcian blue-PAS. X400.

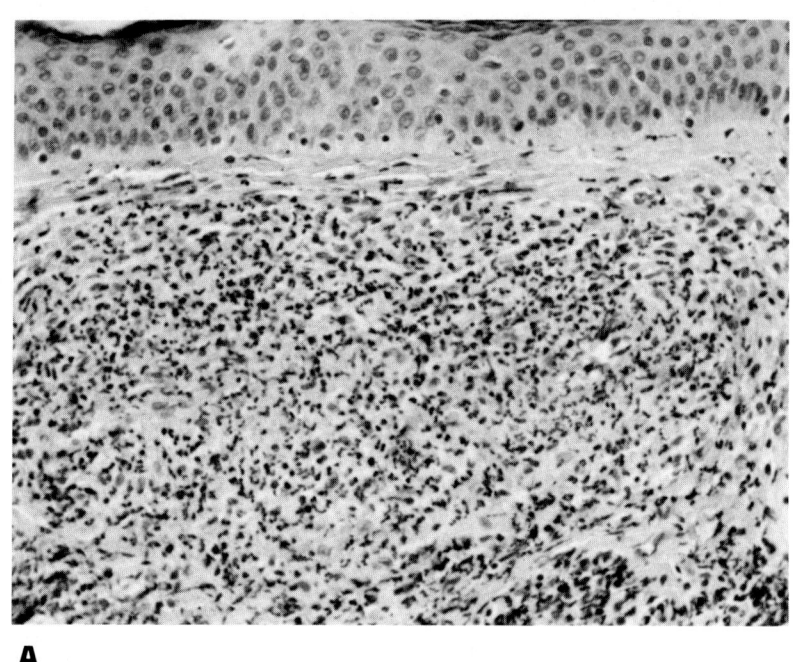

A

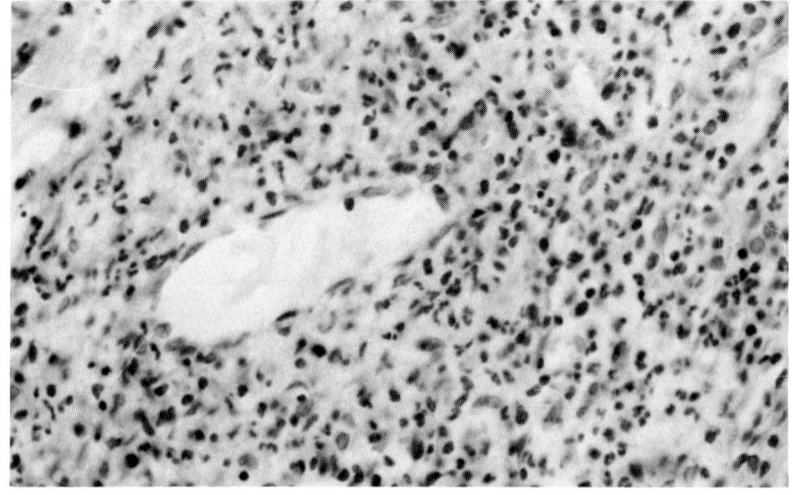

Figure 15–11.
Granuloma faciale. **A.** Superficial portion, illustrating the grenz zone between epidermis and a mixed granulomatous infiltrate. H&E. X225. **B.** Dilated thin-walled vessel surrounded by disintegrating leukocytes in a zone of degenerating connective tissue. Mixed granulomatous infiltrate. H&E. X600.

B

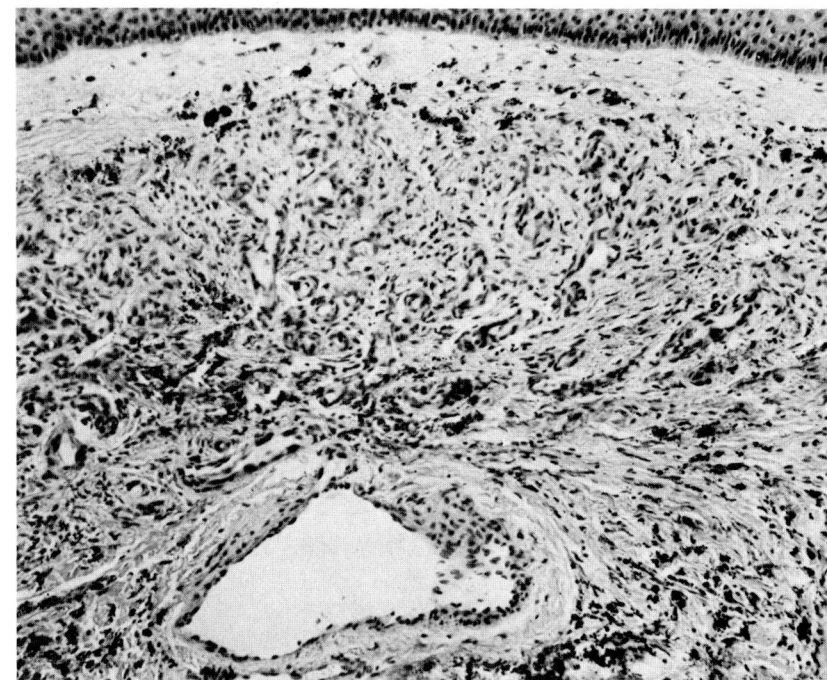

Figure 15–12.
Hypertrophic stasis dermatitis. Diffuse proliferation of superficial blood vessels, whereas the large deeper vessel is intact. Hemosiderotic macrophages are found in this condition and in Kaposi's sarcoma (see Fig. 43–20). H&E. X100.

sarcoma.[63,64] The diffuse character and superficial location of the vascular proliferation are differentiating signs of this *acro-angiodermatitis*.[65]

Atrophie Blanche

White atrophy (atrophie blanche) is at the other end of the clinical spectrum. The chalky white skin is sclerotic and is subject to easy painful ulceration.[66,67] An idiopathic form shows initial pruritic maculopapular lesions with superficial ulceration leading to areas of atrophy telangiectasia and pigmentary changes. Histological examination shows fibrinoid deposition within the superficial dermal blood vessels. A secondary type of atrophie blanche may occur in individuals with arteriosclerosis, connective tissue diseases, diabetes, dysproteinemia, and chronic stasis dermatitis. Occlusion of dermal blood vessels occurs by intimal thickening and fibrin thrombi leading to ulceration and fibrosis.[68]

REFERENCES

1. Ryan TJ: Cutaneous vasculitis. J Cutan Pathol 12: 381, 1985
2. Mackel SE, Jordon RE: Leukocytoclastic vasculitis. Arch Dermatol 118:296, 1982
3. Sanchez NP, Van Hale HM, Su DWP: Clinical and histopathologic spectrum of necrotizing vasculitis. Arch Dermatol 121:220, 1985
4. Callen JP, Ekenstam E: Cutaneous leukocytoclastic vasculitis: Clinical experience in 44 patients. South Med J 80:848, 1987
5. Ekenstam E, Callen JP: Cutaneous leukocytoclastic vasculitis. Clinical and laboratory features of 82 patients seen in private practice. Arch Dermatol 120: 484, 1984
6. Hodge SL, Callen JR, Ekenstam E: Cutaneous leukocytoclastic vasculitis: Correlation of histopathological changes with clinical severity and course. J Cutan Pathol 14:279, 1987
7. Sams WM Jr: Hypersensitivity angiitis. J Invest Dermatol 93:78S, 1989
8. Bonnefoy M, Claudy AL: Etude Prospective De Facteurs Associes Aux Vascularites Leucocytoclasiques. Ann Dermatol Venereol 115:27, 1988
9. Monroe EW: Urticarial vasculitis. J Am Acad Dermatol 5:88, 1981
10. Callen JP, Kalbfleisch S: Urticarial vasculitis: A report of nine cases and review of the literature. Br J Dermatol 107:87, 1982
11. Berg RE, Kantor GR, Bergfeld WF: Urticarial vasculitis. Cleveland Clin Q 27:468, 1988
12. Yasue T, Yasue A: Urticarial vasculitis with circulating immune complexes and mixed cryoglobulins: Studies of pathogenesis. J Dermatol 14:597, 1987
13. Piette WW, Seabury-Stone MD: A cutaneous sign of IgA-associated small dermal vessel leukocytoclastic vasculitis in adults (Henoch–Schoenlein purpura). Arch Dermatol 125:53, 1989

14. Van Hale HM, Gibson LE, Schroeter AL: Henoch–Schoenlein vasculitis: Direct immunofluorescence study of uninvolved skin. J Am Acad Dermatol 15:665, 1986
15. Yevich I: Necrotizing vaculitis with granulomatosis. Int J Dermatol 27:540, 1988
16. Gilhar A, Winterstein G, Turani H, et al: Skin hyperreactivity response (pathergy) in Bechet's disease. J Am Acad Dermatol 21:547, 1989
17. Dicken CH: Bowel-associated dermatosis-arthritis syndrome: Bowel bypass syndrome without bowel bypass. J Am Acad Dermatol 14:792, 1986
18. Shapiro L, Taisch JA, Brownstein MH: Dermatohistopathology of chronic gonococcal sepsis. Arch Dermatol 107:403, 1973
19. Sotto MN, Langer B, Hoshino-Shimizu S, DeBrito T: Pathogenesis of cutaneous lesions in acute meningococcemia in humans. J Infect Dis 133:506, 1976
20. Jorizzo JL, Solomon AR, Zanolli MD, Leshin B: Neutrophilic vascular reactions. J Am Acad Dermatol 19:983, 1988
21. Diaz-Perez JL, Winkelmann RK: Cutaneous periarteritis nodosa. Arch Dermatol 110:407, 1974
22. Meyrick TRH, Black MM: The wide clinical spectrum of polyarteritis nodosa with cutaneous involvement. Clin Exp Dermatol 8:47, 1983
23. Le T, Pierard GE, Lapière CM: Granulomatous vasculitis of Wegener. J Cutan Pathol 8:34, 1981
24. Crotty CP, DeRemee RA, Winkelmann RK: Cutaneous clinicopathologic correlation of allergic granulomatosis. J Am Acad Dermatol 5:571, 1981
25. Chumbley LC, Harrison EG Jr, DeRemee RA: Allergic granulomatosis and angiitis (Churg–Strauss syndrome). Report and analysis of 30 cases. Mayo Clin Proc 52:477, 1977
26. Cooper LM, Patterson JAK: Allergic granulomatosis and angiitis of Churg–Strauss. Case report in a patient with antibodies to human immunodeficiency virus and hepatitis B virus. Int J Dermatol 28: 597, 1989
27. Perniciaro CV, Winkelmann RK, Hunder GG: Cutaneous manifestations of Takayasu's arteritis—A clinicopathologic correlation. J Am Acad Dermatol 17:998, 1987
28. Baum EW, Sams MW Jr, Payne RR: Giant cell arteritis: A systemic disease with rare cutaneous manifestations. J Am Acad Dermatol 6:1081, 1982
29. O'Brien, JP: Vascular accidents after actinic (solar) exposure. An aspect of the temporal arteritis/polymyalgia rheumatica syndrome. Int J Dermatol 26:366, 1987
30. Kahn G: Mucocutaneous lymph node syndrome (Kawasaki's disease). A new disease remarking its debut. Arch Dermatol 114:948, 1978
31. Weston WL, Juff JC: The mucocutaneous lymph node syndrome: a critical reexamination. Clin Exp Dermatol 6:167, 1981
32. Cole WG, Oakes BW: Skin petechiae and fat embolism. Aust NZ J Surg 42:401, 1973
33. Giblin WJ, James WD, Benson PM: Burger's disease. Int J Dermatol 28:672, 1989
34. Johnson WC, Walbrich R, Helwig EB: Superficial thrombophlebitis of the chest wall. JAMA 180:103, 1962
35. Marsch WC, Haas N, Stuttgen G: Mondor's phlebitis—A lymphovascular process. Light and electron microscopic indications. Dermatologica 172:133, 1986
36. Tanii T, Hamada T, Asai Y, Yorifuji T: Mondor's phlebitis of the penis: A study with factor VIII related antigen. Acta Derm Venereol 64:337, 1984
37. Marsch WC, Stuttgen G: Sclerosing lymphangiitis of the penis: A lymphangiofibrosis thrombotica occlusiva. Br J Dermatol 104:687, 1981
38. Lubach D, Schwabe C, Weissenborn K, et al: Livedo racemosa generalisata: An evaluation of thirty-four cases. J Am Acad Dermatol 22:633, 1990
39. Sams WM Jr: Livedo vasculitis—Therapy with pentoxifylline. Arch Dermatol 124:684, 1988
40. Yasue T: Livedoid vasculitis and central nervous system involvement in systemic lupus erythematosus. Arch Dermatol 122:66, 1986
41. Weinstein C, Miller MH, Axtens R, et al: Livedo reticularis associated with increased titers of anticardiolipin antibodies in systemic lupus erythematosus. Arch Dermatol 123:596, 1987
42. Goette DK: Chilblains (Perniosis). J Am Acad Dermatol 23:257, 1990
43. Colman RW, Minna JD, Robboy SJ: Disseminated intravascular coagulation: a dermatologic disease. Int J Dermatol 16:47, 1977
44. Stone MS, Rosen T: Acral purpura: An unusual sign of coumarin necrosis. J Am Acad Dermatol 14:797, 1986
45. Shelley WB, Sayen JJ: Heparin necrosis: an anticoagulant-induced cutaneous infarct. J Am Acad Dermatol 7:674, 1982
46. Rongioletti F, Pisani S, Ciaccio M, Rebora A: Skin necrosis due to intravenous heparin. Dermatologica 178:47, 1989
47. Degos R: Malignant atrophic papulosis. Br J Dermatol 100:21, 1979
48. Su DWP, Schroeter AL, Lee DA, et al: Clinical and histologic findings in Degos' syndrome (malignant atrophic papulosis). Cutis 35:131, 1985
49. Magrinat G, Kerwin KS, Gabriel DA: The clinical manifestations of Degos' syndrome. Arch Pathol Lab Med 113:354, 1989
50. Tribble K, Archer ME, Jorizzo JL, et al: Malignant atrophic papulosis: Absence of circulating immune complexes or vasculitis. J Am Acad Dermatol 15:365, 1986
51. Meunier L, Issautier F, Guillot B, et al: Maladie de Degos neuro-cutanee. Ann Dermatol Venereol 115: 319, 1988
52. Barlow RJ, Heyl T, Simson IW, Schulz EJ: Malignant atrophic papulosis (Degos' disease)—Diffuse involvement of brain and bowel in an African patient. Br J Dermatol 118:117, 1988
53. Okazaki M, Kikuchi I, Narita H, et al: Radioder-

matitis: An analysis of 43 cases. J Dermatol 13:356, 1986
54. Haber H: Erythema elevatum diutinum. Br J Dermatol 67:121, 1955
55. Katz SI, Gallin JI, Hertz KC, et al: Erythema elevatum diutinum: Skin and systemic manifestations, immunologic studies and successful treatment with dapsone. Medicine (Baltimore) 56:433, 1977
56. LeBoit PE, Yen TSB, Wintroub B: The evolution of lesions in erythema elevatum diutinum. Am J Dermatopathol 8:392, 1986
57. Pinkus H: Granuloma faciale. Dermatologica 105:85, 1952
58. Schwitzler L, Verret JL, Schubert B: Granuloma faciale. Ultrastructural study of three cases. J Cutan Pathol 4:123, 1977
59. Velders AJ, Dejong MCJM, Klokke AH: Granuloma eosinophilicum faciale. Z Hautkr 59:1365, 1984
60. Frost FA, Heenan PJ: Facial granuloma. Aust J Dermatol 25:121, 1984
61. Nieboer C, Kalsbeek GL: Immunofluorescence studies in granuloma eosinophilicum faciale. J Cutan Pathol 5:68, 1978
62. Vanscheidt W, Laaff H, Wokalek H, et al: Pericapillary fibrin cuff: a histological sign of venous leg ulceration. J Cutan Pathol 17:266, 1990
63. Caston FX, Denoeux J-P, Remond A, et al: Syndrome de Stewart-Bluefarb. Ann Dermat Venereol 107:919, 1980
64. Marshall ME, Hatfield ST, Hatfield DR: Arteriovenous malformation simulating Kaposi's sarcoma (pseudo-Kaposi's sarcoma). Arch Dermatol 121:99, 1985
65. Strutton G, Weedon D: Acro-angiodermatitis. A simulant of Kaposi's sarcoma. Am J Dermatopathol 9:85, 1987
66. Stiefler RE, Berfeld WF: Atrophie blanche. Int J Dermatol 21:1, 1982
67. Milstone LM, Braverman IM, Lucky P, Fleckman P: Classification and therapy of atrophie blanche. Arch Dermatol 119:963, 1983
68. Priollet P: Atrophie blanche. Ann Dermatol Venereol 114:1005, 1987

16

SUBCUTANEOUS INFLAMMATIONS: PANNICULITIS

Inflammatory processes involving the deepest layers of the dermis and the subcutaneous fat tissue are not rare in a dermatopathologist's material and constitute one of the major diagnostic problems. There are several reasons for the difficulties encountered in differential diagnosis. The ideal way of obtaining an adequate specimen is excisional biopsy of ample size using a sharp knife. Punch biopsies may provide adequate samples in many other dermatoses but often produce inadequate material in these large and deep-seated plaques. The plug of tissue is obtained rather blindly and may or may not include pathognomonic portions of the tissue. If an ample specimen is supplied, the technician must be instructed to cut a considerable number of sections. One of the important points in diagnosis is the presence or absence of a pathologic larger blood vessel, and a conclusion cannot be reached on only a few sections. Another difficulty is the biologic propensity of fat tissue to react in a stereotyped manner to any insult. The response is known by the German term *Wucheratrophie* or *proliferating atrophy*. It means that normal fat tissue disappears and is replaced by fibroblasts and macrophages (Fig. 16–1) associated with a greater or lesser number of inflammatory cells. Once this proliferating atrophy is well established, it is impossible to recognize its cause and origin. It is also obvious that inflammation of the subcutaneous tissue has granulomatous features, so we will not be able to separate simple and granulomatous inflammation in this field.

The border between dermis and subcutis is not sharp. Fat lobes may be found in the dermis, especially around sweat coils, and the large vessels of the deep cutaneous plexus are partly within the dermis, partly below it. The subcutaneous panniculus consists of fat lobes separated by connective tissue septa that usually contain larger vessels, whereas the fat lobes are richly supplied with tiny vessels. All these features must be kept in mind when one analyzes a deep nodose lesion. Since most of these occur on the legs, one should additionally consider the almost invariable presence of some stasis changes even in young persons.

DIFFERENTIAL DIAGNOSIS

A practical approach to differential diagnosis is the following. First, one should decide whether the principal seat of pathologic change, the center of gravity of the lesion, is in the mid-dermis, the cutaneous–subcutaneous border zone, the interlobular septa, or the fat lobes. Inflammatory changes usually involve all of these areas, but a representative section often permits a decision. A center of gravity in the mid-dermis automatically eliminates the lesion from our

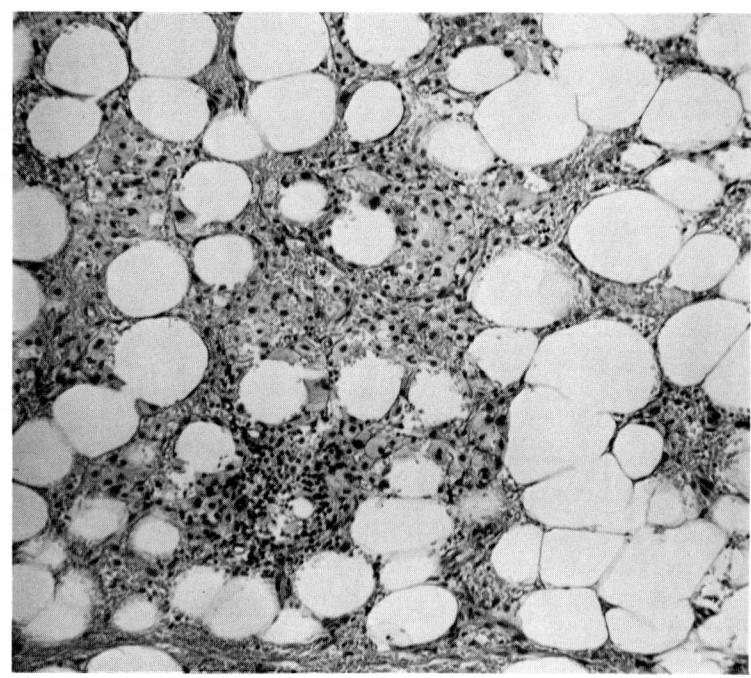

Figure 16–1.
Proliferating atrophy of fat tissue. The relatively large cells having gray-appearing cytoplasm are macrophages containing numerous small lipid droplets. H&E. X135.

present consideration: it might be granuloma annulare, folliculitis, or something else. Center of gravity at the subcutaneous junction strongly suggests primary involvement of a larger vessel, because inflammation of sweat coils is very rare. Primary seat in the interlobar septa is fairly common, and the infiltrate then invades the fat lobes from the periphery. True panniculitis (Fig. 16–2), on the other hand, will show a whole lobe of fat tissue involved with infiltrate and possibly necrosis or liquefaction. Small vessels in the center of the lobe are the primary site of disturbance. Two reviews on panniculitis are published by Eng and Aronson[1] and by Black.[2]

The next point to be considered is the general character of the infiltrate. Well-developed epithelioid cell nodules, associated with round cells, in the absence of granulocytes are almost diagnostic of tuberculosis in the form of erythema induratum or of sarcoidosis or syphilis. The presence of polymorphonuclear leukocytes in a nonulcerated lesion points away from these three granulomatous diseases but may be found in deep fungous infections. Erythema nodosum often shows a peculiar mixture of more acute inflammation around small blood vessels and giant cell reaction of foreign-body type in the interlobar septa. Pure round cell infiltrate suggests lymphoma, and pure polymorphonuclear infiltrate suggests acute infection or allergic reaction.

After ascertaining these parameters, one should institute a careful search for involvement of larger vessels and should remember, as was pointed out in the previous chapter, that vascular structure may be so completely obscured that even a sizable artery or vein resembles a fibrotic or granulomatous nodule in H&E sections. The O&G stain often brings surprises because elastic fibers are usually preserved, at least in part. Immunofluorescent studies may be helpful. A search for microorganisms using PAS and acid-fast methods should be made in doubtful cases.

INDIVIDUAL ENTITIES

Nodular Vasculitis

If a large artery or vein seems to be the center of the process, the diagnosis of nodular vasculitis is appropriate unless a more specific diagnosis suggests itself. One should remember that a relatively small biopsy may not include that vessel or that partial sectioning of a large specimen may miss it. In many cases, the diagnosis of nodular vasculitis is an admission of etiologic ignorance, but only too often it is the best that can be made. Special manifestations of deep vasculitis are *Mondor's disease,* consisting of painful induration of a thrombosed deep chest vein, *temporal arteritis* (giant cell arteritis), a presumably allergic granulomatous vasculitis (Fig. 16–3) that may cause large and deep ulcerations of cranial

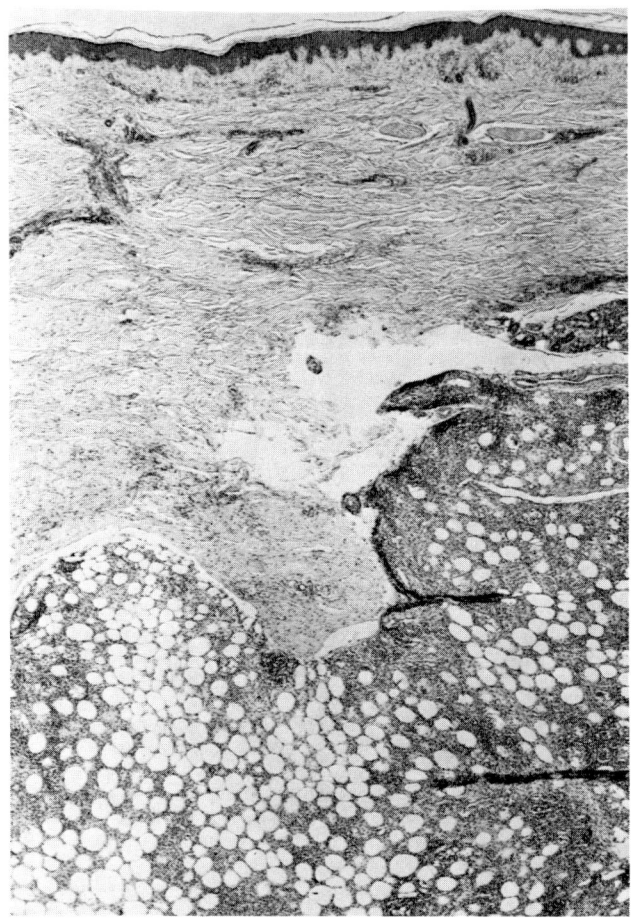

Figure 16–2.
Panniculitis. Entire fat lobes are involved with little change of surrounding connective tissue. H&E. X60.

skin,[3] and *nodular migratory panniculitis* (thrombophlebitis) of the legs,[4,5] which is remarkable for its prompt response to potassium iodide therapy.

Erythema Nodosum

The clinical term *erythema nodosum* lends itself to wide interpretation and has been used indiscriminately for any red or dusky nodosity of the lower legs. The etiology may vary from the classic tuberculosis and leprosy to streptococcal infection or sarcoidosis and many other causes, among which *Yersinia* has been stressed.[6,7] We agree that there is not only the classic subacute form, which runs its course in a few weeks, but that more chronic forms exist. We insist, however, on certain criteria for histologic diagnosis. Erythema nodosum (see Fig. 3–9) involved small and medium-sized blood vessels in deep dermis and the connective tissue septae between the fat lobules preferentially. The latter often show small groups of epithelioid cells and multinucleated giant cells (Fig. 16–4). Inflammatory cells include lymphocytes and at least some polymorphonuclears. Fat lobules are invaded by the infiltrate from the periphery (Fig. 16–5). The small radial granulomatous foci of Miescher are considered pathognomonic,[8] but they are often not present. Definite areas of tissue necrosis rule out erythema nodosum, and so do typical epithelioid tubercles or many plasma cells or numerous eosinophils.

Erythema Induratum and Gummatous Syphilis

In fully developed lesions of Bazin's disease, the combination of tissue necrosis and well-organized tubercles makes a diagnosis of erythema induratum (Chapter 21) easy.[9] The tuberculoid structure, however, may be aped by proliferating atrophy of fat tissue, and, on the other hand, cases of proven tuberculous etiology may show nothing but nonspecific alterations. The theoretically present, deep tuberculous phlebitis is difficult to demonstrate. Clinically, ulcerated lesions may show polymorphonuclear infiltrate and other evidence of secondary infection. Presence of many plasma cells makes gummatous syphilis the more likely diagnosis.

Panniculitis

Panniculitis in the strict sense applies to inflammation of fat lobes rather than of interlobular septa or of large subcutaneous vessels. The fetal development makes each fat lobe a separate organ with a nourishing artery and two draining veins, and explains the sharp limitation of pannicular inflammation (Fig. 16–2). Once fat cells in a lobe are damaged, macrophages are attracted and, by phagocytosis, become foam cells. The mixture of fat atrophy and proliferation of inflammatory cells is called *Wucheratrophie* (Fig. 16–1) and is such a stereotyped response that it soon overshadows all specific processes and makes histopathologic diagnosis difficult.

The prototype of acute or subacute panniculitis was Weber–Christian's *febrile nonsuppurative nodular panniculitis,* but the diagnosis is made less and less frequently as diagnostic acumen increases.[10] The disease is rare. Painful dull-red nodules appear in crops over the thighs and lower legs of middle-aged women in association with fever. The panniculitis is lobular. Although suppuration is ruled out by definition, many cases of the clinical Weber–Christian type undergo liquefaction necrosis and are called "liquefying panniculitis" (Fig. 16–6) on histologic ex-

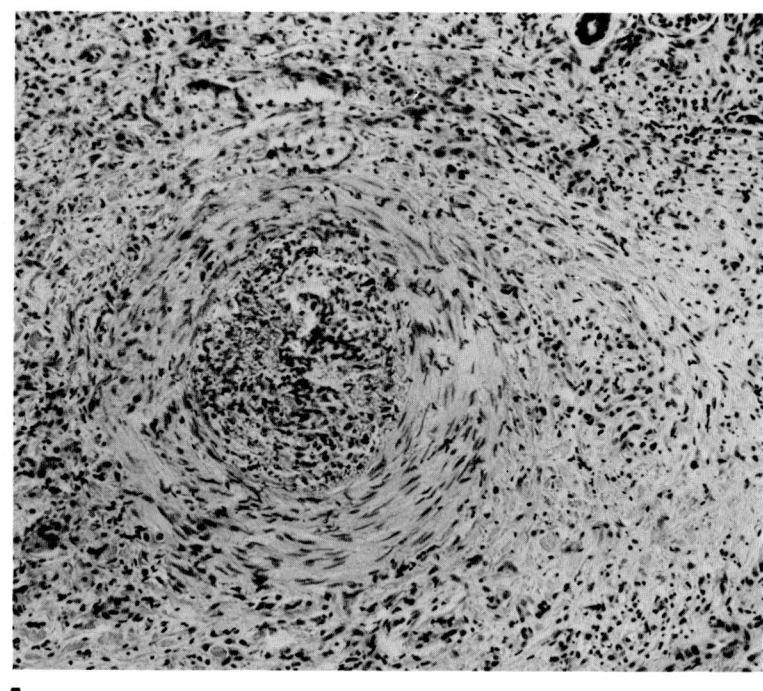

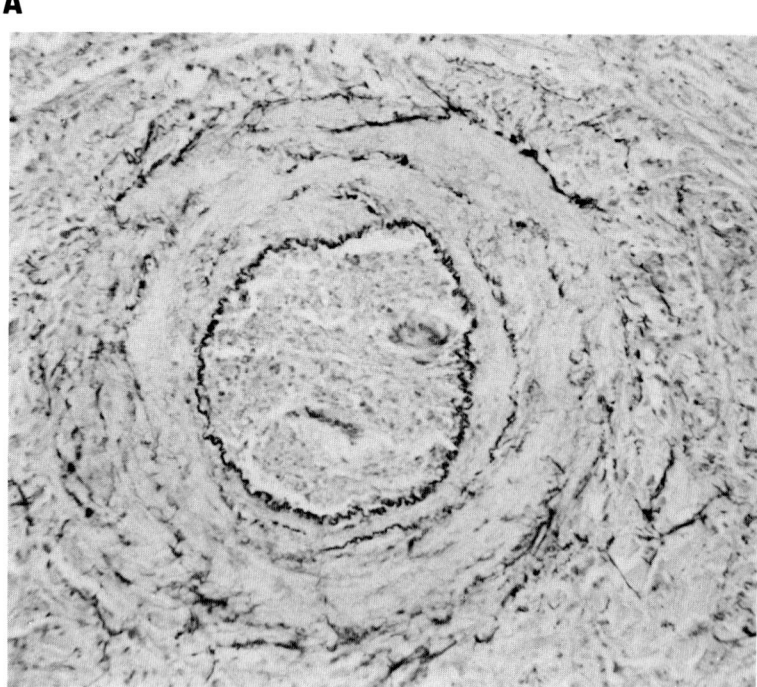

Figure 16–3.
Nodular vasculitis. **A.** The wall of a fairly large vessel of the deep dermal plexus is disrupted by inflammatory infiltrate and its lumen filled by a thrombus. H&E. X120. **B.** Elastic fiber stain permits easier identification of the vessel wall and documents partial destruction of fibers. O&G. X120.

amination. In the acute stage, fat lobules are heavily infiltrated by cells, mostly polymorphonuclears. Later, macrophages and foam cells appear and healing takes place with fibrosis.

In *scleredema neonatorum* waxy hard nodules and plaques appear on the buttocks and spread elsewhere in a debilitated or premature neonate (Fig. 16–7). Subcutaneous fat necrosis appears as nodules and plaques shortly after birth in a healthy infant.[11,12] Both conditions show extensive fat necrosis and granulomatous panniculitis with needle-shaped clefts within foamy multinucleated giant cells.[13,14] Pancreatic panniculitis (Fig. 16–8) is secondary to circulating enzyme (lipases) and shows

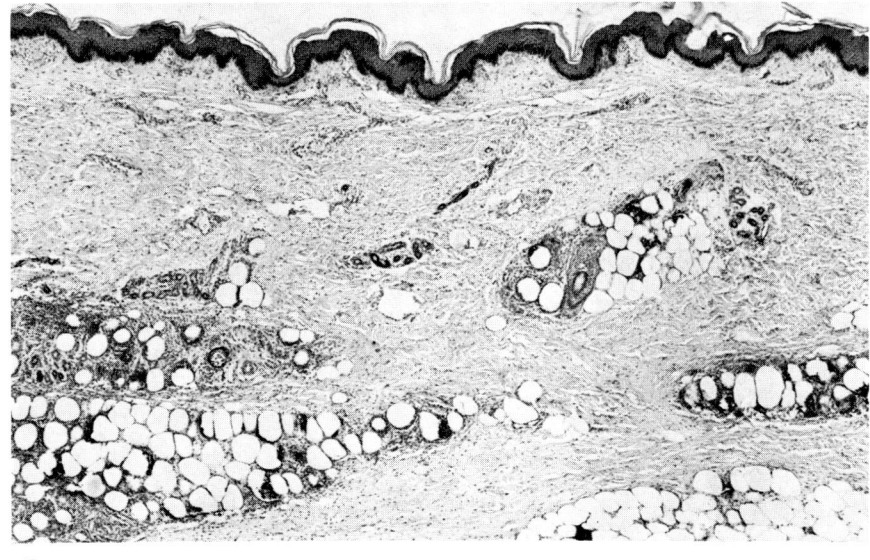

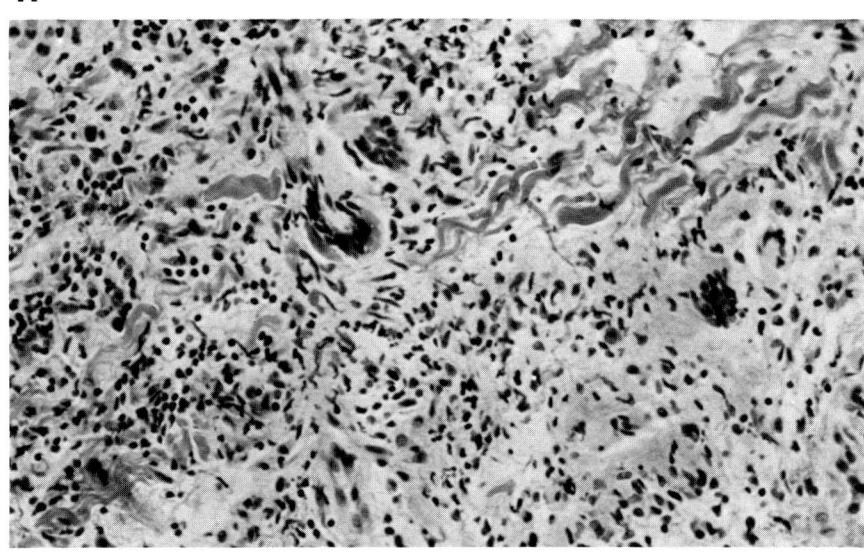

Figure 16-4.
Erythema nodosum. Note deep dermal and subcutaneous fat involvement. **A.** H&E. X90. **B.** H&E. X270.

coagulation necrosis of lipocytes leading to formation ghost cells and foci of calcification.[15]

Cytophagic histiocytic panniculitis is manifested with tender, swollen subcutaneous nodules in patients with fever, hepatosplenomegaly, serosal effusions, ecchymoses, peripheral adenopathy, mucosal ulcers, anemia, leukopenia, elevated liver enzymes, and coagulopathy.[16,17] Histologic sections show extensive infiltration of the subcutaneous fat lobules with benign-appearing histiocytes engulfing lymphocytes, erythrocytes, and platelets. Cytophagia also occurs in other organs. Most patients die of hemorrhagic complications. A nonlethal variety is also recognized.[18]

Severe panniculitis with extensive degeneration of fat cells, edema, and heavy perivascular infiltrate of lymphocytes and histiocytes occurs in association with $alpha_1$-antitrypsin deficiency.[19-21] Another rare and potentially fatal lesion is *necrotizing fasciitis* caused by streptococci and affects the superficial fascia deep to subcutaneous fat tissue with acute necrotizing inflammation.[22]

Panniculitis in Diseases of Connective Tissue

Specific and nonspecific panniculitis may occur in diseases of connective tissue. Lupus panniculitis (lupus erythematosus profundus)[23,24] is discussed in Chapter 14. Other connective tissue diseases associ-

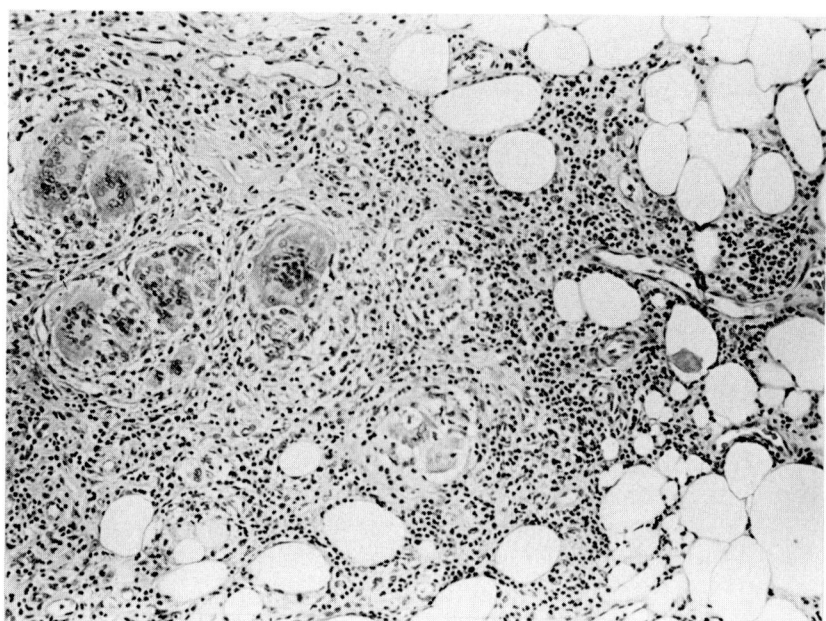

Figure 16–5.
Erythema nodosum. Epithelioid and giant cell granuloma is present within the connective tissue septa between the subcutaneous fat lobules. H&E. X250. (From A. H. Mehregan. In Dermatologic Immunology and Allergy, J. Stone (ed). C. V. Mosby, St. Louis, 1985.)

ated with panniculitis are *scleroderma* and occasionally *dermatomyositis*.[25,26] The inflammation of fat lobules in this type is predominantly lymphocytic. Plasma cells, histiocytes, epithelioid cells, and multinucleated giant cells are also observed.

Deep Fungous Infections

All the granulomatous mycoses, especially sporotrichosis, may have their center of gravity in subcutaneous tissue. They are discussed in Section IV.

Other Inflammatory Entities

The Darier–Roussy type of sarcoid (see Fig. 21–14) may cause deep-seated cutaneous–subcutaneous plaques characterized by typical epithelioid cell tubercles. Spiegler–Fendt sarcoid, on the other hand, is characterized by pure round cell nodes and belongs in the lymphoma group. Deep-seated neoplasm, such as eccrine spiradenoma, glomus tumor, and Kaposi's sarcoma, should be easily ruled out by microscopic examination. Infestation with worms oc-

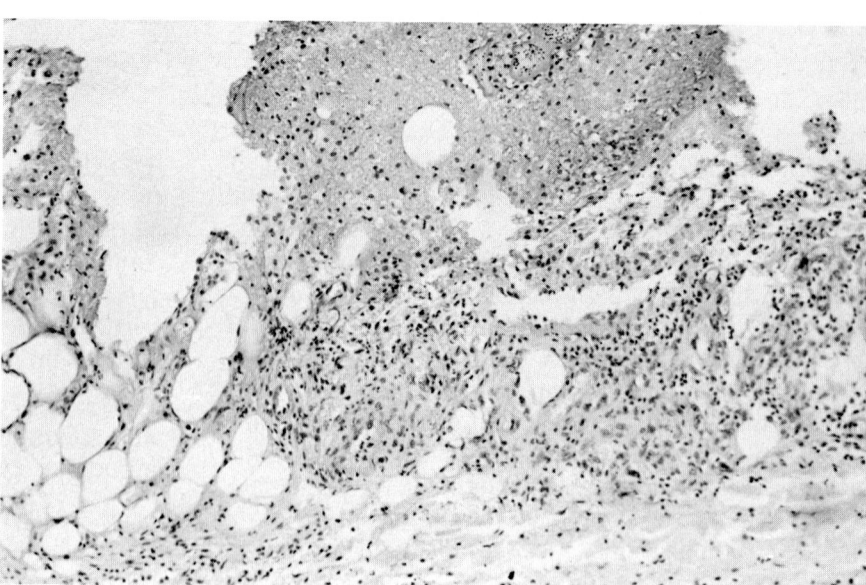

Figure 16–6.
Liquefying panniculitis. The center of the involved fat lobule has undergone necrosis, which is secondarily invaded by relatively small numbers of polymorphonuclear leukocytes. H&E. X125.

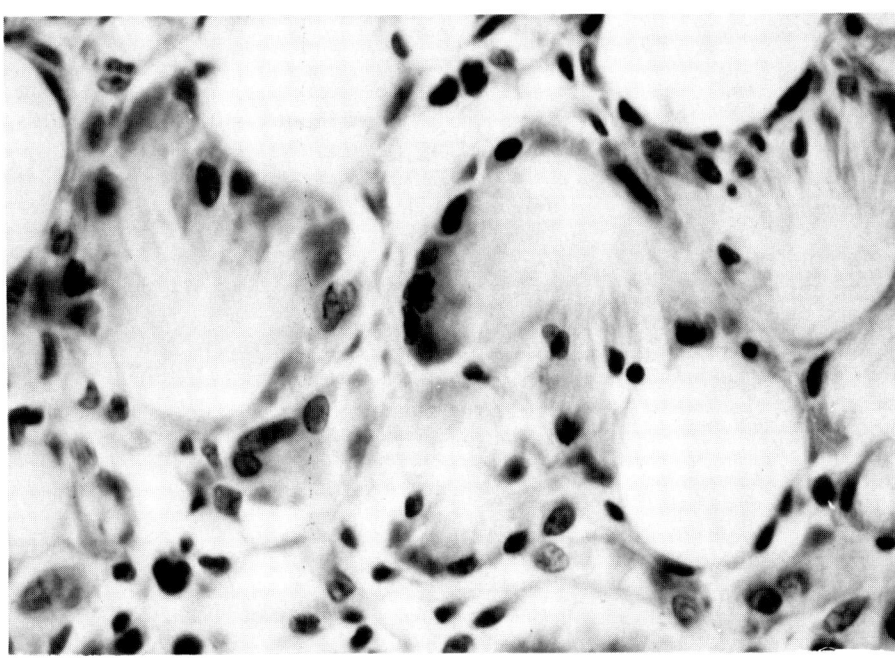

Figure 16–7.
Subcutaneous fat necrosis of newborn shows formation of multinucleated cells and clefts left by fatty acid crystals. H&E. X600.

curs mainly in tropical countries (see Fig. 22–12).

Factitial panniculitis may occur secondary to blunt trauma. The histologic findings of an organizing hematoma and deposition of blood pigment are helpful for diagnosis.[27]

One should not forget that the introduction of foreign matter of various types may produce subcutaneous nodes, which range all the way from infected or sterile abscesses to indolent lipogranulomas. In many cases, only a high rate of suspicion can solve puzzling cases by identifying morphologically or chemically mineral oil, silica, starch, and other substances, to which most recently impure preparations of silicone have been added. Some of these sub-

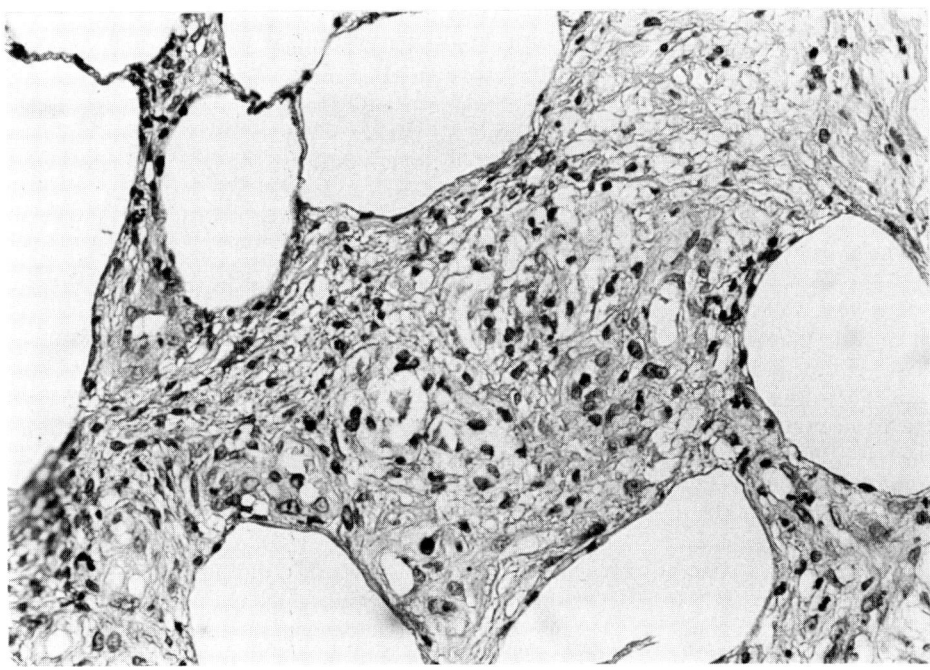

Figure 16–8.
Panniculitis secondary to pancreatitis shows breakdown of fat cells and replacement with foamy histiocytes. H&E. X250.

stances may produce subcutaneous calcifications. For additional data, see Chapter 21 (sarcoid granulomas), Chapter 22 (foreign-body granuloma), and Chapter 28 (foreign bodies).

Equestrian Cold Panniculitis in Women

An affection seen occasionally in female horseback riders in England was described in 1980 and identified as a deep-seated panniculitis caused by insufficient insulation and friction from pants.[28,29]

Noninflammatory Entities

Piezogenic Papules

Under the name piezogenic pedal papules, painful herniations of fat tissue on the soles of the feet have been described, which seem to be provoked by pressure and exhibit degenerative changes of fat tissue, interlobar septa, and overlying dermis.[30,31] Nonpainful, small herniations in similar location are not uncommon and consist of normal fat tissue.

Cellulite

Another, and quite obscure, condition of fat tissue has caused considerable comment in Europe, more in lay circles than in the medical literature. Braun-Falco and Scherwitz,[32] however, felt compelled to investigate the tissue basis of the so-called *cellulite*, which refers to the slight puckering of the skin of the thighs of adipose women and has become a lucrative reason for therapy. They came to the conclusion that this "disease" is a normal phenomenon related to the fibrous retinacula that connect skin and fascia between the fat lobes.[33,34]

REFERENCES

1. Eng AM, Aronson IK: Dermatopathology of panniculitis. Semin Dermatol 3:1, 1984
2. Black MM: Panniculitis. J Cutan Pathol 12:366, 1985
3. Baum EW, Sams MW Jr, Payne RR: Giant cell arteritis: A systemic disease with rare cutaneous manifestations. J Am Acad Dermatol 6:1081, 1982
4. Vilanova X, Piñol Aguadé J: Subacute nodular migratory panniculitis. Br J Dermatol 71:45, 1959
5. De Almeida Prestes C, Winkelmann RK, Su DWP: Septal granulomatous panniculitis: Comparison of the pathology of erythema nodosum migrans (migratory panniculitis) and chronic erythema nodosum. J Am Acad Dermatol 22:477, 1990
6. Murphy EG, Sanchez NP, Flynn TC, et al: Erythema nodosum leprosum: Nature and extent of the cutaneous microvascular alterations. J Am Acad Dermatol 14:59, 1986
7. Ikeya T, Mizuno E, Takama H: Three cases of erythema nodosum associated with *Yersinia enteroclitica* infection. J Dermatol 13:147, 1986
8. Yus ES, Sanz Vico MD, de Diego V: Miescher's radial granuloma—A characteristic marker of erythema nodosum. Am J Dermatopathol 11(5):434, 1989
9. Rademaker M, Lowe DG, Munro DD: Erythema induratum (Bazin's disease). J Am Acad Dermatol 21:740, 1989
10. Aronson IK, West DP, Variakojis D, et al: Fatal panniculitis. J Am Acad Dermatol 12:535, 1985
11. Chen TH, Shewmake SW, Hansen DD, Lajoy HL: Subcutaneous fat necrosis of the newborn. A case report. Arch Dermatol 117:36, 1981
12. Katz DA, Huerter C, Bogard P, Braddock SW: Subcutaneous fat necrosis of the newborn. Arch Dermatol 120:1517, 1984
13. Fretzin DF, Arias AM: Sclerema neonatorum and subcutaneous fat necrosis of the newborn. Pediatr Dermatol 4:112, 1987
14. Friedman SJ, Winkelmann RK: Subcutaneous fat necrosis of the newborn: Light, ultrastructural, and histochemical microscopic studies. J Cutan Pathol 16:99, 1989
15. Haber RM, Assaad DM: Panniculitis associated with a pancreas divisum. J Am Acad Dermatol 14:331, 1986
16. Alegre VA, Winkelmann RK: Histiocytic cytophagic panniculitis. J Am Acad Dermatol 20:177, 1989
17. White JW Jr, Winkelmann RK: Cytophagic histiocytic panniculitis is not always fatal. J Cutan Pathol 16:137, 1989
18. Alegre VA, Fortea JM, Camps C, Aliaga A: Cytophagic histiocytic panniculitis. Case report with resolution after treatment. J Am Acad Dermatol 20:875, 1989
19. Su WPD, Smith KC, Pittelkow MR, Winkelmann RK: Antitrypsin deficiency panniculitis: A histopathologic and immunopathologic study of four cases. Am J Dermatopathol 9(6):483, 1987
20. Smith KC, Pittelkow MR, Su WPD: Panniculitis associated with severe α_1-antitrypsin deficiency. Treatment and review of the literature. Arch Dermatol 123:1655, 1987
21. Smith KC, Su DWP, Pittelkow MR, Winkelmann RK: Clinical and pathologic correlations in 96 patients with panniculitis including 15 patients with deficient level of alpha$_1$-antitrypsin. J Am Acad Dermatol 21:1192, 1989
22. Koehn GS: Necrotizing faciitis. Arch Dermatol 114:581, 1978
23. Sanchez NP, Peters MS, Winkelmann RK: The histopathology of lupus erythematosus panniculitis. J Am Acad Dermatol 5:673, 1981
24. Grob JJ, Villette-Collet AM, Andrac L, Bonerandi JJ: Panniculite lupique fibrosante chez une femme enceinte avec anticorps anti-ro/ssa chez la mere et l'enfant. Ann Dermatol Venereol 114:973, 1987

25. Vincent F, Prokopetz R, Miller RAW: Plasma cell panniculitis: A unique clinical and pathologic presentation of linear scleroderma. J Am Acad Dermatol 21:357, 1989
26. Winkelmann RK: Panniculitis in connective tissue disease. Arch Dermatol 119:336, 1983
27. Winkelmann RK, Barker S: Factitial traumatic panniculitis. J Am Acad Dermatol 13:988, 1985
28. Vickers R: Equestrian cold panniculitis in women. Arch Dermatol 117:315, 1981
29. Boacham BE, Cooper PH, Buchanan CS, Weary PE: Equestrian cold panniculitis in women. Arch Dermatol 116:1025, 1980
30. Dreno B, Renaut J-J, Bureau B, et al: Painful piezogenic pedal papules. Ann Derm Venereol 111:571, 1984
31. Kahana M, Levy A, Ronnen M, et al: Painful piezogenic pedal papules on a child with Ehlers–Danlos syndrome. Pediatr Dermatol 3:45, 1985
32. Braun-Falco O, Scherwitz C: Zur Histopathologie der sogenannten Cellulitis. Hautarzt 23:71, 1972
33. Nürnberger F, Müller G: So-called cellulite: An invented disease. J Dermatol Surg Oncol 4:221, 1978
34. Langeland J: A case of cellulitis generalisata. Dermatologica 166:92, 1983

17

ULCERS

Cutaneous ulceration is one of the secondary manifestations that complicate primary lesions. Ulcers may result from infection, local lack of nutrition, neoplasia, and other causes. It would seem that they need no separate discussion. It was deemed advisable, however, to devote a chapter to ulcers because their clinical diagnosis is difficult, and biopsy specimens have certain nonspecific features in common, as well as some differentiating signs not encountered in nonulcerated lesions.

An ulcer is defined as a loss of tissue that includes at least the epidermis and some superficial dermis. It may imply loss of the entire dermis. If only epidermis or some of its layers are absent, the microscopist speaks of erosion or denudation, but experience proves that the difference may be difficult to tell clinically. Thus, the acantholytic process of pemphigus and even the subepidermal bullae of other blistering diseases lead to denudation, not to ulceration. The uncomplicated syphilitic chancre and the primary lesion of granuloma inguinale may appear ulcerated to the clinician, but they usually retain enough of an epidermal covering to consider them only denuded histologically. Denudations are apt to be reepithelized rapidly without leaving permanent scars. Ulceration will lead to scarring regardless of whether only the papillary layer or the entire dermis was lost.

Biopsy of an ulcer needs special care and may lead to unsatisfactory specimens, even in the hands of experts, because the deep tissue often is friable and the presence of hard crust on the surface may require undue pressure. The specimen should include healthy skin at one margin and extend across the border an adequate distance into the bottom of the ulcer. Punch biopsy, therefore, is rarely adequate. A slice of tissue should be obtained by making two vertical incisions, 2 to 3 mm apart, through the thickness of the skin and into subcutaneous tissue deep enough to secure a coherent block of tissue. The slice is freed by connecting the two long parallel incisions by short cross incisions at either end and carefully undercutting the specimen in the subcutis. When biopsy of an ulcer is indicated, there is no use skimping with tissue. The pathologist should not cut the specimen into smaller pieces but should carefully orient it so that sections are obtained of the entire block.

ULCERS, WOUNDS, AND GRANULATION TISSUE

An ulcer resulting from a pathologic process in or below the skin is different from a tissue defect (wound) resulting from sharp trauma, be it incidental or surgical. A clean wound will exhibit only minor amounts of devitalized tissue in the earliest stages and will show evidence of healing by granulation at later stages. An ucler often will show a combination of the pathologic process that caused it with evidence of a healing effort similar to the granulation tissue of a wound. If the cause of the ulcer has been removed either spontaneously or by therapy, the healing ulcer may become very similar to a healing wound, and no specific diagnosis may be possible.

Granulation tissue (Fig. 17–1) is the simultaneous proliferation of fibroblasts forming young connective tissue and of endothelial sprouts forming capillary blood vessels, which may later acquire the attributes of arteries and veins. Inflammatory cells ranging from neutrophils to lymphocytes to phagocytic histiocytes also are present and may be very numerous if there is infection. The granulations gradually fill the defect, sprouting blood vessels being arranged vertical to the skin surface. Scar formation is discussed in more detail in Chapter 41. In some healing wounds or ulcers, granulation tissue may become excessive (proud flesh) and may simulate granuloma pyogenicum clinically. The histologic differences are clear-cut.

Generic Features of Ulcers

The fact that epidermis and more or less dermis are lost in any ulcer implies that the epidermis ends at its edge. Generally, epidermis has great propensity for coating defects, and it often descends down the rim of an ulcer. Exceptions to this rule have diagnostic significance in some infectious lesions, for example, ecthyma and chancroid, and in some other lesions, for example, pyoderma gangrenosum. Excessive epidermal proliferation at an ulcer's edge, on the other hand, can assume the features of pseudoepitheliomatous hyperplasia, and it may take careful examination to differentiate it from squamous cell carcinoma.

The bottom of the ulcer may be covered with relatively healthy granulations or with debris and inflammatory cells due to secondary infection. It may also present a peculiar lining that combines necrotic material with acute inflammatory and granulomatous features, which is found typically in syphilitic (see Fig. 21–11) and sporotrichotic (see Fig. 22–8) gummas. It is proof that we are looking at the wall of a granulomatous cavity, the contents of which have disintegrated and have been lost. It is, as such, a nonspecific feature and may similarly be found in disintegrating epithelial cysts, around mucoceles, and in other conditions.

Because of the possibility that considerable portions of the pathologic substrate may have become necrotic, may have been completely lost before biopsy was taken, or may have been detached during transport and handling, the technician must embed all fragments that are found in the bottle, and the specific pathologic process, be it inflammatory or neoplastic.

SPECIFIC ENTITIES

Many ulcers are discussed in other chapters, especially under granulomatous inflammation and neoplasia Even the superficial dermatoses discussed in Section II may cause ulceration occasionally, either by themselves, for example, ulcerating lichen planus,[1] or because of secondary infection or mechanical trauma to a denuded area. Pityriasis li-

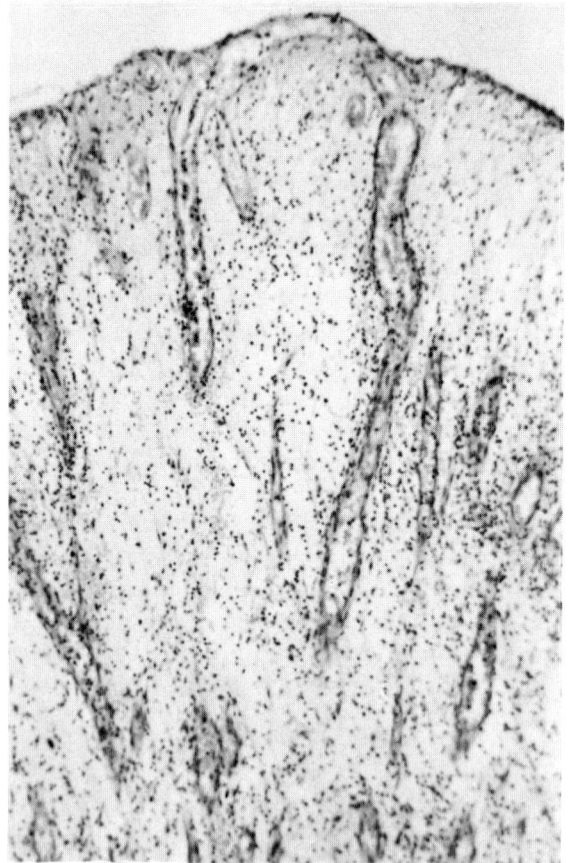

Figure 17–1.
Granulation tissue. Somewhat exuberant granulations fill the wound left by curettage of a basal cell epithelioma a few weeks earlier. Most of the tissue consists of vertical vascular sprouts embedded in loose edematous matrix containing inflammatory cells. Compare with the very different picture of granuloma pyogenicum (see Fig. 43–10). H&E. X70.

chenoides et varioliformis acuta, which typically presents superficial dermal necrosis, may ulcerate in some cases, and herpes zoster, especially in its severe gangrenous form, may cause superficial or deeper ulcers. Ulceration was mentioned several times in the chapters on vasculitides and panniculitis. In all these instances, careful examination for signs of the underlying disease is necessary, although it may not always lead to success. There are, however, some diseases to be considered specifically in this chapter.

Bacterial Infections

Those bacterial infections that produce ulceration as a primary feature exert at least part of their influence through toxins and have certain unifying characteristics, such as absence of epidermal proliferation in the edge of the active lesion and vascular damage expressed either in thrombosis or in disintegration of vascular walls in the bottom of the ulcer. Inflammatory response varies from minimal in the so-called "Buruli ulcer," caused by *Mycobacterium ulcerans*, to more or less noncharacteristic mixed infiltrate in *anthrax*[2] and *ecthyma*, to granulomatous response in *tularemia* (Chapter 21) and others. Meleney's synergistic gangrene is a complication of abdominal and thoracic surgery and is caused by synergistic action of aerobic hemolytic staphylococcus aureus and microaerophilic nonhemolytic streptococcus as well as gram-negative rods.[3] Synergism of aerobic and anaerobic organisms is also involved in formation of tropical ulcers of the lower extremities.[4] Among the differentiating features of bacterial ulcers is presence of identifiable microorganisms, which may be very numerous (anthrax), scarce (chancroid), or demonstrable only by special stains (mycobacteria). The amount of necrosis may vary from extensive (*M. ulcerans*) to moderate with formation of a pseudomembrane (diphtheria) to slight. Some examples follow.

Chancroid

Ducrey's streptobacillus of chancroid (*Haemophilus ducreyi*) always produces an ulcer.[5–8] The epidermis stops abruptly at its edge (Fig. 17–2), giving the appearance of being dissolved. It slightly overhangs a recess in which the gram-negative microorganisms can be demonstrated among necrotic dermal tissue and polymorphonuclear cells. The floor of the rather shallow ulcer is similarly composed of necrotic tissue and a mixture of inflammatory cells exhibiting proliferation and thrombosis of vessels and a deep zone of plasma cells and lymphocytes among which chains of bacilli may be demonstrable.[9] In practice, diagnosis of chancroid, is better secured by using a chalazion curette to obtain a small amount of necrotic tissue from below the overhanging edge of the ulcer, using part of this material for culture and spreading some of it thinly on glass slides for Gram stain. The microorganisms can be seen as gram-negative thin rods forming "schools of fish" (Fig. 17–3).

Ecthyma

Penetration of virulent cocci deeper into the skin than is found in impetigo causes dermal necrosis

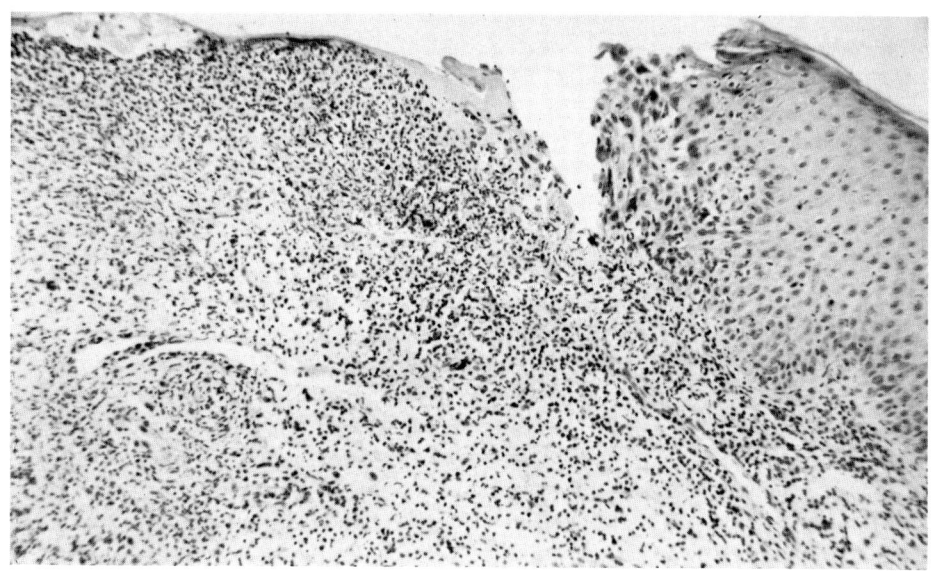

Figure 17–2.
Edge of penile ulcer diagnosed clinically as chancroid and excised as therapeutic measure in preantibiotic ear. The sharp border and partial dissolution of the epidermis are characteristic of chancroid, but the presence of multinucleated epidermal giant cells strongly suggests the coexistence of herpes virus, a not uncommon experience. The nuclei of these cells showed inclusions at higher magnification. Coccobacilli highly suggestive of Ducrey bacilli were demonstrated in a similar section by O&G stain on the surface and in the necrotic base of the ulcer but not deeper in the tissue. H&E. X135.

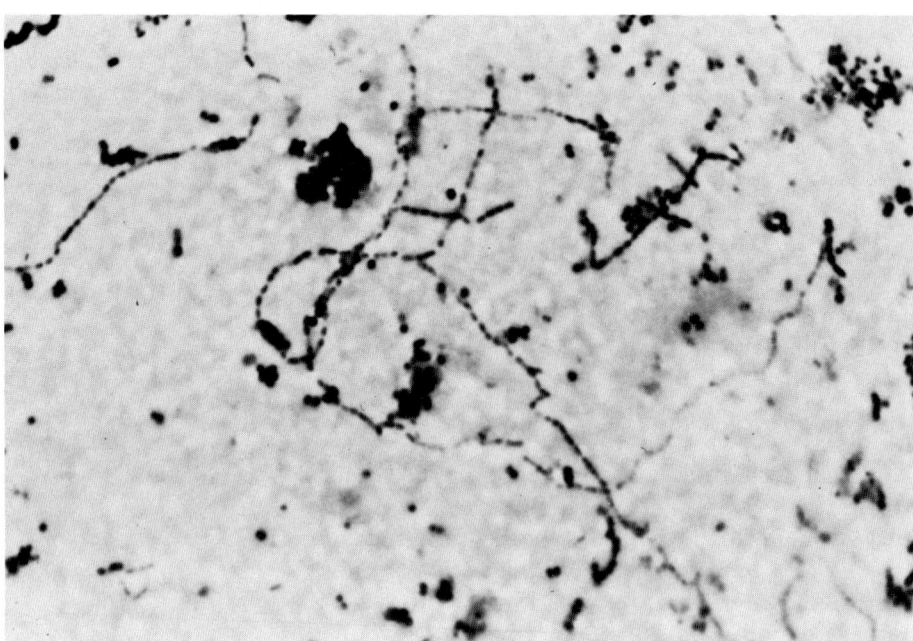

Figure 17–3.
Haemophilus ducreyi. Gram stain. X1100.

and severe inflammatory reaction with neutrophils and round cells. The surface of the ecthyma ulcer usually is covered with a heavy crust consisting of tissue ingredients bound together by dried serum. Colonies of cocci often are present. Ecthyma is apt to heal with irregular scars, which may present pseudoepitheliomatous proliferation of epidermis and adnexal epithelium in the early stages, before the process flattens out. Thus, there may be a temporary resemblance to bromoderma, North American blastomycosis, and other dermatoses producing fibrosis and epithelial hyperplasia.

Diphtheria

Diphtheria of the skin is rare and may produce either noncharacteristic eczematous changes or punched-out ulcers covered with a so-called pseudomembrane of necrotic material, fibrin, and neutrophils.[10] Numerous gram-positive bacilli may be present, but cultures are necessary for indentification.

Disturbances of Immunity

Patients in the last stages of tuberculosis who exhibit weak or no immune reaction to tuberculin might develop ulcerating lesions (tuberculosis orificialis) that are teeming with bacilli but exhibit only a noncharacteristic subacute inflammatory response (Chapter 21). Along somewhat similar lines, malnourished and debilitated individuals may develop destructive ulcerative lesions of secondary syphilis containing numerous treponemes. In recent years a wide spectrum of opportunistic and infectious organisms have been reported producing localized ulcers or progressive disseminated infection in individuals with the acquired immunodeficiency syndrome. In these instances, the tissue reaction is often noncharacteristic and the organisms are present in large number.[11–12]

Pyoderma Gangrenosum

The skin lesions of pyoderma gangrenosum appear initially as inflammatory nodules or pustules over the lower extremities and occasionally elsewhere.[13,14] The lesions may break down rapidly, evolving into painful necrotic ulcers with bluish or gray undermined borders. The ulcers may expand involving large skin areas. Pyoderma gangrenosum is often associated with ulcerative colitis, Crohn's disease, rheumatoid arthritis, or hematologic malignancy.[15–17] Histologic findings in an early lesion consist of a mild to moderate perivascular lymphocytic infiltrate with endothelial swelling (Fig. 17–4). A fully developed lesion shows heavy perivascular lymphocytic infiltrate with fibrinoid deposition, thrombosis, extravasation of erythrocytes, and tissue necrosis.[18,19] Ulceration, infarction, and abscess formation appear in later stages. *Superficial granulomatous pyoderma* is a variant of pyoderma gangrenosum occurring mainly in the head and neck

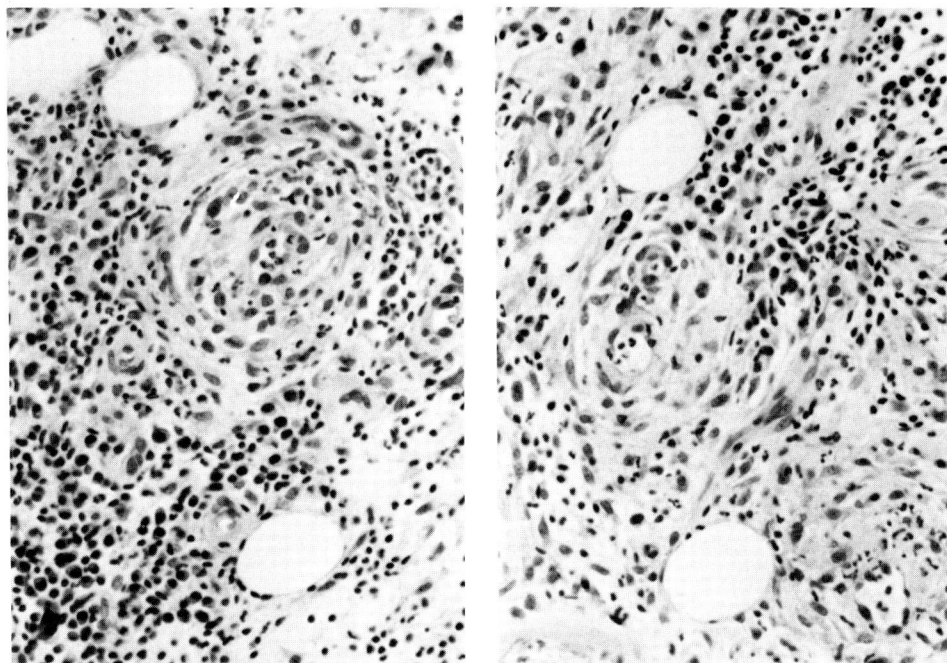

Figure 17-4.
Pyoderma gangrenosum. No necrosis shown in advancing edge of ulcer. Mild vasculitis and mixed cellular infiltrate in subcutaneous fat tissue. H&E. X250.

areas.[20-22] Initial echthyma-like lesions evolve into superficial ulcers with clean base. Histologically, a granulomatous infiltrate with multinucleated giant cells, plasma cells, and eosinophils surround areas of polymorphonuclear abscess formation.[23,24] Pseudoepitheliomatous hyperplasia and epithelial sinus formation may be present.

Other Entities

Leg Ulcers
Leg ulcers secondary to chronic vascular stasis and arteriosclerosis[25] show a bandlike superficial dermal zone of vascular proliferation and various amounts of hemosiderin deposition. A similar picture may be observed in ulcers of lower extremities secondary to arteriovenous malformation.[26] Cutaneous gangrene and ulceration of the lower extremities may occur in association with vascular calcification in individuals with hyperparathyroidism.[27] Sickle cell ulcer also has no characteristic tissue response, but an alert observer can often find the pathognomonic deformed red cells inside or outside of blood vessels. It almost seems that the osmotic changes accompanying tissue fixation provoke sickling (Fig. 17-5). Atrophie blanche and its ulcers are discussed in Chapter 15.

Necrotic Spider Bite
The bite of the brown recluse spider (*Loxosceles reclusa*) produces extensive tissue necrosis followed by ulceration in some individuals,[28,29] whereas it causes only minor reaction in others. The histomechanism has been suggested to be intravascular coagulation.

Coumarin Necrosis
Coumarin and related drugs may cause extensive and deep necrosis, mainly around the buttocks. Histologically, subcutaneous veins contain fibrin thrombi,[30] (see Fig. 15-7) possibly due to direct damage to the endothelium. There is no evidence of immune reaction, and the process may be related to a Shwartzman phenomenon.[31]

Chondrodermatitis Nodularis Chronica Helicis
One characteristic lesion related to cartilage of the ear and the overlying skin, and with the clinical manifestation as a painful nodule of helix or antihelix, is chondrodermatitis nodularis chronica (Fig. 17-6). Histologically, the surface of the lesion shows a small central area of ulceration with the surrounding epidermis exhibiting low-grade pseudoepitheliomatous hyperplasia.[32] Below the ulcer there is

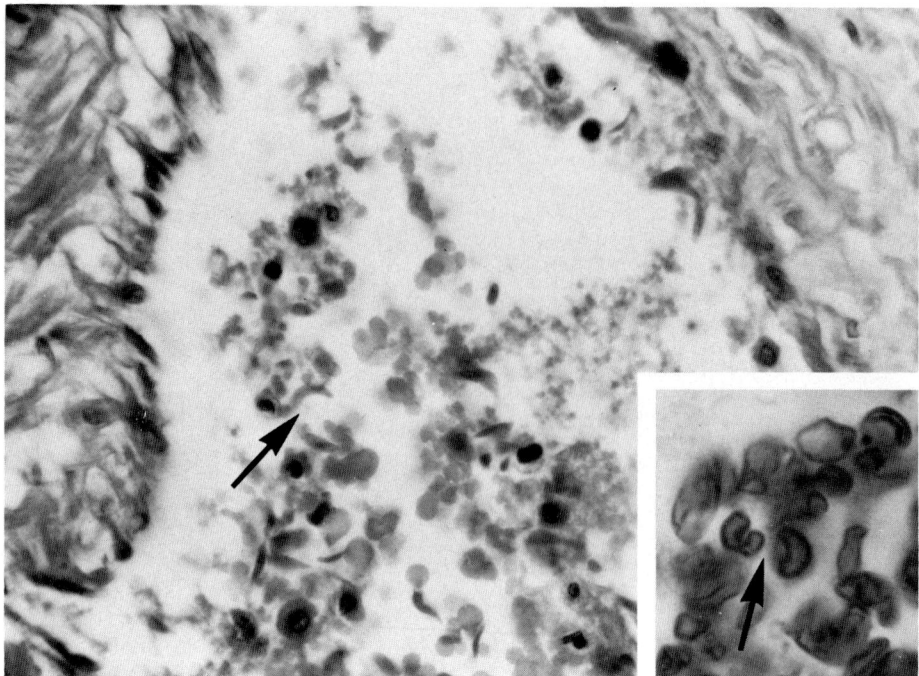

Figure 17–5.
Sickle cells in vessel at base of a leg ulcer. Some of the characteristic cells are indicated by arrows. H&E. X475. Insert, H&E. X1000.

histologic evidence of perichondritis and necrobiotic changes of the collagenous tissue. Chronic inflammation, increased vascularity, and fibrosis are present in the surrounding areas. Elimination of the altered collagenous tissue from the central ulcer or through a channel formed by hyperplastic epidermis has placed this lesion in the group of "perforating dermatoses."[33,34]

Granuloma Fissuratum

An unusual lesion, granuloma fissuratum, probably caused by mechanical irritation in the upper labioalveolar junction of the mouth, has been described by Sutton.[35] Similar lesions have been seen more commonly behind the ears or on the side of the nose, where they are evidently caused by ill-fitting spectacle frames.[36,37] The essential (Fig. 17–7) histologic features consist of a combination of reactive epidermal hyperplasia, dermal chronic inflammation, new formation of capillary blood vessels, and fibrosis. A similar process occurs in the center of the forehead in "prayer's nodule."[38]

Trophic Ulcers and Artifacts

A poorly defined term, trophic ulcer is applied to any nonhealing ulcer, especially on the lower extremi-

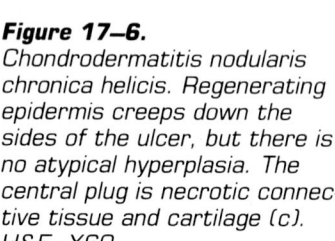

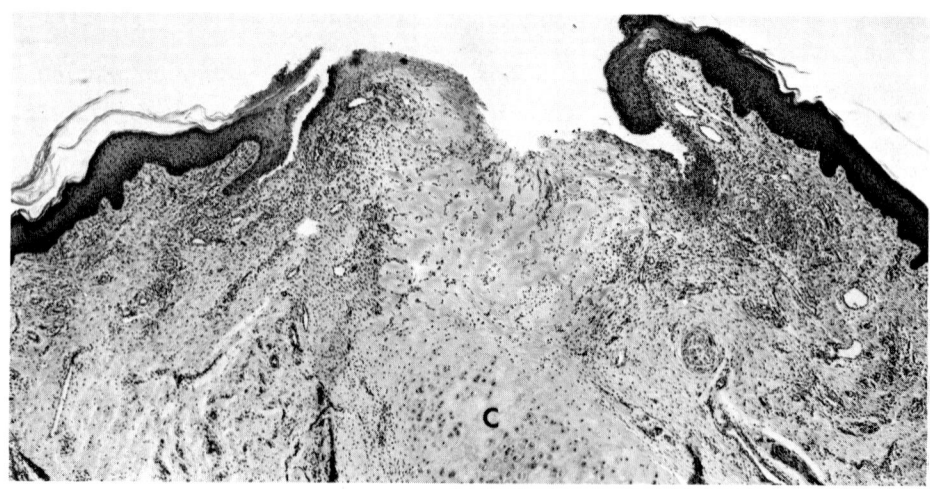

Figure 17–6.
Chondrodermatitis nodularis chronica helicis. Regenerating epidermis creeps down the sides of the ulcer, but there is no atypical hyperplasia. The central plug is necrotic connective tissue and cartilage (c). H&E. X60.

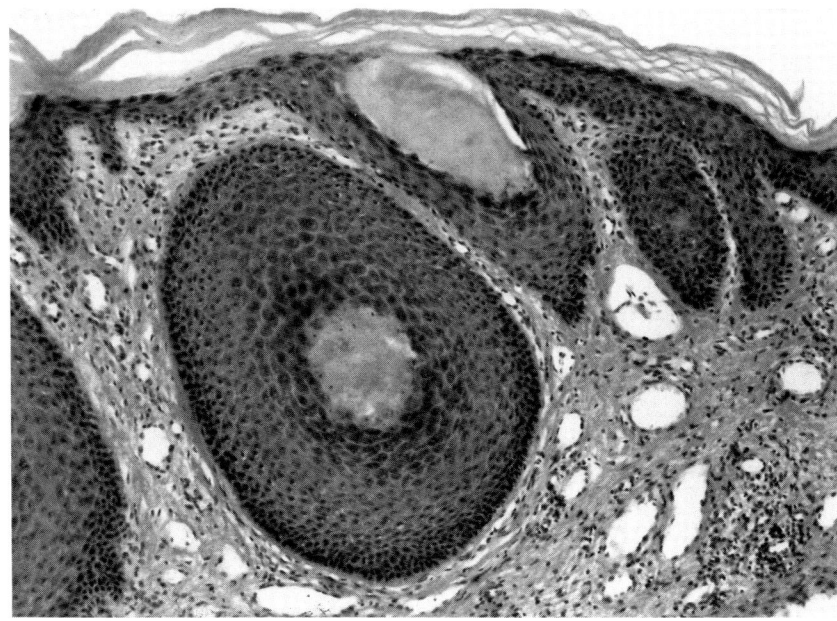

Figure 17–7.
Granuloma fissuratum of postauricular area with slightly acanthotic epidermis and cystic dilated follicles. Dermis shows low-grade chronic inflammation, increased vascularity, and fibrosis. H&E. X125.

ties, which is thought to be caused and maintained by impaired tissue nutrition with or without disturbances of innervation. *Decubitus ulcers*,[39] ulcers in diabetics, and fingertip ulcers of *acrosclerosis* may be included here. None of them have histologic features that permit diagnosis, and examination usually is requested to rule out malignancy or other disorders.

Finally, if no specific diagnosis presents itself, the possibility of the patient's producing ulcers by mechanical or chemical means must be considered. Artifactual ulcerations usually show a disproportionately small amount of inflammatory reaction and sometimes have evidence of tissue destruction by heat or chemical necrosis, as mentioned in Chapter 3.

REFERENCES

1. Connor DH, Lunn HF: Buruli ulceration. Arch Pathol 81:183, 1966
2. Loborich RJ, MacKillip BG, Conboy JR: Cutaneous anthrax. Am J Clin Pathol 13:505, 1943
3. Davson J, Jones DM, Turner L: Diagnosis of Meleney's synergistic gangrene. Br J Surg 75:267, 1988
4. Adriaans B, Hay R, Drasar B, Robinson D: The infectious aetiology of tropical ulcer: A study of the role of anaerobic bacteria. Br J Dermatol 116:31, 1987
5. Fiumara NJ, Rothman K, Tang S: The diagnosis and treatment of chancroid. J Am Acad Dermatol 15:939, 1986
6. Sturm AW, Stolting GJ, Cormane RH, Zanen HC: Clinical and microbiological evaluation of 46 episodes of genital ulceration. Genitourin Med 63:98, 1987
7. Schmid GP, Sanders LL Jr, Blount JH, Alexander ER: Chancroid in the United States: Reestablishment of an old disease. JAMA 258:3265, 1987
8. Orellana-Diaz O, Hernandez-Perez E: Chancroid in El Salvador: Increasing incidence, clinical features and therapeutics. Int J Dermatol 27:243, 1988
9. McCarley ME, Cruz PD Jr, Sontheimer RD: Chancroid: Clinical variants and other findings from an epidemic in Dallas county 1986–1987. J Am Acad Dermatol 19:330, 1988
10. Thomann U, Gasser M, Pietrzak J et al: Cutaneous diphtheria imported from tropical countries. In Sober AJ and Fitzpatrick TB (eds.): Year Book of Dermatology. Chicago: Year Book Medical Publishers, 1989, p 37
11. Toth IR, Kazal HL: Botryomycosis in acquired immunodeficiency syndrome. Arch Pathol Lab Med 11:246, 1987
12. Cohen PR, Bank DE, Silvers DN, Grossman ME: Cutaneous lesions of disseminated histoplasmosis in human immunodeficiency virus-infected patients. J Am Acad Dermatol 23:422, 1990
13. Powell FC, Perry HO: Pyoderma gangrenosum in childhood. Arch Dermatol 120:757, 1984
14. Snyder RA: Pyoderma gangrenosum involving head and neck. Arch Dermatol 122:295, 1986
15. Hickman JG, Lazarus GS: Pyoderma gangrenosum: A reappraisal of associated systemic diseases. Br J Dermatol 102:235, 1980
16. Schoetz DJ Jr, Coller JA, Veidenheimer MC: Pyoderma gangrenosum and Crohn's disease: Eight cases and a review of the literature. Dis Colon Rectum 26:155, 1983

17. Kaplan RP, Newman G, Saperia D: Pyoderma gangrenosum and hairy cell leukemia. J Dermatol Surg Oncol 13:1029, 1987
18. Su WPD, Schroeter AL, Perry HO, Powell FC: Histopathologic and immunopathologic study of pyoderma gangrenosum. J Cutan Pathol 13:323, 1986
19. Bernard P, Amici JM, Catanzano G et al: Pyoderma gangrenosum et vascularite. Discussion pathogenique a propos de 3 observations. Ann Dermatol Venereol 114:1229, 1987
20. Dicken CH: Malignant pyoderma. J Am Acad Dermatol 13:1021, 1985
21. Wernikoff S, Merritt C, Briggaman RA, Woodley DT: Malignant pyoderma or pyoderma gangrenosum of the head and neck? Arch Dermatol 123:371, 1987
22. Malkinson FD: Pyoderma gangrenosum vs malignant pyoderma: Lumpers vs splitters. Arch Dermatol 123: 333, 1987
23. Quimby SR, Gibson LE, Winkelmann RK: Superficial granulomatous pyoderma: Clinicopathologic spectrum. Mayo Clin Proc 64:37, 1989
24. Winkelmann RK, Wilson-Jones E, Gibson LE, Quimby SR: Histopathologic features of superficial granulomatous pyoderma. J Dermatol Tokyo 16:127, 1989
25. Falanga V, Eaglstein WH: A therapeutic approach to venous ulcers. J Am Acad Dermatol 14:777, 1986
26. Matsukawa A, Sakai S: Arteriovenous malformation with an ulcer of the foot. J Dermatol Tokyo 16:154, 1989
27. Mehregan DA, Winkelmann RK: Cutaneous gangrene, vascular calcification, and hyperparathyroidism. Mayo Clin Proc 64:211, 1989
28. Dillaha CJ, Jansen GT, Honeycutt WM, et al: North American loxoscelism. JAMA 188:33, 1964
29. Pennell TC, Babu SS, Meredith WJ: The management of snake and spider bites in the southeastern United States. Am Surg 53:193, 1987
30. Nalbandian RM, Mader JJ, Barrett JL, et al: Petechiae, ecchymoses and necrosis of skin induced by coumarin congeners. JAMA 142:603, 1965
31. Berger RS, Adelstein EH, Anderson RC: Intravascular coagulation: The cause of necrotic arachnidism. J Invest Dermatol 61:142, 1973
32. Santa Cruz DJ: Chondrodermatitis nodularis helicis: A transepidermal perforating disorder. J Cutan Pathol 7:70, 1980
33. Goette DK: Chondrodermatitis nodularis chronica helicis: A perforating necrotic granuloma. J Am Acad Dermatol 2:148, 1980
34. Bard JW: Chondrodermatitis nodularis chronica helicis. Dermatologica 163:376, 1981
35. Sutton RL, Jr: A fissured granulomatous lesion of the upper labio-alveolar fold. Arch Dermatol Syph 26:425, 1932
36. Feinsilber DG, DiFabio NA, Casas JC: Granulom fissuratum Rev Argent Dermatologia 67:129, 1986
37. Cerroni L, Soyer HP, Chimenti S: Acanthoma fissuratum. J Dermatol Surg Oncol 14:1003, 1988
38. Kumar PV, Hambarsoomian B: Prayer nodules: Fine needle aspiration. Cytologic findings. Acta Cytol 32: 83, 1988
39. Versluysen M: New elderly patients with femoral fracture develop pressure sores in hospital. Br Med J 292: 1311, 1986

18

INFLAMMATION INVOLVING THE PILOSEBACEOUS COMPLEX

Follicular inflammations—with the exception of the acrotrichial pustules of impetigo Bockhart, and the superficial lesions of disseminate and recurrent infundibulofolliculitis—are discussed here because they are located in the pars reticularis of the dermis. Inflammatory products may be found inside or outside the follicle and often in both locations. If inflammatory infiltrate is present in perifollicular arrangement only, one has to decide whether it is a response to something present within the follicle, as in certain types of tinea, or results from concentration of small capillaries around follicles, as in follicular exanthems and lichen scrofulosorum. Follicular keratoses are discussed here because they are often accompanied by inflammation. Alopecias are discussed in Chapter 19.

STAPHYLOCOCCAL INFECTIONS

The extent and severity of staphylococcic folliculitis depend on the localization of the cocci, the size of the hair, and the immunologic situation of the host. Although it is not easy to discern these determining factors in histologic sections, there is little doubt that *impetigo Bockhart* (Fig. 18–1) is a superficial infection of a small follicle, and is histologically characterized by spongiform edema and exocytosis of neutrophils and eosinophils that involve the follicular infundibulum and the surrounding epidermis leading to formation of a subcorneal pustule. Furuncle is a deep infection, usually of a larger hair root. In a patient with furunculosis, however, the development of a small folliculitis, a medium or large furuncle, or even a carbuncle probably depends more on the immunologic defensive ability at the particular time than on the exact localization of the cocci. In a fully developed furuncle (Fig. 18–2), a fairly broad column of perifollicular connective tissue becomes necrotic and densely infiltrated with neutrophils to form the clinically characteristic tough green plug. Below the lower end of the follicle, often in the subcutaneous tissue, an abscess containing demonstrable staphylococci develops, which is finally evacuated when the plug has been sequestered. On the other hand, in *sycosis vulgaris* of the beard, it is often only the upper part of the follicle that is involved. The perifollicular inflammation is rather heavy and contains lymphocytes, histiocytes, and plasma cells. The lower follicle and the hair root survive and remain susceptible to the next attack.[1]

ACNE VULGARIS AND RELATED CONDITIONS

In contrast to the hot folliculitis caused by virulent staphylococci and their toxins, the milder, less pain-

250 DEEP INFLAMMATORY PROCESSES

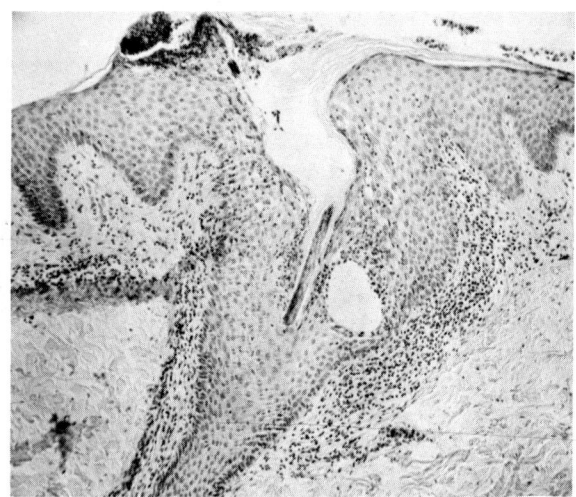

Figure 18–1.
Superficial folliculitis of impetigo Bockhart type. There is eczematous spongiosis and vesiculation of the upper portion of the follicular sheath, in contrast to the mucinous edema of sebaceous gland and sheath in alopecia mucinosa (see Figs. 19–3 and 19–4). H&E. X90.

ful, but more protracted inflammation of an *acne pustule* or *abscess* probably is in a great part caused by chemically irritating sebum in combination with less virulent microorganisms, especially *Corynebacterium acnes*.[2] Histologic examination of very early acne lesions shows infiltration of predominantly helper T lymphocytes at the periphery of the sebaceous ducts (Fig. 18–3). Later, polymorphonuclear leukocytes appear in association with disruption of the ducts.[3] In a fully developed acne lesion a comedonic plug can be recognized within a cystic dilated hair follicle. It may have a wide opening or a very narrow one (closed comedo). Whereas open comedones may persist for several years,[4] the closed ones are likely to rupture (Fig. 18–4), releasing sebaceous and horny material into the dermis.[5] The initial acute inflammation may be followed by foreign body granulomatous reaction and epithelial proliferation that grows around the abscess. In a deep cystic acne lesion, all the features of a mixed granulomatous infiltrate may be present (Fig. 18–5), and differential diagnosis from specific granulomatous disease may be difficult. In such cases, the demonstration of a few keratin flakes or fragments of hair in the granuloma is helpful. Clinical information about age of patient, location of lesion, and other characteristics often helps to confirm the impression that one is dealing with a nonspecific granuloma. In the rare cases of *acne fulminans,* the follicular reaction develops into an extensive, spreading, liquefying necrosis engulfing nearby follicles but shows no evidence of vasculitis or immune processes.[6] Comedonic plugs are also seen in sun-exposed aged skin,[7] especially in the condition outlined by Favre and Racouchot and after application of coal tar[5] and various other substances.

DERMATOPHYTIC FOLLICULITIS

As is well known from superficial fungous infection, dermatophytes usually do not invade living tissues.

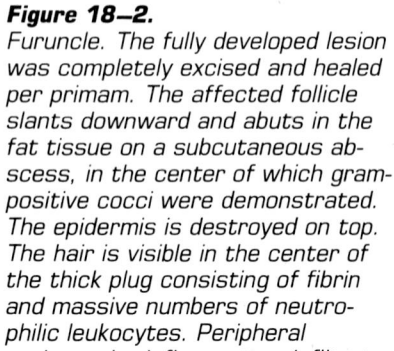
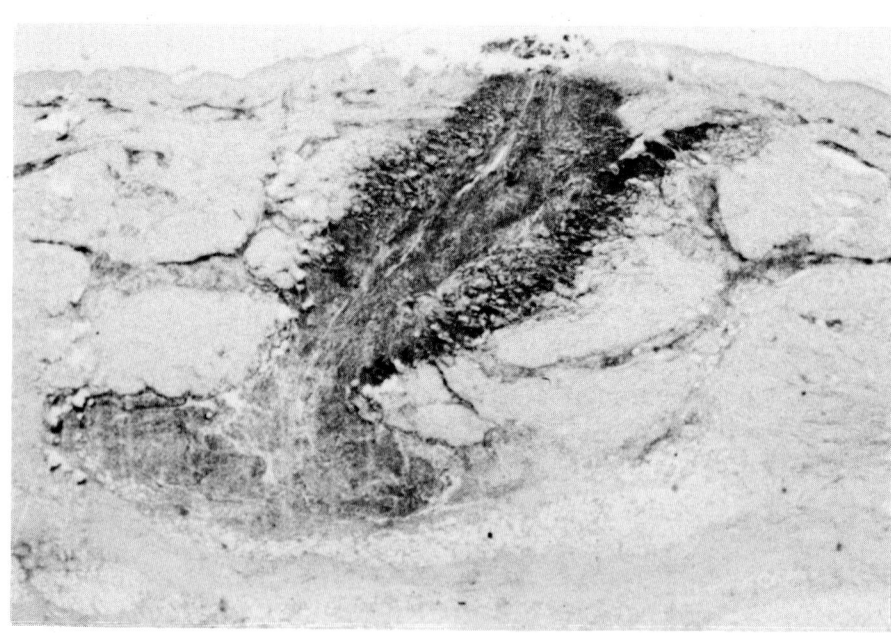

Figure 18–2.
Furuncle. The fully developed lesion was completely excised and healed per primam. The affected follicle slants downward and abuts in the fat tissue on a subcutaneous abscess, in the center of which gram-positive cocci were demonstrated. The epidermis is destroyed on top. The hair is visible in the center of the thick plug consisting of fibrin and massive numbers of neutrophilic leukocytes. Peripheral perivascular inflammatory infiltrate. H&E. X4. (From Pinkus. J Cutan Pathol 6:517, 1979.)

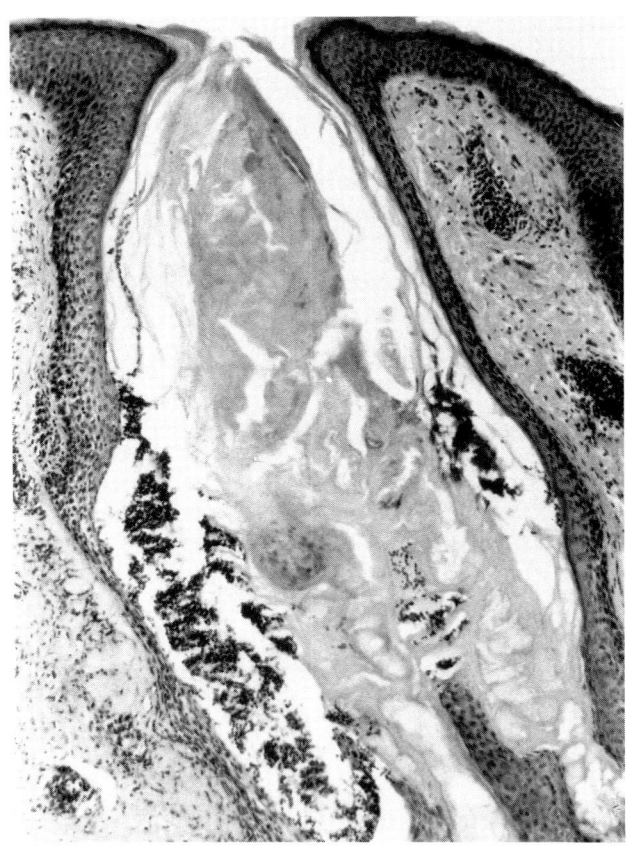

Figure 18–3.
Acne vulgaris shows a dilated hair follicle containing keratin and inflammatory cells. H&E. X125.

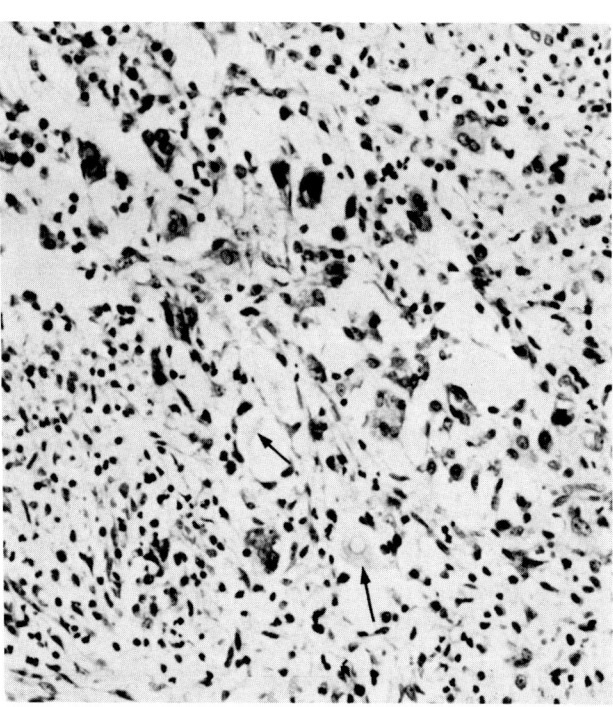

Figure 18–5.
Foreign body type of granulomatous inflammation after rupture of a keratinous cyst. Arrows point to keratin flakes. H&E. X225.

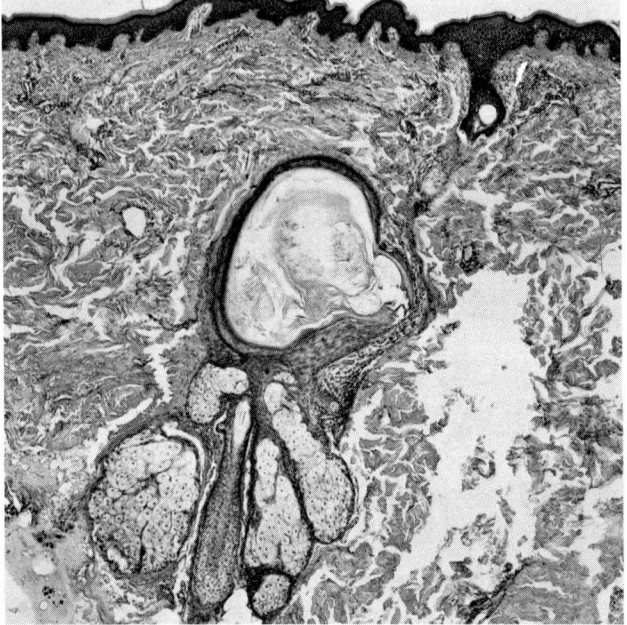

Figure 18–4.
Cystic dilatation of suprasebaceous portion of a follicle and rupture of wall in a relatively noninflammatory lesion of acne vulgaris. H&E. X45.

They produce an inflammatory reaction indirectly. The same is true when a *Trichophyton* or *Microsporon* invades the follicle and possibly the hair. The finer details of *Macrosporum, Microsporum, Ectothrix,* and *Endothrix* infection will not be discussed here. For a thorough discussion, see Graham and Barroso-Tobila.[8] With the exception of *Trichophyton rubrum*,[9] which may enter living tissue in the granulomatous lesions found usually on the legs of women (Fig. 18–6), fungal elements are found almost exclusively in the hair (Fig. 18–7), even in highly inflammatory *kerion* of the scalp or the *Majocchi granuloma*. It is, therefore, necessary to examine a sufficiently large number of sections in suspected cases, and one cannot be content until a hair-containing follicle or remnants of a hair shaft are found within the inflamed zone. Often, only one hair in a specimen is manifestly infected. Follicles quite close to but outside the lesion may be normal, and in the center of the inflammation, hairs and follicles may be completely destroyed. On the other hand, even in a rather superficial tinea, it may be impossible to find mycelia in the scale, whereas close inspection of vellus hair follicles shows hyphae and

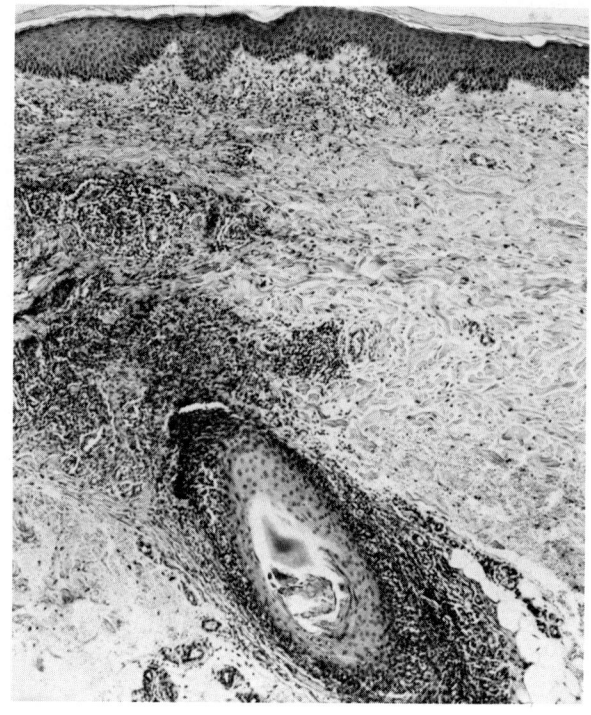
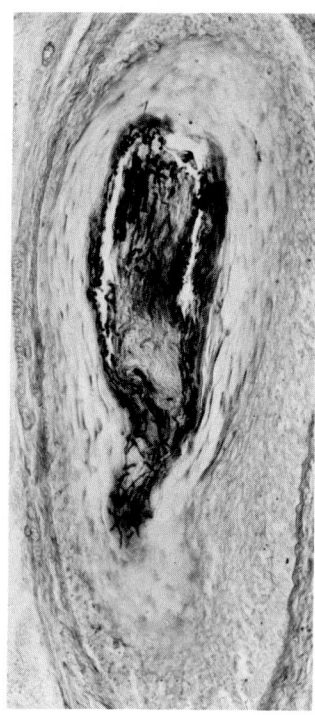

Figure 18–6.
Granulomatous folliculitis due to Trichophyton rubrum. **A.** H&E. X75. **B.** Mycelia and spores in and around the hair. Alcian blue–PAS. X135.

spores in the infundibulum. Tinea infection may lead to formation of superficial follicular pustules containing numerous eosinophils resembling Ofuji's disease.[10]

The inflammatory infiltrate may vary from minor accumulations of round cells, as in *Microsporum audouini* infections, to purulent and mixed granulomatous types in *M. canis* and *Trichophyton* infections.

OTHER DEEP FOLLICULAR INFLAMMATIONS

Perforating Folliculitis

Discrete follicular lesions with keratotic plugging appear over the lower extremities and buttocks. Following a decade in which a large number of cases were observed, the incidence is now decreasing. Per-

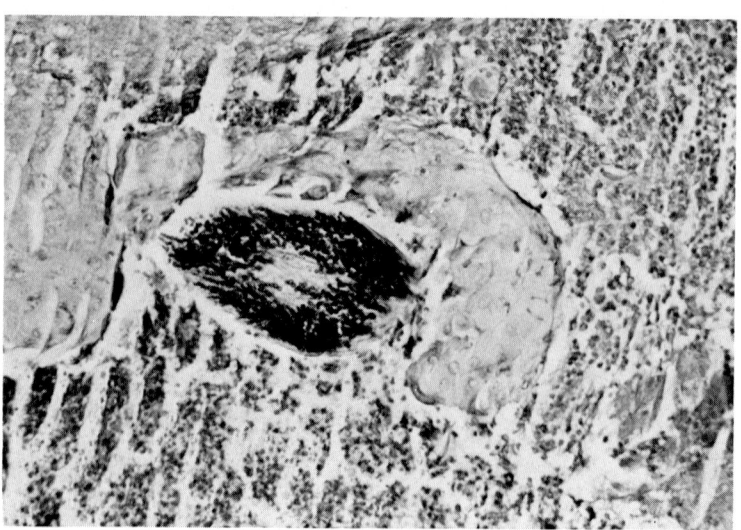

Figure 18–7.
Trichophyton violaceum (endothrix) infection of scalp hair with violent inflammatory reaction that has led to rupture of follicle. PAS–hematoxylin. X185.

forating folliculitis shows some clinical and superficial histologic similarity to Kyrle's extremely rare hyperkeratosis follicularis et parafollicularis in cutem penetrans, and some of the cases published under that name in fact were perforating folliculitis (Fig. 18–8). Biopsy at various stages indicates that the initial lesion is follicular hyperkeratosis with retention of the hair shaft and that the spring action of a rolled-up thin hair produces a break of the follicular wall and causes reactive inflammation and some tissue necrosis lateral to the follicle. The small granulomatous abscess is secondarily surrounded by proliferating follicular epithelium.[11–12] The sequestered mass consisting of pyknotic inflammatory cells, peculiar eosinophilic elastic fibers, and keratinous debris is then evacuated toward the surface within the follicle, a process quite different biologically from that envisioned by Kyrle.

The best histologic criterion is the presence of devitalized elastic fibers, which, being eosinophilic, are easily recognized in O&G sections but not with other elastic fiber stains. Follicles obstructed from other causes and associated with granulomatous inflammation may come into differential diagnosis.

Necrotizing Folliculitis and Pityrosporum Folliculitis

A different clinical and histologic picture has been observed[13] in a number of patients, who presented very pruritic scattered papules not obviously related to hairs. Histologically (Fig. 18–9), a relatively small and sharply defined round cell infiltrate is seen that has destroyed a portion of the middle or deeper part of a vellus follicle without affecting the upper part. The hair root also may survive. *Necrotizing folliculitis* has proved intractable and continues to recur after occasional spontaneous remissions. The histologic picture approaches those seen in pityrosporum folliculitis[14,15] and in topical steroid acne, but the clinical aspects are different inasmuch as there are obvious follicular papules and pustules in pityrosporum folliculitis and comedones in steroid acne.[16] Acne miliaris necrotica of scalp in a very early lesion shows a necrotizing lymphocytic folliculitis. Later, polymorphonuclear leukocytes participate forming a superficial pustular folliculitis.[17]

Disorders Associated with Hair of Blacks

Strongly curved hair brings with it peculiar hazards due to its tendency to be retained in the dermis as an irritating foreign body when the inflamed follicle breaks down or to grow back into the skin when it is shaved. Disorders based on these mechanisms, therefore, are most common in blacks. There are three such disorders: *folliculitis et perifolliculitis suffodiens et abscedens* (Hoffmann's disease), *acne keloidalis,* and *pseudofolliculitis* of the beard.

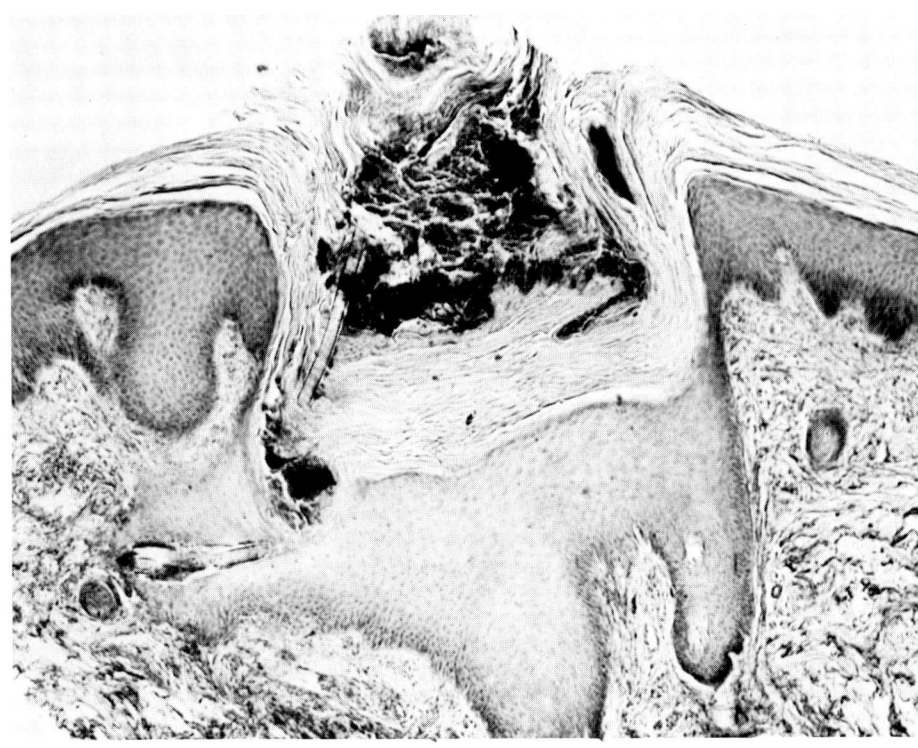

Figure 18–8.
Perforating folliculitis. Note the thin hair in the epithelial channel at left and mixture of keratin, leukocytes, and degenerated dermal fibers in the plug. H&E. X75. (From Mehregan and Coskey. Arch Dermatol 97:394, 1967.)

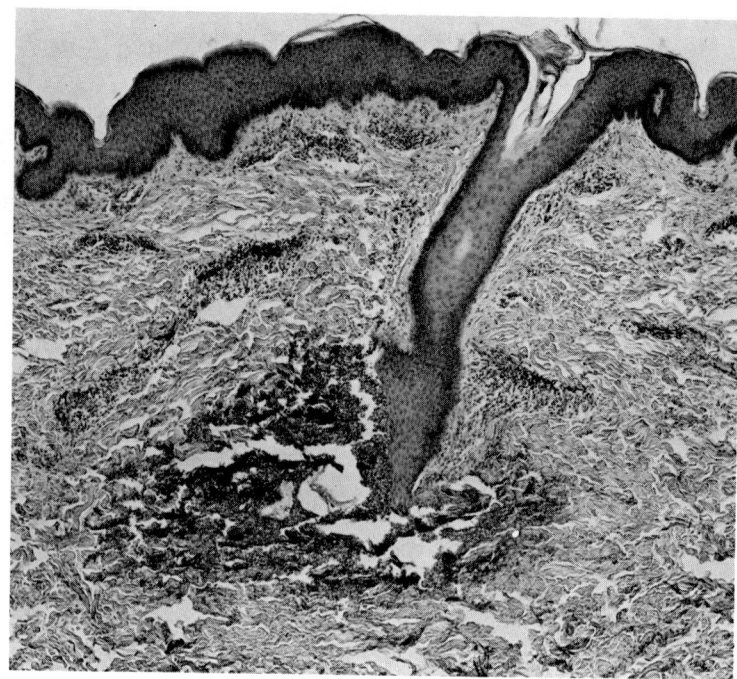

Figure 18–9.
Necrotizing folliculitis. The inflammatory process has destroyed a portion of follicular wall at level of bulge but does not involve entire follicle as in a furuncle. H&E. X75.

Hoffmann's Disease

We have not been impressed with the role of apocrine glands or the association with acne conglobata in Hoffmann's disease, and the simpler name *dissecting cellulitis of the scalp* does not do it justice. The course of the disease is best explained by, and treatment is based on, the assumption that Hoffmann's disease is primarily acute folliculitis and that its progression and chronicity are due to buried dead hairs that produce foreign body inflammation in and below the skin, complicated by recurrent virulent infection. The histologic features bear out this concept and show extensive intradermal formation of sinuses lined with smooth stratified epithelium derived from disrupted follicles. The contents of the sinuses are remnants of hairs, flakes of keratin, and (in an acute attack) inflammatory cells. Cure can be achieved by thorough marsupialization of the burrowing sinuses after antibiotic therapy.

Acne Keloidalis

Buried dead hairs also are largely responsible for dermatitis papillaris capillitii, but infection plays a minor role. Histologically, chronic inflamed hair follicles and fragments of dead hairs are surrounded with chronic inflammation and foreign body granuloma.[18] The surrounding dermis shows proliferation of keloidal scar tissue (Fig. 18–10).

Scarring Pseudofolliculitis

Chronic scarring pseudofolliculitis of the beard is primarily a foreign body reaction around the sharp, shaved ends of curved hairs that grow back into the skin (Fig. 18–11). It is encountered mainly in the beards of black men but may also be seen in the pubic region and on the scalp.[19] Later stages are characterized by scarring and atrophy of hair.[20,21]

Pilonidal Sinus

A pilonidal sinus is a fistulous tract containing hairs surrounded by granulation tissue or sometimes sheathed in stratified epithelium, suggesting a follicle (Fig. 18–12).[22] They are most commonly encountered in the coccygeal area of overweight young men, where it is assumed that dead hairs of this body region have penetrated the epidermis of the fossa coccygea. Basically similar sinuses are encountered in the interdigital webs of barbers and dairymen, where they contain trimmed human hair fragments and cattle hairs, respectively.

SUPERFICIAL LESIONS

The follicular infundibulum, including the acrotrichium and the intradermal portion down to the level of the sebaceous duct, may be involved with spongiosis and inflammatory infiltrate in some cases of eczematous and atopic dermatitis. This is commonly seen in perioral dermatitis and in the follicular forms of seborrheic dermatitis. Mucinous edema may extend upward into this portion in follicular

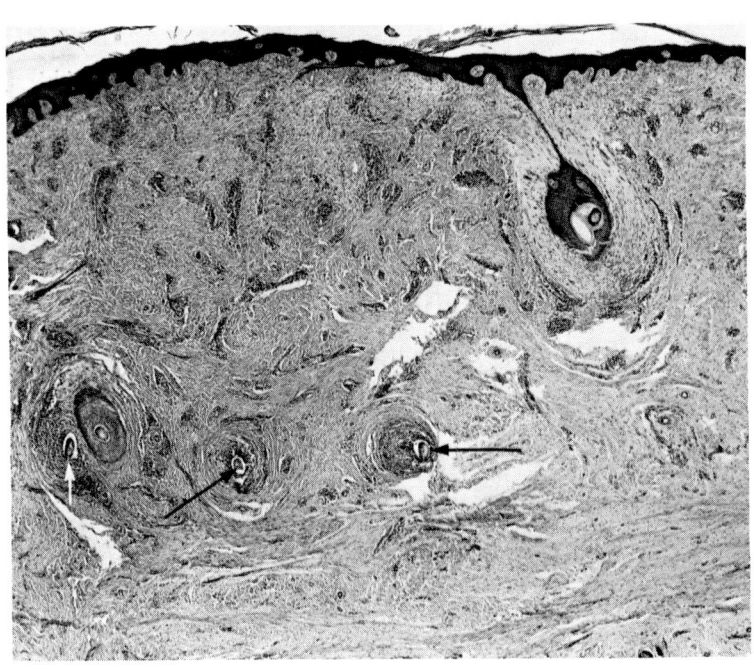

Figure 18–10.
Dermatitis papillaris capillitii. Three dead hairs (arrows) buried deep in skin by keloidal fibrous hyperplasia. Inflammatory reaction is relatively minor, chronic, and partly granulomatous. H&E. X35.

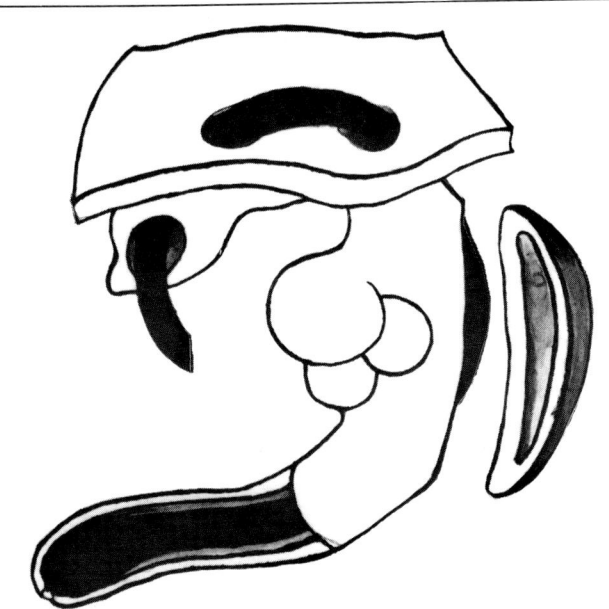

Figure 18–11.
Ingrowing hair in pseudofolliculitis of the beard. Black curved follicle is cut away to expose hair, sharp shaved end of which has reentered skin and is partly surrounded by an epithelial cuff (pseudofollicle). (Drawing by Dr. Felix Pinkus from a three-dimensional model reconstructed from serial sections, 1943.)

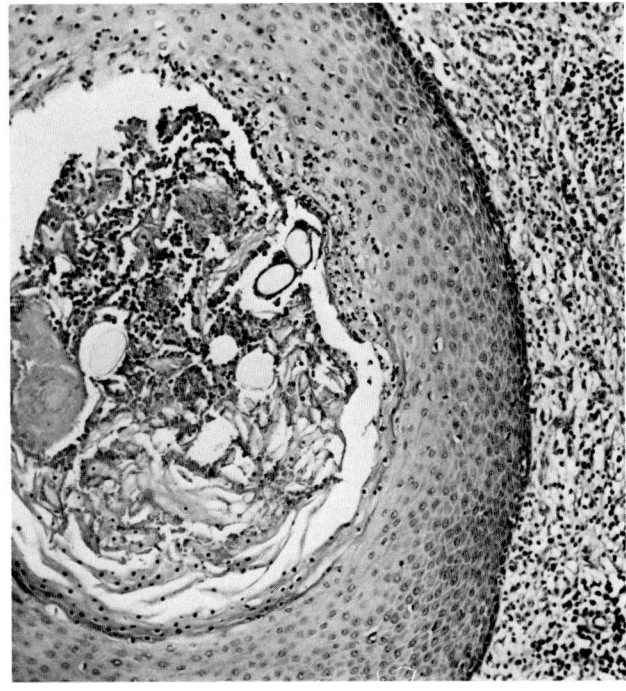

Figure 18–12.
Pilonidal sinus of sacral area. Cross section of a cavity surrounded by stratified epithelium and containing keratinous flakes, debris, leukocytes, and several small hairs. The original hypothesis that the hairs grow from matrices within the sinus as a congenital malformation has been replaced by the concept that dead hairs are sucked into the sinus from surrounding skin. H&E. X100.

mucinosis. There are, however, several clinical entities that specifically localize in the infundibulum. Of these, impetigo Bockhart was mentioned earlier.

Eosinophilic Pustular Folliculitis

This rare affection initially reported exclusively from Japan is now observed in other countries.[23-27] It consists of follicular, tiny red papules with formation of pustules disseminated or within fairly well-defined erythematous plaques involving trunk, limbs, and face. Histologic examination shows destruction of hair follicles by massive infiltration of eosinophils and formation of intrafollicular and subcorneal eosinophilic pustules (Fig. 18–13).[28,29] Blood eosinophilia may be present. Eosinophilic pustular folliculitis has been reported in a number of adults with acquired immunodeficiency syndrome.[30]

Disseminate and Recurrent Infundibulofolliculitis

This now well-recognized entity produces widespread and only slightly pruritic tiny papules, which impress the observer as a gooseflesh-like accentuation of all hair follicles on large areas of the trunk and extremities.[31,32] The histologic picture (Fig. 18–14) of this disseminated eruption includes spongiotic edema of the infundibular portion of the follicle and mild surrounding mononuclear infiltrate. The cause is unknown.

Folliculitis Decalvans

A condition contributing to scarring alopecia shows initially acute inflammation with polymorphonuclear cells found within the hair follicles, usually the upper portion. Perifollicular chronic inflammatory cell infiltrate of lymphocytes, histiocytes, and plasma cells leads to follicular atrophy, scarring, and permanent hair loss. It must be differentiated from pseudopelade of Brocq.

FOLLICULAR KERATOSES

We encountered keratotic plugging of hair follicles as a more or less characteristic by-product of lupus erythematosus and lichen planus. We also find it in lichen sclerosus et atrophicus, lichen scrofulosorum, and Darier's disease. Comedones of acne vulgaris

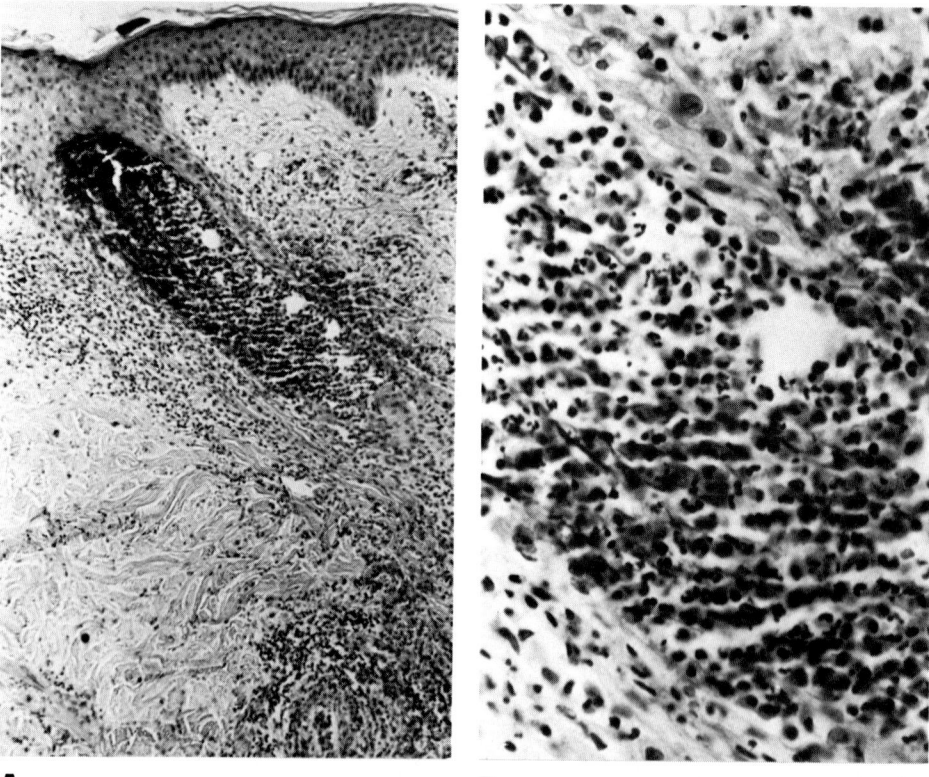

Figure 18–13.
Eosinophilic pustular folliculitis (Ofuji). Extensive involvement of hair follicle resulting in formation of eosinophilic pustule. **A.** H&E. X125. **B.** H&E. X400.

and perivascular-round cell infiltrate. The granulomatous reaction of lichen scrofulosorum (see Fig. 21–2) is absent.

In *phrynoderma* the keratin plug is largely parakeratotic and is situated within a funnel-shaped dilated follicle.[34] The hair follicle is atrophic and is surrounded with patchy lymphocytic infiltrate. *Pellagra* on the other hand, may be associated with the combination of follicular horny spines and large sebaceous glands in the central face, a long-known sign reemphasized by Pons et al.[35]

An inherited condition characterized by follicular plugging, redness, and atrophy is *ulerythema ophryogenes*, which may begin in childhood in the lateral portions of the eyebrows and is gradually progressive. The histologic features bear out the clinical appearance and consist of absence of sebaceous glands, keratotic plugs in hair follicles, der-

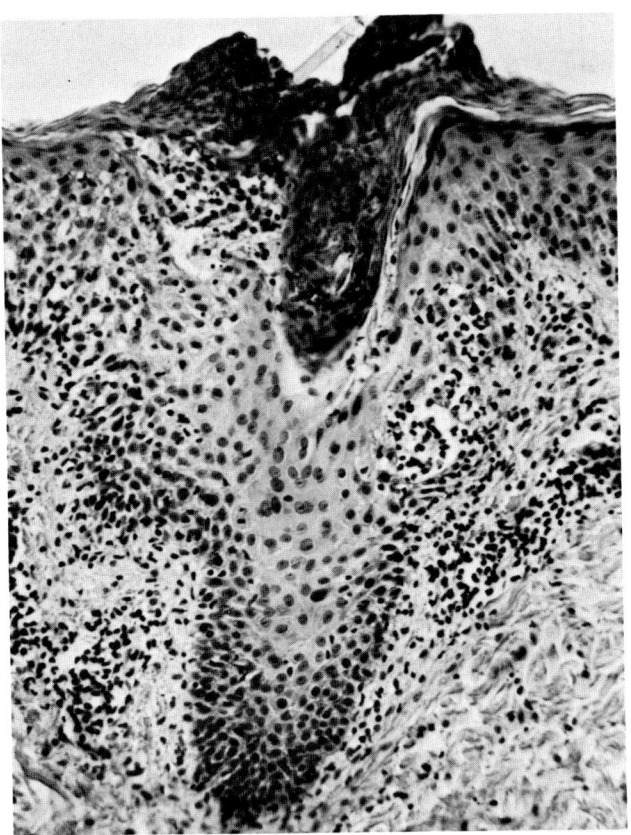

Figure 18–14.
Disseminated and recurrent infundibulofolliculitis. H&E. X180.

were mentioned earlier in this chapter. We now describe some conditions in which keratotic plugs are the outstanding characteristic.

Keratosis Pilaris and Related Conditions

These disorders come to the attention of the pathologist mainly in differential diagnosis from more significant dermatoses. If there is no other disturbance of the skin except a horny plug in the infundibulum (Fig. 18–15), we render a diagnosis of keratosis pilaris. There is some associated round cell infiltrate and telangiectasia in keratosis pilaris rubra. An acne comedo extends deeper into the sebaceous duct region and is more massive.

Lichen spinulosus is most common in black children and resembles lichen scrofulosorum clinically. Histologically, we see a solid infundibular plug (Fig. 18–16), which projects above the skin surface and encases a hair shaft.[33] The follicular wall is apt to be atrophic and the sebaceous gland tiny or absent, and there is a certain amount of perifollicular fibrosis

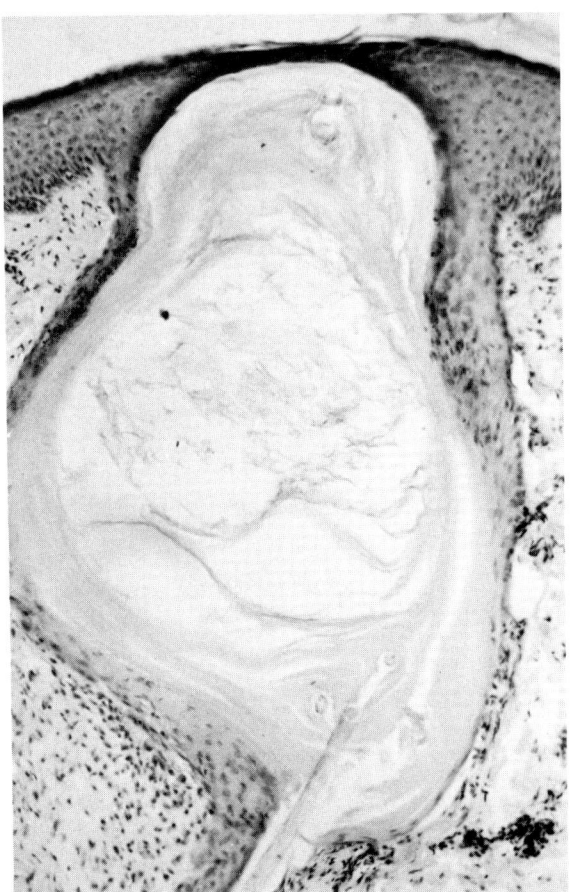

Figure 18–15.
Keratosis pilaris. Infundibular portion of small hair follicle greatly distended by a keratinous plug into which it enters from the bottom. The wall of the follicle is so thin, it is almost ready to rupture, but there is as yet practically no inflammatory reaction. H&E. X125.

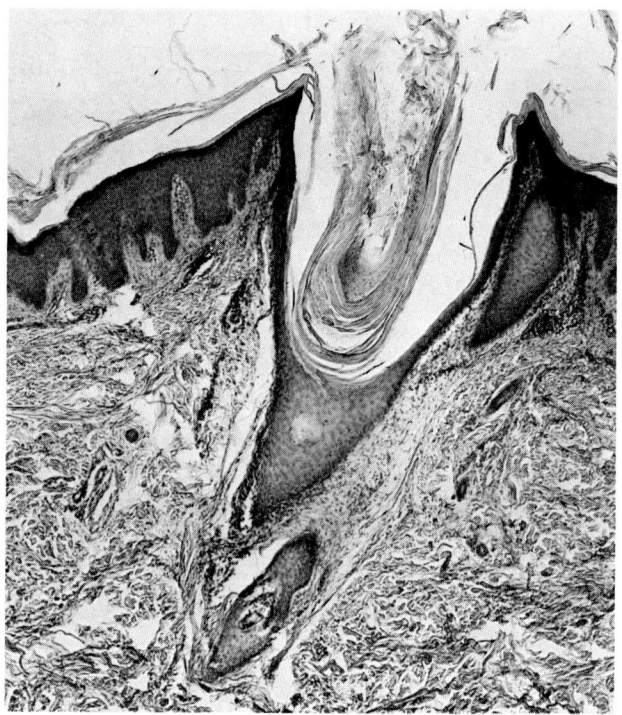

Figure 18–16.
Lichen spinulosus. H&E. X70. Compare with different picture of lichen scrofulosorum in Figure 21–2.

mal fibrosis, and mild chronic inflammatory infiltrate.[36]

Kyrle's Disease

The nature of *hyperkeratosis follicularis et parafollicularis in cutem penetrans* has never been explained satisfactorily. Epidermal biology makes it difficult to consider active penetration of a horny plug into the dermis. Even in a clavus (see Fig. 34–25B), where pressure from the outside forces the hyperkeratotic material downward, and in other instances of keratotic plugs associated with mechanical pressure,[37] there is always a thin epidermal covering around the tip of the conical plug. The only known instances where the living envelope wears away around keratinous material are in the confines of a cystically dilated hair follicle (Fig. 18–15) or other keratinizing cyst. It is noteworthy that some authors do not insist on complete penetration as a pathognomonic feature.[38] Kyrle's disease (Fig. 18–17) has always been extremely rare. Some of the reported cases are examples of perforating folliculitis or the perforating eruption occurring in the individuals with renal failure undergoing dialysis (see Chapter 26).

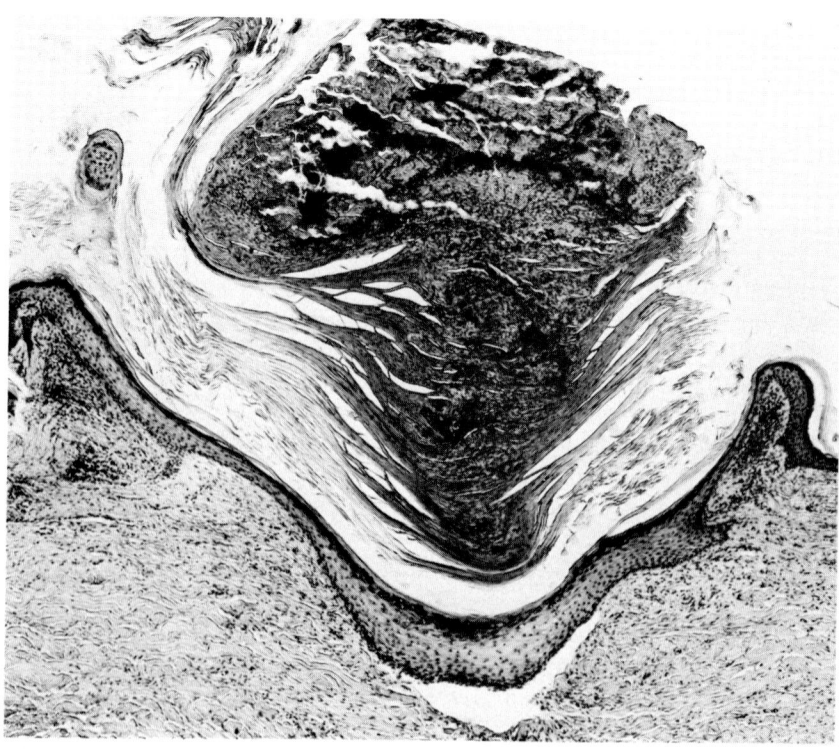

Figure 18–17.
Kyrle's disease. The illustration is taken from a case of perforating folliculitis with a keratotic plug that contains parakeratotic nuclei and pyknotic leukocytes. The epidermis is complete in the picture but is regenerated above scar-like dermis to which it does not closely adhere. Serial sections confirmed the diagnosis. H&E. X70. (From Mehregan. Curr Probl Dermatol 3:144, 1970.)

Pityriasis Rubra Pilaris

Perhaps related to disturbed metabolism of vitamin A is pityriasis rubra pilaris (PRP), which has characteristic features in later stages, when keratotic plugs are well developed, but is easily confused with psoriasis in the early erythrodermic phase (Fig. 18–18), when the mitotic rate is also very high.[39,40] Points for differentiation are the more continuous parakeratosis and the absence of squirting papillae in PRP. The photomicrograph illustrates sebaceous atrophy and hypertrophy of the arrector muscle already in this early stage, but these features are better and more regularly developed in advanced cases. One may say that the skin is in a state of constant cutis anserina. The hypertrophic arrector pili pulls on the follicle, producing an angulation in the bulge region and often eliciting an epithelial tendon (see Fig. 2–31) from the follicular wall. These features may have to be reconstructed from serial sections if the follicles are sectioned obliquely. The fully developed picture (Fig. 18–19) includes conical keratotic plugs in follicular openings and a thick, evenly acanthotic epidermis with accentuated ridges and papillae. The granular layer is thick and the horny layer orthokeratotic, except that, paradoxically, the shoul-

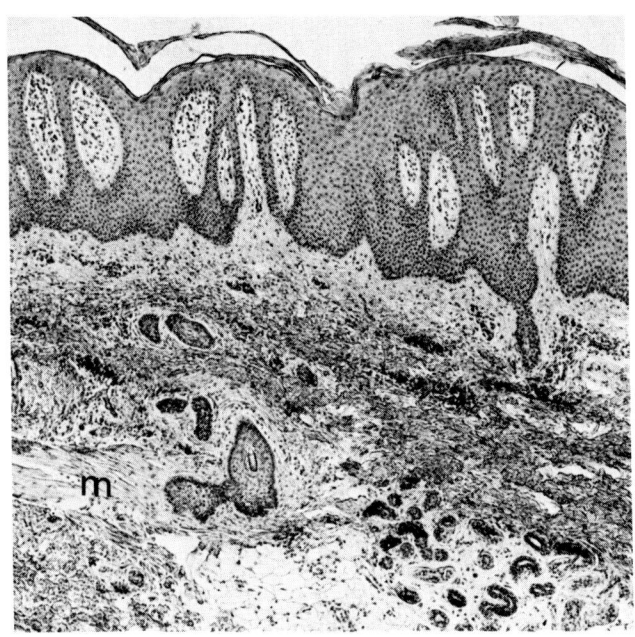

Figure 18–18.
Pityriasis rubra pilaris, early psoriasiform stage in a child. Note absence of suprapapillary exudate in epidermis and hyperplasia of arrector pili muscle (m), for which proliferation of bulge forms an epithelial tendon. H&E. X70.

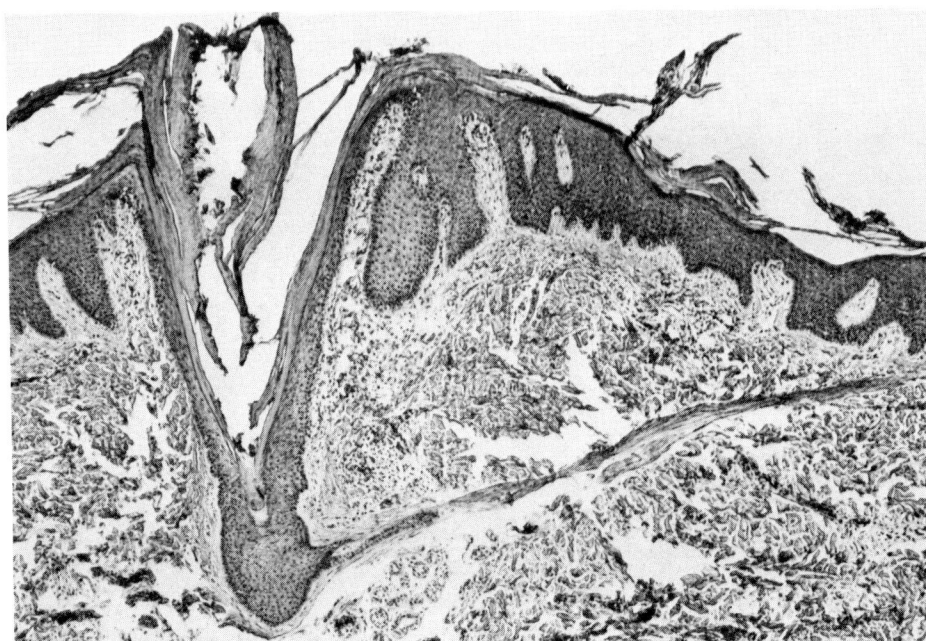

Figure 18–19.
Later stage of pityriasis rubra pilaris. Keratotic plug in a hair follicle that has formed an epithelial tendon for strong arrector muscle. Epidermis is orthokeratotic above a granular layer, except at shoulders of follicle where there is parakeratosis. H&E. X60.

ders of hair follicles show loss of keratohyalin and some parakeratosis.[41] The rete malpighi may show spongiosis in this limited area. Inflammatory infiltrate is moderate or minimal in all stages of PRP. Keratoderma palmare et plantare are common. A peculiar type of dermatomyositis (*type Wong*) has been reported in which PRP-like horny plugs form extensively in hair follicles, due to myositis of the arrector muscles.

ROSACEA, RHINOPHYMA, AND LEWANDOWSKY'S DISEASE

The histologic picture of rosacea varies along with its clinical forms.[42] The epidermis and upper dermis usually show features of seborrheic dermatitis in florid cases. Hair follicles may contain keratotic plugs or pus cells. The sebaceous glands tend to be large. There are variable amounts of interfollicular inflammatory infiltrate, which is mainly lymphocytic but may include neutrophils, some eosinophils, and plasma cells. Marks[43] discounts the primary role of the pilosebaceous apparatus and emphasizes damage to small vessels. Severe cases may show granulomatous reaction (Fig. 18–20), which often has the features of foreign body granuloma but may be of tuberculoid structure.[44] Variable amounts of fibrosis can be expected in the more chronic cases. This is especially true in patients whose condition approaches rhinophyma (Fig. 18–21). In these cases, the sebaceous glands may be tremendous and usually consist of many deep-seated lobes opening into a common sinus that is lined by stratified, keratinizing epithelium. Connective tissue, usually containing wide, thin-walled vessels, fills the spaces in between and may form the greatest volume of the hyperplastic masses. Inflammatory infiltrate may be minor or heavy and often includes features of foreign body granulation tissue.

With some attention, one usually can find *Demodex* (Fig. 18–22) in the follicular channels and even deep in the sebaceous glands of rosacea.[45–47] They are similarly present in normal facial skin in many instances, however.[48,49] It is only when each follicle contains several *Demodex* that one begins to suspect an etiologic role.[50] We also have found dead *Demodex* or its fragments in the center of granulomatous nodules in rosacea (Fig. 18–23), a feature confirmed by Grosshans et al.[51] It appears irrefutable that *Demodex* can cause granulomatous reaction when it gets outside the follicle or gland, as may happen when these structures are destroyed by inflammation.

The peculiar papular affection of the face described by Lewandowsky as rosacea-like tuberculid, but now thought to be *tuberculoid rosacea*, is difficult to differentiate from true micropapular tuberculid (see Chapter 21). One needs serial sections[52] because one has to decide whether the little granulomas are related to follicles or are truly interfollicular, as they ought to be in a tuberculid.

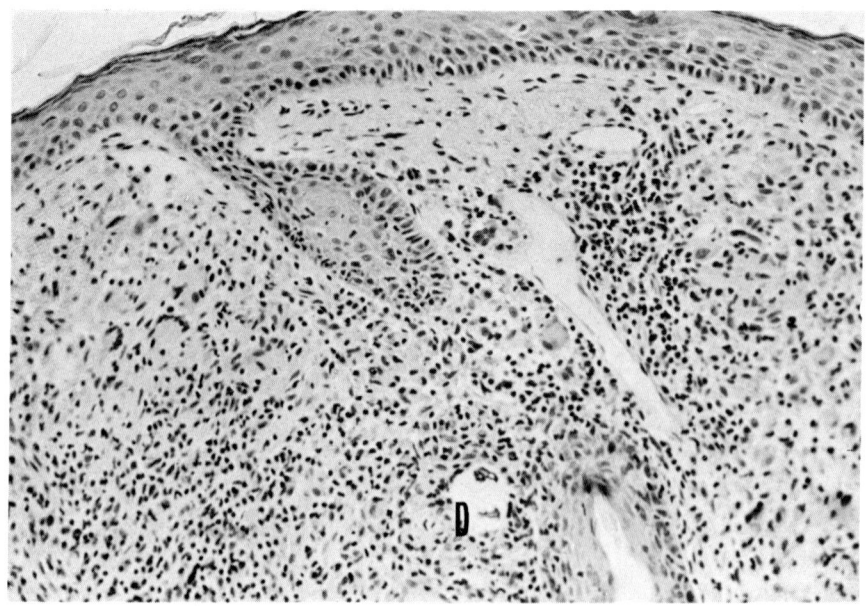

Figure 18–20.
Granulomatous rosacea. Mixed infiltrate with several multinucleated giant cells, telangiectasia, and remnants of hair follicles. Near bottom, a vacuole containing remnants of Demodex (D). H&E. X250.

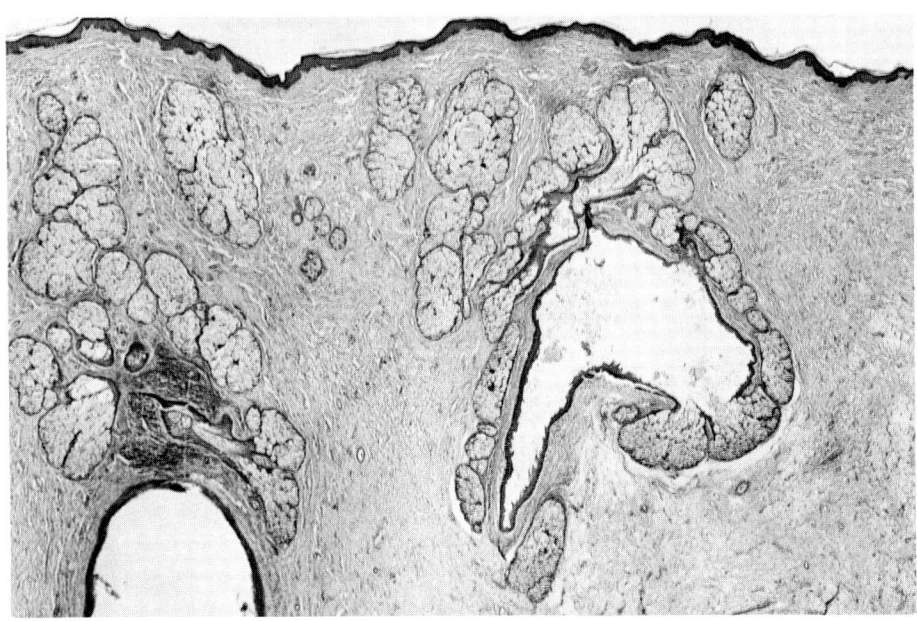

Figure 18–21.
Rhinophyma. Huge sebaceous glands and fibrosis with minor inflammatory infiltrate. H&E. X28.

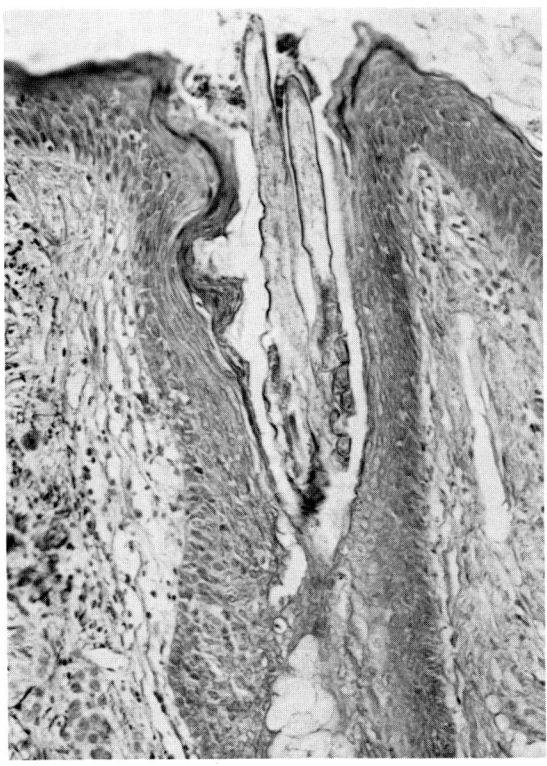

Figure 18–22.
Demodex folliculorum. Two specimens lying head down in a follicular opening. O&G. X180.

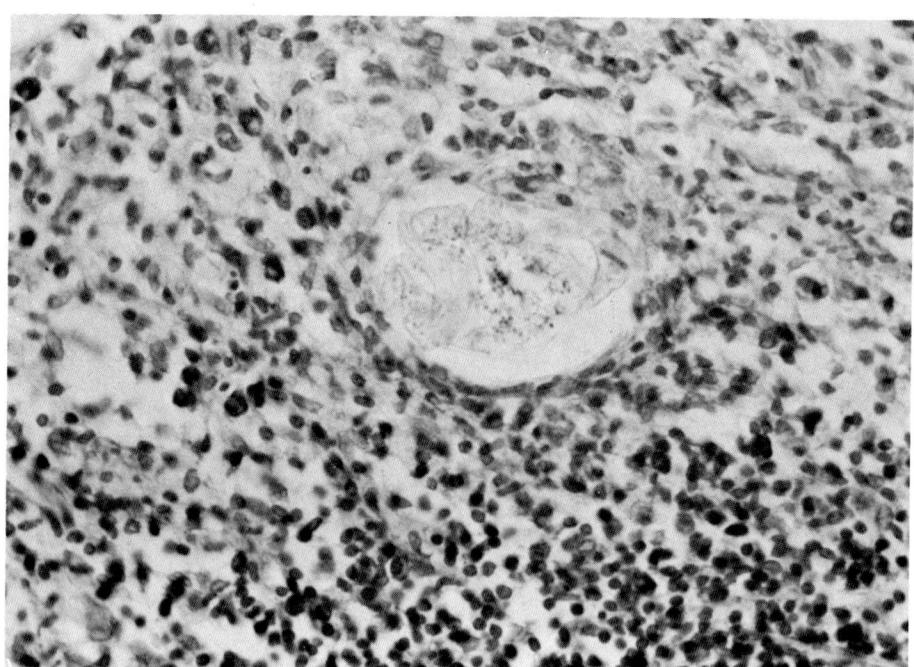

Figure 18–23.
Cross section of dead Demodex folliculorum embedded in dense inflammatory tissue in a case of granulomatous rosacea. O&G. X465.

REFERENCES

1. Pinkus H, Rudner E: Sycosis vulgaris agminata (Lutz). Dermatol Monatsschr 151:628, 1965
2. Montagna W, Bell M, Strauss JS: Sebaceous glands and acne vulgaris. J Invest Dermatol 62:117, 1974
3. Norris JFB, Cunliffe WJ: A histological and immunocytochemical study of early acne lesions. Br J Dermatol 118:651, 1988
4. Leyden JL, Kligman AM: Hairs in acne comedones. Arch Dermatol 106:851, 1972
5. Kaidbey KH, Kligman AM: A human model of coal tar acne. Arch Dermatol 109:212, 1974
6. Goldschmidt H, Leyden JL, Stein KH: Acne fulminans. Investigation of acute febrile ulcerative acne. Arch Dermatol 113:444, 1978
7. Izumi AK, Marples RR, Kligman AM: Senile (solar) comedones. J Invest Dermatol 61:46, 1973
8. Graham JH, Barroso-Tobila C: Dermal pathology of superficial fungus infections. In Baker RD (ed): The Pathologic Anatomy of Mycoses. Handbuch der speziellen pathologischen Anatomie uand Histologie, New York: Springer-Verlag, 1971, vol 3, pt 5
9. Armijo F, Lachapelle J-M: Granulome dermatophytique du derme (A Trichophyton rubrum var. Rhodainii) par envahissement folliculaire. Ann Dermatol Venereol 108:987, 1981
10. Kuo T-T, Chen S-Y, Chan H-L: Tinea infection histologically simulating eosinophilic pustular folliculitis. J Cutan Pathol 13:118, 1986
11. Mehregan AH, Coskey RJ: Perforating folliculitis. Arch Dermatol 97:394, 1968
12. Golitz L: Follicular and perforating disorders. J Cutan Pathol 12:282, 1985
13. Heidelberg RP, Pinkus H: Necrotizing folliculitis. Presented at 1974 Annual Meeting of the National Medical Association
14. Bäck O, Faergemann J, Hörnqvist R: Pityrosporum folliculitis: A common disease of the young and middle-aged. J Am Acad Dermatol 12:56, 1985
15. Oyanguren CJ, Montesinos BE, Sanchez Carazo JL, Boniche AA: Folliculitis por pityrosporum. Med Cutan ILA 13:357, 1985
16. Kaidbey KH, Kligman AM: The pathogenesis of topical steroid acne. J Invest Dermatol 62:31, 1974
17. Kossard S, Collins A, McCrossin I: Necrotizing lymphocytic folliculitis: The early lesion of acne necrotica (varioliformis). J Am Acad Dermatol 16:1007, 1987
18. Dinehart SM, Herzberg AJ, Kerns BJ, Pollack SV: Acne keloidalis: A review. J Dermatol Surg Oncol 15:642, 1989
19. Smith JD, Odom RB: Pseudofolliculitis capitis. Arch Dermatol 113:328, 1977
20. Pinkus H: Chronic scarring pseudofolliculitis of the Negro beard. Arch Dermatol 47:782, 1943
21. Gross KG: Pseudofolliculitis barbae: Shaving bumps of blacks. J Assoc Milit Dermatol 8:4, 1982
22. Bascom J: Pilonidal disease. Long-term results of follicle removal. Dis Colon Rectum 26:800, 1983
23. Ofuji S: Eosinophilic pustular folliculitis. Dermatologica 174:53, 1987
24. Takematsu H, Nakamura K, Igarashi M, Tagami H: Eosinophilic pustular folliculitis. Report of two cases

with a review of the Japanese literature. Arch Dermatol 121:917, 1985
25. Jaliman HD, Phelps RG, Fleischmajer R: Eosinophilic pustular folliculitis. J Am Acad Dermatol 14:479, 1986
26. Meissner K, Kimmig W, Nasemann TH: Folliculite a eosinophiles (maladie d'Ofuji). Ann Dermatol Venereol 115:1207, 1988
27. Malanin G, Helander I: Eosinophilic pustular folliculitis (Ofuji's disease) Response to dapsone but not to isotretinoin therapy. J Am Acad Dermatol 20:1121, 1989
28. Steffen C: Eosinophilic pustular folliculitis (Ofuji's disease) with response to Dapsone therapy. Arch Dermatol 121:921, 1985
29. Lucky AW, Esterly NB, Heskel N, et al: Eosinophilic pustular folliculitis in infancy. Pediatr Dermatol 1:202, 1984
30. Soeprono FF, Shinella RA: Eosinophilic pustular folliculitis in patients with acquired immunodeficiency syndrome. J Am Acad Dermatol 14:1020, 1986
31. Owen WR, Wood C: Disseminated and recurrent infundibulofolliculitis. Arch Dermatol 115:174, 1979
32. Hitch JM, Lund HZ: Disseminate and recurrent infundibulofolliculitis. Arch Dermatol 105:580, 1972
33. Boyd AS: Lichen spinulosus: Case report and overview. Cutis 43:557, 1989
34. Nakjang Y, Yuttanavivat T: Phrynoderma: A review of 105 cases. J Dermatol Tokyo 15:531, 1988
35. Pons S, Ortiz Medina A, Torrez Cortijo A: Disebacéa. Med Cutan Iber Lat Am 7:313, 1973
36. Davenport DO: Ulerythema ophryogenes. Arch Dermatol 89:74, 1964
37. Tapernoux B, Delacrétaz J: Hyperkératose "en bouchons" d'origine mécanique. Dermatologica 143:201, 1971
38. Pajarre R, Alavaikko M: Kyrle's disease. Acta Derm Venereol 53:505, 1973
39. Cohen PR, Prystowsky JH: Pityriasis rubra pilaris: A review of diagnosis and treatment. J Am Acad Dermatol 20:801, 1989
40. Marks R, Griffiths A: The epidermis in pityriasis rubra pilaris. Br J Dermatol 89 (Suppl 9): 19, 1973
41. Niemi KM, Kousa M, Storgårds K, Karvonen J: Pityriasis rubra pilaris. A clinico-pathological study with a special reference to autoradiography and histocompatibility antigens. Dermatologica 152:109, 1976
42. Marks R, Harcourt-Webster JN: Histopathology of rosacea. Arch Dermatol 100:683, 1969
43. Marks R: Histogenesis of the inflammatory component in rosacea. Proc R Soc Med 66:742, 1973
44. Mullanax MG, Kierland RR: Granulomatous rosacea. Arch Dermatol 101:206, 1970
45. Nutting WB: Hair follicle mites (Acari demodicidae) of man. Int J Dermatol 15:79, 1976
46. Norm MS: Demodex folliculorus: Incidence, regional distribution, pathogenicity. Dan Med Bull 18:14, 1971
47. Rufli T, Murncunagli Y: The hair follicle mites Demodex folliculorum and Demodex brevisi biology and medical importance. Dermatologica 162:1, 1981
48. Ramelet A-A, Perroulaz G: Rosacée: Etude histopathologique de 75 cas. Ann Dermatol Venereol 115:801, 1988
49. Forton F: Demodex et inflammation perifolliculaire chez l'homme: Revue et observation de 69 biopsies. Ann Dermatol Venereol 113:1047, 1986
50. Shelley WB, Shelley DE, Burmeister V: Unilateral demodectic rosacea. J Am Acad Dermatol 20:915, 1989
51. Grosshans E, Kremer M, Maleville J, et al: Le rôle des Demodex folliculorum dans l'histogenèse de la rosacêa granulomateuse. Bull Soc Fr Derm Syph 79:639, 1972
52. Michelson HE: Does the rosacea-like tuberculid exist? Arch Dermatol 78:681, 1958

19

ALOPECIAS ASSOCIATED WITH INFLAMMATION

Here we consider as a group all more or less inflammatory processes regularly associated with loss of hair. In most cases, biopsies of this type will have been taken from the scalp, and the most common question asked by the clinician is: What is the prognosis for restoration of hair? Histologic examination pays more attention to the hair follicle and the surrounding dermis than to the hair itself.

Under the microscope we can separate cases into two large groups: those in which hair follicles become smaller but do not disappear and those in which follicles are completely destroyed. The first group comprises patterned alopecia in both sexes, *alopecia areata* and *alopecia mucinosa*. The second comprises the scarring alopecias related to pseudopelade. We defer discussion of pattern alopecia to Chapter 47 because there is little or no inflammation, and examination of the hair itself enters the diagnosis. Trichotillomania and other disturbances due to external causes also are discussed there.

ALOPECIA AREATA

Waves of anagen follicles entering into telogen in a concentric fashion leads to formation of a round patch of alopecia. Apparently anagen follicles in the same stage with high mitotic activity (anagen VI) are affected.[1,2] The shape of the lesion corresponds to the distribution pattern of these hair follicles. In between (Fig. 19–1) hair follicles are transformed into solid cords of undifferentiated basaloid cells surrounded by thickened hyaline sheath and smaller anagen follicles, the so-called miniature type that show signs of trichogenic activity but have a rudimentary papilla and matrix and produce a minuscule hair or just inner root sheath.[3,4] Sebaceous glands usually are reduced in size along with the follicles (Fig. 19–2). Perifollicular (peribulbar) infiltrate may be mild, moderate, or pronounced and consists mainly of helper-inducer T-cell lymphocytes.[5–7]

ALOPECIA MUCINOSA

Loss of hair is actually an incidental but quite regular phenomenon in the disease (Fig. 19–3), characterized by "follicular mucinosis."[8,9] Although in many cases the histologic picture is dominated by inflammatory infiltrate around hair roots, the primary lesion (mucinosis follicularis) is a perversion of metabolism in the sebaceous gland (Fig. 19–4) and the outer root sheath (metaplasia).[10] This leads to the accumulation of much mucinous material and the cells become stellate or rounded. In the earlier stages, the resemblance to a nest of mucinous basal cell epithelioma may be striking. Later, the entire hair follicle may be converted into a bag lined by

266 DEEP INFLAMMATORY PROCESSES

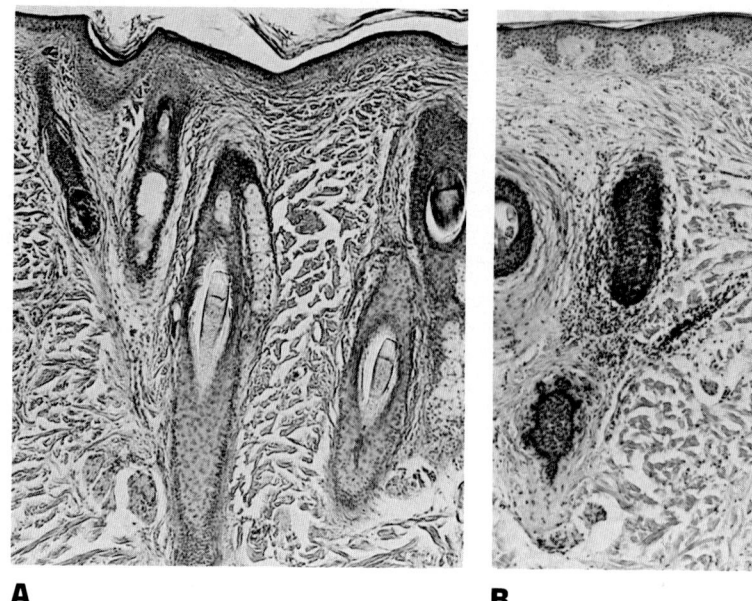

Figure 19–1.
Alopecia areata. **A.** Some relatively normal hair follicles and a miniature follicle often found in alopecia areata. This follicle also has the configuration of a cloaked hair due to sebaceous atrophy. This not too uncommon abnormality has no pathologic significance in itself. H&E. X75. **B.** Inflammatory infiltrate associated with follicles of reduced size containing remnants of inner root sheath but no hairs. H&E. X135.

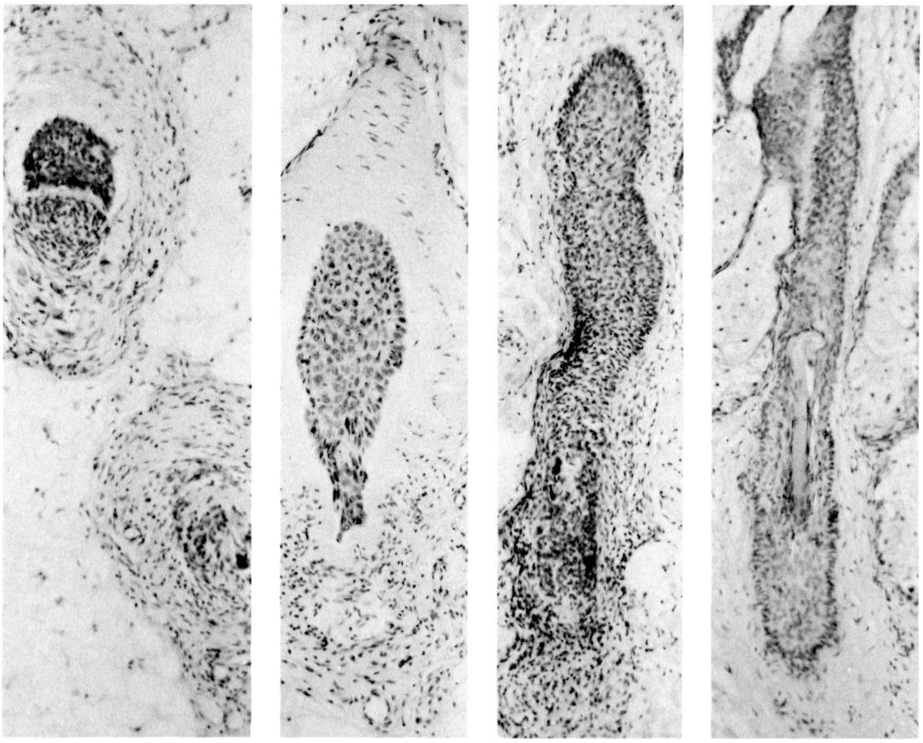

Figure 19–2.
Alopecia areata. Four hair follicles showing variable degrees of inflammatory infiltrate, reduction of epithelial root sheath, and thick fibrous root sheath. **A** and **B.** A dermal papilla below the greatly reduced epithelial matrix (catagen). **C** and **D.** Small hair shaft in follicle at level of sebaceous gland. H&E. X125.

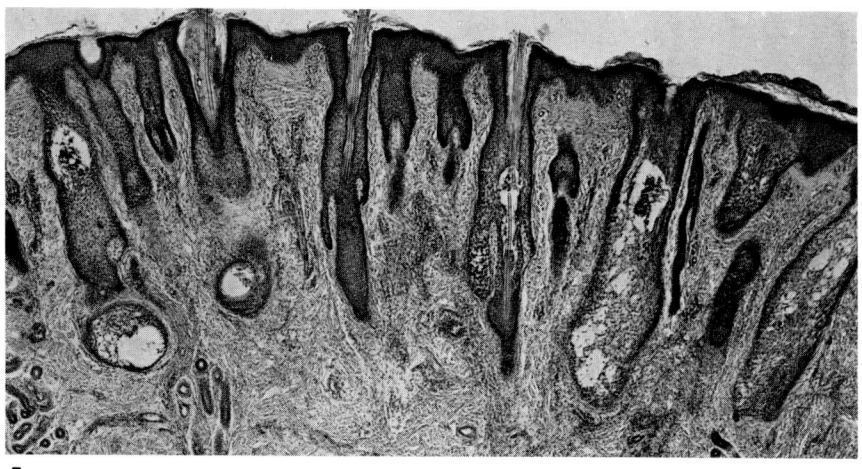

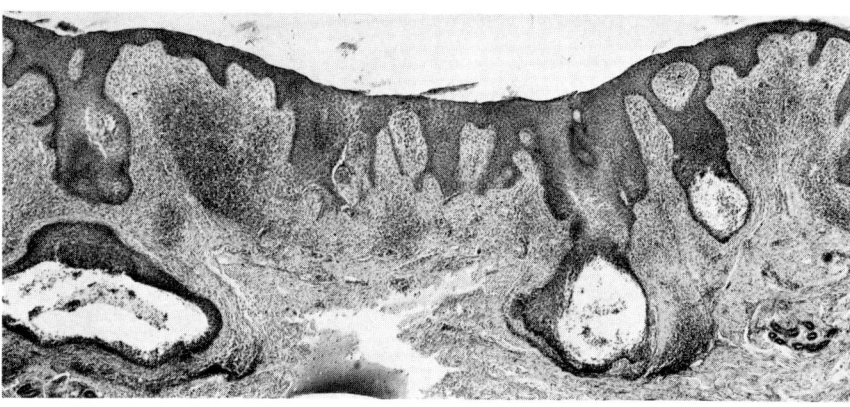

Figure 19–3.
Alopecia mucinosa. Two cases showing varying degrees of inflammatory reaction and cyst formation. H&E. X90.

compressed epithelial cells and filled with a plug of inspissated mucin mixed with less or more horny material.[11–13] The mucin stains slightly bluish in not too highly decolorized H&E sections. It usually is metachromatic and PAS-negative. It stains brilliantly with the Hale procedure or alcian-blue and can be digested by hyaluronidase. The hair, whether large or small, eventually falls out, but the hair root usually survives, and new hair often is formed once the lesion heals. Inflammatory infiltrate may be almost absent, especially in those cases in which the clinical picture is that of follicular papules. In the inflammatory plaques of alopecia mucinosa, infiltrate may be moderate or heavy and often is a mixture of lymphocytes, eosinophils, plasma cells, and some histiocytes.

Once follicular mucinosis has been recognized in a biopsy, one has to decide whether one is dealing with a case of benign alopecia mucinosa or with a case of mycosis fungoides or other lymphoma, in which the follicular mucinosis persists. The occasional transformation of the benign form into lymphoblastoma has been well documented.[14,15] Cytologic features of lymphoblastoma including the presence of atypical cells with hyperchromatic or hyperconvoluted nuclei, absence of eosinophils, and the presence of epidermal involvement should be looked for in the histologic sections. The possibility that mucinous edema of the outer root sheath may occur symptomatically in *staphylococcic follicular keratosis* cannot be denied. It is essential for the diagnosis of alopecia mucinosa to prove the presence of acid mucopolysaccharides in order to differentiate follicular mucinosis from occasional eczematous spongiosis of the root sheath in which mucinous substances are absent.

SCARRING ALOPECIA

Under the term "scarring alopecia" we discuss a group of alopecias characterized by permanent loss of the pilosebaceous structures leaving behind tracers of fibrotic connective tissue and free bundles of

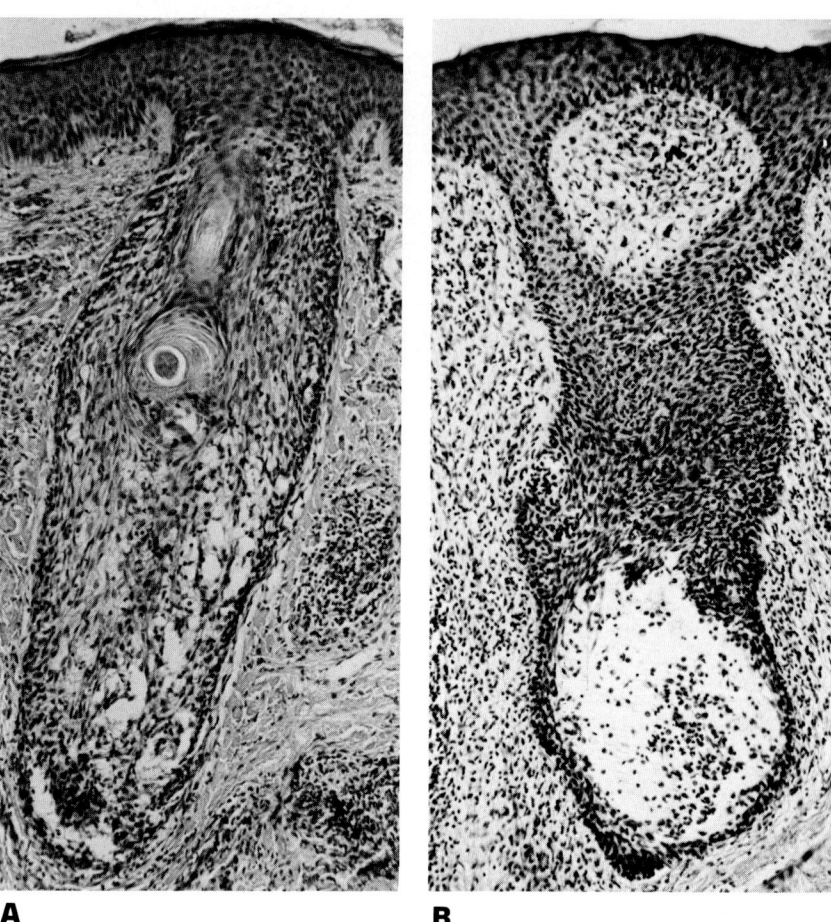

Figure 19–4.
Alopecia mucinosa. **A.** Mucinous degeneration of outer root sheath and a small hair in the center. **B.** Mucin in a cyst filled otherwise with degenerating epithelial and inflammatory cells. Moderately heavy mixed infiltrate in dermis. H&E. X250.

hair muscles. Fibrosis may be minimal or extensive and is associated with loss of elastic fibers.[16] A biopsy of a suspected case of scarring alopecia raises two questions of theoretical and practical significance: Is the loss of hair temporary or permanent? In the latter case, is there evidence of associated nonfollicular disease or is it strictly an atrophying follicular process? Cases of folliculitis decalvans are ruled out by the presence of intrafollicular neutrophils. It will be seen that these questions are answered with greater ease if a good elastic fiber stain is used in the differential diagnosis.[17]

Pseudopelade of Brocq

Ill-defined areas of alopecia with varying degrees of atrophy involve the crown and parietal scalp predominantly in women.[18] The hair loss is initially incomplete and a few normal appearing hairs remain in the area. Histologically, the epidermis usually preserves normal thickness with rete ridges and normal keratinization. There may be some keratotic plugging of hair follicles. The striking abnormality at scanning examination is a total absence of sebaceous glands. The number of hair follicles is diminished in proportion to the stage of the disease. There is moderate perifollicular infiltrate, mainly of T-helper lymphocytes, and the epithelial follicular wall is thinned and eventually disappears (Fig. 19–5). The inflammation is restricted to the upper permanent portion of the follicle, down to the bulge. The lower cyclic portion often is relatively well preserved but perishes, as is shown by one's ability to pull out anagen hairs (cheveux pseudopeladiques[19]). Occasionally, an affected hair may survive and grow back. The space left by the disappearing hair follicle is taken up by the thickened fibrous root sheath on which the surviving hair muscle inserts. There is diffuse loss of the subepidermal fine elastic fibers (Fig. 19–6) without much evidence of inflammation. The thickened fibrous root sheath, which extends into the subcutaneous tissue, is outlined by elastic fibers only in the dermis but not in the subcutis (Fig. 19–7). A peculiar feature observed in a minority of lesions is

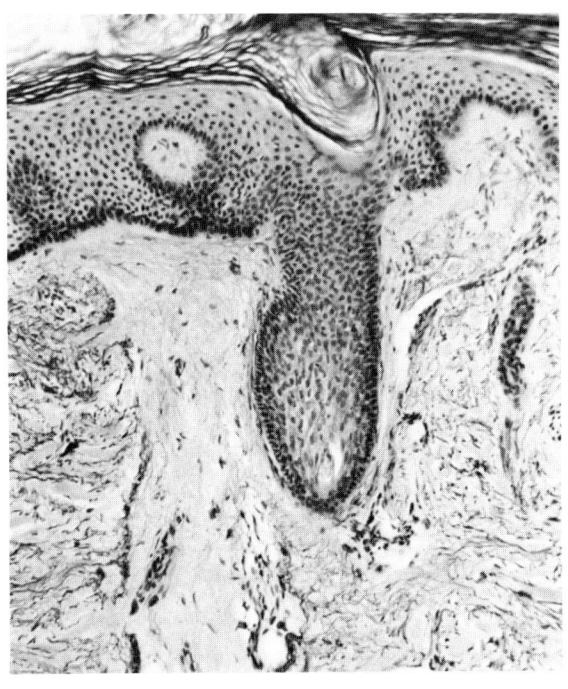

Figure 19–5.
Pseudopelade of Brocq. A reduced hair follicle containing a tiny hair next to the remnant of a completely lost follicle represented by a cord of fibrotic fibrous root sheath. H&E. X250.

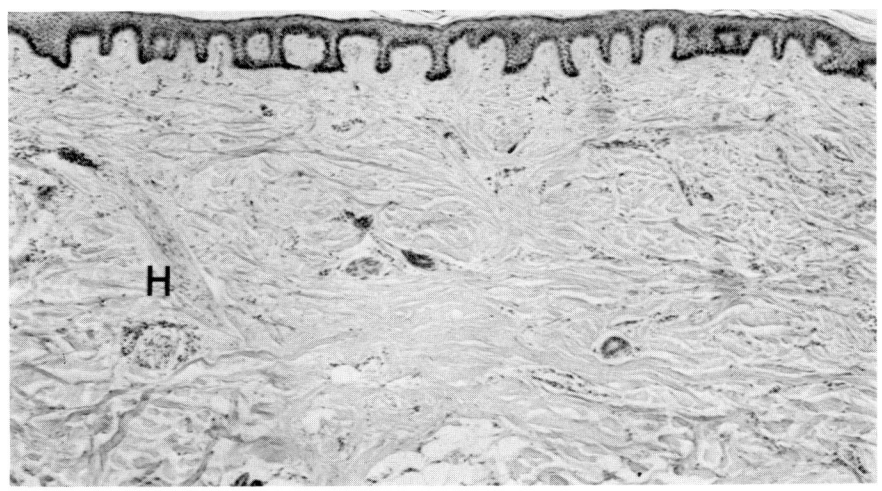

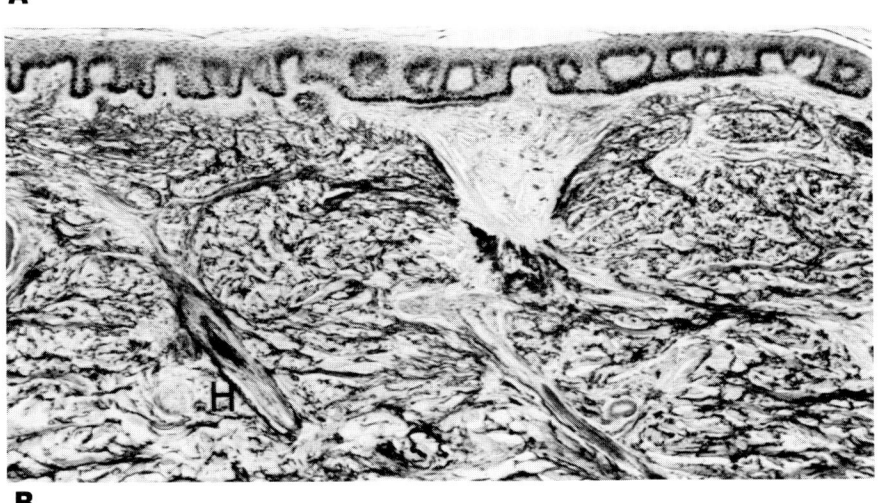

Figure 19–6.
Pseudopelade. Comparison of H&E (**A**) and O&G (**B**) stains shows how much more informative the latter is in this disease. The atrophic follicle (H) is barely discernible in **A** but well-outlined by elastic fibers in **B**, which also shows loss of superficial elastic fibers and nail head appearance of the fibrous remnant of a completely lost follicle. X70.

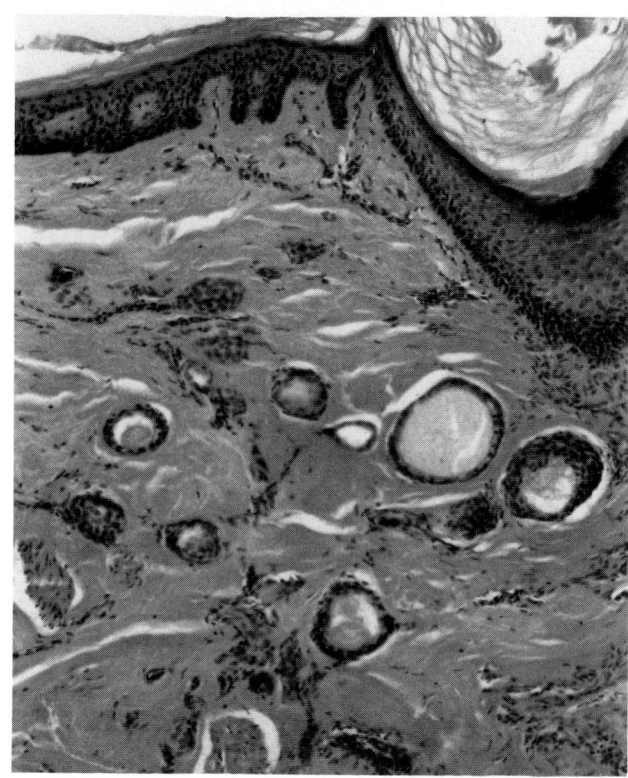

Figure 19–7.
Scarring alopecia of scalp with syringoma-like sweat duct proliferation. H&E. X125.

proliferation of some fairly superficial small eccrine ducts resembling syringoma.[20]

Alopecia Neoplastica

In rare cases, a metastasis from carcinoma of the breast may cause a patch of alopecia without forming a nodule.[21] Hair follicles become atrophic within a dense fibrous stroma surrounding individual large carcinomatous cells or small nests of cells.[22]

REFERENCES

1. Messenger AG, Slater DN, Bleehen SS: Alopecia areata: Alterations in the hair growth cycle and correlation with the follicular pathology. Br J Dermatol 114:337, 1986
2. Tosti A: Alopecia areata: More on pathogenesis and therapy. Dermatologica 178:61, 1989
3. Headington JT, Mitchell A, Swanson N: New histopathological findings in alopecia areata studied in transverse sections. J Invest Dermatol 76:325, 1981
4. Van Scott EJ: Morphological changes in pilosebaceous units and anagen hairs in alopecia areata. J Invest Dermatol 31:35, 1958
5. Perret C, Wiesner-Menzel L, Happle R: Immunohistochemical analysis of T-cell subsets in the peribulbar and intrabulbar infiltrates of alopecia areata. Acta Derm Venereol 64:26, 1984
6. Todes-Taylor N, Turner R, Wood GS, et al: T cell subpopulations in alopecia areata. J Am Acad Dermatol 11:216, 1984
7. Peereboom-Wynia JDR, VanJoost TH, Stolz E, Prins MEF: Markers of immunologic injury in progressive alopecia areata. J Cutan Pathol 13:363, 1986
8. Pinkus H: Alopecia mucinosa. Inflammatory plaques with alopecia characterized by root-sheath mucinosis. Arch Dermatol 76:419, 1957
9. Pinkus H. Alopecia mucinosa (Commentary). Additional data in 1983. Arch Dermatol 119:698, 1983
10. Hempstead RW, Ackerman BA: Follicular mucinosis. A reaction pattern in follicular epithelium. Am J Dermatopathol 7:245, 1985
11. Gibson LE, Muller SA, Peters MS: Follicular mucinosis of childhood and adolescence. Pediatr Dermatol 5:231, 1988
12. Gibson LE, Muller SA, Leiferman KM, et al: Follicular mucinosis: Clinical and histopathologic study. J Am Acad Dermatol 20:441, 1989
13. Lancer HA, Bronstein BR, Nakagawa H, et al: Follicular mucinosis: A detailed morphologic and immunopathologic study. J Am Acad Dermatol 10:760, 1984
14. Sentis JH, Willemze R, Scheffer E: Alopecia mucinosa progressing into mycosis fungoides. A long-term

follow-up study of two patients. Am J Dermatopathol 10:478, 1988
15. Emmerson RW: Follicular mucinosis. A study of 47 patients. Br J Dermatol 81:395, 1969
16. Pinkus H: Alopecia: Clinicopathologic correlations. Int J Dermatol 19:245, 1980
17. Ioannides G: Alopecia: A pathologist's view. Int J Dermatol 21:23, 1982
18. Pinkus H: Differential patterns of elastic fibers in scarring and nonscarring alopecias. J Cutan Pathol 5:93, 1978
19. Braun-Falco O, Imai S, Schmoeckel C, et al: Pseudopelade of Brocq. Dermatologica 172:18, 1986
20. Mehregan AH, Mehregan DA: Syringoma-like sweat duct proliferation. J Cutan Pathol 17:355, 1990
21. Baum EM, Omura EF, Payne RR, Little WP: Alopecia neoplastica—A rare form of cutaneous metastasis. J Am Acad Dermatol 4:688, 1981
22. Velez JR, Ferrando J, Palou J, Mascaro JM: Alopecia neoplastica. Med Cutan Ibero Lat Am 18:185, 1990

20

INFLAMMATION INVOLVING ECCRINE OR APOCRINE GLANDS

Eccrine or apocrine glands are much more rarely the seat of inflammation than is the pilosebaceous complex. A paper by Montgomery et al.[1] points out, on the basis of electron microscopic studies, that the name "eccrine" is not really applicable to the human sweat gland and should be replaced by "atrichial" gland. Another interesting publication reports the existence of a third type of sweat glands (apoeccrine glands) in the human axilla with segmental or diffuse apocrinelike dilated secretory tubules but long and thin ducts that like eccrine glands open into the surface of the epidermis.[2] We continue to use the long-established terms *eccrine* and *apocrine* until this new finding is corroborated by others.

ECCRINE GLANDS

Periporitis, a superficial pustular eruption around sweat pores and analogous to impetigo Bockhart, is almost exclusively found in young babies. Just as with the various types of miliaria of the adult, these lesions will rarely be biopsied. Either dermatosis is easily recognized under the microscope if one is aware of the typical corkscrew shape of the intraepidermal sweat duct unit (the acrosyringium) and keeps in mind that this structure persists uninvolved in most inflammatory dermatoses even in the presence of severe epidermal edema. Disruption of the acrosyringeal wall and presence of leukocytes in the lumen indicate involvement of the unit.[3] In *miliaria crystallina,* as it is often observed a few hours after acute defervescence in bedridden patients, fluid accumulates in the horny layer due to very superficial obstruction of the acrosyringium, and there is little inflammatory reaction. In *miliaria rubra,* a PAS-positive plug is present in the acrosyringium, and inflammation follows the great increase of resident cocci within a few days[4] (Fig. 20–1). We pointed out in Chapter 6 that the dyshidrosiform eruptions are of eczematous character and that the sweat ducts usually pass intact between the intraepidermal vesicles. Erythema toxicum neonatorum (Chapter 7), which may involve eccrine ducts[5] as well as hair follicles, and the toxic erythema with pustules following drug ingestion[6] are characterized by numerous eosinophils in the infiltrate.

Inflammatory involvement of the intradermal duct and the coil are even less frequent, except for the fact that there are numerous small blood vessels associated with these structures, and a more generalized perivascular infiltrate will also involve these vessels. Deep eccrine gland abscesses, formerly a severe and sometimes fatal disease of malnourished infants, have practically disappeared in the United States. The occasional case[7] seems to be associated with immunologic defects in the child. Histologically, a heavy mixed infiltrate of polymorphs and

274 DEEP INFLAMMATORY PROCESSES

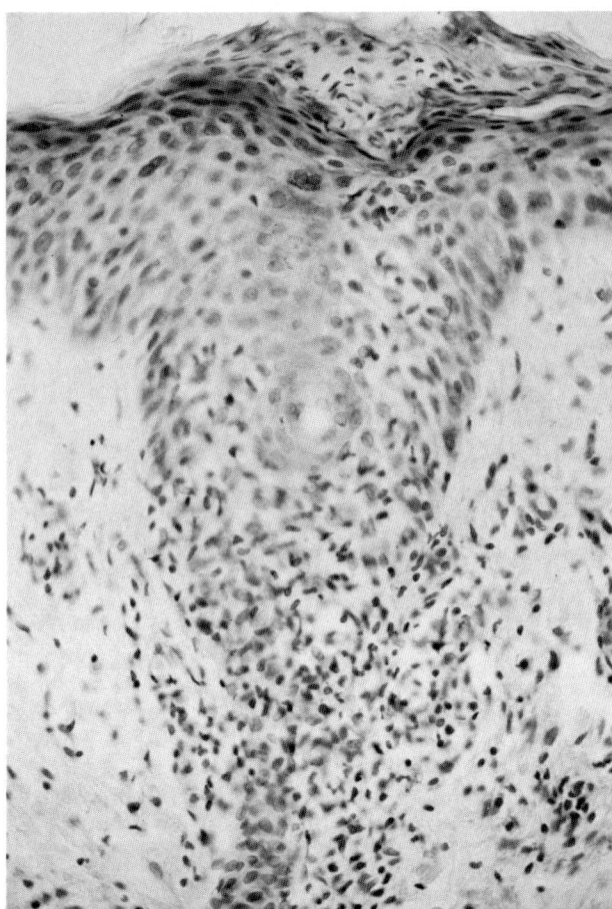

Figure 20–1.
Miliaria rubra. Edema and exocytosis in the sweat duct ridge surrounding the acrosyringium. The lesion is topped by a parakeratotic scale–crust, and there is edema and inflammatory infiltrate in the papillary dermis. That the acrosyringium is, in fact, ruptured in its lower part can be ascertained only in careful serial sections. H&E. X285.

lymphocytes is found deep in the dermis around degenerating sweat coils. Careful examination of multiple sections is needed to rule out primary deep vasculitis. On the other hand, differentiation from a furuncle (Chapter 18) is simple because the thin eccrine duct never becomes the center of a necrotic plug, as is typical of deep follicular inflammation.

Sweat gland necrosis has been described in a case of bullous eruption induced by medicaments[8] and perhaps is more frequent than suspected. *Neutrophilic eccrine hidradenitis* is characterized by infiltration of eccrine coils with neutrophils and necrosis of the secretory epithelium.[9] It occurs in cancer patients undergoing chemotherapy.[10–14] The tissue reaction appears to be unrelated to any specific type of malignancy or any one chemotherapeutic agent.

It may also occur without association with malignancy.[15]

APOCRINE GLANDS

Inasmuch as apocrine glands reach their full development only in puberty, they are rarely diseased in childhood. *Fox–Fordyce disease* and *hidradenitis*

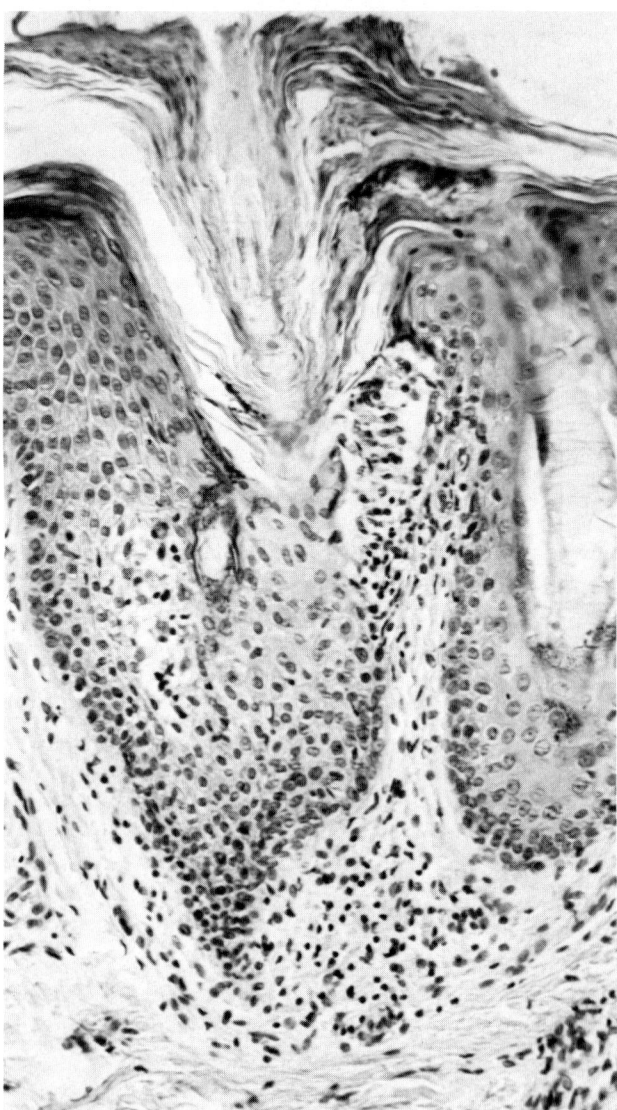

Figure 20–2.
Apocrine miliaria with relatively mild inflammatory infiltrate in Fox–Fordyce disease in a prepubertal girl. Of two hair follicles side by side, the left shows a longitudinal break in the right wall filled with degenerating and inflammatory cells. Some inflammatory cells are also seen in left wall. H&E. X185. (From Mevorah et al. Dermatologica 136:43, 1968.)

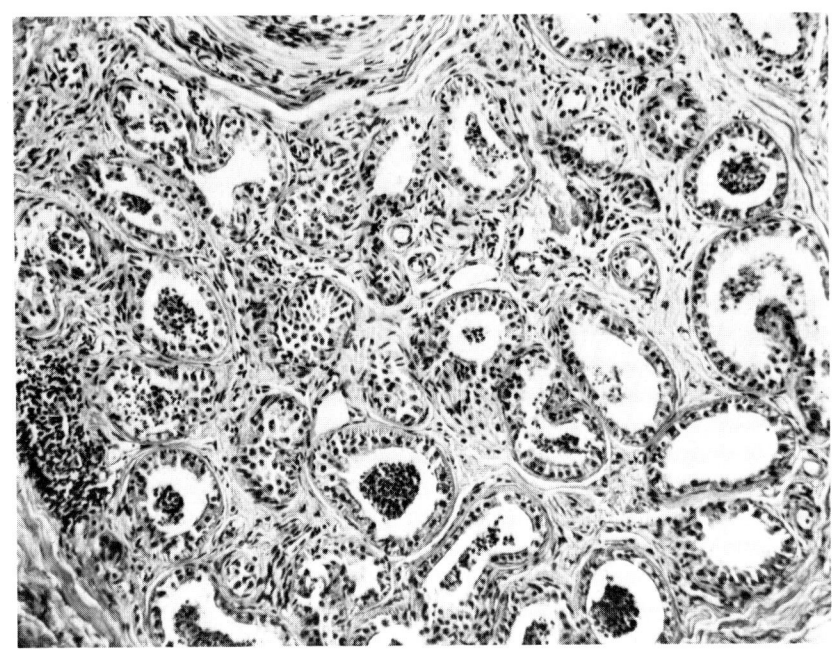

Figure 20–3.
Hidradenitis suppurativa. Well-preserved gland at periphery of lesion shows leukocytes in lumina and mild interstitial inflammation. H&E. X135.

suppurativa are the outstanding examples of inflammation associated with the apocrine apparatus. The histologic basis of Fox–Fordyce disease has been demonstrated to be an obstruction of the apocrine duct (Fig. 20–2) where it enters the follicular wall. Serial sections usually are required to demonstrate this apocrine miliaria.[16,17] In routine diagnostic examination, it is sufficient to show inflammatory infiltrate encircling the upper one third of axillary hair follicles in order to corroborate a diagnosis of Fox–Fordyce disease.

Histologic confirmation of the diagnosis hidradenitis suppurativa is rarely required. Examination of surgical material usually reveals pockets of pus cells between heavy and often granulomatous inflammatory infiltrate in the subcutaneous and deep cutaneous tissue.[18] Sweat glands (Fig. 20–3) may be encountered in various stages of disintegration, and few remain in the late stages of the disease. The solid necrotic plug of the furuncle is absent, just as it is absent in eccrine coil abscesses.[19–22] The changes are those of a deep cellulitis with abscess formation. This explains the clinical features of a slowly enlarging deep swelling, which becomes fluctuant and eventually discharges liquid pus from a relatively small opening at the top of a dome. The process is quite distinct from the pointing of a furuncle and the elimination of the lesion often requires extensive surgical excisions.[23]

We feel that apocrine glands play a minor role in the pathomechanisms of *acne conglobata* and *Hoffmann's disease* (folliculitis et perifolliculitis suffodiens et abscedens). These entities, therefore, are discussed in Chapter 18.

REFERENCES

1. Montgomery I, Jenkinson D McE, Elder HY, et al: The effects of thermal stimulation on the ultrastructure of the human atrichial sweat gland. I. The fundus. Br J Dermatol 110:385, 1984
2. Sato K, Leidal R, Sato F: Morphology and development of an apoeccrine sweat gland in human axillae. Am J Physiol 251:R166, 1987
3. Dobson RL, Lobitz WC Jr: Some histochemical observations on the human eccrine sweat glands. II. The pathogenesis of miliaria. Arch Dermatol 75:653, 1957
4. Hölzle E, Kligman AM: The pathogenesis of miliaria rubra. Role of the resident microflora. Br J Dermatol 99:117, 1978
5. Duperrat B, Bret AJ: Erythema neonatorum allergicum. Br J Dermatol 73:300, 1961
6. Ogino A, Tagumi H, Takahashi C, Higuchi T: Generalized pustular toxic erythema: Pathogenetic relationship between pustule and epidermal appendage (hair follicle or sweat duct). Acta Derm Venereol 58:257, 1978
7. Mopper C, Pinkus H, Iacobell P: Multiple sweat gland abscesses of infants. Arch Dermatol 71:177, 1955
8. Herschtal D, Robinson ML: Blisters of the skin in coma induced by amitryptidine and clorazepate dipotassium. Report of a case with underlying sweat gland necrosis. Arch Dermatol 115:499, 1979
9. Harrist TJ, Fine JD, Berman RS, et al: Neutrophilic

eccrine hidradenitis. A distinctive type of neutrophilic dermatosis associated with myelogenous leukemia and chemotherapy. Arch Dermatol 118:263, 1982
10. Bailey DL, Barron D, Lucky AW: Neutrophilic eccrine hidradenitis: A case report and review of the literature. Pediatr Dermatol 6:33, 1989
11. Beutner K, Packman CH, Markowitch W: Neutrophilic eccrine hidradenitis associated with Hodgkin's disease and chemotherapy. Arch Dermatol 122:809, 1986
12. Katsanis E, Luke K-H, Hsu E, et al: Neutrophilic eccrine hidradenitis in acute myelomonocytic leukemia. Am J Pediatr Hematol Oncol 9:204, 1987
13. Fitzpatrick JE, Bennion SD, Reed OM, et al: Neutrophilic eccrine hidradenitis associated with induction chemotherapy. J Cutan Pathol 14:22, 1987
14. Scallan PJ, Kettler AH, Levy ML, Tschen JA: Neutrophilic eccrine hidradenitis. Evidence implicating bleomycin as causative agent. Cancer 62:2532, 1988
15. Kuttner BJ, Kurban RS: Neutrophilic eccrine hidradenitis in the absence of an underlying malignancy. Cutis 41:403, 1988
16. Shelley WB, Levy EJ: Apocrine sweat retention in man. II. Fox–Fordyce disease (apocrine miliaria). Arch Dermatol 73:38, 1958
17. Mevorah B, Duboff GS, Wass RW: Fox–Fordyce disease in prepubescent girls. Dermatologica 136:43, 1968
18. Hyland CH, Kheir SM: Follicular occlusion disease with elimination of abnormal elastic tissue. Arch Dermatol 116:925, 1980
19. Van Landuyt H, Laurent R: Hidrosadenites suppurees. Ann Dermatol Venereol 117:59, 1990
20. Jemec GBE: The symptomatology of hidradenitis suppurativa in women. Br J Dermatol 119:345, 1988
21. Van Landuyt H, Laurent R: Hidrosadenites suppurees. Ann Dermatol Venereol 117:59, 1990
22. Bhatia NN, Bergman A, Broen EM: Advanced hidradenitis suppurativa of the vulva. A report of three cases. J Reprod Med 29:436, 1984
23. Jemec GBE: Effect of localized surgical excisions in hidradenitis suppurativa. J Am Acad Dermatol 18:1103, 1988

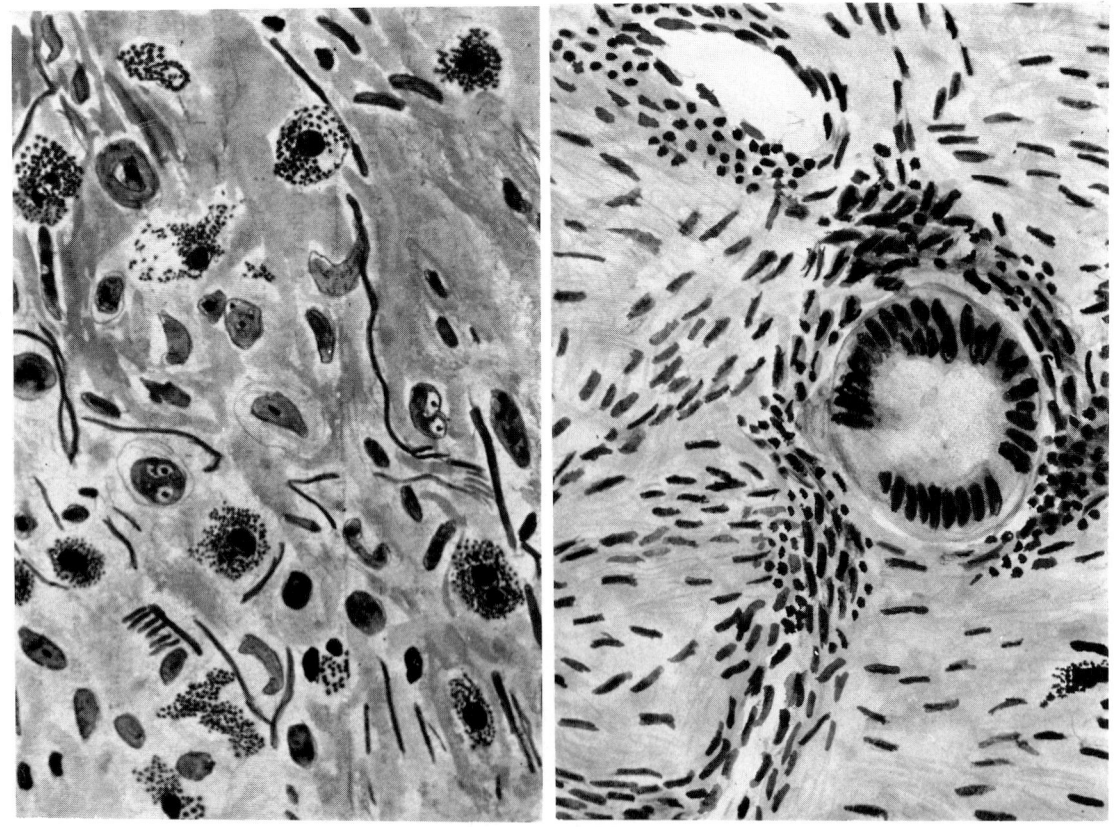

Eosinophils and elastic fibers in O&G (left) stain. Multinucleated giant cells in tuberculosis (right).

SECTION IV

GRANULOMATOUS INFLAMMATION AND PROLIFERATION

The derivation of the term "granulomatous inflammation" is complicated. It is related to granulation tissue, which was given that name originally on the macroscopic clinical basis that a healing wound looks granular. These granulations, of course, correspond to newly formed capillaries and surrounding fibroblasts, histiocytes, and fibrous connective tissue. Always associated are the usual types of inflammatory cells, that is, polymorphonuclear leukocytes, lymphocytes, and perhaps some plasma cells and eosinophils. Masses of microscopically similar tissue in various organs were then called "granulomas" using the suffix meaning a tumor. Similar but now obsolete terms with more specific meaning were "tuberculoma" or "syphiloma," and even today we speak of "lepromatous leprosy." Eventually, when the suffix *-oma* was more specifically reserved for true neoplasms and when the reactive nature of tuberculous and other infiltrates had been recognized, the term *granulomatous inflammation* was preferred. "Granuloma" persists in several dermatologic diagnoses (granuloma annulare), however, and, in fact, has been used for the very purpose of emphasizing the nonneoplastic nature of certain lesions. Thus, "reticulohistiocytoma" has been replaced by *reticulohistiocytic granuloma*.

The simplest definition for the microscopic picture of granulomatous inflammation is "an inflammatory process that contains mononuclear macrophage cells or histiocytes."[1] The word "histiocyte" is used here in the sense of a tissue cell capable of phagocytosis. There is no relation to neoplastic disease. As a matter of fact, disease processes containing histiocytes are stamped thereby as being inflammatory and not malignant.[2]

The cellular infiltrate of all simple inflammatory dermatoses consists predominantly of those cells that come into the skin from the bloodstream or of their modifications: neutrophilic and eosinophilic leukocytes, lymphocytes, and possibly plasma cells. They can disappear again without leaving a trace, either through cell death and absorption or by migration to other parts, such as lymph nodes. Histiocytes present in the tissue may be stimulated to become macrophages and may remain as evidence of past inflammation, for example, the melanophages of postinflammatory pigmentation. If any appreciable number of histiocytes or their various derivatives, especially macrophages, epithelioid cells, and multinucleated giant cells are found in an inflammatory infiltrate, it is assumed that they are derived from reticuloendothelial cells by multiplication at the site of the lesion. Although there is experimental evidence that mononuclear cells in chronic inflammation in small laboratory animals continuously come from the circulation, there is also evidence of cell proliferation in simple inflammatory infiltrates in man,[3,4] and one is entitled to reserve judgment on the cellular dynamics of granulomas in human skin (for reviews see Epstein[5] and Hirsh and

Johnson).[6-9] In any case, development of granulomatous inflammation appears to be a manifestation of cellular rather than humoral immunity. This is exemplified by the development of large epithelioid cell granulomas in patients deficient in circulating antibodies.

It seems preferable to amplify and support the simple criterion of the presence of macrophage histiocytic cells by a few other statements when we are dealing with granulomatous dermatoses. (1) There is production of new blood capillaries and their supporting mesenchymal cells. (2) The formation of granulomatous tissue is practically always associated with destruction of preexisting tissue in the skin. This is easily demonstrated by an elastic fiber stain, which shows absence of elastic fibers in the granulomatous zone. Closer inspection shows that collagenous fibers also are absent, digested, or absorbed. (3) Granulomatous inflammation cannot heal without leaving some trace, either as a defect or, more commonly, in the form of fibrosis and scar formation. These sequelae do not presuppose gross tissue necrosis such as we see in caseation, gummatous liquefaction, or abscess formation. The granulomatous infiltrate itself destroys tissue. The loss is temporarily hidden by the productive inflammation, which actually makes an excess of tissue. The loss becomes obvious only when the granulomatous process heals, either spontaneously or under treatment. Clinical and histologic features of granulomatous dermatoses become more meaningful if these facts are kept in mind.

The details of granulomatous tissue reaction vary widely, and that enables the histopathologist in many cases to make a fairly accurate diagnosis of specific disease even if he cannot demonstrate the responsible agent, be it a microorganism or some nonliving substance. There is considerable overlap between tissue reactions in various diseases, however, and one should always attempt to demonstrate a specific organism or other causative agent in the tissue for definitive diagnosis. On the other hand, in some cases the very absence of a demonstrable agent aids in the classification.

Once one has recognized the histologic picture in a section as being granulomatous inflammation, it is convenient to put it into one of two broad classes. One of these comprises processes that consist almost exclusively of round cells, epithelioid cells, and multinucleated giant cells. In this group are the major three old diseases: syphilis, tuberculosis, and leprosy. To these one must add less common and more recently recognized entities, such as sarcoidosis, leishmaniasis, histoplasmosis, and some foreign body granulomas. The other class is characterized by a mixed infiltrate in which neutrophilic leukocytes and eosinophils are added to round cells and histiocytic elements. In this group are most of the deep fungous infections, granulomatous halogen eruptions, and quite a few foreign body granulomas. Granulomatous lesions associated with large vessels have some special characteristics, and these are touched on in Chapter 15.

In the title of this section, we included granulomatous proliferation: this refers to lesions of almost purely macrophagic histiocytic character to which the concept of inflammation does not really apply. They comprise xanthomas and other processes that are not considered true neoplasms precisely because they consist of histiocytes and are reversible in many cases. From this group has been split off "histiocytosis X."

REFERENCES

1. Van Furth R, Cohn ZA, Hirsch JG, et al: The mononuclear phagocytic system: A new classification of macrophages, monocytes and their precursor cells. Bull WHO 46:845, 1972
2. Ringel R, Moschella S: Primary histiocytic dermatoses. Arch Dermatol 121:1531, 1985
3. Lachapelle JM: Comparative study of ³H-thymidine labelling of the dermal infiltrate of skin allergic and irritant patch test reactions in man. Br J Dermatol 87: 460, 1972
4. Meuret G, Schmitt E, Hagedorn M: Monocytopoiesis in chronic eczematous diseases, psoriasis vulgaris, and mycosis fungoides. J Invest Dermatol 66:22, 1976
5. Epstein WL: The pathogenesis of granulomatous hypersensitivity: Newer observations. J Dermatol Tokyo 9: 335, 1982
6. Hirsh BC, Johnson WC: Pathology of granulomatous diseases. Int J Dermatol 23:237, 1984
7. Hirsh BC, Johnson WC: Pathology of granulomatous diseases. Epithelioid granulomas Part II. Int J Dermatol 23:306, 1984
8. Hirsh BC, Johnson WC: Pathology of granulomatous diseases. Histiocytic granulomas. Int J Dermatol 23: 383, 1984
9. Hirsh BC, Johnson WC: Pathology of granulomatous diseases. Foreign body granulomas. Int J Dermatol 23: 531, 1984

21

PREDOMINANTLY MONONUCLEAR GRANULOMAS

TUBERCULOSIS

Predominantly mononuclear granulomas include disease entities in which the infiltrate consists entirely of purely secretory mononuclear cells, resulting in formation of organized epithelioid cell granuloma. Of the diagnoses listed in Table 21–1, tuberculosis remains didactically most important in spite of the fact that cutaneous tuberculosis is rare in the United States. A change in the pattern of cutaneous tuberculosis has been reported in Asiatic countries.[1] A number of cases with papulonecrotic tuberculids have been reported.[2–4] Another development is the occurrence of tuberculosis among individuals with acquired immunodeficiency syndrome.[5]

Biology

The significance of tuberculosis for biologically based teaching of histopathology rests on several facts. The disease is due to a well-defined organism, which can be cultured and to which a number of animal species are susceptible. It was a very common disease in the days when bacteriology and immunology developed and was intensively studied. Thus, the results of many animal experiments are available in addition to wide clinical experience.

It soon became clear that the result of infection of man or animal with the tubercle bacillus depended on six interacting factors: number and virulence of the bacilli, mode and site of inoculation, and native resistance and immunologic response of the host. Their multifarious combination produces a variety of clinical and histologic pictures.

That the number of bacilli matters can be shown easily in the guinea pig, which is so highly susceptible to human bacilli. More or less virulent strains have been identified by microbiologists, and there is little doubt that the result of an intradermal inoculation will differ from that of an intravenous injection in the animal. The significance of mode and site for cutaneous disease of man is discussed later. It is also well known that animal species vary greatly in their native resistance, and within the human species, individual susceptibility is obviously different even in the same family. Where histopathologic examination is concerned, however, we find again, as in many previous chapters, that tissue response is the basis of our diagnosis, and although tissue response is the product of all the variables mentioned, it depends mainly on the immunologic state of the individual at the time the presenting lesion developed.

The tubercle bacillus does not produce a toxin. Large quantities of dead bacilli can be inoculated into a virgin organism without inflammatory re-

TABLE 21–1. MONONUCLEAR GRANULOMAS

	Histiocytes	Lymphocytes	Plasma Cells	Layering	Caseation	Seat	Identifiable Causative Agents
Infectious diseases						Superficial to deep	Acid-fast bacilli + to 0
Tuberculosis	(+) to +++	+ to +++	−	++	0 to (+)		
Leprosy, lepromatous	++	+	(+)	(+)	0	Variable, perineural	Acid-fast bacilli ++ to ++++
Leprosy, tuberculoid	+++	+	(+)	+	0	Variable, perineural	Acid-fast bacilli (+) to 0
Late syphilis	++	++	++	(+)	+ to +++	Deep	None
Sarcoidosis	++++	0 to +	−	+	(+)	Superficial and deep	None
Histoplasmosis	+++	+	−	−	0	Medium	Intracellular bodies
Leishmaniasis, early	+++	++	+	+	0	Superficial	Intracellular bodies (Donovan)
Leishmaniasis, late	+++	+	−	++	0	Superficial to mid-dermis	None
Tularemia	+++	+	+	+	+	Variable	None
Rhinoscleroma	+	+	++	−	−	Variable	Frisch bacilli
Foreign body Granulomas							
Paraffinoma	++++	(+)	−	−	0	Deep	Empty spaces
Silica granuloma	++++	+	−	−	0	Variable	Polarizing crystals
Zirconium granuloma	++	++	−	+	0 to (+)	Superficial	None
Beryllium granuloma	+++	+	−	+	+++	Variable	None

sponse. A few living bacilli are apt to provoke a response, however. The response develops slowly and depends on the initiation of an immune reaction, usually one of hypersensitivity.

In order to understand this thoroughly, it is pertinent to be aware of Robert Koch's original experiment. If living bacilli are inoculated into a scratch in the skin of an animal that has never been exposed, a barely noticeable traumatic reaction will take place. Otherwise, nothing obvious happens for 1 to 2 weeks. Then, a subacute type of inflammation sets in, and an ulcer develops, which usually persists until the death of the animal. Local lymph nodes become infected, and generalization of the disease into various organs leads to death. If, however, the inoculation is repeated at a different site in an already diseased but not yet marasmic animal, there will be a stormy local reaction with tissue necrosis and acute inflammatory response. This wound will heal in spite of the fact that the animal succumbs to its general infection.

Histologically, after the first few days, the slowly developing primary inflammatory response consists of lymphocytes and increasing numbers of histiocytic macrophages, which engulf the numerous and proliferating bacilli. The histiocytic, granulomatous response to the primary inoculation is never enough to destroy all bacilli, and in the undermining ulcer of the dying animal, bacilli multiply again and may be found in masses among a nonspecific inflammatory infiltrate. Quite in contrast, the second inoculation provokes a massive polymorphonuclear exudate within 24 hours that is associated with tissue necrosis and leads to the mechanical elimination of most of the inoculum. The remaining bacilli are gradually destroyed in tuberculoid granulomatous infiltrate.

This basic experiment of Koch, which was repeated, examined histologically, and interpreted in immunologic terms by Lewandowsky, provides the biologic basis for analysis not only of the many clinical and histologic variants of cutaneous tuberculosis but of other chronic granulomatous infections as well. It plainly shows that the tubercle bacillus is but a bland foreign body to the not previously exposed host. The living bacillus, however, has the power to provoke an immunologic response that may take many forms, from polymorphonuclear exudate to round cell infiltrate, to epithelioid cell response, and to acute tissue necrosis. Jadassohn–Ledwandowsky's law was formulated on this basis: Where microorganisms proliferate in the tissues unchecked by immunologic processes, only nonspecific inflammatory infiltrate will be found. Where immunologic power is strong, development of histiocytic, and particularly of epithelioid, cell response leads to reduction and disappearance of the bacilli. Unusually high sensitivity to bacterial products may lead to primary tissue necrosis with secondary tuberculoid response. It also should be emphasized that anergic nonspecific inflammation is found at the beginning and at the end. It characterizes the tissue reaction before immunity develops in the virgin host and after it has been exhausted in the marasmic host.

Tuberculodermas

On the basis of this discussion, we can tabulate tuberculodermas by correlating their histologic features with the immunologic state of the patient and the site of inoculation, as shown in Table 21–2.

Primary Tuberculosis

As with animals, inoculation of the skin of a noninfected human being results in a chain of events quite different from any caused by superinfection. A primary complex (tuberculous chancre) of local lesion and satellite lymphadenopathy develops similar to that in the lung. There is little doubt that the first histologic stages are just as nonspecific as those in the guinea pig's skin, but biopsies of this type of lesion are usually not taken until lack of healing and swelling of lymph nodes arouse suspicion.[6] At that time, several weeks after inoculation, a more or less well-developed epithelioid cell and lymphocyte response is found similar to that in lupus vulgaris. The tuberculoid response often is associated with ulceration, and acid-fast bacilli may be demonstrable. Congenital tuberculosis may show erythematous papular and necrotic lesions, appearing soon after birth. In very young infants with poor immunologic ability, the ulcer may develop progressively, and death from generalized infection may result just as in the guinea pig. In older individuals the primary site may heal with fibrosis and scarring, or it may turn into and persist as lupus vulgaris.

Lupus Vulgaris

Tuberculosis luposa (Fig. 21–1) is the prototype of chronic tuberculoderma in a previously infected individual. The patient usually has a moderate to high degree of immunity,[7] and it is rare to find lupus vulgaris in tuberculosis sanitaria. The histologic picture is characterized by epithelioid cell nodules embedded in shells of lymphocytes (tubercles).[8] Multinucleated giant cells may be sparse or more numerous and usually are typical Langhans cells. Plasma cells, eosinophils, and neutrophilic polymorphonuclears are absent or rare. The quantitative relation of epithelioid cells and lymphocytes varies. In some cases, one sees only a few histiocytic nodules in the sea of small round cells. In other cases, there are thin rims of lymphocytes around conglomerate tubercles, a picture very similar to *sarcoidosis*.[9] Concentric layering of the tubercles is better developed in tuberculosis than in any of the other granulomatous diseases, but one may encounter a more diffuse scattering of round cells in the nodes. The notorious avascularity of tuberculous infiltrate is difficult to

TABLE 21–2. TUBERCULODERMAS

A. Primary tuberculosis (tuberculous chancre)
B. Chronic lesions in host with relatively high immunity
  1. Lupus vulgaris
  2. Warty tuberculosis
  3. Lupus tumidus
  4. Tuberculosis verrucosa cutis
  5. Scrofuloderma
C. Spontaneously involuting lesions in hypersensitive host (tuberculids)
  1. Lichen scrofulosorum
  2. Papulonecrotic tuberculid
  3. Erythema induratum
D. Progressive lesions in host with low immunity
  1. Acute miliary tuberculosis
  2. Tuberculosis orificialis

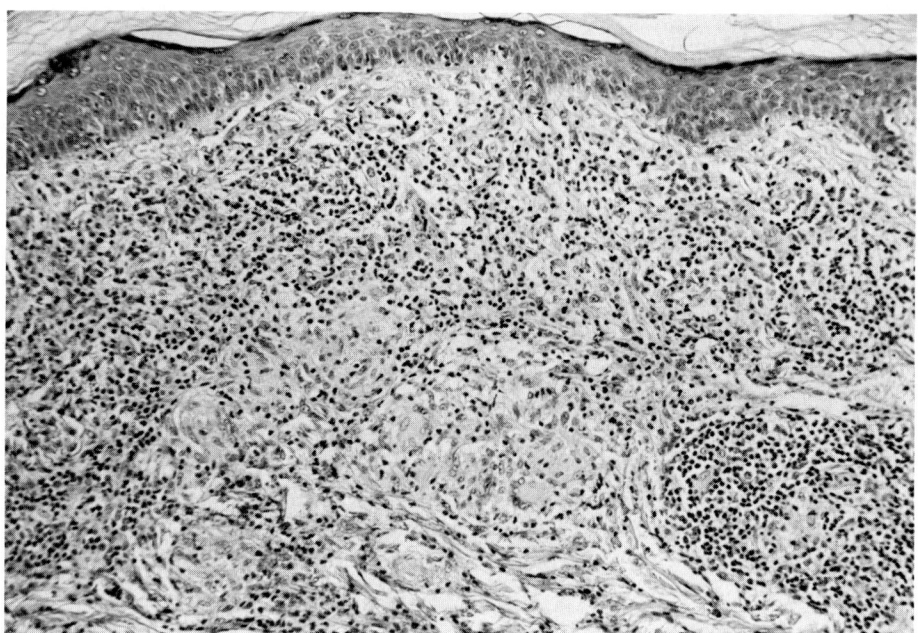

Figure 21-1.
Lupus vulgaris. Nodules of epithelioid cells and small round cells furnish approximately equal portions of the infiltrate that borders on the epidermis. At least one Langhans type giant cell is seen. H&E. X135.

judge in the skin because the mass of tuberculous tissue is not very great, and the rich cutaneous vasculature persists between the nodes. Caseation is practically unheard of in tuberculodermas.

The specific infiltrate usually occupies the upper part of the dermis in lupus vulgaris, but larger or smaller masses may be found deeper. The infiltrate borders on the epidermis from below, often thinning it, but rarely producing ulceration. The superficial seat of the granuloma, which differentiates tuberculosis from syphilis, is the basis of the clinical probe test. Firm pressure will make a blunt probe break through the epidermis and penetrate the soft granulomatous tissue. This test also makes obvious that the normal dermis has been destroyed and replaced by the infiltrate. When lupus vulgaris heals, either spontaneously or under treatment, it leaves a void that is replaced by fibrosis or leads to atrophic scars. Histologically, just as clinically, it is characteristic for the disease to show persistent or recurrent tubercles in the fibrotic areas. It is a thankless task to look for acid-fast bacilli in sections of lupus vulgaris, although modern staining methods may lead to success. Culture and animal inoculation must be used to demonstrate the microorganism, which may be of the bovine type. Differential diagnosis includes the late stage of oriental leishmaniasis.

Lupus Tumidus and Warty Tuberculosis

In contrast to the classic atrophying form leading to the peaked nose, the shrunken lips, and the everted eyelids of the lupus patient's face, there is another form of tuberculosis luposa that is particularly common in the American black. *Lupus tumidus* produces large circumscribed swellings that look like keloids but are peculiarly soft to the touch. Histologically, there are masses of well-layered tubercles. In this form, plasma cells are commonly found between the lymphocytes around and between the epithelioid nodes.

Another form of lupus vulgaris (warty tuberculosis) involves distal parts of the extremities and is histologically associated with significant epidermal hyperplasia forming a verrucous lesion.

Tuberculosis Verrucosa Cutis

This form is usually due to exogenous superinfection in individuals with a high degree of immunity.[10] Butchers' and pathologists' warts are classic examples. Due partly to the immunologic background and partly to the specific terrain of the acral skin, there is a strong tendency to verrucous epidermal hyperplasia and to fibrosis in these lesions. Tuberculoid tissue may have to be searched for and is usually found just below the epidermis. Presence of bacilli must be demonstrated by culture or animal test.

Scrofuloderma

The histologic picture of scrofuloderma is influenced by its peculiar pathomechanism of massive infection by contiguity from underlying lymph nodes. Tuberculoid reaction usually is mixed with nonspecific inflammation in an open and deep sinus. Acid-fast bacilli are more apt to be demonstrable in this tuberculosis cutis colliquativa than in other members of the group.

Tuberculids

The concept of tuberculids was introduced by Darier more than 90 years ago and, in somewhat modified form, was supported by vast clinical evidence over many years, although the clinching postulate of demonstration of the causative agent in the lesion could not be fulfilled. This was attributed to the basic concept that tuberculids are due to the hematogenous lodging of small numbers of bacilli in cutaneous vessels evoking an Arthus reaction in a highly tuberculin-sensitive individual.[11] According to the hypothesis, the embolus of bacilli that either are dead on arrival or are quickly overcome by tissue immunity acts like a tuberculin injection, and the details of the tissue response depend on the site and size of the vessel involved and the balance between sensitivity and immunity of the individual. Criteria for diagnosis of tuberculids include positive tuberculin test, the presence of tuberculosis elsewhere, and good response to antituberculous medications.[12]

Lichen Scrofulosorum

Groups of closely set minute perifollicular lichenoid papules occur mostly over the trunk and heal without scar. The lichenoid tuberculid (Fig. 21–2), results if small perifollicular vessels are involved and the number of bacilli or degree of sensitivity is not large enough to produce tissue necrosis. It has been seen after BCG inoculation in response to the depot of tuberculin that a more or less pronounced tuberculoid granulomatous reaction will develop in perifollicular localization. Early stages may show mainly lymphocytes, fully developed lesions, epithelioid cells, and giant cells, and late stages will show fibrosis. The lesion heals spontaneously in a few weeks, and a biopsy site must be chosen judiciously for best results. Too young a lesion may show noncharacteristic inflammatory infiltrate. Several illustrative cases associated with active tuberculosis and well responding to antituberculous treatment have been reported.[13,14]

Differential diagnosis from papular lesions of late secondary syphilis may not always be possible. Somewhat deeper localization and presence of plasma cells suggest syphilis. Some of the cases reported as micropapular sarcoidosis, lichen scrofulosorum, and lichenoid tuberculid are probably the same condition.[15]

Papulonecrotic Tuberculid

Children and young women are primarily affected with inflammatory papules that become pustular and necrotic forming discrete crusted ulcers. Hands and feet are most common locations.[2,3] There are also a number of cases involving lesions of glans penis.[4] Histologically, when the involved vessel or the number of bacilli is larger and the sensitivity high, the bacillary embolus will produce primary tis-

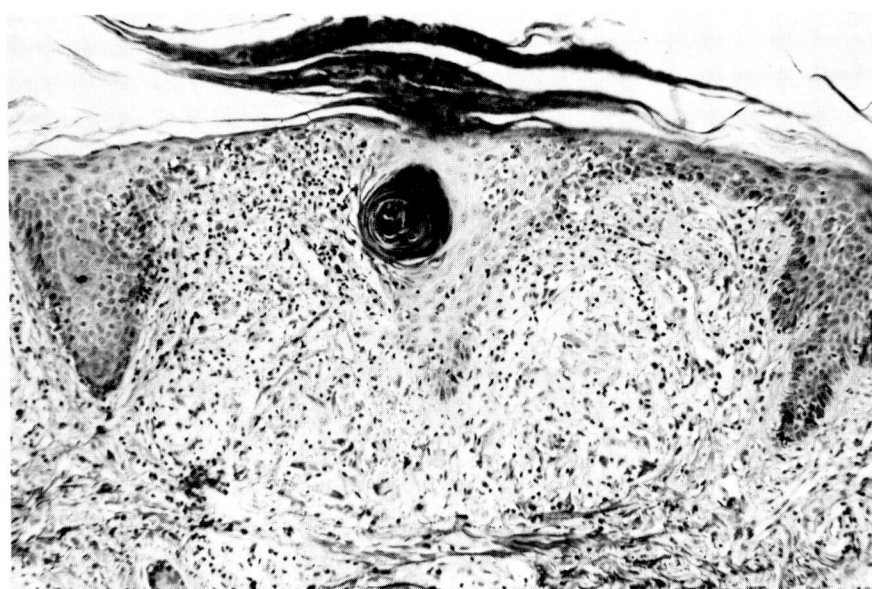

Figure 21–2.
Lichen scrofulosorum. Note destruction of elastic fibers by relatively mild granulomatous infiltrate. The epithelial structures are affected secondarily and have reacted with parakeratosis on the epidermal surface and in the follicular infundibulum. O&G. X135.

sue necrosis similar to that produced by an overdose of intradermal tuberculin. The often wedge-shaped necrotic tissue becomes surrounded by histiocytes and lymphocytes, which usually assume a tuberculoid configuration (Fig. 21–3). Eventually, the necrotic plug is sequestered and eliminated to the outside, and the characteristic punched-out scar results. It is important to realize that necrosis in this case is not caseation but is primary necrosis of healthy tissue. The granuloma develops secondarily. Therefore, an elastic fiber stain will show persistence of elastic fibers in the central necrosis, whereas these are destroyed in the peripheral granuloma. A comparison of Figures 21–3 and 13–7 shows the fundamental difference of the histomechanisms of papulonecrotic tuberculid and acute pityriasis lichenoides, which may come into clinical differential diagnosis, although the random distribution of lesions is quite different from the localization of the tuberculid on the extensor surfaces of the extremities. If necrosis is less complete and granulomatous response less severe, clinical sloughing may be absent, and the histologic picture may be remarkably similar to granuloma annulare.

Erythema Induratum
Bazin's disease has become extremely rare, not only because the prevalence of tuberculosis has decreased but also because better nutrition and change of living habits have almost eliminated the flabby and anemic, pasty young girl who was its principal victim. It is, however, by no means extinct.[16] The term erythema induratum is now often used loosely for chronic nodose lesions of the lower extremities, which histologically belong to the group of nodular vasculitis. The tuberculous form (Bazin's disease) supposedly results from involvement of a subcutaneous vein with a hyperergic tuberculous inflammation. The tissue reaction in erythema induratum is modified by the reaction to damaged fat tissue, the proliferating atrophy discussed in Chapter 16. This stereotyped response of the damaged panniculus often overshadows the typical tuberculoid response. Furthermore, as pointed out in the discussion on panniculitis, it is difficult to find the initial focus in a large and often ulcerated lesion. Unless the pathologist is lucky enough to find typical tubercles, he must be content with calling the changes compatible with erythema induratum and must ask the clinician to validate the diagnosis by the results of other examinations.

Lupus Miliaris Disseminatus Faciei Rosacea-Like Tuberculid (Lewandowsky)
We discuss here a facial eruption that histologically comes into differential diagnosis of tuberculids but is no longer considered as a tuberculoderma because of the constant absence of bacilli and lack of evidence of systemic tuberculosis. The eruption consists of dome-shaped papules with a yellow center giving

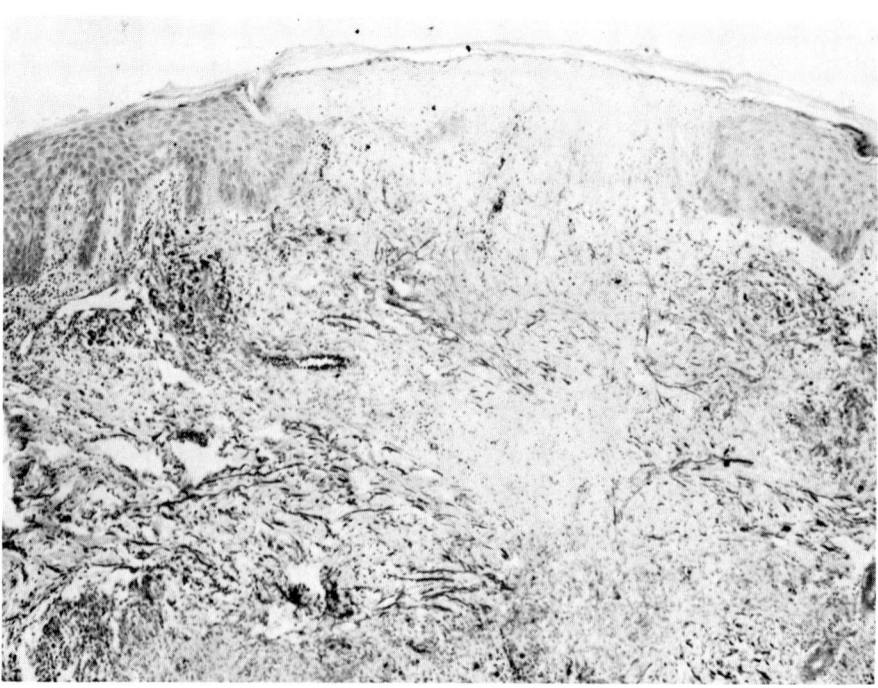

Figure 21–3.
Papulonecrotic tuberculid. Necrosis of epidermis and dermis with preservation of elastic fibers. The latter are partly destroyed in granulomatous infiltrate surrounding primary necrosis. O&G. X75.

the false impression of pustular lesions. The facial lesions heal spontaneously with formation of scars.

The histologic picture is highly characteristic. A combination of a well-developed epithelioid cell granuloma with a number of multinucleated giant cells surrounding a well-defined area of caseation necrosis permits the histologic diagnosis of lupus miliaris disseminatus faciei (Fig. 21–4), and this diagnosis should be made only in the presence of caseation. O&G stain usually will show a neat ring of elastic fibers in the center of the caseous material. It is more likely that this ring is part of the isthmus of a hair follicle that is completely degenerated and is no longer recognized. Relationship between the epithelioid cell granuloma and the pilosebaceous structures has been documented in 43% of the cases.[17]

Progressive Lesions in a Host with Low Immunity

A patient who is anergic as a result of never having been exposed to tubercle bacilli will respond with nonspecific inflammation to proliferating organisms, and a similar response may be all a patient can produce whose immunologic powers have been overwhelmed or exhausted (secondary anergy). A situation of this type develops in miliary tuberculosis or in far-progressed involvement of lungs or bowels when large numbers of bacilli reach the skin through hematogenous dissemination or direct inoculation from infected discharges.

Miliary tuberculosis of the skin does not differ much from that of other organs in its histologic expression. Numerous bacilli can be demonstrated in an infiltrate of lymphocytes with the barest indication of granulomatous reaction.[18]

Tuberculosis orificialis also often presents only polymorphonuclear and round cell infiltrate in the bottom of the ulcers that develop in oral mucosa or anal skin. However, depending on the degree of immunologic resistance left in the patient, a variable amount of epithelioid cell response may be found. The number of demonstrable bacilli varies in inverse relation.

LEPROSY (HANSEN'S DISEASE)

Leprosy, another disease caused by an acid-fast bacillus, is remarkable for the similarities and the differences of the tissue reactions encountered.[19] The immunologically stable *tuberculoid leprosy* follows Lewandowsky's law and exhibits a strong epithelioid cell tissue reaction (Fig. 21–5B), in which few or no bacilli can be demonstrated. The picture of this type of Hansen's disease may be so similar to that of sarcoidosis that it offers diagnostic difficulties. On the other hand, the *lepromatous* type, in which bacilli are numerous and tissue immunity is low, far from having nonspecific inflammatory infiltrate, also shows a highly characteristic picture (Fig. 21–6A) in which nodular accumulations of histiocytes predominate. These, however, do not have the character of epithelioid cells but look foamy (Table 21–3) because they contain large quantities of bacilli (Fig. 21–6B) and also nonpolarizing lipids. "Lepra cells," also called "Virchow cells," may be considered a special type of foreign body reaction rather than an expression of immunity.

The pathogenesis and etiology of the various forms of leprosy are much less clear than those of tuberculosis because of our inability to culture the bacillus in vitro and because of the unavailability of experimental animals. Both of these hindrances seem to be overcome by reports of cultivation of lep-

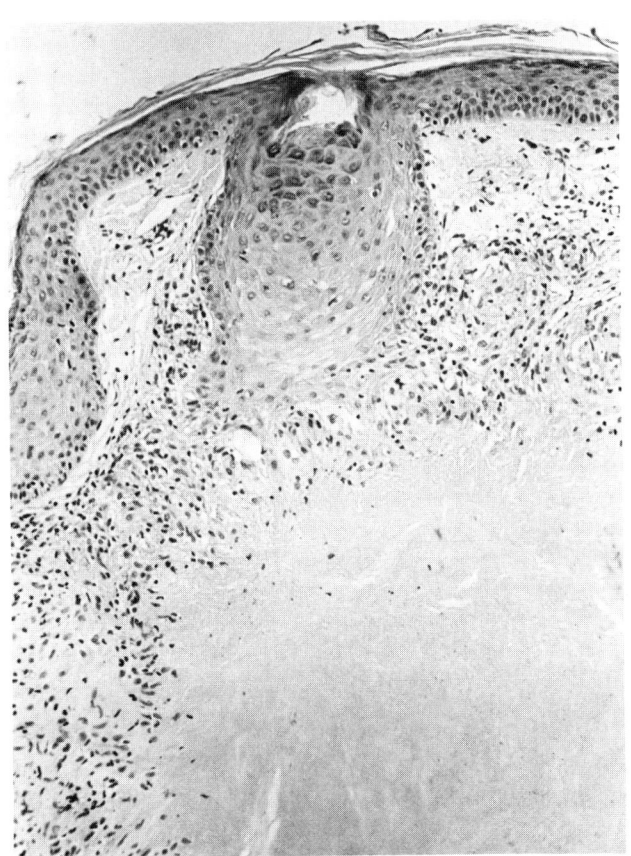

Figure 21–4.
Lupus miliaris disseminatus faciei. H&E. X125.

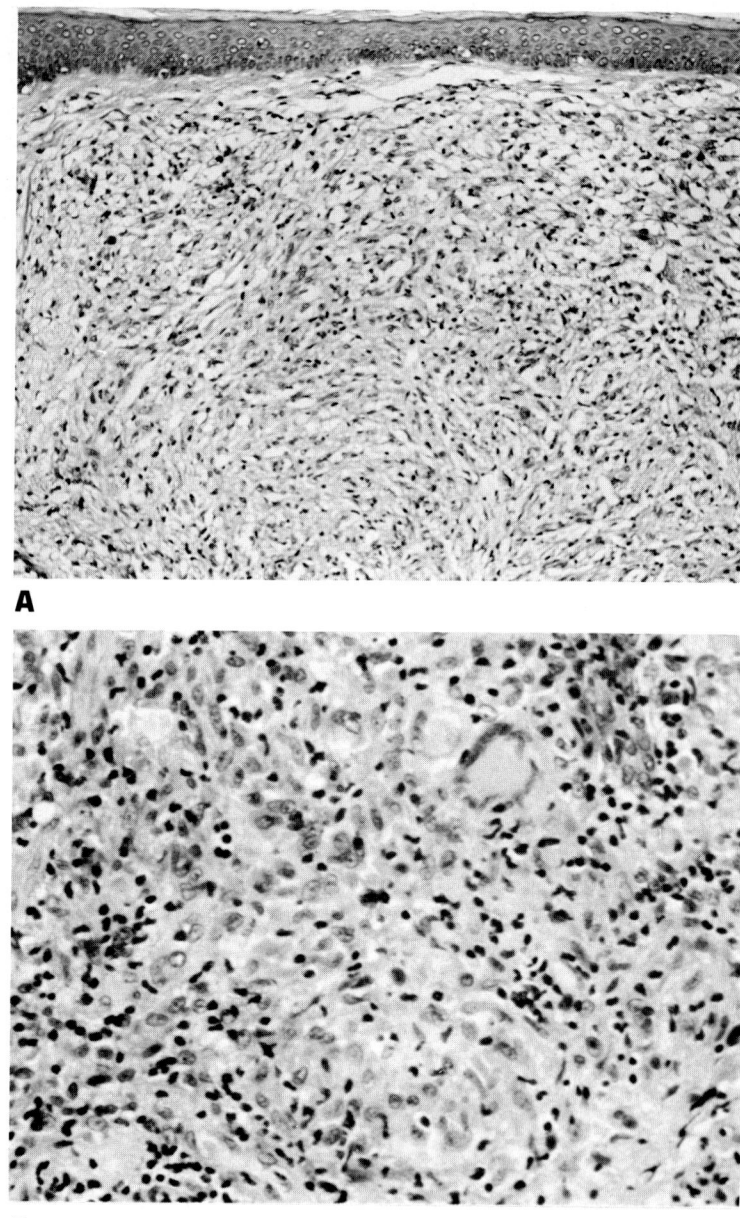

Figure 21–5.
Hansen's disease. **A.** Histoid form consisting of histiocytes between collagenous fibers. **B.** Tuberculoid type. H&E. X250.

rosy bacilli on hyaluronic acid-containing media and by inoculation of mouse footpads and production of the disease in armadillos.[20]

The various classifications of lepromatous lesions also seem to have come to a consensus in recent years[21,22] in the division of the disease into two polar forms, the lepromatous and the tuberculoid, and having these bridged by borderline lesions, which vary from BL (borderline lepromatous) to BB (borderline-borderline) to BT (borderline tuberculid).

Histologically, one can understand the findings better by remembering that the bacillus primarily involves nerves and, in the nerves, Schwann cells, which phagocytize it and harbor it. The rest seems to depend on the ability of the host to react. If cell-mediated immunity remains low and no positive Mitsuda reaction develops in the lepromatous form, tissue macrophages will take up the proliferating rods and will become filled with clusters and globes of bacilli.[23] On the other hand, if tissue immunity develops, histiocytes will destroy bacilli and will

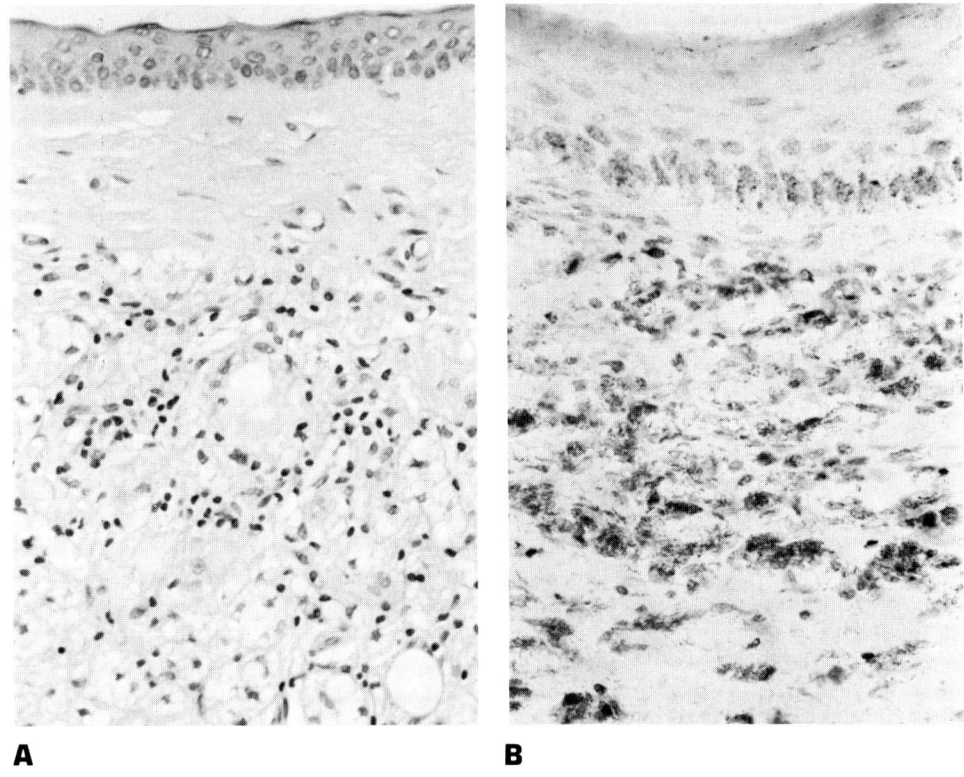

Figure 21-6.
Lepromatous leprosy. **A.** H&E stain shows large foamy histiocytes (Virchow cells) and some lymphocytes. Compare with Figure 24-2, xanthoma cells. **B.** Fite stain shows innumerable acid-fast bacilli clumped in the histiocytes. X800.

form epithelioid tubercles. The aim of the pathologist will have to be to prove or disprove involvement of nerves, and that requires a sizable and deep-reaching biopsy specimen that must include subcutaneous tissue or biopsy of a palpably affected nerve. In lepromatous leprosy, there usually remains a narrow, free, subepidermal grenz zone, whereas the infiltrate presses against the epidermis in tuberculoid cases.

In borderline lesions, all shadings from the lepromatous to the tuberculoid form are represented. It is, of course, often advisable to search for bacilli by scraping incised skin and doing acid-fast stain on the smears. A technical note must be added: to stain for tubercle bacilli by any one of the modifications of the Ziehl–Neelsen method is easy. Hansen's bacilli (Fig. 21–6B) are much less acid-fast, however, and great care must be taken not to decolorize the bacilli in the acid–alcohol bath. Otherwise, false negative results will be obtained. Many modifications and different stains have been developed because of this difficulty. In laboratories that do not have much experience in this field, one must insist that the technician use lepromatous tissue rather than tuberculous tissue as the positive control.

Reactional states seem to be related to shifts of tissue immunity, sometimes in the course of treatment, and involve fairly acute flare-ups of lesions. Exacerbation of the disease process is the so-called "lepra reaction" in lepromatous leprosy. Another manifestation is *erythema nodosum leprosum,* which leads to painful nodular lesions in which many bacilli are granular and degenerating. The histologic picture differs decisively from ordinary erythema nodosum.

The Lucio phenomenon represents a necrotizing vasculitis with many bacilli in cases of diffuse leprosy in which the entire skin is affected.[24,25] It leads to superficial ulcers. *Histoid leprosy* (Fig. 21–5A) has been described as showing tumorous collections of histiocytes separated by dense collagen fibers deep in the dermis. The histiocytes range from unmodified to foamy cells containing many bacilli. The clinical lesions are protuberant nodules, often

TABLE 21–3. MICROORGANISMS FOUND IN MONONUCLEAR CELLS IN GRANULOMAS

Disease	Clinical Type	Organisms	Stain	Size
Leprosy	Lepromatous	Mycobacterium leprae Hansen bacilli in Virchow (foam) cells	Fite modification of acid-fast stain	2–8 μm by 0.2–0.5 μm
Tuberculosis	Scrofuloderma and anergic types	Mycobacterium tuberculosis	Acid-fast	1–4 μm by 0.3–0.6 μm
Rhinoscleroma	Granulomatous ulcer	Klebsiella rhinoscleromatis (Frisch bacilli in Mikulicz cells)	Giemsa, PAS, gram-negative	2–5 μm by 0.5 μm
Granuloma inguinale	Semidenuded granulomas	Donovania granulomatis (Donovan bodies)	H&E, Giemsa gram-negative	1–2 μm
Histoplasmosis	Granulomatous ulcer	Histoplasma capsulatum	H&E, Giemsa, PAS	2–4 μm encapsulated
Histoplasmosis, African	Lymphatic involvement	Histoplasma capsulatum duboisii	H&E, PAS	8–15 μm
Leishmaniasis, Oriental	Early granuloma (oriental sore, Aleppo boil, etc.)	Leishmania tropica (Donovan bodies)	H&E, Giemsa	2–4 μm
Leishmaniasis, American	Granulomatous ulcer	Leishmania braziliensis	H&E, Giemsa	2–4 μm
Leishmaniasis, post-kala-azar	Macular, erythematous, nodular	Leishmania donovani	H&E, Giemsa	2–4 μm
Malakoplakia	Granuloma	Michaelis–Gutmann body	H&E, von Kossa iron stain	10–16 μm

constricted at the base. This variant, found mainly in northern India,[26] is probably not a distinct entity but must be considered in differential diagnosis from neurofibromas.

Atypical Mycobacteria

An ever-increasing number of atypical acid-fast bacilli has been described. They may produce a great variety of inflammatory, purulent, or granulomatous tissue reactions, depending on their antigenicity and the individual immune reaction of the host. One must keep these microorganisms in mind whenever history or atypical clinical and histologic pictures are suggestive.[19,27] Infection by *Mycobacterium ulcerans* is mentioned in Chapter 17. In the United States, the most commonly encountered lesions (Fig. 21–7) are swimming pool or fish tank granulomas, caused by *Mycobacterium balnei* or *Mycobacterium marinum*.[28,29] Histologic findings in an early lesion consist of a nonspecific dermal infiltrate of lymphocytes, histiocytes, and neutrophils. Epithelioid cell granuloma will appear in older lesions. Histologic search for acid-fast organisms should be supplemented by cultures on appropriate media and at different temperatures.

SYPHILIS

The third of the large granulomatous diseases, syphilis, offers its own intriguing peculiarities, in part due to the very different nature of the infectious agent. It is well recognized that the motile *Treponema pallidum* is widely distributed in the body long before any inflammatory tissue reaction sets in. This fact, and the fairly regular sequence of primary, secondary, and tertiary manifestations are eloquent proof of the preeminent role of tissue immunity in the histologic reaction.

The hallmark of the syphilitic tissue reaction is the plasma cell. Otherwise, there is little similarity between massive inflammatory reaction of the chancre, the relatively mild vasculitis of the secondary exanthem, and the gummatous or tuberculoid granuloma of the tertiary stage. Plasma cells may be practically absent in some cases or may not be impressive in number. If, however, a skin lesion contains many plasma cells, the thought of syphilis should enter the examiner's mind and should be dismissed only if a different diagnosis can be established with certainty. At the present time, when the incidence of syphilis is on the rise and the level of

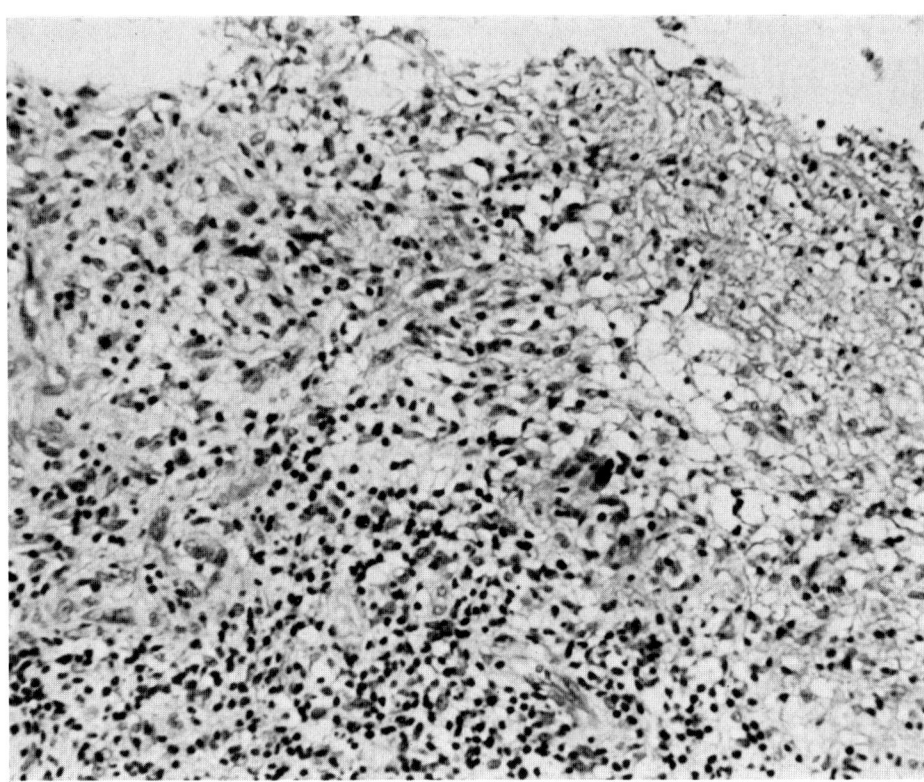

Figure 21-7.
Mycobacterium marinum infection (swimming pool or fishtank granuloma). Ulcerated surface and rather noncharacteristic granulomatous infiltrate H&E. X225.

suspicion of many clinicians is low, it is preferable to consider syphilis too often rather than to overlook it.

Primary Lesion

The primary lesion, the *chancre,* is not an ulcer but an induration.[30] Correspondingly (Fig. 21-8), the epidermis is present and often is acanthotic. It usually is highly edematous, invaded by inflammatory cells, and covered by a parakeratotic crust. This explains the clinical features of oozing and apparent denudation, but true erosion or an ulcer occurs only secondary to trauma or nonspecific infection. The underlying dermis is densely infiltrated with a mixture of lymphocytes and plasma cells. Other cell types may be present. The endothelial and peripheral cells of blood vessels are swollen and increased, and the lesion may assume features of both vasculitis and granulomatous inflammation. Silver stains will reveal treponemes in variable number, more commonly in the epidermis than in the dermis. Organisms, of course, will be absent if antibiotic therapy has been given before biopsy.

Secondary Lesion

Clinical manifestations may be macular, maculopapular, follicular, or psoriasi-form[31,32] (Fig. 21-9).

Depending on the severity of the clinical lesion, secondary syphilitic exanthems may show nothing but perivascular round cell infiltrate, resembling that of a drug eruption, or may present evidence of plasmocytic vasculitis. Invasion of the epidermis by round cells is common, as are edema and acanthosis. A peculiar washed-out appearance of the epidermis due to pale-staining nuclei and cytoplasm is fairly characteristic. Differential diagnosis among a drug eruption, psoriasis, pityriasis lichenoides chronica, reticulosis, and a papule of secondary syphilis may be difficult. A sarcoid tissue reaction[33] and a perifollicular reaction mimicking lichen scrofulosorum may be observed. Nodular lesions with heavy dermal infiltrate may resemble cutaneous lymphoma.[34,35] The presence of plasma cells speaks strongly for syphilis. Treponemes are few [36] and difficult to demonstrate except in condylomata lata, in which histologic reaction includes papillomatous epidermal hyperplasia and perivascular dermal infiltrate of lymphocytes and plasma cells.

Malignant ulcerative lesions develop in the secondary state in malnourished, alcoholic individuals[37] and also in diabetics and sometimes in a seemingly healthy person. Extensive tissue necrosis and deep ulcers may be present. Histologic examination usually reveals severe vasculitis and otherwise the

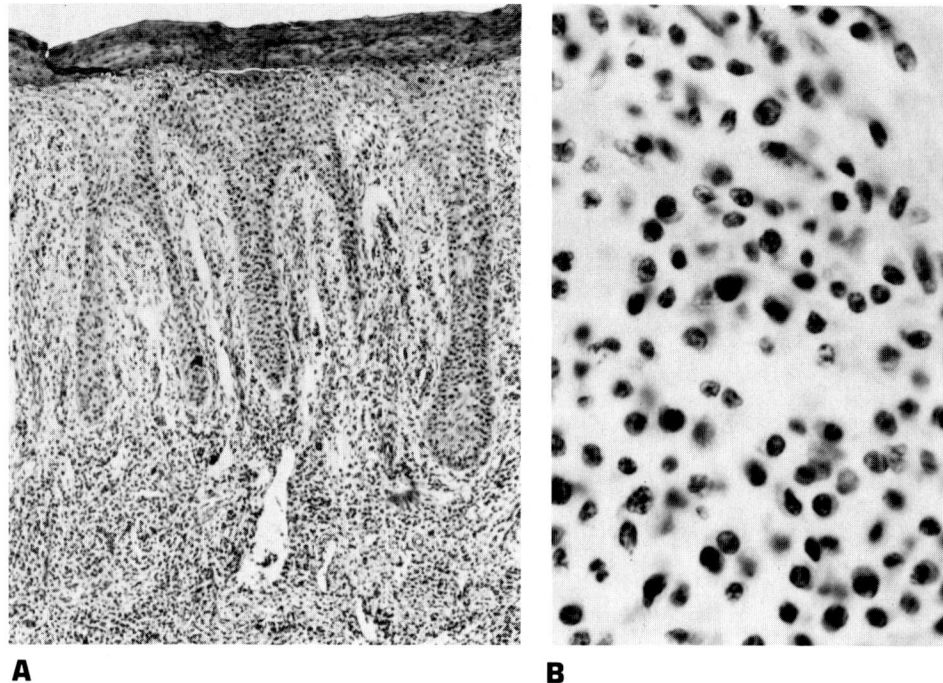

Figure 21–8.
Syphilitic chancre. **A.** H&E. X70. **B.** H&E. X600.

usual plasmocytic infiltrate, modified by tissue necrosis and ulceration. An interesting histologic variant is characterized by necrobiotic dermal changes and palisading granuloma resembling granuloma annulare but with a significant number of plasma cells.[38]

Tertiary Lesion

Later, secondary lesions may show pictures between that of early secondary and granulomatous *tertiary* syphilis. As far as the latter is concerned, the student must remember that the syphilitic gumma is

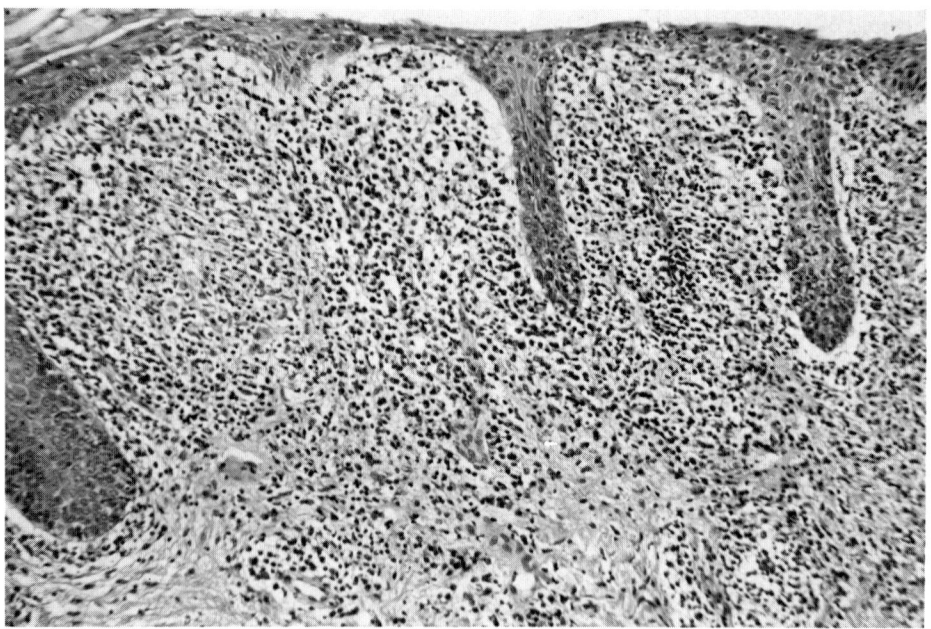

Figure 21–9.
Secondary syphilitic papule. This lesion presents heavier and more diffuse infiltrate than one would find in an early roseola. The large number of plasma cells speaks for syphilis. Note that the epidermis presents general hypoplasia combined with ridge hyperplasia and is invaded by round cells. H&E. X135.

only one, and not the most common, cutaneous manifestation. Superficial nodular and noduloulcerative lesions are encountered more frequently and are histologically characterized by a tuberculoid picture (Fig. 21–10) rather than by that of the gumma.[39] Recognition of the latter under the microscope (Fig. 21–11) actually is not easy because the necrotic center usually has fallen out during biopsy or tissue preparation, and the sections present only part of the granulomatous wall, which may resemble the granulomatous wall around a mucocele or a degenerated epithelial cyst. Again, presence of plasma cells and evidence of vasculitis speak for syphilis. One should also remember that other infections, especially sporotrichosis, produce gummatous lesions, and in differentiation from the latter, even the presence of plasma cells and vascular changes are not helpful.

Tuberculoid tissue reaction is frequently encountered in tertiary cutaneous syphilis.[40] Differentiation from tuberculosis is assisted by several factors. The center of gravity, high in the dermis in lupus vulgaris, is in deep dermis even in clinically superficial-looking syphilids. The neat layering of the tuberculous granuloma is usually absent. Giant cells, epithelioid cells, and round cells are mixed or may occur separated from each other. Plasma cells, common in syphilis, are rare in tuberculosis, except lupus tumidus. Areas of necrosis are much more frequent in syphilis. Perivascular arrangement of granulomatous nodes is of less significance. Epidermal hyperplasia, sometimes of pseudoepitheliomatous character, is often encountered in syphilis and is rare in tuberculosis.

Fibrosis as evidence of scar formation is almost always found in tertiary syphilis and is more evident in O&G stains because of absence of elastic fibers in the granulomatous as well as in fibrotic parts. This stain is helpful in syphilis also because it makes plasma cells stand out much more plainly and assures one of the absence of eosinophils, which are more common in fungous granulomas.

Another cutaneous manifestation of late syphilis, the juxta-articular node, is discussed along with other palisading granulomas in Chapter 23.

Other Treponematoses

Some unusual clinical forms of treponemal infection appear to be due to unfavorable socioeconomic circumstances rather than to different species of treponemes. These nonvenereal endemic types of syphilis are known as bejel and by other names.[41] *Yaws* (frambesia) and *pinta*, however, are caused by *Treponema pertenue* and *Treponema carateum*, respectively. Although morphologically indistinguishable from *T. pallidum*, these organisms are acknowledged as separate species, and tissue reactions present certain differences from syphilis. Lesions of yaws[42] exhibit more excessive epidermal and less definite vascular involvement. Pinta shows peculiar disturbances of melanization associated with basal cell liquefaction and macrophage pigmentation in the primary and secondary stages (Fig. 21–12) and epidermal atrophy in the late stages, thus having features of the poikilodermatous tissue reaction. A mixed infiltrate with a high percentage of plasma cells is found in all these affections.[43]

SARCOIDOSIS AND SARCOID REACTIONS

The word "sarcoid" means sarcoma-like and was used originally for a variety of lesions resembling

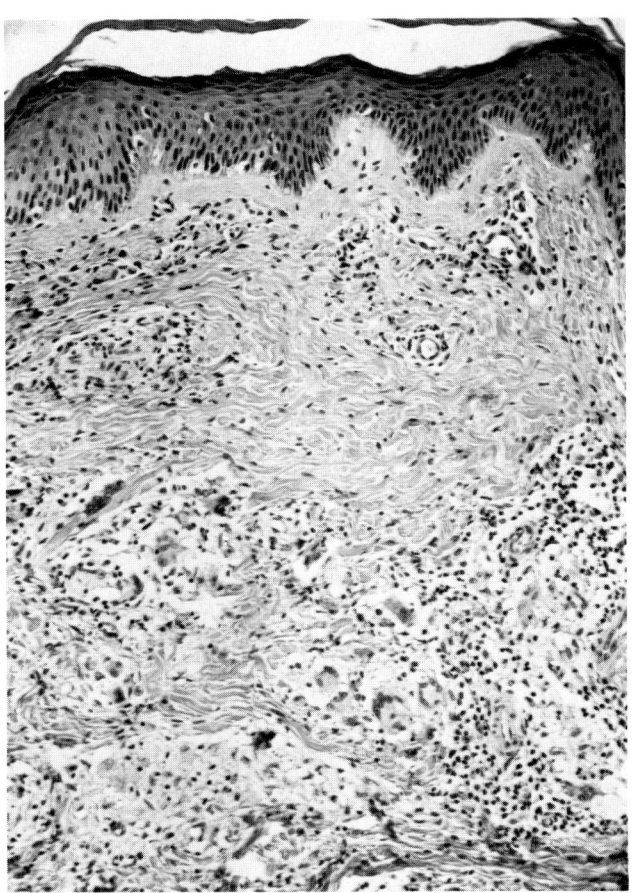

Figure 21–10.
Nodular tertiary syphilis. Disorganized tuberculoid infiltrate, predominantly in deep dermis. H&E. X135.

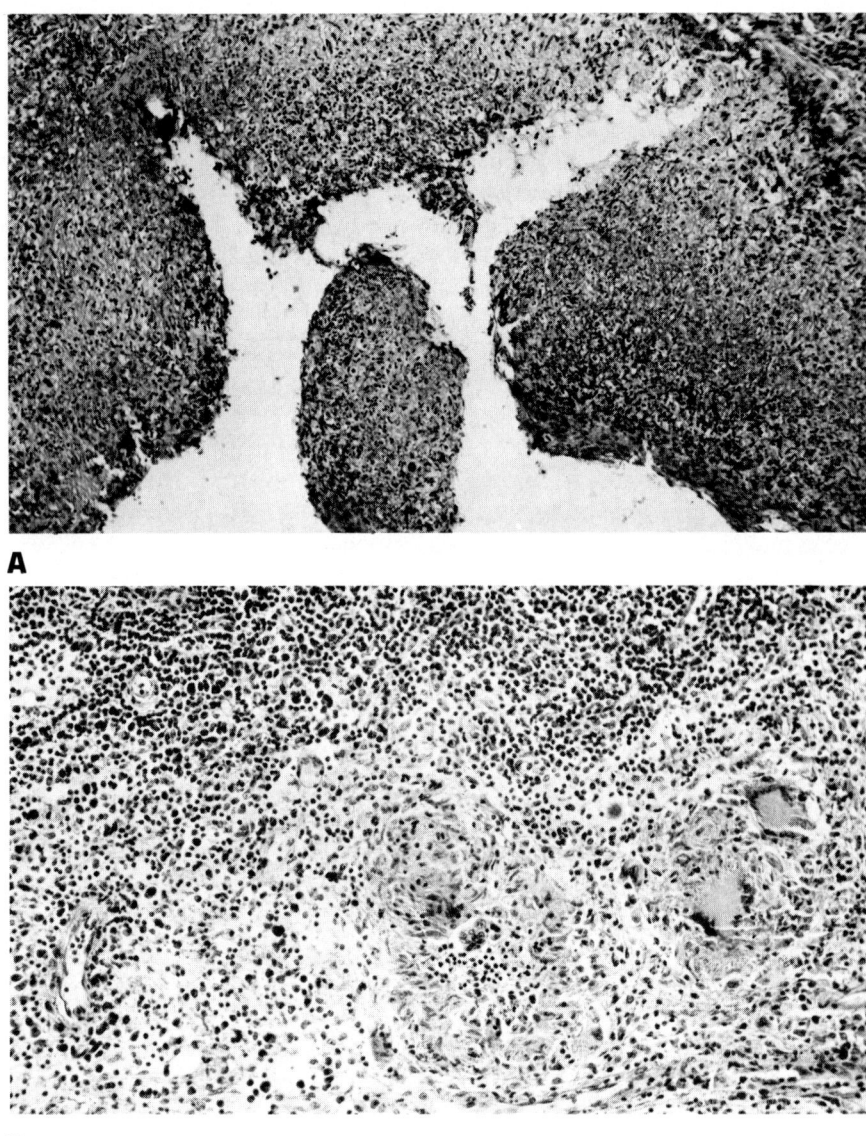

Figure 21–11.
Syphilitic gumma. **A.** Necrotic wall with surrounding granulomatous infiltrate. H&E. X135. **B.** Tuberculoid and plasma cell reaction. H&E. X185.

malignant mesodermal disease. Boeck applied the term to lesions that we now consider the cutaneous manifestations of the generalized disease called "sarcoidosis." Although there is no doubt that sarcoidosis is a distinct disease, it is true that the tissue reaction that we see under the microscope and that seems to be highly specific may actually be due to many different exciting agents ranging from microorganisms to nonliving organic and inorganic substances. The cautious pathologist, therefore, will usually make a diagnosis of sarcoid reaction or noncaseating granuloma unless a specific exciting agent is found in the tissue. It also seems that in this field the specific immunologic or quasi-immunologic status of the host is of utmost importance.

Sarcoid reaction (Fig. 21–13) is characterized by well-defined epithelioid cell nodes that may or may not have multinucleated giant cells of Langhans type. In the purest form, these tubercles lie naked in the tissue, but they may have thin shells of round cells, or round cells may be scattered between the epithelioid cells. Elastic fiber stain makes it obvious that these granulomatous masses have destroyed and replaced normal tissue. Occasionally asteroid bodies are present within multinucleated giant cells, some of which stain like elastotic material.

Sacroid reaction in the skin, if combined with clinical information, can be interpreted as sarcoidosis with reasonable confidence. One must be aware

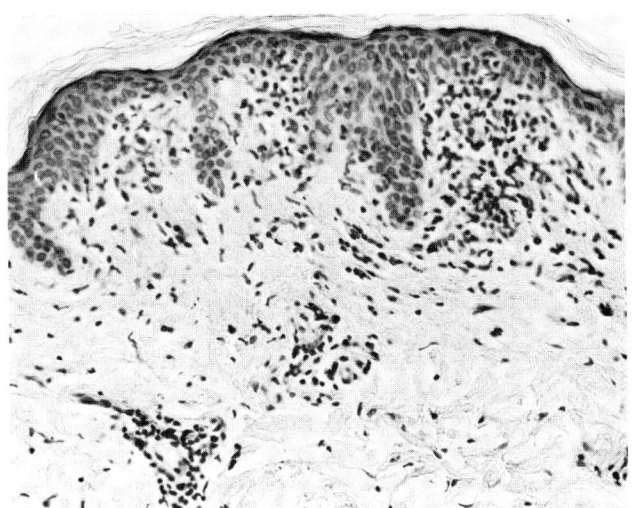

Figure 21–12.
Pinta. Secondary stage showing mild round cell and plasma cell infiltrate invading the epidermis and causing basal cell and melanocyte degeneration. Note resemblance to a lichenoid reaction. H&E. X250.

of pitfalls, however. The histologic pictures of lupus vulgaris and Boeck's sarcoid can merge. If one examines a series containing cases of both diseases, one can find almost any quantitative combination of epithelioid and round cells, and some cases may remain in doubt. Similarly, tuberculoid leprosy and sarcoidosis may look much alike. Involvement of nerves and hair muscles speaks for leprosy, involvement of the epidermis for sarcoidosis. Even syphilis may mimic sarcoidosis.

In order to rule out *silica granuloma,* one should examine every case of sarcoid reaction under polarized light. We have observed, however, cases in which the first biopsy specimen showed double refractile bodies, but the patient had proven sarcoidosis. It was ascertained that old scars had been biopsied, and the embedded silica from dirt probably had acted as localizing factor. Later specimens did not contain the foreign material. Cases of this type have been reported under scar sarcoidosis.[44] Similar observations have also been made in tattoos.[45] It must be remembered that other granuloma-producing substances are not birefringent and are less easily ruled out. The most common substances are beryllium and zirconium.

Cutaneous Sarcoidosis

The clinical picture of sarcoidosis of the skin is so variable that it is taking the place of syphilis in mimicking almost any other skin disease.[46] It ranges from lichenoid lesions to large nodules and may be erythrodermatous[47] and ichthyosiform.[48] It may rarely ulcerate.[49] Hypopigmented lesions in dark skin[50] can be sources of error.

Boeck's sarcoid shows epithelioid cell nodules or sausage-shaped masses mainly in the upper dermis. They usually do not approach the epidermis as massively as the tubercles of lupus vulgaris, but extend often somewhat deeper. Although lymphocytic shells often are present around the superficial nodules, the deeper ones tend to be naked epithelioid cell tubercles. Although in other organs, sarcoidosis is the prototype of noncaseating granuloma formation, in the skin, microscopic foci of central necrosis actually favor a diagnosis of sarcoidosis over lupus vulgaris.

In *Darier–Roussy's sarcoid* (Fig. 21–14), similar granulomas are found deep in the skin and often involve the subcutaneous tissue.[51,52] Variants of sarcoid, rarely seen in the United States, are lupus pernio and angiolupoid, which combine epithelioid cell response with increased vascularity.

The Kveim test, the intradermal injection of sterilized sarcoid tissue, should reproduce the histologic sarcoid reaction faithfully (Fig. 21–15) in order to be considered positive. Granulomas formed in the subcutis are not convincing.

Sarcoidal Foreign Body Granulomas

Metallic compounds containing silicon, beryllium, or zirconium are well-known to produce sarcoid reaction. It seems likely that specific sensitization is necessary for this to happen, although truly allergic reaction has been ruled out for silica granuloma.[53] Silicates (silica), especially talc crystals, sometimes are visible as colorless spicules in giant cells. Polarized light (Fig. 21–16B) is much more apt to show them, however, and this simple type of examination, which requires only two pieces of Polaroid film, should be used in every case of sarcoid reaction, although more elaborate methods are available. Beryllium and zirconium compounds do not polarize light and are not demonstrable in histologic sections. *Beryllium* granulomas (Fig. 21–17) are characterized by massive infiltrates, usually showing central caseation necrosis, and fibrosis. *Zirconium* is more apt to cause tiny superficial tubercles without necrosis,[54] and allergic sensitization is involved in their formation. Accidental barium granuloma from the liquid core of a golf ball has been reported as characterized by the presence of double refractile crystal-like substances and sandlike particles surrounded by foreign body granuloma.[55] Mercury-induced granu-

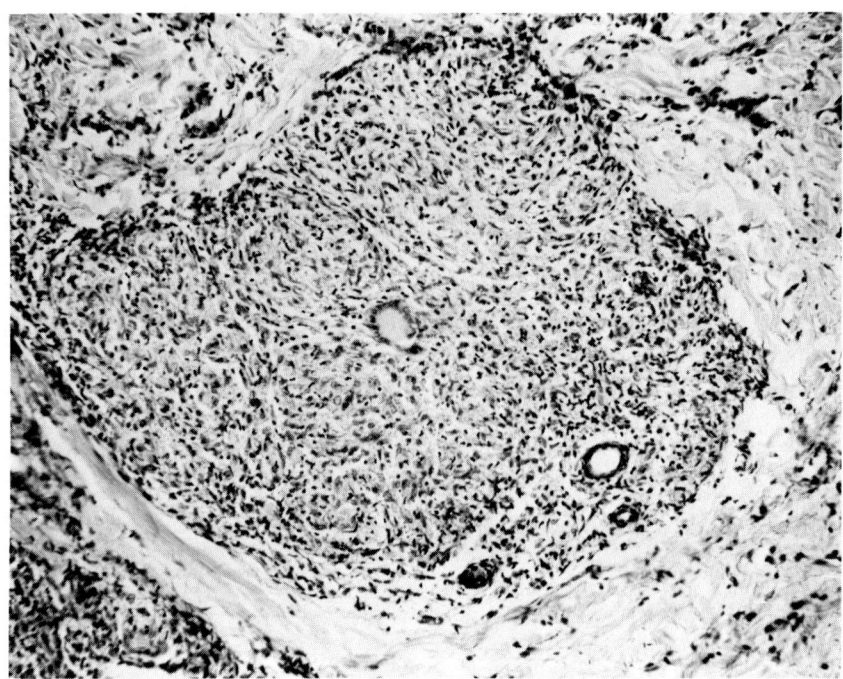

Figure 21–13.
Naked epithelioid cell tubercle representing sarcoid reaction. H&E. X135.

loma is identified by histologic observation of gray to black spherical bodies.[56] Aluminum-induced granuloma has been reported in tattoos and confirmed by electron microscopy and energy dispersive x-ray microanalysis.[57]

If paraffin is deposited in or under the skin, it is apt to be broken up into even tinier particles, which become embedded in diffuse masses of epithelioid and giant cells. In a later stage masses of sclerotic connective tissue show Swiss cheese appearance

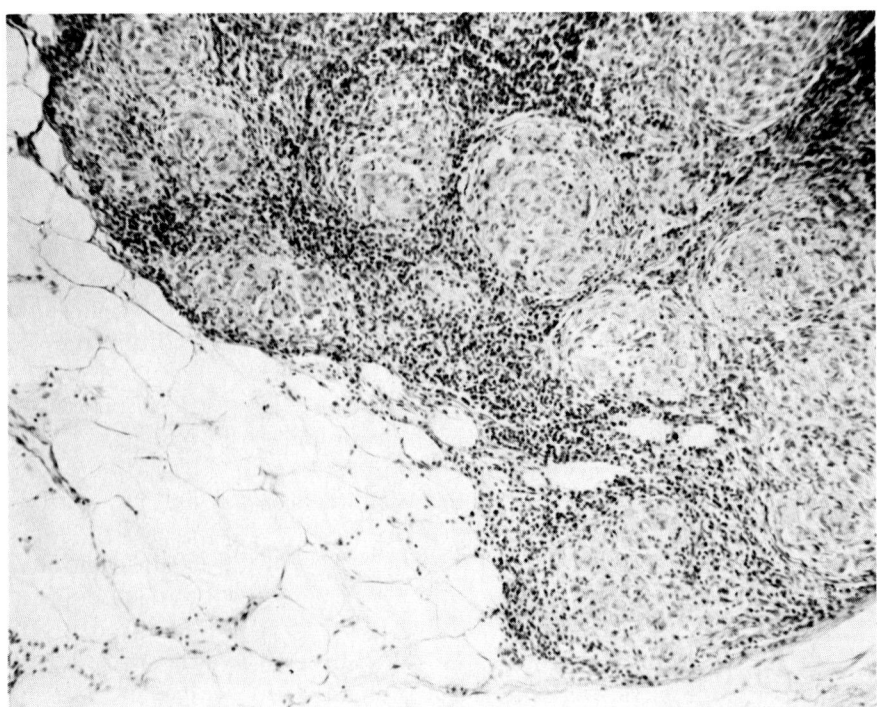

Figure 21–14.
Darier–Roussy sarcoid. Note the difference between this specific granulomatous reaction in the subcutaneous tissue and the nonspecific proliferating atrophy of fat tissue shown in Figures 16–1 and 16–2. H&E. X135.

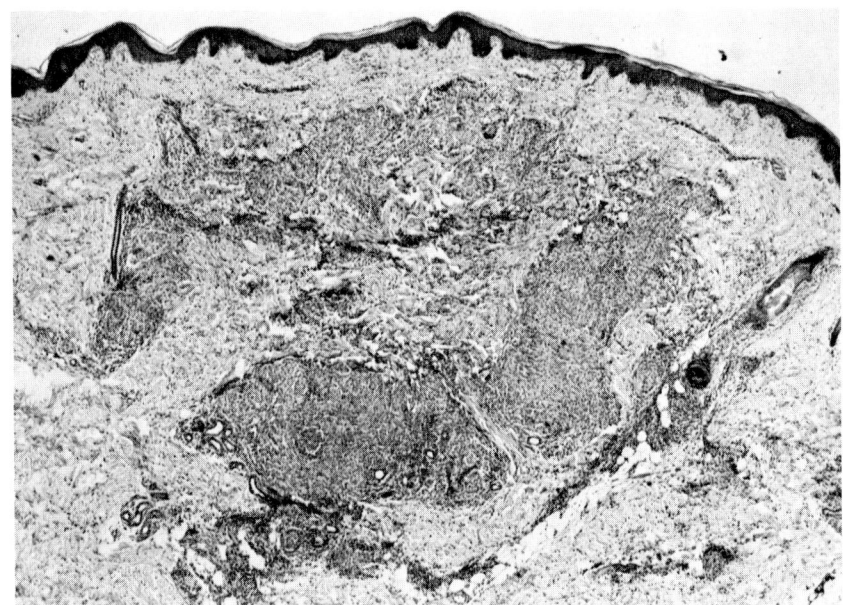

Figure 21–15.
Positive Kveim test. The photo illustrates specific sarcoid reaction to Kveim antigen properly placed in the dermis. If the antigen is deposited too deep (in subcutaneous tissue), proliferating atrophy of fat tissue may cast doubt on histologic interpretation. H&E. X75.

(sclerosing lipogranuloma)[58] (Fig. 21–18). In paraffin-embedded and paraffin-processed sections, only the clefts left by the foreign material remain, but the picture is so characteristic that the diagnosis (paraffinoma) usually can be suspected. Other forms of lipogranulomatous reaction caused by foreign substances are mentioned in Chapter 16. The peculiar sclerosis following parenteral administration of pentazocine is considered in Chapter 26. Hard indurations characterized by fibrosis and histiocytic granulomatous reaction also have been described after the injection of polyvinyl pyrrolidone,[59] used as an excipient for medications of impure silicones[60] for cosmetic purposes, and after accidental inoculation of acrylic and nylon fibers.[61]

Melkersson–Rosenthal Syndrome

A combination of transitory facial paralysis, lingua plicata (scrotal tongue), and fluctuating swelling of the upper lip or, sometimes, other parts of the face constitute the Melkersson–Rosenthal Syndrome.[62] Histologically, the indurated tissues of the lip exhibit sarcoid granulomas (Fig. 21–19), associated with smaller or larger numbers of lymphocytes and plasma cells (Miescher's cheilitis granulomatosa).[63] The cause is unknown.

MALAKOPLAKIA

The occurrence of malakoplakia (derived from the Greek term for "soft") in the skin has been reported.[64] Ordinarily, this is a benign inflammation of the urinary tract presenting distinct inclusion bodies in large histiocytes. These "Michaelis–Gutmann bodies" have been recognized as bacterial in origin and are encrusted with calcium and iron. Most commonly, *Escherichia coli* is associated with the lesions, but *Staphylococcus aureus* and *Pseudomonas* have been found. Most reported cases of cutaneous malakoplakia have occurred in patients who were chronically immunosuppressed and had an underlying systemic disease.[65]

The lesions consist of accumulations of large histiocytes mixed with some other inflammatory cells.

HISTOPLASMOSIS

The cutaneous reaction to *Histoplasma capsulatum* is characterized by the presence of 2 to 4 μm noncapsulated organisms in a large number of histiocytes, often in epithelioid arrangement but usually larger than ordinary epithelioid cells because they contain many organisms that are fairly well demonstrated by Giemsa stain but may require methenamine silver for identification (see Table 21–3).

It takes a high level of suspicion to think of histoplasmosis and to institute a search for the inconspicuous organism. Pulmonary histoplasmosis may be asymptomatic, chronic, or acute with influenzalike symptoms. It is diagnosed by a positive histoplasmin skin test.[66] Disseminated histoplasmosis involves the reticuloendothelial system with granu-

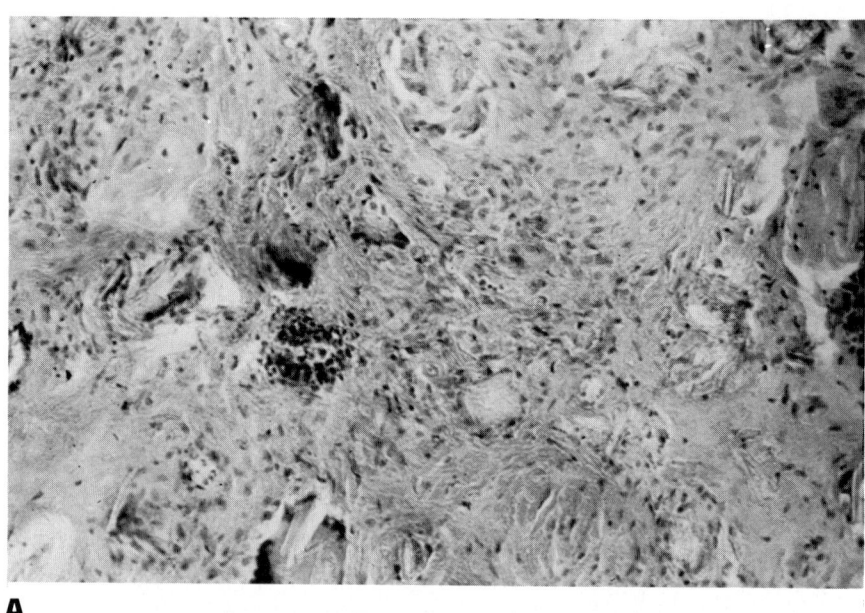
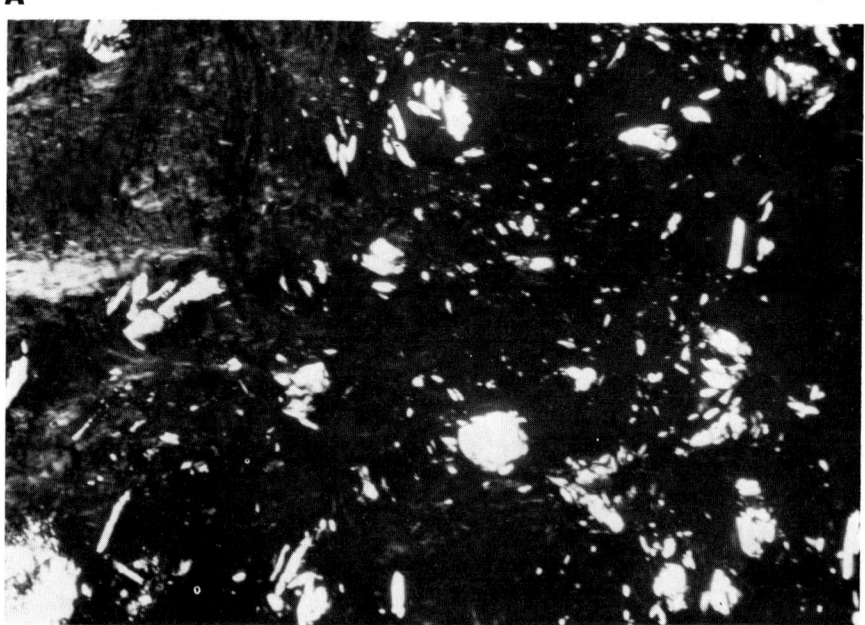

Figure 21-16.
Silica granuloma. **A.** Photographed in bright light. **B.** Photographed in polarized light. H&E. X135.

lomas, necrosis, and calcification in liver, spleen, and bone marrow. In patients with AIDS, a severe septic form occurs. Dissemination to the skin produces papules, plaques, ulcers, and purpuric lesions.[67-69] Skin test may be negative in disseminated disease and in severely immunosupressed patients.

CUTANEOUS LEISHMANIASIS

The recent increase in the incidence of cutaneous leishmaniasis in the endemic Middle East countries and among travelers in this area has renewed interest in investigation of this skin infection.[70-72] There are three species of protozoan leishmaniae causing cutaneous disease. *Leishmania tropica* causes self-limited nodular lesions, known as "Oriental sores" or by other local names, and in some cases late chronic granulomas resembling lupus vulgaris. It is endemic in the eastern Mediterranean and western Asiatic countries. *Leishmania donovani*, the cause of kala-azar in eastern Asia, may produce post-kala-azar granulomas in the skin, and *Leishmania braziliensis* is responsible for slowly extending chronic ulcerations in South and Central America.[73]

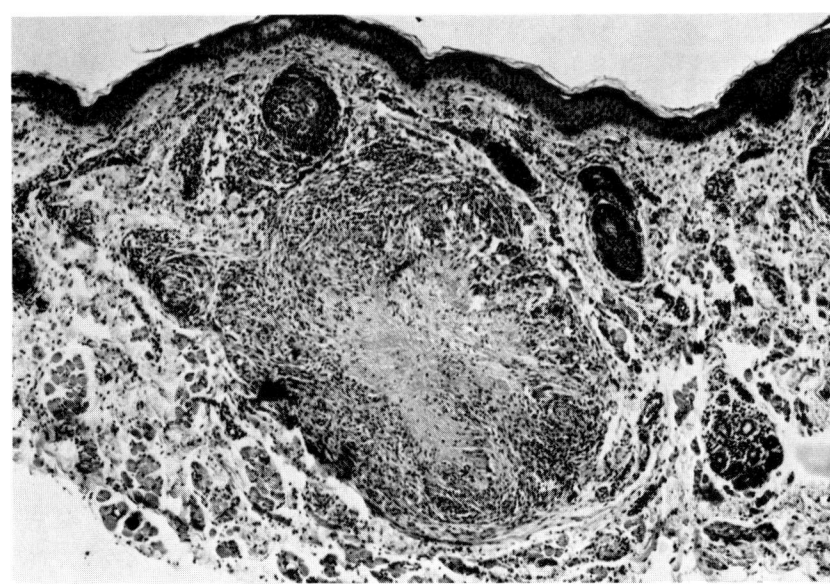

Figure 21–17.
Beryllium granuloma. A relatively small nodule was chosen to show striking similarity to lupus miliaris disseminatus faciei (see Fig. 21–4) owing to central caseation necrosis of a sarcoidal infiltrate. H&E. X60.

The primary inflammatory nodular lesion of Oriental leishmaniasis (Fig. 21–20A) usually shows a combination of histiocytic nodules, lymphocytes, and plasma cells closely associated with acanthotic epidermis. Leishmanial amastigotes (Fig. 21–20B) are easily demonstrated by Giemsa stain.

Disseminated lesions appear all over the body resulting in diffuse infiltrations, hypertrophic and verrucous nodules. Disseminated cutaneous leishmaniasis is characterized by the absence of visceral involvement, minimal or no nasal lesions, specific anergy to leishmanin, chronic progressive course, and poor response to treatment[74,75] (Table 21–3).

The much less common late (lupoid) lesions with chronic and progressive course and areas of scarring show masses of epithelioid cell granuloma and multinucleated giant cells. The histologic picture is so similar to lupus vulgaris that differential diagnosis is impossible.[76] In accordance with Lewandowsky's rule, no leishmaniae or only a few are visible in the tuberculoid tissue. The tissue reactions in post-kala-azar dermal leishmaniasis[77,78] and American leishmaniasis vary in many histologic details and in the number of demonstrable organisms, in reciprocal relation to the formation of tuberculoid granulomas. The three leishmaniae are morpholog-

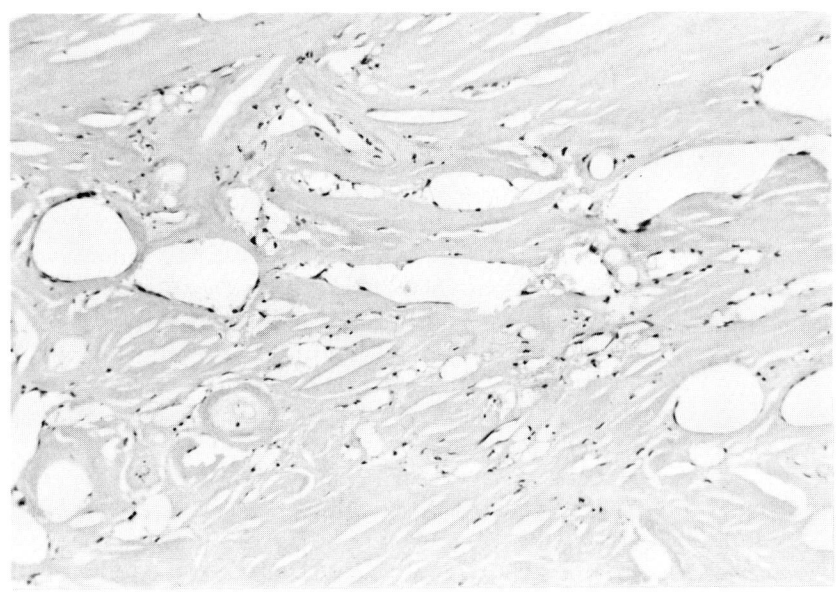

Figure 21–18.
Sclerosing lipogranuloma. Shows hyalinized connective tissue with Swiss cheese appearance. H&E. X250.

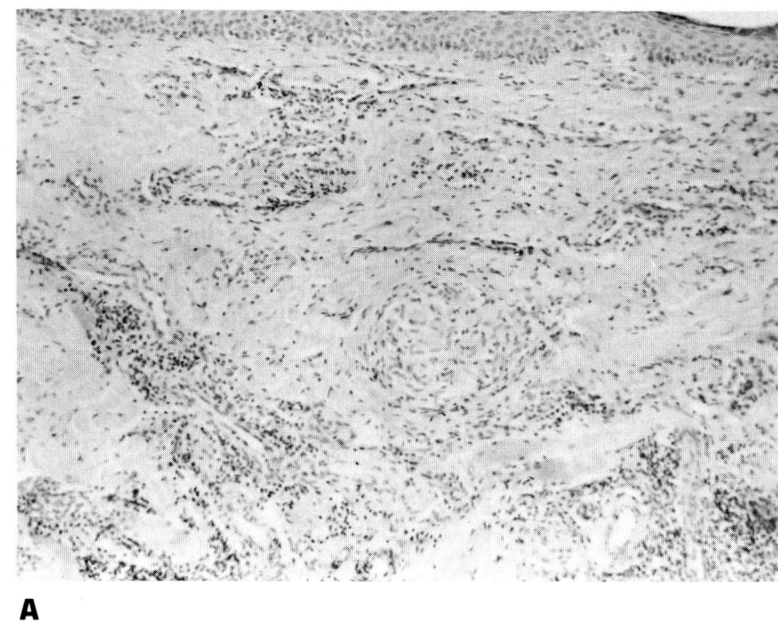

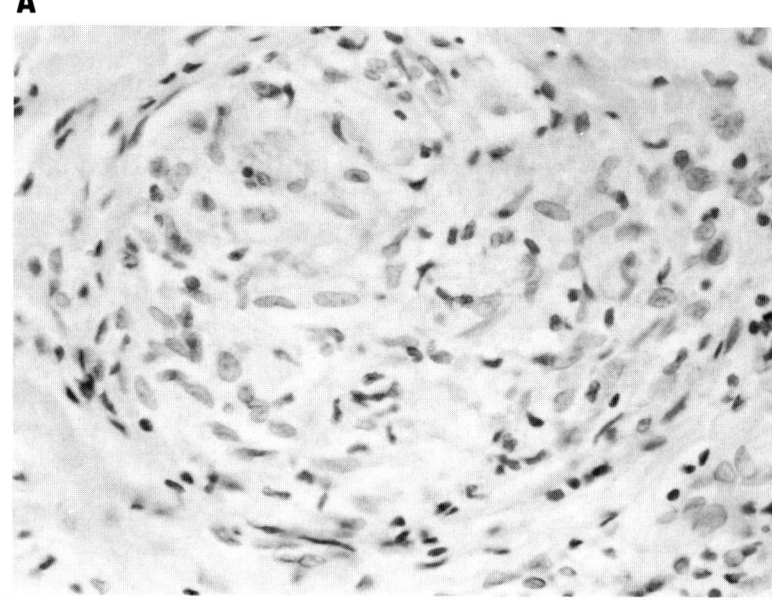

Figure 21–19.
Cheilitis granulomatosa. Fibrosis and infiltrate of epithelioid nodes and small round cells. H&E. **A.** X125. **B.** X400.

ically indistinguishable but can be cultured and differentiated immunologically.

TULAREMIA AND RHINOSCLEROMA

Two other bacterial diseases may occasionally involve the skin with granulomatous ulcers, tularemia and rhinoscleroma. Tularemia, caused by *Francisella tularensis,* may have an ulcerative primary lesion[79] exhibiting a central necrotic zone, an intermediate tuberculoid zone, and an outer zone containing lymphocytes, histiocytes, and plasma cells. Blood vessels of the outer zone show endothelial proliferation and infiltration of the wall by inflammatory cells. Extravasated erythrocytes are often seen in all zones. Later stages may exhibit a sarcoid reaction. Bacilli are not recognizable in tissue sections but may be identified by immunofluorescence.[80] Histologic differentiation from a syphilitic or sporotrichotic gumma may be difficult.

The tissue reaction of rhinoscleroma[81] is characterized by the great number of plasma cells in a granulomatous mononuclear infiltrate and by two specific features: the *Mikulicz cell,* a very large (up

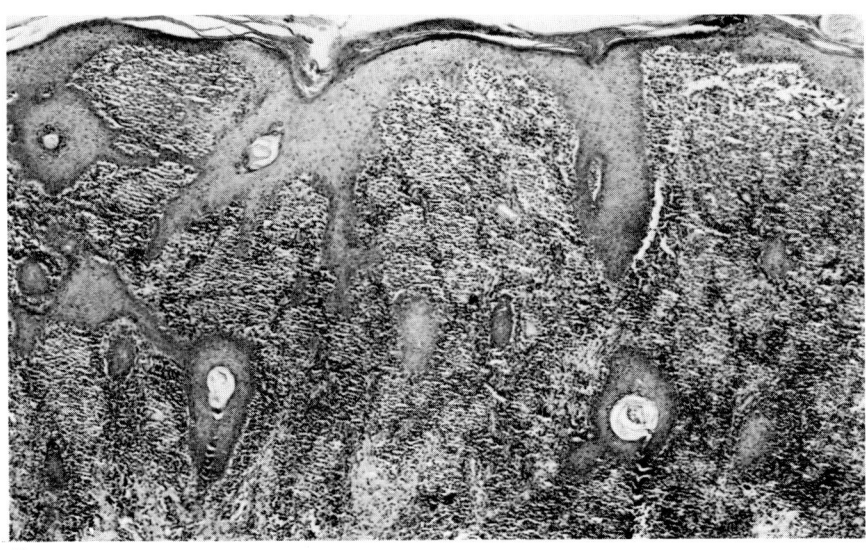

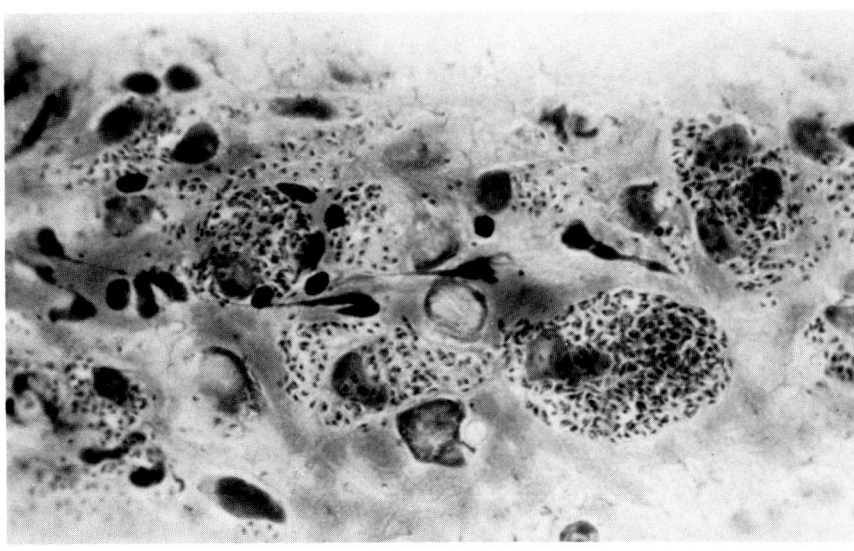

Figure 21-20.
Cutaneous leishmaniasis. **A.** H&E. X75. **B.** Giemsa-stained smear, to show tissue form of Leishmania tropica. X1100.

to 100 μm), roundish cell containing numerous Frisch bacilli (*Klebsiella rhinoscleromatis*), and the *Russell bodies* (see Fig. 5-14), hyaline bodies formed in plasma cells. The latter may also occur in other diseases.

REFERENCES

1. Sehgal VN, Jain MK, Srivastava G: Changing pattern of cutaneous tuberculosis. Int J Dermatol 28:231, 1989
2. Wilson Jones E, Winkelmann RK: Papulonecrotic tuberculid: A neglected disease in western countries. J Am Acad Dermatol 14:815, 1986
3. Ihm CW, Suh JI: Papulonecrotic tuberculid. Report of a case. J Dermatol Tokyo 14:63, 1987
4. Nakamura S, Aoki M, Nakayama K, et al: Penis tuberculid (papulonecrotic tuberculid of the glans penis): Treatment with a combination of Rifampicin and an extract from tubercle bacilli (TB vaccine). J Dermatol Tokyo 16:150, 1989
5. Valle SL: Dermatologic findings related to human immunodeficiency virus infection in high-risk individuals. J Am Acad Dermatol 17:951, 1987
6. Lantos G, Fisher BK, Contreras M: Tuberculous ulcer of the skin. J Am Acad Dermatol 19:1067, 1988
7. Brown FS, Anderson RH, Burnett JW: Cutaneous tuberculosis. J Am Acad Dermatol 6:101, 1982
8. Kakakhel KU, Fritsch P: Cutaneous tuberculosis. Int J Dermatol 28:355, 1989

9. Hirsh BC, Johnson WC: Pathology of granulomatous diseases: Epithelioid granulomas, Part 1. Int J Dermatol 23:237, 1984
10. Buck DC, Dodd HJ, Sarkany I: Tuberculosis verrucosa cutis. Br J Dermatol 119(Suppl 33): 103, 1988
11. Sehgal VN, Srivastava G, Khurana VK et al: An appraisal of epidemiologic, clinical, bacteriologic, histopathologic, and immunologic parameters in cutaneous tuberculosis. Int J Dermatol 26:521, 1987
12. Figuriredo A, Poiares-Baptista A, Branco M, Da Mota CH: Papular tuberculids post-BCG vaccination. Int J Dermatol 26:291, 1987
13. Smith NP, Ryan TJ, Sanderson KV, Sarkany I: Lichen scrofulosorum. A report of four cases. Br J Dermatol 94:319, 1976
14. Graham-Brown RAC, Sarkany I: Lichen scrofulosorum with tuberculous dactylitis. Br J Dermatol 103:561, 1980
15. Ridgway HA, Ryan TJ: Is micropapular sarcoidosis tuberculosis? J R Soc Med 74:140, 1981
16. Wong KC: Erythema induratum: Follow-up study of 46 patients. Dermatol Dig 10:51, 1971
17. Shitara A: Lupus miliaris disseminatus faciei. Int J Dermatol 23:542, 1984
18. Frix CD III, Bronson DM: Acute miliary tuberculosis in a child with anhidrotic ectodermal dysplasia. Pediatr Dermatol 3:464, 1986
19. Saxe N: Mycobacterial skin infections. J Cutan Pathol 12:300, 1985
20. Sehgal VN, Sharma V: Reactions in leprosy—A prospective study of clinical, bacteriological, immunological and histopathological parameters in thirty-five Indians. J Dermatol Tokyo 15:412, 1988
21. Sehgal VN, Jain MK, Srivastava G: Evolution of the classification of leprosy. Int J Dermatol 28:161, 1989
22. Sehgal VN, Joginder, Sharma VK: Immunology of leprosy. A comprehensive survey. Int J Dermatol 28:574, 1989
23. Martinez MI, Sanchez JL: Treatment of leprosy with weekly intravenous infusion of leukocytes. Int J Dermatol 23:341, 1984
24. Pursley TV, Jacobson RR, Apisarnthanarax P: Lucio's phenomenon. Arch Dermatol 116:201, 1980
25. Sehgal VN, Srivastava G, Sharma VK: Contemplative immune mechanism of Lucio phenomenon and its global status. J Dermatol Tokyo 14:580, 1987
26. Sehgal VN, Srivastava G, Status of histoid leprosy—A clinical, bacteriological, histopathological and immunological appraisal. J Dermatol Tokyo 14:38, 1987
27. Murray-Leisure KA, Egan N, Weitekamp MR: Skin lesions caused by *Mycobacterium scrofulaceum*. Arch Dermatol 123:369, 1987
28. Travis WD, Travis LB, Roberts GD, et al: Histopathologic spectrum in *Mycobacterium marinum* infection. Arch Pathol Lab Med 109:1109, 1985
29. Huminer D, Pitlik SD, Block C, et al: Aquarium-borne *Mycobacterium marinum* skin infection. Report of a case and review of the literature. Arch Dermatol 122:698, 1986
30. Drusin L: Syphilis: Clinical manifestation, diagnosis, and treatment. Urol Clin 11:121, 1984
31. Chapel TA: The signs and symptoms of secondary syphilis. Sex Trans Dis 7:161, 1980
32. Jordaan FH: Secondary syphilis. A clinicopathological study. Am J Dermatopathol 10:399, 1988
33. Izumi AK, Navin JJ: Sarcoidal secondary syphilis. Cutis 14:833, 1974
34. Sapra S, Weatherhead L: Extensive nodular secondary syphilis. Arch Dermatol 125:1666, 1989
35. Hodak E, David M, Rothem A, et al: Nodular secondary syphilis mimicking cutaneous lymphoreticular process. J Am Acad Dermatol 17:914, 1987
36. Poulsen A, Kobayasi T, Secher L, Weismann K: *Treponema pallidum* in macular and papular secondary syphilitic skin eruptions. Acta Derm Venereol 66:251, 1986
37. Fisher DA, Chang LW, Tuffanelli DL: Lues maligna. Presentation of a case and a review of the literature. Arch Dermatol 99:70, 1979
38. Green KM, Heilman E: Secondary syphilis presenting as a palisading granuloma. J Am Acad Dermatol 12:957, 1985
39. Pembroke AC, Michell PA, McKee PH: Nodulosquamous tertiary syphilide. Clin Exp Dermatol 5:361, 1980
40. Tanabe JL, Huntley AC: Granulomatous tertiary syphilis. J Am Acad Dermatol 15:341, 1986
41. Wajdi Kanan M, Kaudil E: Bejel or non-venereal endemic syphilis. Br J Dermatol 84:461, 1971
42. Hopkins DR: Yaws in the Americas 1950–1975. J Infect Dis 136:548, 1977
43. Hasselmann CM: Comparative studies on the histopathology of syphilis, yaws, and pinta. Br J Vener Dis 33:5, 1957
44. Rowland Payne CME, Meyrick Thomas RH, Black MM: From silica granuloma to scar sarcoidosis. Clin Exp Dermatol 8:171, 1983
45. Erickson JG, Petko E: Sarcoidal reactions in multiple tattoos with systemic sarcoidosis. Cutis 11:163, 1973
46. Veien NK, Stahl D, Brodthagen H: Cutaneous sarcoidosis in caucasians. J Am Acad Dermatol 16:534, 1987
47. Morrison JGL: Sarcoidosis in a child, presenting as an erythroderma with keratotic spines and palmar pits. Br J Dermatol 95:93, 1976
48. Karch JC, Goody HE, Luscombe HA: Ichthyosiform sarcoidosis. Arch Dermatol 114:100, 1978
49. Saxe N, Benatar SR, Bok L, Gordon W: Sarcoidosis with leg ulcers and annular facial lesions. Arch Dermatol 120:93, 1984
50. Clayton R, Breathnach A, Martin B, Feiwel M: Hypopigmented sarcoidosis in the Negro. Br J Dermatol 96:119, 1977
51. Vainsencher D, Winkelmann RK: Subcutaneous sarcoidosis. Arch Dermatol 120:1028, 1984
52. Kuramoto Y, Shindo Y, Tagami H: Subcutaneous sarcoidosis with extensive caseation necrosis. J Cutan Pathol 15:188, 1988
53. Terzakis JA, Shustak SR, Stock EG: Talc granuloma

identified by x-ray mircoanalysis. JAMA 239:2371, 1978
54. Shelley WB, Hurley HJ: The allergic origin of zirconium deodorant granulomas. Br J Dermatol 70:75, 1958
55. Ishii Y, Inoue S, Kikuchi I, Taketomi I: Barium granuloma. J Dermatol Tokyo 9:153, 1982
56. Lupton GP, Kao GF, Johnson FB, et al: Cutaneous mercury granuloma. A clinicopathologic study and review of the literature. J Am Acad Dermatol 12:296, 1985
57. McFadden N, Lyberg T, Hensten-Pettersen A: Aluminum-induced granulomas in tattoo. J Am Acad Dermatol 20:903, 1989
58. Klein JA, Cole G, Barr RJ, et al: Paraffinomas of the scalp. Arch Dermatol 121:382, 1985
59. Thivolet J, Leung TK, Duverne J, et al: Ultrastructural morphology and histochemistry (acid phosphatase) of cutaneous infiltration by polyvinylpyrrolidone. Br J Dermatol 83:661, 1970
60. Delage C, Shane JJ, Johnson FB: Mammary silicone granuloma. Arch Dermatol 108:104, 1973
61. Cortez Pimentel J: Sarcoid granulomas of the skin produced by acrylic and nylon fibers. Br J Dermatol 96:673, 1977
62. Greene RM, Rogers RS III: Melkersson–Rosenthal syndrome: A review of 36 patients. J Am Acad Dermatol 21:1263, 1989
63. Allen CM, Camisa C, Hamzeh S, Stephens L: Cheilitis granulomatosa: Report of six cases and review of the literature. J Am Acad Dermatol 23:444, 1990
64. Palou J, Torras H, Baradad M, et al: Cutaneous malakoplakia. Report of a case. Dermatologica 176:288, 1988
65. Palazzo JP, Ellison DJ, Garcia IE, et al: Cutaneous malakoplakia simulating relapsing malignant lymphoma. J Cutan Pathol 17:171, 1990
66. Tomecki KJ, Dijkstra JW, Hall GS, Steck WD: Systemic mycoses. J Am Acad Dermatol 21:1285, 1989
67. Mandell W, Goldberg DM, Neu HC: Histoplasmosis in patients with the acquired immune deficiency syndrome. Am J Med 81:974, 1986
68. Dallot A, Monsuez J-J, Chanu B, et al: Localisations cutanees d'une histoplasmose disseminee a histoplasma capsulatum au cours d'une cas d'immunodeficience acquise. Ann Dermatol Venereol 115:441, 1988
69. Greenberg RG, Berger TG: Progressive disseminated histoplasmosis in acquired immune deficiency syndrome: Presentation as a steroid-responsive dermatosis. Cutis 43:535, 1989
70. Walton BC: Leishmaniasis. A worldwide problem. Int J Dermatol 28:305, 1989
71. Lin CS, Wang WJ, Wong CK, Chao D: Cutaneous leishmaniasis. Clinical, histopathologic, and electron microscopic studies. Int J Dermatol 25:511, 1986
72. Kubba R, Al-Gindan Y, El-Hassan AM, Omer AHS: Clinical diagnosis of cutaneous leishmaniasis (Oriental sore). J Am Acad Dermatol 16:1183, 1987
73. Furtado T: Progressos e perspectivas na leishmaniose tegumentar americana. Med Cut ILA 15:105, 1987
74. Kubba R, Al-Gindan Y, El-Hassan AM, et al: Dissemination in cutaneous leishmaniasis. II. Satellite papules and subcutaneous induration. Int J Dermatol 27:702, 1988
75. Sharma VK, Kaur S, Mahajan RC, et al: Disseminated cutaneous leishmaniasis. Int J Dermatol 28:261, 1989
76. Radentz WH: Leishmaniasis: Clinical manifestations, immunologic responses, and treatment. J Assoc Mil Dermatol 13:15, 1987
77. Munro DD: Post-kala-azar dermal leishmaniasis. Br J Dermatol 87:374, 1972
78. Girgla HS, Marsden RA, Singh GM, Ryan TJ: Post-kala-azar dermal leishmaniasis. Br J Dermatol 97:307, 1977
79. Schuermann H, Reich H: Zur Klinik und Histologie des cutan lokalisierten tularämischen Primäraffekts. Arch Dermat Syphilol 190:579, 1950
80. White JD, McGavran MH: Identification of *Pasteurella tularensis* by immunofluorescence. JAMA 194:2940, 1965
81. Kerdel-Vegas F, Convit J, Gordon B, Goihman M: Rhinoscleroma. Springfield, Ill: Thomas, 1963

22
MIXED CELL GRANULOMAS

Mixed cell granulomas result in proliferation of mononuclear cells having a mixed phagocytic and secretory activity.[1] With the exception of histoplasmosis, deep mycotic infections of the skin contain neutrophilic and eosinophilic leukocytes in addition to histiocytes and round cells. Thus, a mixture of all these cells in a granuloma strongly points to fungus infection.[2] There are, however, a number of exceptions including halogen eruptions, especially bromoderma, arthropod bites, lesions caused by worms and larvae, and some types of foreign body granulomas which may also be included in this category. Ulcerated lesions of tuberculosis, leprosy, or syphilis will show neutrophils, but these are usually restricted to the surface layers. Of other chronic infections, granuloma inguinale and lymphogranuloma venereum belong to the mixed cell granulomas.

FUNGAL GRANULOMAS

In most instances, positive diagnosis of a fungal granuloma can be made by finding the characteristic organism in the section. The fungi of North American and South American "blastomycosis," "coccidioidomycosis," "chromomycosis," and "actinomycosis" with its congeners usually can be identified in H&E sections and can be seen better in O&G sections. *Cryptococcus* and *Sporotrichum,* on the other hand, are almost never recognized using these stains. PAS stain after digestion of the tissue sections with amylase (diastase) has made it possible to demonstrate these organisms in many cases. If organisms are not demonstrable, diagnosis becomes much less secure. Although there are characteristic tissue reactions to each one of these fungi, there is enough variation and overlap to be confusing. The following are short descriptions of the more typical features.

Coccidioidomycosis

Primary cutaneous infection is rare.[3] Dissemination into the skin may occur from the bloodstream.[4] Cutaneous manifestations include verrucous granulomas, deep cellulitis and abscesses, papulopustular lesions, ulcers, and formation of sinus tracts.[5] Skin sections show massive granulomatous reaction, almost of foreign body character (Fig. 22–1), with many giant cells containing the characteristic sporangia of *Coccidioides immitis,* measuring from 10 to 80 μm. Some epidermal hyperplasia often is present but rarely as pronounced as in blastomycosis.[6,7]

North American Blastomycosis

Primary lesions are almost always pulmonary.[8,9] Secondary hematogenous spread involves skin forming crusted plaques studded with miliary abscesses,

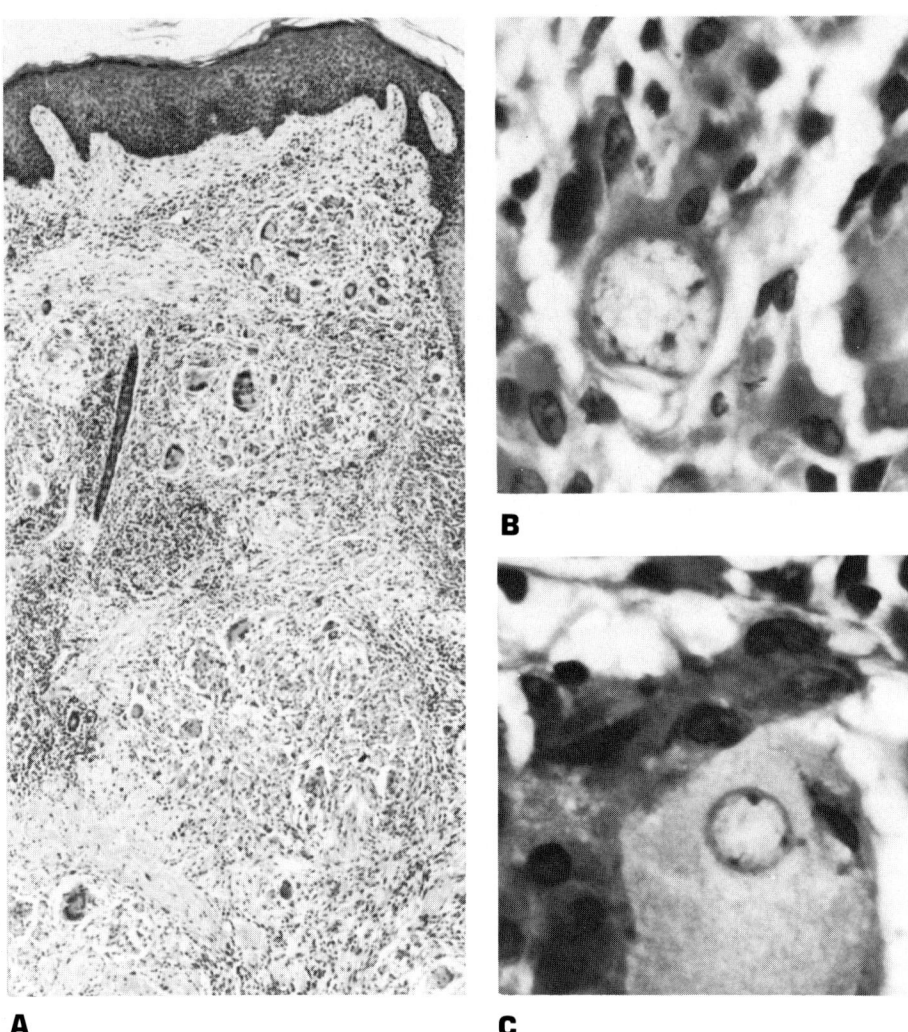

Figure 22–1.
Coccidioidomycosis. **A.** Foreign body type granuloma. H&E. X60. **B.** and **C.** Larger and smaller cysts with endosporulation. H&E. X800.

draining sinuses, and central healing with atrophic scarring. Histologically, a combination of mixed granulomatous infiltrate with pseudoepitheliomatous hyperplasia is the outstanding histologic feature (Fig. 22–2). Intraepithelial abscesses and multinucleated giant cells complete the picture.[10] The characteristic spores (Fig. 22–2B) are generally found in giant cells but may be free in the tissue, especially in intraepidermal-abscesses (see Fig. 5–11D). Search for them is assisted in H&E sections by closing the iris diaphragm of the microscope in order to bring out the refractile thick membrane. The membrane usually stains greenish blue in O&G sections and is dark magenta in PAS stain. *Blastomyces dermatitidis* measures from 8 to 15 μm in diameter. The most important differential diagnosis is bromoderma, and this should be suspected if no multinucleated giant cells are present and careful search reveals no fungi. Pyodermatous lesions also may mimic the pseudoepitheliomatous proliferation of blastomycosis.

South American Blastomycosis

The disease due to *Paracoccidioides braziliensis*[11] has histologic features somewhat similar to other fungous granulomas. Organisms are easily found and measure 10 to 60 μm with one or multiple buds. A remarkable form of South American blastomycosis caused by a related fungus is Jorge Lobo's *keloidal* type.[12,13] The striking histologic picture is illustrated in Figure 22–3. The fungus (*Loboa loboi*) is difficult to culture. It probably persists in macrophages because of defective cellular immunity.

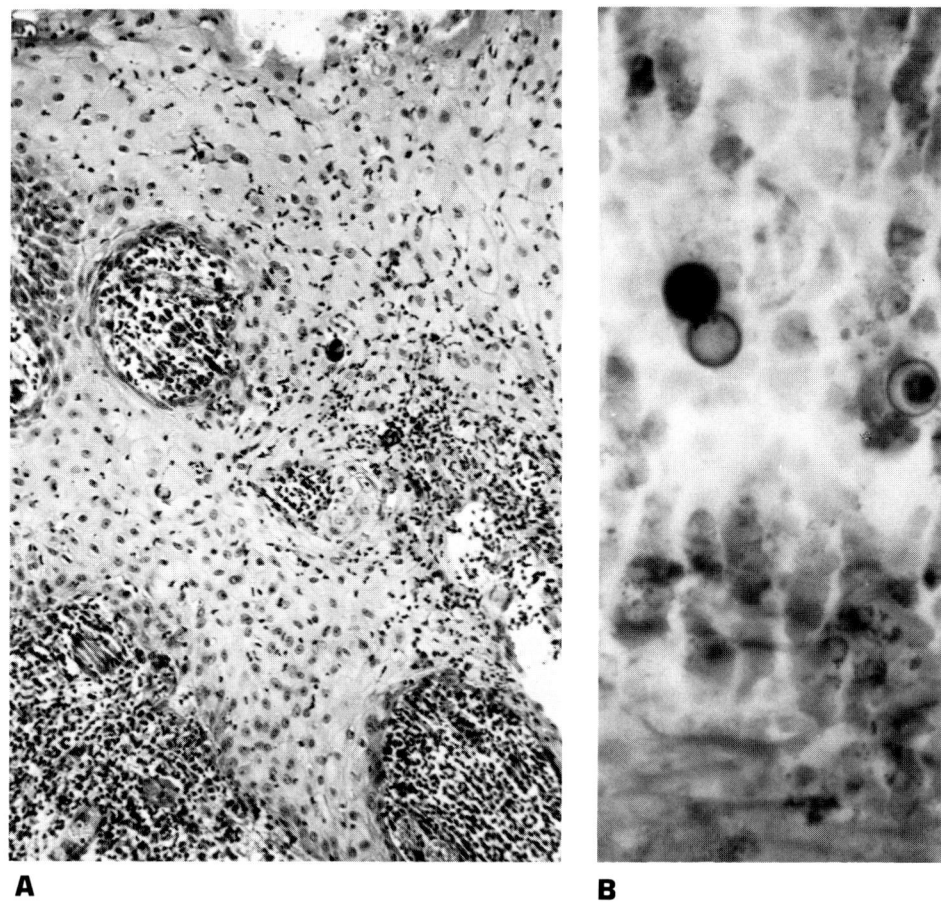

Figure 22–2.
North American blastomycosis. **A.** Pseudoepitheliomatous hyperplasia with intraepidermal abscesses and granulomatous infiltrate. H&E. X135. **B.** Blastomyces dermatitidis. PAS—light green. X800.

Chromomycosis (Chromoblastomycosis)

A mixed granulomatous infiltrate with verrucous epidermal hyperplasia is characteristic of this type of lesion.[14] The naturally dark chestnut-brown, thick-walled organisms[15] (Fig. 22–4), which belong to the genera *Philophora, Cladosporium,* and *Fonsecaea,* are usually sparse and show up better in a lightly stained section than in one overstained with eosin. The cell wall does not change color in either H&E or O&G sections but is tinged by PAS. According to Zaias and Rebell,[16] diagnosis is simplified by identifying in the clinical lesion black dots, which consist of inflammatory products and hemorrhage undergoing transepidermal elimination,[17] and scraping them off and softening them in potassium hydroxide. Round "Medlar bodies" as well as hyphal elements can be identified by this method.

Actinomycosis, Nocardiosis, Botryomycosis

Granulomatous lesions with sinuses discharging pus that contains macroscopically visible granules can be caused by true fungi or by actinomycetes. The former are known as "maduromycosis," and the term "mycetoma" may be applied to all.[18,19] Similar lesions caused by bacteria are known as "botryomycosis." Histologic distinction among the different types is difficult. As a group they have characteristic features. The colonies of organisms are already visible under the scanning lens (Fig. 22–5A). The granules (Fig. 22–5B) usually are present within large accumulations of polymorphonuclear leukocytes (abscesses), surrounded by granulomatous and fibrotic reaction without any distinguishing characteristics.[20] All common stains are suitable for their demonstration. The granules are gram-positive; only oc-

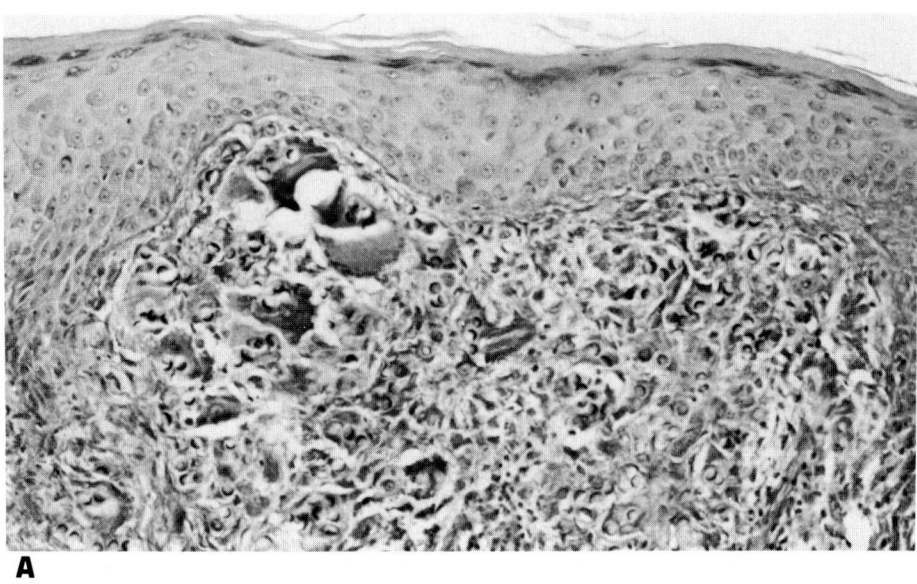
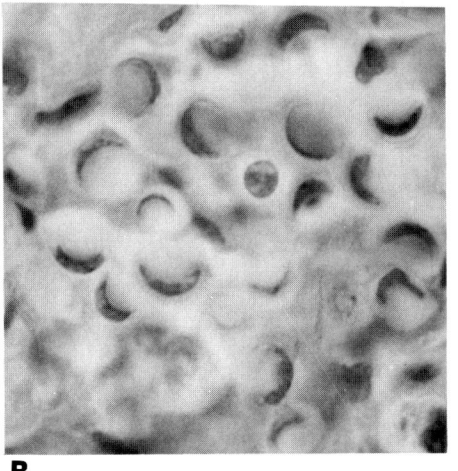
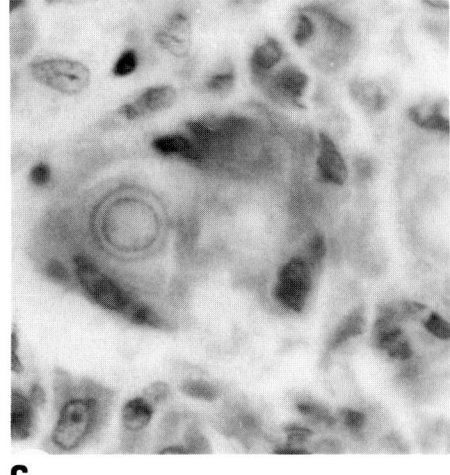

Figure 22–3.
Lobo's type of South American blastomycosis. Numerous organisms are present in large multinucleated giant cells. PAS–hematoxylin. **A.** X250. **B** and **C.** X800.

casionally do they have to be differentiated from similar bacterial colonies found in human botryomycosis.[21,22] The latter, which usually are staphylococcal colonies (Fig. 22–6), do not exhibit filamentous and club-shaped structures, but cultural identification is necessary in every case.[23]

Cryptococcosis

Cryptococcus neoformans is a nonmycelial yeast of 2 to 20 μm in diameter. The infection spread by air and 90 percent of patients have initial pulmonary involvement. Hematogenic dissemination occurs in 10 percent of patients. Cryptococcal antibodies can be demonstrated in 70–90 percent of cases and direct observation of *C. neoformans* in cerebrospinal fluid is made by antigen testing with latex agglutination test in 90 percent of cases.[5] Primary cutaneous cryptococcosis is rare[24,25] but secondary skin lesions are becoming more common in immunosuppressed patients.[26–28] Cutaneous lesions may resemble cellulitis or pyoderma gangrenosum.[29,30] A mixed type granuloma suggest deep fungus infection (Fig. 22–7). Budding yeast form organisms are demonstrated by PAS or silver stains.

Sporotrichosis

Sporotrichosis (Fig. 22–8) should be suspected when one sees a mixed granuloma, including multinucleated giant cells, and cannot find microorganisms even on thorough search. The sporotrichotic lesion has additional characteristics to support the suspicion, however. Just as the clinical lesion represents

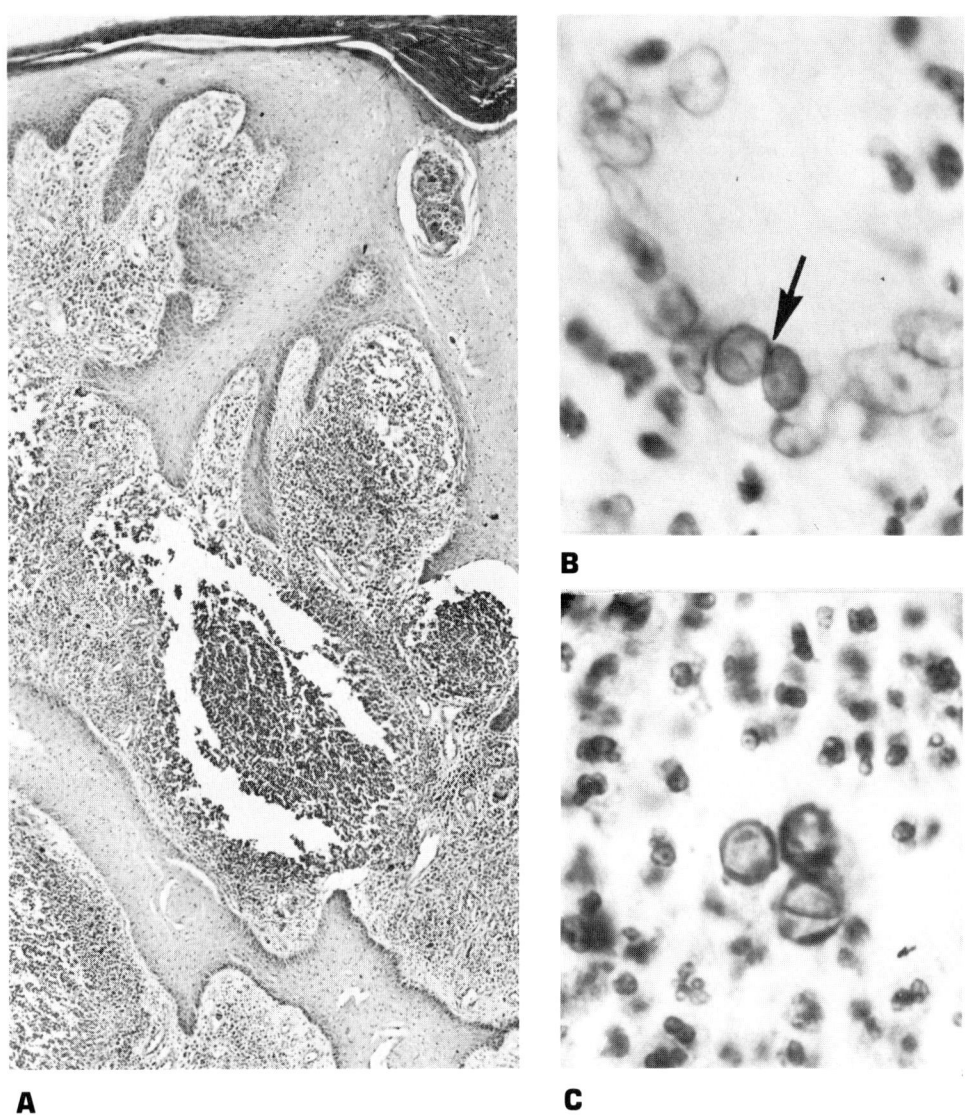

Figure 22–4.
Chromomycosis. **A.** H&E. X135. **B.** Sclerotic cells between nuclei of a multinucleated giant cell. **C.** Fungi free in tissue. H&E. X1100.

a gumma, so one finds necrotic liquefied tissue mixed with polymorphonuclear cells in the center, surrounded by a granulomatous wall. The latter consists of a tuberculoid inner zone with epithelioid nodules, multinucleated giant cells, and round cells and an outer syphiloid zone, in which lymphocytes and plasma cells prevail. Eosinophils are often scattered in considerable numbers or may form small clumps. The epithelioid cell granuloma and multinucleated giant cells may be more prominent in the inflammatory cutaneous plaquelike lesions.[31,32] In sections stained with PAS following amylase digestion, we have been able to identify the organisms in a great majority of cases. One often finds a surprising number of small 3- to 5-μm oval spores, not frequently budding (Fig. 22–9A). Elongated, cigar-shaped bodies may also be seen. Large numbers of organisms are present in some plaquelike lesions,[33] and localized lesions secondary to Feline sporotrichosis[34] and in the disseminated disease.[35] Peculiar large asteroid spores are commonly seen in tropical countries, especially in the southern hemisphere, but only in exceptional cases in the United States. Those observed by us (Fig. 22–9B, C, and D) were lying free in microabscesses surrounded by a histiocytic wall. The wall of the spore takes the PAS stain, whereas the rays do not, in support of the view that the rays are material contributed by the host.

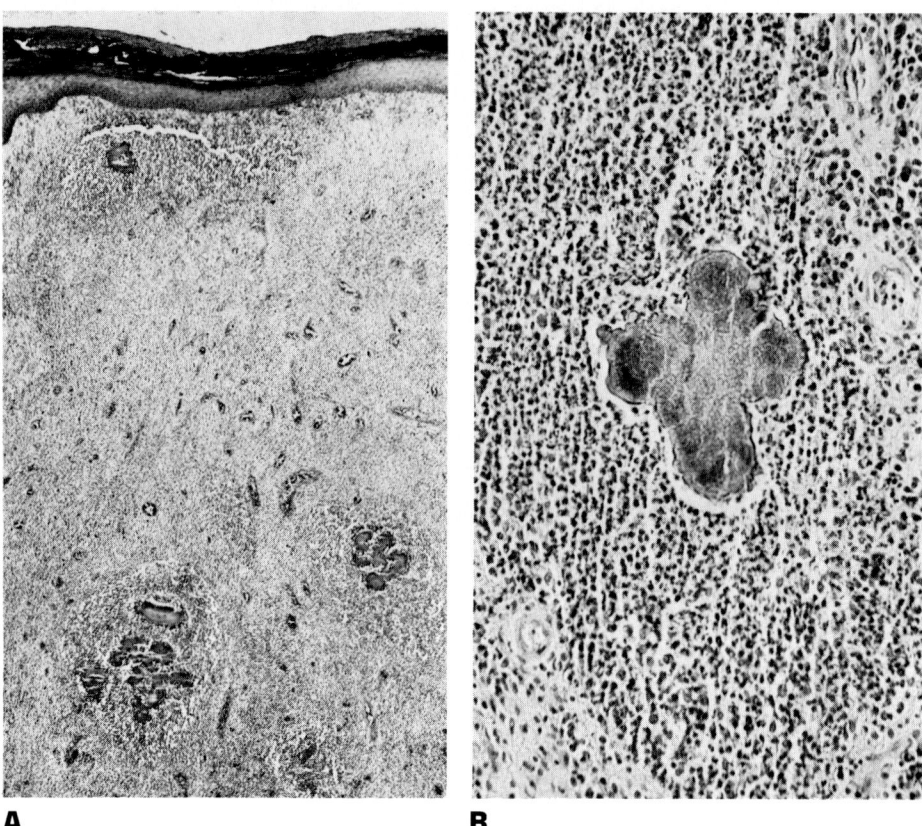

Figure 22–5.
Maduromycosis. **A.** H&E. X30.
B. Granule in abscess. H&E. X225.

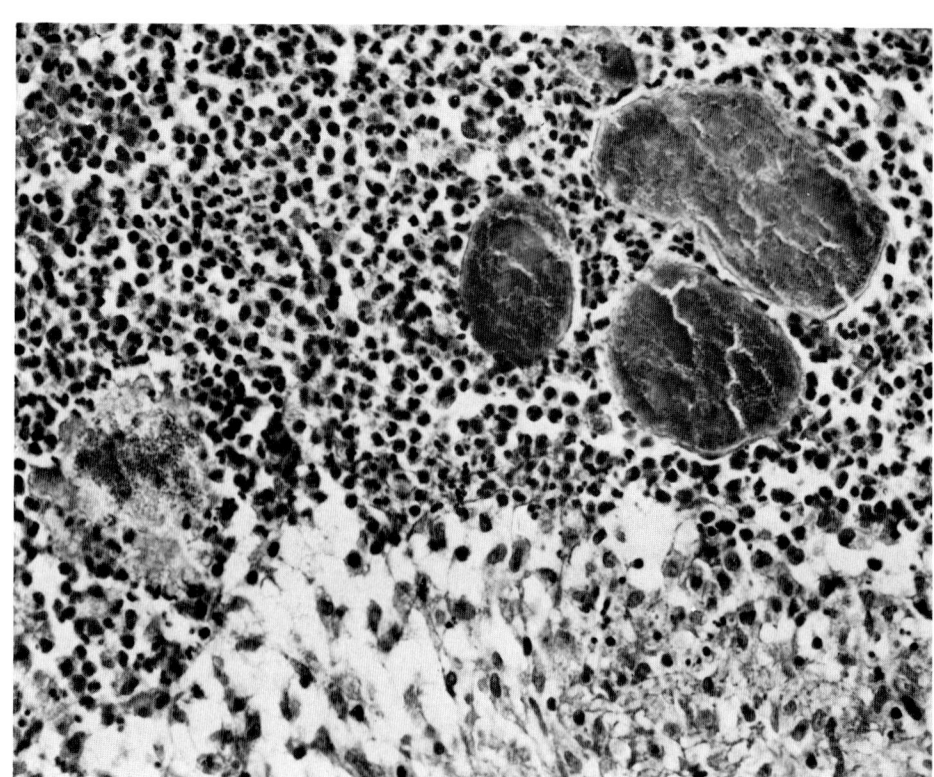

Figure 22–6.
Human botryomycosis. The "granules" are colonies of staphyloccocci embedded in hyaline material. H&E. X370.

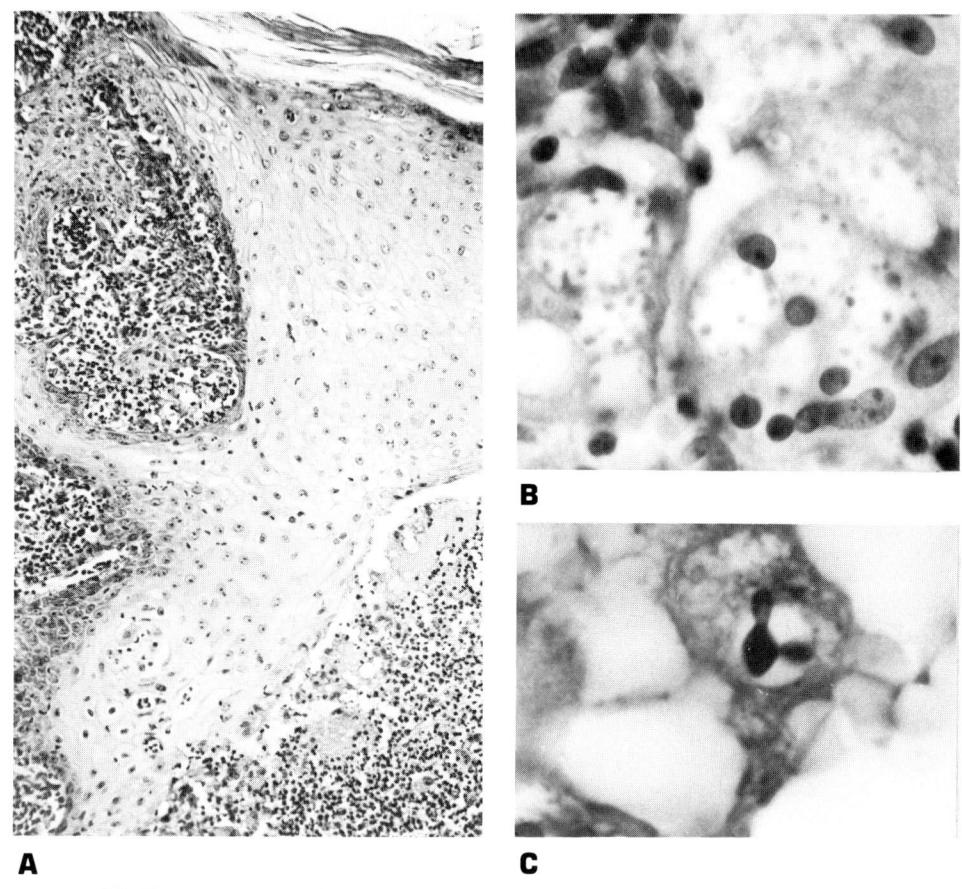

Figure 22–7.
Crytococcosis. **A.** Van Gieson. X135. **B.** Tiny organisms in tissue. Van Gieson. X800. **C.** Budding of yeastlike organism. PAS–picric acid. X2400.

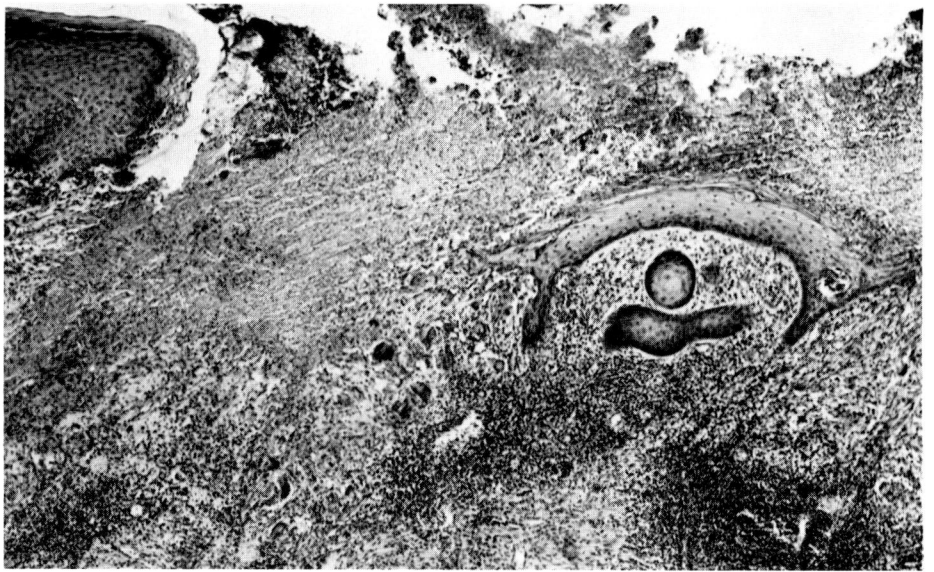

Figure 22–8.
Sporotrichosis. Acanthotic edge of epidermis in upper left corner. Necrotic tissue forms the floor of an ulcer. The granulomatous infiltrate has tuberculoid and syphiloid features. Proliferating epithelium in the tissue is probably derived from hair follicles or sweat glands. Observe similarity of tissue reaction to a syphilitic gumma. (See Fig. 21–11). H&E. X60.

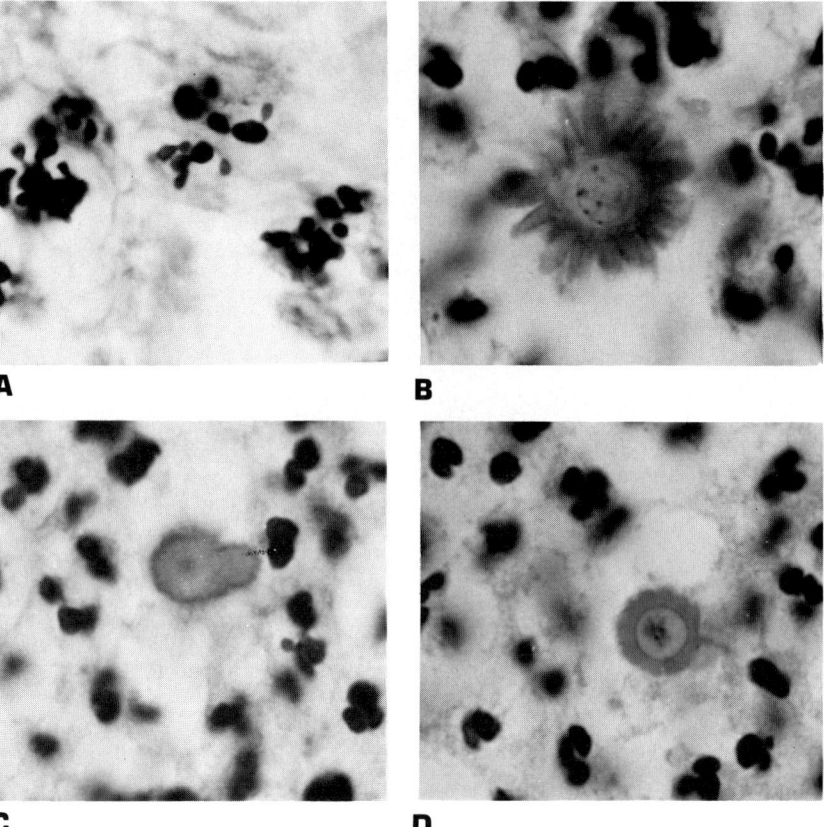

Figure 22–9.
Sporotrichum schenckii. **A.** Oval and round budding spores in human tissue. PAS–light green after amylase digestion. X1100. **B, C,** and **D.** Asteroid spores in small abscesses, a rare observation in a North American case. H&E. X1350. (From Pinkus and Grekin. Arch Dermatol 97:394, 1950.)

Opportunistic Fungi

Prolonged survival of immunodeficient individuals and therapeutic induction of immunodeficiency in many patients have produced cases of unusual infection, not a few due to fungi of low pathogenicity. The common denominator is the occurrence in tissue of typically dematioceous yeastlike cells, pseudohyphal elements, and distorted short or elongated hyphae. Among these are cases with aspergillosis, phaeohyphomycosis,[36] mucormycosis,[37] alternariosis,[38] and rhizopus[39] infection. Among these one may also include the long-known victims of chronic granulomatous candidiasis who are incapable of coping with this ordinary and not highly pathogenic yeast. Tissue reaction may be minimal or absent, of noncharacteristic nature, or more or less granulomatous depending on the immunologic circumstances.

PROTOTHECOSIS

In the last several years, sporadic cases of localized granulomatous inflammation have been recorded in which round bodies forming internal septa were identified within a mixed type of granuloma (Fig. 22–10). The responsible organisms are achloric algae (*Prototheca* spp.). They grow yeastlike on all common media.[40,41]

WORMS AND LARVAE

We make short mention of cutaneous and subcutaneous reactions to parasitic worms and burrowing insect larvae. Most of these are restricted to tropical and subtropical countries.[42] In the United States, only hookworm infestation in the form of creeping eruption (larva migrans) is seen with any frequency, but subcutaneous nodules due to *Cysticercus cellulosae* have been reported.[43] Odd cases of abscesses due to fly larvae[44,45] and sand fleas[46] have been seen. Among the tropical parasitoses, "filiariasis,"[47] "onchocerciasis,"[48] "loaisis," "dirofiliariasis,"[49] and "schistosomiasis"[50,51] may come to the dermatopathologist's attention. Recognition of unfamiliar structures in the tissue as sections of the responsible organism is the most important diagnostic point, as it was in finding the larva of *Gnathostoma spini-*

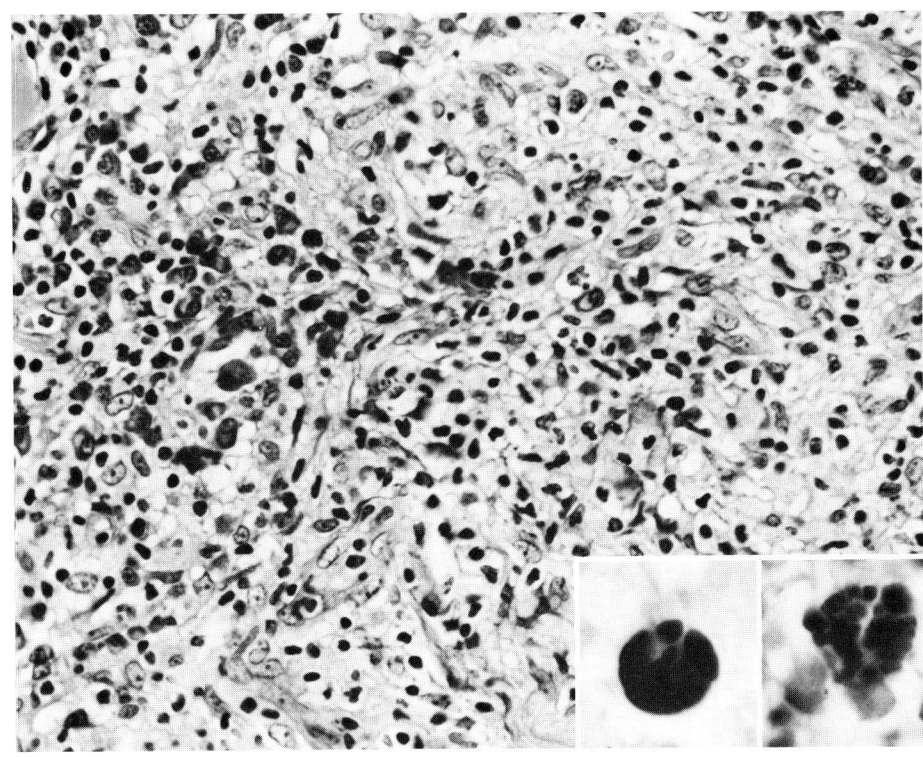

Figure 22–10.
Protothecosis. Granulation tissue harboring large dark-staining cells. H&E. X400. Insets show algae with internal septa between nuclei. X1100. (From Nabai and Mehregan. J Cutan Pathol 1:180, 1974).

gerum (Fig. 22–11) in excisional biopsy specimens of migrating erythematous and nodular lesions of patients in southeast Asian countries.[52-54]

In rare instances *Fasciola hepatica* (liver fluke) may produce human infection in farm workers. Adult flukes are widespread, such as in subcutaneous fat tissue, brain, and bladder (Fig. 22–12).[55] Tissue reaction may vary from lymphangitis to abscess formation and foreign body granulomas. *Schistosoma* is illustrated in Figure 22–13.

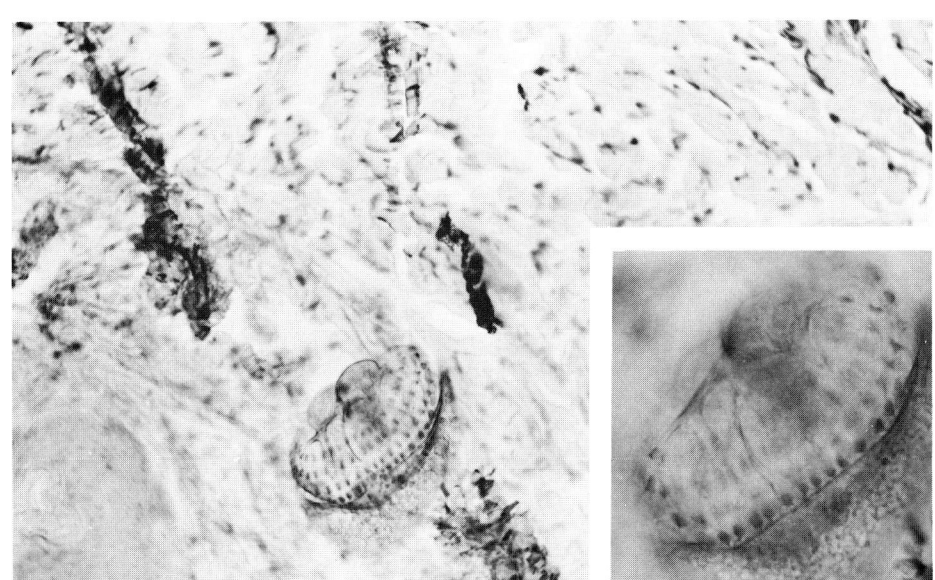

Figure 22–11.
Gnathostoma spinigerum. Head bulb in human skin. Inset shows head bulb with distinctive cuticular spines. O&G. X250. (From Pinkus et al. Int J Dermatol 20: 46, 1981.)

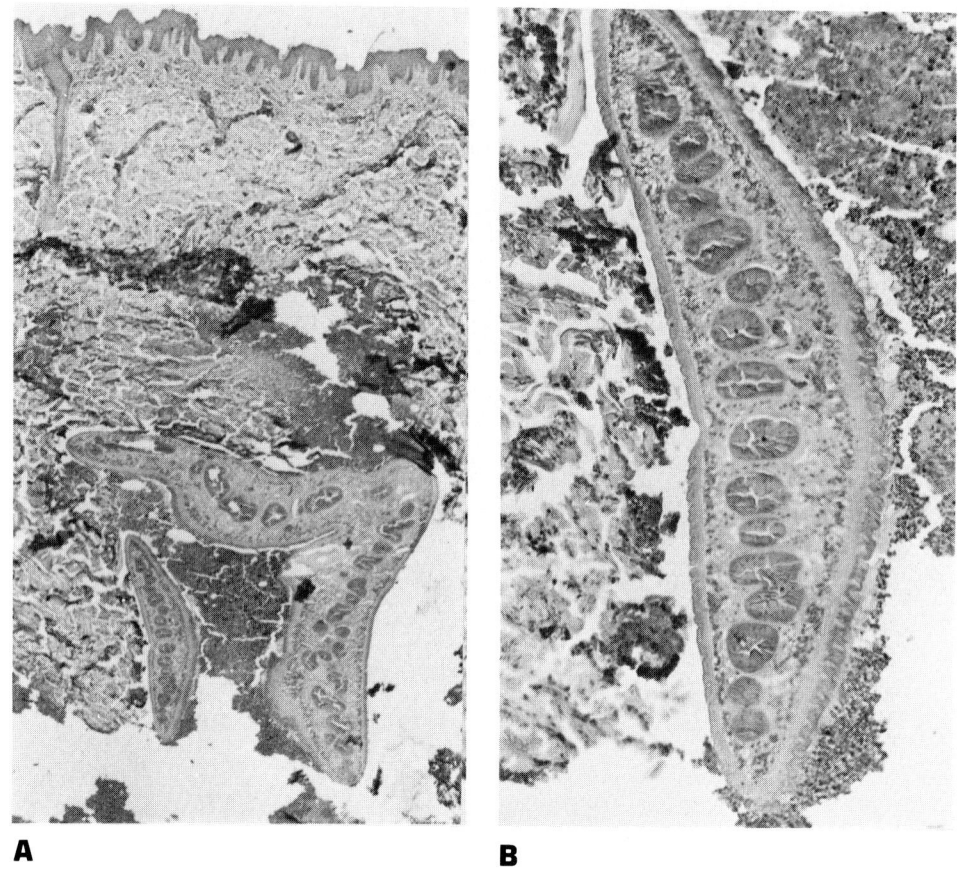

Figure 22-12.
Cutaneous fascioliasis. Cross sections of Fasciola hepatica deep in dermis and subcutaneous fat tissue. H&E. **A.** X45. **B.** X125. (Courtesy of Dr. Y. Dowlati.)

HALOGEN ERUPTIONS

Ingestion of iodides, fluorides, or bromides will produce granulomatous lesions in predisposed patients. The more common side effect of iodide medication is development of small follicular pustules, but in some cases these become furunculoid clinically and granulomatous histologically.[56,57] The infiltrate consists of a mixture of the cells mentioned earlier and is apt to include numerous polymorphonuclear leukocytes. Multinucleated giant cells are rare and are found as a response to disintegrating hair follicles. Papulonodular eruptions have been observed after intraoral application of fluoride-containing gels.

Bromoderma usually is a more chronic, often verrucous lesion, clinically resembling North American blastomycosis. Histologic resemblance (Fig. 22-14) also is striking, the main difference being the absence of multinucleated giant cells. This and the absence of demonstrable organisms in a lesion characterized by much epidermal hyperplasia, intraepithelial abscesses, and a mixed granulomatous infiltrate should arouse strong suspicion of bromoderma. The final diagnosis must be based on result of cultures, blood determination of bromides, and clinical history.

Granuloma Gluteale Infantum

In the bromoderma group may belong vegetating granulomas on the buttocks of babies described as *granuloma gluteale infantum*.[58] They exhibit epidermal acanthosis and hyperkeratosis with a mixed granulomatous infiltrate in the dermis and fibrinoid degeneration of vessel walls. They follow diaper dermatitis and involute spontaneously after several months. Similar eruptions may be found in the aged.[59]

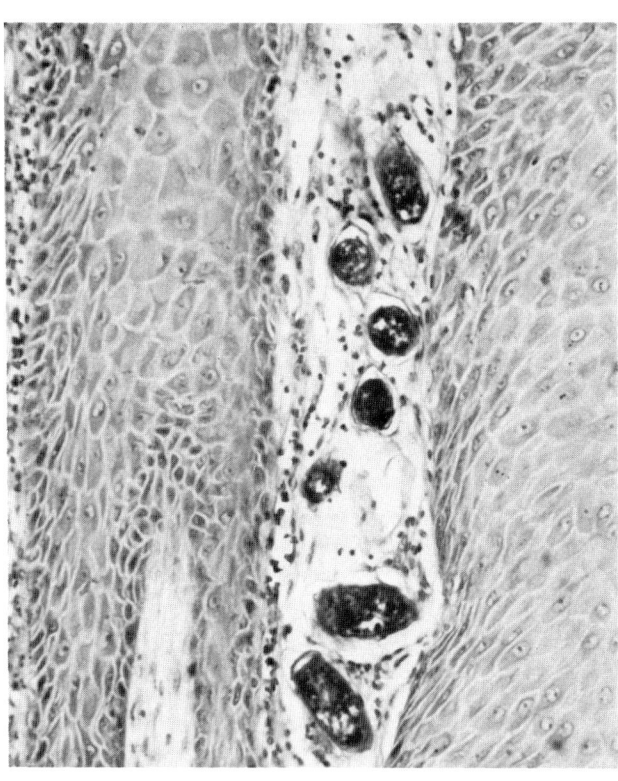

Figure 22–13.
Schistosomiasis. Encapsulated oval sectioned at various angles. H&E. X180. (Courtesy of Dr. H. Z. Lund.)

FOREIGN BODY GRANULOMAS

Whereas lesions due to silica, zirconium, beryllium, and some other substances usually are in the sarcoid reaction group, there are many other instances in which a mixed cell granuloma results from reaction to a foreign body. An outstanding example is formation of massive granulomas and abscesses secondary to an infected and broken down epithelial cyst. In such instances numerous macrophages and multinucleated giant cells contain flakes of keratinous material and foam cells may be present in areas of lipid deposition.

In other cases, granulomas develop around foreign bodies penetrating the skin from the outside. Wood splinters, thorns, cactus spines,[60] and other vegetable matter may be identified by their birefringence, which reveals even tiny particles and their structural characteristics. Old wood splinters may be contaminated with brown hyphae of fungus organisms (Fig. 22–15). Arthropods, stinging and biting insects, and ticks may produce long-lasting

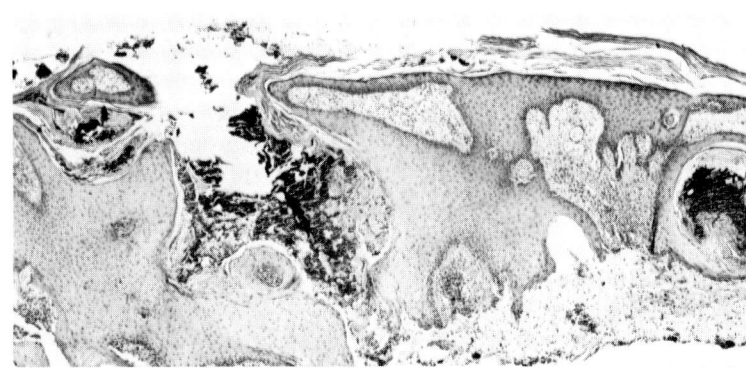

Figure 22–14.
Bromoderma. Pseudoepitheliomatous proliferation of epidermis enclosing necrotic tissue and inflammatory cells. H&E. X75.

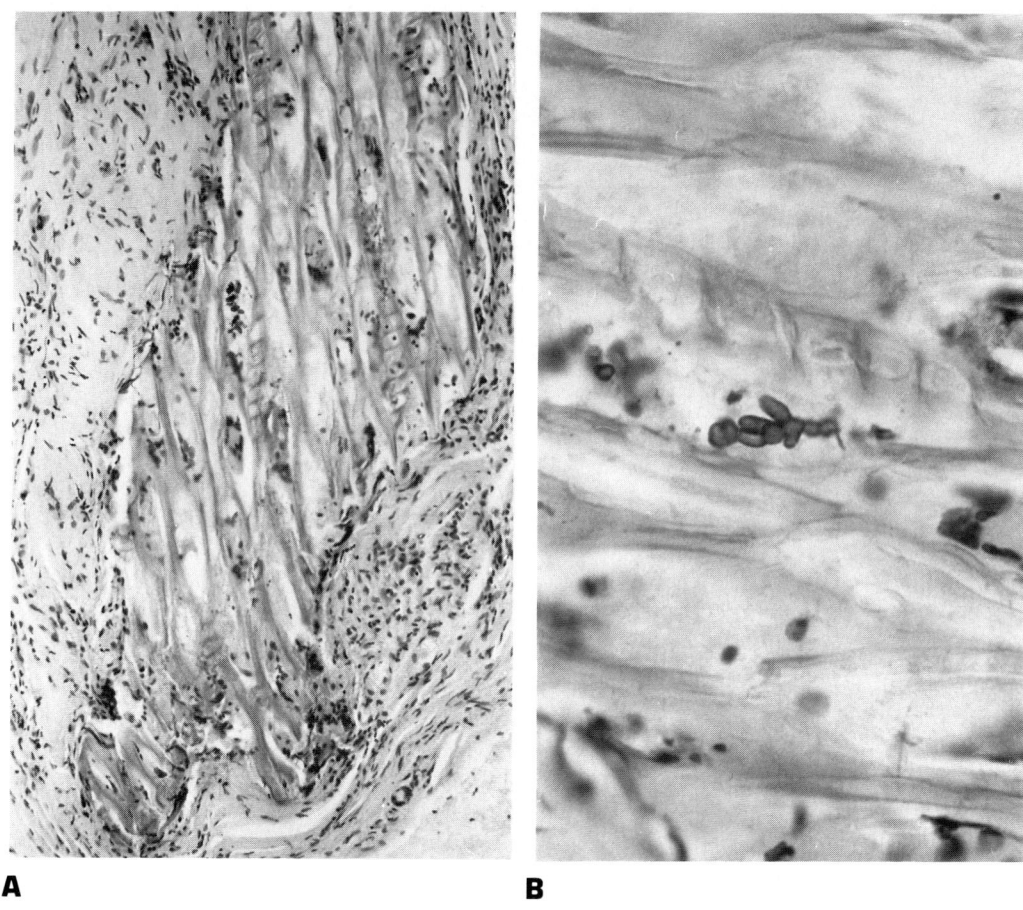

Figure 22-15.
A. Wood splinter embedded in dermis surrounded by foreign body granuloma. H&E. X125. **B.** The wood splinter contains brown budding fungus spores H&E. X400.

mixed cell granulomas, presumably due to the retention of chitinous material, which, however, is not usually demonstrable. Because of their peculiar features, they are discussed under pseudolymphomas. Granulomatous reactions may develop in tattoos containing mercury or other chemicals to which an occasional person may become sensitized.

GRANULOMA INGUINALE

This bacillary disease, assumed to be caused by *Donovania granulomatis*, produces superficial granulomatous lesions, although it may become destructive and mutilating.[61] It shares with the syphilitic chancre the peculiarity that it looks ulcerated clinically, while histologically the epidermis persists for long periods. In fact, the epidermis often is acanthotic (Figs. 22–16 and 22–17) and almost verrucous even though denuded of its surface layers. The granulomatous infiltrate (Fig. 22–16) at low power is dense and amorphous and hugs the epidermis. It usually has a very sharp lower edge in the middermis. Higher power reveals a colorful mixture of cells with little or no organization except around blood vessels. Lymphocytes, plasma cells, neutrophils, and eosinophils are present, in addition to scattered histiocytes. Multinucleated cells are rare. The characteristic cell is a pale-staining macrophage, which contains the diagnostic "Donovan bodies" (Fig. 22–17B and Table 21–3). These cells are more common in the superficial parts of the granuloma.[62] If one prepares smears for diagnosis, one must scrape the lesions, not just wipe superficial purulent matter on the slide.

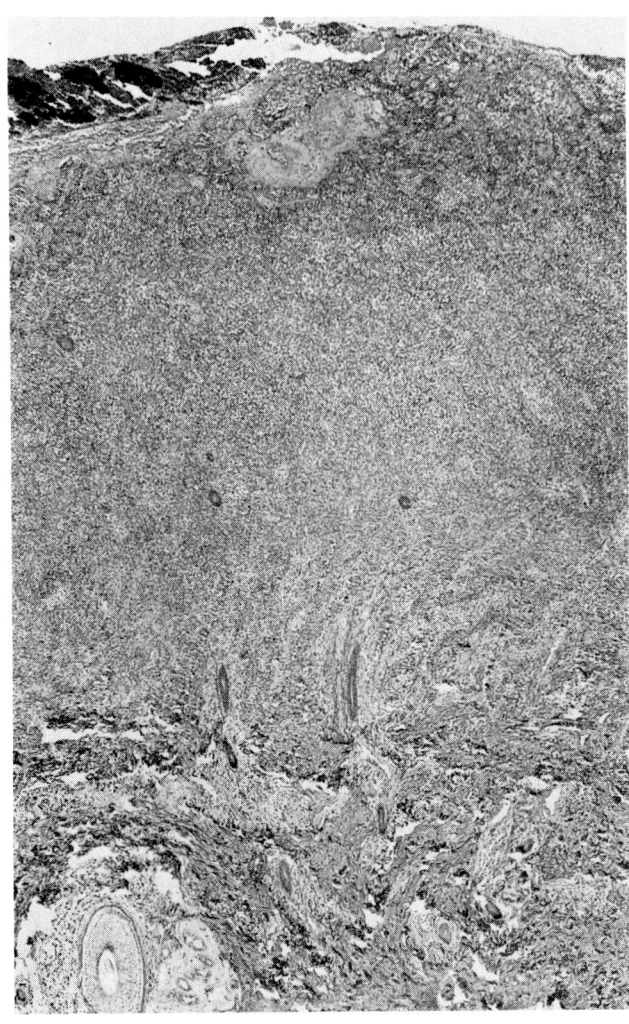

Figure 22–16.
Granuloma inguinale. Diffuse granulomatous infiltrate extends from epidermis into middermis and has a fairly sharp lower border. Note persistence of epidermis below surface crust. H&E. X30.

LYMPHOGRANULOMA VENEREUM

Lymphogranuloma inguinale is mentioned here mainly for the purpose of pointing out that it is not a skin disease but a disorder of lymph nodes. The causative agent is *Chlamydia trachomatis*.[63] The primary lesion in the skin is so small and fleeting that it is rarely biopsied. The late cutaneous changes, called *ésthiomène*, are lymphedematous masses with superimposed infection and ulceration and have no diagnostic features histologically. Lymph node biopsy shows stellate or triangular abscesses surrounded by areas of epthelioid cell granuloma and scattered multinucleated giant cells.[64]

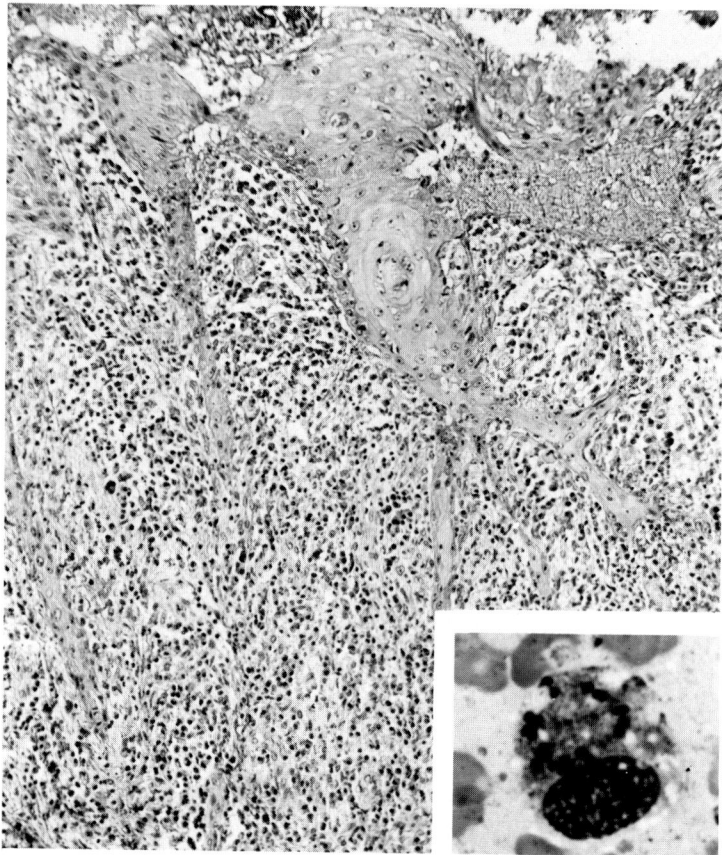

Figure 22–17.
Granuloma inguinale. Epidermis persists and shows some pseudoepitheliomatous proliferation above a diffuse mixed granulomatous infiltrate. H&E. X135. Inset, Donovania granulomatis in a large mononuclear cell. Smear, Wright's blood stain. X1100.

REFERENCES

1. Epstein WL: The pathogenesis of granulomatous hypersensitivity: Newer observations. J Dermatol Tokyo 9:335, 1982
2. Reyes-Flores O: Granulomas induced by living agents. Int J Dermatol 25:158, 1986
3. O'Brien JJ, Gilsdorf JR: Primary cutaneous coccidioidomycosis in childhood. Pediatr Infect Dis J 5:485, 1986
4. Prichard JG, Sorotzkin RA, James RE III: Cutaneous manifestations of disseminated coccidioidomycosis in the acquired immunodeficiency syndrome. Cutis 39: 203, 1987
5. Tomecki KJ, Dijkstra JWE, Hall GS, Steck WD: Systemic mycoses. J Am Acad Dermatol 21:1285, 1989
6. Schwartz RA, Lamberts RJ: Isolated nodular cutaneous coccidioidomycosis. The initial manifestation of disseminated disease. J Am Acad Dermatol 4:38, 1981
7. Hobbs ER, Hempstead RW: Cutaneous coccidioidomycosis simulating lepromatous leprosy. Int J Dermatol 23:334, 1984
8. Klein BS, Vergeront JM, Weeks RJ, et al: Isolation of blastomyces dermatitidis in soil associated with a large outbreak of blastomycosis in Wisconsin. N Engl J Med 134:529, 1986
9. Kantor GR, Roenigk RK, Bailin PL, et al: Cutaneous blastomycosis. Report of a case presumably acquired by direct inoculation and treated with carbon dioxide laser vaporization. Clev Clin J Med 54:121, 1987
10. Murphy PA: Blastomycosis. JAMA 261:3159, 1989
11. Kroll JJ, Walzer, RA: Paracoccidioidomycosis in the United States. Arch Dermatol 106:543, 1972
12. Talhari S, Souza Cunha M De G, Barroso Barros ML, DosReis Gadelha A: Doenca de Jorge Lobo. Estudo de 22 Cases novos. Med Cutan ILA 9:87, 1981
13. Baruzzi RG, Rodrigues DA, Michalany NS, Salomao R: Squamous-cell carcinoma and lobomycosis (Jorge Lobo's disease). Int J Dermatol 28:183, 1989
14. McGinnis MR: Chromoblastomycosis and phaeohyphomycosis: New concepts, diagnosis, and mycology. J Am Acad Dermatol 8:1, 1983
15. Rosen T, Gyorkey F, Joseph LM, Batres E: Ultrastructural features of chromoblastomycosis. Int J Dermatol 19:461, 1980
16. Zaias N, Rebell G: A simple and accurate diagnostic method in chromoblastomycosis. Arch Dermatol 108: 545,1973

17. Batres E, Wolf JE, Rudolph AH, Knox JM: Transepithelial elimination of cutaneous chromomycosis. Arch Dermatol 114:1231, 1978
18. Tsuboi R, Takamori K, Ogawa H, et al: Lymphocutaneous nocardiosis caused by *Nocardia asteroides*. Arch Dermatol 122:1183, 1986
19. Magana M: Mycetoma. Int J Dermatol 23:221, 1984
20. Ndiaye B, Guiraud M, Traore A, et al: Mycetome actinomycosique de la paroi abdominale avec extension viscerale secondaire. A propos d'une obsevation. Nouv Dermatol 8:527, 1989
21. Toth IR, Kazal HL: Botryomycosis in acquired immunodeficiency syndrome. Arch Pathol Lab Med 111:246, 1987
22. Prado de Oliveira ZN, Cuce LC, Salebian A: Botriomicose. Med Cutan ILA 14:49, 1986
23. Tanaka S, Mochizuki T, Watanabe S: Sporotrichoid pyogenic bacterial infection. Dermatologica 178:228, 1989
24. Sussman EJ, McMahon F, Wright D, et al: Cutaneous cryptococcosis without evidence of systemic involvement. J Am Acad Dermatol 11:371, 1984
25. Baes H, Van Cutsem J: Primary cutaneous cryptococcosis. Dermatologica 171:357, 1985
26. Carlson KC, Mehlmauer M, Evans S, Chandrasoma P: Cryptococcal cellulitis in renal transplant recipients. J Am Acad Dermatol 17:469, 1987
27. Geyer SJ, Weber JC: Localized cutaneous cryptococcosis in an immunocompromised man. Int J Dermatol 23:673, 1984
28. Rico MJ, Penneys NS: Cutaneous cryptococcosis resembling molluscum contagiosum in a patient with AIDS. Arch Dermatol 121:901, 1985
29. Bernhardt MJ, Ward WQ, Sams WM: Cryptoccocal cellulitis. Cutis 34:359, 1984
30. Barfield L, Iacobelli D, Hashimoto K: Secondary cutaneous cryptococcosis: Case report and review of 22 cases. J Cutan Pathol 15:385, 1988
31. Dolezal JR: Blastomycoid sporotrichosis. J Am Acad Dermatol 4:523, 1981
32. Bellatorre DL, Latterand A, Buckley HR: Fixed cutaneous sporotrichosis of the face. J Am Acad Dermatol 6:97, 1982
33. Mohri S, Nakajima H, Kurosawa T, et al: Three cases of sporotrichosis with numerous fungal elements. J Dermatol Tokyo 14:382, 1987
34. Dunstan RW, Langham RF, Reimann KA, Wakenell PS: Feline sporotrichosis: A report of five cases with transmission to humans. J Am Acad Dermatol 15:37, 1986
35. Schamroth JM, Grieve TP, Kellen P: Disseminated sporotrichosis. Int J Dermatol 27:28, 1988
36. Boustany Noel S, Greer DL, Abadie SM, et al: Primary cutaneous phaeohyphomycosis. Report of three cases. J Am Acad Dermatol 18:1023, 1988
37. Hall JC, Brewer JH, Reed WA, et al: Cutaneous mucormycosis in a heart transplant patient. Cutis 42:183, 1988
38. Camenen I, De Closets F, Vaillant L, et al: Alternariose cutanee a alternaria tenuissima. Ann Dermatol Venereol 115:839, 1988
39. Hammond DE, Winkelmann RK: Cutaneous phycomycosis. Report of three cases with identification of *Rhizopus*. Arch Dermatol 115:990, 1979
40. Otoyma K, Tomizawa N, Higuchi I, Horiuchi Y: Cutaneous protothecosis. A case report. J Dermatol Tokyo 16:496, 1989
41. Tyring SK, Lee PC, Walsh P, et al: Papular protothecosis of the chest. Immunologic evaluation and treatment with a combination of oral tetracycline and topical amphotricin B. Arch Dermatol 125:1249, 1989
42. Falanga V, Kapoor W: Cerebral cysticercosis: Diagnostic value of subcutaneous nodules. Report of two cases. J Am Acad Dermatol 12:304, 1985
43. King DT, Gilbert DJ, Gurevitch AW, et al: Subcutaneous cysticercosis. Arch Dermatol 115:236, 1979
44. Cogen MS, Hays SJ, Dixon JM: Cutaneous myiaisis of the eyelid due to cuterebra larva. JAMA 258:1795, 1987
45. Grogan TM, Payne CM, Payne TB, et al: Cutaneous myiasis. Immunohistologic and ultrastructural morphometric features of a human botfly lesion. Am J Dermatopathol 9:232, 1987
46. Goldman L: Tungiasis in travelers from tropical Africa. JAMA 236:1386, 1976
47. Jung RC, Harris FH: Human filiarial infection in Louisiana. Arch Pathol 69:371, 1960
48. Kpodzro K, Menning G, Bitho M, Vovor M: Onchocercomes. A propos de 41 cas au C.H.U. de Lomé. Castellania (Berlin) 4:187, 1976
49. Payan HM: Human infection with dirofiliaria. Arch Dermatol 114:593, 1978
50. Torres VM: Dermatological manifestations of schistosomiasis mansoni. Arch Dermatol 112:153, 1976
51. Walther RR: Chronic papular dermatitis of the scrotum due to schistosoma Mansoni. Arch Dermatol 115:869, 1979
52. Pinkus H, Fan J, DeGiusti D: Creeping eruption due to *Gnathostoma spinigerum* in a Taiwanese patient. Int J Dermatol 20:46, 1981
53. Kagen CN, Vance JC, Simpson M: Gnathostomiasis. Infestation in an Asian immigrant. Arch Dermatol 120:508, 1984
54. Ollague Torres JM, Ollague Loaiza W: Cronologia histologica de la paniculitis nodular migratoria eosinofilica (gnathostomiasis). Med Cutan ILA 15:85, 1987
55. Hardman EW, Jones RLH, Davies AH: Fascioliasis— A large outbreak. Br Med J 3:502, 1970
56. O'Brien TJ: Iodic eruptions. Austr J Dermatol 28:119, 1987
57. Burnett JW: Iodides and bromides. Cutis 43:130, 1989
58. Bonifazi E, Garofalo L, Lospalluti M, et al: Granuloma gluteale infantum with atrophic scars: Clinical and histological observations in eleven cases. Clin Exp Dermatol 6:23, 1981
59. Bluestein J, Furner BB, Phillips D: Granuloma gluteale infantum: Case report and review of the literature. Pediatr Dermatol 7:196, 1990

60. Schreiber MM, Shapiro SI, Berry CZ: Cactus granuloma of the skin. Arch Dermatol 104:374, 1971
61. Davis CM: Granuloma inguinale, a clinical, histological, and ultrastructural study. JAMA 211:632, 1970
62. Sehgal VN, Shyam Prasad AL: Donovanosis. Current concepts. Int J Dermatol 25:8, 1986
63. Becker LE, Charles CR, Babcock WS: Electron microscopic diagnosis of lymphogranuloma venereum. J Assoc Mil Dermatol 7:5, 1981
64. Becker LE: Lymphogranuloma venereum. Int J Dermatol 15:26, 1976

23
PALISADING GRANULOMAS

A palisading granuloma exhibits a primary focus of localized damage to the dermis that affects the cells more than the fibers and is accompanied by deposits of abnormal substances. This area of "necrobiosis" is surrounded by a granulomatous reaction in which rather loosely arranged histiocytes have a tendency to point radially toward the center of degeneration.[1] Lymphocytes and altered blood vessels usually are found more peripherally. Immunologic studies have shown evidence of vasculitis, suggesting that the central area of necrobiosis may be related to vascular occlusion.[2,3] This finding reminds us of the concept of papulonecrotic tuberculid, in which primary tissue necrosis is supposed to be due to an embolus of bacteria occluding small vessels, with resulting toxic necrosis of the surrounding tissue in a host with high immune reaction to tuberculin. The histologic changes of papulonecrotic tuberculid are indeed very similar to those of granuloma annulare.

The primary cause of the vascular occlusion may vary and in some cases remains unknown. Granuloma annulare, actinic granuloma, granulomatosis disciformis of miescher, necrobiosis lipoidica, rheumatic and rheumatoid nodules, and the juxta-articular nodes of syphilis are in this group. The latest additions are granulomatous slack skin, necrobiotic xanthogranuloma and cat-scratch disease. Lesions of this group must be sharply differentiated from lesions in which a granulomatous wall surrounds a central area of necrosis, which is secondary to the granuloma. Outstanding examples of the latter category are lupus miliaris faciei (see Fig. 21–4), gummatous syphilis (see Fig. 21–11), and sporotrichotic gumma (see Fig. 22–8). Beryllium granuloma (see Fig. 21–17) exemplifies a somewhat different process in which tissue has probably been damaged by the presence of foreign material. Deposition of urates in a gouty tophus produces a palisading granuloma, and so does degeneration of eosinophils in eosinophilic cellulitis and perhaps in the Churg–Strauss syndrome, in which the involvement of blood vessels is likely.

GRANULOMA ANNULARE

The most characteristic representative of the palisading granuloma is granuloma annulare. Just as the clinical lesion usually is a ring, so does the annular shape dominate the histologic picture. Each of the small papules that often compose the clinical ring-shaped rim is made up of one or several palisading granulomas. These are more often ovoid (Fig. 23–1) than round and are commonly located in the upper half of the pars reticularis. They may sit higher or lower, however, and usually are small and are either single or multiple. Occasionally, a large lesion may occupy almost the entire width of the dermis.

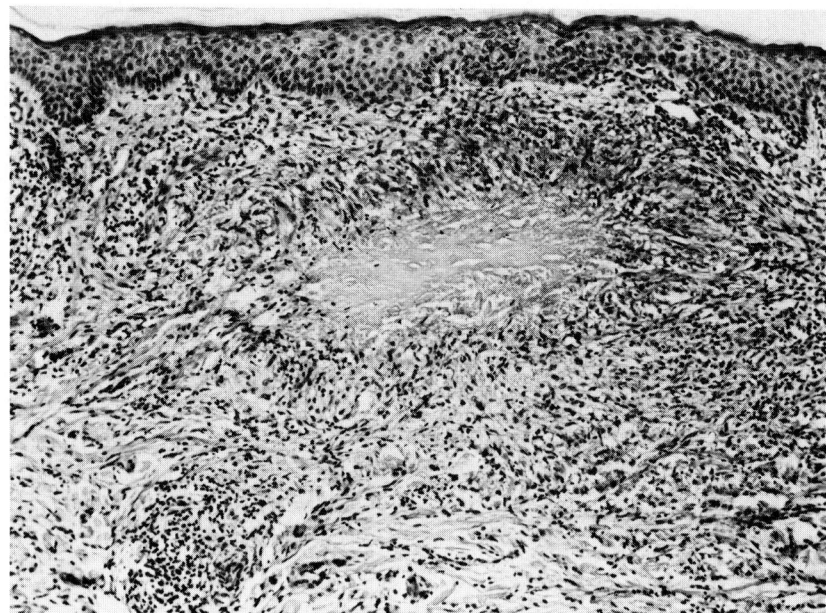

Figure 23-1.
Granuloma annulare. Note absence of cell nuclei in the central necrobiotic area. H&E. X75.

The histologic diagnosis of granuloma annulare is best made under low power because it is the peculiar configuration that counts rather than details of the lesion. An ovoid area of lymphohistiocytic infiltrate in the mid dermis should arouse suspicion. If the necrobiotic center is small, it may be missed in some sections, and multiple sections must be examined. The size and degree of degenerative change vary widely. It ranges from a small focus of stringy hematoxylinophilic material between well-preserved and pink staining connective tissue bundles to sizable areas of complete necrosis. The most typical expression is an ovoid area in which one sees only traces of nuclear dust between normal-appearing collagen bundles and some amorphous mucoid material that stains bluish in H&E sections and metachromatic with toluidine blue reaction indicating the presence of acid mucopolysaccharide. Microdroplet lipid deposition may be demonstrated by lipid stain. The acid orcein–giemsa stain however, reveals persistence of elastic fibers and thus testifies to primary tissue damage. Elastic fibers persist even if the center is more definitely necrotic (Fig. 23–2) and the collagen bundles are fragmented and assume a washed-out or ground-glass appearance.[4] In such cases, small vessels and sweat ducts running through the area will also undergo necrosis.

The granulomatous wall varies considerably in quantity and composition. Typical is a loose, almost reticular arrangement of fusiform or stellate histiocytic cells that fill the interfascicular spaces and more or less point their ends toward the center.

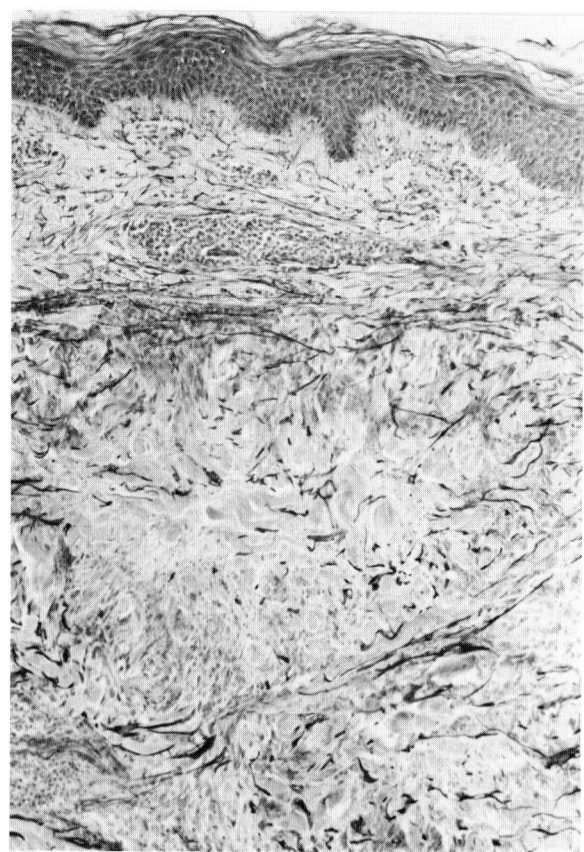

Figure 23-2.
Granuloma annulare showing persistence of many elastic fibers in central necrobiotic zone, their absence in granulomatous wall. O&G. X135.

Multinucleated giant cells (Fig. 23–3) are found if the infiltrate is more massive. Phagocytosis of elastic fibers by multinucleated giant cells can be demonstrated in O&G sections.[5–7] Epithelioid cell lobules are present in only a small percentage of lesions.[8] Lymphocytes surround blood vessels in the periphery. Although they are not numerous in typical cases, they may occasionally overshadow the histiocytic ovals and their necrobiotic centers. Eosinophils are present in a good number of lesions.[9] O&G sections show considerable destruction of elastic fibers in the granulomatous wall, but in general this stain is not favorable for diagnosis because the presence of elastic fibers in the center is more impressive than their lack in the thin wall. Immunofluorescent studies have demonstrated deposition of IgM, complement, and fibrinogen on blood vessels of the granulomatous wall and fibrinogen in the necrobiotic center.[2,3]

More advanced immunopathologic studies suggest that cell-mediated immune response producing cytokines may be important in the pathogenesis of granuloma annulare.[3]

The great variability in the details of the lesion is the reason for the advice to train one's eye for diagnosis of granuloma annulare under the low-power lens by recognizing its general configuration and location in the pars reticularis.

Major deviations from this localization occur in two directions and give rise to interesting diagnostic deliberations. In rare cases, granuloma annulare may develop in the subcutaneous fat tissue. Because of the lack of tough collagen in this area, central necrosis is apt to be more complete, and the granulomatous wall is heavier (Fig. 23–4). In these lesions, large numbers of eosinophils may be found, often disintegrating and leaving eosinophilic dust in the center. It is important to know of this variant because it is indistinguishable histologically from rheumatic or rheumatoid nodes. The diagnosis becomes obvious if the patient, usually a child, also has typical cutaneous lesions, but cases are on record where a diagnosis of rheumatic fever was made mistakenly on the strength of histologic examination. Cases of this type should be examined thoroughly for any other evidence of rheumatic fever. If none is found, the isolated subcutaneous nodules can be accepted as harmless granuloma annulare.

Association of granuloma annulare with necrobiosis lipoidica and rheumatic nodules is rare.[10,11] The relationship with diabetes mellitus may be more than coincidence and may indicate an underlying personal or familial predisposition.[12]

The necrobiotic area may develop unusually high in dermis, especially on the fingers or extremities. It may then involve the epidermis, with necro-

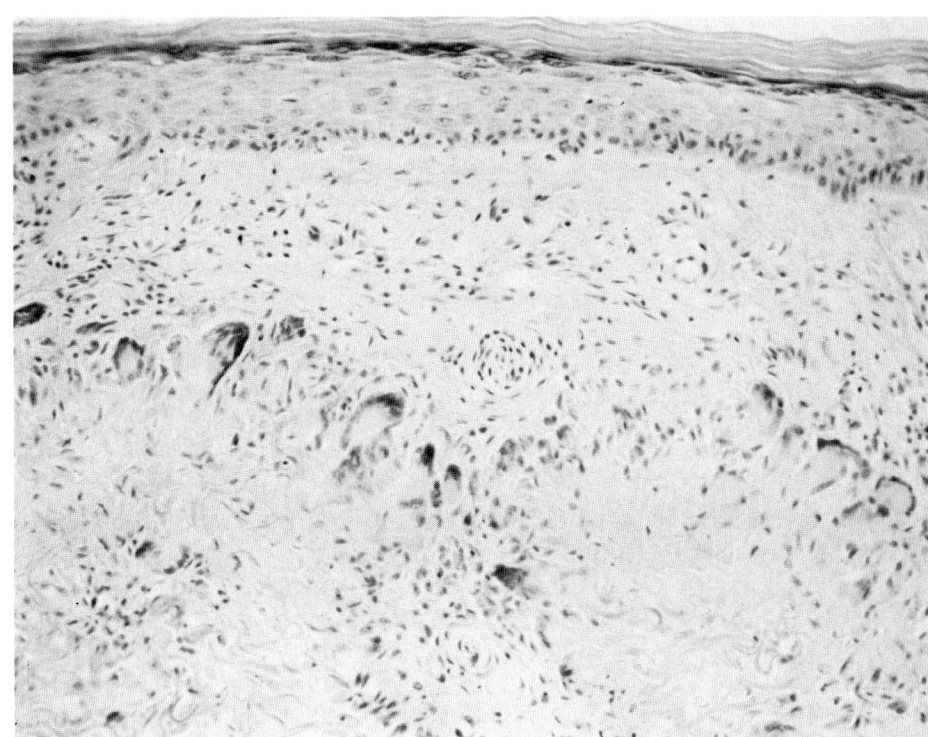

Figure 23–3.
Granuloma annulare containing an unusual number of multinucleated giant cells. H&E. X180.

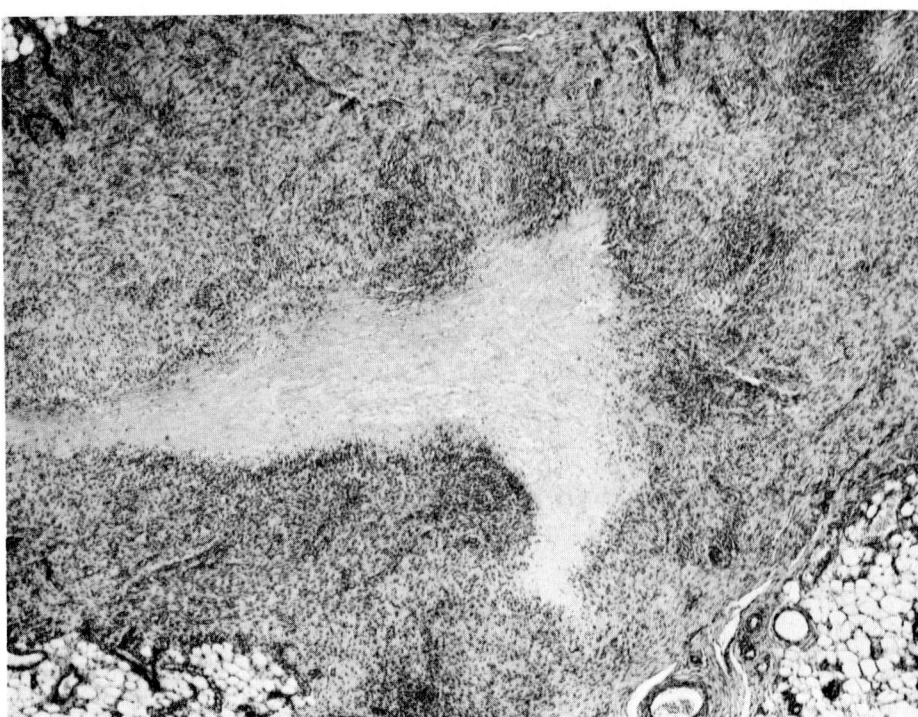

Figure 23–4.
Subcutaneous granuloma annulare. Complete central necrosis and heavy granulomatous wall make lesion morphologically indistinguishable from a rheumatic node. H&E. X45.

sis forming an umbilicated (perforating) lesion. This phenomenon is observed most commonly in the generalized papular variety[13–16] (Fig. 23–5). Perforation occurs immediately above the area of necrobiosis and shows altered collagenous tissue being extruded into the surface of the lesion. In the underlying dermis, the necrobiotic area is surrounded by palisading granuloma.

A histologic picture similar to granuloma annulare, but with heavier granulomatous infiltrate, is encountered in an African disease called "granuloma multiforme"[17] and in an occasional case of cutaneous "schistosomiasis."[18] Necrobiotic areas surrounded by palisading granulomas are also observed in test sites of bovine collagen injections.[19]

ACTINIC GRANULOMA

Ring-shaped or circinate and slowly expanding papular plaques are seen occasionally on the neck or dorsa of hands of heavily sun-exposed individuals.[20–23] A few cases with lesions in covered areas have also been reported.[24,25] Histologic changes are initiated by extracellular and intracellular destruction of elastic fibers and a rather heavy granulomatous infiltrate in which a number of macrophages and multinucleated giant cells contain fragments of elastotic material.[26] O'Brien[27] has suggested four different histologic patterns. (1) The giant cell pattern shows small foci of giant cell granulomas at the advancing border of the annular lesion. The center shows atrophy and loss of elastic tissue. (2) The histiocytic pattern shows a number of histiocytes scattered between the actinic elastic fibers. Giant cells are few and the elastolysis is mild. (3) In the necrobiotic vascular pattern, prominent vascular involvement with single or multiple foci of ischemic necrosis is present in the advancing border. (4) The sarcoidal pattern shows masses of epithelioid cells and collections of multinucleated giant cells some containing asteroid bodies. Remnants of elastic fibers are present within the central atrophic and fibrotic area.

Granulomatosis Disciformis (Miescher)

A condition very likely related to actinic granuloma, Miescher's granulomatosis disciformis is characterized by slowly progressing gray brown rings and plaques on forehead and scalp which leaves slightly atrophic skin in the center.[28,29] (Fig. 23–6). Histologically it is distinguished by the absence of necrobiosis and diffuse dermal infiltrate of lymphocytes, histiocytes, and multinucleated giant cells, some

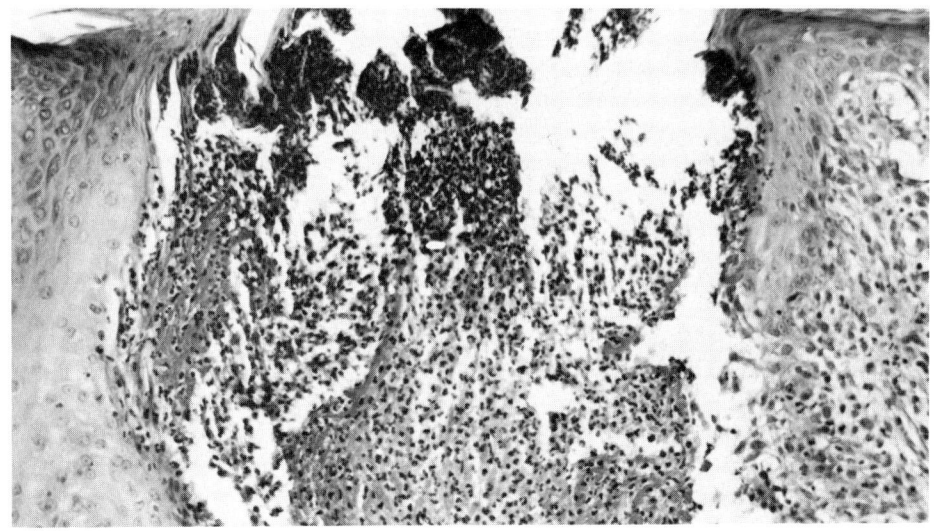

A

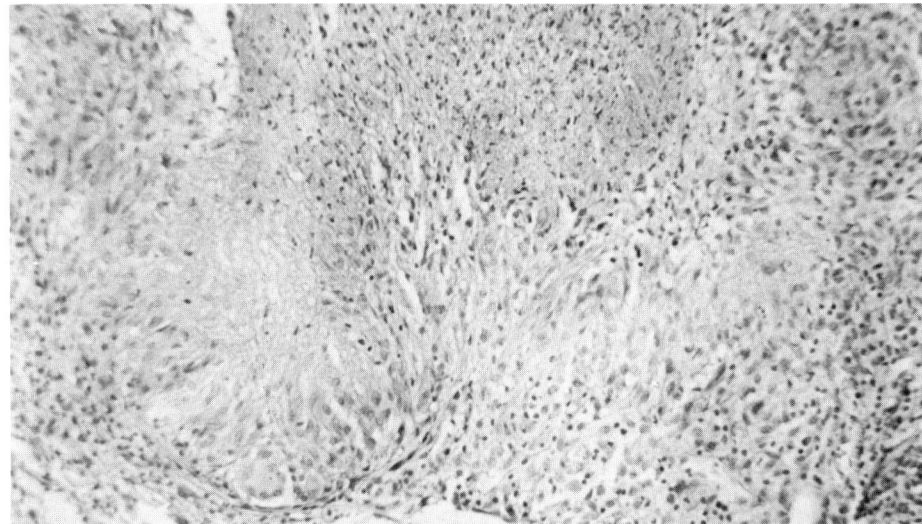

B

Figure 23–5.
Perforating granuloma annulare. Upper and lower portions are shown. Lesion of finger where the necrobiotic focus lies close to thick epidermis. Epidermis has disintegrated above the necrobiosis and shows some proliferative activity at the sides. Many polymorphs are present in the necrotic tissue being discharged to the surface. The picture has some similarity to chondrodermatitis nodularis helicis (see Fig. 17–6), and both diseases may be classified as transepithelial elimination. H&E. X135. (From A. Mehregan. Curr Prob Dermatol 3:144, 1970.)

containing elastotic asteroid bodies. There is patchy loss of elastic fibers and mild dermal fibrosis.

NECROBIOSIS LIPOIDICA

We purposely list necrobiosis lipoidica without the addition of *diabeticorum*. Although there is much evidence for an association of the skin disease with diabetes,[30,31] there is no definite difference in the histologic picture between patients having overt diabetes mellitus and those who do not have even laboratory evidence at the time the biopsy is taken.

In routine histologic sections, the features of necrobiosis lipoidica (Fig. 23–7) are similar in principle to granuloma annulare, the main difference being that the areas of necrobiosis are less focal. Instead of closed rings, one finds more often a sandwiching effect of alternating zones of tissue degeneration and infiltrate. Usually, the latter is heavier and more definitely granulomatous. Multinucleated giant cells and epithelioid nodules are frequently found. Occasionally lymphoid structures are present in deep dermis and the subcutaneous fat tissue.[32] Thickening of the vascular walls and narrowing of lumina are more pronounced. Immunofluorescence shows globulins in vascular walls and fibrinogen in

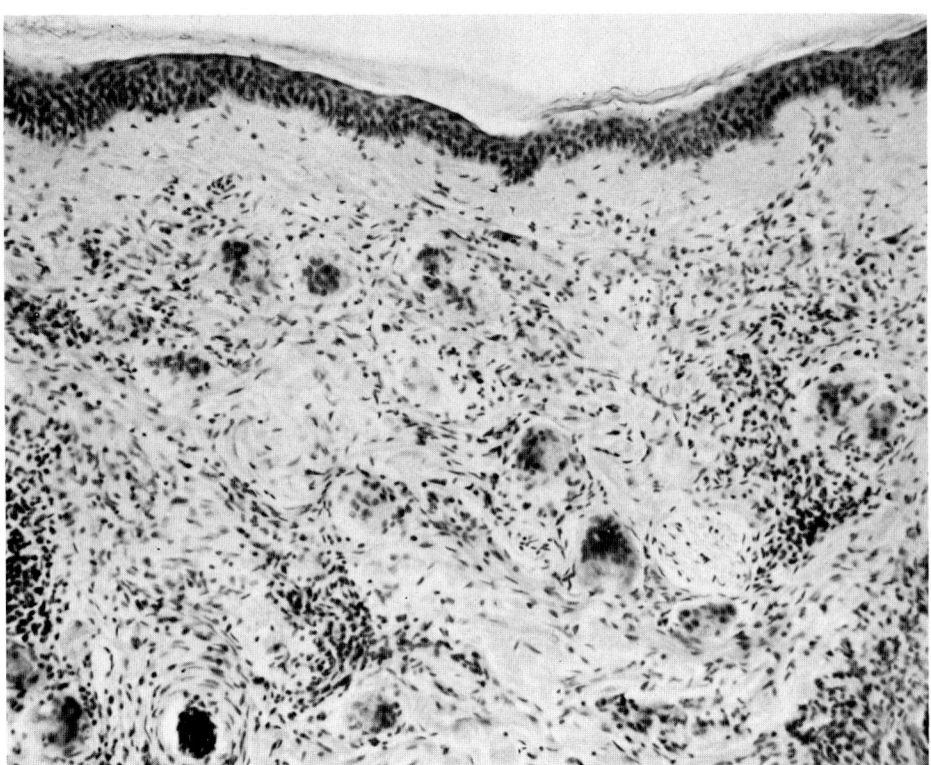

Figure 23–6.
Miescher's granuloma of forehead. Disorganized granulomatous infiltrate without areas of necrobiosis. Note similarity of histologic picture to nodular tertiary syphilis (see Fig. 21–10). H&E. X180.

the necrotic areas.[33] Electron microscopy shows loss of cross-striation, variation in diameter of collagen fibrils, and total reduction in concentration of collagen.[34] The histopathologic changes are similar to granuloma annulare. The crucial differentiating test is demonstration of extracellular lipids in the necrobiotic areas. This, however, requires frozen sections of fresh tissue, and the clinician must alert the laboratory to do these before the specimen is embedded in paraffin. Actually, fat stain is not necessary for diagnosis in most cases. Metachromatic substances may also be present in necrobiosis lipoidica and are not an exclusive feature of granuloma annulare.

RHEUMATIC AND RHEUMATOID NODES

Palisading granulomas associated with rheumatic fever or rheumatoid arthritis usually develop in the subcutaneous tissue but may be found in the skin (Fig. 23–8). The histologic findings are similar to those of subcutaneous granuloma annulare, however, they often exhibit a more extensive, eosinophilic, and homogeneous necrobiosis and no significant deposition of acid mucopolysaccharide. There are more giant cells within the surrounding granuloma and there is significant stromal fibrosis.[35]

Juxta-articular Nodes of Syphilis

Whereas the nodes of rheumatoid arthritis may be found close to joints but may occur elsewhere, similar lesions in old syphilitics are practically always situated near elbows and knees and may reach large size. Histologically, syphilitic juxta-articular nodes resemble the other palisading granulomas and are differentiated from gummas by their hard fibrotic centers. These centers grow by deposition of fibrous tissue and contain only remnants of elastic fibers. The granulomatous wall may be relatively thin and often contains plasma cells as a clue to syphilitic origin.

GRANULOMATOUS SLACK SKIN

Bulky erythematous and folded lesions with loose skin giving the impression of a localized cutis laxa occur near the axilla or groin. Extensive granulomatous inflammation is present in the dermis and subcutaneous fat tissue with a number of macrophages and multinucleated giant cells phagocytizing lymphocytes and fragments of elastic tissue.[36] The etiology is unknown. Lymphoproliferative nature has been proposed.[37]

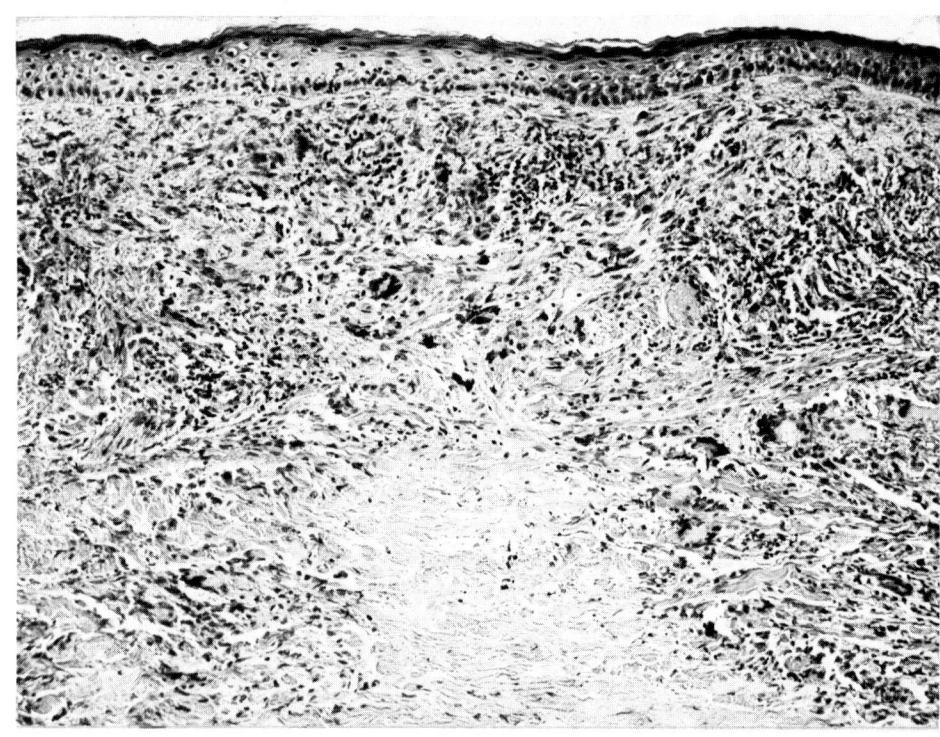

Figure 23–7.
Necrobiosis lipoidica, showing the upper rim of necrobiosis and granuloma, both of which extend downward into the dermis. H&E. X135.

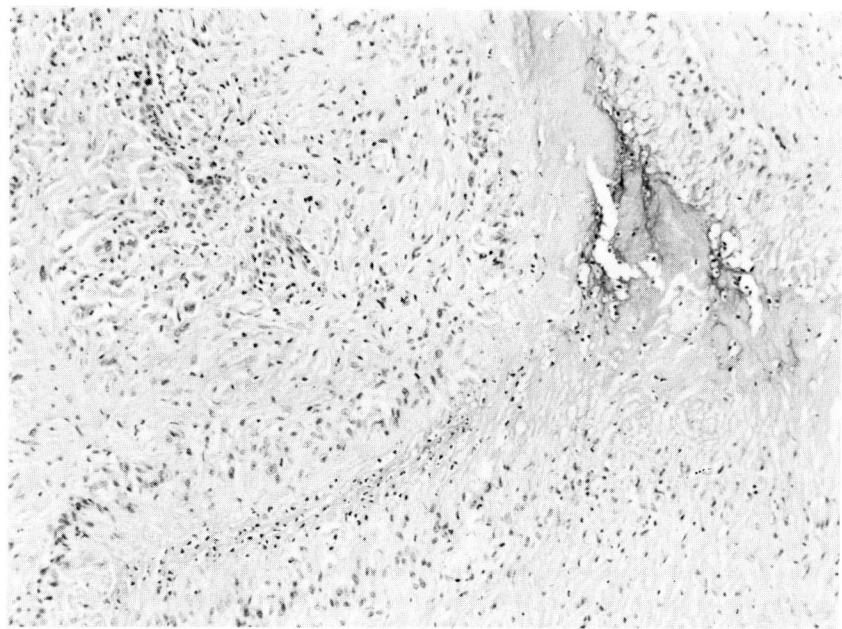

Figure 23–8.
Rheumatoid nodule. Note resemblance to subcutaneous granuloma annulare (Fig. 23–4). Necrobiotic center shows more fibrinoid degeneration. H&E. X60.

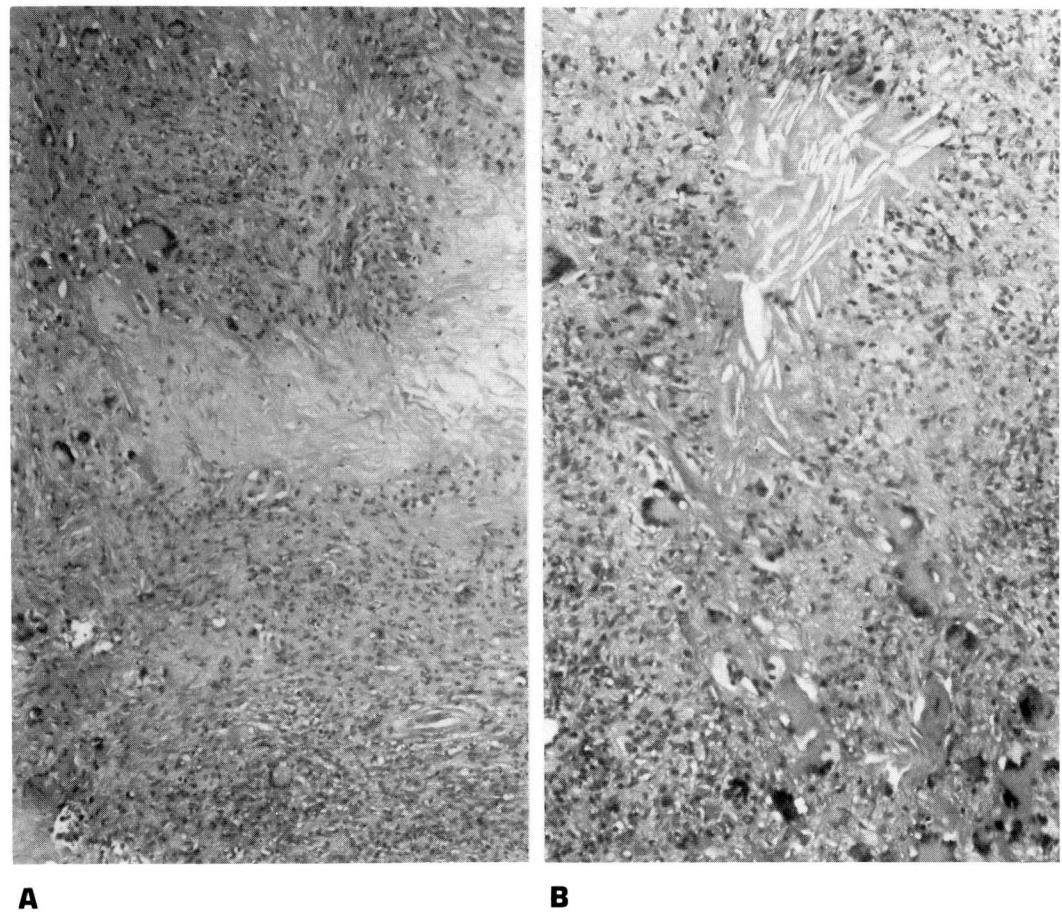

Figure 23–9.
Necrobiotic xanthogranuloma. **A.** Central necrobiotic areas and surrounding granuloma. **B.** Cholestrol clefts and multinucleated giant cells. H&E. X125. (Courtesy of Dr. David Mehregan.)

NECROBIOTIC XANTHOGRANULOMA

Indurated yellow-red nodules and plaques involve trunk and extremities in association with paraproteinemia.[38-40] Extensive periorbital involvement with ulceration and scarring is present in majority of cases (Fig. 23–9). Granulomatous masses consisting of sheets of histiocytes, multinucleated giant cells of both Touton and foreign body types, and a lesser number of lymphocytes are present in the full thickness of dermis and extend into the subcutaneous fat tissue. Broad bands of hyalin necrobiosis give a lobulated appearance to the granuloma. Foci of plasma cells and cholestrol crystals complete the picture.[41-42]

CAT-SCRATCH DISEASE

Cat-scratch disease is caused by a small gram-negative pleomorphic bacillus best demonstrated in the tissue sections of Warthin–Starry silver impregnation.[43] Skin manifestations include inoculation papules, pustules, and, rarely, vesicles. Five percent of the patients may develop generalized macular or maculopapular morbiliform eruptions.[44]

The primary inoculation site,[45] as well as the reaction to Hangor–Rose's skin test,[46] shows a palisading granuloma that may lead to necrosis of the overlying epidermis. It is similar to the granulomas formed in lymph nodes and exhibits necrosis of cells without deposition of acid mucous substances in the center and histiocytes, giant cells, and a mantle of lymphocytes in the periphery. Eosinophils are often scattered in the surroundings.

REFERENCES

1. Johnson WC: Necrobiotic granulomas. J Cutan Pathol 12:289, 1985
2. Dahl MV, Ullman S, Goltz RW: Vasculitis in granu-

loma annulare. Histopathology and direct immunofluorescence. Arch Dermatol 113:463, 1977
3. Modlin RL, Horwitz DA, Jordan RR, et al: Immunopathologic demonstration of T lymphocyte subpopulations and interleukin 2 in granuloma annulare. Pediatr Dermatol 2:26, 1984
4. Dabski K, Winkelmann RK: Generalized granuloma annulare: Histopathology and immunopathology. Systematic review of 100 cases and comparison with localized granuloma annulare. J Am Acad Dermatol 20:28, 1989
5. Burket JM, Zelickson AS: Intracellular elastin in generalized granuloma annulare. J Am Acad Dermatol 14:975, 1986
6. Nakagawa K, Tsuji T, Chanoki M, et al: Phagocytosis of elastic fibers by macrophage and giant cell in granuloma annulare: Immunohistochemical and ultrastructural studies. J Invest Dermatol 92:488, 1989
7. Yanagihara M, Kato F, Mori S: Extra- and intracellular digestion of elastic fibers by macrophages in annular elastolytic giant cell granuloma. J Cutan Pathol 14:303, 1987
8. Friedman-Birnbaum R, Weltfriend S, Munichor M, Lichtig C: A comparative histopathologic study of generalized and localized granuloma annulare. Am J Dermatopathol 11:144, 1989
9. Silverman RA, Rabinowitz AD: Eosinophils in the cellular infiltrate of granuloma annulare. J Cutan Pathol 12:13, 1985
10. Burton JL: Granuloma annulare, rheumatoid nodules and necrobiosis lipoidica. Br J Dermatol 97 (Suppl): 52, 1977
11. Schwartz ME: Necrobiosis lipoidica and granuloma annulare. Simultaneous occurrence in a patient. Arch Dermatol 118:192, 1982
12. Muhlemann MF, Williams DRR: Localized granuloma annulare is associated with insulin-dependent diabetes mellitus. Br J Dermatol 111:325, 1984
13. Wright AL, Buxton PK, Mclaren KM: Perforating granuloma annulare. Int J Dermatol 28:466, 1989
14. Dos Reis Gadelha A, Talhan S: Granuloma anular perforante. Med Cutan ILA 9:101, 1981
15. Aliaga A, Serrano G, De La Cuadra J, Fortea JM: Perforating granuloma annulare and vitamin D. Dermatologica 164:62, 1982
16. Husz S, Szabo E, Hunyadi J, et al: Disseminated atypical granuloma annulare. J Dermatol Tokyo 14:67, 1987
17. Meyers WM, Connor DH, Shannon R: Histologic characteristics of granuloma multiforme (Mkar disease); including a comparison with leprosy and granuloma annulare; report of first cases from Congo (Kinshasa). Int J Lepr 38:241, 1970
18. Findlay GH, Whiting DA: Disseminated and zosteriform cutaneous schistosomiasis. Br J Dermatol 85 (Suppl 7):98, 1971
19. Barr RJ, King FD, McDonald RM, Bartlow GA: Necrobiotic granulomas associated with bovine collagen test site injections. J Am Acad Dermatol 6:867, 1982
20. Moulin G, Moyne G, Franc M-P, Barrut D: Le granulome actinique de O'Brien. Ann Dermatol Venereol 109:135, 1982
21. Moreno A, Salvatella N, Guix M, De Moragas JM: Actinic granuloma. An ultrastructural study of two cases. J Cutan Pathol 11:179, 1984
22. Moulin G: Le granulome actinique. Ann Dermatol Venereol 114:269, 1987
23. McGrae JD: Actinic granuloma. A clinical, histopathologic and immunocytochemical study. Arch Dermatol 122:43, 1986
24. Ishibashi A, Yokoyama A, Hirano K: Annular elastolytic giant cell granuloma in covered areas. Dermatologica 174:293, 1987
25. Muramatsu T, Shirai T, Yamashina Y, Sakamoto K: Annular elastolytic giant cell granuloma: An unusual case with lesions arising in non-sun-exposed areas. J Dermatol Tokyo 14:54, 1987
26. Steffen C: Actinic granuloma (O'Brien). J Cutan Pathol 15:66, 1988
27. O'Brien: Actinic granuloma: The expanding significance. An analysis of its origin in elastotic ("aging") skin and a definition of necrobiotic (vascular), histiocytic, and sarcoid variants. Int J Dermatol 24:473, 1985
28. Mehregan AH, Altman J: Miescher's granuloma of the face. A variant of the necrobiosis lipoidica-granuloma annulare spectrum. Arch Dermatol 107:62, 1973
29. Wilson-Jones E: Necrobiosis lipoidica presenting on the face and scalp. Trans St Johns Hosp Dermatol Soc 57:202, 1971
30. Muller SA, Winkelmann RK: Necrobiosis lipoidica diabeticorum. Histopathologic study of 98 cases. Arch Dermatol 94:1, 1966
31. Boulton AJM, Cutfield RG, Abouganem D, et al: Necrobiosis lipoidica diabeticorum: A clinicopathologic study. J Am Acad Dermatol 18:530, 1988
32. Alegre VA, Winkelmann RK: A new histopathologic feature of necrobiosis lipoidica diabeticorum: Lymphoid nodules. J Cutan Pathol 15:75, 1988
33. Ullman S, Dahl MV: Necrobiosis lipoidica. An immunofluorescence study. Arch Dermatol 113:1671, 1977
34. Oikarinen A, Mortenhumer M, Kallioinen M, Savolainen ER: Necrobiosis lipoidica: Ultrastructural and biochemical demonstration of a collagen defect. J Invest Dermatol 88:227, 1987
35. Patternson JW: Rheumatoid nodule and subcutaneous granuloma annulare. A comparative histologic study. Am J Dermatopathol 10:1, 1988
36. Alessi E, Crosti C, Sala F: Unusual case of granulomatous dermohypodermitis with giant cells and elastophagocytosis. Dermatologica 172:218, 1986
37. LeBoit PE, Beckstead JH, Bond B, et al: Granulomatous slack skin: Clonal rearrangement of T-cell receptor B gene is evidence for the lymphoproliferative nature of a cutaneous elastolytic disorder. J Invest Dermatol 89:183, 1987
38. Finan MC, Winkelmann RK: Necrobiotic xanthogranuloma with paraproteinemia. A review of 22 cases. Medicine 65:376, 1986
39. Holden CA, Winkelmann RK, Wilson Jones E: Necro-

biotic xanthogranuloma: A report of four cases. Br J Dermatol 114:241, 1986
40. Finan MC, Winkelmann RK: Histopathology of necrobiotic xanthogranuloma with paraproteinemia. J Cutan Pathol 14:92, 1987
41. Bourlond A, Pirard C, Eggers S: Xanthogranulome necrobiotique et myelome. Dermatologica 179:139, 1989
42. Scupham RK, Fretzin DF: Necrobiotic xanthogranuloma with paraproteinemia. Arch Pathol Lab Med 13:1389, 1989
43. English CK, Wear DJ, Margileth AM, et al: Cat-scratch disease: Isolation and culture of the bacterial agent. JAMA 259:1347, 1988
44. Margileth AM: Dermatologic manifestations and update of cat-scratch disease. Pediatr Dermatol 5:1, 1988
45. Johnson WT, Helwig EB: Cat-scratch disease. Histopathologic changes in the skin. Arch Dermatol 100:148, 1969
46. Czarnetzki BM, Pomeranz JR, Khanderka PK, et al: Cat-scratch disease skin test. Studies of specificity and histopathologic features. Arch Dermatol 111:736, 1975

24

PREDOMINANTLY HISTIOCYTIC LESIONS

Since the presence of histiocytes is the essential feature of granulomatous inflammation, a lesion consisting entirely of histiocytes should be the prototype of this form of tissue reaction. However, simple inspection makes one feel that pure accumulations of histiocytes belong rather in the field of tumors, of neoplastic lesions. This is how they had been classified. "Xanthoma" is the outstanding example and "histiocytoma" is another. Xanthomas, histiocytomas, and others, however, are now considered reactive lesions. Some xanthomas regress without a trace and others through fibrosis and scarring.

While histiocytes predominate in the lesions discussed here, other cells may be present. The histiocytes may occur in a nonphagocytic state or may appear as foam cells (lipophages) or macrophages containing hemosiderin and other substances. Differentiation from epithelioid tubercles of sarcoid reactions and from lepromatous leprosy sometimes is based more on configuration of the entire lesion than on cytologic characteristics.

Recently a new population of cells called "dermal dendrocytes" have been identified in normal skin by electron microscopy and by positive reaction to factor XIII in immunostaining. In histiocytomas 70–100 percent of cells, especially at the periphery of the lesions, are factor XIII positive. It has been proposed that histiocytomas are tumors of dermal dendrocytes.[1]

XANTHOMA

A more or less pure accumulation of histiocytic cells with pale foamy cytoplasm is characteristic of all clinical forms of xanthoma. If fresh tissue is available, frozen sections stained with scarlet red or other lipid stains (Fig. 24–1) will confirm the diagnosis, but this is neither feasible nor necessary in routine diagnosis.

The metabolic and genetic disorders leading to xanthoma formation have been well defined.[2] They must be investigated in every case, whether we recognize clinically tuberous, eruptive, or plane xanthomas. Various types of lipids are taken up from the bloodstream by primitive dermal mesenchymal cells that become macrophages.[3,4] An outstanding characteristic of all xanthoma cells is that they contain birefringent substances.

Histologic differentiation of the various clinical types of xanthoma is difficult and is based on ancillary features. For instance, if the foam cells are distributed in small clusters in the dermis and between striated muscle bundles, one is entitled to make a diagnosis of xanthelasma (Fig. 24–2) of the eyelid. Large accumulations of foam cells (Fig. 24–1) suggest tuberous xanthoma rather than the eruptive type. The former may become quite fibrotic, and the latter is apt to show evidence of cellular disintegration so that some lipid may be free in the tissue.

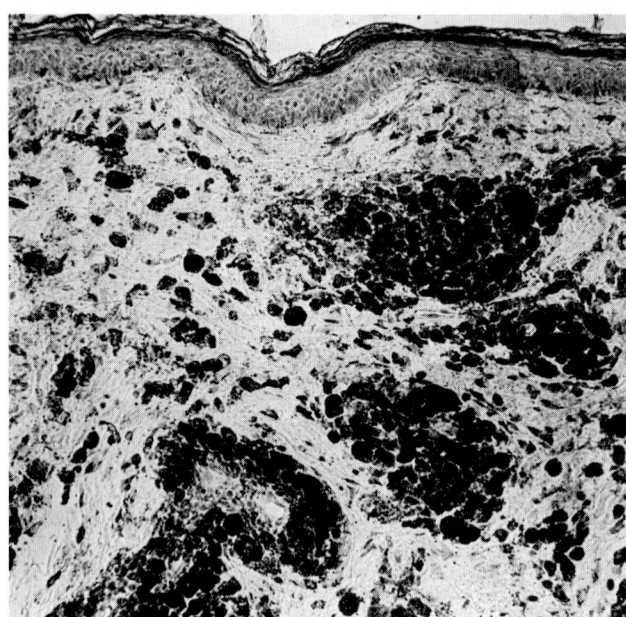

Figure 24–1.
Xanthoma, frozen section stained with Sudan IV and hematoxylin. Foam cells appear black in photograph. X135.

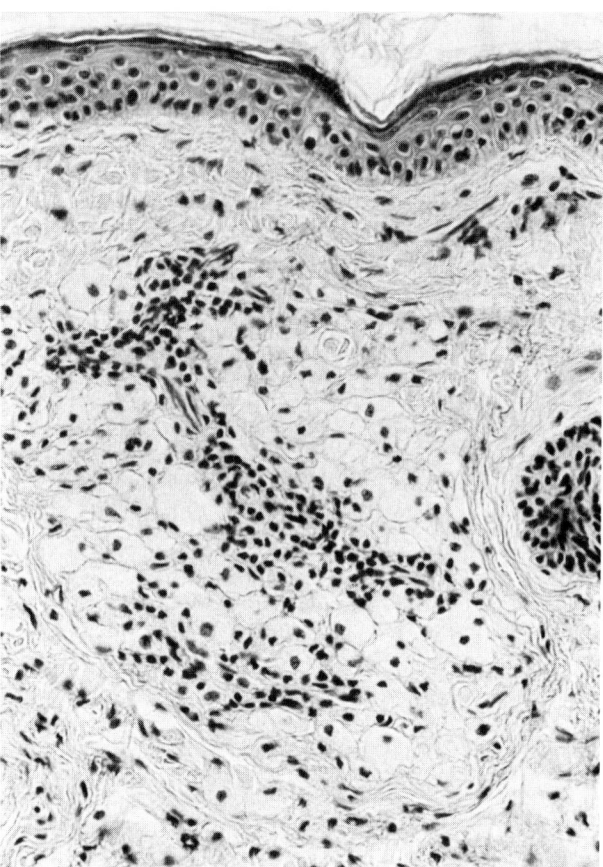

Figure 24–2.
Xanthelasma of eyelid. Note small collections of foamy histiocytes. H&E. X125.

Paraffin sections show empty cleftlike spaces in addition to foam cells. In normolipemic plane xanthomatosis, foam cells are present in large areas of skin, and there may be associated paraproteinemia.[5] The characteristic Touton giant cell may be found in all forms of xanthoma, but usually in small numbers.

Although other disturbances of lipid metabolism (Gaucher's disease, Niemann–Pick's disease) may produce foam cells in other organs, the skin is usually spared.

Verruciform Xanthoma

Hyperkeratotic verrucous lesions over the genital area[6] or developing within an epidermal nevus[7,8] have been described as verruciform xanthoma (Fig. 24–3). Collections of xanthomatous foam cells are present within the papillary dermis beneath an area of verrucous epidermal hyperplasia.[9]

JUVENILE XANTHOGRANULOMA

This lesion,[11] formerly called "nevoxanthoendothelioma" appears most commonly during infancy and childhood and is also found in adults,[10] usually can be differentiated histologically from other xanthomas. It often presents (Fig. 24–4) a relatively large number of multinucleated cells, some of which may be of the Touton type, but good foam cells are relatively rare, and in many cases the lesion consists of compact histiocytes. Only high-power study reveals vacuolation of the cytoplasm. Most cells display positive reaction for lysozyme and alpha$_1$-antichymotrypsin suggesting derivation from the mononuclear phagocyte system.[11] There is also a minor population of S-100 positive dendritic cells.[12] Lymphocytes, plasma cells, and a variable number of eosinophils are often present. The picture may closely resemble that of xanthoma disseminatum, one of the manifestations of histiocytosis X (Langerhans cell granuloma), which is discussed in Chapter 25. An important difference is the absence of epidermal invasion by mononuclear cells in the juvenile xanthogranuloma. Under the electron microscope, the cytoplasmic Birbeck granules are absent.

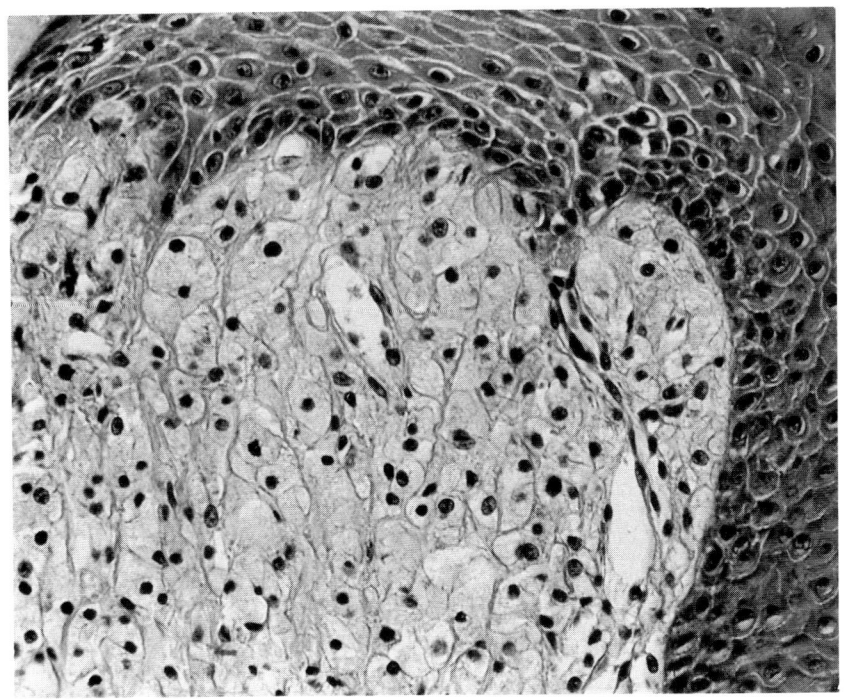

Figure 24–3.
Verruciform xanthoma shows numerous foam cells below an acanthotic epidermis. H&E. X225.

HISTIOCYTOMA (FIBROUS HISTIOCYTOMA)

Nature

There is fairly general agreement that the histiocytomas are not true tumors but reactive accumulations of cells. The nature of the predominant cell is debated, however, and this doubt is expressed in the designations *fibroma durum, histiocytoma, subepidermal nodular fibrosis,* and *fibrous histiocytoma.*[13] It seems likely that many of these lesions start as reactions to mosquito bites or other minor trauma. Keeping in mind the pluripotentiality of mesenchymal cells, one might rationalize the histologic features by the assumption that histiocytes accumulate in response to injury, that some may become macrophages, and that later many become fibroblasts. Fibroblasts may also be of perivascular origin. A variable degree of vascular proliferation, one of the common features of productive inflammation, adds to the colorful spectrum of histologic findings. However, there is little to support the contention that histiocytomas are "sclerosing hemangiomas." A last feature, which is discussed in some detail here, is the pronounced tendency of the epidermis and pilar complexes to undergo reactive changes.

Histology

The histologic picture (Fig. 24–5) of a typical histiocytoma has two components. There is a roughly lenticular accumulation of fixed-tissue-type cells in the midcorium, and there is perivascular round cell infiltrate around the periphery of the lesion. The latter feature is quite constant and serves in the differentiation from dermatofibrosarcoma protuberans. Sudan-stained frozen sections are apt to reveal fine lipid droplets in the perivascular cells. The main lesion has no sharp border and certainly has no capsule, and fusiform or stellate cells are present between the collagen bundles of the periphery. In this respect, the lesion differs from *keloid*. On the other hand, there is no shelf effect such as we shall encounter with dermatofibrosarcoma protuberans.

The cells of the main lesion are fusiform or stellate and usually are arranged in whorls or bending streams rather than in straight intersecting bundles such as are seen in *leiomyomas*. Occasionally, nuclear palisading may be present with formation of Verocay-like bodies.[14] Multinucleated giant cells are common findings (Fig. 24–6). Large cells with irregularly shaped and hyperchromatic nuclei are present in rare occasions.[15] Variable amounts of collagen fibers and bundles are present. Some of these are old dermal tissue with associated remnants of

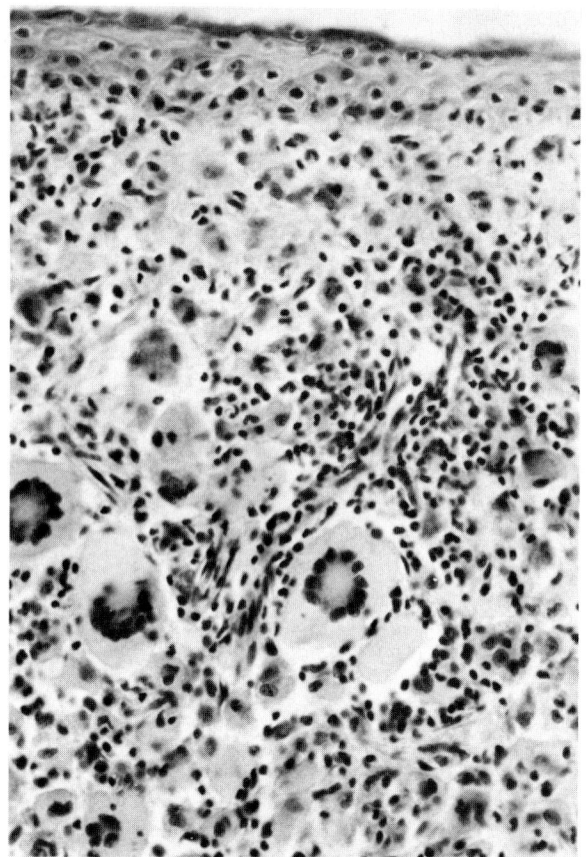

Figure 24–4.
Juvenile xanthogranuloma. Touton giant cells and histiocytes with rather solid cytoplasm mixed with small round cells. No invasion of epidermis. H&E. X90.

elastic fibers. Others are hyalinized fibers newly formed by fibroblasts in the lesion and are free of elastic fibers. In these respects, histiocytoma also differs from leiomyoma, in which new elastic fibers frequently are formed. Blood vessels usually are small in number and size, but they may become prominent and then often are the source of small hemorrhages followed by macrophage formation.

The view that most of the constituent cells are histiocytes is based mainly on experiments[16] that showed that locally injected colloidal iron is taken up by the tumor cells, thereby revealing their phagocytic nature. In routine histologic examination, one may find single or clustered foam cells and other cells containing hemosiderin.

Variants

Variants of the typical picture occurs in several directions. Old lesions may become very fibrotic, and they then really deserve the title "subepidermal nodular fibrosis." Other lesions are more cellular than average, may grow to considerable size, and may involve subcutaneous fat tissue. These often have a more pronounced cartwheel pattern (Fig. 24–7), and the differentiation from dermatofibrosarcoma protuberans may become difficult. Attention should be paid to the presence of perivascular infiltrate of lymphocytes and plasma cells at the periphery and deep-seated areas of lymphoid follicle formation[17] in histiocytoma, and absence of the deep fibroblastic shelf, which we shall find as a feature of dermatofibrosarcoma. Another variant is the *hemosiderotic histiocytoma*. These are lesions, more vascular than usual, which may grow to large size due to a vicious cycle of repeated small hemorrhage and reactive proliferation of histiocytes that engulf blood pigment and lipid. Thus, macrophages, multinucleated giant cells, and thin-walled blood vessels dominate the picture. Factor VIII stain is, however, negative, ruling out the endothelial origin of these lesions.[18] The nodular lesions may look almost black and clinically arouse suspicion of malignant melanoma. H&E sections (Fig. 24–8) may at first sight support this suspicion due to the presence of large quantities of brown pigment. O&G sections reveal the nonmelanin nature of the pigment, thus making stain for hemosiderin unnecessary, especially when the foamy cytoplasm of many cells is appreciated. Another modification is the *xanthomatized histiocytoma*, in which most of the cells contain lipid. These lesions may reach a size of several centimeters, are often located on the legs, and may be sessile or pedunculated. Many look yellow on gross section, but true foam cells may be surprisingly few because the lipid is present as very fine droplets. In epithelioid cell histiocytoma large epithelioid-type cells show prominent eosinophilic cytoplasm. Most cells are binucleated or trinucleated. There is some resemblance to a fibrotic lesion of Spitz nevus. Fifty percent of the tumor cells are factor VIII-positive.[19]

Associated Epithelial Changes

Of great practical and theoretical significance are epithelial changes associated with histiocytomas. They are present in more than half of the cases[18] and take three principal forms. The simplest is general acanthosis and hyperkeratosis of the epidermis, resembling that of lichenification. It may be mentioned that epidermal atrophy can be encountered, especially after trauma and scarring. More complicated and interesting are two other changes, one of which simulates seborrheic verruca, the other

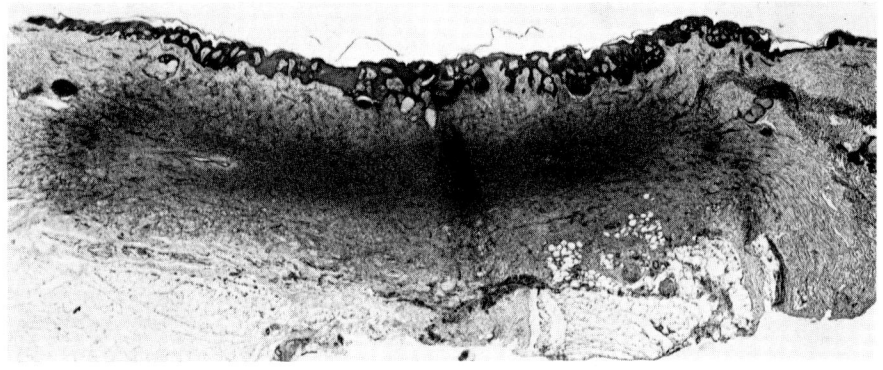

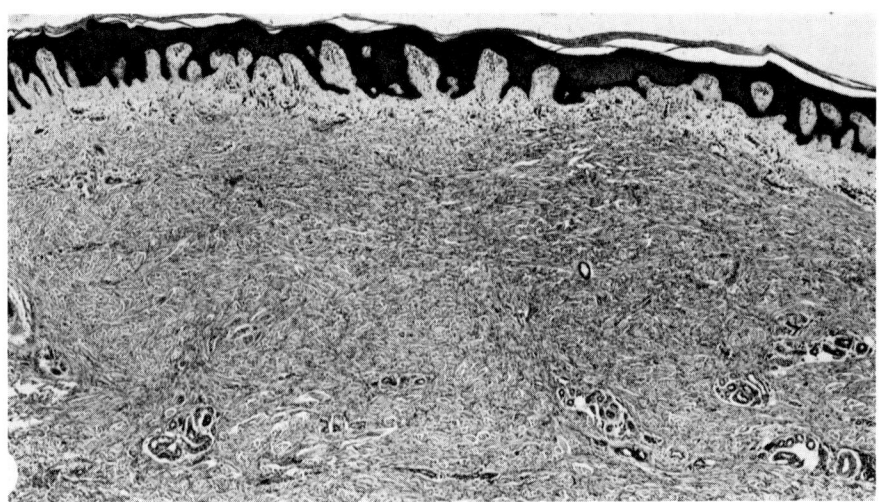

Figure 24–5.
Histiocytoma: **A.** Low-power view shows seat of roughly lenticular lesion in middermis, absence of a distinct border, and reactive epidermal proliferation that is papillomatous in some areas, while other areas simulate superficial basal cell epithelioma. H&E. X9. **B.** Less cellular lesion at higher magnification. Shows whorled arrangement of fibrous bundles. Note persistence of sweat coils below benign lesion and cross section of a duct traversing the lesion. H&E. X60.

one basal cell epithelioma. Papillomatous hyperplasia of the epidermis exhibiting horny pearls and retarded maturation of prickle cells, and thus resembling seborrheic verruca, is not uncommon. The question of whether such changes constitute a true seborrheic verruca associated with the histiocytoma is theoretically intriguing but of no great practical importance. Considerable theoretical and practical importance attaches to the question of whether basal cell epithelioma is associated with the benign mesodermal pseudotumor in as high as 8 percent of cases, however.[20]

Thorough examination of serial sections of well over a thousand histiocytomas has convinced us[21] that pictures as illustrated in Figure 24–9 mimic superficial basal cell epithelioma and are the result of peculiar regressive and proliferative changes of hair follicles (Fig. 24–10) but are not true neoplasia. In most lesions foci of basaloid cell proliferations remain small and do not progress into nodular or ulcerating basal cell epitheliomas.

True basalioma may be found in rare cases.[22] Attentive study of histiocytomas reveals that hair follicles and eccrine glands are affected in a different manner by the slow accumulation of cells and fibers in the middermis. The sweat coil is fixed deep to the tumor. The duct continues to make its way through the tumor to the surface unless it is eventually choked off and disappears. In that case, the entire eccrine unit atrophies. The roots of vellus or terminal hairs, on the other hand, are mobile. With each hair change, about twice a year, the lower follicle disintegrates, and the dermal papilla moves upward close to the sebaceous gland, which usually is situated above or in the upper portion of the histiocytoma. With the onset of the next anagen, the hair root tries to grow down but finds its path blocked. The entire follicle is foreshortened and will form a new hair above the tumor. As the latter expands and presses closer to the epidermis, hair matrices, often still associated with sebaceous glands, can be found almost immediately below the

336   GRANULOMATOUS INFLAMMATION AND PROLIFERATION

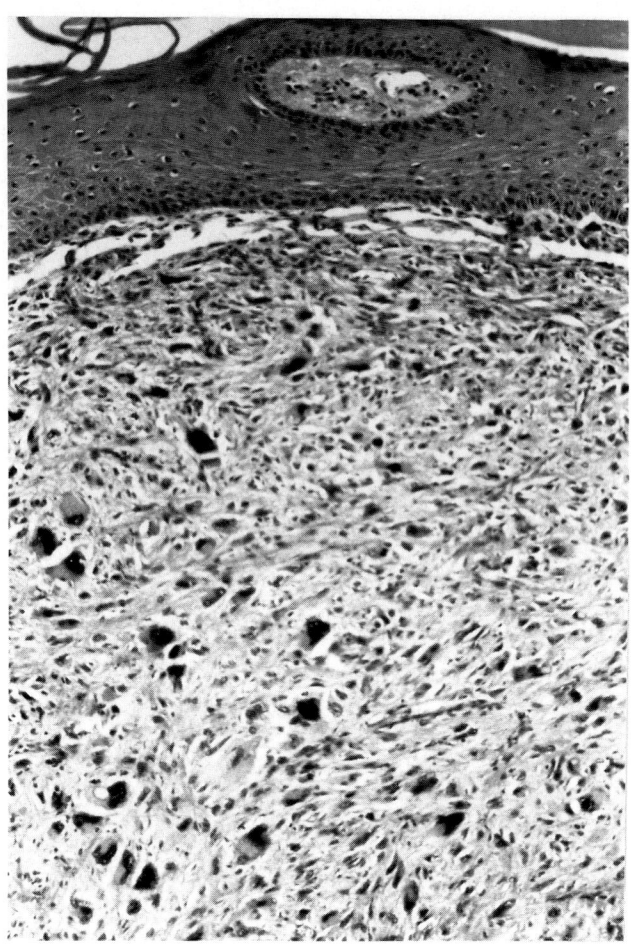

Figure 24–6.
Histiocytoma with numerous atypical multinucleated giant cells.

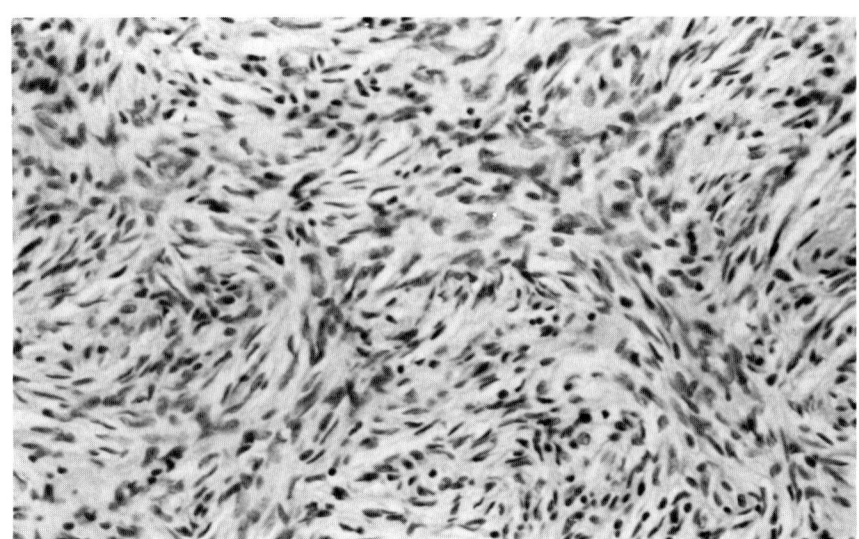

Figure 24–7.
Cartwheel pattern approximated in a histiocytoma. Compare with Figure 42–18 (dermatofibrosarcoma protuberans). H&E. X250.

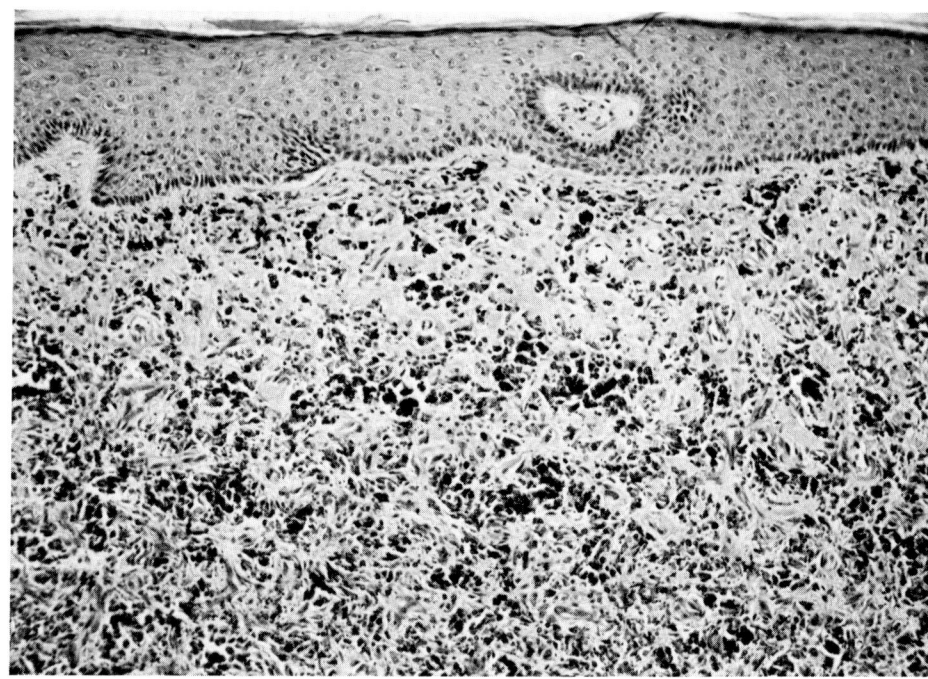

Figure 24—8.
Hemosiderotic histiocytoma. Dark masses are clumps of hemosiderin in histiocytes transformed into macrophages. H&E. X135.

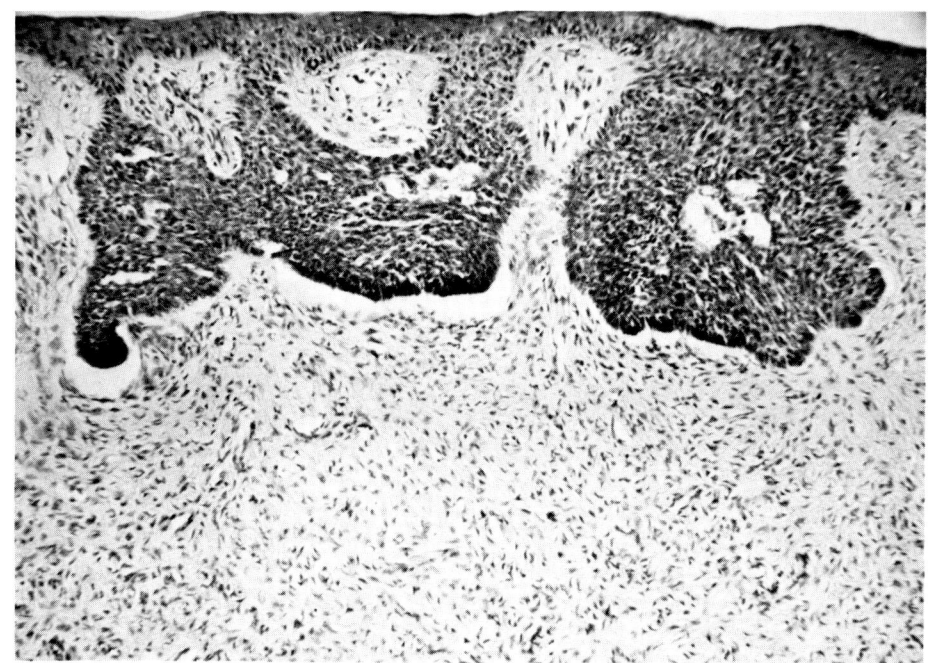

Figure 24—9.
Basalioma-like epithelial proliferation above a histiocytoma. H&E. X135.

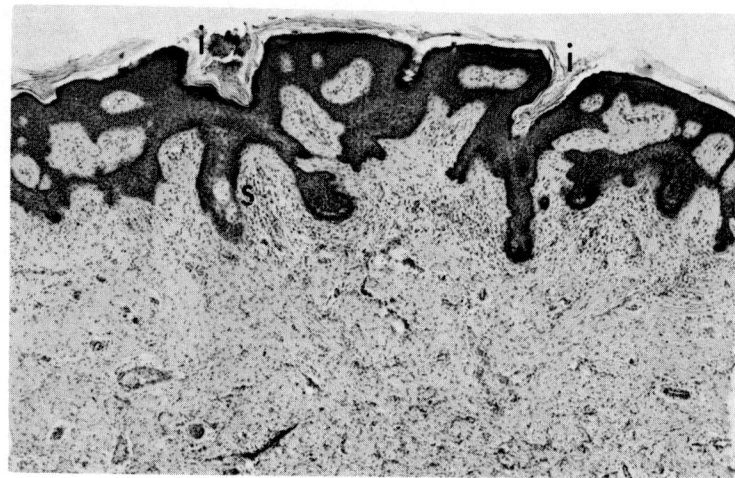

Figure 24-10.
Regressive changes of pilary complexes above histiocytoma. **A.** Tiny sebaceous gland (s) associated with rudimentary hair root and infundibulum (i). Three other rudimentary hair roots, one connected with infundibulum (i), at right. Note similarity to Figure 24-9. H&E. X90. **B.** Two foreshortened hair follicles resembling cloaked hairs. H&E. X135.

epidermis.[23] The final step seems to be a diffuse spreading of the material of epithelial matrix and mesodermal papilla along the lower surface of the epidermis. This process gives rise to multiple foci (Fig. 24-10) strongly resembling fetal hair germs or the rudimentary matrix-papilla complexes found in organoid nevi and trichoepitheliomas. That they still represent a pilar complex often is documented by the presence of a keratinizing channel in the epidermis and the occasional presence of a tiny but mature sebaceous gland. Whether a picture as shown in Figure 24-9 is the final state of this process or now truly represents neoplasia is a question one cannot decide in the histologic section. The overwhelming biologic evidence seems to be in favor of a reactive hyperplasia.

RETICULOHISTIOCYTOMA

Lesions of a type perhaps better called "reticulohistiocytic granuloma" are encountered as small single papules or in multicentric and diffuse forms.[24-29] In the latter cases, there are associated involvements of the joints of the hands and other evidence of multisystem disease. Histologically, (Fig. 24-11), they are composed of massive dermal infiltration of histiocytes and multinucleated giant cells of foreign body type. The histiocytic and the giant cell cytoplasm is eosinophilic and either shows a finely granular, ground-glass appearance or is foamy and vacuolated. The histiocytic cell cytoplasm is PAS-positive and diastase resistant. There are also scattered lymphocytes and eosinophils (Fig. 24-12).

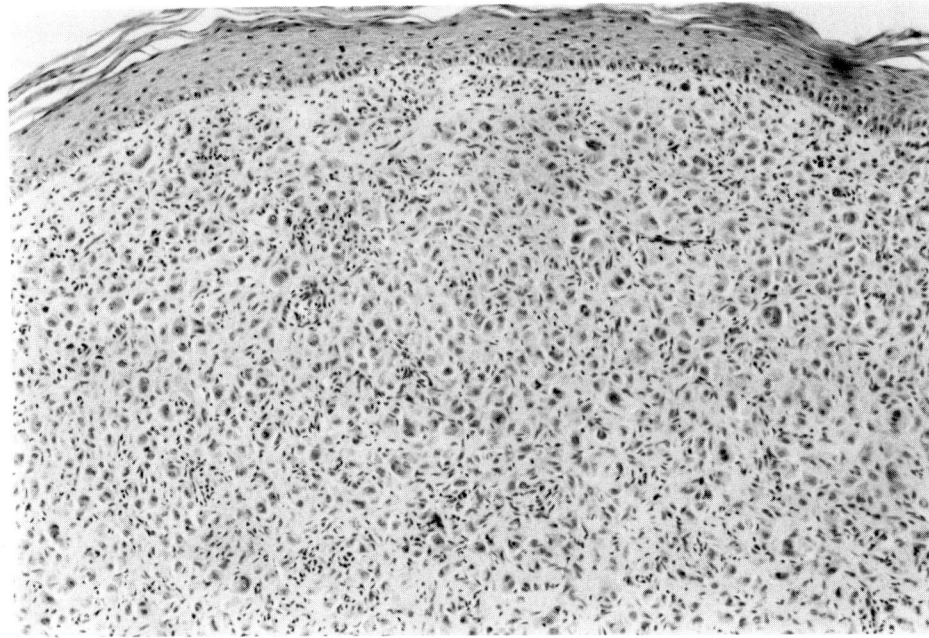

Figure 24–11.
Multicentric reticulohistiocytoma. Massive dermal infiltrate of histiocytes and multinucleated giant cells. H&E. X125.

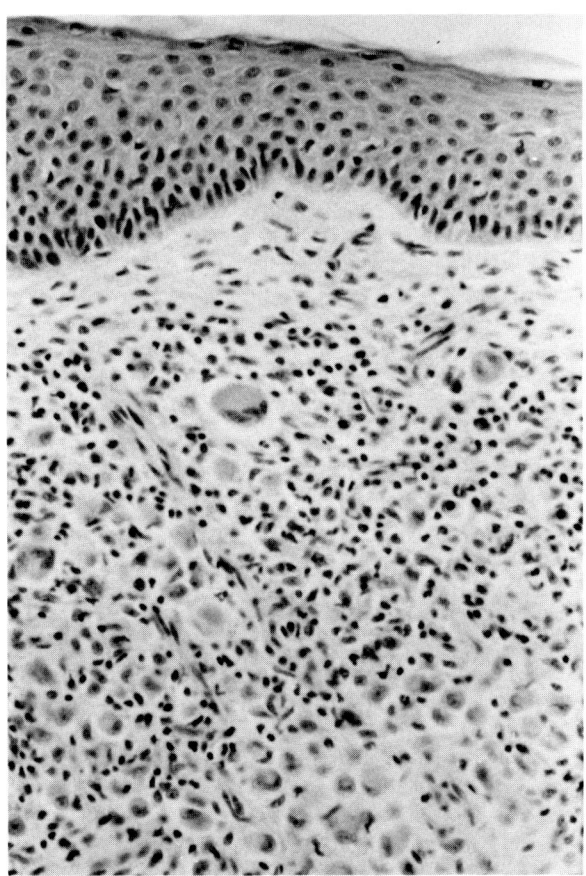

Figure 24–12.
Multicentric reticulohistiocytoma. Histiocytes and small multinucleated giant cells are mixed with small round cells. H&E. X250.

GENERALIZED ERUPTIVE HISTIOCYTOMA

Winkelmann and Muller identified a self-healing form of histiocytoma affecting adults with successive crops of discrete 3- to 10-mm dark red or bluish papules in symmetrical distribution.[30,31] The lesions last several years and disappear spontaneously. Histologically, massive proliferation of monomorphous histiocytic cells in upper and middermis are shown. Foam cells or giant cells are not present and stains for lipid or S-100 protein are negative.[32]

BENIGN CEPHALIC HISTIOCYTOSIS

Described by Gianotti et al. it occurs in the first year of life with 2- to 3-mm erythematous and yellowish papular lesions of face, occipital and neck areas.[33] Histological examination shows a well-defined infiltrate in the upper dermis involving the lower surface of the epidermis, which is often atrophic. The infiltrate consists of histiocytes with pleomorphic nuclei and light-staining and sometimes glassy cytoplasms. Scattered lymphocytes and occasional eosinophils are also present. Twenty percent of the histiocytic cells show intracytoplasmic clusters of comma-shaped bodies in electron microscopy. Langerhans granules are absent.[34]

REFERENCES

1. Cerio R, Spaull J, Wilson Jones E: Histiocytoma cutis: A tumor of dermal dendrocytes (dermal dendrocytoma). Br J Dermatol 120:197, 1989
2. Brewer BH Jr, Fredrickson DS: Dyslipoproteinemias and xanthomatoses. In Fitzpatrick TB, et al (eds): Dermatology in General Medicine, 3rd ed, New York: McGraw Hill, p 1722, 1987
3. Bulkley BH, Buja LM, Ferrans VJ, et al: Tuberous xanthoma in homozygous type II hyperlipoproteinemia: Histologic, histochemical and electron microscopic study. Arch Pathol 99:293, 1975
4. Braun-Falco O: Struktur und Morphogenese von Xanthomen bei Hyperlipoproteinämie von Type III. Eine morphologische, histochemische und elektronenmikroskopische Untersuchung. Hautarzt 27:122, 1976
5. Weber G, Pilgrim M: Contribution to the knowledge of normolipemic plane xanthomatosis. Br J Dermatol 90:465, 1974
6. Kimura S: Verruciform xanthoma of the scrotum. Arch Dermatol 120:1378, 1984
7. Grosshans E, LaPlanche G: Verruciform xanthoma or xanthomatous transformation of inflammatory epidermal nevus. J Cutan Pathol 8:382, 1981
8. Palestine RF, Winkelmann RK: Verruciform xanthoma in an epithelial nevus. Arch Dermatol 118:686, 1982
9. Chyu J, Medenica M, Whitney DH: Verruciform xanthoma of the lower extremity: Report of a case and review of the literature. J Am Acad Dermatol 17:695, 1987
10. Nakamura S, Izawa R, Nakayama K, et al: Xanthogranuloma in the adult. J Dermatol Tokyo 10:151, 1983
11. Sonoda T, Hashimoto H, Enjoji M: Juvenile xanthogranuloma. Clinicopathologic analysis and immunohistochemical study of 57 patients. Cancer 56:2280, 1985
12. Tahan SR, Pstel-Levy C, Bhan AK, Mihm MC: Juvenile xanthogranuloma. Clinical and pathologic characterization. Arch Pathol Lab Med 113:1057, 1989
13. Vilanova JR, Flint A: The morphological variations of fibrous histiocytomas. J Cutan Pathol 1:155, 1974
14. Schwob VS, Santa Cruz DJ: Palisading cutaneous fibrous histiocytoma. J Cutan Pathol 13:403, 1986
15. Tamada S, Ackerman BA: Dermatofibroma with monster cells. Am J Dermatopathol 9:380, 1987
16. Senear FE, Caro MR: Histiocytoma cutis. Arch Dermatol 33:209, 1936
17. Barker SM, Winkelmann RK: Inflammatory lymphadenoid reactions with dermatofibroma/histiocytoma. J Cutan Pathol 13:222, 1986
18. Kanitakis J, Hermier C, Mauduit G, Thivolet J: Negative immunolabelling for factor VIII-related antigen in the so-called "sclerosing hemangiomas" (histiocytofibromas) of the skin. J Dermatol Tokyo 14:326, 1987
19. Wilson-Jones E, Cerio RC, Smith NP: Epithelioid cell histiocytoma—a new entity. Br J Dermatol 119(Suppl 33):35, 1988
20. Bryant J: Basal cell carcinoma overlying longstanding dermatofibromas. Arch Dermatol 113:1445, 1977
21. Pinkus H: Pathobiology of the pilary complex. Jpn J Dermatol (B) 77:304, 1967
22. Goette DK, Helwig EB: Basal cell carcinomas and basal cell carcinoma-like changes overlying dermatofibromas. Arch Dermatol 111:589, 1975
23. Rahbari H, Mehregan AH: Adnexal displacement and regression in association with histiocytoma (dermatofibroma). J Cutan Pathol 12:94, 1985
24. Catterall MD: Multicentric reticulohistiocytes a review of eight cases. Clin Exp Dermatol 5:267, 1980
25. Tani M, Hori K, Nakanishi T: Multicentric reticulohistiocytosis. Arch Dermatol 117:495, 1981
26. Lesher JL, Allen BS: Multicentric reticulohistiocytosis. J Am Acad Dermatol 11:713, 1984
27. Green CA, Walker DJ, Malcolm AJ: A case of multicentric reticulohistiocytosis: Uncommon clinical signs and a report of T-cell marker characteristics. Br J Dermatol 115:623, 1986

28. Peteiro C, Fernandez-Redondo V, Zulaica A, et al: Reticulohistiocytosis multicentrica: Estudio clinico y ultrastructural de un caso. Med Cutan ILA 15:435, 1987
29. Finelli LG, Tenner LK, Ratz JL, Long BD: A case of multicentric reticulohistiocytosis with thyroid involvement. J Am Acad Dermatol 15:1097, 1986
30. Winkelmann RK, Muller SA: Generalized eruptive histiocytoma: A benign papular histiocytic reticulosis. Arch Dermatol 88:586, 1963
31. Bobin P, Carsuzaa F, Seurat P, Lucas D: Histiocytome eruptif generalise. A propos d'un cas, Revue de la litterature. Ann Dermatol Venereol 110:817, 1983
32. Caputo R, Ermacora E, Gelmetti C, et al: Generalized eruptive histiocytoma in children. J Am Acad Dermatol 17:449, 1987
33. Gianotti F, Caputo R, Ermacora E, Gianni E: Benign cephalic histiocytosis. Arch Dermatol 122:1038, 1986
34. De Luna ML, Glikin I, Goldberg J, et al: Benign cephalic histiocytosis: Report of four cases. Pediatr Dermatol 6:198, 1988

25
HISTIOCYTOSIS X (LANGERHANS CELL GRANULOMAS)

Lichtenstein was responsible for pulling together three manifestations of a "peculiar inflammatory histiocytosis" and integrating them into a single nosologic entity that he called "histiocytosis X."[1] Previously, Pinkus et al,[2] had used the term "reticulogranuloma" for cases when the specific cells seemed to be of reticuloendothelial origin capable of phagocytosis and when the lesions were neither simple inflammatory proliferations nor truly malignant sarcomas. They possessed the essential features of a granuloma consisting of histiocytes invading and destroying tissues. Then introduction of electron microscopy showed that the large cells, which together with eosinophils are the major component of the infiltrate, contain the specific racket-shaped Birbeck granules found in the epidermal Langerhans cells.[3,4] Langerhans cells derive from mononuclear stem cells in the bone marrow but are a specialized subpopulation of the mononuclear phagocyte system, different from histiocytes and macrophages. The ultrastructural demonstration of racket-shaped Birbeck granules is needed for identification of Langerhans cells. Langerhans cells can also be identified in tissue sections by immunostaining with OKT-6 or S-100 protein antibodies.[5,6]

SKIN MANIFESTATIONS

Skin lesions are often present in all three forms of histiocytosis X.[7,8] *Letterer–Siwe disease* is an acute and disseminated malignant form of histiocytosis X, which begins in infancy and may be present at birth. It is rare in adults.[9] Skin lesions are present in 80 to 100 percent of cases, consisting of scaly papular eruptions resembling seborrheic dermatitis and involving scalp and postauricular, perianal, and axillary areas. Reddish or purpuric papules and nodules may be present. Gingivitis and oral ulceration may be observed in rare instances.

Hand–Schuller–Christian disease is a chronic multifocal type of histiocytosis X in children 2 to 6 years of age or older or in young adults. The classic triad includes osteolytic bone lesions, diabetes insipidus, and exophthalmos.[10] Cutaneous manifestations are similar to those of Letterer–Siwe disease. *Eosinophilic granuloma* is a benign localized form of histiocytosis X with osteolytic bone lesions similar to those seen in *Hand–Schuller–Christian* disease affecting older children and adults. Cutaneous lesions are rare and include infiltrated nodules or areas of periorificial ulceration.[11–13]

HISTOPATHOLOGY

Histologic changes in histiocytosis X may be proliferative, granulomatous, or xanthomatous in type. Proliferative pattern is characterized by massive infiltration of well-differentiated histiocytes and Langerhans cells with no foam cells or multinucleated giant cells (Fig. 25–1). Langerhans cells are

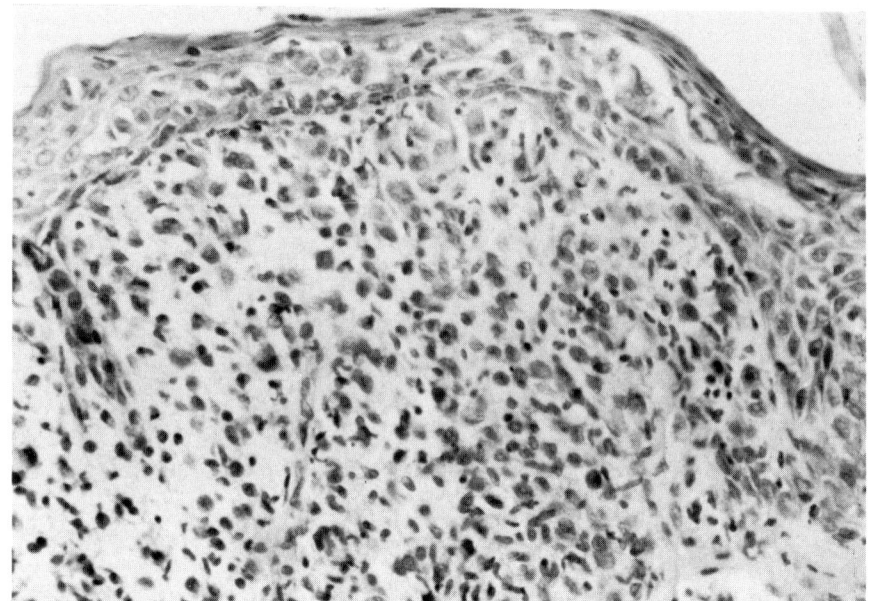

Figure 25—1.
Histiocytosis X. Heavy dermal infiltrate with atypical histiocytic cells and epidermal invasion. H&E. X250.

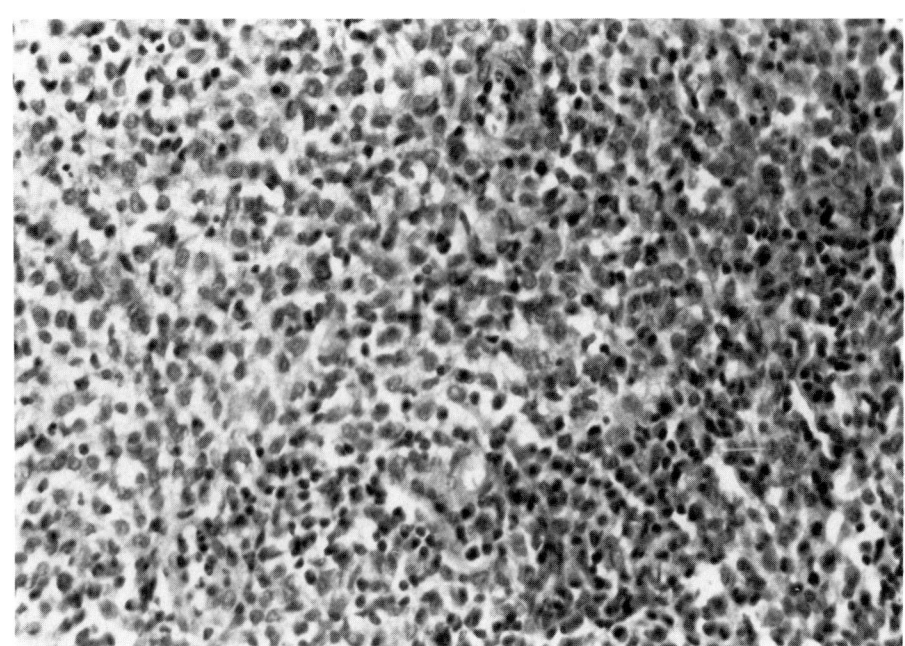

Figure 25—2.
Skin involvement of eosinophilic granuloma in a patient with underlying bone involvement. (Courtesy of Dr. Y. Dowlati) H&E. X400.

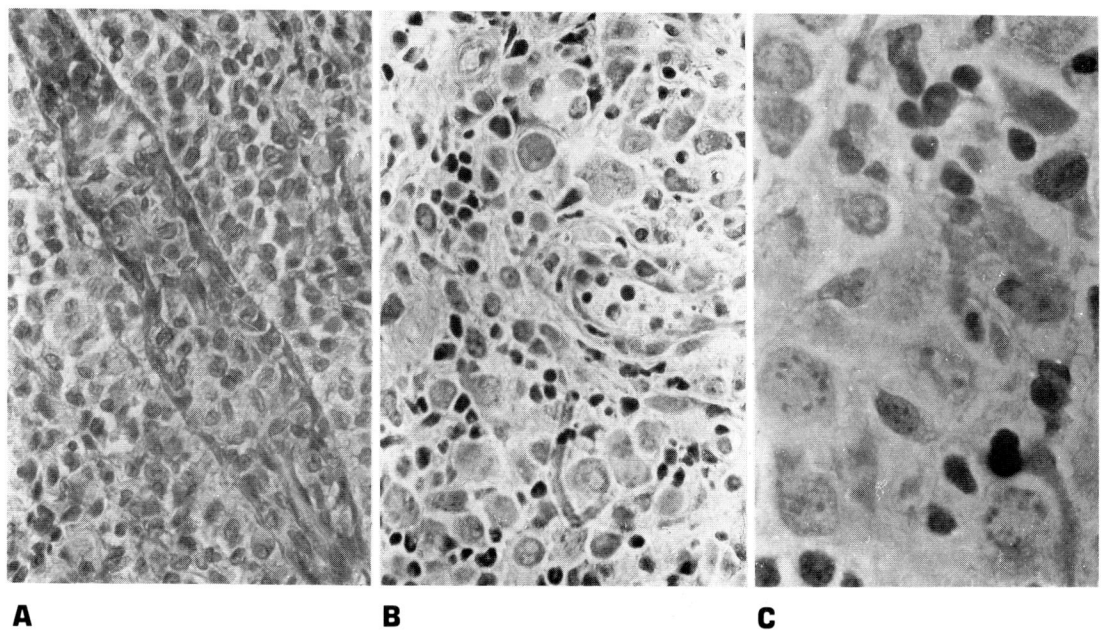

Figure 25–3.
Self-healing reticulohistiocytosis. **A.** Massive proliferation of histiocytic cells involving a central eccrine sweat duct. H&E. X400. **B.** Large histiocytic cells with eosinophilic cytoplasms. H&E. X600. **C.** Large histiocytes containing PAS-positive inclusions. PAS.

large with pale-staining ovoid or kidney-shaped vesiculated nuclei and abundant eosinophilic cytoplasm. Upward transmigration of infiltrating cells within the overlying epidermis is observed in scaly papules or seborrheic dermatitis-like lesions. Approximately one third or one half of the cells can be identified as Langerhans cells. In the granulomatous lesions, irregularly multinucleated giant cells are mixed with histiocytes and Langerhans cells. Xanthomatous type shows a number of Touton and foreign-body-type multinucleated giant cells. This pattern is observed in yellowish papular chronic lesions (Fig. 25–2). The skin manifestation of eosinophilic granuloma shows extensive dermal infiltrate of histiocytes, Langerhans cells, and large numbers of polymorphonuclear eosinophils.

CONGENITAL SELF-HEALING RETICULOHISTIOCYTOSIS

Another entity earlier described by Hashimoto and Pritzker is a cutaneous reticulohistiocytosis present at birth and disappearing within a few months.[14–16] Newborns show single or multiple pink or dusky red nodules ranging in size from 0.2 to 2.5 cm in diameter and with no specific distribution pattern[17–19] (Fig. 25–3). The dermis is infiltrated with numerous large histiocytic cells with eosinophilic cytoplasms containing PAS-positive and diastase-resistant inclusions and some eosinophils.[20,21] The epidermis is infiltrated and may show superficial ulceration (Fig. 25–4). Electron microscopy shows 10 to 25 percent of large cells are Langerhans cells having Birbeck granules and staining positive with S-100 protein antibody.[22,23]

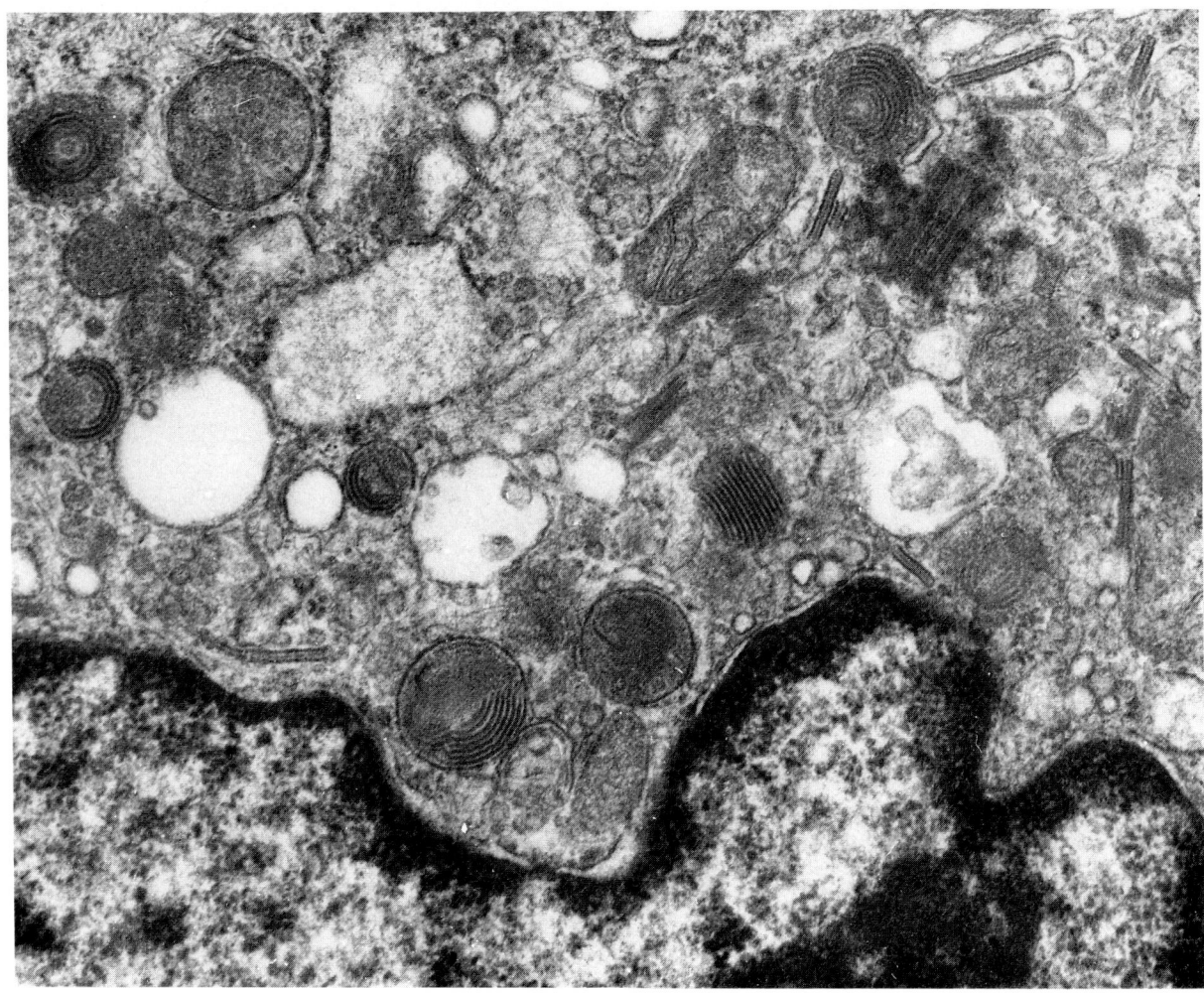

Figure 25-4.
Self-healing reticulohistiocytosis shows Langerhans cell granules and dense bodies with myelinlike lamination. X45,000.

REFERENCES

1. Lichtenstein L: Histiocytosis X: Integration of eosinophilic granuloma of bone, "Letterer-Siwe disease," and "Schüller–Christian disease" as related manifestations of a single nosologic entity. Arch Pathol 56:84, 1953
2. Pinkus H, Copps LA, Custer C, et al: Reticulogranuloma: Report of a case of eosinophilic granuloma of bone associated with nonlipid reticulosis of skin and oral mucosa under the clinical picture of Hand–Schüller–Christian disease. Am J Dis Child 77:503, 1949
3. Gianotti F, Caputo R: Histiocytic syndromes: A review. J Am Acad Dermatol 13:383, 1985
4. Ringel E, Moschella S: Primary histiocytic dermatoses. Arch Dermatol 121:1531, 1985
5. Rowden G, Connelly EM, Winkelmann RK: Cutaneous histiocytosis X. The presence of S-100 protein and its use in diagnosis. Arch Dermatol 119:553, 1983
6. Watanabe S, Nakajima T, Shimosato Y, et al: Malignant histiocytosis and Letterer–Siwe disease. Neoplasms of T-zone histiocyte with S-100 protein Cancer 51:1412, 1983
7. Esterly NB, Maurer HS, Gonzales-Crussi F: Histiocytosis X: A seven-year experience at a children's hospital. J Am Acad Dermatol 13:481, 1985
8. Roper SS, Spraker MK: Cutaneous histiocytosis syndromes. Pediatr Dermatol 3:19, 1986
9. Novice FM, Collison DW, Kleinsmith DM, et al: Letterer–Siwe disease in adults. Cancer 63:166, 1989
10. Villaret E, Dorcier D, Brucher C, et al: Histiocytose langerhansienne chronique de l'adulte. Ann Dermatol Venereol 116:873, 1989

11. Verret J-L, Hadet M, Brunet A, et al: Histiocytose X avec granulome éosinophile perianovulvaire. Ann Dermatol Venereal 112:165, 1985
12. Pareek SS, Haeass N: An unusual presentation of histiocytosis X. Int J Dermatol 24:126, 1985
13. Gnassia AM, Gnassia RT, Bonvalet D, et al: Histiocytose X avec "granulome eosinophile vulvaire" effet spectaculaire de la thalidomide. Ann Dermatol Venereol 114:1387, 1987
14. Hashimoto K, Pritzker MS: Electron microscopic study of reticulohistiocytoma. An unusual case of congenital, self-healing reticulohistiocytosis. Arch Dermatol 107:263, 1973
15. Hashimoto K, Griffin D, Kohsbaki M: Self-healing reticulohistiocytosis: A clinical, histologic, and ultrastructural study of the fourth case in the literature. Cancer 49:331, 1982
16. Hashimoto K, Takahashi S, Lee RG, Krull EA: Congenital self-healing reticulohistiocytosis. Report of the seventh case with histochemical and ultrastructural studies. J Am Acad Dermatol 11:447, 1984
17. Berger TG, Lane AT, Headington JT, et al: A solitary variant of congenital self-healing reticulohistiocytosis: Solitary Hashimoto–Pritzker disease. Pediatr Dermatol 3:230, 1986
18. Ofuji S, Tachibana S, Kanato M, Horiguchi Y: Congenital self-healing reticulohistiocytosis (Hashimoto–Pritzker): A case report with a solitary lesion. J Dermatol Tokyo 14:182, 1987
19. Timpatanapong P, Rochanawutanon M, Siripoonya P, Nitidandhaprabhas P: Congenital self-healing reticulohistiocytosis: Report of a patient with strikingly large tumor mass. Pediatr Dermatol 6:28, 1989
20. Kapila PK, Grant-Kels JM, Allred C, et al: Congenital, spontaneously regressing histiocytosis: Case report and review of the literature. Pediatr Dermatol 2:312, 1985
21. Jordaan FH, Drusinsky SF: Congenital self-healing reticulohistiocytosis: Report of a case. Pediatr Dermatol 3:473, 1986
22. Kanitakis J, Zambruno G, Schmitt D, et al: Congenital self-healing histiocytosis (Hashimoto–Pritzker) an ultrastructural and immunohistochemical study. Cancer 61:508, 1988
23. Herman LE, Rothman KF, Harawi S, Gonzalez-Serva A: Congenital self-healing reticulohistiocytosis. Arch Dermatol 126:210, 1990

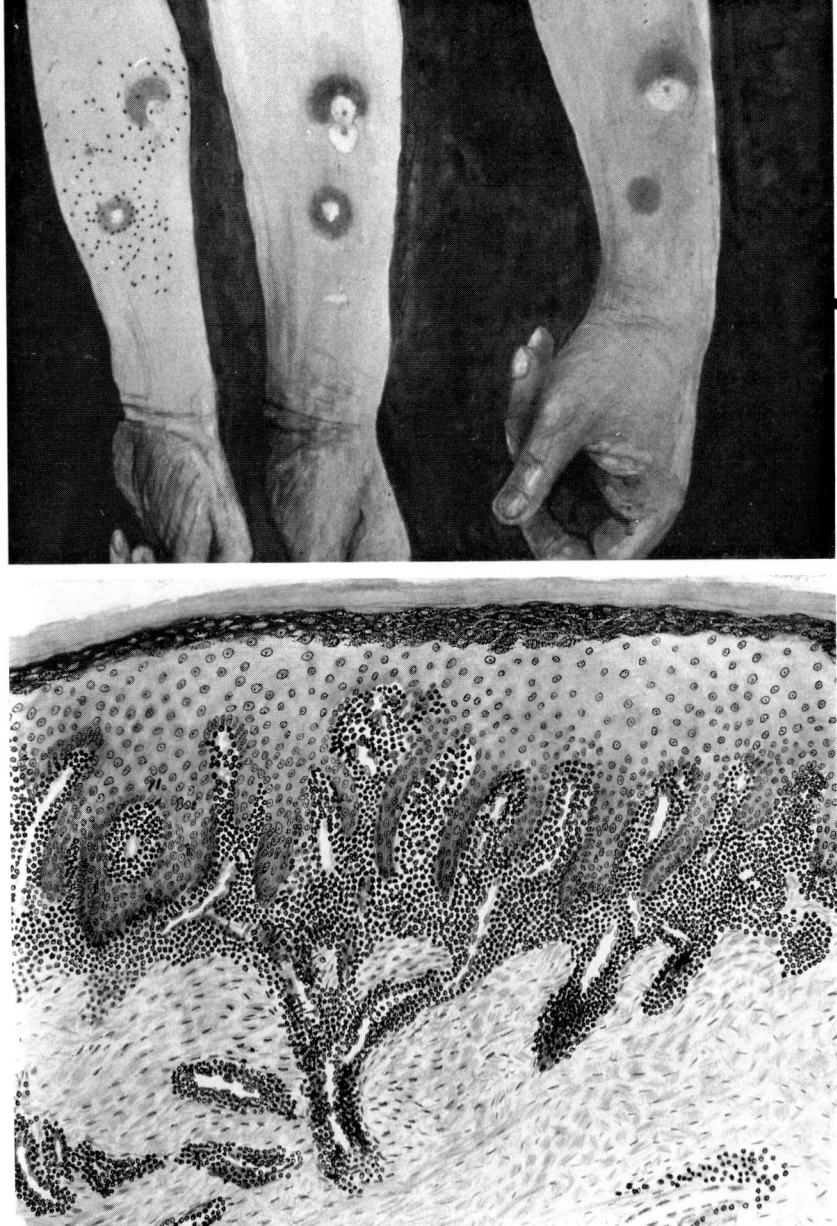

Insect bite reaction in three stages (*top*). Lichen urticatus (*bottom*).

SECTION V

METABOLIC AND OTHER NONINFLAMMATORY DERMAL DISEASES

Obviously, there can be no strict division between inflammatory and noninflammatory dermatoses. Just as obviously, all skin diseases are accompanied by changed metabolism, and in some of those discussed in this section we only presume that metabolic derangement is the primary cause. Yet there are a number of nonneoplastic skin diseases in which inflammatory changes are minor or are overshadowed by alterations of the fibrous constituents and ground substance. In others, deposition of various abnormal substances is the diagnostic feature. In these groups, we encounter even greater diagnostic difficulties if we rely merely on H&E stain. The O&G procedure, especially when its results are compared with H&E-stained sections, is informative in many cases, but special stains are needed in some instances, and a high level of suspicion is advisable so that the proper stains will be employed. For additional information we refer our readers to a symposium on structural elements of the dermis published as a supplement to the *Journal of Investigative Dermatology* in 1982[1] and two books on genodermatoses.[2,3]

REFERENCES

1. Wuepper KD, Holbrook KA, Pinnell SR, Uitto J: Structural elements of the dermis. J Invest Dermatol 79 (Suppl):1, 1982
2. Der Kaloustian VM, Kurban AK: Genetic Diseases of the Skin. New York: Springer-Verlag, 1979
3. Alper JC: Genodermatoses in Dermatologic Clinics. Vol 5, Philadelphia: WB Saunders Co, 1987.

26

CHANGES OF COLLAGEN AND GROUND SUBSTANCE

Destruction, new formation, and other changes of the collagen fibers and bundles were encountered in granulomatous inflammatory diseases. Changes in ground substance are to be assumed in any skin section exhibiting edema. In this chapter we deal mainly with scleroderma in the localized and general forms, sclerodermoid processes, scleredema, various forms of myxedema, and lymphedema. Lichen sclerosus et atrophicus and atrophodermas and lipodystrophies are put here for convenience and differential diagnosis. Reactive perforating collagenosis and the Ehlers–Danlos syndrome also find their legitimate place in this chapter.

SCLERODERMA

Generalized

Generalized scleroderma has a variable but well-defined clinical symptomatology.[1] The histologic diagnosis of generalized scleroderma (*systemic sclerosis*) is unsatisfactory in the early stages and not too secure in late stages. Whatever it is that gives the skin the hidebound consistency and the glistening aspect is poorly expressed in stained paraffin sections. In any case, one has to have a fairly large and deep biopsy extending well into the subcutaneous tissue in order to evaluate all changes completely. Some of the features that must be weighed in differential diagnosis from clinically similar conditions are indeed negative ones: the epidermis preserves its normal configuration for a long time, the elastic fibers are preserved, and there is no or little inflammatory infiltrate. The most impressive changes in a well-developed case (Fig. 26–1) are that the collagen bundles of the pars reticularis are thick, homogeneous, and eosinophilic and the interfascicular spaces are narrow or almost absent.[2] Structural differences between pars reticularis and papillaris are blurred because the latter also looks dense. Fixed-tissue-type cells are few, giving a desert-like look to the dermis. It has been suggested that sclerodermatous fibroblasts in tissue culture produce more collagen than normal ones.[3]

Small blood vessels, especially those of the papillary and subpapillary layers, are generally few and narrow, although excessive telangiectasia may be a prominent clinical feature. More significant vascular changes are observed by electron microscopy, including gaps, vacuolization, destruction of endothelial cells, reduplication of basal lamina, and perivascular fibrosis.[4] The width of the dermis is increased, not only because the collagen bundles are thicker but also because new dermal tissue replaces part of the subcutaneous fat tissue. All these points are subject to individual judgment and may be influenced by technical differences in tissue preparation. This is particularly true for the width of inter-

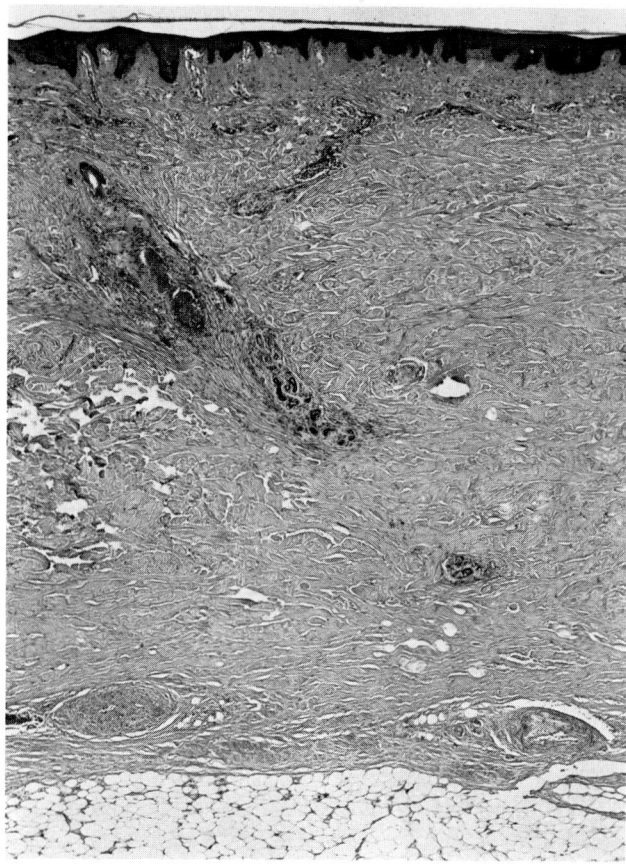

Figure 26–1.
Diffuse, generalized scleroderma. H&E. X45.

subepidermal bullae encountered in lichen sclerosus et atrophicus.

The internist often seeks help from a skin biopsy in early and questionable cases of systemic sclerosis. He must be told that the microscopic examination of a skin specimen, usually obtained from a finger or the wrist, is apt to be less informative than clinical judgment. Its main value is in ruling out other skin diseases and in establishing a record for comparison with later biopsies.

Morphea and Linear Scleroderma

Histologic diagnosis is more satisfactory[8] in *localized scleroderma* or *morphea* (Fig. 26–2), which has a variety of morphologic manifestations and usually has to be differentiated from lichen sclerosus, atrophoderma, and other dermatoses with which it may be confused clinically.[9] Most of the description given for generalized scleroderma is applicable. The epidermis usually is relatively normal, elastic fibers are preserved (Fig. 26–3), the dermis looks dense,

fascicular spaces. If inflammatory infiltrate is present, it is usually of lymphohistiocytic cell type with a few plasma cells[5] and is located in the deep dermis. Mast cells are found in the vicinity of blood vessels or sweat glands.[6] Special attention should be given to the eccrine coils, which are apt to show signs of atrophy earlier than hair follicles and often seem to be situated in the middermis, owing to the new formation of collagen bundles below them. One has to realize, however, that there are deeper and more superficial coils in normal skin and that the coils are apt to lie within the dermis in thick-skinned areas, such as the back of the trunk. To judge the size of sweat coils is impossible unless one examines a considerable number of sections. A somewhat more reliable feature is flattening of secretory cells and corresponding widening of the lumen.

In rare cases of systemic sclerosis as well as widespread morphea, the development of vesicles and bullae has been observed. They seem to be due to obstruction of superficial lymphatics by the sclerodermatous process[7] and are different from the

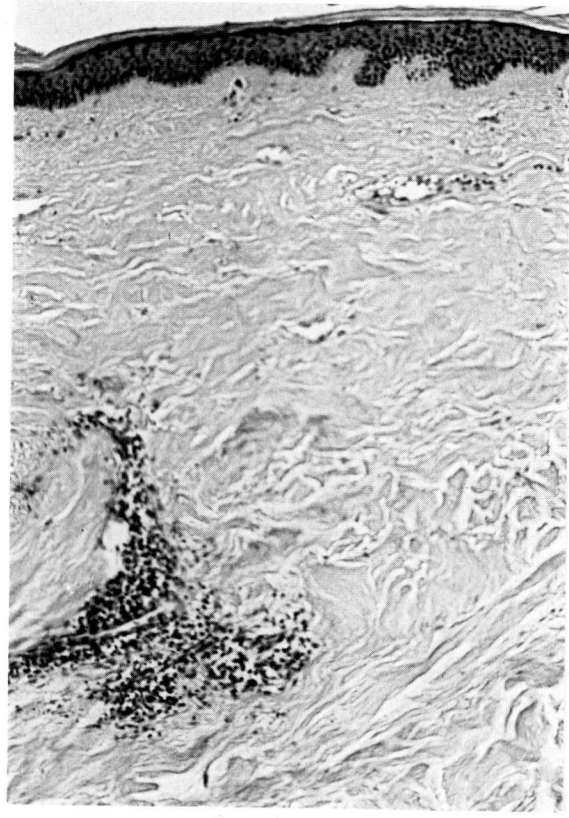

Figure 26–2.
Morphea exhibiting thickening and homogenization of collagen bundles and perivascular lymphocytic infiltrate. H&E. X125.

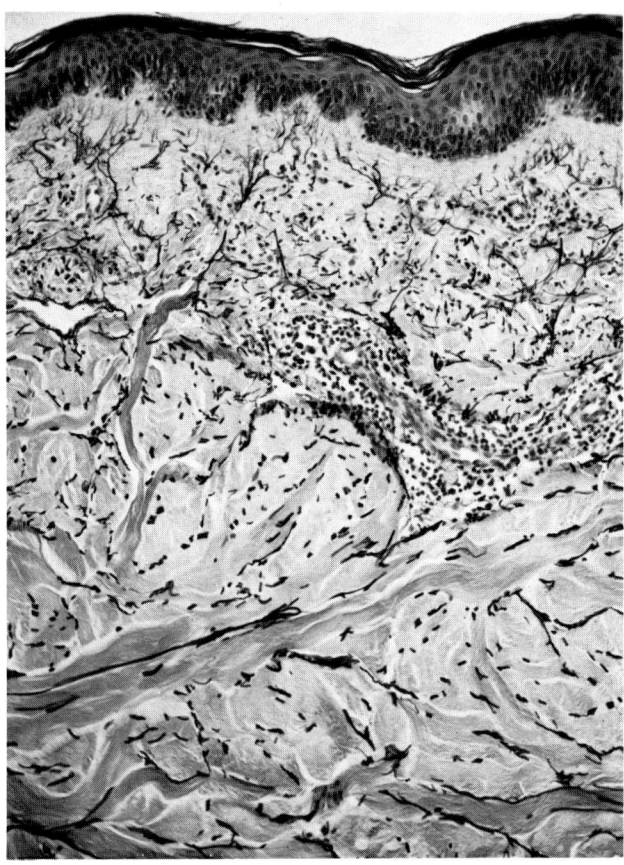

Figure 26–3.
Morphea at higher magnification. Structure of epidermis and distribution of connective tissue fibers are quite normal. Elastic fibers are chopped into pieces of different lengths by a microtome knife. There is no fragmentation of elastic fibers. The collagen bundles are thick and dense, interfascicular spaces narrow. O&G. X135.

and fibrocytes are sparse. While pars papillaris and reticularis are involved equally in some cases and the structural differences between them are obliterated, there are cases in which the subpapillary layer looks more sclerotic than the deeper portions, or the sclerosis may spare the upper dermis and involve mainly the deep dermis and even the subcutaneous tissue. Inflammatory infiltrate is more regularly found (Fig. 26–4) than in generalized scleroderma. It usually involves deep dermal vessels and may be spotty and mild or rather pronounced and almost continuous. Both multiple level sclerosis, with deep lymphocytic inflammation, and hyaline panniculitis are observed in children with generalized morphea and also in morphea profunda.[10–12] The histologic features of morphea profunda are very similar to those seen in eosinophilic fasciitis.*

Nothing of special note can be said about *linear scleroderma*[13] except that it may involve the deeper tissue along with the skin. *Linear melorheostotic scleroderma* is a rare event encountered in association with, but probably not secondary to, specific bone lesions and also involving the subcutaneous tissue.[14] The calcifying form, so-called CRST syndrome, will be mentioned in Chapter 28.

Sclerodermoid Disorders

Attention is directed here to the prior discussion of pseudosclerodermatous artifact (Chapter 3, Fig. 3–5).

Sclerodermoid changes are encountered in the Winchester syndrome,[15] in which an abnormal function of fibroblasts is suspected. Scleroderma may be imitated by *pachydermoperiostosis,* which affects both skin and bones of extremities and face and exhibits thickened dermis and thick fibrous bands extending into the subcutis.[16] In contrast to scleroderma, however, there is an increase of fibroblasts and ground substance.[17] Sclerodermoid hardening of exposed skin occurs in porphyria cutanea tarda and is difficult to distinguish from scleroderma histologically,[18] except that it usually does not involve subcutaneous tissue and is associated with actinic elastosis and possibly some evidence of scar formation from preceding blistering. On the other hand, Fleischmajer and Nedwich[19] found the subcutaneous tissue replaced by hyalinized connective tissue in a sclerodermoid plaque of Werner syndrome. Severe and extensive sclerodermoid change of skin and subcutaneous tissue has been observed after pentazocine injections[20] and following injection of silicone for augmentation mammoplasty.[21] There is extensive collagenous fibrosis, and the elastic fibers are correspondingly reduced. *Acroosteolysis* may produce sclerodermoid histology in both its spontaneous[22] and occupational forms.[23] Graft-vs-host reaction may assume sclerodermoid aspects in the chronic stage both clinically and histologically.[24]

Eosinophilic Fasciitis

Patients with Shulman's[25] eosinophilic fasciitis develop an inflammatory scleroderma-like illness without Raynaud's phenomenon or internal organ involvement. The clinical course is characterized by spontaneous remission, relapses, and recurrences. Corticosteroid therapy leads to complete resolution. Histologic examination shows extensive involvement of panniculus with sclerotic fibrous tissue and collections of lymphocytes[26] (Fig. 26–5). Laboratory

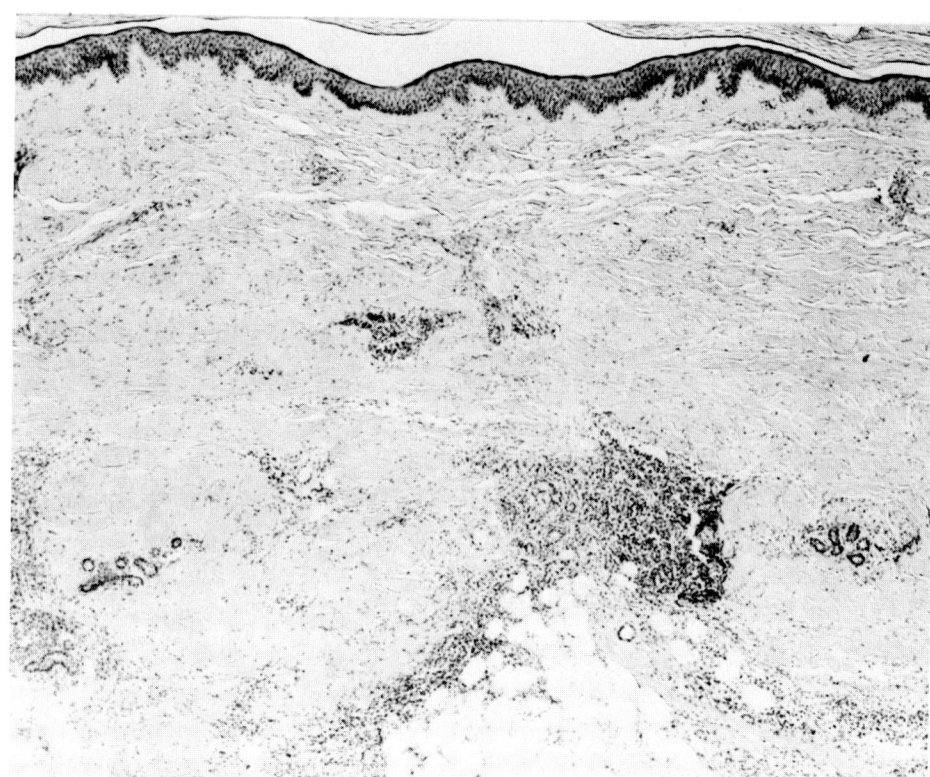

Figure 26–4.
Morphea. Lesion shows somewhat more inflammatory infiltrate than average case. Note obliteration of differences between pars papillaris and pars reticularis of dermis and extension of dense fibrous tissue below sweat coils, which seem atrophic. H&E. X60.

findings include blood eosinophilia, and in half of the cases elevated sedimentation rate and hypergammaglobulinemia. There are histologic similarities between eosinophilic fasciitis and inflammatory form of morphea or scleroderma. Blood eosinophilia may also be present in a small number of patients with morphea and scleroderma.[27] The possibility exists that eosinophilic fasciitis is a subset of morphea or morphea profunda.

ATROPHODERMAS AND LIPODYSTROPHIES

Atrophoderma of Pasini and Pierini

In pure cases of idiopathic atrophoderma of Pasini and Pierini,[28–30] none of the histologic features of scleroderma or any other alteration are present except that epidermis and dermis are somewhat thinner than the normal surrounding area and the subcutaneous fat tissue is located closer to the surface. This feature (Fig. 26–6) can be recognized only by comparison. Examination requires either a fairly long strip of skin extending from normal across the shoulder into the depressed area, or two punch biopsies, one taken outside, the other inside the lesion. Both must include a considerable portion of the subcutaneous panniculus and should be processed together and mounted side by side for comparison. Relation between atrophoderma of Pasini and Pierni and morphea is not clear. Both conditions may occur in the same patient.[31]

Senile Atrophy

In pure senile atrophy unrelated to climatic influences or disease, the thickness of the epidermis is reduced by one or two cell layers and rete ridges and papillae tend to be effaced. The dermis exhibits progressive loss of papillary capillaries and some general thinning that does not strikingly alter the proportion of collagenous and elastic fibers, although aged skin probably contains relatively more elastin than does young adult skin. The lobes of the subcutaneous fat tissue may become smaller because fat cells are reduced in size.

Progeria

A generalized form of atrophy is progeria,[32,33] in which all elements of skin and subcutaneous tissue

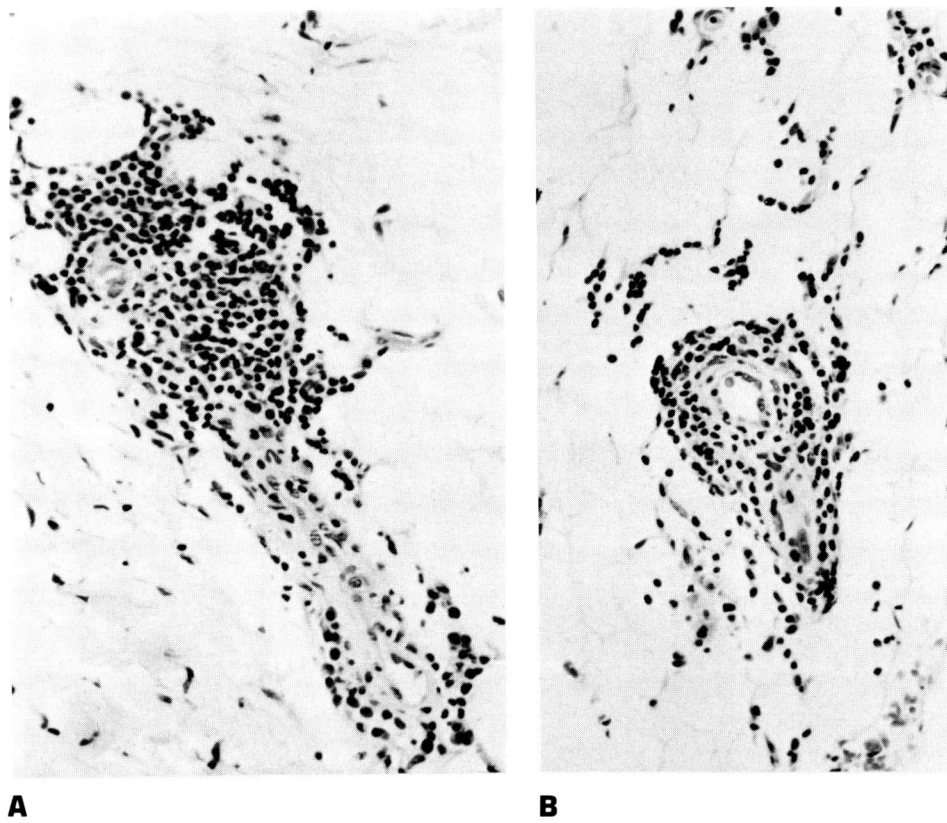

Figure 26–5.
Eosinophilic fasciitis. Perivascular infiltrate in fat tissue near deep fascia. **A** and **B**, H&E. X400.

are atrophic. The deeper parts of the dermis may show hyalinization.

Corticosteroid Atrophy

Atrophy caused by local application of corticosteroid preparations, whether fluorinated or not, can be most disturbing and must be considered in many skin biopsy specimens of chronic disease. Epidermal atrophy of varying degree occurs early.[34] The visible and palpable thinning of the skin is due mainly to a decrease of collagen, leading to a crowding together of elastic fibers, which, however, do not exhibit the changes of actinic elastosis. Sweat coils are found much closer to the epidermis than in normal skin.

Acrodermatitis Chronica Atrophicans

Acrodermatitis chronica atrophicans can lead to extreme degrees of cutaneous and subcutaneous atrophy but is the end result of a characteristic inflammatory process, which probably is due to the tick-borne spirochete *Borrelia burgdorferi* endemic in parts of the Old World.[35] In the early stages, the dermis is edematous and contains focal infiltrate of lymphocytes, plasma cells, and some histiocytes.[36] Elastic fibers are destroyed early, and epidermis and pilosebaceous complexes undergo atrophy, while eccrine glands are apt to persist. In later stages, the inflammatory component disappears, but the extensive loss of elastic fibers differentiates the lesion from primary atrophies.

Lipodystrophy

Several clinical forms of lipodystrophy exist. A *congenital* form is characterized by the absence of subcutaneous fat tissue at birth and development in the second decade of life of insulin-resistant diabetes mellitus.[37] An *acquired* form of lipodystrophy may appear following bacterial or acute viral infection. In both the congenital or the acquired forms, lipodystrophy is characterized by absence of subcutaneous fat tissue with no disturbances of dermis or

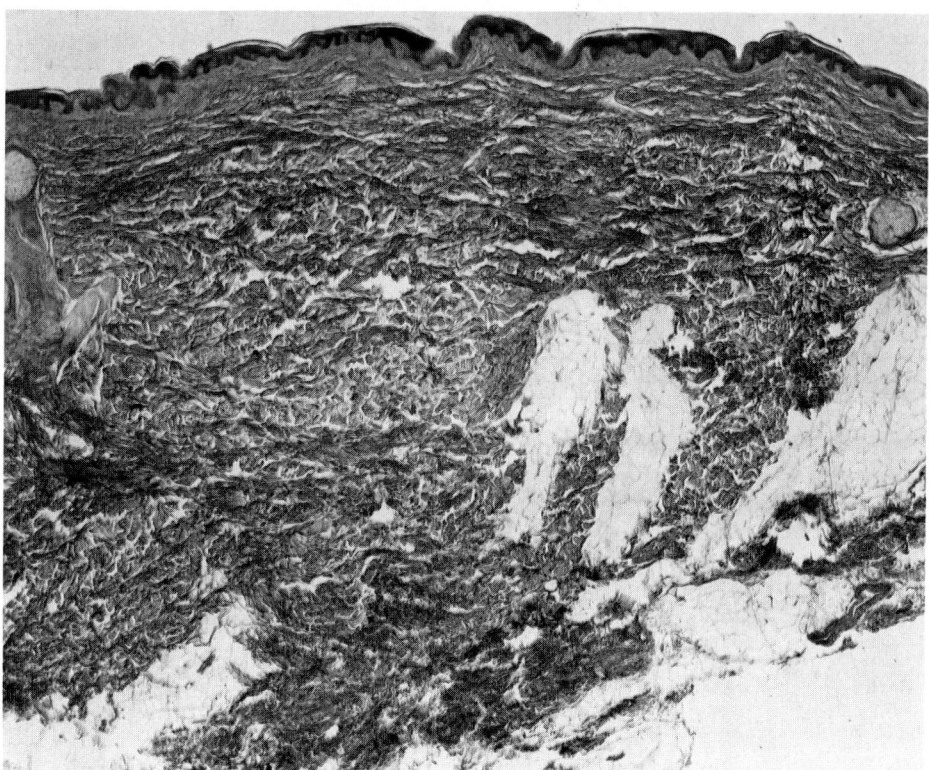

Figure 26–6.
Idiopathic atrophoderma (Pasini and Pierini). Normal dermis at left is almost twice as thick as atrophic dermis at right, as indicated by distribution of subcutaneous fat tissue. Skin presents no other structural or inflammatory changes. H&E. X45. (From Mehregan and Pinkus. Dermatol Dig 7:49, 1968.)

epidermis. *Localized* lipoatrophy occurs following injections or trauma. Idiopathic panatrophy of Gower's is a localized lesion located over the deltoid area. In localized lipoatrophy lobules of small lipocytes are embedded in hyalinized connective tissue.[38,39] Lipodystrophia centrifugalis abdominalis reported in children shows localized depression of the abdominal skin with an erythematous, scaling, and centrifugally advancing border. Histologically, it shows loss of the subcutaneous fat tissue surrounded by areas of heavy lymphohistiocytic infiltrate.[40–44]

Aplasia Cutis Congenita

The most extreme instances of cutaneous atrophy or defective development are cases of aplasia cutis congenita.[45–48] Both isolated instances and cases occurring among successive generations in multiple families have been reported.[49] These defects are most often seen on the scalps of newborn infants and gradually heal with formation of granulation tissue and an atrophic scar devoid of cutaneous adnexa. They have been interpreted as aplastic (minus) nevi (Fig. 26–7). Another type of congenital localized ab-

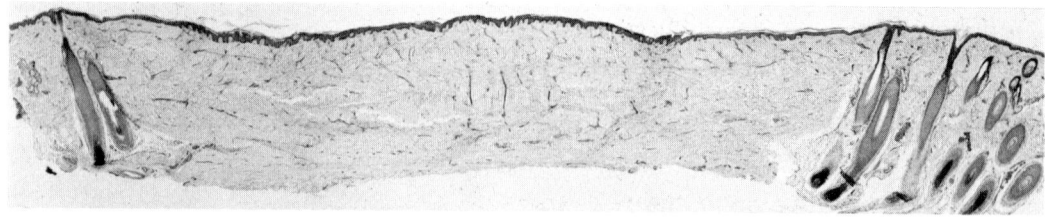

Figure 26–7.
Aplasia cutis congenita. Absence of cutaneous adnexa and dermal replacement with scar tissue. H&E. X30.

sence of skin with other associated abnormalities was described by Bart et al.[50] This particular lesion is often localized in the legs and has some features of epidermolysis bullosa. It is inherited in autosomal dominant fashion, although it may be encountered as a solitary case.[51]

LICHEN SCLEROSUS ET ATROPHICUS

In contrast to morphea, lichen sclerosus et atrophicus (see Figs. 5-2, 26-8) exhibits marked changes not ony of collagen but of epidermis and elastic fibers as well. The rete malpighi is thinned, and ridges and papillae are flattened or lost. Basal cells are flat, often vacuolated. The horny and granular layers are thick and are partly responsible for the chalky white clinical appearance.[52-54] Hair follicles and sweat glands undergo atrophy, and their ostia are dilated with keratin corresponding to the black comedo-like plugs of the typical early lesion. Later, they may disappear completely. The most characteristic feature is a peculiar homogenization of the upper dermis, which on closer analysis is quite different from sclerosis.[55] The collagen bundles seem to become diffused within the markedly increased ground substance, which gives the impression of edema in H&E and O&G sections, and stains positive for hyaluronic acid. In pronounced cases, especially in the genital

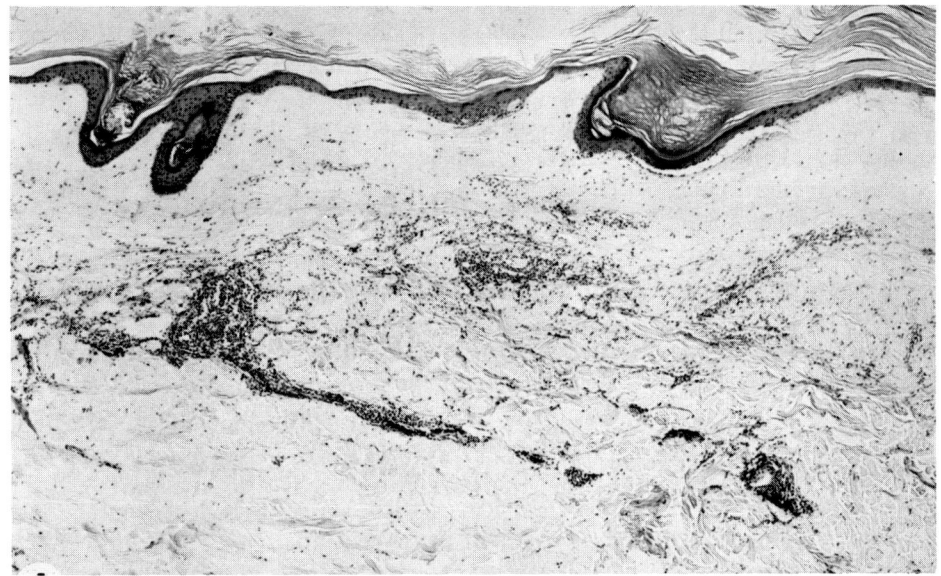

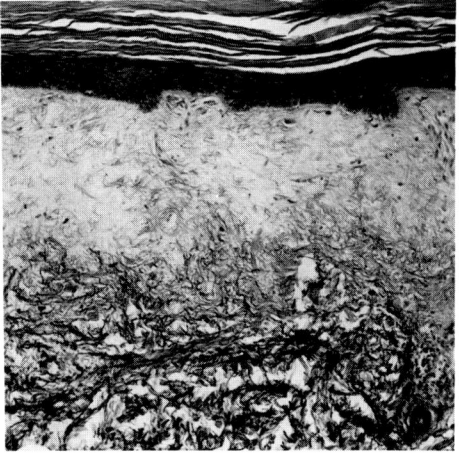

Figure 26–8.
Lichen sclerosus et atrophicus. **A.** *Dense hyperkeratosis, epidermal atrophy, and keratotic plugging of hair follicles and sweat ducts above a zone of edematous dermis and deep infiltrate. The subepidermal cleft is probably a technical artifact but indicates diminished adhesion between epidermis and dermis. H&E. X45.* **B** *and* **C.** *Sections of another specimen stained H&E and O&G, respectively, to show edematous homogenization and loss of elastic fibers of pars papillaris and upper pars reticularis. X75.*

area of children, this change leads to subepidermal bullae through rarefication of the fibers. Within this zone, a few ectatic thin-walled vessels are seen which may rupture and produce hemorrhage. O&G stains (see Fig. 26–8C) show interesting phenomena. Even though the homogenized zone may be narrow, it always involves the pars reticularis, the pars papillaris frequently being just as atrophic as the epidermis. Elastic fibers are markedly diminished or are completely absent. O&G stain also emphasizes loss of epidermal pigment and presence of melanin-filled macrophages in the upper dermis.

Below the involved zone, there is round cell infiltrate which may be focal or continuous. Below it, the dermis is normal. Sections through an entire small papule show the infiltrate beginning at either side just at the epidermis and curving below the homogenized zone. If the infiltrate is fairly heavy, the similarity to atrophying lichen planus (see Fig. 9–7) may be striking in H&E sections. O&G sections, however, show that all the changes in lichen planus are in the widened pars papillaris, while they are in the pars reticularis in lichen sclerosus. If the infiltrate is minor, and one is dealing with a small portion of a larger plaque, differential diagnosis from morphea may be difficult. Epidermal atrophy and loss of elastic fibers speak for lichen sclerosus.[56]

Lichen sclerosus et atrophicus may affect any part of the skin surface, including palms and soles, but has a predilection for the female anogenital region, where it has been confused with leukoplakia and often is called *kraurosis vulvae*. It has also been mentioned as a common and distinctive cause of phimosis in boys.[57] Lesions on the glans penis were given the appellation *balanitis xerotica obliterans*. These localizations are discussed in Chapter 46.

REACTIVE PERFORATING COLLAGENOSIS

A remarkable histobiologic phenomenon involving dermal collagenous tissue was described in children as reactive perforating collagenosis.[58] Adult and familial cases have been reported and an autosomal dominant trait has been suggested. The lesions appear following superficial trauma or exposure to cold in the form of pinpoint keratotic papules that grow in size and become centrally umbilicated.[62–64] The lesions may occur in linear fashion suggesting Koebner's phenomenon.[59–61] Initially an area of basophilic degeneration of collagenous tissue is observed within the papillary dermis (Fig. 26–9). This is followed by reactive pseudoepitheliomatous hyperplasia of the epidermis and transepithelial elimination of the altered connective tissue in an umbilicated lesion.[65] The extruded collagen bundles mixed with parakeratotic and inflammatory cells form a dense plug situated within the center of umbilicated lesion. The process subsides completely within a 6- to 8-week period.

Perforating Lesions in Chronic Renal Failure

Hyperkeratotic and umbilicated papular and nodular lesions occur over the extensor aspect of the extremities in 5 to 10 percent of patients undergoing hemodialysis for chronic renal failure secondary to diabetes.[66–69] Histologically, the lesions have been categorized as Kyrle-like (Fig. 26–10), perforating folliculitis and reactive perforating collagenosis.[70–72] The perforating channel is unrelated to the hair follicles and contains collagen bundles, inflammatory cells, and nucleated keratinocytes.

EHLERS–DANLOS SYNDROME

Cutis hyperelastica or Ehlers–Danlos syndrome is due to a disturbance in collagen rather than in elastic fibers.[73,74] Several abnormalities of collagen biosynthesis have been described. Based on clinical manifestations, mode of inheritance, and the underlying biochemical defects, nine types of Ehlers–Danlos syndrome are recognized[75–78] (Table 26–1).

The skin of patients with Ehlers–Danlos syndrome is soft to touch, easily stretched, and shows tendency for easy bruising, delayed wound healing, and abnormal scar formation.[79] Histologic findings are peculiarly disappointing. Abnormality of collagen bundles is not detectable in histologic sections. There may be a relative abundance of elastic tissue in proportion to the collagen.[80,81] No structural abnormality is seen in elastic tissue. Secondary lesions such as hematomas or fibrotic scars will, of course, show definite histologic changes.

SCLEREDEMA, LYMPHEDEMA, AND MYXEDEMA

The wooden hard indurations of *scleredema adultorum* are histologically disappointing because they are due to increased hyaluronic acid in the ground

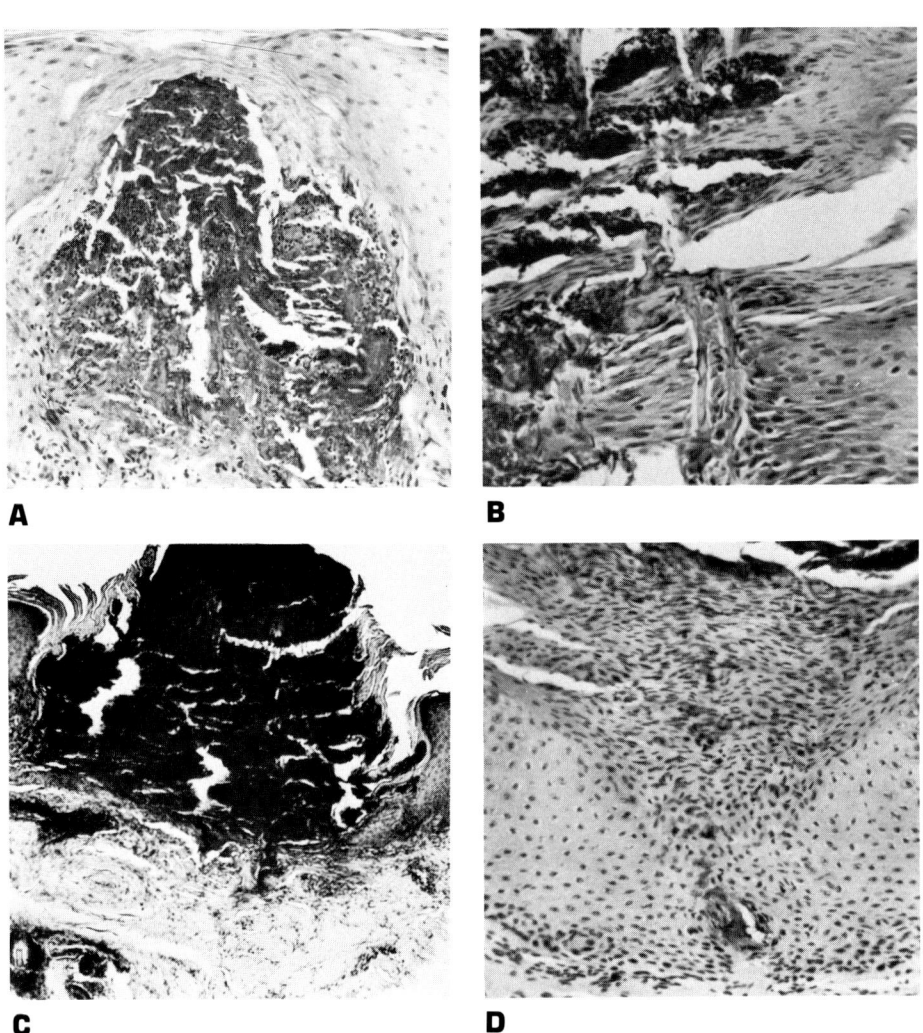

Figure 26–9.
Reactive perforating collagenosis. **A** and **C**. Early and late stages of the process. H&E. **B** and **D**. Details of thin collagen bundles being eliminated transepidermally. H&E. **A**. X135. **B**. X135. **C**. X45. **D**. X90.

substance. Routine H&E and O&G sections show little, inasmuch as edema is difficult to see in fixed tissue sections. Mucopolysaccharide stains are needed.[82–84] Lymphedema also is hard to recognize, but pronounced cases show such excessive fraying and separation of collagen bundles that a spectacular picture results. Dilated lymph vessels, so inconspicuous in H&E sections, often stand out nicely in O&G sections due to their elastic coat. Cases of *verrucous lymphedema* (Fig. 26–11) show an even more spectacular configuration. It is worth remembering that most cases clinically suspected to be pyoderma vegetans turn out to be verrucous lymphedema with some secondary inflammation.

Myxedema of the generalized and tuberous types shows essentially similar features (Fig. 26–12), except that the changes are fairly sharply localized in the second form. H&E and O&G sections show widened interfascicular spaces as in simple edema but also show separation of the elastic fibers and fraying of collagen bundles, which may become almost as extreme as in lymphedema. The mucin,[85] being mainly hyaluronic acid, stains bright blue with Hale method or alcian blue stain and may entirely obscure the collagen in such sections.

Mucopolysaccharidoses

We must mention here *Hurler syndrome* and other mucopolysaccharidoses and mucolipidoses,[86] in which various unusual metachromatic substances are deposited in many types of cells, including dermal fibrocytes and epidermal cells. These deposits may appear as cytoplasmic vacuoles in routine sections and may require fixation in alcohol because of their water solubility. An electron microscopic study

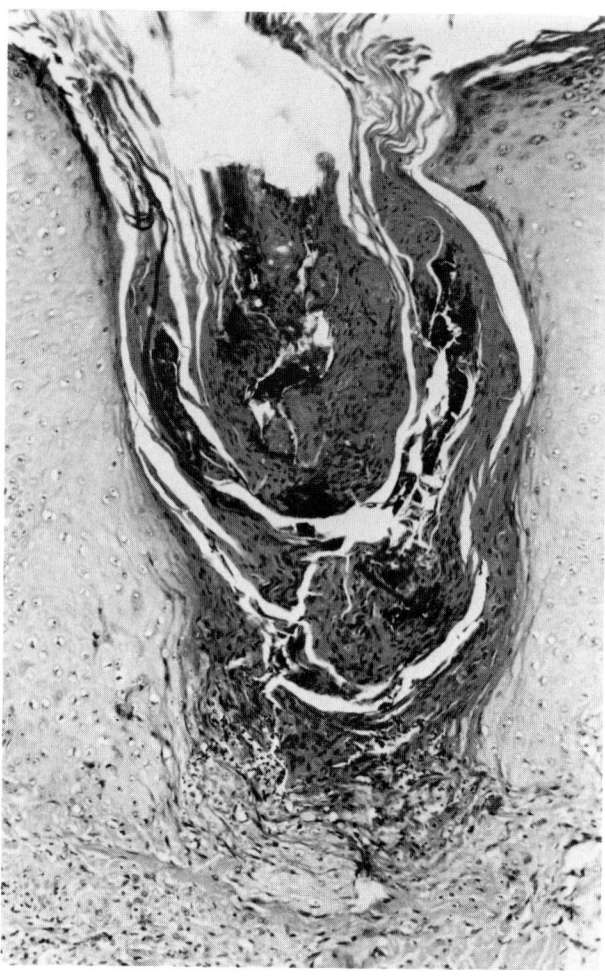

Figure 26–10.
Perforating eruption in a patient with diabetes mellitus and chronic renal failure undergoing dialysis. Central perforating channel contains fragments of collagen bundles mixed with keratinocytes and inflammatory cells. H&E. X125.

of the specific subscapular papulosis of Hunter syndrome was offered by Larrègne et al.[87]

Lichen Myxedematosus: Papular Mucinosis and Scleromyxedema

Accumulation of mucin substances, especially hyaluronic acid, is characteristic of two conditions: papular mucinosis and scleromyxedema. These have been often lumped together under the name "lichen myxedematosus," but deserve to be considered separately because there are considerable differences in the clinical picture, prognosis, histologic changes, and pathogenesis.

The clinical manifestations of *papular mucinosis*,[88] grouped papules which come and go over a period of months or years, and may show persistent acral involvement, are represented by myxomatous histologic changes.[89,90] There is an ill-defined area in which collagen bundles are frayed and stellate fibrocytes are suspended in the meshes filled with hyaluronic acid (Fig. 26–13).

Scleromyxedema, on the other hand, is clinically characterized by extensive skin involvement by numerous papular lesions coalescing to form areas of sclerodermoid thickening and infiltration.[91] Histologically, the first impression is a fibroma because of massive proliferation of fibrocytes with a relatively small amount of ground substance (Fig. 26–14). Metachromatic or mucin stains are needed to show deposition of acid mucopolysaccharides, a major portion of which is hyaluronic acid.[92] A specific paraprotein has been found in the serum of patients with scleromyxedema.[93,94]

In this area we must also mention multiple papular and nodular mucinous lesions developing in patients with lupus erythematosus. The histologic changes are very similar to papular mucinosis.[95,96]

REM Syndrome

An erythematous reticular maculopapular eruption encountered usually on the backs of women was described by Steigleder et al.[97] as reticular erythematous mucinous syndrome. This condition appears to be identical to the "plague-like form of cutaneous mucinosis" described by Perry et al.[98,99] previously. Histologic sections show perivascular and perifollicular lymphocytic infiltrate in addition to dermal deposition of alcian blue reactive acid mucopolysaccharide (hyaluronic acid).[100] Although the eruption is aggravated by sun exposure, phototesting shows no abnormal response. The eruption responds to administration of hydroxychloroquine sulfate.

SYNOVIAL LESIONS AND MYXOID CYSTS

Isolated papules and nodules consisting of myxomatous tissue may occur anywhere on the skin, but there is a typical localization on the distal phalanx of the finger, just proximal to the nail fold. These lesions clinically resemble cysts and are known as synovial lesions or myxoid cysts.[101] They discharge mucinous fluid or jelly periodically and then fill again. Histologically, a central cystic cavity is lined by a layer of connective tissue (Fig. 26–15) with

TABLE 26-1. CLINICAL, GENETIC, AND BIOCHEMICAL CLASSIFICATION OF EHLERS-DANLOS SYNDROME

Type	Inheritance	Clinical Manifestations	Biochemical Defects
Gravis	Autosomal dominant	Hyperextensibility of skin, marked fragility, atrophic scars, and molluscoid	Unknown
Mitis	Autosomal dominant	Hyperextensibility of skin, hypermobility of joints, bleeding problems	Unknown
Benign hypermobile	Autosomal dominant	Marked joint hypermobility, minimal skin manifestations	Unknown
Ecchymotic	Autosomal recessive	Hypermobility limited to digits, skin fragility with ecchymoses, arterial rupture	Deficiency of type III collagen
X-linked	X-linked recessive	Minimal joint hypermobility, hyperextensibility of skin with bruising, skeletal disorders	Lysyl oxidase deficiency
Ocular	Autosomal recessive	Hyperextensibility of skin, hypermobility of joints, scleral and corneal fragility	Lysyl hydroxylase deficiency
Arthrocalasis multiplex congenita	Autosomal recessive	Hyperextensibility and fragility of skin, hypermobility of joints, short stature, multiple dislocations	Defective conversion of procollagen to collagen
Periodontitis	Autosomal dominant	Minimal skin hyperextensibility, hypermobility of joints, advanced periodontitis	Unknown
Fibronectin type	Autosomal recessive	Striae, moderate skin extensibility, joint hypermobility, platelet aggregation defect	Dysfunction of plasma fibronectin

fibrotic and myxomatous areas depending on the stage of the lesion.[102,103] It is fairly characteristic that the epidermis is very thin though hyperkeratotic, and sometimes one finds layers of inspissated mucus alternating with keratinous lamellae. The connection that these lesions often have with joint or tendon sheath usually cannot be demonstrated in a section of excised skin lesion.[104]

AFFECTIONS OF EAR CARTILAGE

The elastic cartilage of the ear is so close to the skin that lesions affecting it must be considered. The most common, *chondrodermatitis nodularis chronica helicis*, is discussed in Chapter 17.

Long-continued traumatic injury to the ears of professional boxers leads to the so-called cauliflower ear. A nodular lesion with smooth surface and without history of trauma is known as *pseudocyst of the auricle*.[105] It was found to consist of eosinophilic hyalinized material deposited between the superficial and deep portions of the ear cartilage and including cystic spaces and scattered chondroblasts and fibroblasts. A potentially more serious disease is *relapsing polychondritis* (Fig. 26–16). The disease, most likely of autoimmune etiology, affects individuals between 20 to 60 years of age. The most common clinical manifestation is bilateral auricular chondritis followed by arthritis, nasal chondritis, and involvement of the cartilage in the upper respiratory tract.[106,107] Histologically, the involved cartilage loses its basophilic staining and exhibits focal degeneration of chondrocytes and inflammatory cells, initially neutrophils and later lymphocytes and plasma cells.[108]

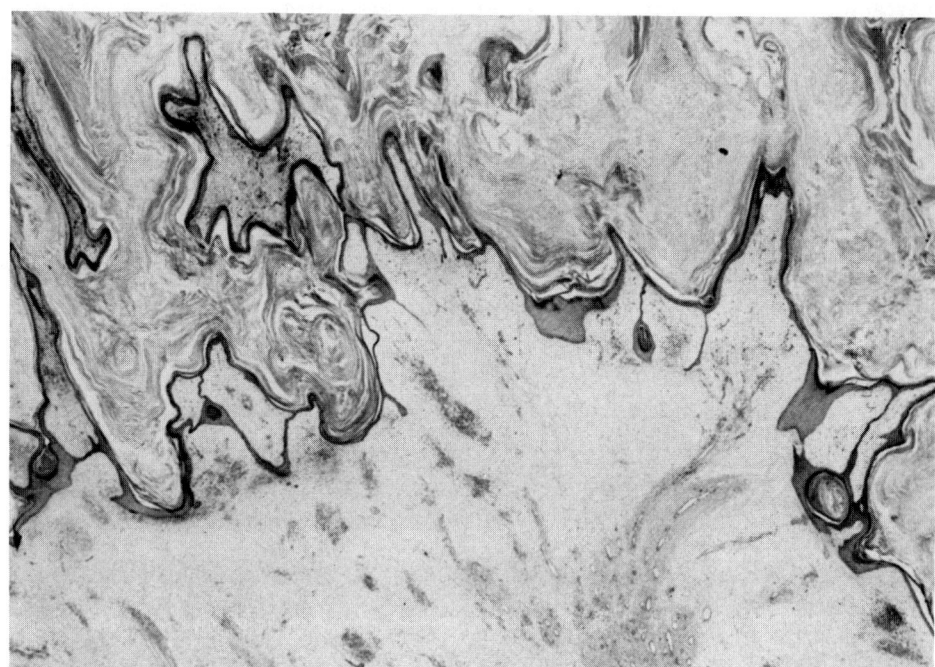

Figure 26–11.
Verrucous lymphedema. Extreme rarefication of collagenous substance of dermis, which, however, is rich in blood vessels. Voluminous papillae have elevated the thin and hyperkeratotic epidermis to produce a highly papillomatous pattern. H&E. X28.

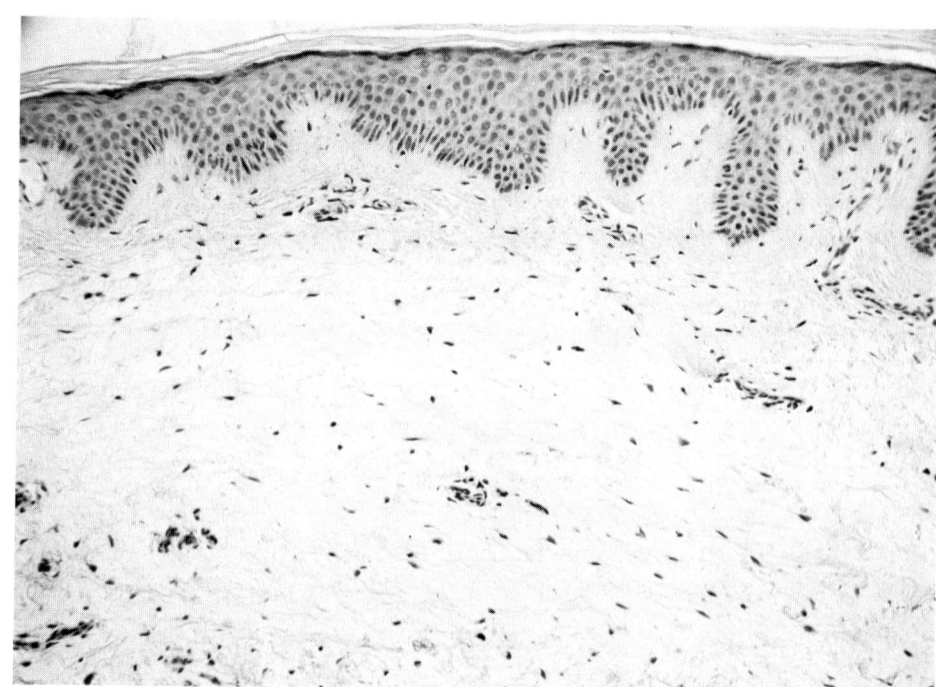

Figure 26–12.
Pretibial myxedema. The increased mucinous content of the ground substance is not evident in either H&E or O&G sections and must be confirmed by methods for demonstration of hyaluronic acid. H&E X135.

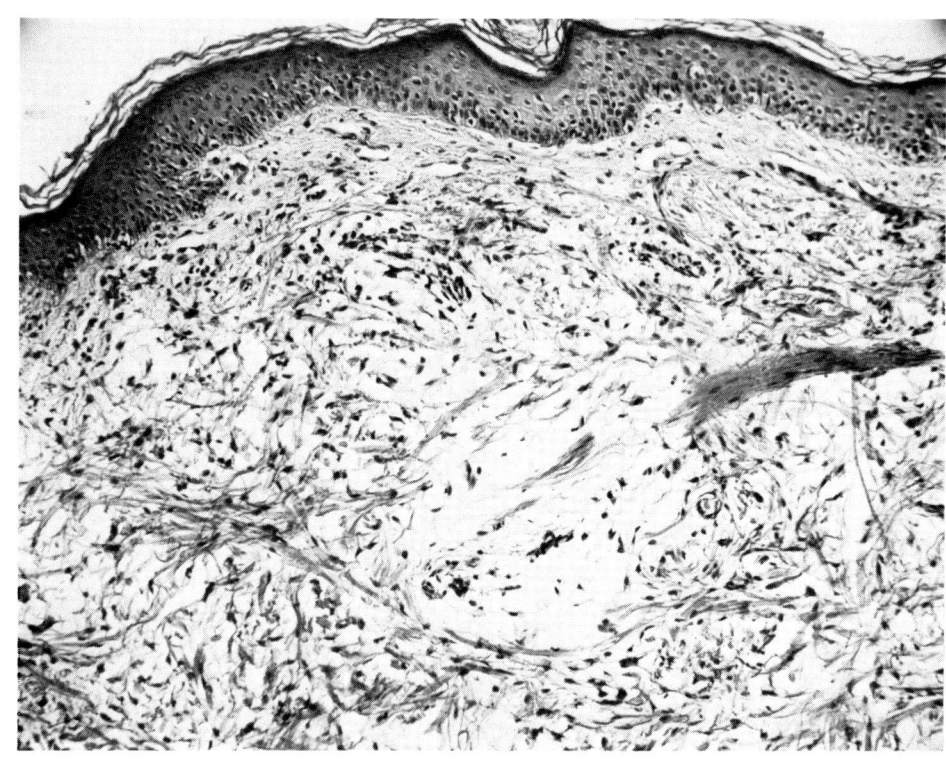

Figure 26–13.
Papular mucinosis. Note myxomatous aspect due to stellate fibroblasts. H&E. X135.

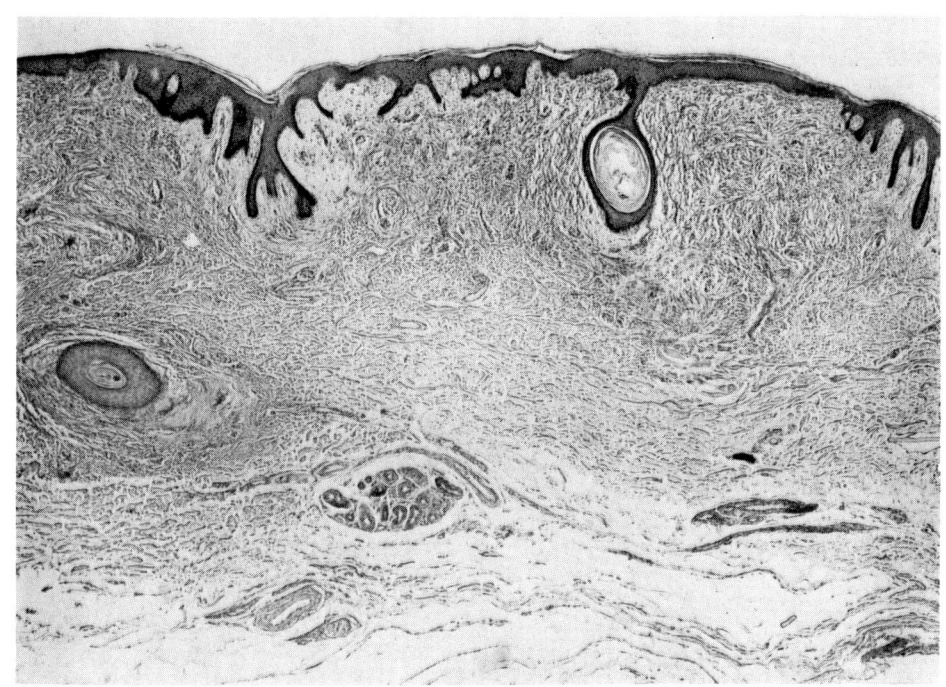

Figure 26–14.
Scleromyxedema. Overall impression is that of a fibroma. In some of these lesions it requires a high level of suspicion to recognize mucinous change. Note general thickening of skin. H&E. X30. (From Rudner et al. Arch Dermatol 93:3, 1966.)

METABOLIC AND OTHER NONINFLAMMATORY DERMAL DISEASES

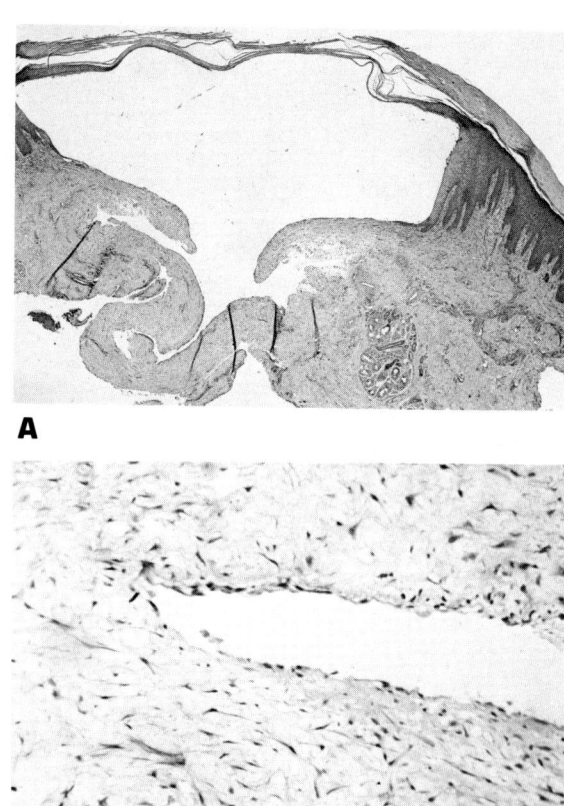

Figure 26-15.
Synovial lesion of finger. **A.** Note extension into deep tissue, pressure atrophy of epidermis, and absence of cyst wall. H&E. X30. **B.** Myxomatous aspect of the surrounding connective tissue. H&E. X250.

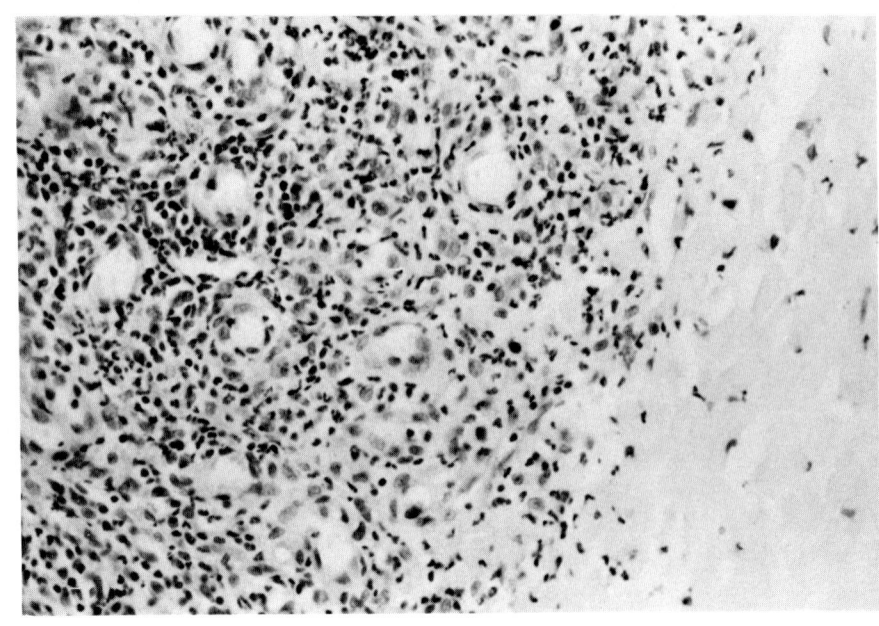

Figure 26-16.
Relapsing polychondritis. Devitalized cartilage on right. Vascular granulation tissue with infiltrate containing polymorphs, both neutrophilic and eosinophilic, on left. H&E. X250.

REFERENCES

1. Asboe-Hansen G: Scleroderma. J Am Acad Dermatol 17:102, 1987
2. Krieg T, Meurer M: Systemic scleroderma. Clinical and pathophysiologic aspects. J Am Acad Dermatol 18:457, 1988
3. Fleischmajer R, Perlish JS, Duncan M: Scleroderma. A model for fibrosis. Arch Dermatol 119:957, 1983
4. Fleischmajer R, Perlish JS: Capillary alterations in scleroderma. J Am Acad Dermatol 2:161, 1980
5. Pierard GE, Perard-Franchimont C, Lapiere CM: Les compartiments conjonctifs dans les sclerodermis. Etude de la structure et des propriétés biomécaniques. Dermatologica 170:105, 1985
6. Nishioka K, Kobayashi Y, Katayama I, Takijiri C: Mast cell numbers in diffuse scleroderma. Arch Dermatol 123:205, 1987
7. Synkowski DR, Lobitz WC Jr, Provost TT: Bullous scleroderma. Arch Dermatol 117:135, 1981
8. Fleischmajer R, Nedwich A: Generalized morphea: Histology of the dermis and subcutaneous tissue. Arch Dermatol 106:509, 1972
9. Falanga V, Medsger TA, Reichlin M, Rodnant P: Linear scleroderma: Clinical spectrum, prognosis, and laboratory abnormalities. Ann Intern Med 104:849, 1986
10. Su DWP, Person JR: Morphea profunda. A new concept and a histopathologic study of 23 cases. Am J Dermatopathol 3:251, 1981
11. Doyle JA, Connoly SM, Winkelmann RK: Cutaneous and subcutaneous inflammatory sclerosis syndromes. Arch Dermatol 118:886, 1982
12. Nakamura T, Ono T, Yamashita N, et al: Morphea profunda—A cutaneo-pulmonary variant with profuse sweating. J Dermatol Tokyo 16:122, 1989
13. Larregue M, Ziegler JE, Lauret P, et al: Sclerodermie en bande chez l'enfant (a propos de 27 cas). Ann Dermatol Venereol 113:207, 1986
14. Miyashi Y, Horio T, Yamada A, et al: Linear melorheostotic scleroderma with hypertrichosis. Arch Dermatol 115:1233, 1979
15. Nabai H, Mehregan AH, Mortezai A, et al: Winchester syndrome: Report of a case from Iran. J Cutan Pathol 4:281, 1977
16. Vogl A, Goldfischer S: Pachydermoperiostosis. Am J Med 33:166, 1962
17. Hambrick GW, Carter DM: Pachydermoperiostosis. Arch Dermatol 94:504,1966
18. Friedman SJ, Doyle JA: Sclerodermoid changes of porphyria cutanea tarda: Possible relationship to urinary uroporphyrin levels. J Am Acad Dermatol 13:70, 1985
19. Fleischmajer R, Nedwich A: Werner's syndrome. Am J Med 54:111, 1973
20. Parks DL, Perry HO, Muller SA: Cutaneous complications of pentazocine injections: Arch Dermatol 104:231, 1971
21. Spiera H: Scleroderma after silicone augmentation mammoplasty. JAMA 260:236, 1988
22. Meyerson, LB, Meier GC: Cutaneous lesions in acroosteolysis. Arch Dermatol 106:224,1972
23. Markowitz SS, McDonald CJ, Fethiere W, et al: Occupational acroosteolysis. Arch Dermatol 106:219, 1972
24. Graham-Brown RAC, Sarkany I: Scleroderma-like changes due to chronic graft-versus-host disease. Clin Exp Dermatol 8:531, 1983
25. Coyle HE, Chapman RS: Eosinophilic fasciitis (Shulman syndrome) in association with morphoea and systemic sclerosis. Acta Derm Venereol 60:181, 1980
26. Michet CJ Jr, Doyle JA, Ginsburg WW: Eosinophilic fasciitis. Report of 15 cases. Mayo Clin Proc 56:27, 1981
27. Falanga V, Medsger TA: Frequency, levels, and significance of blood eosinophilia in systemic sclerosis, localized scleroderma and eosinophilic fasciitis. J Am Acad Dermatol 17:648, 1987
28. Canizares O, Sachs PM, Jaimovich L, et al: Idiopathic atrophoderma of Pasini and Pierini. Arch Dermatol 77:42, 1958
29. Pierini LE, Abulafia J, Mosto SJ: Atrophodermie idiopathique progressive et états voisins. Ann Dermatol Syphiligr 97:391, 1970
30. Miller RF: Idiopathic atrophoderma. Arch Dermatol 92:653, 1965
31. Kee CE, Brothers WS, New W: Idiopathic atrophoderma of Pasini and Pierini with coexistent morphea. Arch Dermatol 82:100, 1960
32. DeBusk FL: The Hutchinson–Gilford progeria syndrome. J Pediatr 80:697, 1972
33. Fleischmajer R, Nedwich A: Progeria (Hutchinson–Gilford). Arch Dermatol 107:253, 1973
34. Polano MK, et al (eds): Advances in topical cortosteroid therapy. Dermatologica 152 (Suppl 1) 1976
35. Abele DC, Anders KH: The many faces and phases of borreliosis II. J Am Acad Dermatol 23:401, 1990
36. Asbrink E, Brehmer-Andersson E, Hovmark A:Acrodermatitis chronica atrophicans-A spirochetosis. Clinical and histopathological picture based on 32 patients; course and relationship to erythema chronicum migrans Afzelius. Am J Dermatopathol 8:209, 1986
37. Huntley A: The cutaneous manifestations of diabetes mellitus. J Am Acad Dermatol 7:427, 1982
38. Peters MS, Winkelmann RK: The histopathology of localized lipoatrophy. Br J Dermatol 114:27, 1986
39. Perrot H: Les lipo-strophies localisees. Ann Dermatol Venereol 115:523, 1988
40. Mizoguchi M, Nanko S: Lipodystrophia centrifugalis abdominalis infantilis in dizygotic twins. J Dermatol Tokyo 9:139, 1982
41. Giam YC, Rajan VS, Hock OB: Lipodystrophia centrifugalis abdominalis infantilis. Br J Dermatol 106:461, 1982
42. Lee S, Houh W, Kim YK, et al: Lipodystrophia centrifugalis abdominalis juvenilis. Dermatologica 164:95, 1982
43. Zachary CB, Wells RS: Centrifugal lipodystrophy. Br J Dermatol 110:107, 1984

44. Rongioletti F, Rebora A: Annular and semicircular lipoatrophies. J Am Acad Dermatol 20:433, 1989
45. Frieden IJ: Aplasia cutis congenita: A clinical review and proposal for classification. J Am Acad Dermatol 14:646, 1986
46. Prigent F: Aplasies cutanees congenitales. Ann Dermatol Venereol 110:933, 1983
47. Sanchez-Pedreno Guillen P, Rodriguez-Pichardo A, Camacho Martinez F: Aplasia cutis congenita. J Am Acad Dermatol 13:429, 1985
48. Sybert VP: Aplasia cutis congenita: A report of 12 new families and review of the literature. Pediatr Dermatol 3:11, 1985
49. Itin P, Pletscher M: Familial aplasia cutis congenita of the scalp without other defects in 6 members of three successive generations. Dermatologica 177:123, 1988
50. Bart BJ, Gorlin RJ, Anderson VE, et al: Congenital localized absence of skin and associated abnormalities resembling epidermolysis bullosa. Arch Dermatol 93:296, 1966
51. Smith SZ, Crain DL: A mechanobullous disease of the newborn. Bart's syndrome. Arch Dermatol 114:81, 1978
52. Garcia-Bravo B, Sanchez-Pedreno P, Rodriguez-Pichardo A, Camacho F: Lichen sclerosus et atrophicus. A study of 76 cases and their relation to diabetes. J Am Acad Dermatol 19:482, 1988
53. Pelisse M: Lichen sclereux. Ann Dermatol Venereol 114:411, 1987
54. Tremaine RDL, Miller RAW: Lichen sclerosus et atrophicus. Int J Dermatol 28:10, 1989
55. Romppanen U, Rantala I, Lauslahti K, Reunala T: Light and electron-microscopic findings in lichen sclerosus of the vulva during etretinate treatment. Dermatologica 175:33, 1987
56. Rahbari H: Histochemical differentiation of localized morphea—scleroderma and lichen sclerosus et atrophicus. J Cutan Pathol 16:342, 1989
57. Chalmers RJG, Burton PA, Bennett RF, et al: Lichen sclerosus et atrophicus. A common and distinctive cause of phimosis in boys. Arch Dermatol 120:1026, 1984
58. Mehregan AH, Schwartz OD, Livingood CS: Reactive perforating collagenosis: Arch Dermatol 96:277, 1967
59. Kanan MW: Familial reactive perforating collagenosis and intolerance to cold. Br J Dermatol 91:405, 1974
60. Woo Ty, Rasmussen JE: Disorders of transepidermal elimination. Int J Dermatol 24:267, 1985
61. Patterson JW: The perforating disorders. J Am Acad Dermatol 10:561, 1984
62. Berlin C, Goldberg LH: Reactive perforating collagenosis and phototraumatism. Dermatologica 171:255, 1985
63. Battan VJ, Planas-Giron G: Collagenosis perforante reactiva. A proposito de un caso y revision de la literatura. Med Cutan ILA 14:120, 1986
64. Kumar Bhatia K, Kumar S, Narang A: Reactive perforating collagenosis. A case report. J Dermatol Tokyo 14:70, 1987
65. Fretzin DF, Beal DW, Jao W: Light and ultrastructural study of reactive perforating collagenosis. Arch Dermatol 116:1054, 1980
66. Hood AF, Hardegen GL, Zarate AR: Kyrle's disease in patients with chronic renal failure. Arch Dermatol 118:85, 1982
67. Stone R: Kyrle-like lesions in two patients with renal failure undergoing dialysis. J Am Acad Dermatol 5:707, 1981
68. Hurwitz RM, Weiss J, Melton ME, et al: Perforating folliculitis in association with hemodialysis. Am J Dermatopathol 4:101, 1982
69. Poliak SC, Lebwohl MG, Parris A: Reactive perforating collagenosis associated with diabetes mellitus. N Engl J Med 306:81, 1982
70. Bank DE, Cohen PR, Kohn SR: Reactive perforating collagenosis in a setting of double disaster: Acquired immunodeficiency syndrome and end-stage renal disease. J Am Acad Dermatol 21:371, 1989
71. Beck HI, Brandrup F, Hagdrup HK, et al: Adult, acquired reactive perforating collagenosis. Report of a case including ultrastructural findings. J Cutan Pathol 15:124, 1988
72. Berger RS: Reactive perforating collagenosis of renal failure/diabetes responsive to topical retinoic acid. Cutis 43:540, 1989
73. Krieg T, Ihme A, Weber L, et al: Molecular defects of collagen metabolism in the Ehlers–Danlos syndrome. Int J Dermatol 20:415, 1981
74. Pinnell SR: Molecular defects in the Ehlers–Danlos syndrome. J Invest Dermatol 79:90, 1982
75. Rizzo R, Contri MB, Micali G, et al: Familial Ehlers–Danlos syndrome type II: Abnormal fibrillogenesis of dermal collagen. Pediatr Dermatol 4:197, 1986
76. De Paepe A, Nicholls A, Narcisi P, et al: Ehlers–Danlos syndrome type I: a clinical and ultrastructural study of a family with reduced amounts of collagen type III. Br J Dermatol 117:89, 1987
77. Boullie MC, Venencie PY, Thomine E, et al: Syndrome d'Ehlers–Danlos type IV a type d'acrogeria. Ann Dermatol Venereol 113:1077, 1986
78. Nelson DL, King RA: Ehlers–Danlos syndrome type VIII. J Am Acad Dermatol 5:297, 1981
79. Pinnell SR: The skin in Ehlers–Danlos syndrome. J Am Acad Dermatol 16:399, 1987
80. Pierard GE, Pierard-Franchimont C, Lapiere CM: Histopathological aid at the diagnosis of the Ehlers–Danlos syndrome, gravis and mitis types. Int J Dermatol 22:300, 1983
81. Holzberg M, Hewan-Lowe KO, Olansky AJ: The Ehlers–Danlos syndrome: Recognition, characterization, and importance of a milder variant of the classic form. A preliminary study. J Am Acad Dermatol 19:656, 1988
82. Carrington PR, Sanusi ID, Winder PR, et al: Scleredema adultorum. Int J Dermatol 23:514, 1984
83. McNaughton F, Keczkes K: Scleredema adultorum

and diabetes mellitus (scleredema diutinum). Clin Exp Dermatol 8:41, 1983
84. Venencie PY: Le scleroedeme de Buschke. Ann Dermatol Venereol 114:1291, 1987
85. Truhan AP, Roenigk HH Jr: The cutaneous mucinoses. J Am Acad Dermatol 14:1, 1986
86. Greaves MW, Inman PM: Cutaneous changes in the Morquio syndrome. Br J Dermatol 81:29, 1969
87. Larrègne M, Debray H, Père CC, et al: Papulose sous-scapulaire systématisée avec corps anhistes en microscopie électronique: Signes cutanés specifiques de la maladie de Hunter. Ann Dermatol Venereol 105:57, 1978
88. Coskey RJ, Mehregan AH: Papular mucinosis. Int J Dermatol 16:741, 1977
89. Rongioletti F, Rebora A: Acral persistent papular mucinosis: A new entity. Arch Dermatol 122:1237, 1986
90. Flowers SL, Cooper PH, Landes BH: Acral persistent papular mucinosis. J Am Acad Dermatol 21:293, 1989
91. Rudner EJ, Mehregan AH, Pinkus H: Scleromyxedema, a variant of lichen myxedematosus. Arch Dermatol 93:3, 1966
92. Ishii M, Furukawa M, Okada M, Hamada T: The use of improved ruthenium red staining for the ultrastructural detection of proteoglycan aggregates in normal skin and lichen myxedematosus. J Cutan Pathol 11:292, 1984
93. Lang E, Zabel M, Schmidt H: Scleromyzödem Arndt–Grotton und assoziierte Phänomene. Dermatologica 160:29, 1984
94. Harris AO, Altman AR, Tschen JA, Wolf JE Jr: Scleromyxedema. Int J Dermatol 28:661, 1989
95. Lamberts RJ, Lynch PJ: Nodular cutaneous mucinosis associated with lupus erythematosus. Cutis 28:294, 1981
96. Revier J, Kienzler JL, Blanc D, et al: Mucinose papuleuse et lupus erythemateux. A propos d'un cas, avec revue de la litterature. Ann Dermatol Venereol 109:331, 1982
97. Steigleder GK, Kuchmeister B: Cutaneous mucinous deposits. J Cutan Pathol 12:334, 1985
98. Perry HO, Kierland RR, Montgomery H: Plaquelike form of cutaneous mucinosis. Arch Dermatol 82:980, 1960
99. Braddock SW, Davis CS, Davis RB: Reticular erythematous mucinosis and thrombocytopenic purpura. Report of a case and review of the world literature, including plaquelike cutaneous mucinosis. J Am Acad Dermatol 19:859, 1988
100. Cohen PR, Rabinowitz AD, Ruszkowski AM, DeLeo VA: Reticular erythematous mucinosis syndrome: Review of the world literature and report of the syndrome in a prepubertal child. Pediatr Dermatol 7:11, 1990
101. Johnson WC, Graham JH, Helwig EB: Cutaneous myxoid cyst. JAMA 191:15, 1965
102. Armijo M: Mucoid cysts of the fingers. J Dermatol Surg Oncol 7:317, 1981
103. Salasche SJ: Myxoid cysts of the proximal nail fold. J Dermatol Surg Oncol 10:35, 1984
104. Newmeyer WL, Kilgore ES Jr, Graham WP III: Mucous cysts: The dorsal distal interphalangeal joint ganglion. Plast Reconstr Surg 53:313, 1974
105. Botella-Anton R, Matos Mula M, Jimenez Martinez A, et al: Pseudo-kystes du pavillon auriculaire. Etude clinique et histologique de trois cas. Ann Dermatol Venereol 111:919, 1984
106. Foidart JM, Katz SI: Relapsing polychondritis. Am J Dermatopathol 1:257, 1979
107. Cohen PR, Rapini RP: Relapsing polychondritis. Int J Dermatol 25:280, 1986
108. Crivellato E, Trevisan G, Mallardi F: Relapsing polychondritis: A histopathological and electron microscope study on the inflammatory infiltrate. Ann Ital Dermatol Clin Sper 37:149, 1983

27

DISORDERS OF ELASTIC FIBERS

NORMAL PROPERTIES

The elastic fibers of the skin form a three-dimensional network in the pars reticularis and around the subpapillary vascular plexus. They have a brushlike arrangement in the upper portion of the pars papillaris. Their function is to prevent overstretching of the skin and to return the stretched skin to its normal configuration. Loss of thin vertical fibers within the papillary dermis leads to formation of superficial wrinkles over the sun protected skin of old individuals.[1] Similar superficial wrinkles are also found over superficial scars or mild atrophic spots following lichen planus or some other skin conditions. Loss of fibers in the pars reticularis leads to bulging and buttonhole-type loss of resistance in the affected area (stria, anetoderma) unless the skin is at the same time hardened by collagenous fibrosis.

In electron microscopy, elastic fibers are made up of two distinct components. The major component, elastin, has an amorphous ultrastructural appearance of light density. The amorphous elastin is surrounded by the second component, microfibrils, ranging from 10 to 12 nm in diameter and with a moderate electron density.[2] In contrast collagen fibers are made up of bundles of tightly packed fibrils. The fibrils are 30 to 60 nm in diameter and are moderately electron dense, showing cross striations appearing at 64- to 78-nm intervals.

It was pointed out in Chapters 5 and 6 that thorough knowledge of the normal configuration and distribution of elastic fibers and routine examination for elastic fiber pathology is of great value in a variety of dermatoses ranging from inflammation to neoplasia. We point out again that many elastic fibers are chopped into short pieces by the microtome knife and that these fragments should not be mistaken for pathologic fragmentation (Fig. 5–17). Tinctorial properties were discussed in Chapter 3. Here we recall that elastic fibers are practically unidentifiable in H&E-stained sections. Acid orcein is the most satisfactory stain for elastic fibers and permits qualitative and quantitative appraisal of this important constituent of the skin in every case. Biochemical essays are also applicable. Desmosine and isodesmosine are cross-linking structures that are unique to the elastic tissue. The determination of desmosine is directly proportional to the amount of tissue elastic fibers.[3]

DISTURBANCES

Diseases and conditions specifically characterized by alterations and disturbances of the elastic tissue are shown in Table 27–1. These were reviewed in a symposium published as a supplemental issue in the

TABLE 27–1. DISTURBANCES OF ELASTIC TISSUE

Congenital
Circumscribed
    Nevus elasticus, Lewandowsky type (minus nevus)
    Juvenile elastoma; nevus elasticus (plus nevus)
Generalized
    Cutix laxa (generalized elastolysis)
    Pseudoxanthoma elasticum

Acquired
Idiopathic
    Elastosis perforans serpiginosa
    Anetoderma, primary
Induced
    Actinic elastosis and related conditions
    Anetoderma, secondary
    Stria distensa

Journal of Investigative Dermatology in 1982,[4] by Hashimoto and Niizuma in 1983.[5]

Congenital

Nevus Elasticus

Nevoid disturbances of elastic tissue that manifest themselves clinically as papules or plaques of pale or yellowish color may be on the minus or plus side.[6] Lewandowsky's *nevus elasticus regionis mammariae* actually is a collagenous nevus in which elastic fibers are distributed in an uneven manner. Other lesions, described as *juvenile elastoma* or nevus elasticus en tumeurs disséminés, show a marked increase (Fig. 27–1) in number and diameter of elastic fibers.[7,8] There may also be increased vascularity. In Buschke–Ollendorff's syndrome (*dermatofibrosis lenticularis disseminata*) multiple papular and plaque-like skin lesions occur in association with osteopoikilosis.[9,10] Skin lesions show localized elastic tissue hyperplasia that is almost indistinguishable from nevus elasticus.[11]

Pseudoxanthoma Elasticum

Although this disease is an inherited systemic disorder of connective tissue, expression of the trait is peculiarly patchy even in the skin. Neck, axilla, and periumbilical areas are often involved with papular lesions and yellow discoloration. The specific histologic changes (Fig. 27–2) are seen in the middermis, while pars papillaris and deep dermis usually show normal elastic morphology. In the affected foci, the fibers stain more strongly with hematoxylin because they contain calcium hydroxyapatite, and thus they become more visible in H&E sections, having a tinge

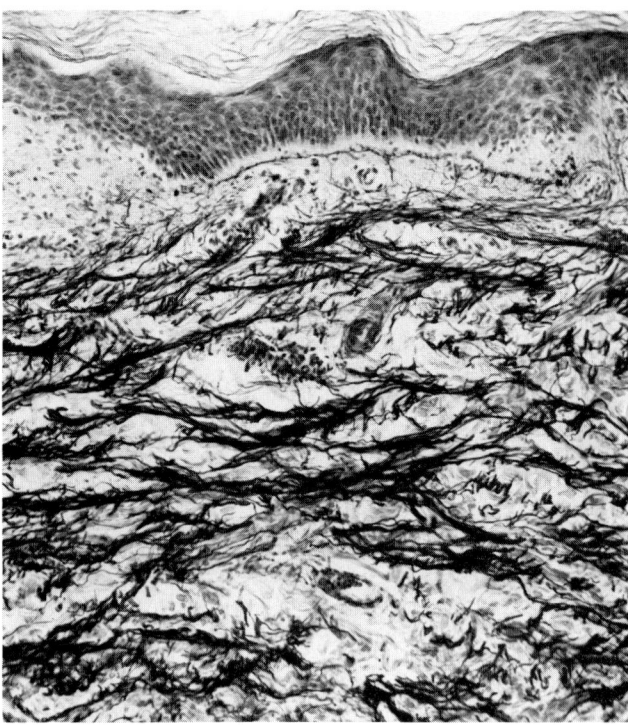

Figure 27–1.
Nevus elasticus (juvenile elastoma) shows hyperplasia of morphologically normal elastic fibers O&G. X135.

similar to basophilic degeneration seen in actinic elastosis.

The peculiar morphology of the affected fibers has been described as broken, frayed, or curled. The best comparison seems to be that of raveled wool. The increased calcium content, which makes the Von Kossa stain a favorite means of identification, is very obvious in the quantitative studies of the affected areas.[12] Sometimes massive calcification and secondary foreign-body granuloma lead to the formation of intrafollicular or transepidermal perforating channels.[13,14] Acid mucopolysaccharides demonstrable by the Hale method or alcian blue stain also are increased.[15] Electron microscopic studies show primary depositions of calcium salts in the homogeneous matrix of the elastic fibers in addition to minor abnormalities of the collagen fibrils.[16] Cutaneous changes clinically similar and histologically indistinguishable from pseudoxanthoma have been reported in farmers exposed to saltpeter during land fertilization.[17,18] Pseudoxanthoma elasticum-like changes associated with skin fragility are also complications of long-term penicillamine therapy.[19,20]

Generalized Elastolysis Cutis Laxa

Cutis laxa is a relatively rare disorder of elastic fibers that occurs in inherited and acquired forms. In

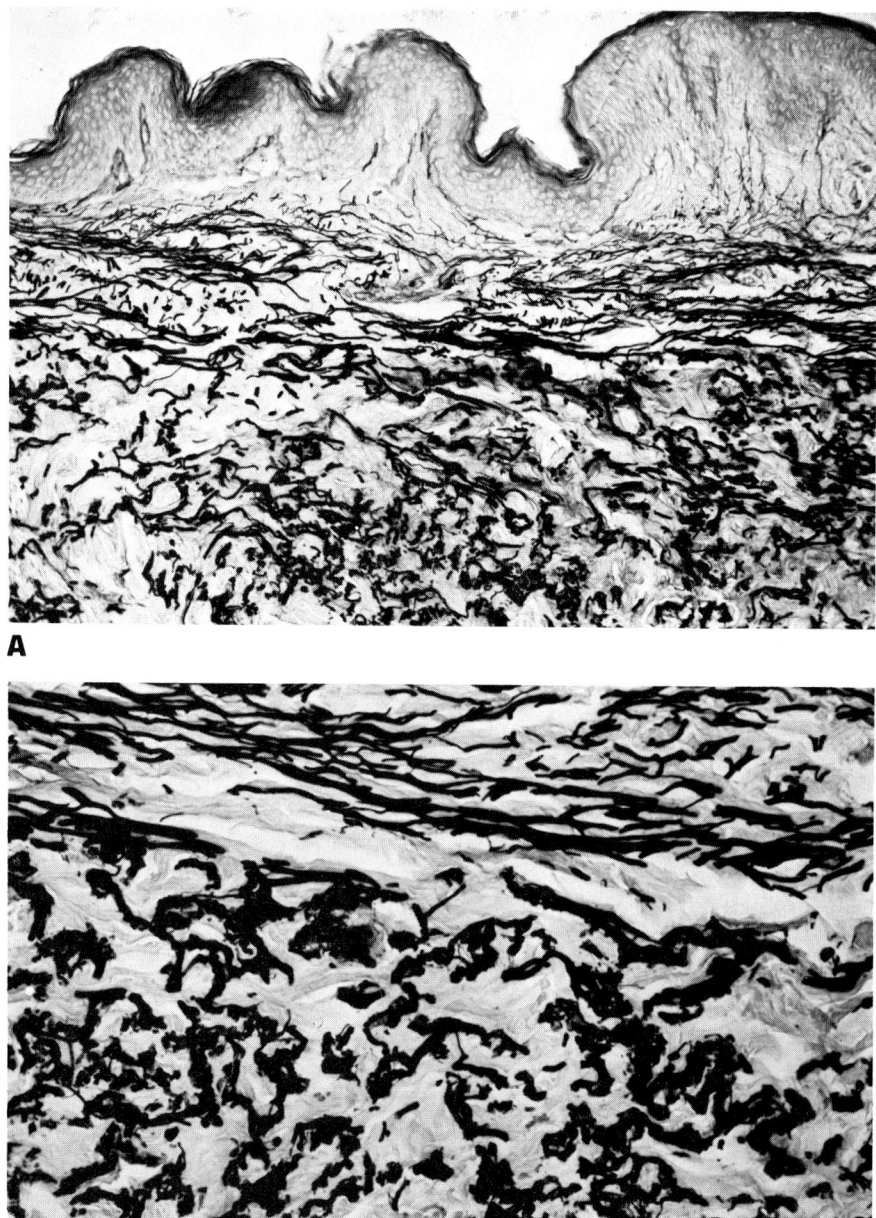

Figure 27–2.
Pseudoxanthoma elasticum.
Raveled-wool appearance of elastic
fibers in middermis only. Aldehyde
fuchsin. **A.** X135. **B.** X225.

the case of inheritance, autosomal dominant, autosomal recessive, and X-linked recessive patterns have been described.[21] "Generalized elastolysis" is a good term to describe the clinical and histologic features of this disease. The soft and inelastic skin, which hangs in thick folds and seems much too large for the infant's body (*dermatomegaly*), shows a breakdown of elastic fibers (Fig. 27–3) into small fibrous particles or dustlike granules.[22–25] The severity of the changes varies topographically, and some areas of skin may look quite normal. In association with the breakdown of elastic fibers, there may be marked deposition of acid mucopolysaccharides forming small lakes between the connective tissue fibers. Systemic manifestations of cutis laxa include pulmonary emphysema, cardiovascular abnormalities, various types of hernia, and multiple diverticula of the urinary bladder.[26–28]

The acquired form of cutis laxa appears later in life. Occasionally, a stage of generalized erythema or urticarial edema precedes the development of loose skin changes.[29,30] Generalized elastolysis has also

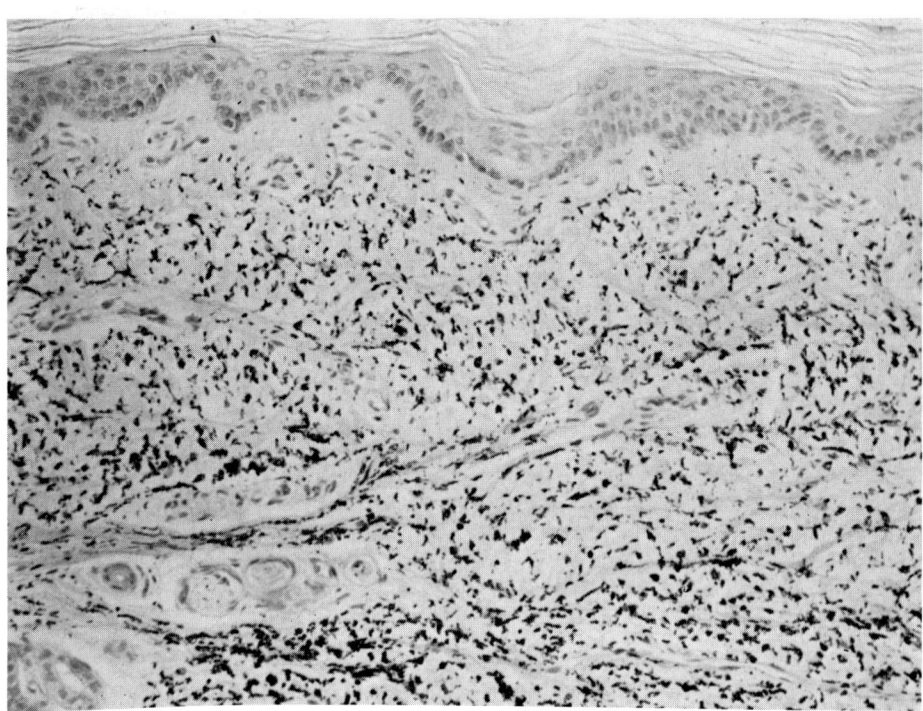

Figure 27–3.
Cutis laxa exhibits true fragmentation of elastic fibers (elastolysis). O&G. X225.

followed eruption of systemic lupus erythematosus.[31] The acquired form is not heritable but can be associated with emphysema and digestive tract abnormalities.[32]

Acquired

Elastosis Perforans Serpiginosa

The clinical picture of keratotic papules arranged in a ring or in serpiginous configuration around an atrophic center can be shown histologically (Figs. 27–4 and 27–5) to arise in a skin that has an overabundance of elastic fibers.[33–36] These cases may be otherwise normal or genetically defective, as in instances associated with Ehlers–Danlos syndrome, osteogenesis imperfecta, or Marfan syndrome.[37] Elastosis perforans serpiginosa may occur together with a generalized defective vascular system.[38,39] Elastosis perforans serpiginosa has appeared in patients with Down syndrome under treatment with penicillamine. In these instances, abnormal elastic fibers exhibiting serrated outline (bramble bush fibers) can be demonstrated in the skin and respiratory system[40,41] (Figs. 27–6 and 27–7). Outside the ringlike lesions of elastosis perforans serpiginosa, the superficial elastic fibers are coarser than normal and, in some areas, overlap with the lower border of the epidermal basal cells. In H&E sections, epithelial changes catch the eye (see Fig. 27–4). There is epidermal thickening, sometimes resembling pseudoepitheliomatous proliferation, around single or multiple perforating channels. These canals extend from the corium to the skin surface either in a straight line or in wavy or corkscrew fashion.[37] They contain loose parakeratotic flakes peripherally and a central dense mass of bluish-staining necrobiotic material made up of exfoliating keratinocytes and degenerating inflammatory cells with which are mixed brightly eosinophilic fibers. The latter may resemble fungal mycelia if KOH preparations are examined. Small streams of connective tissue fibers mixed with degenerating leukocytic nuclei enter the perforating channels from below, and O&G stain shows that the elastic fibers lose their orceinophilia and become brightly eosinophilic. There may be foci of foreign-body granuloma, and the upper dermis inside the ring has lost its elastic fibers and resembles a fibrotic scar.

Anetoderma

The three clinical types of *idiopathic macular atrophy*—described by Jadassohn, the form named after Schweninger and Buzzi, and the Pelizzari type—share with each other and with secondary anetoderma one decisive histologic feature, that is, complete absence of elastic fibers (Fig. 27–8) in the involved areas.[42]

In an early stage, anetoderma will show significant perivascular infiltrate of lymphocytes and occasionally plasma cells. Histiocytes and multinucleated giant cells may form small granulomas.[43] The fully developed lesions, however, are undiagnosable in H&E sections, while O&G stain reveals a sharply limited area of elastic fiber defect.[44] New formation of very thin elastic fibers may take place in older lesions. Some thinning of epidermis and dermis may be present, but this feature is difficult to judge in routine biopsy material and, in any case, is not diagnostic. Similar changes associated with hair follicles have been described as "perifollicular elastolysis."[45] Patchy loss of elastic fibers may be manifested as superficial wrinkles,[46] atrophic plaques,[47,48] or linear lesions[49] resembling striae distensa. Blephrochalasis is another manifestation of loss of dermal elastic fibers in localized skin areas. An eruptive form of elastolysis may occur in patients with pancreatic carcinoma.[50]

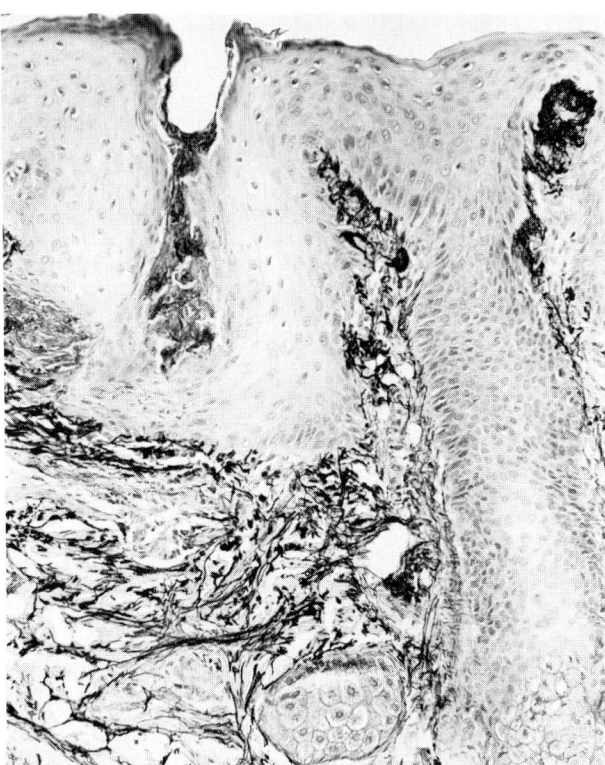

Figure 27–5.
Elastosis perforans serpiginosa. Note hyperplasia of elastic fibers in upper dermis and a perforating channel. O&G. X125. (From Mehregan. Arch Dermatol 97:381, 1968.)

Actinic Elastosis

Skin changes due to aging can be discussed in two categories. The cutaneous changes secondary to chronologic aging occur in all skin areas and consist of epidermal atrophy, loss of rete ridges, flattening of the dermoepidermal interface, reduction in thickness of dermis, decreased vascularity, and reduction in the number of pilosebaceous structures and eccrine sweat glands.[51-54] The changes are relatively mild and may not be well appreciated in routine histologic sections.[55] On the other hand, photoaging in light-exposed skin areas shows characteristic alterations unless the skin is protected by heavy pigmentation.[56] The facial skin of individuals with poor tanning ability who lead an outdoor life in the southern United States may show beginning "senile elastosis" or "basophilic degeneration" of the corium before the end of the second decade. These two terms are used here only to point out that they are inappropriate. The changes are characteristic not of old age but of sun-exposed skin, and there is no good evidence that elastotic skin is functionally inferior. On the contrary, the replacement of collagen by elas-

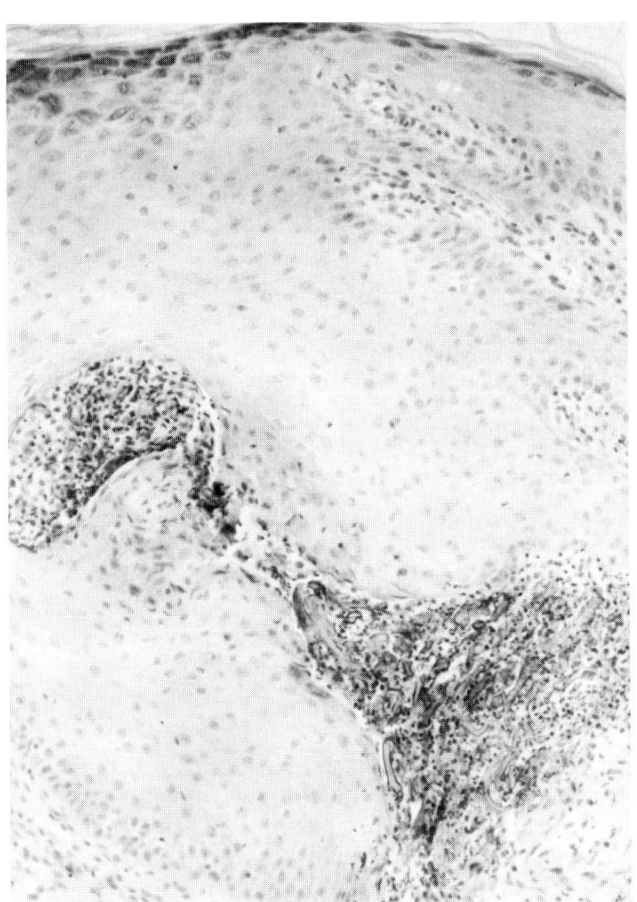

Figure 27–4.
Elastosis perforans serpiginosa. Perforating channel in proliferating epidermis contains connective tissue including refractile elastic fibers and leukocytes. H&E. X135.

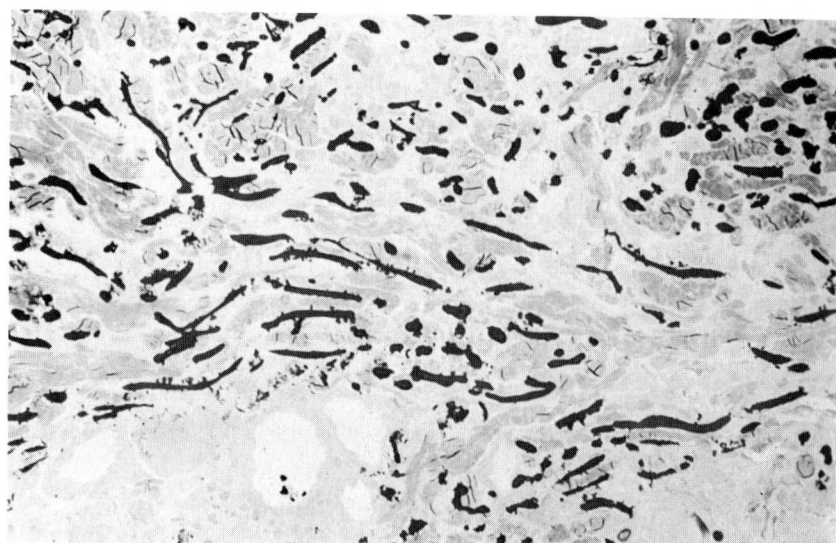

Figure 27–6.
Elastosis perforans serpiginosa. Penicillamine-induced lesion shows bramble-bush appearance of dermal elastic fibers. Verhoeff. X250. (Courtesy of Dr. K. Hashimoto.)

tin may well be adaptive, enabling the integument to survive under adverse conditions.

Early stages of actinic elastosis are characterized by a relative increase and thickening of elastic fibers. Later (Fig. 27–9), the fibers appear curled and conglomerated, and eventually amorphous masses may be formed. At the same time, orceinophilia gradually decreases, and in more advanced stages the fibers may stain a pale gray-brown. They also acquire affinity for hematoxylin and, thus, show gray or bluish in H&E sections.[57–59] Only in severe cases do they become truly basophilic and stain blue in O&G sections. This feature may be due to an increase in acid mucopolysaccharides, which can be demonstrated by AB–PAS stain. Sudanophilic substances also are present and may be plentiful (imbibitio lipoidica telae elasticae).

Characteristically, elastotic changes are confined to the upper third or half of the dermis and spare a narrow subepidermal grenz zone as an indication that we are dealing with a biologic process rather than with a simple physicochemical effect. The grenz zone, being the immediate support of, and interacting constantly with, the epidermis, behaves differently from the deeper layers. The elastotic zone usually is well vascularized, and silver impregnation reveals a net of reticulum fibrils. Both features speak against considering actinic elastosis as a degenerative process. Electron microscopy of severely actinic, exposed skin areas shows depletion of collagen fibrils. The affected elastic fibers contain large masses of electron-dense grains or many large holes leading to widening of their diameter. In erythema ab igne (Fig. 27–10) the initial histologic findings include epidermal atrophy, telangiectasia of the superficial capillary blood vessels, and perivascular inflammatory cell infiltrate.[60–61] Older lesions show depletion of collagen fibers and increased elastic tissue with the presence of macrophages containing melanin pigment granules.

Acrokeratoelastoidosis (Costa) and Keratoelastoidosis Marginalis of Hands

Acrokeratoelastoidosis of Costa involves periphery of palms and soles and dorsa of fingers with small hyperkeratotic papules.[62,63] Histologically it shows regular epidermal acanthosis with orthokeratotic hyperkeratosis and a minor decrease and fragmentation of dermal elastic fibers.[64] Keratoelastoidosis marginalis[65] also known as "degenerative collagenous plaques"[66] involves the periphery of both palms with wrinkled slightly hyperkeratotic areas (Fig. 27–11). Histologically the epidermis appears normal. The dermis shows extensive changes resembling severe actinic elastosis with massive deposition of thickened and homogeneous elastotic material and collagen bundles.

Special Forms Related to Personal Predisposition

The elastotic material is not always evenly distributed and may even form circumscribed tumorlike nodules, which arouse clinical suspicion of basal cell epithelioma or other neoplasia.[67] *Nodular elastosis with cysts and comedones,* as described by Favre and Racouchot,[68] seems to affect predisposed individuals, especially elderly men, whose faces had considerable exposure to the sun. Histologically, it shows a

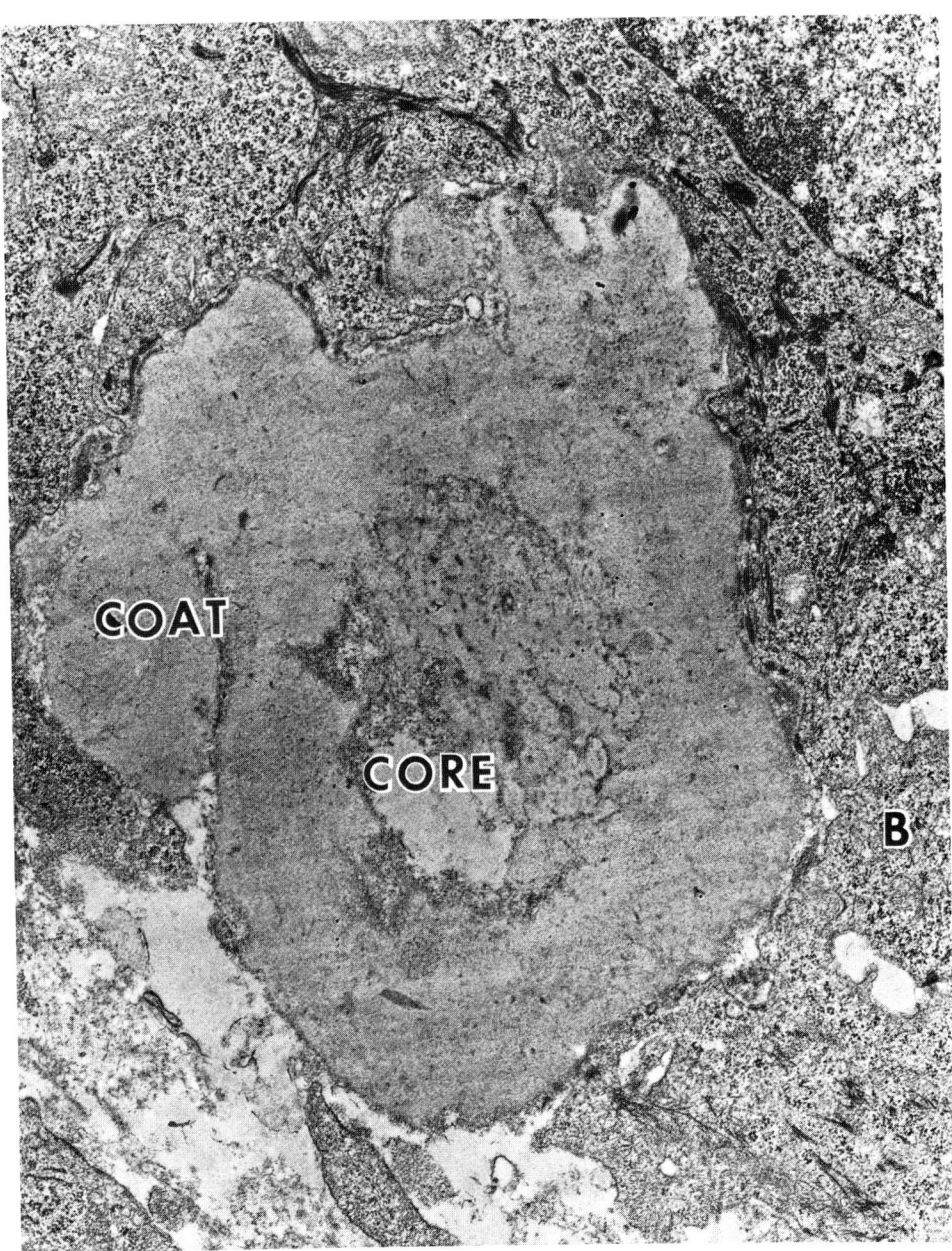

Figure 27–7.
Elastosis perforans serpiginosa. Penicillamine-induced lesion shows an abnormal elastic fiber entering the epidermis (B, epidermal basal cell). Central core of the fiber appears normal. Outer coat shows serrated border. X23,100. (Courtesy of Dr. K. Hashimoto.)

combination of the features mentioned in the name with mild inflammatory changes.

Peculiarly localized to forearms and arms of elderly individuals, especially women, is the condition described as *stellate spontaneous pseudoscars*.[69] The clinical combination of atrophic skin with senile purpura, bizarre stellate scars, and possibly small ulcers and crusts often arouses suspicion of dermatitis factitia but seems to be due to a combination of factors leading to increased fragility of the skin.[70] Histologically (Fig. 27–12), there is a combination of actinic elastosis with spotty round cell infiltrate and focal loss of elastic fibers. Extravasation of red blood cells and epidermal and dermal atrophy complete the picture.

Another disorder that seems to require the combination of actinic influence and individual predisposition is "colloid" milium.[71] The dome-shaped translucent papules seen clinically correspond to dilated and confluent papillae filled with chunks of an amorphous material (Fig. 27–13) that stains a pale gray with a tinge of blue in O&G sections but is PAS positive and gives other staining reactions similar to amyloid. It may border directly on the epidermis,

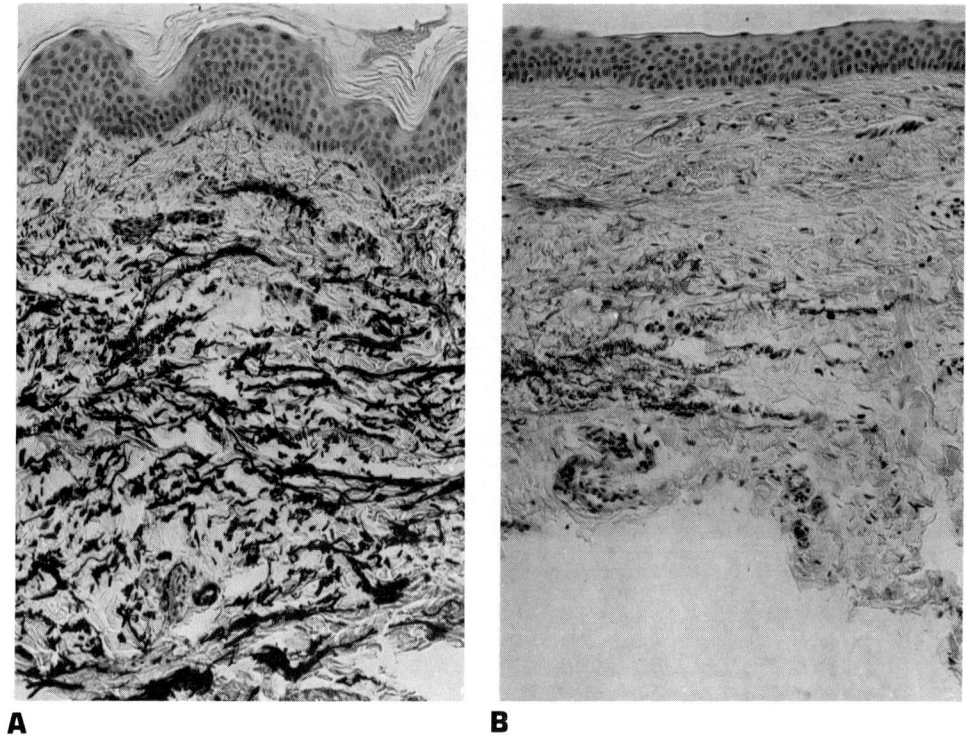

Figure 27–8.
Anetoderma. Schweninger–Buzzi type. **A.** Normal skin. **B.** Lesion. O&G. X135.

leaving no grenz zone. Below the colloid, the dermis shows a high degree of actinic elastosis. In electron microscopy, colloid milium is made up of tightly packed, filamentous bundles.[72] Individual filaments are 8 to 10 nm wide and form wavy and whorled fascicles. Recent ultrastructural studies have suggested that colloid material is at least partially produced by sequential degenerative changes of elastic fibers in chronic actinic-exposed skin areas.[73,74]

Stria Distensa

While the topography and direction of striae are related to mechanical stress, their occurrence and severity depend on damage to elastic fibers under the influence of hormones related to physiologic stress. The fresh stria, which clinically may look red or bluish, exhibits actual breakage and retraction of the thick elastic fibers of the reticular portion of the dermis, whereas the collagen bundles appear stretched across the width of the stria parallel to the skin surface.[75] The red or livid clinical color is due to engorgement of blood vessels and some inflammatory infiltrate. The ends of broken elastic fibers are curled up at both sides of the stria. Fibers of the pars papillaris retain normal configuration. Older, white, and sunken striae exhibit new formation of thin elastic fibers (Fig. 27–14) in the upper half of the dermis parallel to the stretched collagen bundles, a feature that gave rise to the inaccurate interpretation that elastic fibers are stretched and thinned in a stria.[76,77] Elastic tissue usually remains defective in the lower half of the dermis, and the entire skin, epidermis as well as corium, usually remains thinner.

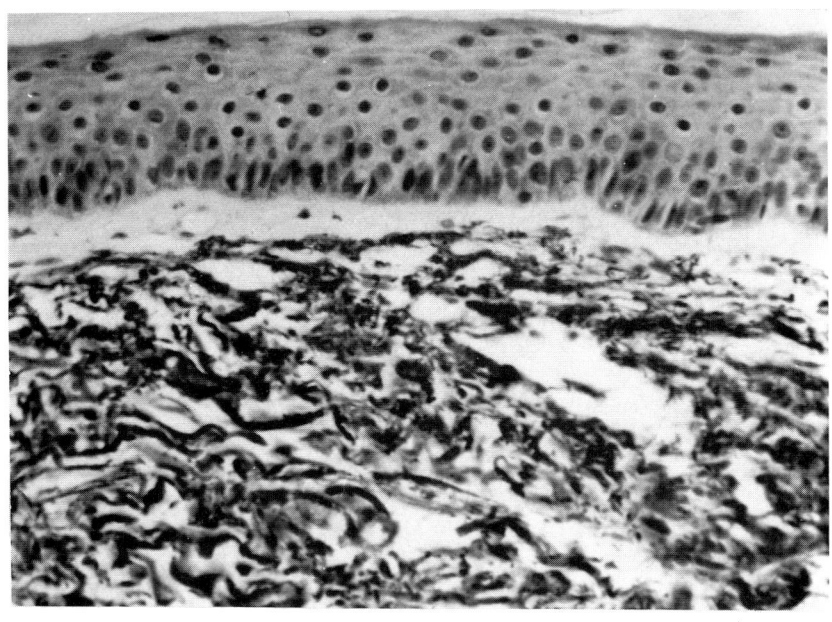
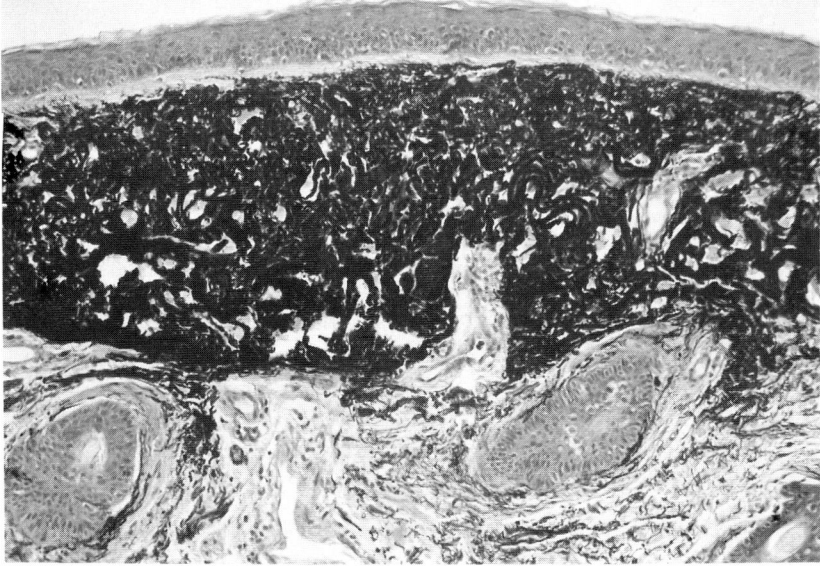

Figure 27–9.
Actinic elastosis of face. **A.** Moderate hyperplasia and thickening of the elastic fibers. **B.** Severe actinic elastosis with massive deposition of elastotic material. Note narrow subepidermal grenz zone. O&G. X185.

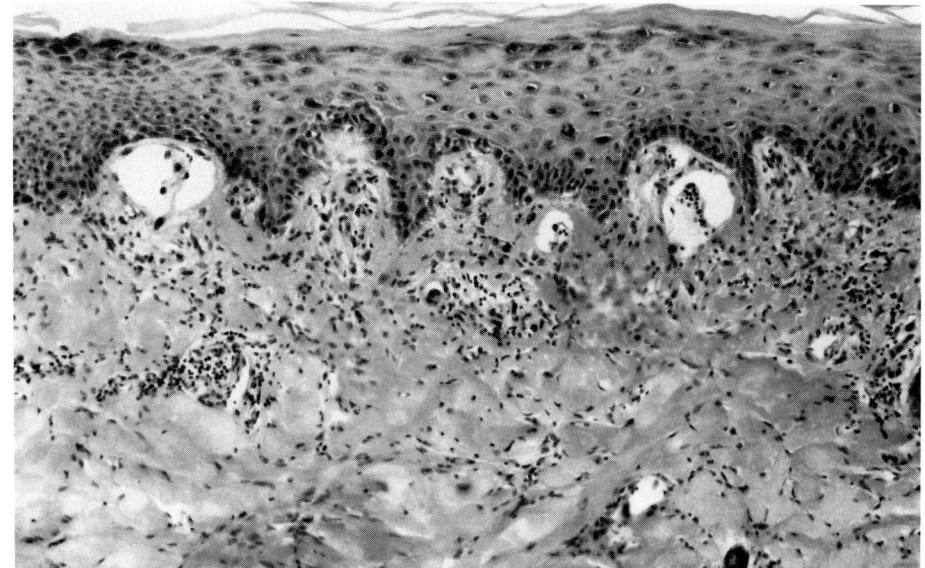

Figure 27–10.
Erythema ab igne shows low-grade epidermal atrophy, superficial telangiectasia, and perivascular lymphocytic infiltrate. H&E. ×185.

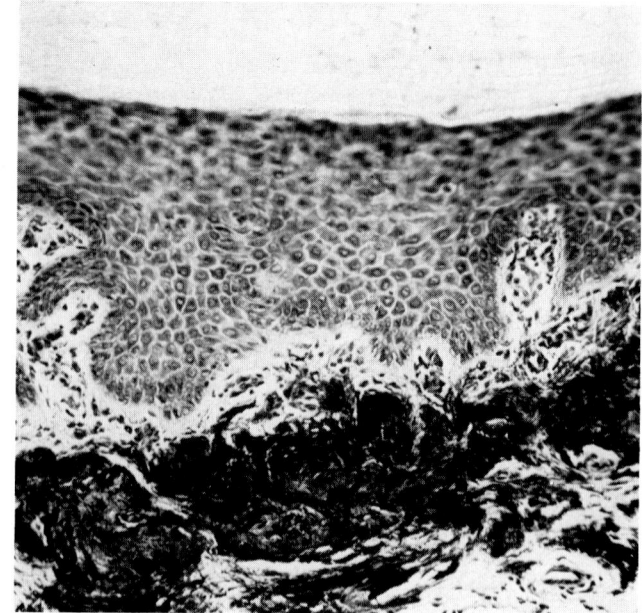

Figure 27–11.
Degenerative collagenous plaque of hand (Burks). This type of lesion, also called keratoelastoidosis marginalis (Kocsard), is characterized by acanthosis with hyperkeratosis and dermal changes, which may be due to a combination of mechanical trauma (tool handling) and actinic exposure (farming). O&G. ×135. (From Mehregan. Arch Dermatol 93:633, 1966.)

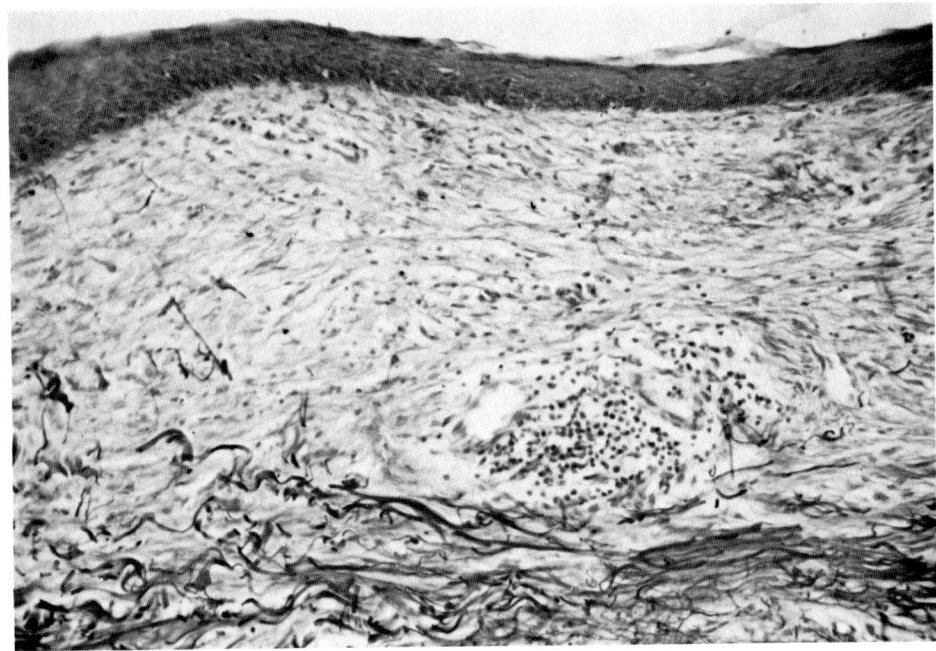

Figure 27–12.
Stellate spontaneous pseudoscar. Scarlike fibrosis and loss of elastic fibers in upper dermis, mild perivascular round cell infiltrate. Degenerating erythrocytes scattered between collagen fibers. O&G. X180.

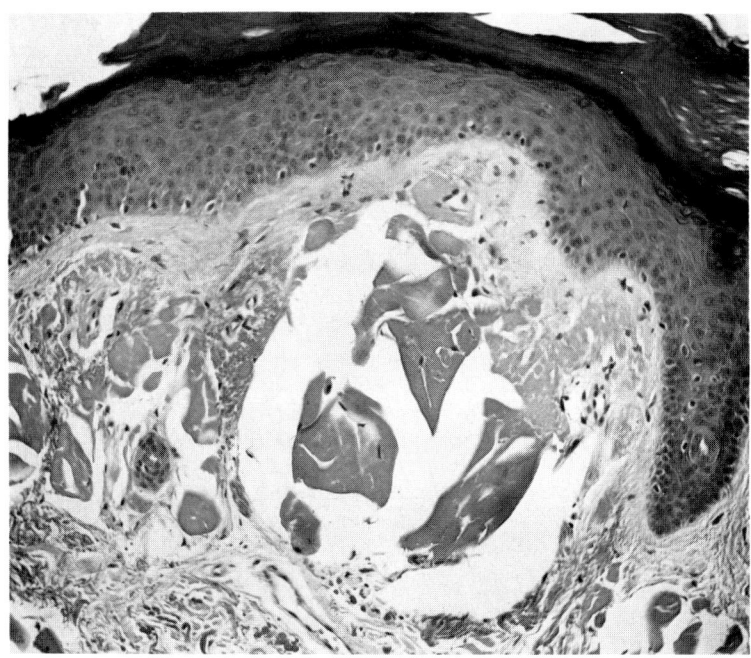

Figure 27–13.
Colloid milium. Fragmentation and retraction of brittle amorphous material is artifact. H&E. X135.

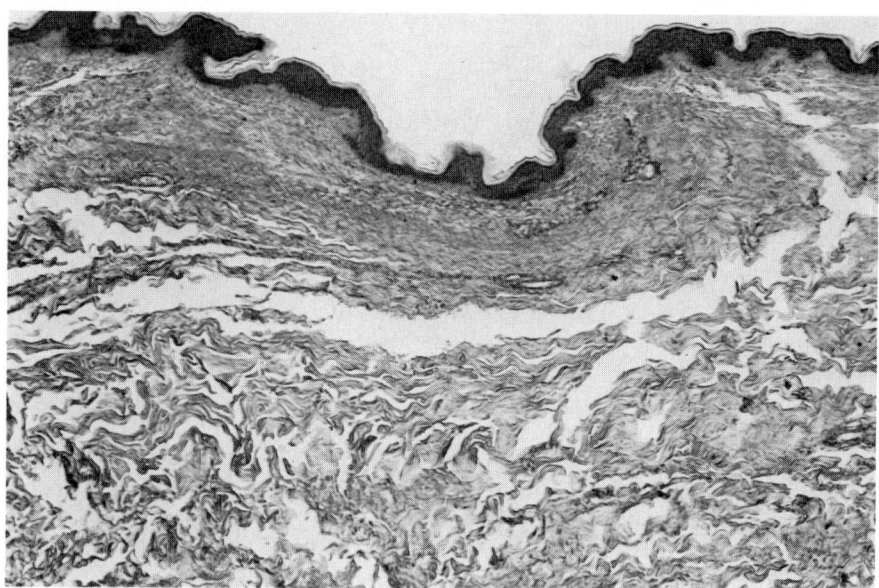

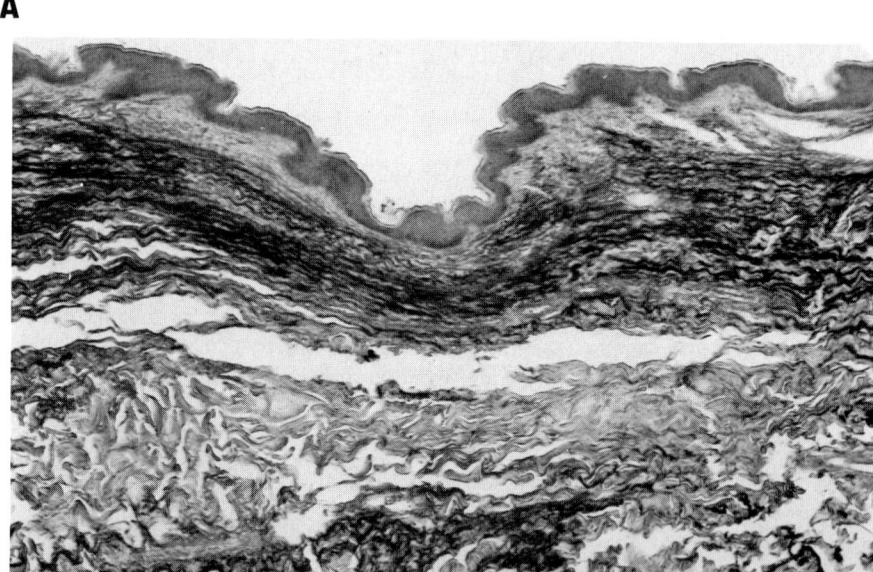

Figure 27–14.
Stria distensa. This is a quiescent older lesion. Note retracted and truly fragmented original elastic fibers to both sides and below stria, while new thin fibers have been formed parallel to the collagen bundles but only in upper dermis. **A.** H&E. X60. **B.** O&G. X60.

REFERENCES

1. Tsuji T, Yorifuji T, Hayashi Y, Hamada T: Light and scanning electron microscopic studies on wrinkles in aged persons' skin. Br J Dermatol 114:329, 1986
2. Uitto J, Ryhänen L, Abraham PA, Perejda AJ: Elastin in diseases. J Invest Dermatol 79:160, 1982
3. Flotte TJ, Seddon JM, Zhang Y, et al: A computerized image analysis method for measuring elastic tissue. J Invest Dermatol 93:358, 1989
4. Wurpper KD, Holbrook KA, Pinnell SR, Uitto J: Structural elements of the dermis. J Invest Dermatol 79(Suppl 1), July 1982
5. Hashimoto K, Niizuma K: Skin Pathology by Light and Electron Microscopy. New York: Igaku-Shoin Publisher 1983
6. Uitto J, Santa-Cruz DJ, Eisen AZ: Connective tissue nevi of the skin. Clinical, genetic, and histopathologic classification of hamartomas of the collagen, elastin and proteoglycan type. J Am Acad Dermatol 3:441, 1980
7. Ledoux-Corbusier M, Achten G, Dobbeleer G: Juvenile elastoma (Weidman): An ultrastructural study. J Cutan Pathol 8:219, 1981
8. Crivellato E: Disseminated nevus anelasticus. Int J Dermatol 25:171, 1986

9. Decroix J, Frankart M, Pollet J-C. Bourlond A: Syndrome de Buschke–Ollendorff. Six observations dans une famille. Ann Dermatol Venereol 115:455, 1988
10. Dahan S, Bonafe JL, Laroche M, et al: Iconographie du syndrome de Buschke–Ollendorff: Etude tomodensitometrique et en resonance magnetique nucleaire de l'osteopoecilie. Ann Dermatol Venereol 116:225, 1989
11. Reymond JL, Stoebner P, Beani JC, Amblard P: Buschke–Ollendorf syndrome. An electron microscope study. Dermatologica 166:64, 1983
12. Reeve EB, Neldner KH, Subryan V, Gordon SG: Development of calcification of skin lesions in thirty-nine patients with pseudoxanthoma elasticum. Clin Exp Dermatol 4:291, 1979
13. Kazakis AM, Parish WR: Periumbilical perforating pseudoxanthoma elasticum. J Am Acad Dermatol 19:384, 1988
14. Patterson JW: The perforating disorders. J Am Acad Dermatol 10:561, 1984
15. Yamamura T, Sano S: Ultrastructural and histochemical analysis of thready material in pseudoxanthoma elasticum. J Cutan Pathol 11:282, 1984
16. Walker ER, Frederickson RG, Mayes MD: The mineralization of elastic fibers and alterations of extracellular matrix in pseudoxanthoma elasticum. Arch Dermatol 125:70, 1989
17. Christensen OB: An exogenous variety of pseudoxanthoma elasticum in old farmers. Acta Derm Venereol 58:319, 1978
18. Nielsen AO, Christiansen OB, Hentzer B, et al: Saltpeter-induced dermal changes electron microscopically indistinguishable from pseudoxanthoma elasticum. Acta Derm Venereol 58:323, 1978
19. Light N, Meyrick Thomas RH, Stephens A, et al: Collagen and elastin changes in D-penicillamine-induced pseudoxanthoma elasticum-like skin. Br J Dermatol 114:381, 1986
20. Burge S, Dalziel K, Mowat A, Ryan TJ: Elastic fibre damage with low dose penicillamine—A review of 18 patients with rheumatoid arthritis. Br J Dermatol 119(Suppl 33):50, 1988
21. Lambert D, Beer F, Jeannin-Magnificat C, et al: Cutis laxa généralisée congénitale. Ann Dermatol Venereol 110:129, 1983
22. Oku T, Nakayama F, Imaizumi S, et al: Congenital cutis laxa. Dermatologica 179:79, 1989
23. Ledoux-Corbusier M: Les cutis laxa generalisees. Nouv Dermatol 8:427, 1989
24. Koch SE, Williams ML: Acquired cutis laxa: Case report and review of disorders of elastolysis. Pediatr Dermatol 2:282, 1985
25. Kitano Y, Nishida K, Okada N, et al: Cutis laxa with ultrastructural abnormalities of elastic fibers. J Am Acad Dermatol 21:378, 1989
26. Mehregan AH, Lee SC, Nabai H: Cutis laxa (generalized elastolysis). A report of four cases with autopsy findings. J Cutan Pathol 5:116, 1978
27. Ledoux-Corbusier M: Cutis laxa, congenital form with pulmonary emphysema: An ultrastructural study. J Cutan Pathol 10:340, 1983
28. Bechelli LM, Pagnano PMG, De Souza NM, et al: Cutis laxa congenitale generalisee associee a des lesions viscerales. Ann Dermatol Venereol 112:835, 1985
29. Lewis PG, Hood AF, Barnett NK, Holbrook KA: Postinflammatory elastolysis and cutis laxa. A case report. J Am Acad Dermatol 22:40, 1990
30. Kerl H, Burg G, Hashimoto K: Fatal penicillin induced, generalized postinflammatory elastolysis (cutis laxa). Am J Dermat Pathol 5:267, 1983
31. Randle HW, Muller S: Generalized elastolysis associated with systemic lupus erythematosus. J Am Acad Dermatol 8:869, 1983
32. Koch SE, Williams ML: Acquired cutis laxa: Case report and review of disorders of elastolysis. Pediat Dermatol 2:282, 1985
33. Moreno-Gimenez JC, Escudero-Ordonez J, Rodriguez-Pichardo A, Camacho-Martinez F: Elastose perforante serpigineuse de Lutz-Miescher Ann Dermatol Venereol 113:339, 1986
34. Van Joost TH, Vuzevski VD, Ten Kate FJW, et al: Elastosis perforans serpiginosa: Clinical, histomorphological and immunological studies. J Cutan Pathol 15:92, 1988
35. Ueda K, Matsubara M, Horie J, Kusaba K: A case of elastosis perforans serpiginosa: An ultrastructural study. J Cutan Pathol 10:217, 1983
36. Ayala F, Donofrio P: Elastosis perforans serpiginosa. Report of a family. Dermatologica 166:32, 1983
37. Mehregan AH: Elastosis perforans serpiginosa, a review of the literature and report of eleven cases. Arch Dermatol 97:381, 1968
38. London ID, Givhan EG, Garrick J, Mehregan A: Elastosis perforans serpiginosa with systemic involvement. South Med J 67:225,1974
39. Eide J: Elastosis perforans serpiginosa with widespread arterial lesions: a case report. Acta Derm Venereol 57:553, 1977
40. Sfar Z, Lakhoua M, Kamoun MR, et al: Deux cas d'elastomes verruciformes après administration prolongée de D-penicillamine. Ann Dermatol Venereol 109:813, 1982
41. Reymond JL, Stoebner P, Zambelli P, et al: Penicillamine induced elastosis perforans serpiginosa: An ultrastructural study of two cases. J Cutan Pathol 9:352, 1982
42. Venencie PY, Winkelmann RK, Moore BA: Anetoderma. Clinical findings, associations, and long term follow-up evaluations. Arch Dermatol 120:1032, 1984
43. Venencie PY, Winkelmann RK: Histopathologic findings in anetoderma. Arch Dermatol 120:1040, 1984
44. Oikarinen AI, Palatsi R, Adomian GE, et al: Anetoderma: Biochemical and ultrastructural demonstration of an elastin defect in the skin of three patients. J Am Acad Dermatol 11:64, 1984
45. Lemarchand-Venencie F, Venencie P-Y, Foix C, et al: Elastolyse perifolliculaire. Discussion du role d'un sta-

phylocoque epidermidis secreteur d'elastase. Ann Dermatol Venereol 112:735, 1985
46. Shelley WB, Wood MG: Wrinkles due to idiopathic loss of dermal elastic tissue. Br J Dermatol 97:441, 1977
47. Heudes A-M, Boullie M-C, Thomine E, Lauret PH: Elastolyse acquise nappe du derme moyen. Ann Dermatol Venereol 115:1041, 1988
48. Fisher BK, Page E, Hanna W: Acral localized acquired cutis laxa. J Am Acad Dermatol 21:33, 1989
49. Burket JM, Zelickson AS, Padilla SR: Linear focal elastolysis (elastotic striae). J Am Acad Dermatol 20:633, 1989
50. Slater DN, Messenger A: Eruptive elastolysis: A new manifestation of pancreatic carcinoma. J R Soc Med 79:237, 1986
51. Uitto J, Fazio MJ, Olsen DR: Cutaneous aging: Molecular alterations in elastic fibers. J Cutan Aging Cosmet Dermatol 1:13, 1988
52. Fenske NA, Lober CW: Structural and functional changes of normal aging skin. J Am Acad Dermatol 15:571, 1986
53. Herzberg AJ, Dinehart SM: Chronologic aging in black skin. Am J Dermatopathol 11:319, 1989
54. Balin AK, Pratt LA: Physiological consequences of human skin aging. Cutis 43:431, 1989
55. Smith L: Histopathologic characteristics and ultrastructure of aging skin. Cutis 43:414, 1989
56. Gilchrest BA: Skin aging and photoaging: An overview. J Am Acad Dermatol 21:610, 1989
57. Chen VL, Fleischmajer R, Schwartz E, et al: Immunochemistry of elastotic material in sun-damaged skin. J Invest Dermatol 87:334, 1986
58. Lavker RM, Zheng P, Dong G: Aged skin: A study by light, transmission electron, and scanning electron microscopy. J Invest Dermatol 88:44, 1987
59. Mera SL, Lovell CR, Russell Jones R, Davies JD: Elastic fibres in normal and sun-damaged skin: An immunohistochemical study. Br J Dermatol 117:21, 1987
60. Dover JS, Phillips TJ, Arndt KA: Cutaneous effects of therapeutic use of heat with emphasis on infrared radiation. J Am Acad Dermatol 20:278, 1989
61. Shahrad P, Marks R: The wages of warmth: Changes in erythema ab igne. Br J Dermatol 97:179, 1977

62. Korc A, Hansen RC, Lynch PJ: Acrokeratoelastoidosis of Costa in North America. A report of two cases. J Am Acad Dermatol 12:832, 1985
63. Daniel F, Foix C, Leblond P, et al: Acrokeratoelastoidose. A propos de 2 observations. Ann Dermatol Venereol 113:956, 1986
64. Handfield-Jones S, Kennedy CTC: Acrokeratoelastoidosis treated with etretinate. J Am Acad Dermatol 17:881, 1987
65. Rahbari H: Acrokerato-elastoidosis and keratoelastoidosis marginalis—any relation? J Am Acad Dermatol 5:348, 1981
66. Mehregan AH: De generative collagenous plaques of hands. Arch Dermatol 93:633, 1966
67. Degos R, Civatte J. Belaïch S: L'élastome en nappe du nez. Arch Belg Dermatol 26:247, 1970
68. Helm F: Nodular cutaneous elastosis with cysts and comedones (Favre-Racouchot syndrome). Arch Dermatol 84:666, 1961
69. Colomb D: Stellate spontaneous pseudoscars: Senile and presenile forms, especially those forms caused by prolonged corticoid therapy. Arch Dermatol 105:551, 1972
70. Björnberg A, Mobacken H: "Spontaneous stellate pseudoscars" of the arms caused by increased skin fragility. Acta Derm Venereol (Stockh) 52:151, 1972
71. Hashimoto K, Nakayama H, Chimenti S, et al: Juvenile colloid milium. Immunohistochemical and ultrastructural studies. J Cutan Pathol 16:164, 1989
72. Hashimoto K: Diseases of amyloid, colloid, and hyalin. J Cutan Pathol 12:322, 1985
73. Kobayashi H, Hashimoto K: Colloid and elastic fiber: Ultrastructural study on the histogenesis of colloid milium. J Cutan Pathol 10:111, 1983
74. Matsuta M, Kunimoto M, Kosegawa G, et al: Electron microscopic study of the colloid-like substance in solar elastosis. J Dermatol (Tokyo) 16:191, 1989
75. Zheng, Lavker RM, Kligman AM: Anatomy of striae. Br J Dermatol 112:185, 1985
76. Pinkus H, Keech MK, Mehregan AH: Histopathology of striae distensae, with special reference to striae and wound healing in the Marfan syndrome. J Invest Dermatol 46:283, 1966
77. Tsuji T, Sawabe M: Elastic fibers in striae distensae. J Cutan Pathol 15:215, 1988

28
VARIOUS EXTRACELLULAR DEPOSITS

Having dealt with accumulations of excessive ground substance (mucin) in Chapter 26, we will consider here substances of a less physiologic nature: lipids, calcium, hyaline substances, amyloid, pigments, and foreign bodies.

LIPIDS

Extracellular deposits of lipid derive from four principal sources: disintegration of xanthomatous foam cells, blood, fat cells, and metabolic accumulation. Thus, in many cases lipid becomes extracellular secondarily. It was mentioned in Chapter 24 that the cells of eruptive xanthomas have a tendency to rupture, with release of lipids into the tissue. It also was mentioned that in vascular histiocytomas, foam cells result from ingestion of blood lipids derived from repeated small hemorrhages. It is possible that foam cells in histiocytosis X are due to similar mechanisms. Free lipids can be demonstrated in these and other cases of hemorrhage if proper stains are done. Of greater diagnostic significance is free lipid in various cases of fat necrosis. This chapter will cover sclerema neonatorum, fat necrosis in pancreatic disease, and various forms of panniculitis. The first two lead to the formation of crystals recognized in paraffin sections as clefts (see Fig. 16–7), often fan shaped. The last, whether they are of the purulent or liquefying type, usually do not have this feature.

While deranged metabolism does play a part in xanthomas and other accumulations of lipid in skin, there are some processes in which sudanophilic material is deposited without provoking an inflammatory or granulomatous reaction. One of these is actinic elastosis, especially the severe form seen as cutis rhomboidalis nuchae. The pronounced yellow tinge of this type of skin is partly due to the yellow color of elastic tissue and partly to lipids that can be demonstrated in frozen section (imbibitio lipoidica telae elasticae, Chapter 25). Lipoid proteinosis is mentioned in this chapter. Three other disorders exhibiting extracellular deposits of lipids are necrobiosis lipoidica, necrobiotic xanthogranuloma (Chapter 23), and extracellular cholesterosis, the latter considered to be a variant of erythema elevatum diutinum (Chapter 15). Although there is inflammatory infiltrate present in all, this probably is not caused by lipid material.

CALCIUM

The presence of insoluble calcium salts is easily seen in H&E sections because nothing except masses of pyknotic nuclei and keratohyalin is tinged in the same dark purple color. Confirmation is offered by

384 METABOLIC AND OTHER NONINFLAMMATORY DERMAL DISEASES

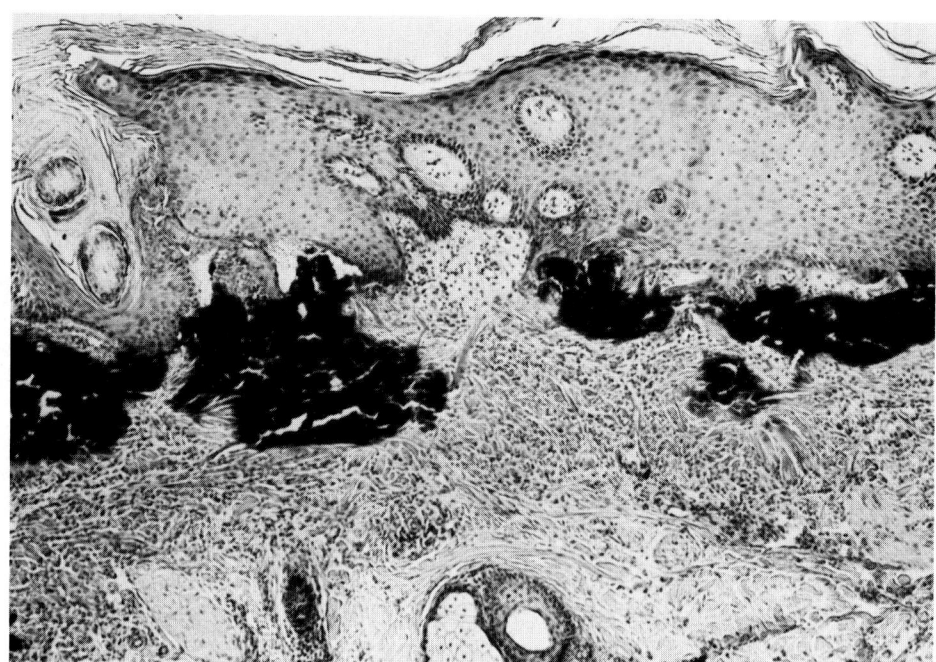

Figure 28–1.
Calcification of superficial dermis after electroencephalography due to the calcium chloride content of the electrode paste. H&E. X75.

O&G stain in a negative manner: the deposits of calcium do not stain, but nuclei do. On the other hand, O&G stain permits one to analyze the matrix on which calcium was deposited, for example, elastic fibers and shadow cells of pilomatricoma. Special stains (von Kossa and Alizarin red) were discussed in Chapter 3. That only insoluble forms of calcium are shown in sections is just as true as with many other substances, since all soluble salts are removed in processing. A vivid demonstration of this fact is found in traumatic tissue necrosis from application of strong calcium chloride to slightly abraded skin.[1] In this condition (Fig. 28–1), calcium is not seen in the epidermis, and it becomes stainable only after it

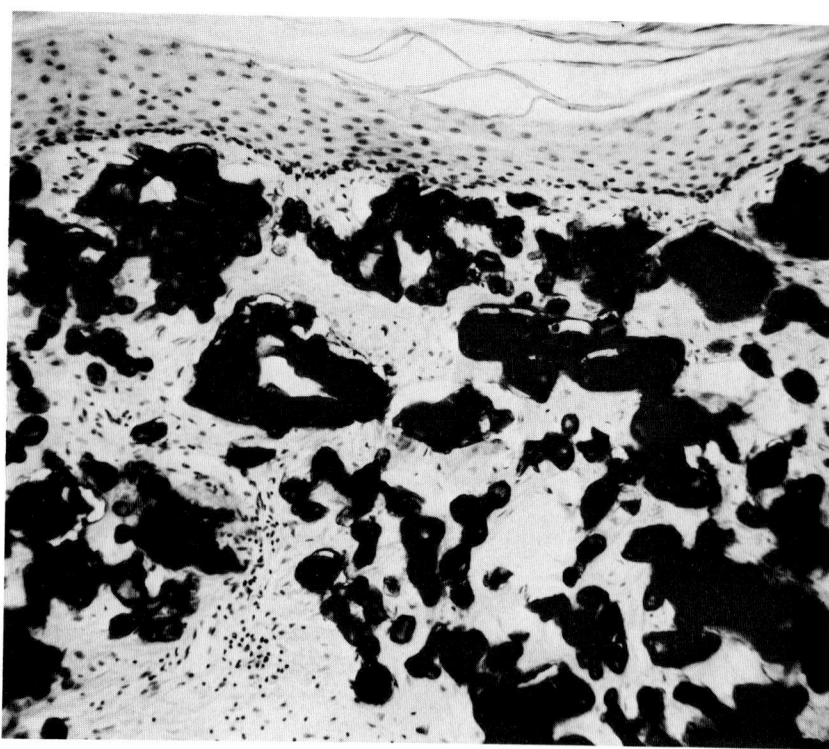

Figure 28–2.
Nodular calcinosis of children. H&E. X135.

has been precipitated as carbonate or phosphate in the dermis.[2]

One must remember that calcium usually is deposited on a pathologic substrate, and it is important to identify this if possible. Calcium may be found in collagenous tissue in scleroderma (CRST syndrome) and juvenile dermatomyositis, in elastic fibers in pseudoxanthoma elasticum, in faded epithelium in pilomatricoma, and in keratinized material in epidermoid and trichilemmal cysts. Other clinical manifestations of calcinosis cutis include the solitary nodular calcinosis (Fig. 28–2) of Winer,[3] calcinosis cutis of scrotum,[4–8] auricular calcification,[9] calcification of heel in newborns undergoing intensive care,[10] and massive tumoral calcinosis.[11] Solitary calcified nodules in young children probably result from calcification of nests of nevus cells or hamartomatous structures.[12] Free calcium globes are not infrequently present in trichoepitheliomas, basal cell epithelioma, and other benign hamartomatous conditions later in life, and such globes may secondarily be transformed into bone. It seems likely that, in these cases, calcium was originally deposited on the horny materials of milia and other cysts. Admittedly, it is not always possible to demonstrate the primary substrate morphologically, but even in cases of so-called metastatic calcinosis, where calcium is probably precipitated in the ground substance, and in such metabolic disorders as Albright's hereditary osteodystrophy,[13] one may presuppose precipitating factors in the connective tissue.

Metastatic calcinosis cutis develops when the serum calcium level is elevated due to various conditions including primary hyperparathyroidism, hypervitaminosis D, osteomyelitis, and bone tumors. Hyperphosphatemia due to a chronic renal failure causes secondary hyperparathyroidism and calcium deposition.[14–16]

BONE

Small globes of a bony tissue are found infrequently beneath old pigmented nevi or in adnexal tumors.[17] Osteomas are often secondary to inflamed and broken down hair follicles or epithelial cysts but may also be primary. Calcification often precedes development of bony tissue. Distinctive varieties include multiple skin color or bluish nodules in longstanding acne vulgaris[18] and extensive calcification of abdominal skin areas[19–20] during infancy (Fig. 28–3). Albright's hereditary osteodystrophy may manifest at birth or later in life. No definite predilection sites or sizes of deposits are known. In addition to multiple bone deformities absence of several knuckles is noted when patient makes a fist. Subungual exostoses (Fig. 28–4) are outgrowths of normal bony tissue or calcified cartilagenous remains.[21] These may be single or multiple and are usually asymptomatic unless traumatized or secondarily infected.[22]

URIC ACID

Gouty tophi are due to deposits of urates to which the tissues react with granulomatous inflammation. The histologic picture (Fig. 28–5) is that of a palisading granuloma (Chapter 23), especially when formalin fixation has converted the characteristic needle-like crystals into an amorphous mass. When urate crystals are preserved in ethanol fixation, they stain moderately with hematoxylin or appear gray. Under the polarized light they demonstrate beauti-

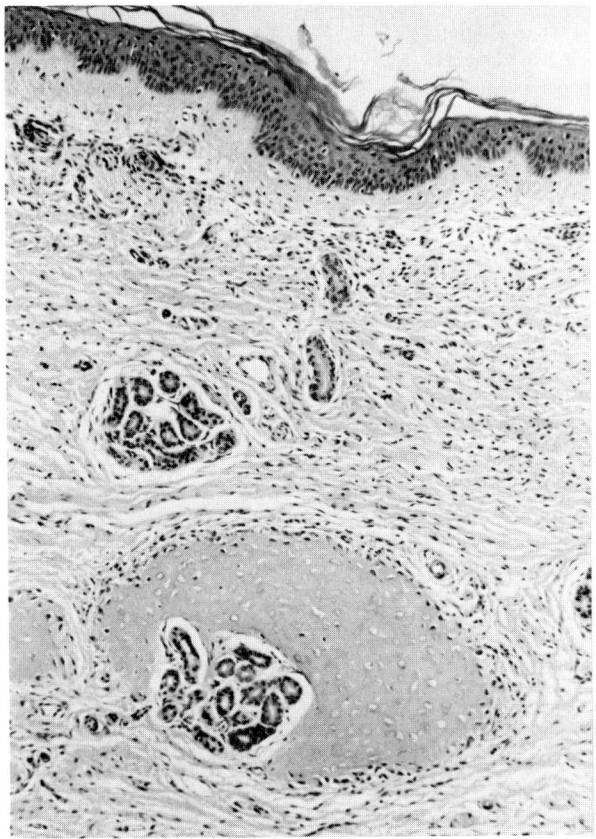

Figure 28–3.
Osteoma cutis in a child. The ossification involves the connective tissue associated with one sweat coil. There was no indication of any predisposing cause. H&E. ×125.

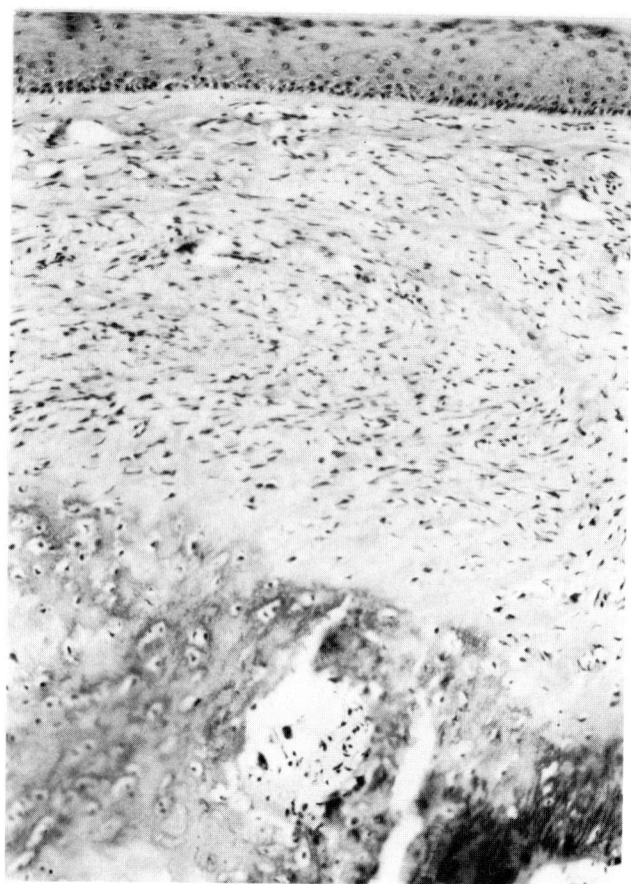

Figure 28–4.
Subungual exostosis. Fragment of bone embedded in a fibrotic tissue. H&E. X125.

ful multicolor birefringence in hematoxylin and eosin stained tissue. Special stain is rarely needed for their identification because of their grayish color and intense foreign body reaction in the vicinity. One should remember that tophi calcify secondarily.

HYALIN

The term "hyalin" has vaguely been applied to many ill-defined, amorphous insoluble substances in the skin. All hyaline substances stain pink in H&E and O&G sections, with the exception of amyloid, which will be discussed separately. All of them react with the PAS stain. Some contain lipids, which can be demonstrated in frozen sections.[23,24]

Extensive hyalinization, beginning as a coating of papillary vessels and progressing to large masses filling papillae and subpapillary layer, is seen in lipoid proteinosis (hyalinosis cutis et mucosae),[25–27] erythropoietic protoporphyria[28,29] (Fig. 28–6), and colloid milium. In lipoid proteinosis (hyalinosis cutis et mucosae), hyalin deposition initially occurs in the superficial network of capillary blood vessels, in eccrine sweat coils, and in hair muscles.[30] Hyalin is PAS positive and diastase resistant. It is argyrophilic, weakly reactive with colloidal iron, and stains positive with Sudan III for fat. It is most likely composed of neutral mucopolysaccharide with some hyaluronic acid, tryptophan, neutral fat, and cholesterol. In electron microscopy, it shows 8- to 10-nm fibrillar structures forming bundles and whorls.[31] Massive deposition of hyalin and fibroblasts occurs in juvenile hyalin fibromatosis in childhood (Chapter 42). In erythropoietic protoporphyria (EPP), endothelial cells of superficial capillary blood vessels are primary targets of the photodynamic reaction.[32] Electron microscopy shows multiplication of the basement membrane surrounding small vessels in the upper dermis. Each layer of multilayered basement membrane reflects consecutive reparative processes following endothelial cell injuries. The number of layers, therefore, relates to the duration and severity of the skin lesions. Foamy exudate of plasma and cell debris seen in early lesions provides the basic substrate for the formation of fibrillar material that characterizes hyalin deposits in chronic lesions. Final diagnosis of EPP is made by demonstration of fluorescent erythrocytes or excess protoporphyrin in blood or feces.[32]

AMYLOID

Skin Limited Types

Amyloid occurs in the skin as purely cutaneous lichen amyloidosis (lichenoid amyloidosis) and as macular amyloidosis, which may be a variant of the lichenoid form.[33–36] In the diffuse biphasic variety, generalized macular eruption is associated with the lichenoid papular lesions of the pretibial area.[37] Macular and lichenoid lesions also occur together in the familial form.[38–40] Poikiloderma-like eruptions and Riehl's melanosis-associated amyloid are other morphologic variations. These purely cutaneous varieties are caused by degeneration of epidermal or appendageal keratinocytes through apoptotic dropping off into the dermis. Thus, keratin amyloid or amyloid K is the proper designation.[41] Actinic damage of the epidermal keratinocytes also produces amyloid K in juvenile colloid milium,[42] amyloidosis

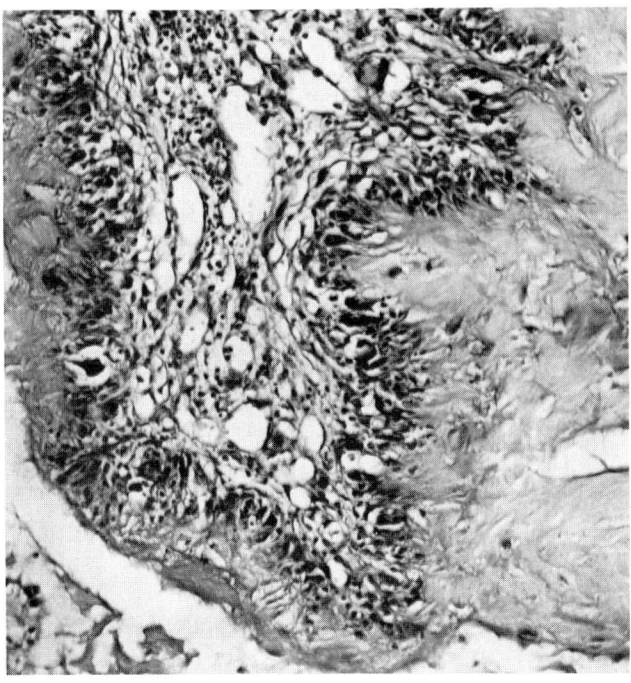

Figure 28–5.
Gouty tophus presenting features of a palisading granuloma. Most of crystalline structure of urates has been lost due to formalin fixation. H&E. X135.

of auricular concha,[43] actinic keratosis,[44] and in PUVA-treated skin.[45] Mechanical damage of keratinocytes may induce amyloid transformation and in susceptible individuals it causes friction amyloidoses.[46,47] In long-standing lesions of actinic keratosis, seborrheic keratosis, basal cell epitheliomas, and particularly in Bowen's disease and premalignant fibroepithelial tumor of Pinkus, amyloid or filamentous degeneration of tumor keratinocytes results in depositions of amyloid K. The proofs that these amyloids are of keratinocyte derivation comes from several studies such as the demonstrations in these amyloids of the presence of keratin epitopes by antikeratin autoantibodies,[48,49] disulfide bonds, and admixture of basal lamina components in addition to ultrastructural evidence of the presence of a tonofilament–amyloid mixture, melanosomes, hemidesmosomes, and desmosomes.[50]

Systemic Amyloidosis

Cutaneous manifestations of primary systemic- or multiple myeloma-associated amyloidosis may be purpura, waxy papules, tumors, plaques, alopecia, and rarely bullous lesions.[51–53] Myeloma-associated systemic amyloidosis can be diagnosed by rectal biopsy or the presence of Bence-Jones protein in urine. Serum immunoelectrophoresis shows elevated immunoglobulin light chains, either λ or κ. The predominance of one chain indicates a monoclonal proliferation of plasma cells in bone marrow and biopsy or bone survey often demonstrates the presence of multiple myeloma. In those cases that lack the evidence of plasma cell dyscrasia, a long-term follow-up often detects the development of multiple myeloma. The designation for this type of systemic amyloidosis is "AL amyloid." Nodular

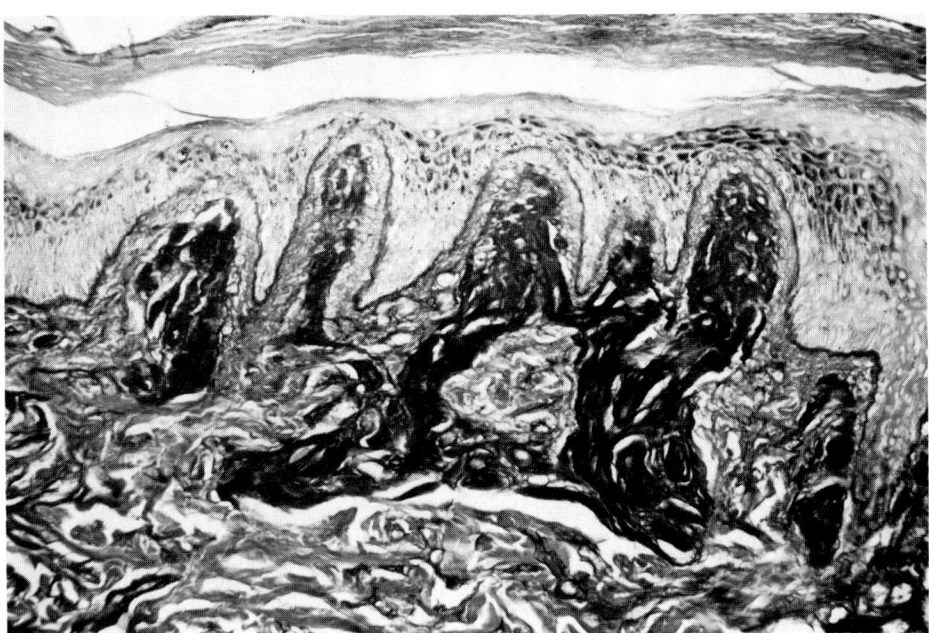

Figure 28–6.
Erythropoietic protoporphyria. Hyaline masses in dermis and glycogen in acanthotic epidermis appear dark in this alcian blue–PAS-stained section. Histologic picture is very similar to that of lipoid proteinosis. X135.

amyloidosis of the skin also belongs to this group, although multiple myeloma is not necessarily always detectable.[54,55]

Secondary Systemic Amyloidosis

Although the skin is spared in secondary systemic amyloidosis, deposits were found as rings around subcutaneous fat cells in biopsies from lower abdomen in eight cases.[56] This type of amyloidosis occurs secondary to chronic infections or inflammation such as chronic osteomyelitis and rheumatoid arthritis. The designation for this type of amyloid is "AA protein," which is derived from serum alpha-globulin. Congo red staining of AA protein can be eliminated by potassium permanganate treatment and, thus, can be differentiated from AL protein, which is resistant to this procedure.

While deposits may be massive in the systemic form (AL amyloids), the lichenoid papules (amyloid K) often contain only minute quantities of amyloid in individual papillae. It takes a high level of suspicion to locate amyloid in H&E sections, because it either does not stain differently from collagen or may be slightly bluish to gray at best. A suspicion-arousing feature in lichenoid and macular types is the association of a few melanophages with pink-staining material in a widened papilla, epidermal lichenification, and the presence in the epidermis of globes of amorphous eosinophilic material. Many special stains have been recommended for amyloid, but they are unnecessary if O&G stain is done. It stains amyloid (Fig. 28–7) a light sky blue (or grayish blue if the section was decolorized too much), a hue that no other substance will take. While no claim is made for the specificity of this staining reaction, it has proved its value in skin sections. The only other amorphous substances that stain similarly are fibrin and some forms of fibrinoid, but the hue is a colder greenish blue as a rule.

Cotton dyes stain all types of amyloid specifically in a bright orange-red color[57] (see Fig. 4, Color Plate II). Electron microscopy of all types of amyloid shows short, straight, and nonbranching filaments measuring 6 to 10 nm[58,59] in diameter (Fig. 28–8).

BLOOD AND BLOOD PIGMENT

Extravasation of blood may be due to trauma or various pathologic conditions affecting vascular walls or the blood itself. With the exception of leukemia, where the number of white cells is relatively large, evidence of hemorrhage in the tissue sections exists in the presence of free erythrocytes in the tissue. It was pointed out in Chapter 5 that biopsy trauma must be suspected if only fresh red cells are seen. It

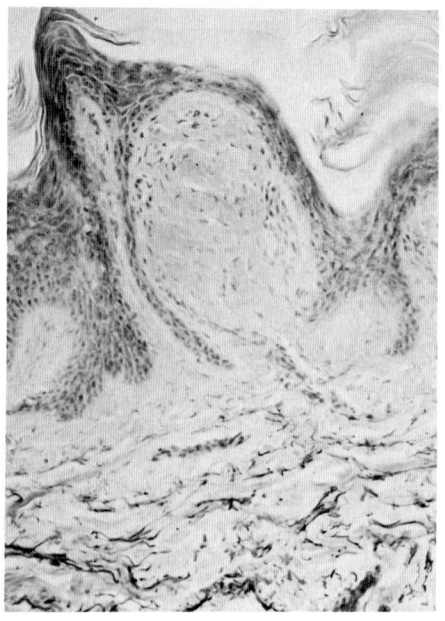
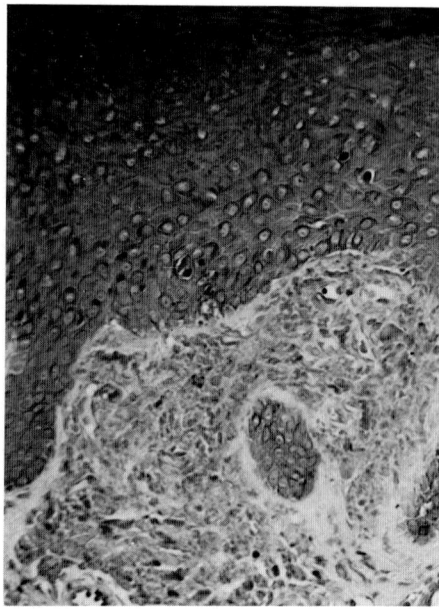

Figure 28–7.
Lichen amyloidosus. **A.** Amyloid deposits in widened papillae. O&G. X135. **B.** Amyloid below acanthotic epidermis. Crystal violet. X180.

A B

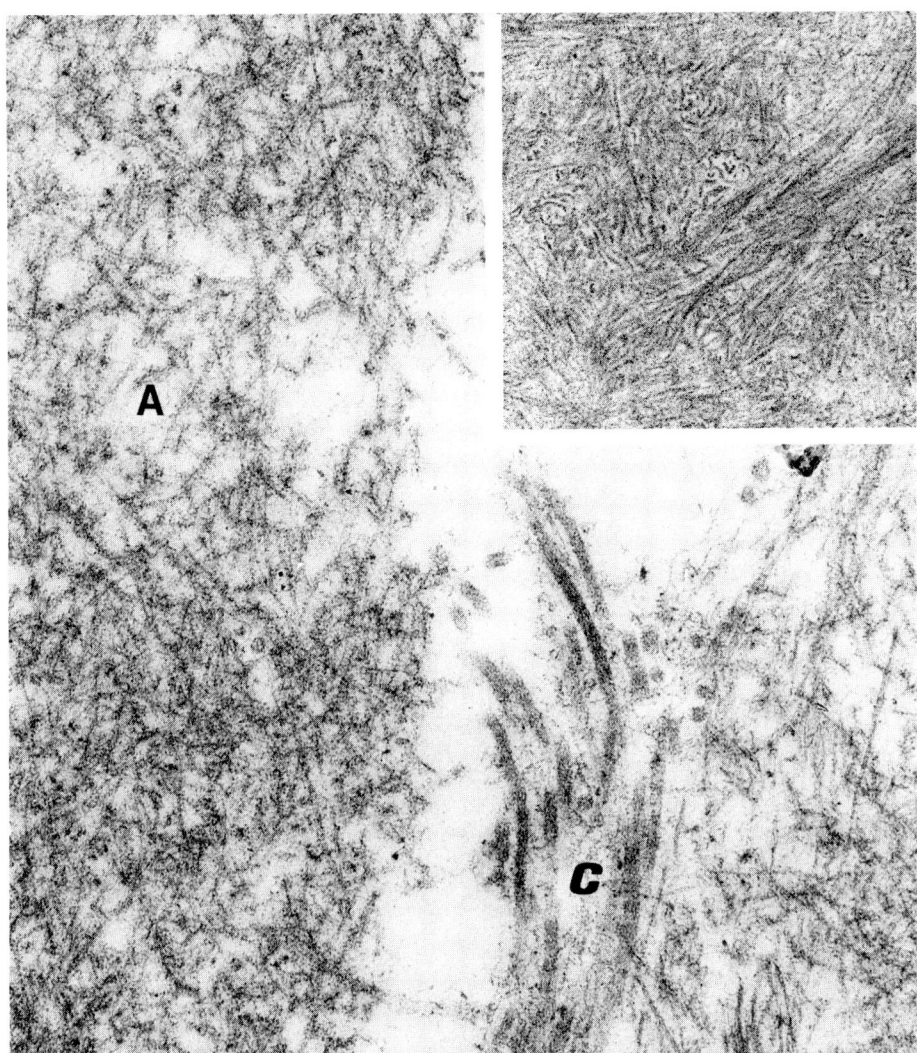

Figure 28–8.
Lichenoid amyloidosis. Straight wirelike amyloid filaments (A) are shown on the left side and in the inset. Compare with the collagen fibers (C) in the right lower portion of the figure ×62,400.

takes, however, several days before appreciable numbers disintegrate, and fresh spontaneous purpura cannot be ruled out by this criterion. In many cases of purpura, an inflammatory reaction sets in soon, but it may be absent in others such as scurvy or senile purpura. The formation of hemosiderin takes even longer, and it was mentioned in the discussion of pigmented purpuric eruptions that hemosiderin is rarely seen because the biopsy usually is taken of fresh purpuric papules. On the other hand, hemosiderin may be present in a large quantity in specimens taken from the lower legs of older persons for a variety of reasons, especially if the characteristic yellow-brown to brown-black discoloration informs the clinician of long-standing stasis damage. These hemosiderin deposits may provoke the thought of Kaposi's sarcoma if they are associated with considerable vascular proliferation.

FOREIGN BODIES

Foreign materials are discussed in Chapter 31. Of colorless materials, the easiest to recognize is silica (Fig. 21–16), owing to its birefringence. It was mentioned in Chapter 21 that any sarcoid granuloma should be examined in polarized light to rule out silica. On the other hand, skin biopsy sections examined for confirmation of fiberglass dermatitis have not been informative. Spicules of fiberglass are difficult to identify even in an early lesion. Dirt tattooed into skin through an abrasion usually consists in part of silica and in part of nonpolarizing particles, which may be colored.[60] Other substances, such as plant fibers (usually birefringent), sutures, and parts of arthropods, are found occasionally. Starch granules (Fig. 3–19) and silica needles (talc) were identified in a subcutaneous granuloma resulting from injection of face powder, the most common material containing a mixture of these two ingredients. The starch granules were seen in a PAS stain.

REFERENCES

1. Shoenfeld RJ, Grekin JN, Mehregan AH: Calcium deposition in the skin. A report of four cases following electroencephalography. Neurology 15:477, 1965
2. Wheeland RG, Roundtree JM: Calcinosis cutis resulting from percutaneous penetration and deposition of calcium. J Am Acad Dermatol 12:172, 1985
3. Mehregan AH: Calcinosis cutis: A review of the clinical forms and report of 75 cases. Semin Dermatol 3:53, 1984
4. Swinehart JM, Golitz LE: Scrotal calcinosis. Dystrophic calcification of epidermoid cysts. Arch Dermatol 118:985, 1982
5. Nakamura S, Imai T, Nakayama K: Idiopathic calcinosis of the scrotum. J Dermatol Tokyo 12:369, 1985
6. Song DH, Lee KH, Kang WH: Idiopathic calcinosis of the scrotum: Histologic observations of fifty-one nodules. J Am Acad Dermatol 19:1095, 1988
7. Dare AJ, Axelsen RA: Scrotal calcinosis: Origin from dystrophic calcification of eccrine duct milia. J Cutan Pathol 15:142, 1988
8. Melo CR, Schmitt FC, Melo IS, et al: Calcinosis del escroto relato de un caso asociado a calcificaciones de quistes epidermoides. Med Cutan ILA Ibero Lat Am 16:355, 1988
9. Chadwick JM, Downham TF: Auricular calcification. Int J Dermatol 17:799, 1978
10. Sell EJ, Hansen RC, Struck-Pierce S: Calcified nodules on the heel: A complication of neonatal intensive care. J Pediatr 96:473, 1980
11. Pursley TV, Prince MJ, Chausmer AB, Raimer SS: Cutaneous manifestations of tumoral calcinosis. Arch Dermatol 115:1100, 1979
12. Shmunes E, Wood MG: Subepidermal calcified nodules. Arch Dermatol 105:593, 1972
13. Brook CGD, Valman HB: Osteoma cutis and Albright's hereditary osteodystrophy. Br J Dermatol 85:471, 1971
14. Barranco VP: Cutaneous ossification in pseudohypoparathyroidism. Arch Dermatol 104:643, 1971
15. Putkonen T, Wangel GA: Renal hyperparathyroidism with metastatic calcification of the skin. Dermatologica 118:127, 1959
16. Laurent R, Thiery F, Saint-Hillier Y, et al: Panniculite calcifiante associee a une insuffisance renale: Un syndrome de calciphylaxie tissulaire. Ann Dermatol Venereol 114:1073, 1987
17. Coskey JR, Mehregan AH: Metaplastic bone formation in an organoid nevus. Arch Dermatol 102:233, 1970
18. Basler RSW: Calcifying acne lesions. Int J Dermatol 16:755, 1977
19. Rotteleur G, Becquart P, Piette F, Blankaert D: Osteomatose cutanée diffuse du nourrisson. Arch Fr Pediatr 37:397, 1980
20. Perez Lopez M, De Moragas JM: Osteoma cutis. Gaceta Dermatol 2:147, 1981
21. Bendl BJ: Subungual exostosis. Cutis 26:260, 1980
22. Lebowitz SS, Miller OF, Dickey RF: Subungual exostosis. Cutis 13:426, 1974
23. Bauer EA, Santa-Cruz DJ, Eisen AZ: Lipoid proteinosis: In vivo and in vitro evidence for a lysosomal storage disease. J Invest Dermatol 76:119, 1981
24. Bravo-Piris J, Unamuno Perez P, Armijo M: Hylinose cutanéo-muqueuse chez des jumelles monzygotes. Ann Dermatol Venereol 112:235, 1985
25. Hashimoto K: Diseases of amyloid, colloid and hyalin. J Cutan Pathol 12:322, 1985
26. Lin J, Hurng JJ, Wong C-K: Hyalinosis cutis et mucosae. A case report. J Dermatol Tokyo 14:497, 1987
27. Lebbe C, Blanchet-Bardon C, Mariano A, et al: Hyalinose cutaneomuqueuse: Polymorphisme clinique. Ann Dermatol Venereol 116:794, 1989
28. DeSelys R, Decroix J, Frankart M, et al: Protoporphyrie erythropoietique. Ann Dermatol Venereol 115:555, 1988
29. Marcoux C, Bourlond A: Protoporphyrie erythropoietique. Ultrastructure du complexe basal pericapillaire dans le jerme superficiel. Ann Dermatol Venereol 115:561, 1988
30. Ishibashi A: Hyalinosis cutis et mucosae. Defective digestion and storage of basal lamina glycoprotein synthesized by smooth muscle cells. Dermatologica 165:7, 1982
31. Fleischmajer R, Krieg T, Dziadek M, et al: Ultrastructure and composition of connective tissue in hyalinosis cutis et mucosae skin. J Invest Dermatol 82:252, 1984
32. Poh-Fitzpatrick MB: Erythropoietic protoporphyria. Int J Dermatol 17:359, 1978
33. Breathnach SM: The cutaneous amyloidosis. Pathogenesis and therapy. Arch Dermatol 121:470, 1985
34. Grossin M, Crickx B: Amylose. Ann Dermatol Venereol 113:869, 1986
35. Breathnach SM: Amyloid and amyloidosis. J Am Acad Dermatol 18:1, 1988
36. Leonforte J-F: Sur l'origine de l'amyloidose maculeuse. A propos de 160 cas. Ann Dermatol Venereol 114:801, 1987
37. Piamphongsant T, Kullavanijaya P: Diffuse biphasic amyloidosis. Dermatologica 153:243, 1976
38. De Pietro WP: Primary familial cutaneous amyloido-

sis. A study of HIA antigens in a Puerto Rican family. Arch Dermatol 117:639, 1981
39. LeBoit PE, Greene I: Primary cutaneous amyloidosis: Identically distributed lesions in identical twins. Pediatr Dermatol 3:244, 1986
40. Moulin G, Cognat T, Delaye J, et al: Amylose disseminee primitive familiale.(Nouvelle forme clinique?). Ann Dermatol Venereol 115:565, 1988
41. Hashimoto K: Progress on cutaneous amyloidoses. J Invest Dermatol 82:1, 1984
42. Hashimoto K, Nakayama H, Chimenti S. et al: Juvenile colloid milium: Immunohistochemical and ultrastructural studies. J Cutan Pathol 16:164, 1989
43. Hicks BC, Weber PJ, Hashimoto K, et al:Primary cutaneous amyloidosis of the auricular concha. J Am Acad Dermatol 18:19, 1988
44. Hashimoto K, King LE Jr: Secondary localized cutaneous amyloidosis associated with actinic keratosis. J Invest Dermatol 61:293, 1973
45. Hashimoto K, Kohda H, Kumakiri M, et al: Ultrastructural changes in a psoralen–UVA treated psoriatic lesion: Ultrastructure of PUVA-treated psoriasis. Arch Dermatol 114:711, 1978
46. Hashimoto K, Ito K, Kumakiri M, Headington J: Nylon brush macular amyloidosis. Arch Dermatol 123:633, 1987
47. Wong C-K, Lin C-S: Friction amyloidosis. Int J Dermatol 27:302,1988
48. Yoneda K, Watanabe H, Yanagihara M, Mori S: Immunohistochemical staining properties of amyloids with anti-keratin antibodies using formalin-fixed, paraffin-embedded sections. J Cutan Pathol 16:133, 1989
49. Kitano Y, Okada N, Kobayashi Y, et al: A monoclonal anti-keratin antibody reactive with amyloid deposit of primary cutaneous amyloidosis. J Dermatol Tokyo 14: 427, 1987
50. Hashimoto K, Yamanishi Y, Dabbous M: Collagenolytic activities of basal cell epithelioma. J Invest Dermatol 58:251, 1972
51. Bieber T, Ruzicka T, Linke RP, et al: Hemorrhagic bullous amyloidosis. Arch Dermatol 124:1683, 1988
52. Schmutz JL, Barbaud A, Cuny JF, et al: Amylose bulleuse. Ann Dermatol Venereol 115:295, 1988
53. Johnson TM, Rapini RP, Hebert AA, et al: Bullous amyloidosis. Cutis 43:346, 1989
54. Ito K, Hashimoto K, Kambe N, Van S: Roles of immunoglobulins in amyloidogenesis in cutaneous nodular amyloidosis. J Invest Dermatol 89:415, 1987
55. Masuda C, Mohri S, Nakajima H: Histopathological and immunohistochemical study of amyloidosis cutis nodularis atrophicans—Comparison with systemic amyloidosis. Br J Dermatol 119:33, 1988
56. Westermark P: Occurrence of amyloid deposits in the skin in secondary systemic amyloidosis. Acta Pathol Microbiol Scand 80A:718, 1972
57. Yanagihara M, Mehregan AH, Mehregan DR: Staining of amyloid with cotton dyes. Arch Dermatol 120: 1184, 1984
58. Kobayasi T, Asboe-Hansen G: Ultrastructure of skin in primary systemic amyloidosis. Acta Derm Venereol 59:407, 1979
59. Hashimoto K: Electron microscopy for diagnosis of selected dermatoses. Semin Dermatol 3:36, 1984
60. Mehregan AH, Faghri B: Implantation dermatoses. Acta Derm Venereol 54:61, 1974

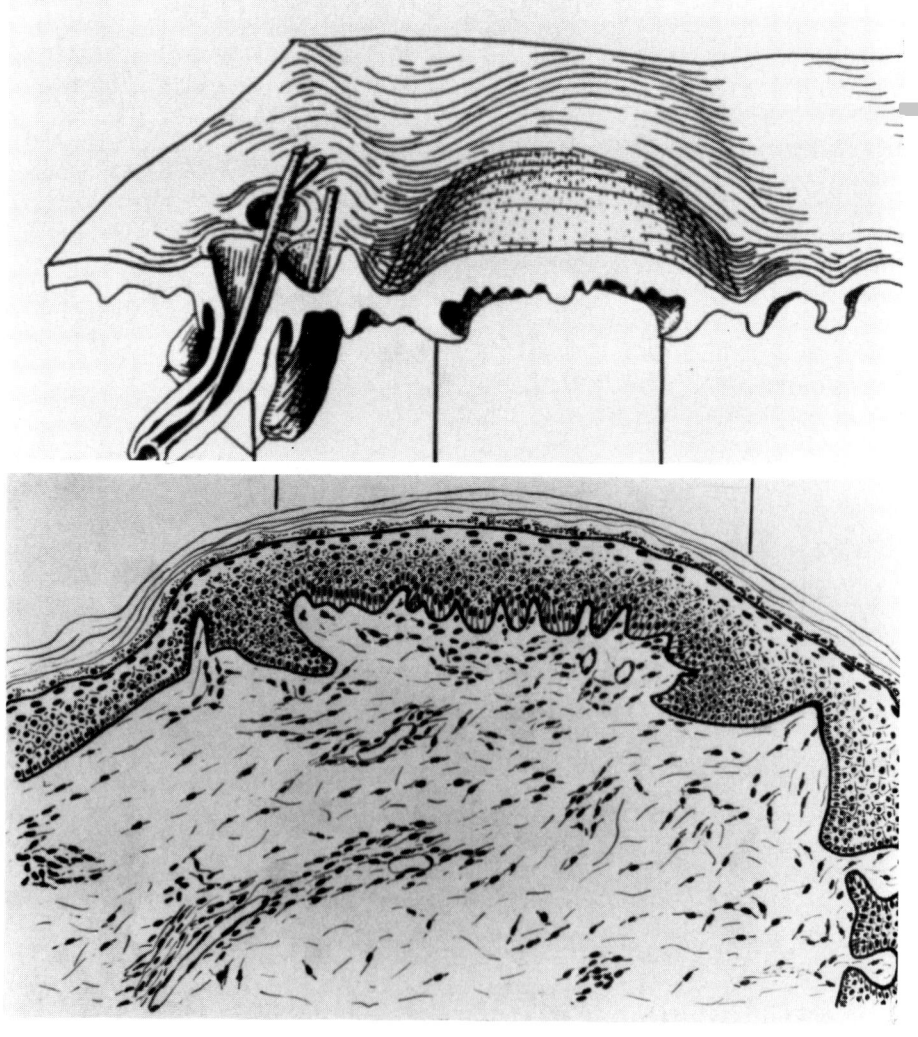

Hairdisk

SECTION VI

NONNEOPLASTIC EPITHELIAL AND PIGMENTARY DISORDERS

We have discussed a great variety of changes of epidermis and adnexal epithelium associated with inflammatory disease in the widest sense. We will discuss epithelial nevi and neoplasms in Section VII. In between these large groups of disorders, there are some that seem to fit neither definition. The epidermis appears to be abnormal in itself, without depending on dermal stimuli.[1] Thus, epidermis from cases of lamellar ichthyosis transplanted into athymic nude mice[2] retained its abnormal properties for long times. Removal of epidermis and superficial dermis in Darier's disease resulted in long-lasting remissions, an indication that the epidermis was inherently abnormal.[3] The changes tend to be generalized or at least widespread, are often inconstant in their expression, and seem to be due to inborn metabolic derangement rather than to inflammation, malformation, or neoplasis.[4] Then there are the virus epidermoses, which are neither inflammatory nor neoplastic in the usual sense. And finally, it seems convenient to discuss here various disturbances of skin color, which also are not definitely related to inflammation or neoplasia.

REFERENCES

1. Burgdorf WHC, Alper JC, Goldsmith LA: Genodermatoses. J Am Acad Dermatol 16:1045, 1987
2. Briggaman RA, Wheeler CE Jr: Lamellar ichthyosis: Long-term graft studies on congenitally athymic nude mice. J Invest Dermatol 67:567, 1976
3. Dellon AL, Chretien PB, Peck GL: Successful treatment of Darier's disease by partial-thickness removal of skin. Plast Reconstr Surg 59:823, 1977
4. Sybert VP, Dale BA, Malbrook KA: Ichthyosis vulgaris: Identification of a defect in synthesis of filaggrin correlated with an absence of keratohyalin granules. J Invest Dermatol 84:191, 1985

29
DARIER'S, HAILEY–HAILEY'S, AND GROVER'S DISEASES

Keratosis follicularis, chronic benign familial pemphigus, and transient acantholytic dermatosis have in common the basic histologic feature of acantholysis leading to suprabasal cleft formation.[1] They share this feature with the acantholytic diseases of the pemphigus group (Chapter 11). For histologic differential diagnosis it is often necessary to take into consideration all available clinical features and morphology, as well as the general course of the disease. On that basis, pemphigus vulgaris and vegetans, Hailey–Hailey's disease, Darier's disease, and Grover's disease are well definable. Difficulties of histologic differentiation, which do exist in some cases, should make us admit our diagnostic limitations rather than postulate the identity of diseases. While suprabasal acantholysis is the common feature, most cases present sufficiently diagnostic differences in other respects. These are listed in Table 29–1, which clearly shows variable, but rather characteristic, combinations for each disease.

KERATOSIS FOLLICULARIS (DARIER)

The histologic picture of the average case of Darier's disease (Fig. 29–1) presents relatively small foci of dry suprabasal clefting that give the impression of being largely due to retraction during tissue processing. The same areas usually show a minor degree of basal layer budding and exhibit individual cell keratinization, so that a smaller or larger number of dyskeratotic cells are mixed with normally keratinizing cells in the granular and horny layers. The clefting thus extends from the basal layer through the granular layer, and there is no coherent roof except the stratum corneum.

The dyskeratotic cells were morphologically divided into "corps ronds" and "grains" (See Fig. 5–9) by Darier, and this division has been maintained and supported by recent electron microscopic work, which suggests a somewhat different cytogenesis for either form.[2,3] In routine histologic sections, corps ronds are large roundish cells with a central vesicular nucleus and are separated by an empty cleft from the surrounding prickle cells. They have a dense outer rim and may contain keratohyalin granules.[4] Grains are smaller, eosinophilic, and presumably cornified bodies of round, elongated, or irregular shape and may or may not contain remnants of a nucleus. They are usually found in the stratum corneum, and there is no obvious reason for not assuming that corps ronds and grains are consecutive stages in the process of individual cell keratinization leading from a prickle cell without prickles through a granular stage to a shrunken, nonnucleated, keratinized body.

If the lesion is more severe, all these features increase in proportion, but variations may occur. For instance, in the moist creases of the skin, suprabasal

TABLE 29–1. DIFFERENTIAL FEATURES OF SOME ACANTHOLYTIC DISEASES

	Pemphigus Vulgaris	Pemphigus Vegetans	Hailey–Hailey	Darier	Grover
Suprabasal acantholysis	+	+	+	+	+
Dry cleft	–	+	–	+	–
Lake or bulla	+	+	+	–	+
Tombstone basal cells	+	+	–	–	–
Degeneration of acantholytic cells	+	+	–	–	–
Dyskeratosis	–	–	±	+	+
Basal layer budding	–	+	+ +	+ to + + +	+
Pseudoepitheliomatous proliferation	–	+	–	+	–
Acantholysis affecting follicular sheath	±	+	–	+	–
Inflammatory infiltrate	+	+ + +	± to +	± to + +	+

clefting (Fig. 29–2) may become much more extensive, while individual cell keratinization decreases. These cases resemble Hailey–Hailey's disease, and differential diagnosis may require more than one biopsy.[5,6] It should be remembered that benign familial pemphigus is a chronically recurrent disease in which plaques of vesicular or crusted lesions come and go over the intertriginous areas and usually respond to antibiotic therapy, while keratosis follicularis is a progressive disease that begins with discrete keratotic papules over the chest and back and, in typical cases, builds up over the years to more and more severe horny and verrucous foci responding, if at all, only to high doses of vitamin A[7] or retinoic acid preparations.

Focal abnormality of cell adhesion has been demonstrated in the clinically normal and perilesional skin of patients with Darier's disease.[8] The histologic features of Darier's disease are remarkably constant, while the clinical picture may vary from zosteriform arrangement,[9] resembling ichthyosis hystrix, to papular or macroscopically inapparent single or multiple lesions,[10] in addition to the typical generalized form. Darier's disease may in-

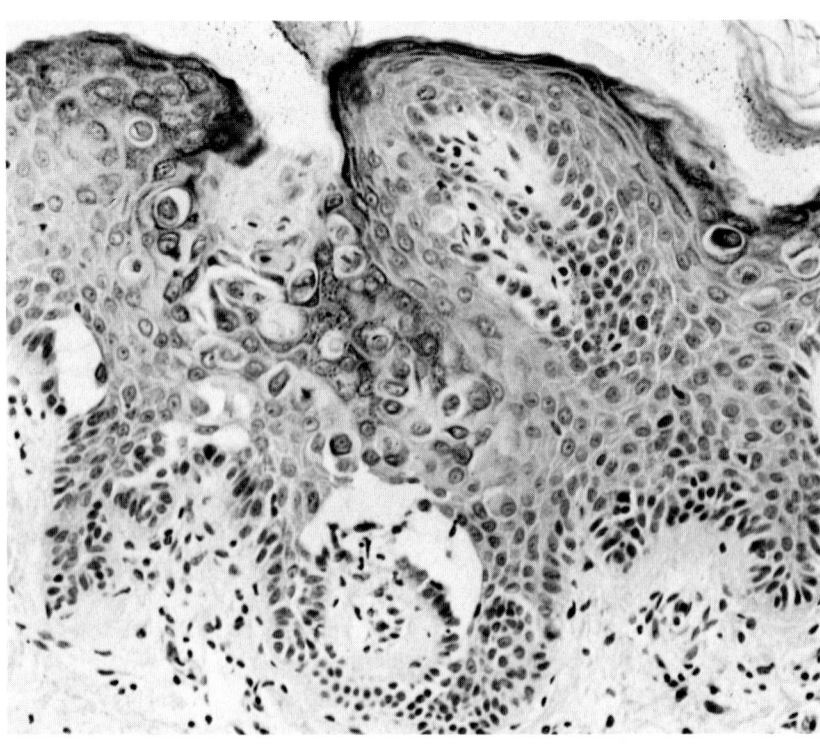

Figure 29–1.
Darier's keratosis follicularis. Suprabasal clefts and corps ronds are evident. Grains with or without pyknotic nuclei are discernible in the horny plug. H&E ×135. (From Sutton. Diseases of the Skin, 11th ed. 1956. Courtesy of Dr. R.L. Sutton, Jr. Contributed by H. Pinkus.)

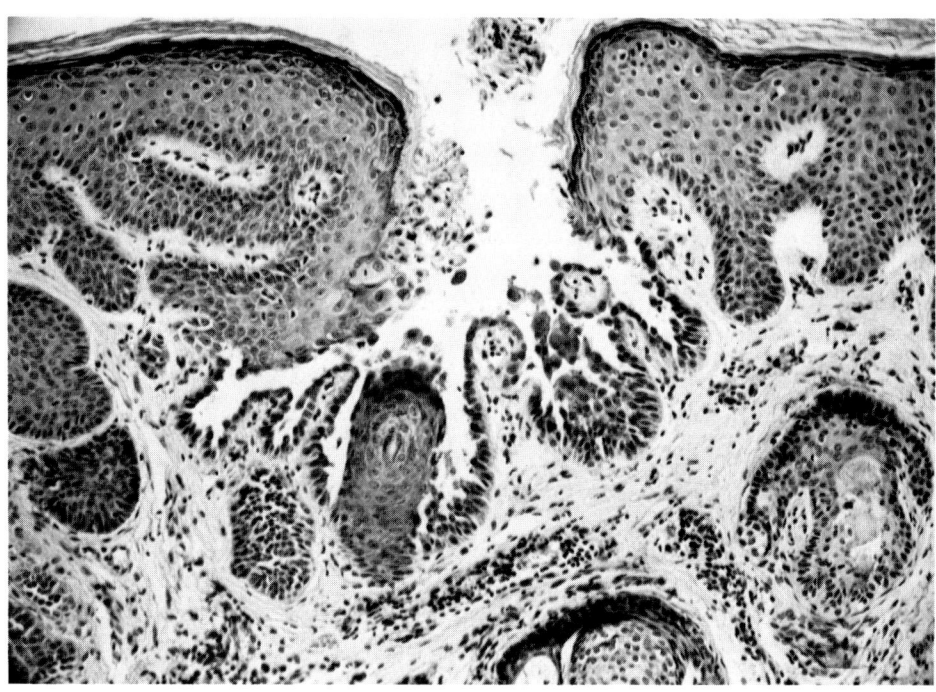

Figure 29–2.
Basal budding and extensive clefting due to acantholysis in Darier's disease. Eccrine keratinocytes in wall of sweat duct are not affected. H&E. X135.

volve the mucous membranes. The principal histologic variation is excessive downward budding of acantholytic epithelium (Fig. 29–3), which leads to convoluted masses. These structures, on cross section, consist of two rows of basal cells separated by a cleft.[11] In some cases, however, their thickness builds up, and the central cells assume prickle cell character and may even form horn pearls. Such *pseudoepitheliomatous proliferation* should not be mistaken for squamous cell carcinoma. High degrees

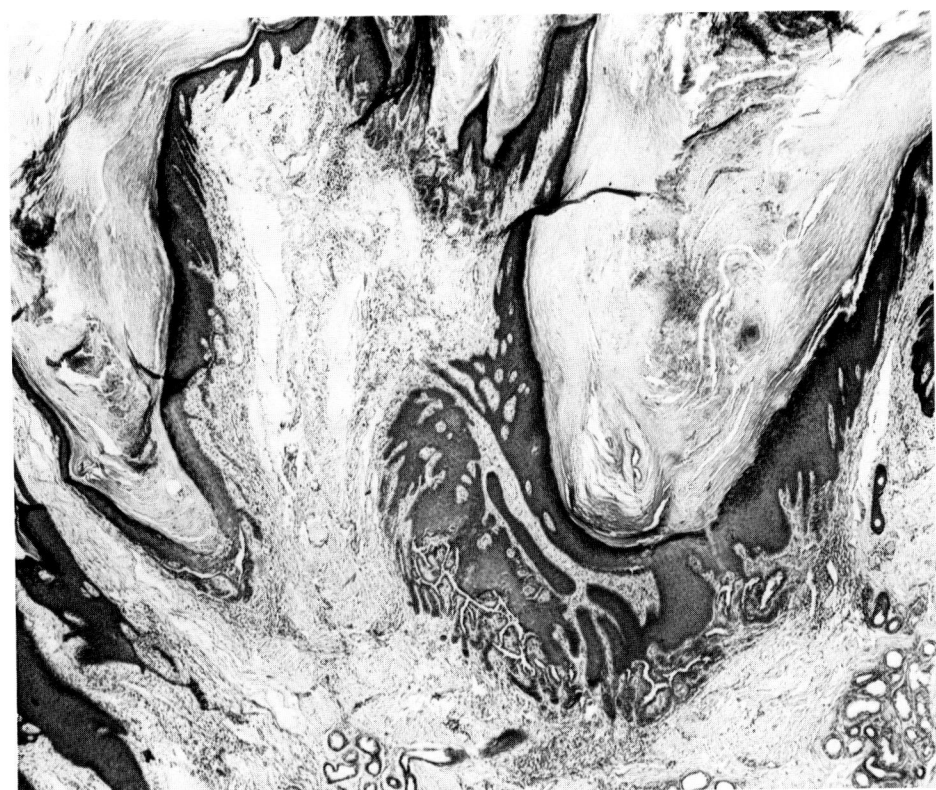

Figure 29–3.
Hypertrophic, verrucous, and pseudoepitheliomatous form of Darier's disease. Epidermis extends down to level of sweat coils. H&E. X28.

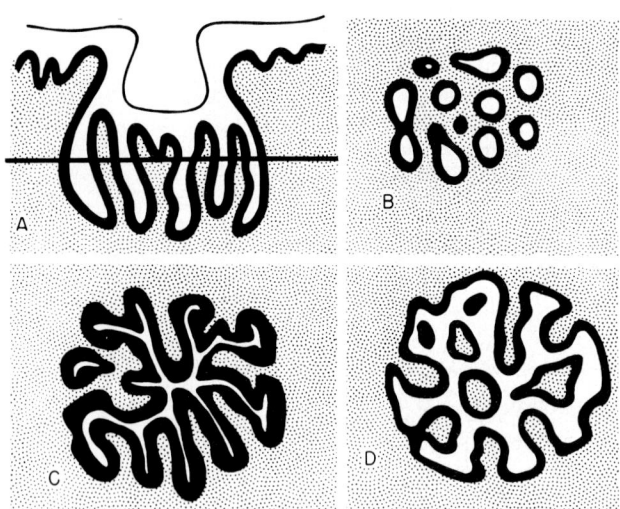

Figure 29–4.
Diagram illustrating structural differences between a tubular adenoma **(B)**, the cerebriform convolutions of hypertrophic Darier's disease **(C)**, and a papilliferous cystadenoma **(D)**, all of which may look deceptively similar in a vertical section **(A)**. The heavy line in **A** designates the level at which a transverse section would reveal the three different configurations shown in **B, C,** and **D**. (From Pinkus. Arch Dermatol 82:681, 1960.)

of proliferating clefting epidermis may mislead the casual observer to the assumption that he is dealing with a *syringadenoma papilliferum*.[12] Figure 29–4 tries to elucidate the three-dimensional structural differences between the gyrated epithelial mass of Darier's disease, with sections cut at different angles, and the hidradenomatous cyst (see Fig. 39–7), which is filled with papilliform projections. Closer examination reveals the quite different character of the cells that line the clefts: a simple layer of basal cells in Darier's disease, a double layer of columnar and flat cells in syringadenoma. Dyskeratotic cells occur only in keratosis follicularis.

Inflammatory dermal infiltrate plays no significant role in Darier's disease, although it may become heavier in macerated or secondarily infected lesions. This is in contrast to the heavy infiltrate usually encountered in pemphigus vegetans and in syringadenoma papilliferum, both characterized by plasma cells, and in pemphigus vegetans by eosinophils.

Warty Dyskeratoma

Isolated keratosis follicularis or warty dyskeratoma appears most commonly over the head and neck as an open comedone.[13–15] Mucosal involvement is rare.[16] The lesion is made up of a cystic dilated hair follicle containing soft keratin and dyskeratotic cells. The follicular epithelium is hyperplastic and shows basaloid budding into the surrounding areas (Fig. 29–5), many foci of suprabasal cleft formation, and a number of dyskeratotic cells.

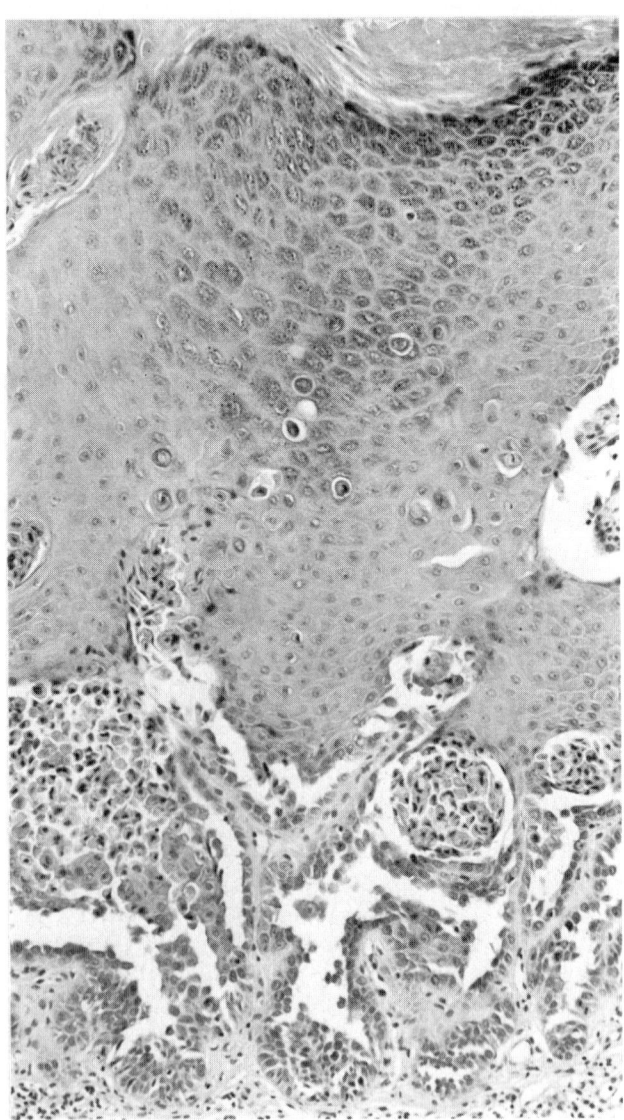

Figure 29–5.
Warty dyskeratoma. The follicular epithelium shows downward budding of basal cells, acantholysis, and suprabasal cleft formation. H&E. X125.

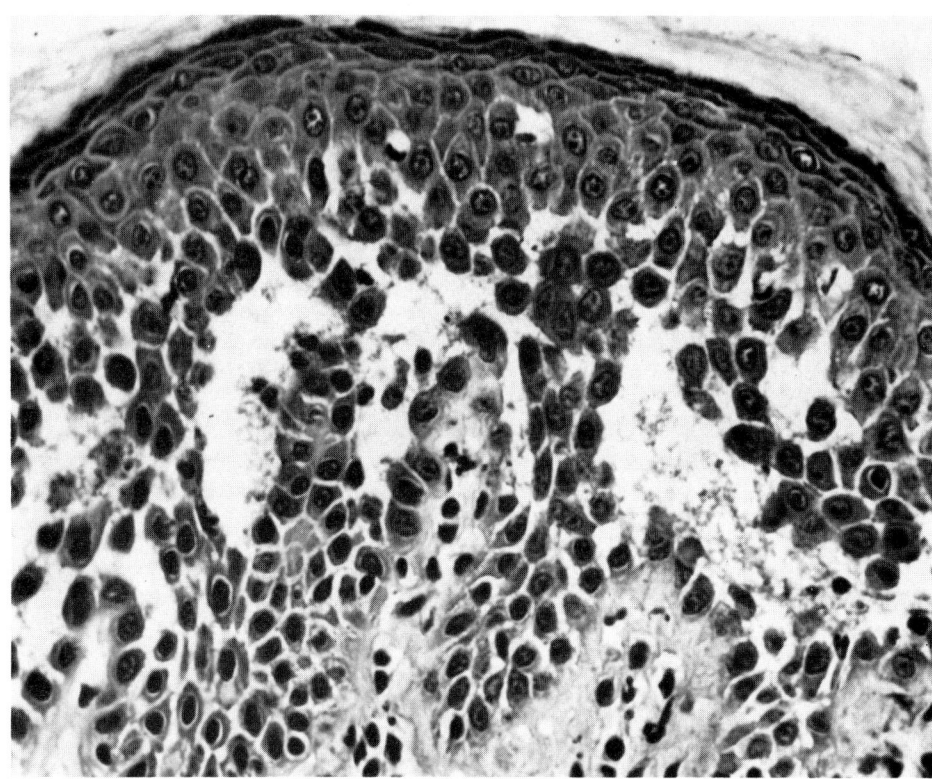

Figure 29-6.
Hailey–Hailey's disease. Acantholysis without dyskeratosis. H&E. X185. (From Sutton. Diseases of the Skin, 11th ed, 1956. Courtesy of Dr. R.L. Sutton, Jr. Contributed by H. Pinkus.)

BENIGN FAMILIAL CHRONIC PEMPHIGUS (HAILEY–HAILEY)

In contrast to the dry, open dyskeratotic cleft of Darier's disease, the benign familial pemphigus lesion (Fig. 29–6) shows extensive suprabasal splits, which are usually covered by coherent upper epidermal layers. These lakes (lacunae) commonly show evidence of having contained fluid in which isolated round prickle cells float.[17,18] Electron microscopic observations suggest that the desmosomes split in early lesions and are then retracted into the cells.[19] The acantholytic cells have well defined nuclei and sharply outlined cytoplasm, in contrast to the degenerating cells of pemphigus vulgaris or vegetans, and only occasionally show keratohyalin granules or a tendency to keratinize. They are acantholytic but generally not dyskeratotic. Basal layer budding often is pronounced, though never pseudoepitheliomatous. Hair follicles are spared by the process. In more acute or older lesions, the upper epidermal layers degenerate into a parakeratotic crust, and several such layers may be one on top of the other, somewhat resembling pemphigus foliaceus. Inflammatory infiltrate is variable but not significant. Patients with Hailey–Hailey's disease appear to have increased tendency to develop contact hypersensitivity.[20]

A very astounding occurrence is the coexistence in the same patient, and even in the same lesion, of the acantholytic changes of benign familial pemphigus and of psoriasis.[21,22] Another observation is the histologic findings of Hailey–Hailey's disease in a patient with immunologically confirmed bullous pemphigoid.[23]

Grover's Disease

In transient acantholytic dermatosis[24] of Grover, discrete papules and vesicobullous lesions, usually very pruritic, occur over a period of several months or up to a few years and subside spontaneously.[25] Persistent form has been described as related to the actinic damage.[26] The histologic picture (Fig. 29–7) shows similarity to Hailey–Hailey's disease as well as to pemphigus vulgaris or Darier's disease (Fig. 29–8). Immunofluorescence studies have failed to demonstrate a persistent pattern.[27]

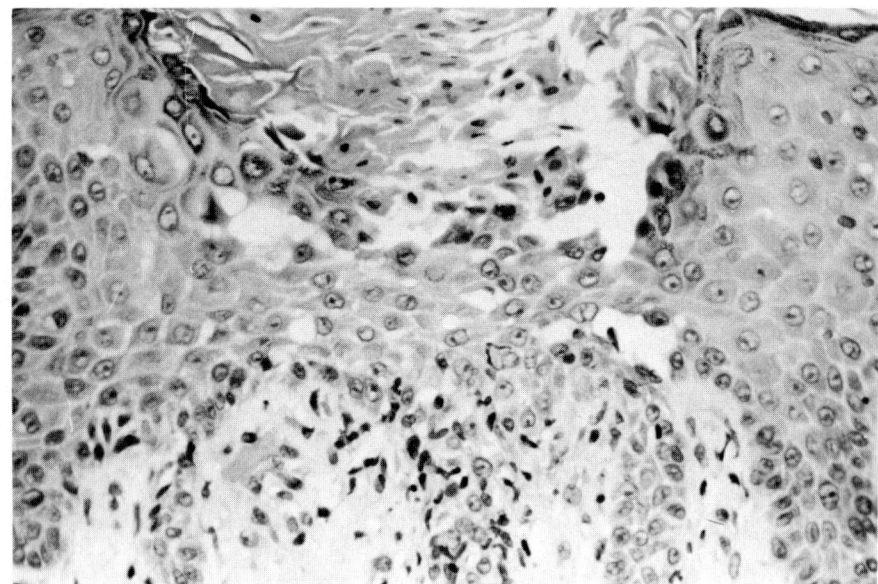

Figure 29-7.
Grover's disease. In this instance, the histologic picture is very similar to Darier's disease, and clinical information must give the definitive diagnosis. H&E. X250.

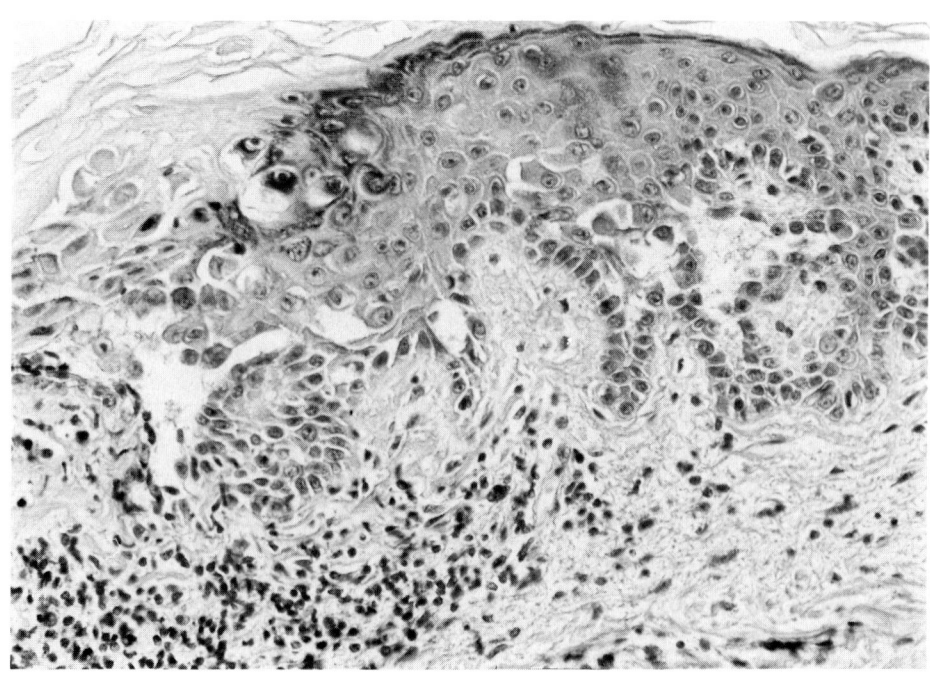

Figure 29-8.
Grover's disease combining features of Darier's and Hailey–Hailey diseases. H&E. X250.

REFERENCES

1. Pierard-Franchimont C, Pierard GE: Suprabasal acantholysis. Am J Dermatopathol 5:421, 1983
2. Gottlieb SK, Lutzner MA: Darier's disease: An electron microscopic study. Arch Dermatol 107:225, 1973
3. Sato A, Anton-Lamprecht I, Schnyder UW: Ultrastructure of dyskeratosis in Morbus Darier. J Cutan Pathol 4:173, 1977
4. Ishibashi Y, Kajiwara Y, Andoh I, et al: The nature and pathogenesis of dyskeratosis in Hailey–Hailey's disease and Darier's disease. J Dermatol Tokyo 11:335, 1984
5. Hori Y, Tsuru N, Niimura M: Bullous Darier's disease. Arch Dermatol 118:278, 1982
6. Schanne R, Burg G, Braun-Falco O: Zur nosologischen beziehung der dyskeratosis follicularis (Darier) und des pemphigus benignus chronicus familiaris (Hailey–Hailey). Hautarzt 36:504, 1985
7. Ayres S Jr: Darier's disease. Update on an effective new therapy. Arch Dermatol 119:710, 1983
8. Burge SM, Millard PR, Wojnarowska F, Ryan TJ: Darier's disease: a focal abnormality of cell adhesion. J Cutan Pathol 17:160, 1990
9. Starink Th M, Woerdeman MJ: Unilateral systematized keratosis follicularis. A variant of Darier's disease or an epidermal naevus (acantholytic dyskeratotic epidermal naevus)? Br J Dermatol 105:207, 1981
10. Ackerman AB: Focal acantholytic dyskeratosis. Arch Dermatol 106:702, 1972
11. Wheeland RG, Gilmore WA: The surgical treatment of hypertrophic Darier's disease. J Dermatol Surg Oncol 11:420, 1985
12. Beerman H: Hypertrophic Darier's disease and nevus syringocystadenomatosus papilliferus. Arch Dermatol 60:500, 1949
13. Graham JH, Helwig EB: Isolated dyskeratosis follicularis. Arch Dermatol 77:377, 1958
14. Tanay A, Mehregan AH: Warty dyskeratoma. Dermatologica 138:169, 1969
15. Szymanski FJ: Warty dyskeratoma. Arch Dermatol 75:567, 1957
16. Harrist TJ, Murphy GF, Mihm MC: Oral warty dyskeratoma. Arch Dermatol 116:928, 1980
17. Defresne C, Adam C, Marneffe K: Pemphigus chronique benin familial de Hailey–Hailey. Dermatologica 165:624, 1982
18. Galimberti RL, Kowalczuk AM, Bianchi O, et al: Chronic benign familial pemphigus. Int J Dermatol 27:495, 1988
19. De Dobbeleer G, Achten G: Disrupted desmosomes in induced lesions of familial benign chronic pemphigus. J Cutan Pathol 6:418, 1979
20. Remitz A, Lauerma AI, Stubb S, et al: Darier's disease, familial benign chronic pemphigus (Hailey–Hailey disease) and contact hypersensitivity. J Am Acad Dermatol 22:134, 1990
21. Heaphy MR, Winkelmann RK: Coexistence of benign familial pemphigus and psoriasis vulgaris. Arch Dermatol 112:1571, 1976
22. Fisher I, Orkin M, Bean S: Familial benign chronic pemphigus and psoriasis vulgaris in the same patient. Acta Derm Venereol 47:111, 1967
23. Mehregan DA, Umbert IJ, Peters MS: Histologic findings of Hailey–Hailey disease in a patient with bullous pemphigoid. J Am Acad Dermatol 21:1107, 1989
24. Chalet M, Grover R, Ackerman AB: Transient acantholytic dermatosis. A re-evaluation. Arch Dermatol 113:431, 1977
25. Heenan PJ, Quirk CJ: Transient acantholytic dermatosis. Br J Dermatol 102:515, 1980
26. Fawcett HA, Miller JA: Persistent acantholytic dermatosis related to actinic damage. Br J Dermatol 109:349, 1983
27. Bystryn J-C: Immunofluorescence studies in transient acantholytic dermatosis (Grover's disease). Am J Dermatopathol 1:325, 1979

30

ICHTHYOSIFORM DERMATOSES

The field of ichthyosiform dermatoses[1] can be best understood by realizing that *ichthyosis* is one of those diagnostic terms that cover quite unrelated disorders and that it is a purely clinical designation for chronically hyperkeratotic skin.[2] The term also covers the even wider field of epidermal dysplasia. Histologically, biologically, and genetically, it includes a variety of disorders of keratinization.[3] If one considers that specific disturbances of hair keratinization in mice are due to individual gene mutations and that the number of known mutations keeps increasing, it is not unreasonable to presume that there are many gene mutations in man which directly or indirectly affect epidermal keratinization in a manner that is clinically expressed as ichthyosis. Future progress in this field seems to depend, therefore, on the cloning of the genes that encode keratin proteins and the identification of the loci of abnormal genes on the chromosomes. Various histologic features of ichthyotic state are listed in Table 30–1. If these qualities of the epidermis are related to the involvement of follicular and eccrine ostia, abnormal features of hairs, presence or atrophy of sebaceous glands and if exact mode of inheritance is established[4] and clinical development from infancy to adulthood is recorded,[5,6] a considerable number of combinations result. Table 30–2 lists entities that are recognized at the present time.

ICHTHYOSIS VULGARIS

Ichthyosis vulgaris, the most prevalent clinical form of ichthyoses, is inherited by an autosomal dominant trait and shows manifestations soon after birth, with involvement of the extensor surfaces of the extremities with adherent scales (fish scales) and keratosis pilaris. Palms and soles may be thick. There are often increased folds and creases. Nonhereditary forms of the disease may occur as a case of spontaneous mutation, and ichthyosis-vulgaris-like skin changes may result from lymphoma, carcinoma, and sarcoidosis.[7–9]

The epidermis in ichthyosis vulgaris has a rather thin stratum malpighii and a thick and compact horny layer without parakeratosis (Fig. 30–1). The granular layer is very thin or defective.[10] Hyperkeratosis may extend into the hair follicles. Mitotic figures are scarce and kinetic studies show normal rate of keratinocyte production. Scaliness, therefore, results from a retention or slow desquamation of corneocytes.

X-LINKED ICHTHYOSIS

X-linked ichthyosis is relatively rare and shows a recessive mode of inheritance. Full expression of skin

TABLE 30-1. HISTOLOGIC PICTURES FOUND IN ICHTHYOSIFORM DISORDERS

Orthokeratotic
  Granular layer thin or absent, horny layer compressed (superkeratinization) or thick
  Granular layer thick, epidermis acanthotic, horny layer stratified
  Granular cells ballooning, horny layer thick, verrucous (epidermolytic type)

Parakeratotic
  Granular layer absent, epidermis psoriasiform
  Granular layer present, nuclei preserved in horny layer

changes appear only in the male infant, usually in the first few months of life. The involvement of the extensor as well as flexural aspects of the extremities, ears, sides of neck, and scalp are common. Scales are large and darkly pigmented[11] (dirty appearance). Corneal opacity may be detected in affected male patients. Keratosis pilaris is not seen. The epidermis shows thickened stratum corneum with normal or slightly thick granular layer, acanthosis, and prominent rete ridges. Kinetic studies show normal epidermal transit time.[12] As in ichthyosis vulgaris, detachment of corneocytes is delayed due to a deficiency of steroid sulfatase that hydrolyzes cholesteryl sulfate, an adhesive cellular cement[13] derived from lamellar granules or cementosomes. The gene for steroid sulfatase is located at terminal part of the short arm of X chromosome (Xp 22.3–PTER) and a complete deletion of this gene was confirmed in 89% of patients from 45 different families.[14]

LAMELLAR ICHTHYOSIS

The autosomal recessive ichthyosis may present as two separate entities, *lamellar ichthyosis* and *nonbullous congenital ichthyosiform erythroderma*.[15,16] Lamellar ichthyosis is usually manifested at birth. The newborn is encased in a thick membrane of stratum corneum (collodion baby). This membrane is shed within several weeks and is replaced with areas of scaling erythema involving even the intertriginous areas. Flexure surface and palms and soles are involved. Hairs may be matted down with scales. Nails may show ridges and grooves. Ectropion is almost always present (Fig. 30–2). Lamellar ichthyosis shows epidermal acanthosis with slight thickening of the granular layer, hyperkeratosis, and focal parakeratosis. Kinetic studies show increased mitotic activity and reduced transit time. Nonbullous congenital ichthyosiform erythroderma shows fine white scales, easily discernible parakeratotic areas, and increased labeling index.

In *Chanarin–Dorfman syndrome*, a rare autosomal recessive ichthyosis, a neutral lipid storage is seen in the basal cells and granular cells of the epidermis and in many dermal connective tissue cells. Lipid vacuoles are also present in blood leukocytes. Cementosomes are vacuolated and lamellar structures are distorted.[17]

EPIDERMOLYTIC HYPERKERATOSIS

Epidermolytic hyperkeratosis (formerly known as "bullous congenital ichthyosiform erythroderma," a term that should be discontinued) is inherited as an autosomal dominant trait.[18] At birth the skin is erythematous, moist, and tender; subsequently, it becomes dry and scaly. Thick, gray, and verrucous areas may develop over the elbows and knees. Bullous lesions occur in neonates and may continue to be present for a few years particularly over the lower extremities.

Histopathology of epidermolytic hyperkeratosis is distinctive in the presence of upper epidermal cell vacuolization, hypergranulosis, and hyperkeratosis (Fig. 30–3). The keratohyalin granules are large and irregularly shaped. Vacuolization of the epidermal cells is marked in the upper stratum malpighii and granular layer. Severe vacuolization of epidermal keratinocytes may lead to intraepidermal blister formation.

Ichthyosis Hystrix and Ichthyosiform Nevi

Severe cases of the diffuse epidermolytic hyperkeratosis may show patches and streaks of heavy verrucous hyperkeratosis of the porcupine type. In other cases the epidermal malformation is entirely localized in segmental fashion and may be classified as an epidermal nevus (Chapter 34). These are usually called ichthyosis hystrix (Fig. 30–4). In some families both the diffuse and segmental forms have occurred. There are also occasional cases in which a small localized epidermal nevus is found to have the same histologic picture. These observations and the concept of epidermolytic hyperkeratosis as a histobiologic entity, put forward in the first edition of this volume, have been substantiated by several authors in subsequent years.[19] They have been extended to include cases with hereditary palmoplantar kerato-

TABLE 30-2. MAJOR FORMS AND SOME RARE TYPES OF ICHTHYOSIFORM DERMATOSES

	Inheritance	Presence at Birth	Histology
Ichthyosis vulgaris	Autosomal dominant	No	Compressed orthokeratosis, decreased granular layer, average epidermal thickness
Sex-linked ichthyosis	Sex-linked recessive	Yes	Stratified orthokeratosis, normal or slightly thickened granular layer and rete malpighi, perivascular dermal infiltrate
Lamellar ichthyosis	Autosomal recessive	Yes (collodion baby)	Hyperkeratosis with focal parakeratosis, thickened granular and spinous layers, dermal infiltrate
Epidermolytic hyperkeratosis	Autosomal dominant	Yes	Marked thickening of all epidermal layers, vacuolar degeneration of granular cells
Harlequin fetus	Autosomal recessive	Yes	Extreme orthokeratotic hyperkeratosis, average granular layer, diffuse acanthosis
Psoriasiform ichthyosis (congenital psoriasis?)	Psoriasis in family	Yes	Parakeratosis, loss of granular layer, acanthosis with thin suprapapillary plate, Munro abscesses?
Sjögren–Larsen syndrome	Autosomal recessive	Yes	Lamellated orthokeratosis, normal or diminished granular layer, acanthosis with papillomatosis
Netherton's syndrome (ichthyosis linearis circumflexa with bamboo hairs)	Autosomal recessive?	Soon after	Orthokeratosis and parakeratosis depending on stage of eruption, variable granular layer, acanthosis, changes may be obscured by coexisting eczematous dermatitis, trichorrhexis invaginata
Erythrokeratodermia variabilis	Autosomal dominant	Sometimes	Hyperkeratosis with focal parakeratosis, average granular layer, acanthosis and papillomatosis, all depending on stage of disease
Biphasic ichthyosiform dermatosis (ichthyosis hystrix Curth–Macklin)	Autosomal dominant	No	Orthokeratotic hyperkeratosis above an incomplete granular layer, acanthosis and papillomatosis with binucleate prickle cells and "intracellular edema"
Refsum's disease	Autosomal recessive	No	Moderate acanthosis, hypergranulosis, hyperkeratosis, lipid vacuoles in basal cells
Acquired ichthyosis	None	No	Similar to ichthyosis vulgaris

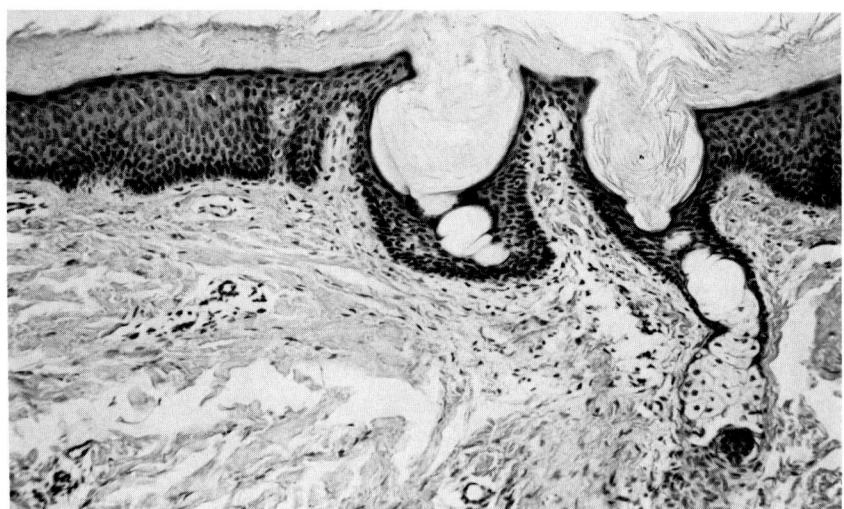

Figure 30–1.
Ichthyosis vulgaris. Compact orthokeratotic layer above a thin or defective granular layer. Rete malpighi usually is thinner than in this case. Sweat ducts and hair follicles have keratotic plugs. Sebaceous glands are small. H&E. X135.

derma (Chapter 34)[20–23] and subclinical lesions.[24] Recently, cases of disseminated palmoplantar keratoderma have been described, one of which was associated with truncal lesions.[25] Thus, somewhat similar to Darier's disease, a peculiar metabolic derangement of the epidermis can occur in a small island, in one or several dermatomes, or be more or less widespread or diffuse.

Collodion Baby

Collodion baby is not a single genetic disease. At birth the infant is encased in a shiny, brown-yellow membrane that has fissures and peels off within several weeks.[26] Affected infants most commonly develop lamellar ichthyosis. Some collodion babies clear and remain free of ichthyosis.[27]

Harlequin Fetus

Harlequin fetus is often born premature. The newborn is covered with a thick "armor plated" skin, which is split by fissures into polygonal plates. Respiratory movements are restricted, secondary infection is common, and death occurs within the first few weeks of life. It is probably inherited by an autosomal recessive trait.[28] Histologically, there is massive and dense hyperkeratosis with an average

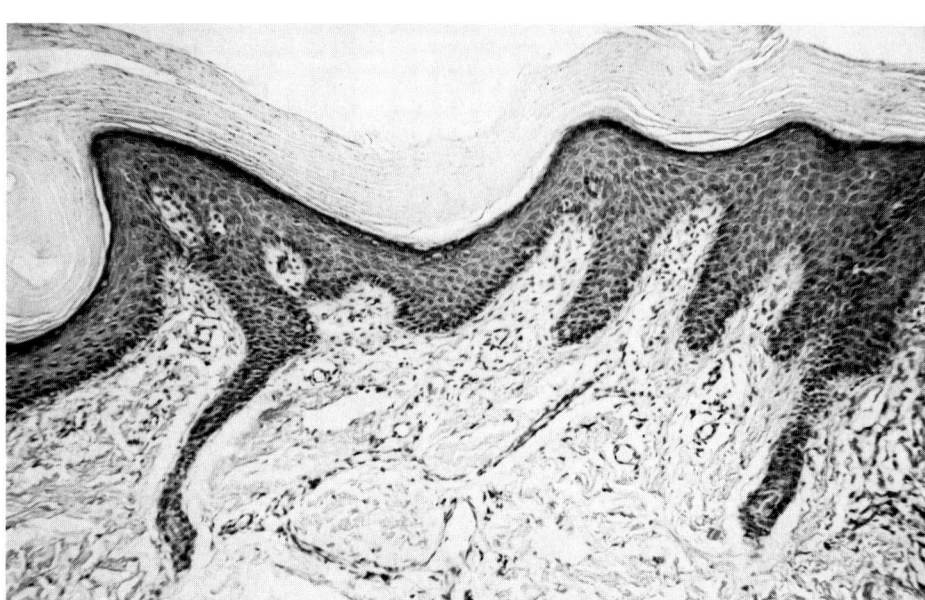

Figure 30–2.
Lamellar ichthyosis. Orthokeratotic horny layer rests on acanthotic epidermis with thick granular layer. Horny layer contains some melanin due to genetic pigmentation. H&E. X135.

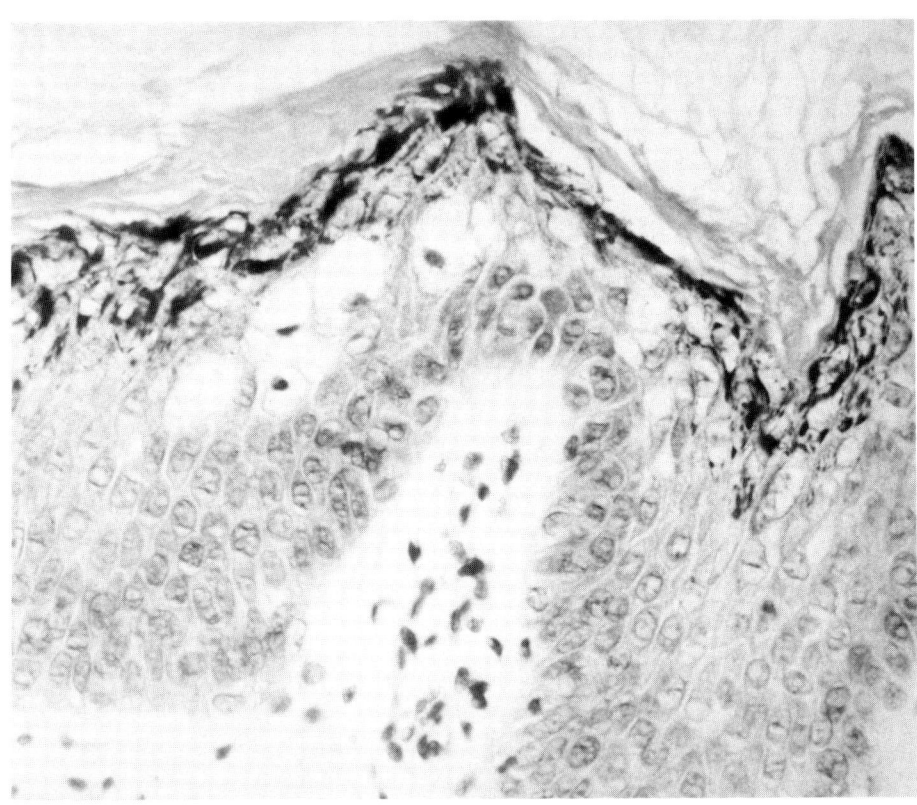

Figure 30—3.
Epidermolytic hyperkeratosis (so-called bullous type of ichthyosiform erythroderma). Ballooning pregranular and granular cells without signs of acantholysis predispose this epidermis to formation of bullae. H&E. X185.

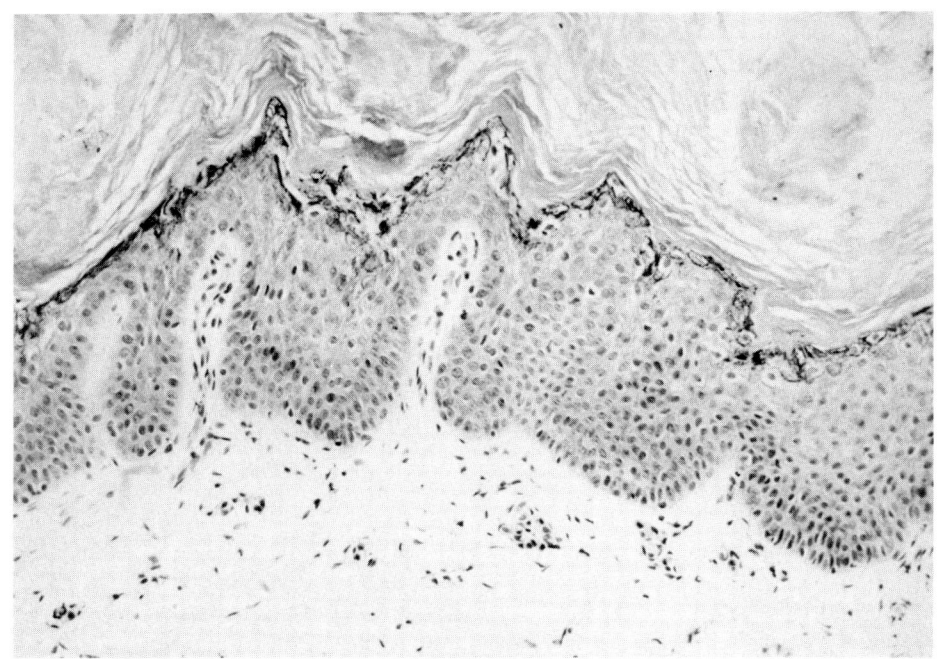

Figure 30—4.
Ichthyosis hystrix shows changes identical with epidermolytic hyperkeratosis. H&E. X135.

408   NONNEOPLASTIC EPITHELIAL AND PIGMENTARY DISORDERS

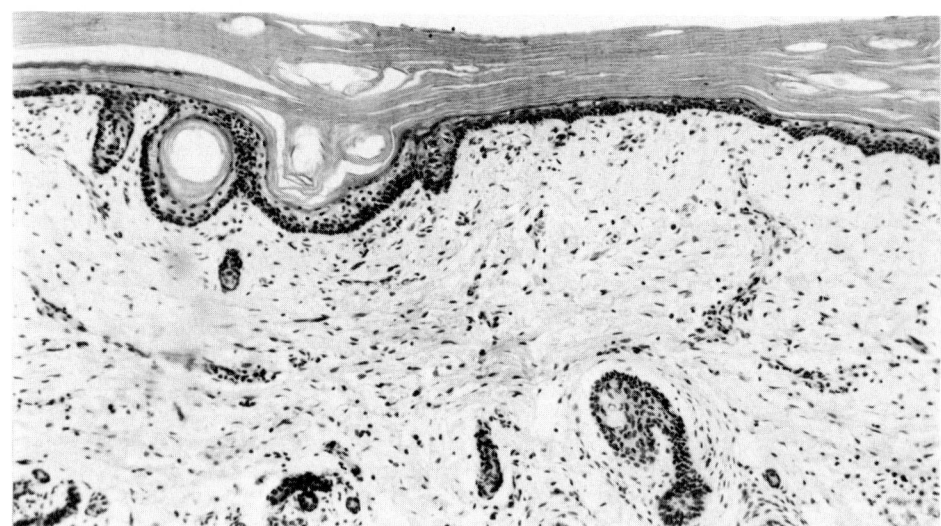

Figure 30–5.
Harlequin ichthyosis. Thick horny layer extends into the follicular orifices. H&E. X125.

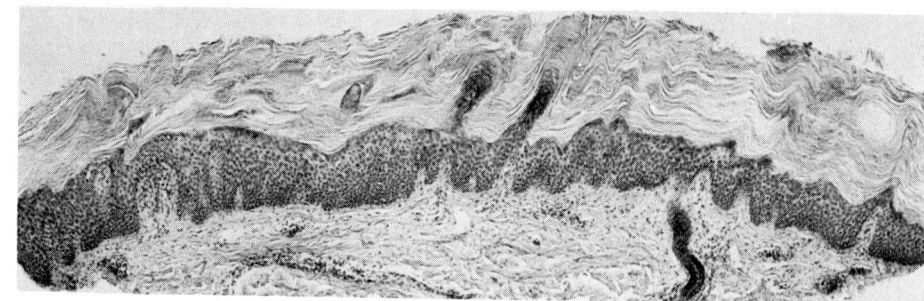

A

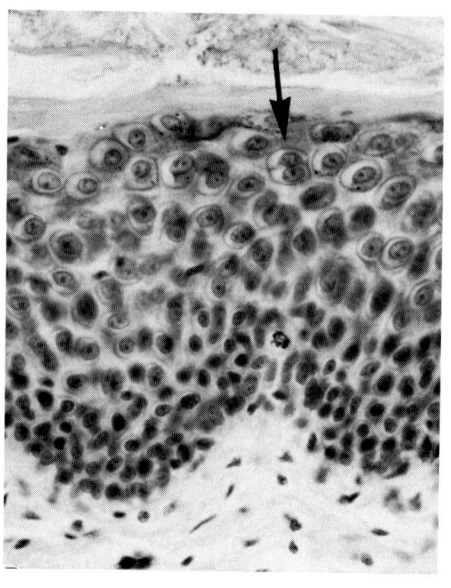

B

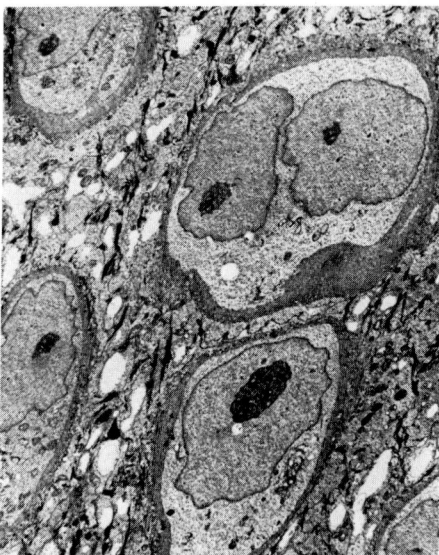

C

Figure 30–6.
Biphasic ichthyosiform dermatosis. **A.** Thick epidermis without keratohyalin layer and very thick orthokeratotic horny layer into which individual long papillae project. H&E. X45. **B.** At higher power, epidermis shows several mitoses and exhibits peculiar rings at some distance around nuclei. Note one binucleated cell (arrow). A few keratohyaline granules are visible. Cells flatten out into stratum corneum. H&E. X370. **C.** Electron Micrograph shows the biphasic structure of the cytoplasm. Mitochondria in inner phase, tonofilaments in outer realm separated by a shell. One binucleated cell. X4,500. (From Pinkus and Nagao. Arch Klin Exp Dermatol 237:737, 1970.)

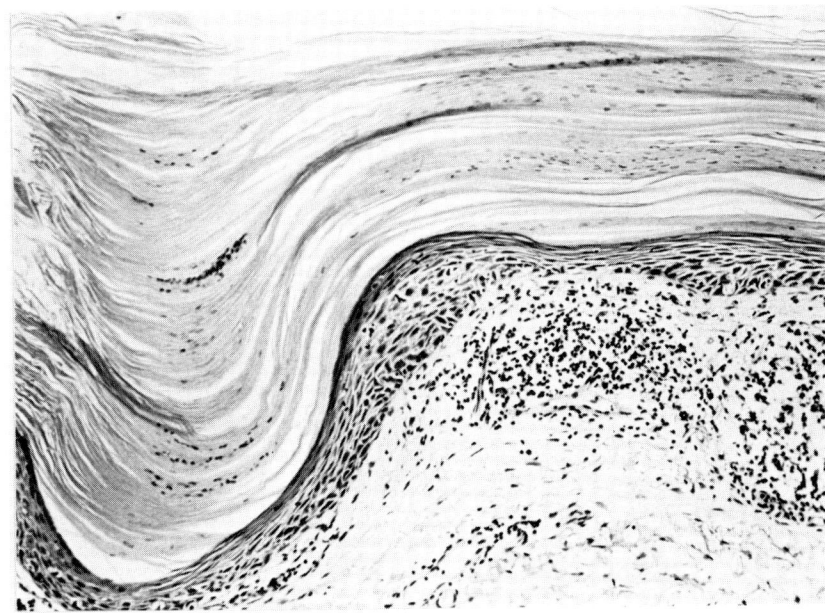

Figure 30–7.
Hyperkeratosis lenticularis perstans (Flegel's disease). A bandlike lymphocytic infiltrate below an atrophic and hyperkeratotic epidermis. H&E. X125.

thickness of granular layer[29,30] (Fig. 30–5). The granular layer may be reduced or even absent.[31]

Rare Forms of Ichthyoses

Erythrokeratodermia variabilis, a rare autosomal dominant disease, begins during infancy. Erythematous and hyperkeratotic plaques with polycyclic or circinate configuration occurs over the limbs, buttocks, and face.[32,33] Histopathologic changes are nonspecific and consist of epidermal acanthosis, hyperkeratosis, and some inflammatory cell infiltrate.

Ichthyosis linearis circumflexa, a rare autosomal recessive disease, has been associated with bamboo hairs (see Fig. 47–8) and other abnormalities such as atopic dermatitis.[34] In a personally observed case of biphasic ichthyosiform dermatosis,[6] an unusual clinical course was combined with unusual cytologic abnormalities (Fig. 30–6), consisting of a separation of the cytoplasm of prickle cells into edematous inner zones, tonofibril-rich outer zones, and thick orthokeratosis, in spite of defective keratohyalin formation. Similar hereditary cases were analyzed by Anton–Lamprecht et al.[35] Such observations make one feel that more variants of the ichthyotic process await identification.

Acquired Ichthyosis

Acquired ichthyosis applies to ichthyotic states that develop later in life as a symptom of malignancy.[36] Malnutrition has been implied as a cause as dry ichthyotic skin is not infrequently seen on the lower legs in marasmic patients. The diagnosis should be reserved for severe generalized conditions,[37] however. The histologic picture resembles that of ichthyosis vulgaris.

Hyperkeratosis Lenticularis Perstans (Flegel's Disease)

A genetic disease of autosomal-dominant type, Flegel's disease manifests itself as hyperkeratotic papules, mainly on the lower extremities.[38,39] The histologic picture consists of a bandlike inflammatory infiltrate in the papillary dermis and an epidermis that alternates between atrophy and acanthosis with peculiar tentlike elevations of the skin surface (Fig. 30–7).[40] Frank and Tapernoux[41] found a complete absence of lamellar bodies or cementosomes below the hyperkeratotic lesions, an observation confirmed by other groups.[42,43]

REFERENCES

1. Rand RE, Baden HP: The ichthyoses—A review. J Am Acad Dermatol 8:285, 1983
2. Williams ML: The ichthyoses-pathogenesis and prenatal diagnosis: A review of recent advances. Pediatr Dermatol 1:11, 1983
3. Burgdorf WHC, Alper JC, Goldsmith LA: Genodermatoses. J Am Acad Dermatol 16:1045, 1987

4. Harper PS: Genetic heterogeneity in the ichthyoses. In Marks R, Dykes PJ (eds): The Ichthyoses. New York: Spectrum, 1978, p 127
5. Lentz CL, Altman J: Lamellar ichthyosis: The natural clinical course of collodion baby. Arch Dermatol 97:3, 1968
6. Pinkus H. Nagao S: A case of biphasic ichthyosiform dermatosis: Light and electron microscopic study. Arch Klin Exp Dermatol 237:737, 1970
7. Stevanovic DV: Hodgkin's disease of the skin. Arch Dermatol 82:96, 1960
8. Flint GL, Flam M, Soter NA: Acquired ichthyosis. A sign of nonlymphoproliferative malignant disorder. Arch Dermatol 111:1446, 1975
9. Kauh YC, Goody HE, Luscombe HA: Ichthyosiform sarcoidosis. Arch Dermatol 114:100, 1978
10. Sybert VP, Dale BA, Malbrook KA: Ichthyosis vulgaris: Identification of a defect in synthesis of filaggrin correlated with an absence of keratohyalin granules. J Invest Dermatol 84:191, 1985
11. Shapiro LJ: X-linked ichthyosis. Int J Dermatol 20:26, 1981
12. Shapiro LJ, Weiss R, Buxman MM, et al: Enzymatic basis of typical X-linked ichthyosis. Lancet 2:756, 1978
13. Epstein EH Jr, Williams ML, Elias PM: Editorial: Steroid sulfatase, X-linked ichthyosis, and stratum corneum cohesion. Arch Dermatol 117:761, 1981
14. Bonifas JM, Epstein EH: Detection of carriers for X-linked ichthyosis by southern blot analysis and identification of one family with de novo mutation. J Inest Dermatol 95:16, 1990
15. Hazell M, Marks R: Clinical, histologic, and cell kinetic discriminants between lamellar ichthyosis and nonbullous congenital ichthyosiform erythroderma. Arch Dermatol 121:489, 1985
16. Williams ML, Elias PM: Heterogeneity in autosomal recessive ichthyosis. Clinical and biochemical differentiation of lamellar ichthyosis and nonbullous congenital ichthyosiform erythroderma. Arch Dermatol 121:477, 1985
17. Elias PM, Williams ML: Neutral lipid storage disease with ichthyosis. Arch Dermatol 121:1000, 1985
18. Holbrook KA, Dale BA, Sybert VP, Sagebiel RW: Epidermolytic hyperkeratosis: Ultrastructure and biochemistry of skin and amniotic fluid cells from two affected fetuses and a newborn infant. J Invest Dermatol 80:222, 1983
19. Ackerman AB: Histopathologic concept of epidermolytic hyperkeratosis. Arch Dermatol 102:253, 1970
20. Kanitakis J, Tsoitis G, Kanitakis C: Hereditary epidermolytic palmoplantar keratoderma (Vorner type). Report of a familial case and review of the literature. J Am Acad Dermatol 17:414, 1987
21. Larregue M, Bardy-Decrion I, Bonvalet D, et al: Keratodermie palmoplantaire de type epidermolytique. Experience therapeutique sur 13 ans. Ann Dermatol Venereol 114:1418, 1987
22. Hamm H, Happle R, Butterfass T, Traupe H: Epidermolytic palmoplantar keratoderma of Vorner: Is it the most frequent type of hereditary palmoplantar keratoderma? Dermatologica 177:138, 1988
23. Moriwaki S, Tanaka T, Horiguchi Y, et al: Epidermolytic hereditary palmoplantar keratoderma. Histologic, ultrastructural, protein-chemical and DNA analyses in two patients. Arch Dermatol 124:555, 1988
24. Mehregan AH: Epidermolytic hyperkeratosis. Incidental findings in the epidermis and in the intraepidermal eccrine sweat duct units. J Cutan Pathol 5:76, 1978
25. Mutasim D, Kurban AK: Disseminate palmoplantar keratodermia with truncal lesions. Dermatologia 168:296, 1984
26. Larregue M, Ottavy N, Bressieux J-M, Lorette J: Bebe collodion. Trente deux nouvelles observations. Ann Dermatol Venereol 113:773, 1986
27. Frenk E: A spontaneously healing collodion baby: A light and electron microscopic study. Acta Derm Venereol 61:168, 1981
28. Lawlor F, Peiris S: Harlequin fetus successfully treated with atretinate. Br J Dermatol 112:585, 1985
29. Buxman MM, Goodkin PE, Fahrenbach WH, et al: Harlequin ichthyosis with epidermal lipid abnormality. Arch Dermatol 115:189, 1979
30. Baden HP, Kubilus J, Rosenbaum K, Fletcher A: Keratinization in the harlequin fetus. Arch Dermatol 118:14, 1982
31. Unamuno P, Pierola JM, Fernandez E, et al: Harlequin foetus in four siblings. Br J Dermatol 116:569, 1987
32. Gewritzman GB, Winkler NW, Dobson RL: Erythrokeratodermia variabilis. A family study. Arch Dermatol 114:259, 1978
33. Hacham-Zadeh S, Evan-Paz Z: Erythrokeratodermia variabilis in a Jewish Kurdish family. Clin Genet 13:404, 1978
34. Greene SL, Muller SA: Netherton's syndrome. Report of a case and review of the literature. J Am Acad Dermatol 13:329, 1985
35. Anton-Lamprecht I, Curth HO, Schnyder UW: Zur Ultrastruktur hereditärer Verhornungsstörungen II. Ichthyosis hystrix Typ Curth-Macklin. Arch Dermatol Forsch 246:77, 1973
36. Humbert PH, Dupond J-L, Aqache P: L'ichtyose acquise. Ann Dermatol Venereol 115:937, 1988
37. Dykes PJ, Marks R: Acquired ichthyosis: Multiple causes for an acquired generalized disturbance in desquamation. Br J Dermatol 97:327, 1977
38. Sanchez-Jacob I, Miranda A, Perez Oliva N, Quinones PA: Hiperqueratosis lenticularis perstans (Flegel). Med Cutan ILA 17:321, 1989
39. Pearson LH, Graham Smith J Jr, Chalker DK: Hyperkeratosis lenticularis perstans (Flegel's disease). Case report and literature review. J Am Acad Dermatol 16:190, 1987
40. Price ML, Wilson Jones E, MacDonald DM: A clinicopathologic study of Flegel's disease (hyperkeratosis

lenticularis perstans) Br J Dermatol 116:681, 1987
41. Frenk E, Tapernoux B: Hyperkeratosis lenticularis perstans (Flegel): A biological model for keratinization occurring in the absence of Odland-bodies? Dermatologica 153:253, 1976
42. Ikai K, Murai T, Oguchi M, et al: An ultrastructural study of the epidermis in hyperkeratosis lenticularis perstans. Acta Derm Venereol 58:363, 1978
43. Tidman MJ, Price ML, MacDonald DM: Lamellar bodies in hyperkeratosis lenticularis perstans. J Cutan Pathol 14:207, 1987

31

PIGMENTARY DISORDERS

Pigmentary disorders not related to nevi or neoplasms manifest themselves clinically as either lightening or darkening of the skin. The histologic possibilities of producing these effects are manifold and are listed in Table 31–1.

The quantity of melanin is difficult to judge in H&E sections, especially when they are deeply stained with eosin. Here, the O&G stain proves its worth because melanin granules, having a proteinaceous base, turn greenish black and appear much darker against the light blue background of the epidermal cells. In the dermis, the same reaction permits one to differentiate melanin from hemosiderin and other pigments that do not change color. For additional data on identification of various colored substances, see Chapters 3 and 28.

DECREASE AND INCREASE OF EPIDERMAL MELANIN

Changes in quantity of epidermal pigmentation can be judged only when normal tissue is available for comparison. The untanned skin of whites can resemble that of an albino or can contain considerable melanin in the basal layer, depending on complexion. Visible melanin granules are usually restricted to basal cells, except in suntan and other forms of hyperpigmentation. Again depending on complexion, the epidermis of blacks may resemble brunet white skin but usually contains variable amounts of dark melanin granules in higher strata, including the horny layer. Oriental epidermis often contains a surprising amount of melanin granules, which, however, have a lighter hue in an unstained condition.

Depigmentation

If visible melanin is completely absent in epidermal cells, one must ascertain the condition of the junctional melanocytes. These may contain a few pigment granules even in very blond skin and in some conditions of hypopigmentation or may appear as clear cells of Masson, indistinguishable by light microscopy from similarly situated Langerhans cells.

Clear cells (nonkeratinocytes) are present in normal number in *total* and *partial albinism* but their ability to produce melanin is either reduced or is absent. In the tyrosinase negative form of oculocutaneous albinism there is complete lack of tyrosinase activity.[1] Some other forms show only reduced activity of this enzyme. Depigmented skin in all clinical forms of *vitiligo* show no recognizable melanocytes or melanin pigmentation.[2] Quantitative studies in vitiligo, using the electron microscope,[3] have shown that melanocytes are gradually replaced by indeterminate cells, containing neither melanosomes nor Langerhans granules, and that eventu-

TABLE 31–1. HISTOLOGIC SUBSTRATES OF LIGHTENED OR DARKENED SKIN

Clinical lightening
    Absence of epidermal melanin (leukoderma, vitiligo, nevus depigmentosus, albinism)
    Reduction of epidermal melanin (hypopigmentation, tinea versicolor achromians)
    Increased granular layer (lichen sclerosus et atrophicus, Wickham's striae)
    Increased dermal fibrosity (scars, lichen sclerosus et atrophicus, morphea)
    Diminished amount of blood (scars, nevus anemicus, Raynaud's phenomenon)

Clinical darkening
    Increase of epidermal melanin (suntanning, chloasma, freckles, lentigines, nevus spilus, nevus Ota, nevus Becker, chronic inflammation)
    Increase of subepidermal melanin (postinflammatory pigmentation, incontinentia pigmenti, lichen planus, lupus erythematosus, Mongolian spot, nevus Ota, blue nevus)
    Increased horny layer (acanthosis nigricans, papillomas, tinea versicolor, ichthyosis)
    Blood in horny layer (thrombosed angiomas, warts, black heel)
    Increased amount of blood in dermis (various hemangiomas and angiectasias, superficial hemorrhage)
    Hemosiderin (hemosideroses)
    Other pigments in dermis (tattoos, ochronosis, apocrin cystadenoma)

ally Langerhans cells take the place of melanocytes at the junction.

In repigmenting vitiligo, it is commonly seen that pigment arises and spreads from hair follicles. This mechanism has been confirmed by histoenzymatic studies in patients under oral photochemotherapy.[4] Follicular melanocytes become active, migrate up the length of the follicle, and spread laterally in the epidermis in a manner comparable to the repigmentation of burn wounds. Varying degrees of damage of keratinocytes are observed by electron microscopy at the periphery of depigmented skin areas.[5]

Another phenomenon seen occasionally in vitiligo is an erythematous infiltrated border.[6] Histologically, there is noncharacteristic inflammatory infiltrate with epidermal invasion by polymorphs and lymphocytes. It is questionable whether the inflammatory infiltrate is an indication of autoimmune mechanism. Increased frequency of antithyroid antibodies and association with autoimmune and endocrine diseases in patients with vitiligo tend to support an autoimmune etiology.[7-9] Depigmentation secondary to contact with chemical agents (occupational vitiligo) shows histologic changes identical to those of idiopathic vitiligo in light and electron microscopy.[10] In the Vogt–Koyanagi syndrome, which is certainly related to autoimmune processes, association of depigmenting melanocytes with lymphocytes has been reported.[11] In Chediak–Higashi syndrome,[12,13] melanocytes have abnormal, incompletely melanized granules which may be very large. Leukocytes in blood smears also contain large granules. The leaf-shaped hypopigmented spots of the tuberous sclerosis syndrome have melanocytes exhibiting weak tyrosinase reaction and incompletely melanized melanosomes.[14] *Nevus depigmentosus* is usually present at birth. Clinical patterns include isolated plaque, dermatomal and systematized forms with whorls and streaks in unilateral distribution.[15] Histologically, there are normal melanocytes containing normal-appearing melanosomes. The defect is in the transfer of melanosomes from melanocytes to the keratinocytes. Idiopathic guttate hypomelanosis is an acquired leukoderma consisting of numerous 2- to 8-mm hypopigmented macular spots over the extensor surfaces of arms and legs.[16] Histologically there is a sharply defined area of decreased melanin pigmentation of the basal layer and a diminished number of dopa-positive melanocytes.

So-called *incontinentia pigmenti achromians* (hypomelanosis of Ito)[17] is properly classified as a systematized hypochromic nevus and may be associated with mental, ocular, and osseous manifestations. It differs from vitiligo in the presence of vacuolated epidermal cells and normal melanocytes with decreased melanogenesis.[18,19]

A peculiar situation exists in epidermis that has regenerated after a burn or other denudation. The new epidermis usually carries a few melanocytes with it as it migrates over the wound surface. It is repopulated with melanocytes secondarily some weeks later[20] by migration from hair follicles and from the wound border and by local multiplication. Linear hypopigmentation may occur following intraarticular corticosteroid injection.[21]

Epidermal pigment is reduced in all forms of *tinea versicolor,* but this effect becomes clinically visible only in the *achromians* type, or after treatment of the disease in tanned skin. It seems to be due to inhibition of melanin production, disturbance in melanin transfer to keratinocytes, and vacuolar degeneration of melanocytes.[22] The depigmentation of Sutton's halo nevus and related phenomena is discussed in Chapter 33.

Hyperpigmentation

Sharply localized increase of epidermal melanin is seen in freckles (ephelis), chloasma (melasma), nevus spilus, solitary pigment spots of the lips and volar surfaces, and the various forms of lentigo. All these lesions are discussed in Chapter 33.

Generalized

General increase of epidermal melanization is responsible for the dark skin of Addison's disease and hemochromatosis.[23] In the latter, hemosiderin appears in the integument much later than the clinical bronzing, which is due to epidermal hyperpigmentation with melanin, and one should advise internists to take liver biopsies rather than skin biopsies for early diagnosis. Topically limited epidermal hyperpigmentation, is encountered in sun tanning. In this condition, all layers of the epidermis contain visible granules during the active phase of melanin production.[24] If exposure is discontinued, the melanin content of the outer layers gradually diminishes, but basal cell pigment may persist for many months. The combined effect of oral methoxsalen and external long wave ultraviolet (PUVA) therapy will result in generalized tanning and a number of irregularly pigmented lentiginous spots, some showing atypical melanocytes.[25,26]

Localized

Erythromelanosis follicularis faciei et colli is a fairly common condition.[27,28] It owes its clinically poikilodermatous features to a combination of focal epidermal hyperpigmentation with large sebaceous glands and telangiectasia and is confined to sun-exposed areas of the face and neck. In *linear and whorled nevoid hypermelanosis* streaks of macular hyperpigmentation occur in the pattern of Blaschko's line.[29] Histologically there is increased pigmentation of the basal layer and prominent vacuolization of melanocytes. Other types of hyperpigmentation are restricted to the acra of the extremities and are also better sorted out on the basis of their clinical appearance than on the histologic substrate of epidermal melanization. Reticulate acropigmentation of Kitamura,[30] zosteriform reticulate hyperpigmentation,[31] and acropigmentation of Dohi (acromelanosis albo-punctata[15]) are examples.

Melanin Block

Many types of chronic inflammation induce some epidermal hyperpigmentation, while others produce hypopigmentation. These phenomena were mentioned in their respective chapters. A paradoxic situation exists in black skin in chronic eczematous and other forms of dermatitis. Clinical darkening in these cases is due to increased blood supply and increased pigmentation. However, under the low power of the microscope, the acanthotic and spongiotic epidermis actually appears lighter. Close examination reveals that the keratinocytes contain less or no melanin. On the other hand, melanocytes appear highly dendritic (see Fig. 2–43B) and stuffed with pigment granules. This phenomenon of "melanin block" (see Fig. 2–45), or disruption of the functional epidermal melanin unit, spreads melanin over a larger area and dilutes it as far as tissue sections are concerned. On the other hand, it produces a clinical darkening effect similar to the one a frog produces by spreading melanin in its dermal melanophores.

INCREASE OF SUBEPIDERMAL MELANIN

Subepidermal melanin may be found in macrophages or in dermal melanocytes, only rarely free in the tissue. Barring histochemical demonstration of acid phosphatase in macrophages or tyrosinase in melanocytes, the best available criterion for differentiation of these cell types is the size and distribution of the granules, which are of small, even size and diffusely distributed in the melanin-forming cell, with the nucleus plainly visible. They are of uneven size and clumped in the macrophage and often obscure the nucleus by their great quantity. In these respects, macrophages containing melanin resemble those containing hemosiderin. The Giemsa stain will differentiate the two pigments without recourse to special measures. Subepidermal pigmentation due to dermal melanocytes is discussed in Chapter 33.

Subepidermal macrophage pigmentation is found in many chronic inflammatory diseases and may be associated either with epidermal hyperpigmentation or with epidermal pigment loss. The latter condition often exhibits focal damage to basal cells and melanocytes and melanosomes phagocytized by macrophages,[32] and is designated as "incontinentia pigmenti." It is present in the disease of that name (see the following heading) or as symptomatic incontinence in lichenoid tissue reactions, lupus erythematosus, lichen sclerosus et atrophicus, and poikilodermatous states. The leukomelanoderma of the chronically irritated skin in vagabond's disease also deserves mention here.[33]

Subepidermal melanophages are found without obvious basal layer derangement and often associated with some epidermal hyperpigmentation in *postinflammatory pigmentation* (Fig. 5–12). The pigment usually is retained for many months and may thus remain after all evidence of active disease, such as lichen planus or lupus erythematosus, has subsided. It is most prominently found in fixed drug eruptions. Its amount depends on the natural pigmentation of the skin and therefore is greatest in blacks, who exhibit the phenomenon of postinflammatory pigmentation following a variety of dermatoses which would not lead to appreciable deposition of pigment in macrophages in a light-complexioned skin. Postinflammatory pigmentation, therefore, is not diagnostic, although one may venture suggestions if there are associated remnants of a specific dermatosis or signs of acute flare-up of inflammation, as in a fixed drug eruption.

In cases in which neither clinical history nor histologic evidence suggests specific inflammatory disease, one may consider two rare dermatoses. One is the so-called Naegeli type of incontinentia pigmenti (*reticular pigmented dermatosis*), in which, according to Whiting,[34] transitory fragility of the epidermal melanin unit leads to loading of macrophages along the venous network. The other one was described in Japan as *pigmentatio maculosa multiplex* and is characterized clinically by brownish gray or bluish gray macules measuring from a few millimeters to 1 cm in diameter. Histologically, there is macrophage pigmentation with or without epidermal hyperpigmentation, but no evidence of significant inflammation.[35]

The diffuse melanosis secondary to malignant melanoma is probably due to perivascular deposition of melanin granules[36] but was found in one case[37] to be caused by diffuse spread of melanoma cells in the dermis.

Incontinentia Pigmenti

Further investigations of Bloch–Sulzberger's disease have shown that the characteristic streaky pigmentation is only the end stage of a chain of processes, which in the fully developed case start with blisters in the newborn period and often have an intermediate verrucous stage.[38] Incontinentia pigmenti is assumed to present an X-linked dominant mutation and is usually lethal in affected hemizygous males. Increased chromosomal instability has been reported in several families.[39]

Babies born with, or developing, vesicles or bullae soon after birth should be suspected to have incontinentia pigmenti, especially if they are female. The bulla, on histologic examination, shows accumulation of eosinophilic leukocytes (Fig. 31–1A) in the stratum spinosum. By the time the bullous stage subsides, the epidermis may become acanthotic and hyperkeratotic in a verrucous manner (Fig. 31–1C)

The epidermis usually contains large vacuolated cells (Fig. 31–1B), which electron microscopists have interpreted as degenerating melanocytes[40] or as macrophages.[41] The most characteristic feature is the presence of many small foci of whorling of prickle cells with central keratinization, which simulates cross sections of intraepidermal sweat ducts in individual sections but may be shown in serial sections to be independent of acrosyringia. These first stages are variable in their clinical expression and usually subside by the time the baby is 1 year old. It is only then that pigmentation becomes clinically apparent. Histologically, the disease develops gradually and presents the contrast (Fig. 31–1D) between dermal melanophages and a practically nonpigmented epidermis. A histologic picture somewhat similar to that illustrated in Figure 31–1B may be seen in the unrelated *pseudoatrophoderma colli*.[42]

OTHER INTRADERMAL COLORED MATTER

Hemosiderin is a common cause of dermal pigmentation, as described in Chapter 28. It should not be confused with the artifactual formalin pigment sometimes observed in blood-rich tissue sections (Chapter 3). Practically all other colored granular material present in the skin, is either due to "tattooing" (intentional or accidental) or to long-continued internal uptake of metals or certain modern drugs. Carbon particles are used for blue tattoos and may get into the skin accidentally, mainly as a professional hazard of miners. They are recognized in sections because they are truly black. Other granules may appear black in transillumination, for example, cinnabar and other pigments used in tattooing. Cinnabar crystals have a characteristic rounded shape, and examination with oil immersion usually brings out their red color. Sometimes examination in incident light may give a clue. White powders (such as the material contained in golf balls, paints, and other substances[43]), which have been accidentally tattooed into the skin, appear black in transmitted light but chalky in incident light.

Metal pigmentation is most commonly due to

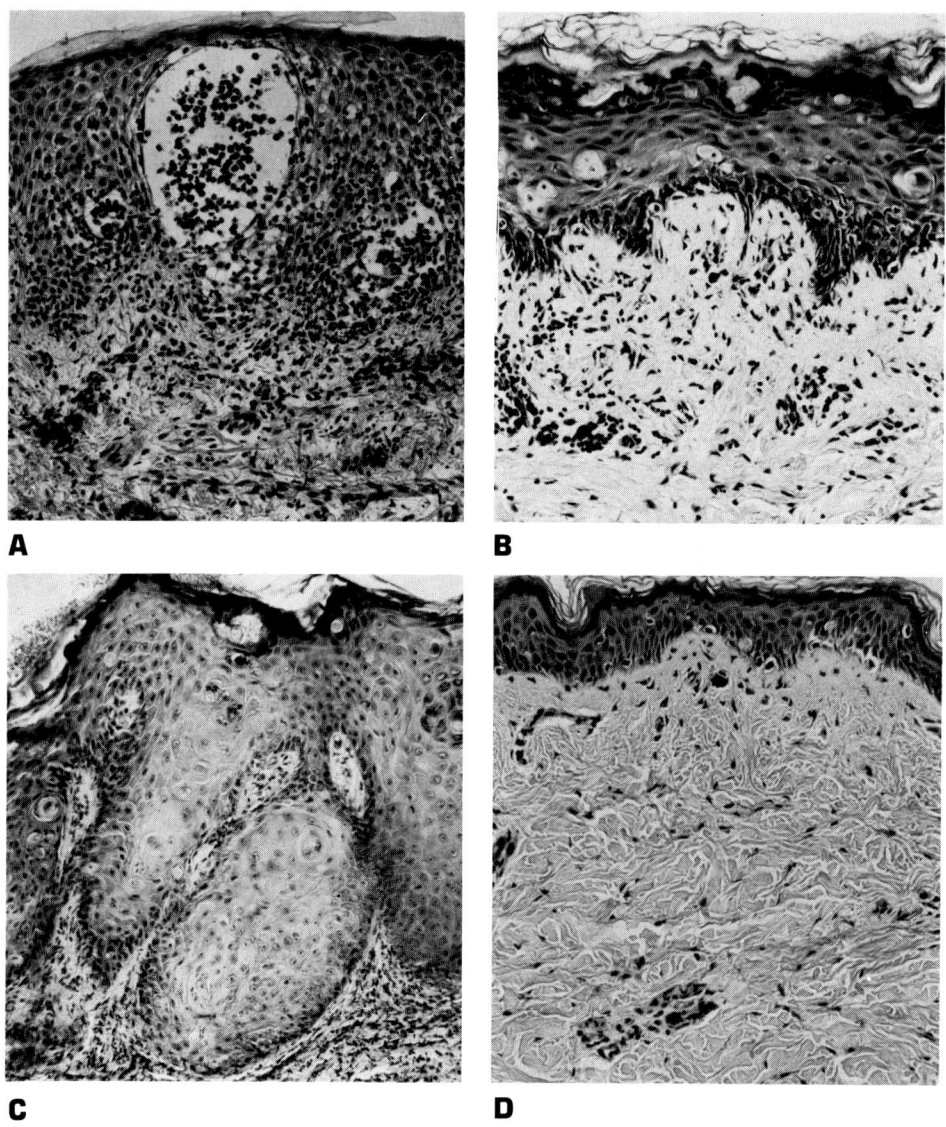

Figure 31–1.
Four stages of incontinentia pigmenti. **A.** Intraepidermal vesicles filled with eosinophils in newborn period. **B.** Hyperkeratotic and dyskeratotic phase often preceding verrucous stage shown in **C. D.** End stage of macrophage pigmentation below a nonpigmented, but otherwise fairly normal, epidermis. All H&E. X135.

silver (argyria), which may be seen as tiny black granules (Fig. 31–2) deposited in dermal tissue cells, fibers, and on the basement membrane of sweat coils, if it is present in profusion.[44] It is startlingly demonstrated, even in small amounts, by darkfield illumination x-ray microprobe, and electron microscopy[45] (Chapter 3). Localized argyria may occur on earlobes after wearing silver earrings.[46] Histologic changes similar to argyria is also observed secondary to gold (auriasis) and mercury.[47,48] Amalgam is sometimes introduced into oral tissues by the slip of a dental drill.

Peculiar discoloration of light-exposed skin has been observed after long-continued intake of certain tranquilizers, cardiac drugs, and other modern medicaments, notably minocycline and amiodarone.[49–51] Macrophages containing coarse pigment are found in the vicinity of dermal capillary blood vessels. The nature of the responsible pigments is not fully elucidated, but they are not necessarily melanin. The specific pigment of ochronosis[45] occurs more commonly in cartilage, but masses of it may be found in the skin (Fig. 31–3) and stain specifically dark with methylene blue. Exogenous cutaneous ochronosis occurs fol-

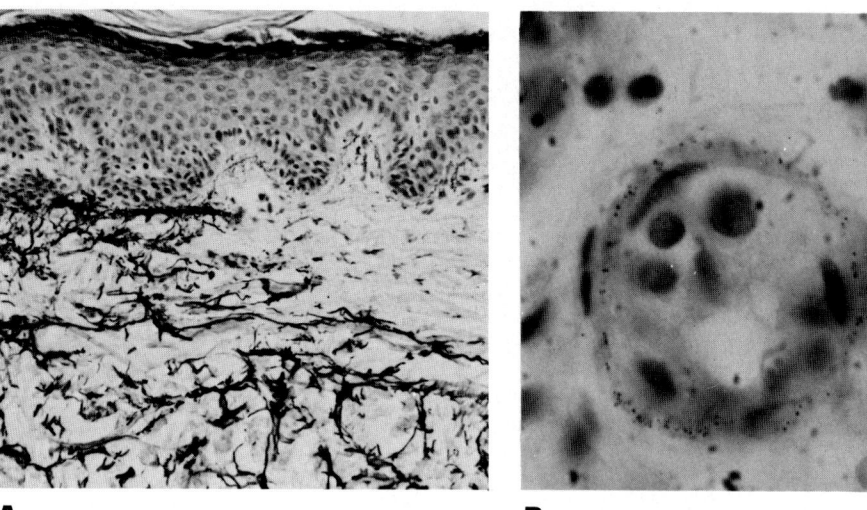

Figure 31–2.
Argyria. **A.** Silver amalgam inoculated into oral mucosa. Metal preferentially deposited on elastic fibers. H&E. X125. **B.** Argyria caused by ingestion. Silver granules preferentially deposited on basement membrane of eccrine secretory tubule. H&E. X540.

lowing prolonged use of strong hydroquinone bleaching creams.[52,53] The contents of epithelial cysts or apocrine cystadenomas may impart a dark blue hue to the overlying skin.

OTHER DERMAL CHANGES AFFECTING COLOR

Just as excessive blood makes the skin redder or darker, so does reduced content of blood make it look paler, as we can observe in cold weather when fingers and hands turn white. Permanently contracted vessels seem to be the only substrate in *nevus anemicus*,[54,55] while melanin, dermal structure, and structure of vessels appear normal in histologic section. Relative lack of vessels, together with increased density of collagen bundles, is the reason that scars remain lighter than surrounding skin long after the epidermis has regained its ability to pigment. The white color of lichen sclerosus et atrophicus and of atrophie blanche also is in part due to these factors. It takes a sharp eye and an open mind to recognize such rather subtle changes in tissue sections. Distinctly yellow color may be imparted to the skin not only by lipids but also by elastic tissue, as in pseudoxanthoma elasticum and actinic elastosis.

COLOR CHANGES DUE TO HORNY LAYER

On gross examination, thickened stratum corneum may look any hue from pale yellow (keratoderma

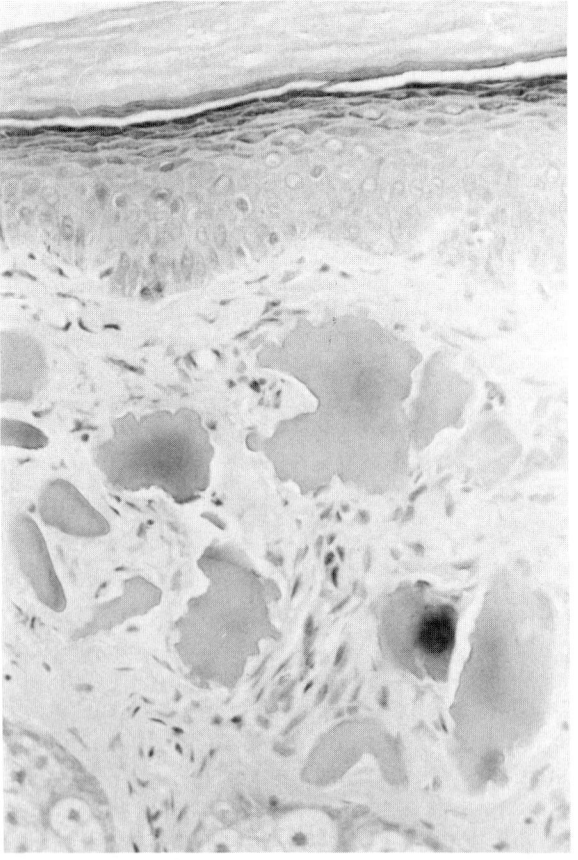

Figure 31–3.
Ochronosis. Irregular masses of brown material not related to cells in upper dermis of face. Unusually thick stratum granulosum and stratum corneum for this part of body. H&E. X250.

palmare) to grayish black (ichthyosis). It may express the color of contained melanin but often owes its tinge to other, ill-defined substances. In *acanthosis nigricans* one is often surprised by the small amount of melanin contained in a clinically very dark epidermis. Similarly, other verrucous papillomas, and particularly seborrheic verruca, may owe their dark color to keratin rather than melanin. The varied hues of *tinea versicolor* are due to a combination of erythema and thick horny layer, even in the presence of diminished melanization.[56] That the peculiar orange-yellow color in *carotinemia* is most pronounced in volar skin indicates that it resides mainly in the horny layer. These and other possibilities must be kept in mind when the clinically evident color of the skin seems to have no substrate in histologic sections.

Intrakeratinous traumatic hemmorrhage (Fig. 31–4) has been found to be the substrate of *black heel*, a condition encountered in young athletes.[57]

On the other hand, one has to remember that a thick stratum granulosum reflects and diffuses light. It can hide or change the color of underlying blood or melanin, giving it a bluish tinge. This was mentioned under lichen planus. Keratohyalin may even give the surface a chalky white color, as in lichen sclerosus et atrophicus or leukoplakia of the mucous membranes.

REFERENCES

1. Bolognia JL, Pawelek JM: Biology of hypopigmentation. J Am Acad Dermatol 19:217, 1988
2. Koga M, Tango T: Clinical features and course of type A and type B vitiligo. Br J Dermatol 118:223, 1988
3. Mishima Y, Kawasaki H, Pinkus H: Dendritic cell dynamics in progressive depigmentations: Distinctive cytokinetics of dendritic cells revealed by electron microscopy. Arch Dermatol Forsch 243:67, 1972
4. Ortonne J-P, Macdonald DM, Micoud A, et al: La repigmentation du vitiligo induite par la photochimiothérapie orale: Étude histoenzymologique (Split-Dopa) et ultrastructurale. Ann Dermatol Venereol 105:939, 1978
5. Bhawan J, Bhutani LK: Keratinocyte damage in vitiligo. J Cutan Pathol 10:207, 1983
6. Ortonne J-P, Baran R, Civatte J: Vitiligo à bordure inflammatoire: A propos de 2 observations avec revue de la littérature (18 cas). Ann Dermatol Venereol 106:613, 1979
7. Grimes PE, Halder RM, Jones C, et al.: Autoantibodies and their clinical significance in a black vitiligo population. Arch Dermatol 119:300, 1983
8. Sanchez JL, Vazquez M, Sanchez NP: Vitiligolike macules in systemic scleroderma. Arch Dermatol 119:129, 1983
9. Koranne RV, Derm D, Sachdeva KG: Vitiligo. Int J Dermatol 27:676, 1988
10. Stevenson CJ: Occupational vitiligo: Clinical and epidemiological aspects. Br J Dermatol 105(Suppl 21):51, 1981
11. Bazex A, Balas D, Bazex J, et al: Maladie de Vogt–Koyanagi–Harada. A propos de 2 observations. Ann Dermatol Venereol 104:849, 1977
12. Blume RS, Wolff SM: The Chediak–Higashi syndrome: Studies in four patients and a review of the literature. Medicine 51:247, 1972
13. Deprez P, Laurent R, Griscelli C, et al: La maladie de Chédiak–Higashi. A propos d'une nouvelle observation. Ann Dermatol Venereol 105:841, 1978
14. Denoeux J-P, Cesarini J-P, Carton F-X: Les mélanocytes dans l'épiloia: Aspects ultrastructuraux (à propos de 7 cas). Ann Dermatol Venereol 104:845, 1977

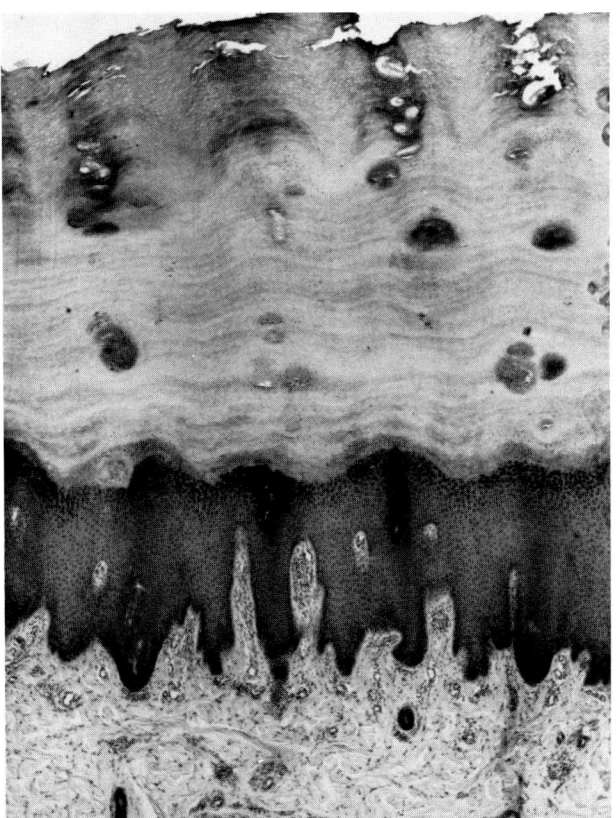

Figure 31–4.
Intrakeratinous hemorrhages of black heel (pseudochromidrosis). Dark areas in horny layer consist of inspissated erythrocytes, some of which are inside sweat ducts. Others result from capillary hemorrhage and enter the stratum corneum by transepidermal elimination. H&E. X45. (From Mehregan. Can Med Assoc J 95: 584, 1966.)

15. Foldes C, Wallach D: Les dyschromies congenitales. Ann Dermatol Venereol 114:1267, 1987
16. Falabella R, Escobar C, Giraldo N, et al: On the pathogenesis of idiopathic guttate hypomelanosis. J Am Acad Dermatol 16:35, 1987
17. Cambazard F, Hermier C, Thivolet J, Perrot H: Hypomelanose de Ito. Revue de la literature a propos de 3 cas. Ann Dermatol Venereol 113:15, 1986
18. Takematsu H, Sato S, Igarashi M, Seiji M: Incontinentia pigmenti achromians (Ito). Arch Dermatol 119: 391, 1983
19. Sybert VP: Hypomelanosis of Ito. Pediatr Dermatol 7:74, 1990
20. Staricco RG: Mechanism of migration of the melanocytes from the hair follicle into the epidermis following dermabrasion. J Invest Dermatol 36:99, 1961
21. McCormack PC, Ledesma GN, Vaillant JG: Linear hypopigmentation after intra-articular corticosteroid injection. Arch Dermatol 120:708, 1984
22. Charles CR, Sire DJ, Johnson BL, et al.: Hypopigmentation in tinea versicolor: A histochemical and electron microscopic study. Int J Dermatol 12:48, 1973
23. Chevrant-Breton J, Simon M, Bourel M, et al: Cutaneous manifestations of idiopathic hemochromatosis. Arch Dermatol 113:161, 1977
24. Langner A, Kligman AM: Tanning without sunburn with aminobenzoic acid-type sunscreen. Arch Dermatol 106:338, 1972
25. Senff H, Reinel D, Schaeg G: Puva-induced disseminated lentigines. Cutis 41:199, 1988
26. Rhodes AP, Harrist TJ, Momtaz-TK: The PUVA-induced pigmented macule: A lentiginous proliferation of large, sometimes cytologically atypical, melanocytes. J Am Acad Dermatol 9:47, 1983
27. Mishima Y, Rudner E: Erythromelanosis follicularis faciei et colli. Dermatologica 132:269, 1966
28. Colomb D, Racouchot J, Gho A, et al.: L'erythrosis interfollicularis colli de Leder. Ann Dermatol Venereol 104:238, 1977
29. Kalter CD, Griffiths AW, Atherton DJ: Linear and whorled nevoid hypermelanosis. J Am Acad Dermatol 19:1037, 1988
30. Wallach D, Dronne Ph, Foldes C, Cottenot F: Acropigmentation reticulee de Kitamura. Ann Dermatol Venereol 114:14600, 1987
31. Iijima S, Naito Y, Naito S, Uyeno K: Reticulate hyperpigmentation distributed in a zosteriform fashion: A new clinical type of hyperpigmentation. Br J Dermatol 117:503, 1987
32. Onoda S: The mechanisms of histological incontinence of pigment: Light and electron microscopic studies of lesions and patch test sites in female facial melanosis and DNCB reactions in guinea pigs. J Dermatol Tokyo 14:449, 1987
33. Grosshans E, Stoebner F, Basset A: La leukomélanodermie des vagabonds: Étude anatomopathologique et ultrastructurale. Ann Dermatol Syphiligr 99:141, 1972
34. Whiting DA: Naegeli's reticular pigmented dermatosis. Br J Dermatol 85 (Suppl 7): 71, 1972
35. Degos R, Civatte J, Belaïch S: La pigmentation maculeuse eruptive idiopathique. Ann Dermatol Venereol 105:177, 1978
36. Sexton M, Snyder CR: Generalized melanosis in occult primary melanoma. J Am Acad Dermatol 20:261, 1989
37. Konrad K, Wolff K: Pathogenesis of diffuse melanosis secondary to malignant melanoma. Br J Dermatol 91: 635, 1974
38. Garcia-Bravo B, Rodriguez-Pichardo A, Camacho-Martinez F: Incontinentia pigmenti. Etude de trois familles. Ann Dermatol Venereol 113:301, 1986
39. Roberts MW, Jenkins JJ, Moorhead EL, Douglass EC: Incontinentia pigmenti, a chromosomal instability syndrome, is associated with childhood malignancy. Cancer 62:2370, 1988
40. Wong CK, Guerrier CJ, MacMillan DC, et al: An electron microscopical study of Bloch–Sulzberger syndrome (incontinentia pigmenti). Acta Derm Venereol 51:161, 1971
41. Schaumburg-Lever G, Lever WF: Electron microscopy of incontinentia pigmenti. J Invest Dermatol 61:151, 1973
42. Kanan MW, Kendil E: Pseudoatrophoderma colli in a male. Br J Dermatol 81:65, 1969
43. Macaulay JC: Occupational high-pressure injection injury. Br J Dermatol 115:379, 1986
44. Pezzarossa E, Alinovi A, Ferrari C: Generalized argyria. J Cutan Pathol 10:361, 1983
45. Shelley WB, Shelley DE, Burmeister V: Argyria: The intradermal "photograph," a manifestation of passive photosensitivity. J Am Acad Dermatol 16:211, 1987
46. Van den nieuwenhuijsen IJ, Calame JJ, Bruynzeel DP: Localized argyria caused by silver earrings. Dermatologica 177:189, 1988
47. Pelachyk JM, Bergfeld WF, McMahon JT: Chrysiasis following gold therapy for rheumatoid arthritis: Ultrastructural analysis with x-ray energy spectroscopy. J Cutan Pathol 11:491, 1984
48. Bergfeld WF, McMahon JT: Identification of foreign metallic substances inducing hyperpigmentation of skin: Light microscopy, electron microscopy, and X-ray energy spectroscopic examination. In Callen JP, et al (eds): Advances in Dermatology, Vol 2. Chicago, Ill: Year Book Med Publishers, page 171, 1987
49. Serwatka LM: Minocycline-associated cutaneous pigmentation. J Assoc Mil Dermatol 14:10, 1988
50. Argenyi ZB, Finelli L, Bergfeld WF, et al: Minocycline-related cutaneous hyperpigmentation as demonstrated by light microscopy, electron microscopy and X-ray energy spectroscopy. J Cutan Pathol 14: 176, 1987
51. Rappersberger K, Honigsmann H, Ortel B, et al: Photosensitivity and hyperpigmentation in amiodarone-treated patients: Incidence, time course, and recovery. J Invest Dermatol 93:201, 1989

52. Phillips JI, Isaacson C, Carman H: Ochronosis in black South Africans who used skin lighteners. Am J Dermatopathol 8:14, 1986
53. Lawrence N, Bligard CA, Reed R, Perret WJ: Exogenous ochronosis in the United States. J Am Acad Dermatol 18:1207, 1988
54. Greaves MW, Birkett D, Johnson C: Nevus anemicus: A unique catecholamine-dependent nevus. Arch Dermatol 102:172, 1970
55. Daniel RH, Hubler WR, Wolf JE, et al: Nevus anemicus: Donor dominant defect. Arch Dermatol 113:53, 1977
56. Dotz WI, Henrikson DM, Yu GSM, Galey CI: Tinea versicolor: A light and electron microscopic study of hyperpigmented skin. J Am Acad Dermatol 12:37, 1985
57. Mehregan AH: Black heel: A report of two cases. Can Med Assoc J 95:584, 1966

32

VIRUS EPIDERMOSES

This chapter discusses proliferative epidermal lesions for which an infectious viral etiology is well established. These lesions are molluscum contagiosum and infectious warts.

MOLLUSCUM CONTAGIOSUM

The agent of molluscum contagiosum belongs to the large intracytoplasmic viruses of the pox group.[1] The umbilicated clinical papule is represented histologically in Figure 32–1 by an orderly, lobulated mass of stratified epithelium, which hangs down from the epidermis like a small septate tomato. Occasionally, the lesion may develop within a dilated hair follicle or in the wall of an epidermoid cyst and assume a large nodular dimension.[2,3] The keratinizing products of the thick wall of the molluscum are discharged into a central chamber, which opens to the surface through a relatively narrow pore. It is characteristic that only a certain percentage of the epithelial elements show evidence of viral infection, leaving a majority of cells to keratinize fairly normally. The altered cells (Fig. 32–1B) become recognizable in the low layers of the stratum spinosum. They exhibit a small hazy mass in their cytoplasm, which increases in size in the higher layers, compressing the nucleus and dislodging it to the periphery, where it is seen as a thin sickle in cross section.

The cells assume large ovoid shape as they enter the keratohyaline layer and are transformed into basophilic ellipsoid bodies of hyaline appearance in the horny layer. These "molluscum bodies" are seen in fresh unstained preparations of the material that can be squeezed from the pore of the molluscum. Special stains can demonstrate the "virus elementary bodies" in the intracytoplasmic mass. They are at the borderline of light microscopic visibility. Their cubelike shape has been demonstrated by electron microscopy.

Ordinarily, the molluscum is surrounded by a thin shell of finely woven connective tissue, and this permits the epithelial ball to be shelled out easily by firm lateral pressure. Occasionally, a lesion will become clinically inflamed. Histologically, there is then found a heavy mixed infiltrate that has granulomatous features and even may simulate lymphoma. This infiltrate, which is most likely an immune-mediated reaction, may lead to spontaneous disappearance of the lesion.[4,5] This inflamed type of lesion often is biopsied without the clinician's suspecting molluscum contagiosum. Inasmuch as the epithelial part may have been largely destroyed by the time the specimen is obtained or may have been dislodged and lost during surgery, such lesions offer considerable diagnostic difficulties, and in some cases only the identification of a few molluscum bodies in the purulent surface crust solved the riddle.

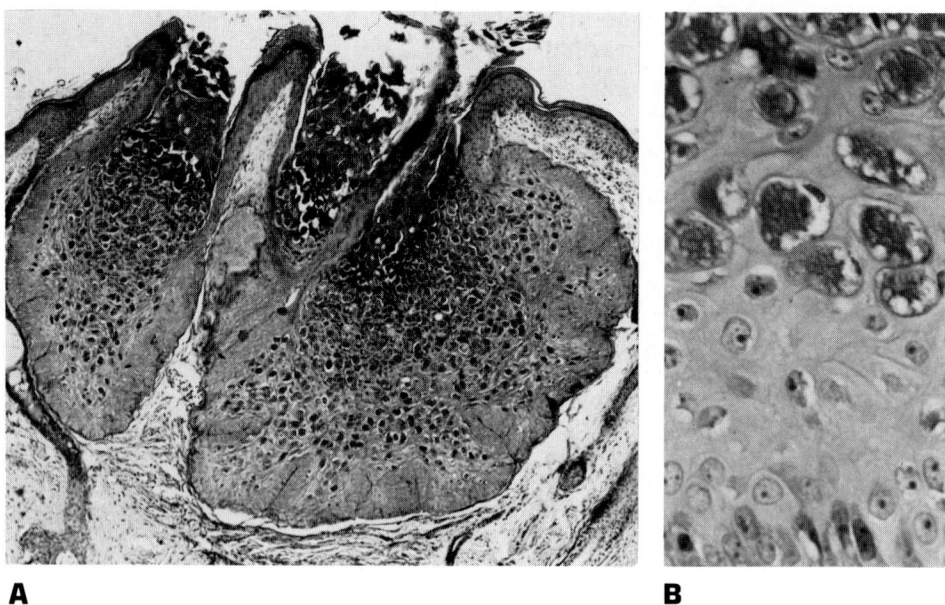

Figure 32–1.
Molluscum contagiosum. **A.** Aggregate of three mollusca. H&E. X60. **B.** Formation of molluscum bodies in hyperplastic epithelium. H&E. X280.

VIRUS WARTS

Under the general heading of virus warts we discuss the variants of verruca plana juvenilis, verruca plana, verruca vulgaris, verruca filiformis, verruca digitata, verrucae of the plantar type, condyloma acuminatum, epidermodysplasia verruciformis, and focal epithelial hyperplasia (Heck's disease). The virus or viruses of warts belonging to the papova group are very small and intranuclear. More than 50 types of human papilloma viruses (HPV) have been identified, each observed predominantly in one of the clinical manifestations.[6–9] The terminology in this field is changing rapidly. Table 32–1 lists various clinical forms of human papillomavirus infection and the types of HPV with which they are associated.

Human papilloma viruses manifest themselves in routine sections only by the presence of stainable nuclei in the horny layer above a thick granular layer. Although it has been shown by immunostaining that the stainable material is viral DNA rather than nuclear chromatin, it is their spheric shape (Fig. 32–2) that distinguishes these masses from ordinary flat parakeratotic nuclei in routine stains (Fig. 32–3).[10,11] Often, they are not present, and histologic diagnosis of the various types of virus warts must rely on other criteria.

TABLE 32–1. CUTANEOUS AND MUCOSAL MANIFESTATIONS OF HUMAN PAPILLOMAVIRUSES

	Clinical manifestation	Human papillomavirus type
Skin	Common verruca vulgaris	1, 2, 4
	Plantar warts	1, 4
	Palmar warts	2, 4, 7
	Verruca plana	3, 10
	Epidermodysplasia verruciformis	
	Verruca plana	3, 10
	Macular lesions	5,8,9,12,14, 15,17,19,25, 36,37,38
	Squamous cell carcinoma	5, 8, 14
Mucosa	Condyloma acuminata	6, 11
	Buschke–Loewenstein	6
	Bowenoid papulosis	6,18,31,33, 35,39,41,45, 51,56
	Focal epithelial hyperplasia (Heck's disease)	13,32
	Genital squamous cell carcinoma	16, 18

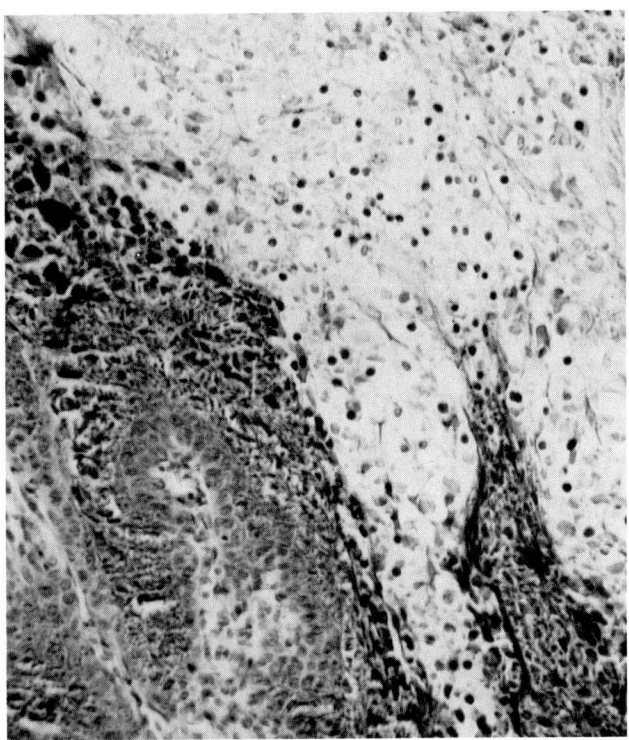

Figure 32–2.
Verruca vulgaris. Keratohyalin hyperplasia and spherical DNA inclusion bodies in horny layer simulating parakeratotic nuclei. H&E. X185.

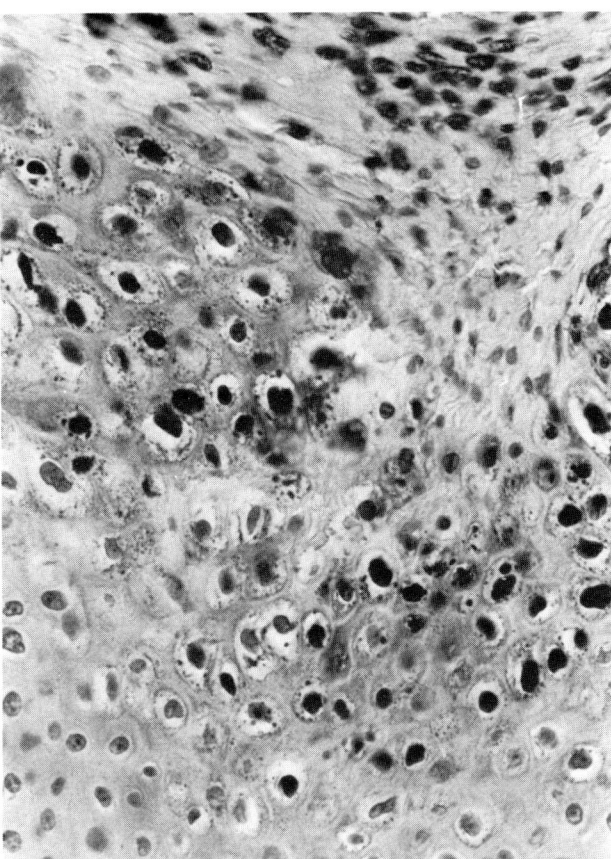

Figure 32–3.
Verruca vulgaris stained for papillomavirus common antigen by immunoperoxidase technique shows positive cells within stratum granulosum. Diaminobenzidine–hematoxylin X250.

One can put diagnosis on a more rational basis by remembering that all warts are verrucous papillomas and that cellular maturation is not impeded or grossly altered, in contrast to certain other epidermal papillomas and dysplastic precanceroses. That a flat wart should be a papilloma may sound surprising. Papilloma means circumscribed combined hyperplasia of epidermis and papillae, however, and one can usually find, even in a flat verruca (Fig. 32–4), one or two papillae that project so high that the suprapapillary plate is thin or elevated. In most viral warts, elongation of papillae is a prominent feature of diagnostic value.

Verruca Vulgaris

The prototype of all virus warts (Fig. 32–5) consists of thickened acanthotic epidermis, the mass of which greatly exceeds that of the thin, compressed, but elongated papillae. These cause the surface of the lesion to be elevated into cone-shaped projections covered with thin and often parakeratotic epithelium. While the granular layer is hyperplastic in the valleys, it becomes thinner on the slopes of the projections and is often absent at their tips, which appear covered with a stack of inverted hollow parakeratotic cones. The center contains scant connective tissue and a blood-filled capillary. The granular layer in the valleys is not only hyperplastic but contains unusually large and often angular blobs of keratohyalin, a very characteristic but not pathognomonic feature. In between, especially in young warts, there are large vacuolated cells with a central nucleus but few keratohyalin granules. Occasionally, a few of the above-mentioned spheric nuclei are seen in the thick, regularly lamellated, and otherwise orthokeratotic horny layer that fills the valleys. The living portion of the epidermis consists of large prickle cells in regular array, and the basal layer is well formed and shows a single row of cuboid or columnar cells. Inflammatory infiltrate is not a characteristic feature of common warts.

A very important feature is the centripetal di-

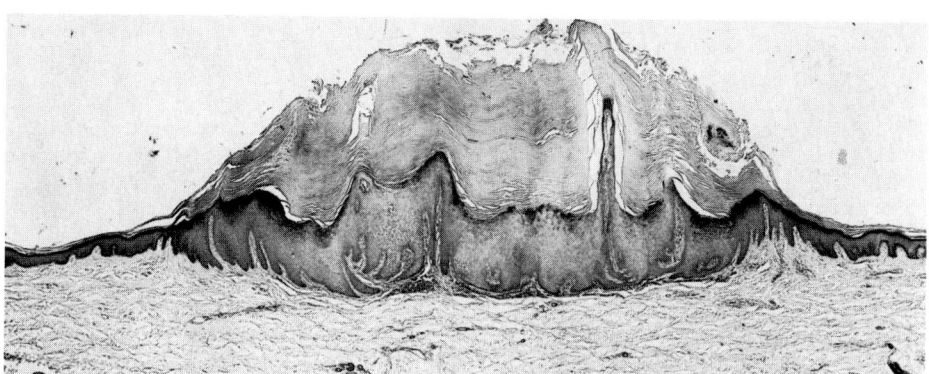

Figure 32–4.
Verruca vulgaris plana. Individual long papillae attest to papillomatous nature of lesion. Convergence of rete ridges is well shown. H&E. X35.

rection of the tips of rete ridges (Fig. 32–4). This is due to the expansive growth of the upper layers, which have become voluminous and have displaced the surrounding normal structures, while the lowest point of the ridges and the corresponding bases of the papillae remain fixed near the site of origin of the lesion. This convergence of the ridges, which actually is a sign that the vascular papillae diverge like the stamens of a flower, is in contrast to the divergence of any invasive epithelial tumor and a valuable sign in differential diagnosis.

The foregoing detailed description of the common wart was given for two reasons. It is the basis for differential diagnosis from other types of verrucous and papillomatous lesions and from malignant tumors. It is also the basis for understanding the variable features of other virus warts. Those of oral mucosa will be mentioned in Chapter 46.

Verruca Plana

Reduction of the papillomatous features of the common wart makes the surface smoother and gives the aspect of *verruca vulgaris plana* (Fig. 32–4). Hypergranulosis, elongation of some papillae, and convergence of rete ridges are characteristic features. *Verruca plana juvenilis* (Fig. 32–6) may show compressed papillae in a platelike thickened epidermis. Vacuolated cells, hypergranulosis, and the basketweave type of horny layer are the outstanding features. The latter is due to intracellular edema of prickle cells and is an exaggeration of an aspect of normal stratum corneum. In both cases, it is the walls of the keratinized cells that stain. The cells of the wart remain more bulky but look empty. It is not always easy to be sure of the border between normal and abnormal in this respect.

Plane warts occasionally undergo involution associated with clinical signs of inflammation. Histologically, the epidermis is infiltrated with inflammatory cells (Fig. 32–7), suggesting cell-mediated immunity.[12,13] Vacuolization is minimal and spotty parakeratosis may occur.[14]

Verruca Filiformis and Verruca Digitata

Exaggeration of the papillomatous features and extremely elongated papillae are found preferentially on the face and neck and around elbows and knees. If only a single papilla is involved, a filamentous growth results, and only this should properly be called *verruca filiformis*. If several papillae are forming long, fingerlike protrusions, we deal with *ver-*

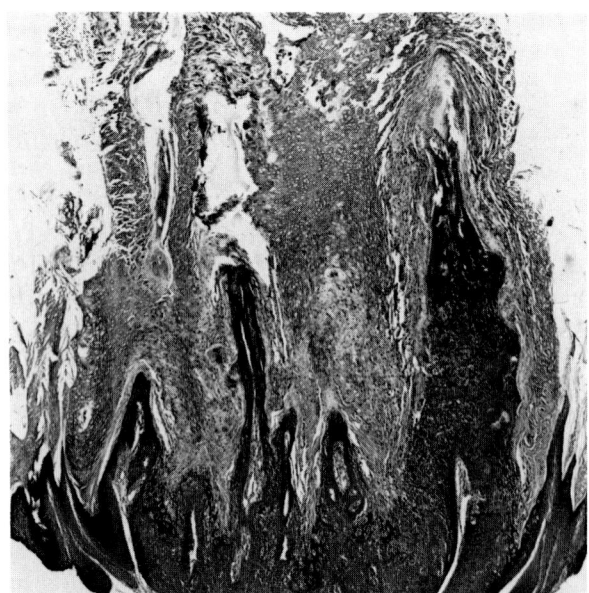

Figure 32–5.
Manifestly papillomatous verruca vulgaris combining features of digitate form with so much coherent hyperkeratosis that cutaneous horn results. H&E. X14.

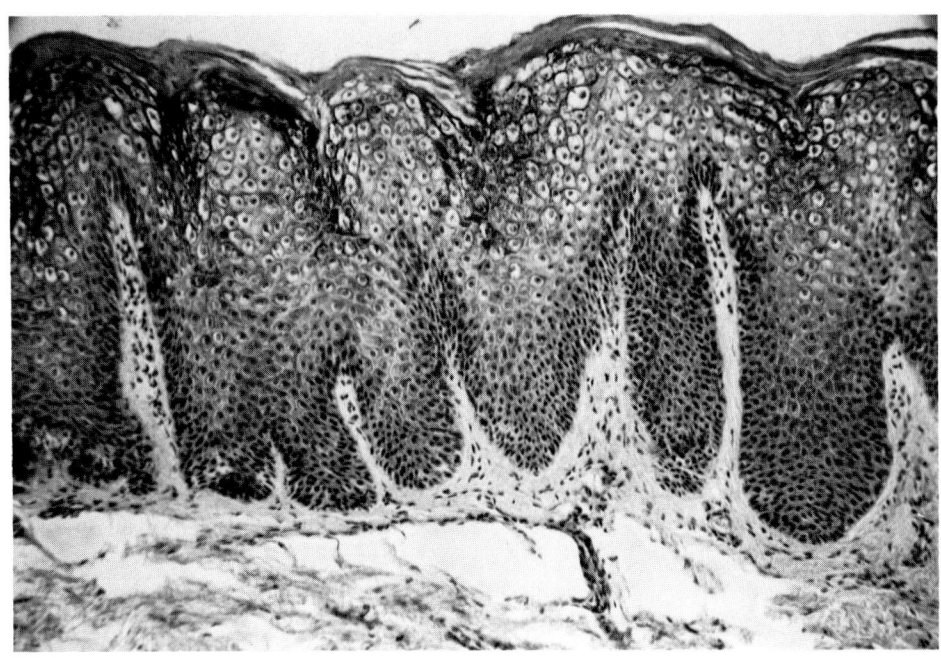

Figure 32–6.
Verruca plana. In this case, intracellular edema of the upper malpighian layers sets the stage for a basket-weave horny layer, but alteration has not reached stratum corneum. H&E. X135.

ruca digitata. In both cases, the papillae may branch, and their terminal portions, including the engorged capillaries, often become dehydrated in the thick horny layer, making the tips look black due to inspissated blood.

Verrucae of Plantar Type

Lesions with the histologic features of *verruca plantaris* (Fig. 32–8) may also be found on the volar surface of the hand, and even in the thickly keratinized dorsal portions of feet, hands, elbows, and knees. They represent an extreme degree of thickening of all epidermal layers above the stratum basale and grotesque exaggeration (see Fig. 32–2) of the keratohyalin formation already described for verruca vulgaris. In addition, virus-laden nuclei are prominent in the horny layer, and thin papillae become extremely long and form columns of dehydrated blood in the upper strata. The resulting picture, with

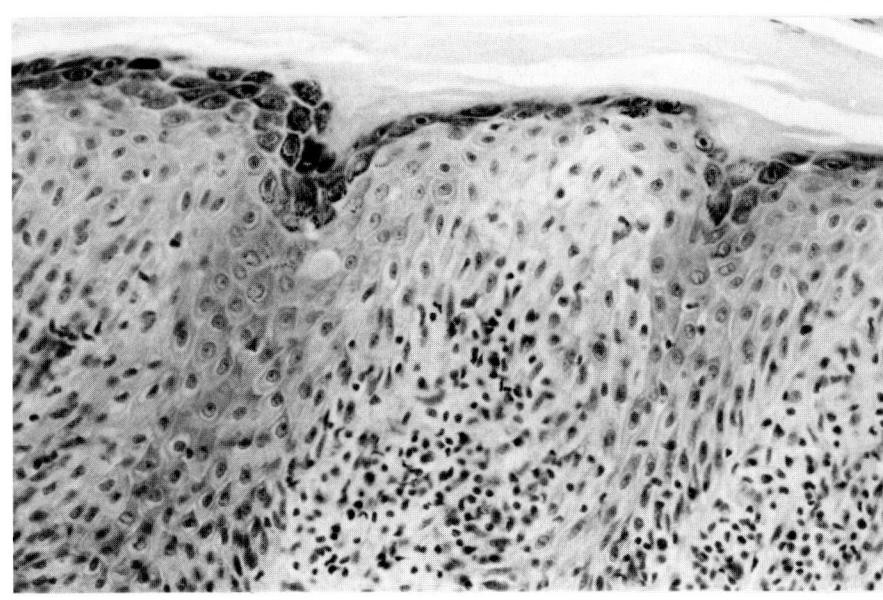

Figure 32–7.
Inflamed regressing verruca plana juvenillis. Keratinocytes of epidermis have small fading nuclei, and some vacuolated cells are left as the only characteristic of verruca. Cells of acrosyringium stain normally dark, have normal nuclei with nucleoli, and keratinize. H&E. X375.

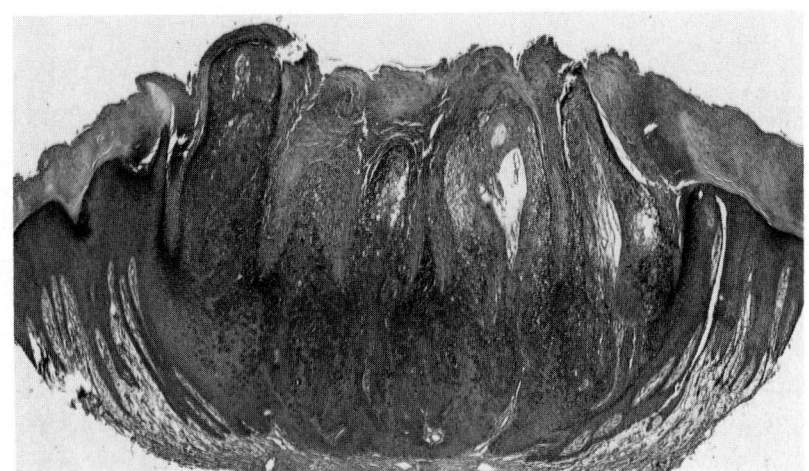

Figure 32–8.
Verruca vulgaris plantaris. Convergence of rete ridges makes possible removal of entire lesion with sharp curette without appreciable damage to underlying dermis. H&E. X14.

alternating columns of nucleated and nonnucleated horny layer, is highly characteristic but quite confusing to the uninitiated, especially if the sections were not cut vertically to the skin surface. A common error is to declare the large keratohyalin-filled cells as molluscum bodies. Close examination shows that they contain a spheric nucleus near the center rather than a compressed sickle-shaped one at the periphery, however, and that the stainable intracytoplasmic material consists of irregular masses of keratohyalin rather than of homogeneous globes of molluscum virus particles. The dehydrated blood in the long papillae is the basis for the diagnostic black dots that one sees when shaving a plantar wart, and deeper shaving leads to fairly profuse bleeding from the exposed capillaries. The convergent rete ridges cause a plantar wart to have a smooth lower contour, and a sharp-spoon curette can shell out the entire lesion as a glistening ball, with minimal damage to connective tissue. Knowledge of histopathology thus aids in diagnosis and rational treatment.

Condyloma Acuminatum

The question of whether warts in the moist skin of the genitoanal region owe their specific character to a different virus or just to the terrain in which they develop seems to be resolved in favor of a specific HPV-6 infection.[15–18] Actually, genital warts only rarely (Fig. 32–9) exhibit histologic evidence of the virus but are the purest example (Fig. 32–10A) of a cutaneous papilloma. The core consists of fairly loose collagenous tissue having a good blood supply and no or just a few thin elastic fibers. There is branching of papillae, and the epidermis is acanthotic with a variable amount of keratinization. There is no unusual hypergranulosis. The horny layer is orthokeratotic unless maceration causes parakeratosis. The prickle cells are large, show a well-developed system of tonofibrils and intercellular bridges, and a few vacuolated keratinocytes are present close to the surface of the lesion. The peculiar cytologic features caused by the therapeutic application of podophyllin are shown in Fig. 32–10B.

Differential Diagnosis

It may be difficult to differentiate condyloma acuminatum histologically from a papillomatous epidermal nevus, especially when the lesion is situated in a relatively dry area, such as the shaft of the penis. Lesions on the female genitalia are more often macerated and superinfected and exhibit inflammatory infiltrate and parakeratosis. On the other hand, it is usually easy to rule out malignancy if one pays attention to the presence of large stratified prickle cells above a single layer of basal cells. Mitoses often are seen in the basal layer, but rarely in great number. Nuclei are evenly sized and normochromatic. Difficulty arises in cases of *giant condylomata acuminata* (Buschke–Loewenstein type), which develop in a preputial sac and break through the foreskin. Although these are as a rule clinically benign, malignant behavior and metastasis have been recorded, and histologic differentiation from verrucous carcinoma of mucous membranes[19] must be based on examination of ample material from the borders as well as the depth of the lesion (Chapter 46).

A follow-up study of 746 cases with condyloma acuminatum in Rochester, Minnesota, revealed subsequent development of anaplastic genital lesions in 42 instances. There appears to be an association be-

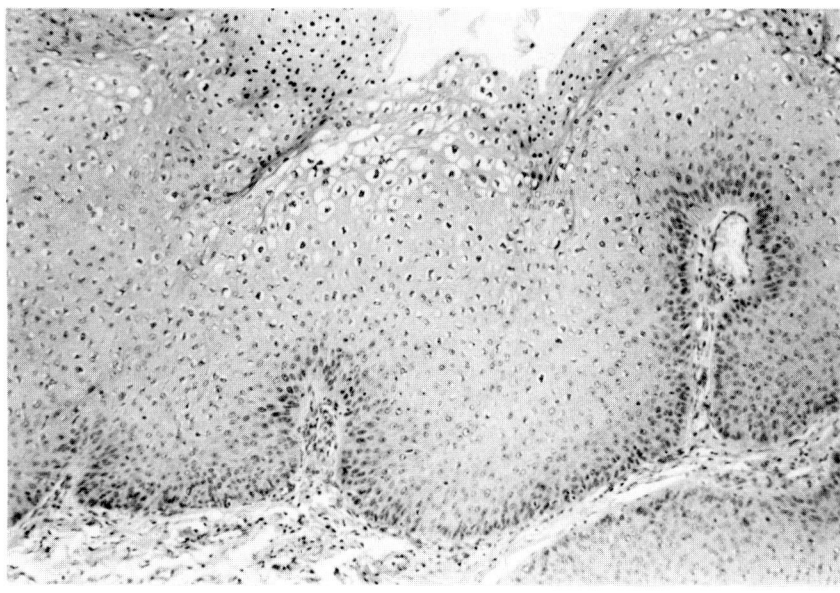

Figure 32–9.
Condyloma acuminatum showing vacuolated cells and viral inclusion bodies resembling parakeratotic nuclei. H&E. X135.

tween condyloma acuminatum and genital malignant neoplasms.[20-21]

Bowenoid Papulosis

The importance of clinical information in interpretation of histologic findings is highly exemplified in the lesion of bowenoid papulosis. The lesions are often multiple papules resembling lichen planus, psoriasis, or flat type of condyloma acuminatum involving the penis or vulva of young individuals (Fig. 32–11). Histologically, the acanthotic epidermis shows marked dysplasia with the presence of cells

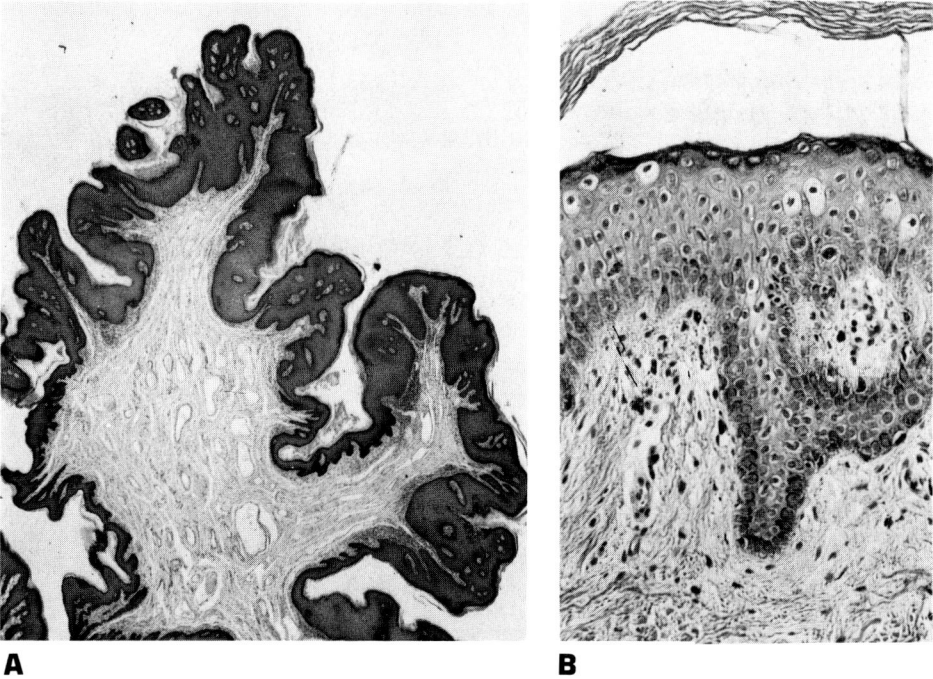

Figure 32–10.
Condyloma acuminatum. **A.** Relatively dry lesion shows fibroepithelial, papillomatous character. H&E. X13. **B.** Shows effects of podophyllin treatment (podophyllin cells). H&E. X209.

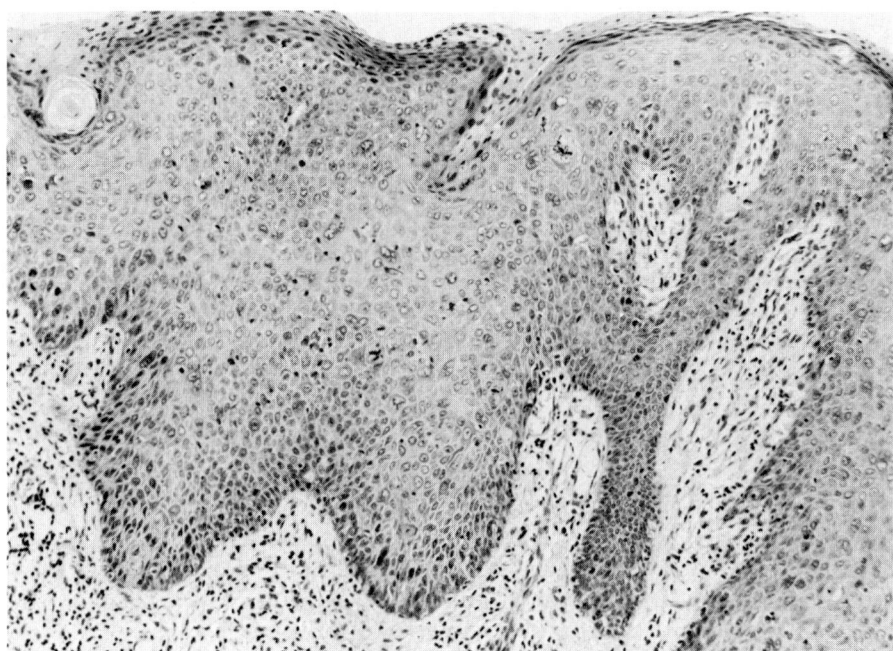

Figure 32–11.
Bowenoid papulosis. The general unrest of the acanthotic epidermis, the presence of multinucleated epidermal cells and many scattered mitotic figures sets this lesion apart from the large but regular appearance of prickle cells in condyloma acuminatum. H&E. X125.

with large and hyperchromatic nuclei, multinucleated cells, and scattered mitotic figures closely resembling Bowen's disease.[22–24] There may be associated typical lesions of condyloma acuminatum. Some lesions may disappear spontaneously. Virus-like particles have been demonstrated by electron microscopy and human papillomavirus antigens are located by immunostaining.[25–27]

An increased incidence of cervical neoplasia in females or sexual partners of male patients with bowenoid papulosis has been reported.[28]

Epidermodysplasia Verruciformis

It has been long recognized that flat warts and macular lesions of epidermodysplasia verruciformis show changes similar to those of verruca plana.[29] Moderate epidermal acanthosis with hypergranulosis, vacuolization, and basket-weave hyperkeratosis are present. A partial defect of cell-mediated immunity has been reported.[30] Electron microscopy has demonstrated papillomavirus in the nuclei of keratinocytes. The histologic findings of large epidermal cells with hyperchromatic nuclei and dyskeratotic cells indicate the beginning malignant transformation (Fig. 32–12).[31,32]

Focal Epithelial Hyperplasia (Heck's Disease)

Another papillomavirus-induced lesion is Heck's focal epithelial hyperplasia, which was initially re-

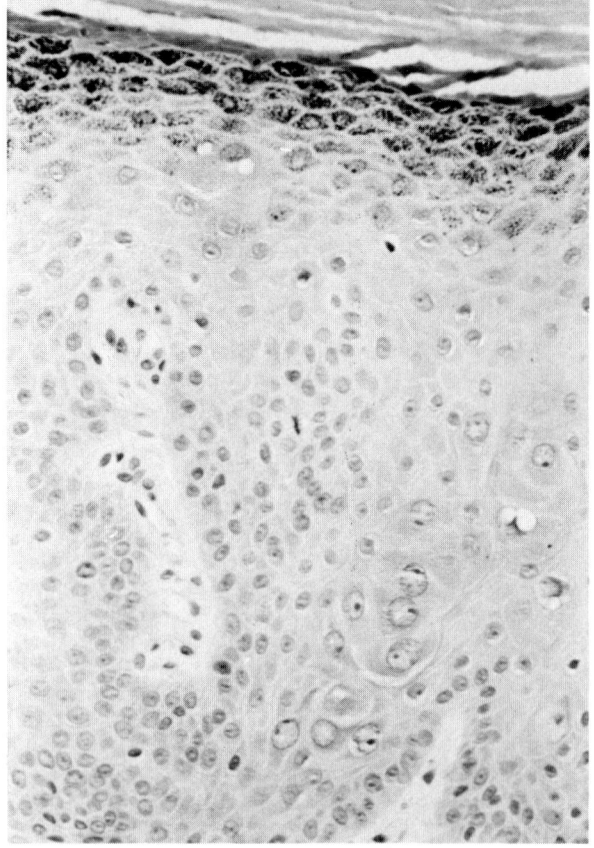

Figure 32–12.
Epidermodysplasia verruciformis exhibiting nests of large cells with large nuclei and prominent nucleoli suggesting transformation into malignant neoplastic cells. H&E. X400.

ported among Eskimos and Canadian Indians but also occurs elsewhere.[33,34] Usually multiple white papular and nodular lesions are situated anywhere within the oral mucosa, including the tongue. Histologically, the mucosal epithelium is markedly acanthotic and shows many large vacuolated cells. HPV-13 and HPV-32 have been identified as the causative agents.[35,36]

REFERENCES

1. Becker TM, Blount JH, Douglas J, Judson FN: Trends in molluscum contagiosum in the United States 1966–1983. Sex Trans Dis 13:88, 1986
2. Aloi FG, Pippione M: Molluscum contagiosum occurring in an epidermoid cyst. J Cutan Pathol 12:163, 1985
3. Brandrup F, Asschenfeldt P: Molluscum contagiosum-induced comedo and secondary abscess formation. Pediatr Dermatol 6:118, 1989
4. Pinkus H, Frisch D: Inflammatory reactions to molluscum contagiosum, possibly of immunologic nature. J Invest Dermatol 13:289, 1949
5. Kipping HF: Molluscum dermatitis. Arch Dermatol 103:106, 1971
6. Cobb MC: Human papillomavirus infection. J Am Acad Dermatol 22:547, 1990
7. Gross G, Ikenberg H, Gissmann L, et al: Papilloma virus infection of the anogenital region: Correlation between histology, clinical picture, and virus type. Proposal of a new nomenclature. J Invest Dermatol 85:147, 1985
8. Lynch PJ: Warts and cancer: The onchogenic potential of human papilloma virus. Am J Dermatopathol 4:55, 1982
9. Koutsky LA, Galloway DA, Holmes KK: Epidemiology of genital human papillomavirus infection. Epidemiol Rev 10:122, 1988
10. Penneys NS, Mogollon RJ, Nadji M, Gould E: Papillomavirus common antigens: Papillomavirus antigen in verruca, benign papillomatous lesions, trichilemmoma, and bowenoid papulosis: An immunoperoxidase study. Arch Dermatol 120:859, 1984
11. Eng AM, Jin Y-T, Matsuoka LY, et al: Correlative studies of verruca vulgaris by H&E, PAP immunostaining and electronmicroscopy. J Cutan Pathol 12:46, 1985
12. Aiba S, Rokugo M, Tagami H: Immunohistologic analysis of the phenomenon of spontaneous regression of numerous flat warts. Cancer 58:1246, 1986
13. Iwatsuki K, Tagami H, Takigawa M, Yamada M: Plane warts under spontaneous regression. Immunopathologic study on cellular constituents leading to the inflammatory reaction. Arch Dermatol 122:655, 1986
14. Berman A, Winkelmann RK: Involuting common warts: Clinical and histopathologic findings. J Am Acad Dermatol 3:356, 1980
15. Brescia RJ, Jenson BA, Lancaster WD, Kurman RJ: The role of human papillomaviruses in the pathogenesis and histologic classification of precancerous lesions of the cervix. Human Pathol 17:552, 1986
16. Turner MLC: Human papillomavirus infection of the genital tract. Prog Dermatol 23(2):1, 1989
17. Cassenmaier A, Hornstein OP: Presence of human papillomavirus DNA in benign and precancerous oral leukoplakia and squamous cell carcinoma. Dermatologica 176:224, 1988
18. Rudlinger R, Grab R, Buchanan P, et al: Anogenital warts of the condyloma acuminatum type in HIV-positive patients. Dermatologica 76:277, 1988
19. Dawson, DF, Duckworth JK, Bernhardt H, et al: Giant condyloma and verrucous carcinoma of the genital area. Arch Pathol 79:225, 1965
20. Chuang TY, Perry HO, Kurland LT, Ilstrup DM: Condyloma acuminatum in Rochester, Minn., 1950–1978: I. Epidemiology and clinical features. Arch Dermatol 120:469, 1984
21. Chuang T-Y: Condyloma acuminata (genital warts). An epidemiologic view. J Am Acad Dermatol 16:376, 1987
22. Rudlinger R, Grob R, Yu YX, Schnyder UW: Human papillomavirus-35-positive bowenoid papulosis of the anogenital area and concurrent human papillomavirus-35-positive verruca with bowenoid dysplasia of the periungual area. Arch Dermatol 125:655, 1989
23. Patterson JW, Kao GF, Graham JH, Helwig EB: Bowenoid papulosis. A clinicopathologic study with ultrastructural observations. Cancer 57:823, 1986
24. Steffen C: Concurrence of condyloma acuminata and bowenoid papulosis. Confirmation of the hypothesis that they are related conditions. Am J Dermatopathol. 4:5, 1982
25. Gross G, Hagedorn M, Ikenberg H, et al: Bowenoid papulosis. Presence of human papillomavirus (HPV) structural antigens and of HPV 16-related DNA sequences. Arch Dermatol 121:858, 1985
26. Guillet GY, Braun L, Masse R, et al: Bowenoid papulosis. Demonstration of human papillomavirus (HPV) with anti-HPV immune serum. Arch Dermatol 120:514, 1984
27. Gross G, Hagedorn M, Ikenberg H, et al: Bowenoid papulosis. Presence of human papillomavirus (HPV) structural antigens and of HPV 16-related DNA sequences. Arch Dermatol 121:858, 1985
28. Obalek S, Jablonska S, Beaudenon S, et al: Bowenoid papulosis of the male and female genitalia: Risk of cervical neoplasia. J Am Acad Dermatol 14:494, 1986
29. Jablonska S, Orth G, Jarzabek-Chorzelska M, et al: Epidermodysplasia verruciformis versus disseminated verrucae planae: Is epidermodysplasia verruciformis a generalized infection with wart virus? J Invest Dermatol 72:114, 1979
30. Majewski S, Skopinska-Rozewska E, Jablonska S, et al: Partial defects of cell-mediated immunity in pa-

tients with epidermodysplasia verruciformis. J Am Acad Dermatol 15:966, 1986
31. Orth G, Jablonska S, Jarzabek-Chorzelska M, et al: Characteristics of the lesions and risk of malignant conversion associated with the type of human papilloma virus involved in epidermodysplasia verruciformis. Cancer Res 39:1074, 1979
32. Yabe Y, Yashi M, Yoshino N, et al: Epidermodysplasia verruciformis: Viral particles in early malignant lesions. J Invest Dermatol 71:225, 1978
33. Samson J, Fiore-Donno G, Avizara N: L'hyperplasie epitheliale focale: Premiers cas suisse et revue de la litterature. Dermatologica 171:308, 1985
34. Beaudenon S, Praetorius F, Kremsdorf D, et al: A new type of human papillomavirus associated with oral focal epithelial hyperplasia. J Invest Dermatol 88:130, 1987
35. Civatte J, Jaubert A, Orth G, Cavelier-Balloy B: Hyperplasie focale epitheliale de Heck associee a HPV 32. Ann Dermatol Venereol 113:945, 1986
36. Cobb MW: Human papillomavirus infection. J Am Acad Dermatol 22:547, 1990

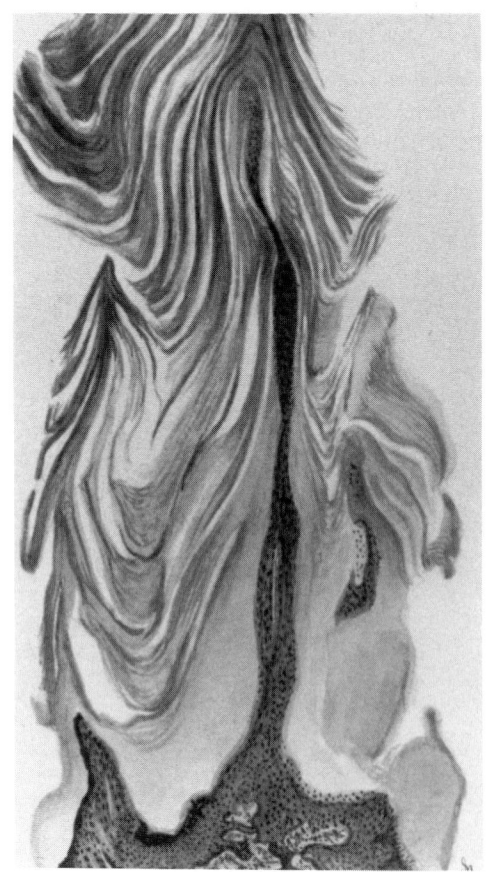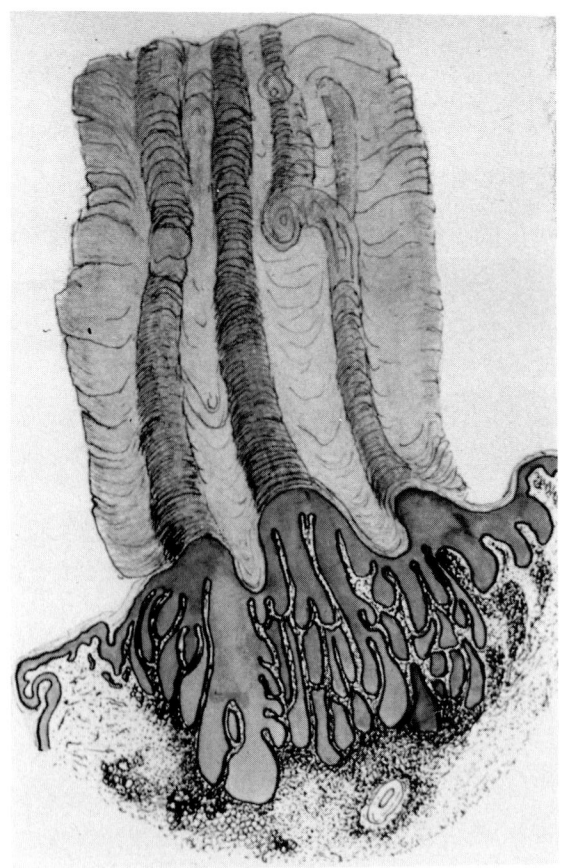

Digitate verruca vulgaris (*left*). Cutaneous horn (*right*).

SECTION VII

MALFORMATION AND NEOPLASIA

In those chapters dealing with inflammatory diseases in the widest sense, we are concerned with normal cells reacting to certain stimuli and either dying or returning to normal when the disease heals. Even though healing of the skin organ might take place with scar formation or atrophy, there is no permanent derangement of the tissue cells. When discussing certain epithelial diseases, such as Darier's or ichthyosis, we assume that the metabolism of all epidermal cells is genetically deranged but that the clinical and histologic expression of the derangement depends on internal or external regulatory factors and can be reversed or suppressed temporarily. Similarly, when the metabolism of mesodermal cells is deranged, as in angiokeratoma of Fabry or the mucopolysaccharidoses, we can expect to overcome the general but specific enzymatic deficiency by supplying the missing enzyme, withholding the substrate that cannot be metabolized, or administering the lacking end product.

We discuss virus epidermoses as tumorlike but different from neoplasia because of the presence of an identifiable virus and because of known immunologic reactions that lead to spontaneous destruction or involution of the epidermal derangement. Possibility of progression from a viral papilloma to a true neoplasm underlines the distinction.

We now come to disorders that are localized, since only a local focus of cells is deranged, but that can be cured only by removal or destruction of the cells involved because the derangement is *permanent* and its expression more or less *independent* of regulatory influences. The cellular derangement may be present at birth, due to either inheritance or prenatal events, or it may occur at any time in life due to internal or external factors (e.g., radiation). Once it has occurred, the change is permanent and is transmitted to the offspring of the deranged cell.

It is important, for diagnostic interpretation, to keep these concepts clearly in mind, even though there are borderline cases in which a decision is difficult. Exact definitions and distinct terminology take us further than a denial that limits can be drawn. Having defined the field of this section as localized disturbances due to heritable derangement of specific tissue cells, we subdivide it into malformations and neoplasias. A *malformation* is stable, or relatively so. It consists of excess or deficiency of one or several of the normal constituents of the skin and usually is designated as a "nevus." We shall, however, have to discuss the nevus concept in more detail later. A *neoplasm* consists of cells that not only are present in excess but also are retarded in their maturation and often deviate from normal cells in other morphologic or functional characteristics. One of the basic features of a neoplasm is that it is not stable but increases in size due to either excessive proliferation or delayed death of its constituent cells. A neoplasm may be benign or malignant, depending on the ability of its cells to destroy normal tissue and to metastasize. There are neoplasms that fit into neither the benign nor the malignant classification, as we shall discuss later.

In this section we do not describe in detail every malformation or neoplasm that occurs in the skin. We give, rather, a conceptual framework into which the known nevi and tumors fit and into which unusual cases, and even as yet unclassified lesions, can be fitted. We have done this in previous publications when eccrine poroma, apocrine cystadenoma, tumor of follicular infundibulum, pilar sheath acanthoma, and melanoacanthoma were recognized as entities worth identifying within the larger categories of benign sweat apparatus tumor (hidradenoma), benign follicular tumor, and benign epidermoid tumor.

NEVUS

The term "nevus" has been used and misused in so many ways that it has become almost meaningless. It deserves, however, to be preserved because, if properly defined, it describes one category of skin lesions for which no better name is available. The present confusion has its basis in history and stems from a time when the nature of the nevus cell was unknown and nevus was used for almost any inborn circumscribed mark on the skin. It came to mean what we call a "pigmented mole" just as well as a nevus sebaceus, epidermal nevus, or strawberry mark. We recommend a return to the classic concept outlined by Jadassohn[1] and Darier[2] and prefer to make their definition even more precise, as follows. "A nevus is a circumscribed stable malformation of the skin, not due to external causes and, therefore, thought to be of congenital origin. It consists of local excess of one or several of the normal mature constituents of the skin organ. Minus nevi are similarly defined as local deficiency due to underdevelopment of one or several constituents (aplasia cutis congenita, nevus depigmentosus, nevus anemicus)." Jadassohn pointed out that a supernumerary digit is a malformation, but not a neoplasm (tumor) or a hyperplasia, and that, similarly, a localized excessive accumulation of sebaceous glands is not a neoplasm, nor is it described sufficiently as hyperplasia, but it deserves the name "nevus sebaceus," which implies congenital origin, stability, and maturity. The words "hamartoma" and "phakoma" are not suitable substitutes because they are formed with the suffix -oma, indicating neoplasia, and they do not include the concept of mature tissue. We must, however, recognize that nevus as defined here includes tissue nevi and organoid nevi but excludes the melanocytic *nevus* or *nevus cell nevus*, which is a benign tumor consisting of peculiar abnormal cells and undergoing evolution and involution. The definition also separates nevi from *nevoid tumors*, lesions that are thought to arise on a congenital basis but exhibit retarded maturation of cells, deviate in essential points from normal histologic structures, and show continued growth, even though this may be slow. For these nevoid tumors, the term "hamartoma" is well suited. We shall see later that these distinctions have practical as well as theoretical significance.

BENIGN VERSUS MALIGNANT TUMORS

Benign and malignant are old clinical terms that are not even restricted to the field of neoplasia. Malignant hypertension and Degos' malignant atrophic papulosis are examples. When a modern pathologist tries to define benign and malignant tumors, considerable difficulties are encountered. The borderline is not sharp (Fig. VII–1), and malignant transformation may progress by steps. Features such as rapid growth, cellular atypiae, invasion, and metastasis

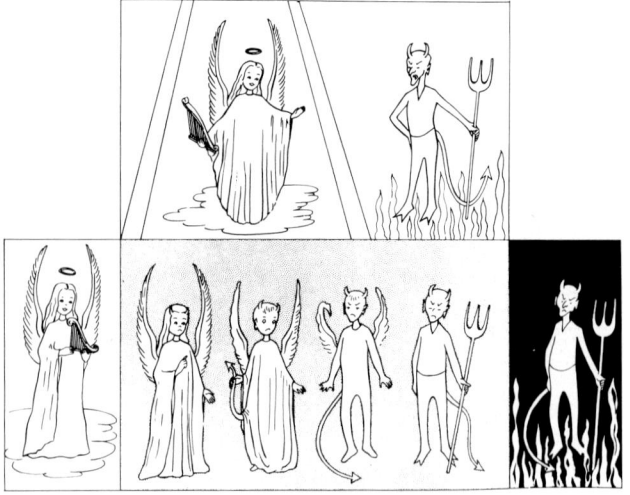

Figure VII–1.
The borderline between benign and malignant is not sharp; there is a broad, gray border zone. (Adapted from Fig. 183 in Hamperl: Lehrbuch der allgemeinen Pathologie und der pathologischen Anatomie, 28th ed. New York, Springer-Verlag, 1968.)

usually are named as characteristic of malignant tumors. One needs only to think of keratoacanthoma, lymphomatoid papulosis, and nodular fasciitis to find cutaneous lesions that have one or several of these attributes but are not biologically malignant. The only absolute proof of malignancy in the sense of modern oncologic knowledge is metastasis, because it proves the existence of a self-perpetuating and relatively autonomous cancer cell. Metastasis, however, is a clinical phenomenon and, as far as skin tumors are concerned, does not help the histopathologist in the evaluation of a given primary tumor.

It has become quite clear that as dermatopathologists we must include in our considerations not only quite benign tumors and definitely malignant tumors, but in-between categories of which there are three: precanceroses, pseudocancers, and basaliomas.[3] We must also keep in mind that our diagnosis includes prognostication and implied advice to the clinician on what to expect and how to handle a given tumor. We thus exceed the pathologist's basic task of doing morphologic interpretation, and we become partners in patient care. We must, therefore, know the therapeutic philosophy of the clinician in regard to a certain diagnosis. It is not wise to give a diagnosis of carcinoma in situ instead of actinic keratosis or of basal cell carcinoma instead of very superficial basal cell epithelioma to a practitioner to whom the word "carcinoma" is the trigger for extensive surgery.

A general classification of epithelial nevi and neoplasms is given in Table VII–1. The table is based on degree of maturation (morphologic differentiation) of the constituent cells and on the direction in which they are determined (embryologic differentiation). The question of histogenesis needs to be reviewed in the light of new information. Traditionally, the origin of adnexal tumors has been credited to the pluripotential matrix cells of the epidermis and the adnexal structures. The theory of pluripotentiality was advanced by experimental data obtained in the process of wound healing and dermabraision. It was observed that the epidermis and the lost portions of various structures are replaced by proliferation of cells of the surrounding epidermis and the residual portions of the underlying adnexa. It was postulated that the matrix cells of the epidermis and the cutaneous adnexa are able to undergo modulation (return to a quasi-embryonic state) and later to differentiate in other directions. These cells are therefore pluripotential and are equally capable of giving rise to a variety of adnexal neoplasms.

On the other hand, different classes of adnexal tumors appear predominantly within areas where those specific structures are most concentrated. Follicular tumors are most commonly located over the head and neck areas, eccrine tumors on the palms and soles, and the apocrine neoplasms within the apocrine triangle. In addition, the adnexal tumor cells retain significant portions of the enzyme histochemical patterns, ultrastructural features, and antigenic properties of their normal counterparts.[4] These features have been used for identification and proper classification of the adnexal tumors. It appears, therefore, that we cannot eliminate the possibility that adnexal tumors originate from cells of cutaneous adnexa, toward which they are differentiated and with which they share enzyme histochemical pattern, ultrastructural characteristics, and antigenic properties.[5]

The use of the word "differentiation" in the two very different meanings of determination (embryologists) and maturation (pathologists) has caused considerable confusion, because the undifferentiated (immature) cell of a malignant tumor is actually more highly differentiated (determined), being incapable of producing anything but more tumor cells of its own kind. It cannot be contended that maturation of a squamous carcinoma cell into a keratinized flake means return to a more normal state. Certainly, a keratinizing cell that has left the mitotic pool is no longer malignant, but only because it is committed to death, just as other cancer cells that die as mucinous blobs or just fade away. This example cannot be used to raise false hopes of our ability to revert malignant cells to viable normal ones. An exceptional situation seems to exist in the field of basaliomas[6] and is discussed in Chapter 40.

The classification of epithelial lesions shown in Table VII–1 has been compared with Mendeléeff's Periodic Table of the Elements. This classification actually has made it possible to predict the existence of certain tumors, which had not been identified previously. The vertical arrangement, however, represents a spectrum rather than a set of pigeonholes. Not infrequently tumors are encountered that do not exactly fit any of the slots. Classification, after all, is an ordering process of the human mind. The classification presented here has been the most satisfactory one in our work, but nature is apt to come up with exceptions that do not fit human rules, and it is not necessary to give new names to all minor variants.

Classifications of lesions of pigment-forming

TABLE VII–1. CLASSIFICATION OF FIBROEPITHELIAL NEVI AND NEOPLASMS

Level of Maturation	Epidermis	Direction of Differentiation			
		Sebaceous Gland	Hair Follicle	Apocrine Gland	Eccrine Gland
Hyperplasia (nevi)	Verrucous epidermal nevus	Organoid nevus	Hair nevus	Apocrine nevus	Eccrine nevus
			Hair follicle nevus		Eccrine angiomatous nevus
	I.L.V.E.N. Ichthyosis hystrix Becker's nevus Melanoacanthoma	Senile sebaceous hyperplasia	Nevus comedonicus Trichofolliculoma Trichoadenoma	Apocrine cystadenoma Syringocystadenoma papilliferum	Hidroacanthoma simplex Eccrine poroma Dermal duct tumor
			Dilated pore	Hidradenoma of vulva	Syringoma
	Clear cell acanthoma	Sebaceous trichofolliculoma	Pilar sheath acanthoma		Papillary eccrine adenoma
Adenomatous	Seborrheic verruca	Sebaceous adenoma	Trichilemmoma	Tubular apocrine adenoma	Eccrine spiradenoma
			Tumor of follicular infundibulum	Erosive adenomatosis of nipple	Chondroid syringoma
			Inverted follicular keratosis Proliferating trichilemmal cyst Pilomatricoma		Clear cell hidradenoma (Eccrine acrospiroma)
Epitheliomatous	Palmar pit	Sebaceous epithelioma	Trichoepithelioma		Aggressive digital papillary adenoma
			Desmoplastic trichoepithelioma Basaloid follicular hamartoma	Cylindroma	
		Basal cell epithelioma			

cells and mesodermal cells will be given in their respective chapters.

REFERENCES

1. Jadassohn J: Bemerkungen zur Histologie der systematisierten Naevi und über "Talgdrüsen-Naevi." Arch Dermat Syph (Berlin) 33:355, 1895
2. Darier J, Civatte A. Tzanck A: Précis de Dermatologie. Paris: Masson et Cie, 1947
3. Hashimoto K, Mehregan AH: Tumors of the epidermis. Butterworths: Boston, 1990
4. Hashimoto K, Mehregan AH, Kumakiri M: Tumors of the skin appendages. Boston: Butterworths, 1987
5. Mehregan AH: The origin of the adnexal tumors of the skin: A viewpoint. J Cutan Pathol 12:459, 1985
6. Cooper M, Pinkus H: Intrauterine transplantation of rat basal cell carcinoma as a model for reconversion of malignant to benign growth. Cancer Res 37:2544, 1977

33

MELANOCYTIC TUMORS AND MALFORMATIONS

It is now generally accepted that the normal junctional melanocyte is a neuroectodermal derivative and that its stem cell, the melanoblast, arrives at the dermoepidermal junction during fetal life by migrating there from the neural crest through the dermis. Dermal melanocytes, which form so-called Mongolian spots, are thought to be of similar origin and to complete their migration within the reticular portion of the corium. The origin of nevus cells is the junctional melanocyte and therefore a neuroectodermal derivation is accepted by most authors. We do not have to decide here whether all nevus cells are derived from adult junctional melanocytes, whether some of them are derived from Schwann cells of cutaneous nerves, or whether they are embryonically misdirected cells, although this last hypothesis (Fig. 33–1) explains many data most satisfactorily.[1] Our task is to identify benign nevus cells and to differentiate them from normal and pathologic melanocytes and from malignant melanoma cells. This task is interrelated with giving diagnostic criteria for the various forms of nevus cell nevi, dermal melanocytic lesions, and malignant melanomas. The lesions discussed in this chapter are listed in Table 33–1. It is to be noted that some of these disorders were listed also in Chapter 31 as causing visible color changes of the skin.

HOW TO RECOGNIZE MELANOCYTES, NEVUS CELLS, AND MELANOPHAGES

The terminology for vertebrate melanin-containing cells, their precursors, and related cells based on electron microscopic features and enzyme and immunohistochemical findings is listed in Table 33–2. For our purposes, we will have to rely mostly on what we can see in paraffin sections and routine stains. If, in a particular case, fresh material is available, histochemical reactions for tyrosinase, and cholinesterase or electron microscopy, are useful. Immunostaining for S-100 protein, HMB-45, and other markers can be used for identification of melanocytic cells in fresh or in paraffin-embedded tissue sections.[2,3]

Melanophages contain acid phosphatase activity and collect phagocytized melanin in lysosomal vacuoles. In routine sections, the pigment forms clumps of uneven sizes. Often the cell has gorged itself to the point where the nucleus becomes obscured. In H&E sections, melanophages resemble macrophages containing similar clumps of hemosiderin. O&G stain easily distinguishes the two pigments.

Epidermal Melanocytes

The normal junctional or epidermal melanocyte has a small, dark-staining, and often shrunken-looking

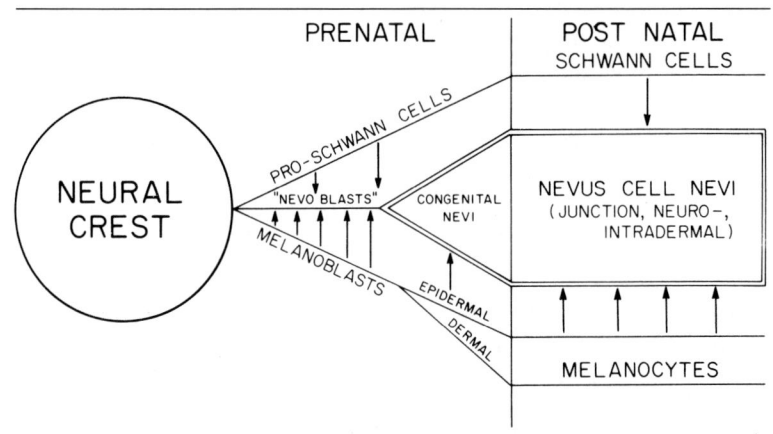

Figure 33–1.
Direct and indirect derivation of nevus cells from neural crest. Nevus cells, the benign neoplastic cells forming nevocytic nevi, may be derived early from neural crest cells as immature nevoblasts or later during fetal life from melanoblasts or pro-Schwann cells, or still later in postnatal life from melanocytes or Schwann cells.

nucleus, in which a nucleolus is not easily recognized. Its cytoplasm, when not occupied by melanin granules, stains pale and appears retracted from the surrounding keratinocytes, so that the cell seems to sit in a hole. Occasionally, thin dendritic processes are seen to insert themselves between prickle cells.

These should not be mistaken for intercellular bridges. The cell usually is situated between the lower halves of neighboring basal cells, its lower border resting on the basement membrane, but it may sit a little higher, or it may bulge down and may actually seem to be attached to the lower epidermal

TABLE 33–1. MALFORMATIONS AND TUMORS OF PIGMENT-FORMING CELLS

Epidermal melanocytes
  Malformation (nevi)
    Ephelis
    Pigmented macules of lip and volar skin
    Nevus spilus
    Nevus depigmentosus and partial albinism
  Neoplasia
    Lentigo simplex
    Lentigo senilis
    Melanoacanthoma
    Lentigo maligna
    Acral lentiginous melanoma
    Malignant melanoma

Dermal melanocytes
  Malformation
    Persistent Mongolian spot
    Nevi of Ota and Ito
    Blue nevus
  Neoplasia
    Cellular blue nevus
    Malignant blue nevus

Nevus cells
  Neoplasia
    Junction nevus
    Compound nevus
    Intradermal nevus
    Spitz nevus
    Congenital (Bathing-trunk type) nevus
    Superficial spreading malignant melanoma
    Nodular malignant melanoma

TABLE 33–2. TERMINOLOGY FOR VERTEBRATE MELANIN-CONTAINING CELLS, THEIR PRECURSORS, RELATED CELLS, AND SPECIFIC PARTICLES

Melanocyte	A cell that synthesizes a melanin-containing organelle, the melanosome.
Melanophore	A type of melanocyte that participates with other chromatophores in the rapid color changes of amphibians and reptiles by intracellular displacement (aggregation and dispersion) of melanosomes.
Melanoblast	A hypothetical precursor cell of melanocyte that is capable of mitosis.
Langerhans cell	An epidermal dendritic cell with phagocyte/histiocyte functions as well as helper T-cell (CD 4) marker. It is derived from mononuclear stem cell in bone marrow and contains distinctive Birbeck granules. Its functions include immune surveillance and primary antigen processing. It may be found in dermis.
Melanosome	A discrete, melanin-forming organelle of melanocyte. Following maturation (stage IV) melanosomes are transferred into basal keratinocytes.
Premelanosome	Immature melanosome (stage I or less mature).

surface like a spider. The melanocyte may contain a few or many evenly sized pigment granules, which, if numerous, outline the dendrites. These then can be followed for many micrometers along the basal membrane or upward between keratinocytes. The nucleus usually is not obscured by the melanin granules, although it may be tightly surrounded by them. Most normal melanocytes give a positive dopa reaction if the test is done on fresh or properly fixed tissue.

DIAGNOSIS OF SPECIFIC LESIONS

Lesions Involving Epidermal Melanocytes

Ephelis
Freckles or ephelides may be considered a malformation because they consist of localized areas of functionally overactive melanocytes. It has been shown that the junctional melanocytes are larger and somewhat more widely spaced in the freckle, and it has been suggested that, at least in red-haired, white-skinned people, these melanocytes are the only mature ones, those in the normal skin being functionally deficient. Histologic examination shows a structurally normal epidermis with a sharply defined area in which the basal cells contain more pigment. Junctional melanocytes are present in approximately normal number.

Pigmented Macules of Lip, Genitalia, and Volar Skin
The *solitary labial lentigo*[4] shows deep pigmentation of the basal keratinocytes (Fig. 33–2) and a fairly normal or slightly increased number of junctional melanocytes. Some pigmented macrophages are present in the uppermost dermis. It is unexplained why the prickle cells remain quite free of pigment.

Atypical pigmented penile macules[5,6] are single or multiple macular lesions with irregular borders and variegated pigmentation involving glans penis. Histologically, there is prominent hyperpigmentation of the basal layer and some increase in the number of junctional melanocytes.[7] *Pigmented macules* (Fig. 33–3) found commonly on the lightly pigmented palms and soles of blacks and orientals usually show an area of increased epidermal pigmentation and the presence of pigment-laden dendritic melanocytes involving mainly the epidermal rete ridges especially in the crista profunda intermedia.[8,9] *Melasmas* are patchy areas of hyperpigmentation with ill-defined borders occurring over the sun-exposed facial skin of women and occasionally in men.[10] Histologically there is marked increase in pigmentation of the basal layer and occasional mac-

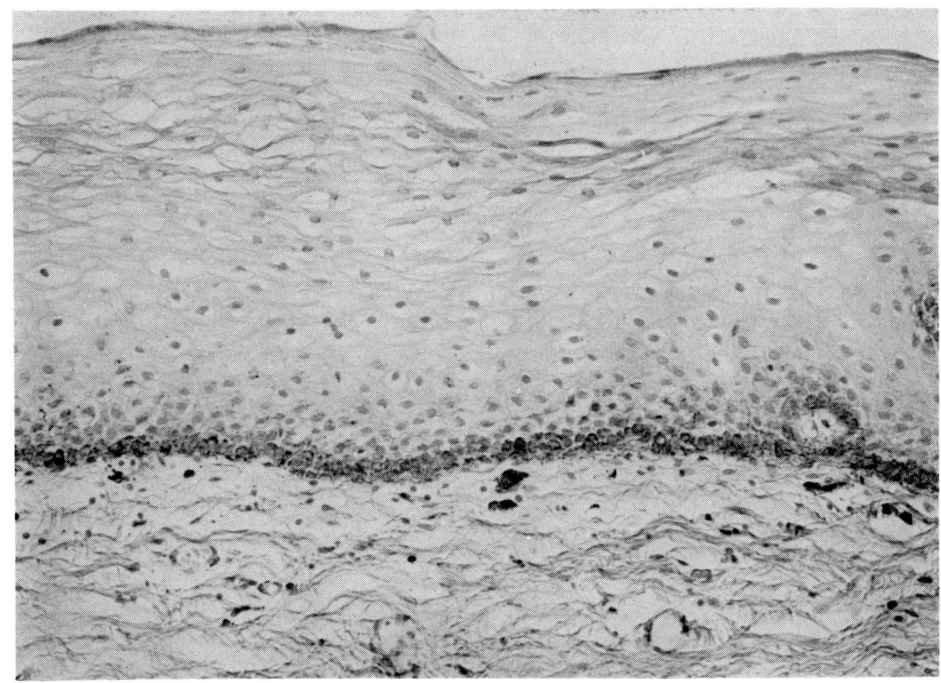

Figure 33–2.
Solitary labial lentigo. Increased basal cell pigmentation due to increased activity of local melanocytes. A few pigmented macrophages in upper dermis. H&E. X185.

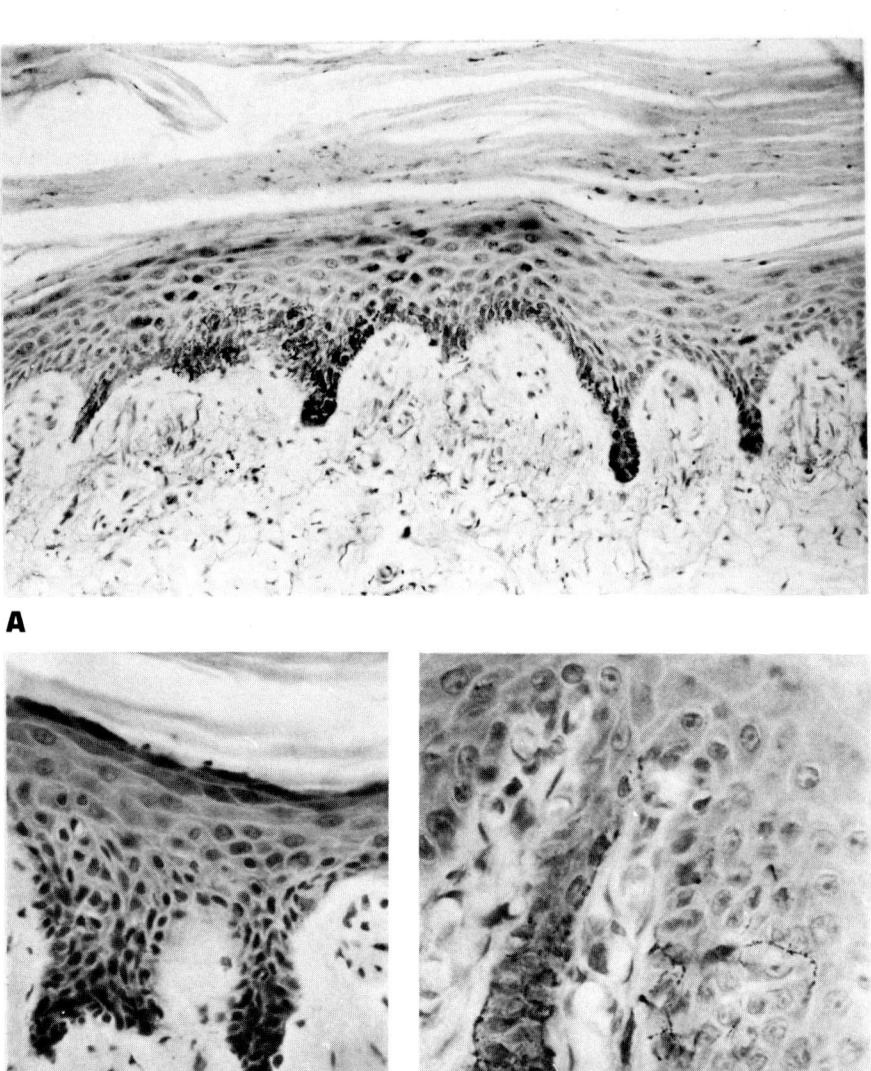

Figure 33–3.
Volar melanotic macules. **A.** Pigment distribution similar to lentigo simplex in all epidermal layers including stratum corneum. O&G. **B.** Pigment concentrated in basal layer. Some rete ridges have a squared-off lower border that is very conspicuous in some lesions. H&E. **C.** Pigment block prevents melanin from being accepted by keratinocytes and remains in large dendritic melanocytes. H&E. Various magnifications. (From Chapel et al. Int J Dermatol 18:222, 1979.)

rophages containing melanin pigment in the upper dermis.

Nevus Spilus

Nevus spilus is a well-established term for macular hyperpigmented areas that are permanent and may be a few millimeters or several centimeters in diameter. Smaller macules often are grouped. That the hyperpigmentation is permanent and independent of insolation differentiates nevus spilus from freckles. Histologically, they are identical. Larger areas of hyperpigmentation, especially if they have light brown color, are also known as *café au lait spots,* a term used mainly for those associated with neurofibromatosis and the Albright syndrome. It has been shown by light and electron microscopy that the melanocytes in von Recklinghausen's disease contain giant melanosomes,[11] while those in the Albright syndrome do not.[12] These are large round melanin granules, up to 5 μm in diameter.

The term "nevus spilus" has been applied to lesions containing deeply pigmented papular nevus cell nevi on a light brown macular background. These often segmental lesions are better differentiated as *speckled lentiginous nevus*.

Nevus Depigmentosus and Partial Albinism

Histologic diagnosis of these conditions and the related *hypomelanosis of Ito*, all of which are minus nevi, is rather unsatisfactory in routine sections and should be investigated with dopa reaction or even electron microscopic melanocyte counts[13] in properly prepared specimens. According to Jimbow et al.,[14] decreased synthesis and abnormal transfer of melanosomes are involved in nevus depigmentosus.

Lentigo Simplex

The histologic borderline between an ephelis and a lentigo simplex, which is the simplest form of melanocytic neoplasia, is not always sharp (Fig. 33–4). We use the term lentigo *simplex* in preference to lentigo juvenilis because it may persist unchanged into old age. In a typical lentigo simplex, melanin is present not only in the basal layer, but also in the upper layers of the epidermis, and some of these lesions present the most extreme degree of epidermal pigmentation, every cell including those of the horny layer being stuffed with brown granules. In addition, there is usually some acanthosis and accentuation of rete ridges, which may be bulbous. Deeply pigmented junctional melanocytes appear to be increased in number but are difficult to see, and there may be pigmented macrophages in the upper dermis. Inflammatory infiltrate in the papillary layer also is not uncommon and probably constitutes a reaction to melanin. Lentigines usually develop in the first years of life, and there is probably no human being who does not have at least one or several.

Leopard syndrome[15] is transmitted by an autosomal dominant trait and includes multiple lentigines, electrocardiographic conduction defects, ocular hypertelorism, pulmonary stenosis, abnormalities of genitalia, retardation of growth, and deafness. In Peutz–Jeghers syndrome[16] numerous 1- to 10-mm circular to ovoid lentigines occur over the vermilion border of the lower lip, in the oral cavity, and on the fingers and toes in association with gastrointestinal polyposis. Another syndrome is characterized by the association of cutaneous lentigines, cutaneous myxomas, bilateral atrial myxomas, and possibly central nervous system aneurysm.[17,18] Inherited patterned lentigines[19] have been reported in blacks with involvement of face, lips, buttocks, and extremities including palms and soles. Lentigines may also be the consequence of long term sun-bed light exposure or PUVA treatment.[20–22]

Lentigo Senilis

Small light-brown pigmented spots of senile lentigines appear most commonly over the light exposed facial skin and dorsa of hands and eventually elsewhere. Small lesions may coalesce to form plaques of one or more centimeters. Histologically, lentigo senilis has a rather diagnostic picture (Fig. 33–5). The epidermis is slightly acanthotic and shows club-shaped budding of the basal layer with hyperpigmentation.[23] Lentigo senilis differs from lentigo simplex by the more irregular epidermal budding,

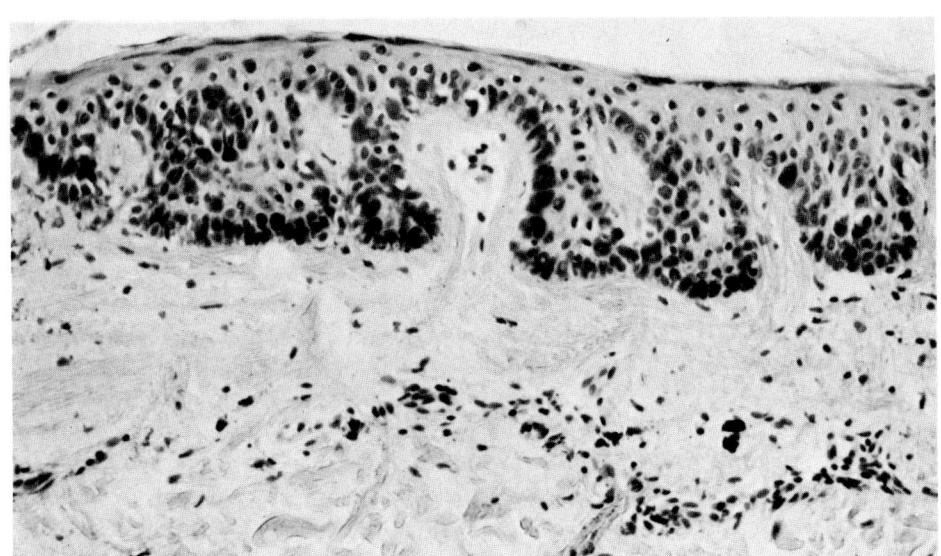

Figure 33–4.
Lentigo simplex. Rete ridges elongated and broadened at their tips. Increased amount of melanin in melanocytes, basal cells, and, to less degree, in prickle cells. Note dense collagen bundles in papillae, some melanized macrophages in subpapillary layer. H&E. X225.

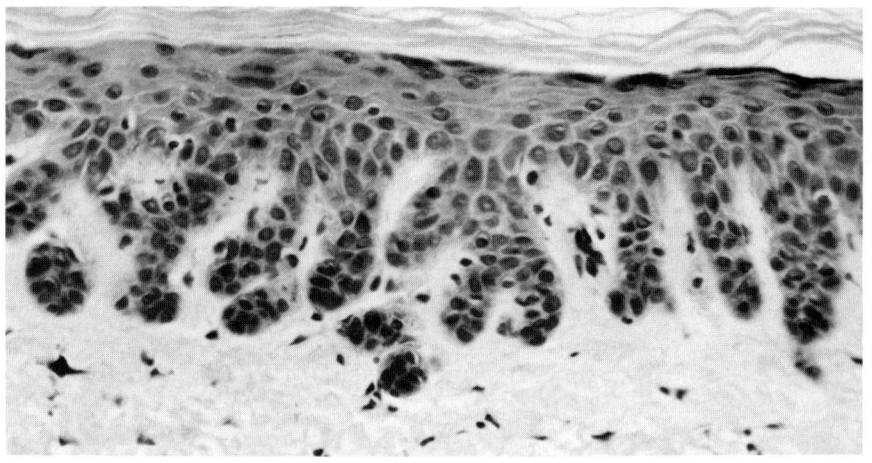

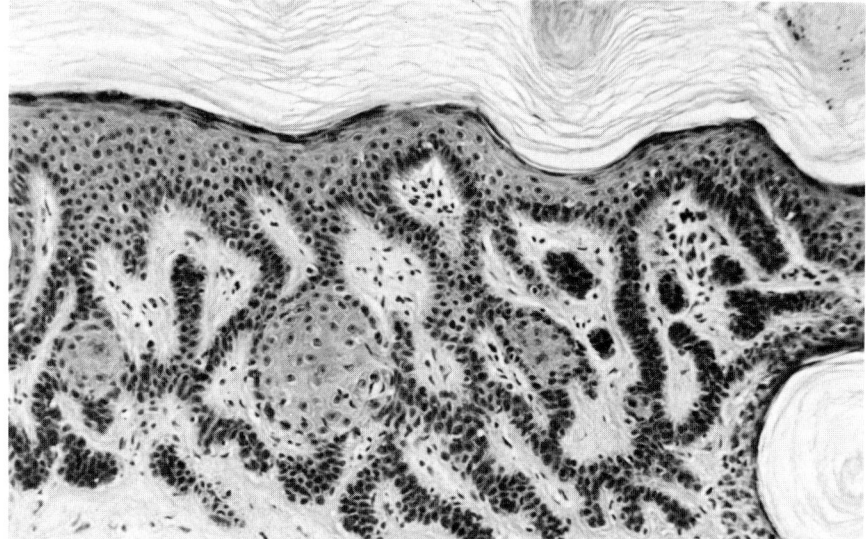

Figure 33–5.
Lentigo senilis. **A.** Distorted budding rete ridges embedded in dense papillary stroma. No noticeable increase of melanocytes; pigment confined to tips of ridges. H&E. X225. **B.** More pronounced budding of narrow epidermal ridges approaches the picture of the reticulated type of seborrheic verruca (Fig. 34–12). Maturation of basal cells into prickle cells and horny cyst formation also points in that direction. H&E. X180.

which is not simple lengthening of the rete ridges, by the tendency of pigmentation to be heaviest in the tips of the buds, and by the presence of a dense, eosinophilic band of connective tissue separating buds of pigmented basaloid cells from the zone of actinic elastosis. Relationship of this lesion to solitary lichen planuslike keratosis and reticulated seborrheic verruca is discussed in Chapters 9 and 34.

Pigmented Nevus Cell Nevi

Nevus cells are variants of melanocytes and are a specific human characteristic. Nevus cell nevi in animals are extremely rare. The animal malignant melanomas are mainly derived from dermal melanocytes. The nevus cell differs in important points from normal melanocyte, as outlined in Table 33–3. The most important difference is its ethologic behavior. Normal melanocytes are dendritic, individualistic cells, each occupying its own territory, as can be seen well in split skin preparations (see Fig. 2–44). Nevus cells have a herd instinct: they crowd together in theques. This indicates specific differences in cell membrane constituents. The nevus cells are abnormal cells, not a normal tissue component. Whether we consider them a derivative of normal melanocytes, Schwann cells, or of embryonically misdirected nevoblasts (Fig. 33–1), lesions composed of nevus cells are neoplasms and not malformations. On the other hand, nevus cells can occur in congenital lesions which otherwise satisfy the definition of a nevus, as will be discussed under bathing-trunk

TABLE 33-3. BENIGN MELANOGENIC CELLS: THE MELANOCYTE VERSUS THE NEVUS CELL

	Melanocytes	Nevus Cells
Cell shape	Epidermal: dendritic Dermal: fusiform, ameboid	Round-oval, fusiform, rarely dendritic
Nucleus	Dark-staining, shrunken	Vesicular with nucleolus
Enzymes	Dopa-oxidase-positive, cholinesterase- and S-100-negative	Dopa- and/or cholinesterase-positive or negative, S-100-positive
Ethology	Solitary, territorial even when crowded	Sociable, herd instinct, forming nests (theques)
Habitat	Epidermal: junction, basal layer, hair matrix Dermal: reticular dermis	All layers of epidermis and dermis

nevus. These paradoxes must be kept in mind. The nevus cell nevus or melanocytic nevus, is a peculiar tumor. It develops some time after birth, grows, then may remain stable for many years or show renewed spurts of growth, and it often fibroses or atrophies late in life. It rarely undergoes malignant transformation.

Nevus Incipiens

In its first stage nevus incipiens either is, or strongly resembles, a lentigo simplex. While some lentigines persist indefinitely in their macular form, many become clinically palpable, and that coincides with the appearance of nests of nevus cells at the junction.

This nevus incipiens (Fig. 33–6), in which features of lentigo and junction nevus are combined, gradually transforms into the common *junction nevus,* or the latter may arise de novo. One may encounter lesions in which all stages from lentigo to intradermal nest formation are present simultaneously. Inflammatory infiltrate in the papillae and subpapillary layer is not uncommon in nevus incipiens, seems to be related to the amount of melanin discharged into the dermis, and, like the presence of occasional mitosis, does not signify malignancy.

Junction Nevus and Compound Nevus

In a pure junction nevus (Fig. 33–7A), theques or single nevus cells are intraepidermal,[24] or their lower portion bulges downward, but there is no connective tissue between keratinocytes and nevus cells (Fig. 33–7B). Electron microscopy shows that the basement membrane may be thin or absent around the lower border of the junctional nests. Immunostaining for type IV collagen and laminin, however, demonstrates variable degrees of continuity of basement membrane.[25,26]

Although there is no doubt that junctional nests are transformed into intradermal nests, Unna's classic concept of *Abtropfung,* meaning dropping down of nevus cells into the dermis, describes the process misleadingly. Actually, as the nests of nevus cells bulge into the dermis reticulum and, later, collagen fibers and elastic fibers envelop the nests, pushing the epidermis away from them. This corresponds to the clinical phenomenon that a junction nevus becomes elevated when it transforms into a compound nevus (Fig. 33–8). The nevus cell nests do not migrate into preformed dermis but become surrounded by new connective tissue, which forms the stroma of

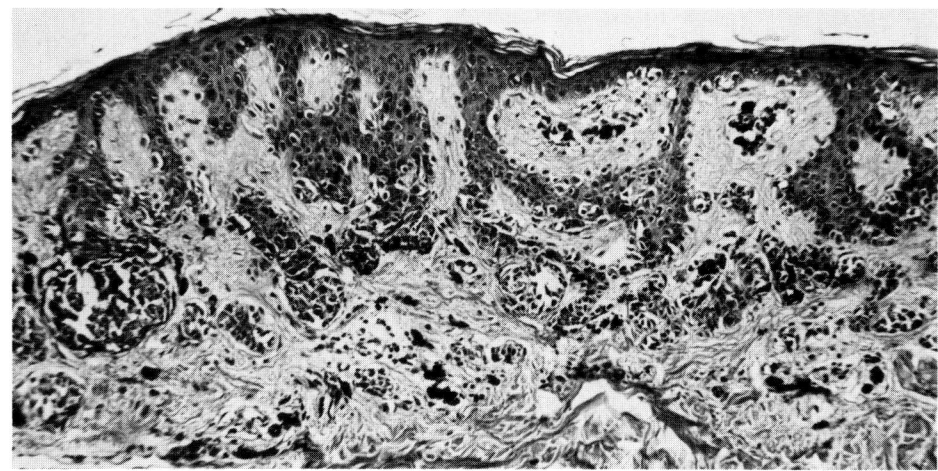

Figure 33–6.
Nevus incipiens. Theques of junctional nevus cells and individual large clear cells in a lesion which otherwise has characteristics of lentigo simplex (see Fig. 33–4). H&E. X135.

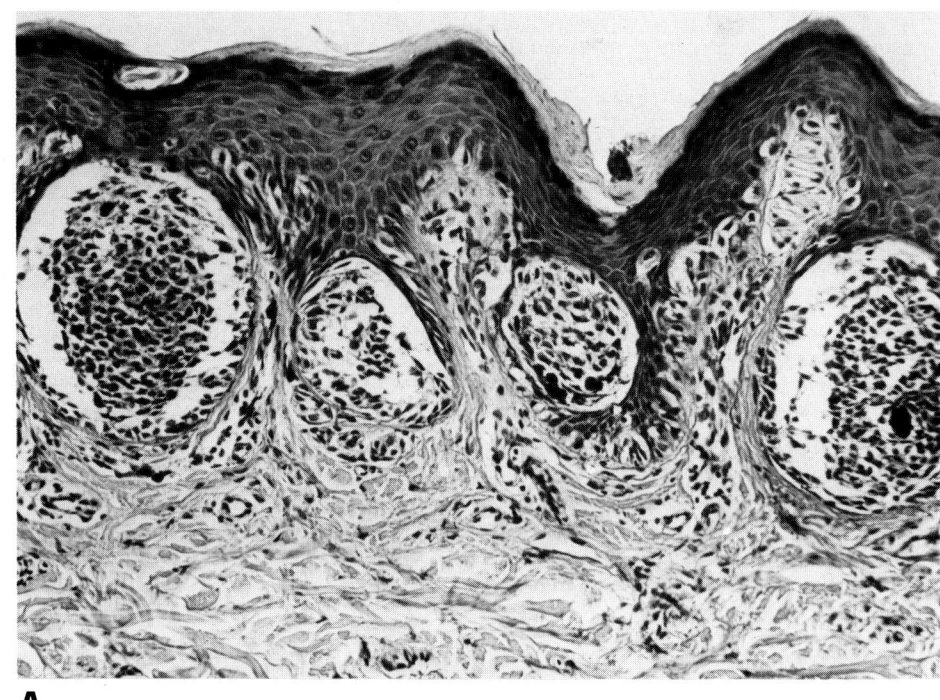

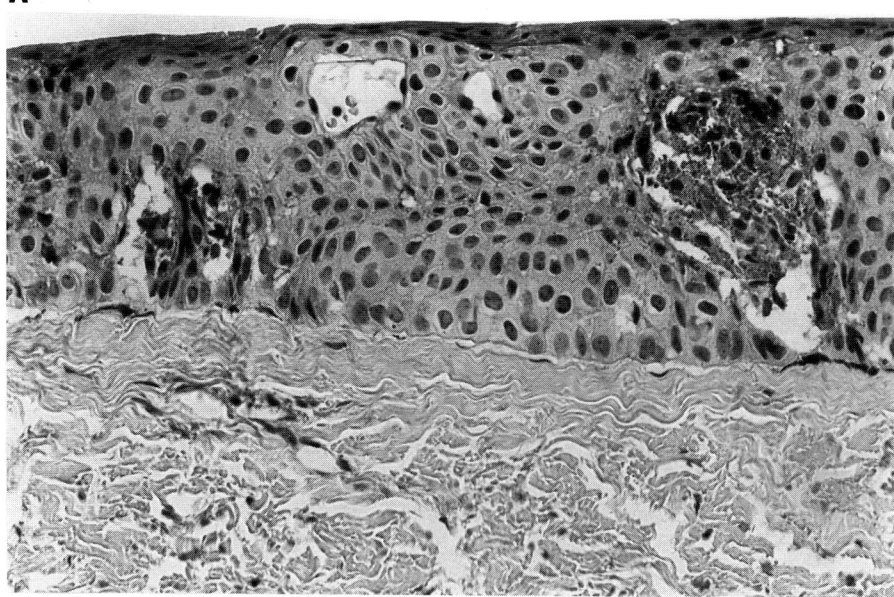

Figure 33–7.
A. Junction nevus of sole. Note Meissner's corpuscle, identifying hairless skin, in upper right corner. H&E. X185.
B. Junction nevus of nail matrix. H&E. X250.

the tumor. In superficial dermis the nevus cell nests display a more continuous basement membrane.[26] Nevi that extend deeper usually contain hairs, and one often sees nevus cell nests arising at the junction of follicular epithelium and fibrous root sheath. In rare cases, eccrine sweat ducts may serve as centers.[24] Every benign cellular nevus beyond the junction stage is a well-organized neuroectodermal–mesodermal tumor. With increasing distance from the epidermis, the nevus cells lose their melanin granules, and the dopa reaction becomes weaker. This does not mean that the cells become quiescent. It has been shown[27] that they maintain metabolic activity and that thymidine incorporation as an indication of mitotic activity persists at all levels of a mole.

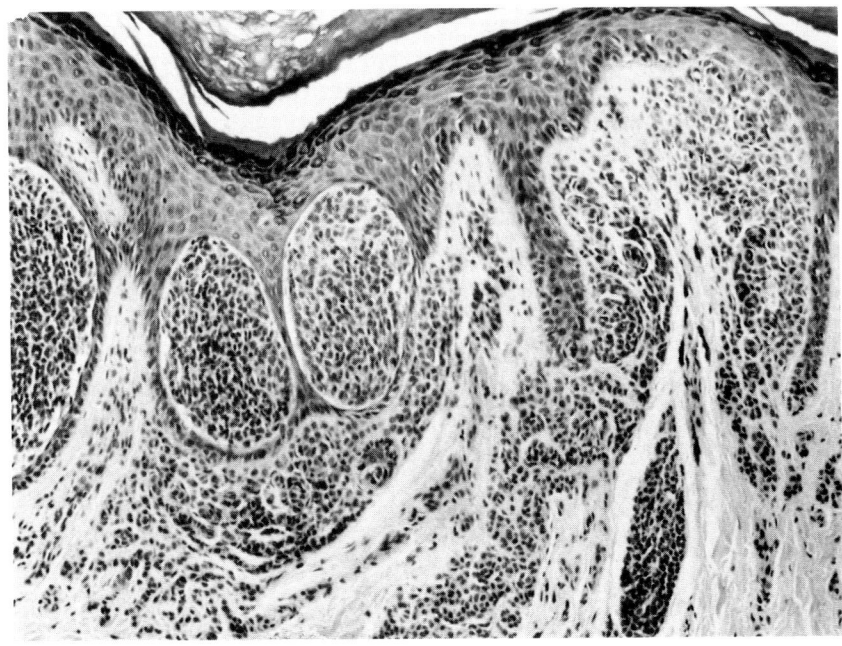

Figure 33–8.
Compound nevus. Well-defined nests of nevus cells at the dermoepidermal junction. The intradermal nests are of small (B type) variety. H&E. X125.

Intradermal Nevus

We favor the designation intradermal over dermal nevus because the latter term may give rise to confusion with the blue nevus, which consists of dermal melanocytes. In most nevi, the new formation of theques at the epidermodermal junction subsides after some years, and all nests become intradermal (Fig. 33–9). Most cellular nevi of postadolescent age are intradermal nevi, but new junction nevi may spring up in adult life and go through all the stages of their natural history without indication of malignancy. On the other hand, nevi in certain locations,

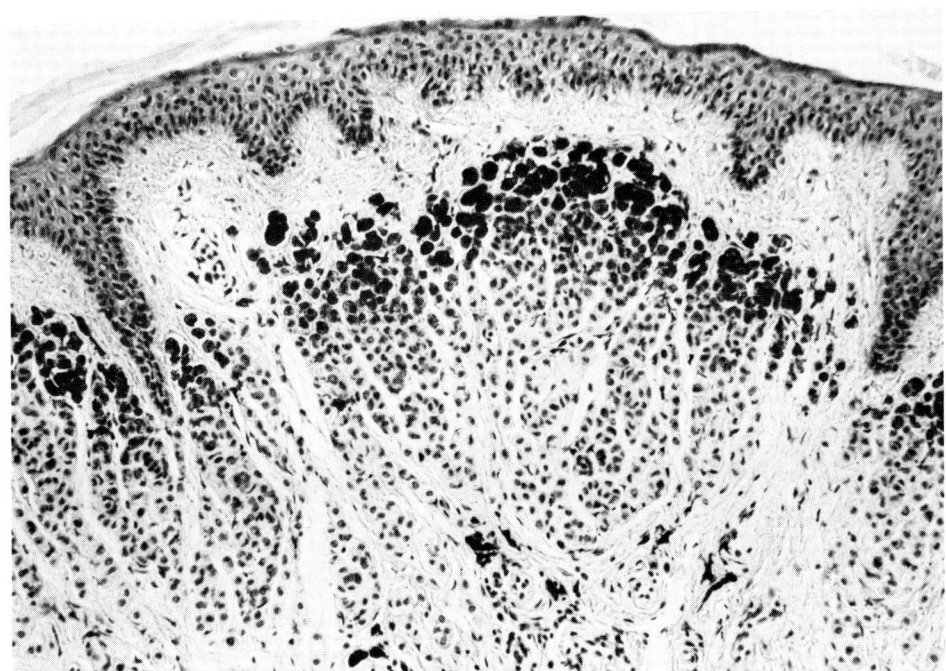

Figure 33–9.
Intradermal nevus. Majority of nevus cells are of pigmented epithelioid (A type) variety. H&E. X185.

especially on the hands and feet, may persist as junction or compound nevi throughout life. Finding a junction nevus on the sole of an elderly person does not imply malignancy unless there is cytologic evidence.

In many of the common brown moles of the face, new formation of junctional nests never ceases completely. Their prevalence in any pathologist's material depends on the number of sections of individual moles examined. It is likely that complete serial sections would reveal a few junctional nests in almost every mole. Thus, the presence of occasional nests and of single junctional nevus cells above an intradermal nevus does not indicate activity and certainly not malignancy. Nevus cell nevi having papillomatous configuration (Fig. 33–10), especially the type resembling a raspberry clinically, never lose their junctional element; they keep growing outward all the time. Therefore, the line between the diagnosis of compound and intradermal nevus is not sharp, and terminology depends somewhat on personal preference. The diagnosis "predominantly intradermal nevus," perhaps with the added notation "no unusual activity at the junction," seems to offer an acceptable compromise in many cases.

Nevus cells in the dermis are of three types, designated "A," "B," and "C" by Miescher and Albertine[28] and "epithelioid," "lymphocytoid," and "neuroid," by others. These are illustrated in Figures 33–8, 33–9, and 33–15. Other descriptive terms, such as "large," "small," and "fusiform," also have been used. The A-type cells have nucleus and cytoplasm similar to junctional nevus cells, usually form nests in the papillary and subpapillary layer, and may or may not be pigmented. B-type cells are smaller, with a dark-staining nucleus and small amount of cytoplasm and usually occupy the middermis. They rarely contain melanin. C-type cells are found still deeper. These are larger, light staining cells with plenty of cytoplasm, may form Meissner corpuscle-like aggregates, and practically never contain pigment. Nevus cells, unless they contain melanin, are characterized mainly by their negative attributes; they do not contain other visible granulations or fibers and have no intercellular connections. They may lie singly in the dermis but, more commonly, form nests of a few to many cells. Nests may be surrounded by flattened elements (*thequocytes*), producing the impression of nevus cells lying in an endothelium-lined space.[29] In some cases, larger masses may resemble basal cell epithelioma in H&E sections. O&G stain, however, usually reveals elastic fibrils (Fig. 33–11) which surround smaller aggregates within the larger masses, and if need be, a reticulum stain will always show fine fibrils spun around small nests or even individual cells.[30] When intradermal nevus cells contain melanin, it is present in evenly sized and fairly small granules.

The uppermost row generally contains melanin granules, and these may be present in somewhat deeper nests. Melanization of nevus cells deep in the dermis arouses suspicion of malignant melanoma but may be related to the origin of nevus cells from

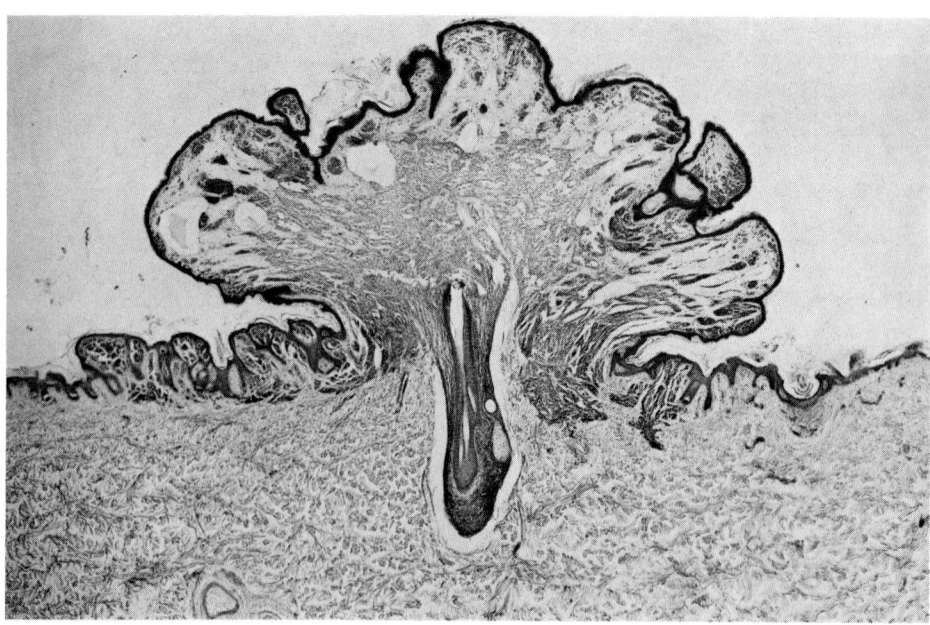

Figure 33–10.
Papillomatous nevus cell nevus with flat halo. Tumor is predominantly intradermal, but some nevus cell nests are present at the junction. Note involvement of perifollicular tissue. The superficial nests are surrounded by fat cells, producing the impression of lymph spaces. H&E. X30.

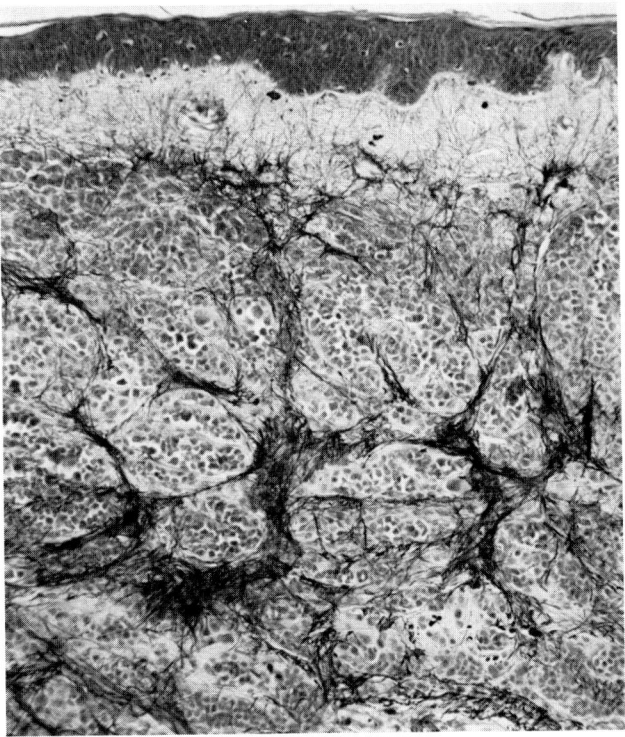

Figure 33–11.
Intradermal nevus with network of elastic fibers. Note difference in size between large superficial (type A) and smaller (type B) cells in the deep portions of the nevus. O&G. X135.

hair roots. Cytologic analysis and evaluation of the entire lesion are necessary in every case. Old quiescent nevi not infrequently contain multinucleated giant cells (Fig. 33–12), which have no clinical significance. Occasional association of intradermal nevus cell nests with dermal melanocytes, that is, of a nevus cell nevus with a blue nevus, can be observed.

Eruptive Nevi

New nevi may appear in crops. They may seem to be quite spontaneous in some persons. In other cases, an eruption of new nevi followed an attack of toxic epidermal necrolysis, erythema multiforme, or as the consequence of cancer chemotherapy.[31,32] In these instances, the newly formed nevi follow the ordinary course from junctional to compound and intradermal, and they become stable.

Speckled Lentiginous Nevus (Naevus sur Naevus)

Nevi appearing early in life in a zonal arrangement consist of numerous small dark pigmented lesions over a light tan and uniformly pigmented area.[33,34] The histopathology of lightly pigmented background is similar to lentigo simplex. The small dark spots show junctional, compound, and rarely blue nevi. Secondary development of malignant melanoma has been reported in a few cases.[35,36]

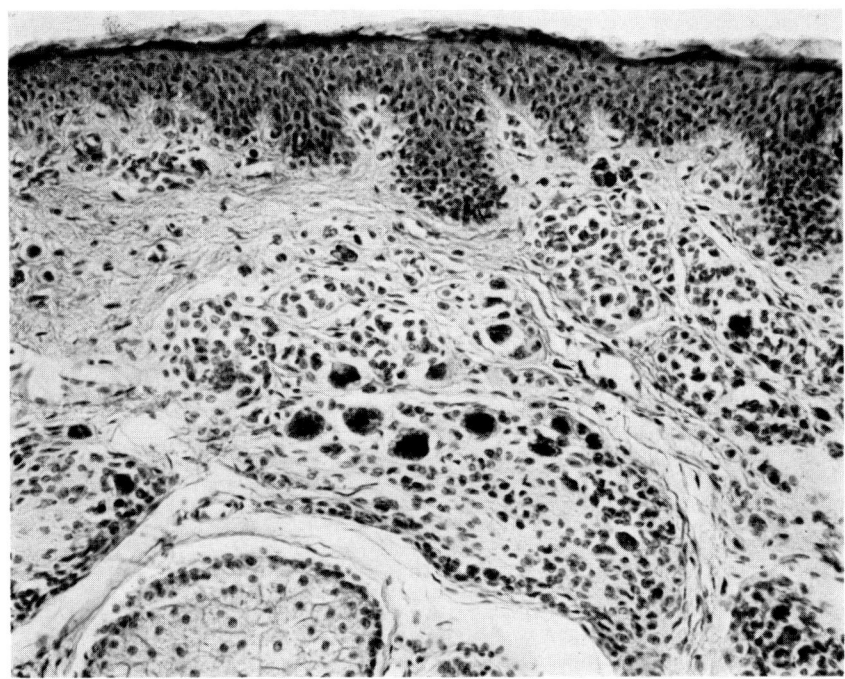

Figure 33–12.
Variability of nevus cells in benign intradermal nevus. Nevus giant cells. H&E. X180.

Dysplastic Nevi

Diagnosis of dysplastic nevus requires clinical and histopathologic correlation. Clinically, individuals with dysplastic nevi may have 100 or more lesions that exhibit variation in color ranging from orange to light brown and black.[37-39] The majority of nevi are centrally slightly elevated and are surrounded by a macular tan zone with an irregular border that fades out into the surrounding skin areas. Most lesions are 0.5 cm or larger and are located over the trunk, limbs, or face with greater concentration over sun-exposed skin areas. Irregular border, variation in pigmentation, and accentuated skin marking is better appreciated when the lesions are examined by surface macroscopy.[40] Histologically (Fig. 33-13), the epidermis shows mild to moderate acanthosis and hyperpigmentation. The epidermal rete ridges are often elongated and their tips interconnected.[41] Diffuse junctional melanocytic hyperplasia involves the epidermal rete ridges predominantly. Junctional nests occur in scattered fashion and are irregularly spaced.[42] Junctional nests may be round or elongated and appear in connection with multiple neighboring rete ridges[43,44] (Fig. 33-14). The cells may be elongated and spindle shaped or may have a slightly irregular nuclei and abundant clear cytoplasm with dustlike pigment granules. Mitotic figures are rare and upward transmigration of melanocytic cells within the overlying epidermis is not observed. A bandlike zone of fibroplasia is present immediately beneath the epidermis. This zone shows lamellated eosinophilic collagen bundles and fine elastic fibers (Fig. 33-15). A few or large number of nevus cell nests may be present in the upper dermis. These are populated with small melanocytes having round or ovoid nuclei and small amounts of cytoplasm. Areas of junctional melanocytic hyperplasia and foci of junctional activity may extend out at the periphery of the lesion. The border is often ill-defined. Other features include the presence of pigmented macrophages in the upper dermis and a patchy or diffuse lymphocytic inflammatory cell infiltrate. Electron microscopic studies have demonstrated abnormally shaped melanosomes, uneven melanization, and transfer of abnormal melanosomes to keratinocytes.[45,46] Dysplastic nevi may occur in members of families or sporadically with no family history.[47] The incidence may be as high as 2 to 5 percent in predominantly white populations. Individuals with dysplastic nevi are in a higher risk group for development of malignant melanoma.[48-50] Family members of heritable melanoma who harbor multiple dysplastic nevi have an estimated 100% risk over their life span of developing malignant melanoma.[51] Over 90% of cases with heritable malignant melanoma were also found to have dysplastic nevi.

Neuronevus

A special form of intradermal nevus, most commonly found about the head and neck, is *Masson's neuronevus*. The neuroid formations (Fig. 33-16) usually occupy the deep portion or the center of a long-standing lesion. The cells composing this part of a nevus are the type C cells of Miescher and Albertini

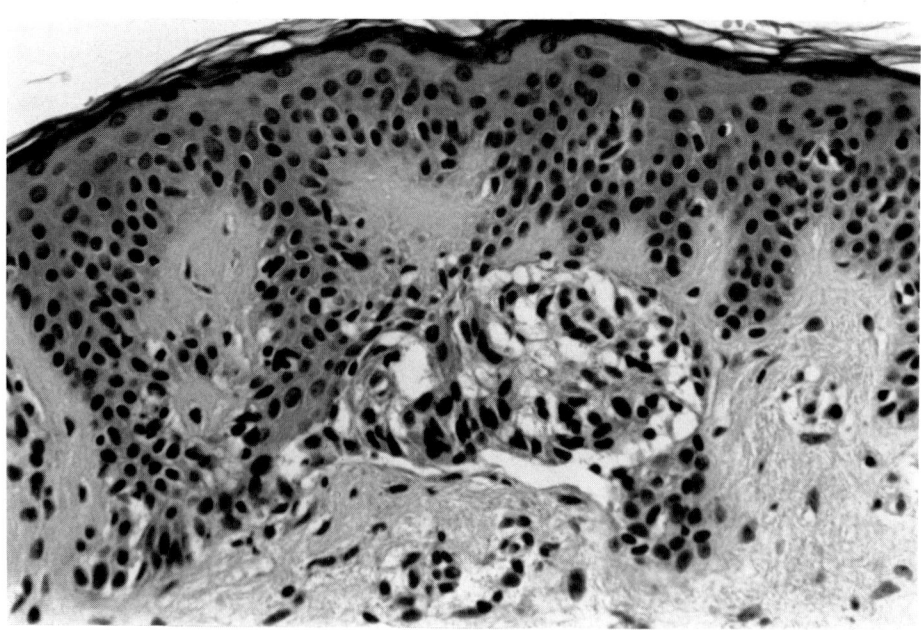

Figure 33-13.
Dysplastic nevus. Elongated junctional nest is connected with several epidermal rete ridges. H&E. X400.

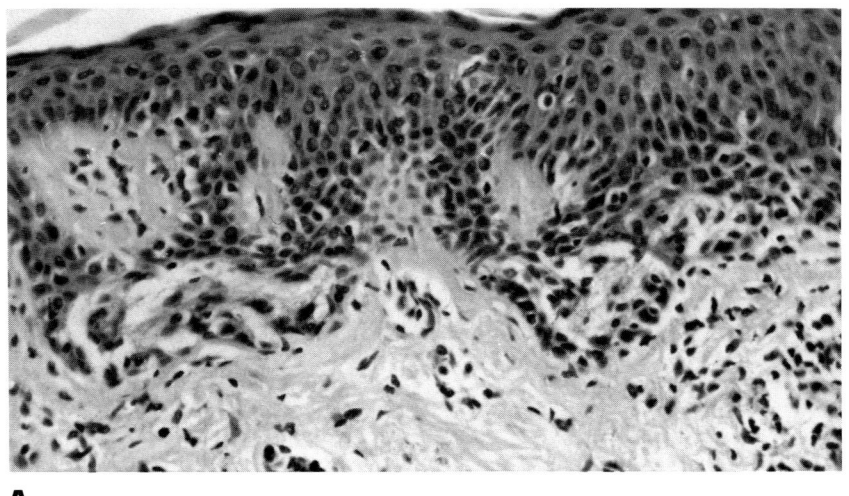

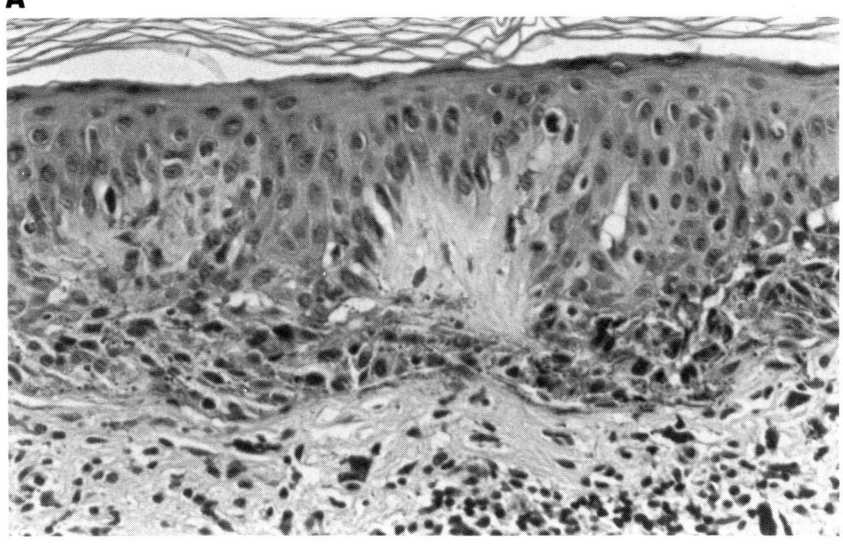

Figure 33-14.
Dysplastic nevus. **A.** Two junctional nests are connected with several epidermal rete ridges. H&E. X225. **B.** A small plate of junctional activity in connection with the lower surface of the epidermis. H&E. X225.

and have been thought to be derived from neural Schwann cells rather than from melanocytes. Positive reactivity for Schwann-cell-associated antigen has been demonstrated by immunostaining.[52] Enzyme histochemistry has shown that they contain the nonspecific cholinesterase characteristic of sensory corpuscles.[53] Electron histochemistry has also been able to find tyrosinase and cholinesterase activity in the same nevus cell, thus suggesting unitarian origin rather than strict dichotomy of nevus histogenesis and supporting the concept that all nevus cells are deranged neuroectodermal elements distinct from melanocytes. Beginners are greatly helped in recognizing neuronevi in routine sections when they examine O&G sections. Here the neuroid structures, being of cellular nature, stain blue and are distinct from eosinophilic collagen. Mast cells, common in many nevi, and especially in this type, add to the distinctive appearance in O&G sections.

Balloon Cell Nevus

An always surprising and occasionally misleading histologic variant of nevus cell is the balloon cell (Blasenzelle). Balloon cells (Fig. 33-17) are up to 10 times larger than ordinary nevus cells and have a centrally or eccentrically placed vesicular nucleus and empty-appearing or foamy cytoplasm which stains faintly with PAS and Nile blue sulfate and perhaps contains phospholipids.[54] It may contain fine particles of melanin granules. Balloon cells may be sparse or many, and some nevi consist entirely of these elements.[55] They are now acknowledged to be functional cells[56] capable of mitosis. Malignant forms have been recorded[57,58] but, in general, pres-

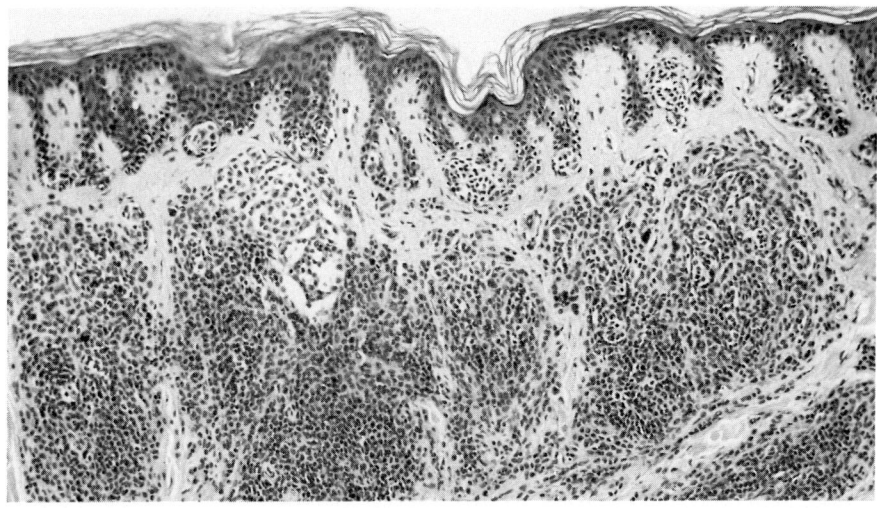

Figure 33-15.
Dysplastic compound nevus. **A.** The intradermal nests are of small (B type) cells. The overlying epidermis shows lentiginous melanocytic hyperplasia and foci of junctional nest formation. H&E. X70. **B.** Foci of junctional activity extending at the periphery of the lesion. H&E. X125.

ence of balloon cells does not alter either diagnosis or prognosis of a benign nevus.

Benign Juvenile Melanoma (Nevus of Spitz)

The benign juvenile melanoma is an outstanding example of the fact that the pathologist must constantly refine the diagnostic criteria in correlating them with the clinical experience. When Spitz[59] first reviewed malignant melanomas in children because of their favorable course, she could histologically identify a certain pattern common to those lesions that were clinically benign. Subsequently, it was found that similar lesions occur in adults.[60] In the following years, particularly based on detail histologic investigation in large series of cases, we became more confident in our ability to differentiate benign and malignant lesions under the microscope regardless of the age of the patient. While the initial term "benign juvenile melanoma" is generally accepted, other designations include "spindle or epithelioid cell" nevus or simply "spitz" nevus. The lesion is usually single, located over the head, trunk, or extremities. Multiple Spitz nevi may be diffuse, linear, or aggregated within a localized normal skin area or scattered over an area of lentiginous macular hyperpigmentation.[61-63]

The outstanding histologic feature of benign juvenile melanoma is the large size of its cells, but it shares this sign with most malignant melanomas.[64,65] Many lesions consist predominantly of spindle-shaped cells (Fig. 33-18). Others may show cells with round or ovoid nuclei and abundant cytoplasm (epithelioid type, Fig. 33-19). Multinucleated giant cells may be present (Fig. 33-20) and mitoses

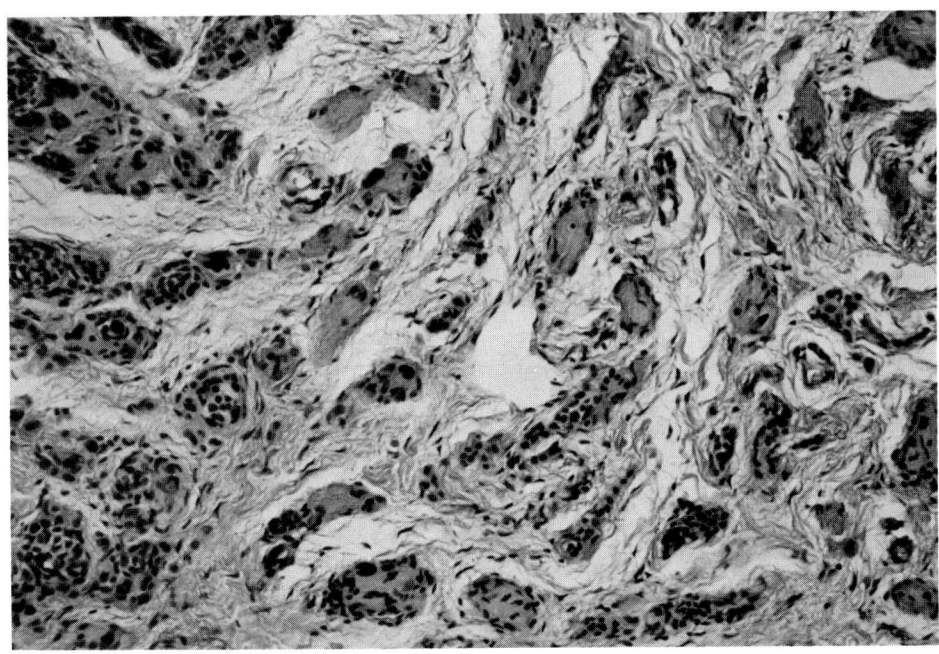

Figure 33–16.
Neuroid formations in an intradermal nevus. Type C cells usually exhibit nonspecific cholinesterase activity. H&E. X225.

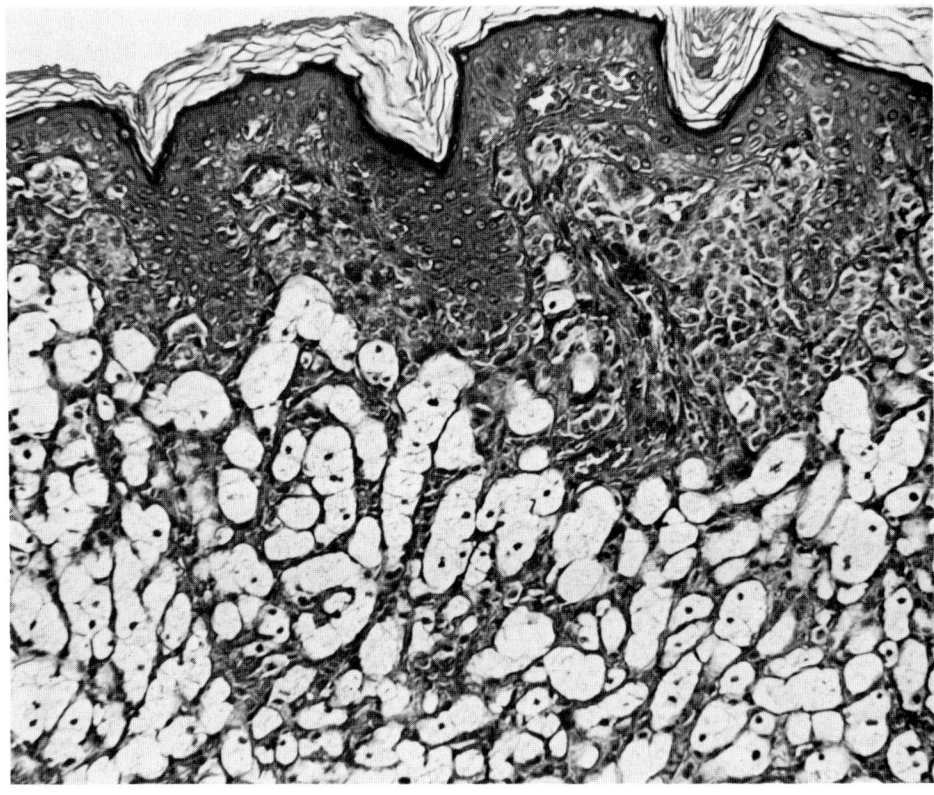

Figure 33–17.
Balloon cell nevus. Compare the type A nevus cells below the epidermis with the extraordinary size of the balloon cell bodies, while nuclei are reduced in size. H&E. X180.

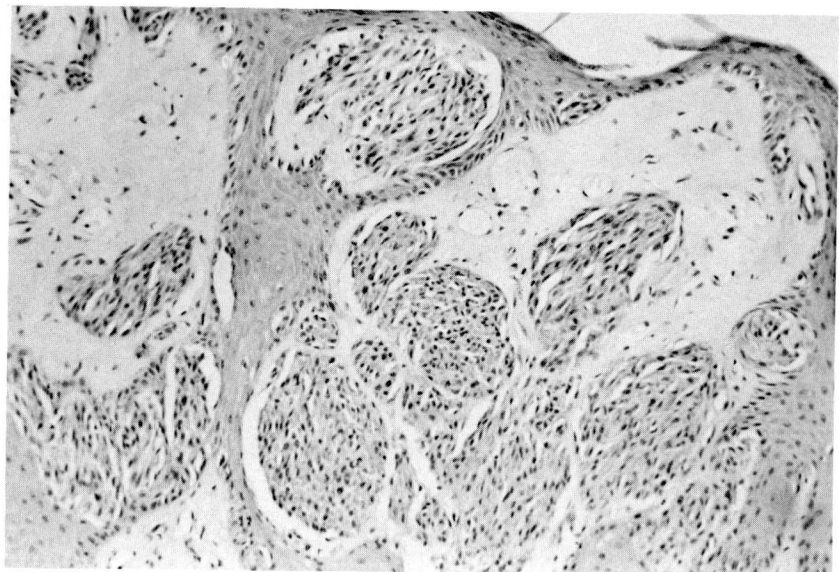

Figure 33–18.
Spitz nevus. The large nevus cells contain no melanin and are arranged in the epidermis, at the junction, and in the dermis. They have fusiform shape in this lesion. H&E. X125.

are not uncommon, but are usually restricted to the nests at the dermoepidermal junction. Telangiectasia and inflammatory cell infiltrate are observed. Most lesions contain little or no melanin; deeply pigmented lesions are rare. The most significant histologic feature is the well-circumscribed nature of the lesion. Peripheral spread of junctional activity similar to that seen in superficial spreading malignant melanoma does not occur. Epidermal acanthosis is variable and may approach low grade pseudoepitheliomatous hyperplasia.[66] Hyperkeratotic lesions of extremities are often clinically diagnosed as verruca vulgaris. Upward transmigration of epithelioid or spindle cells within the acanthotic epidermis is minimal. Degenerated cells forming globular eosinophilic bodies (Kamino bodies)[67] are found in a majority of lesions, but their diagnostic significance is questionable (Fig. 33–21).[68] Older lesions show diminished junctional activity and may be completely intradermal (Fig. 33–22). Fibrotic intradermal Spitz nevus (desmoplastic nevus) needs to be differentiated from fibrous histiocytoma.[69]

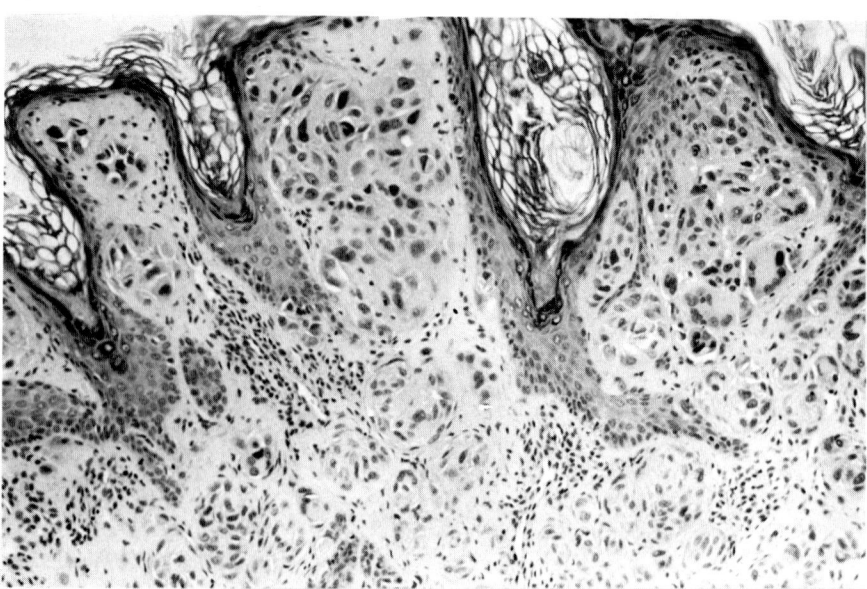

Figure 33–19.
Spitz nevus. Numerous nests of epithelioid nevus cells extending from the dermoepidermal junction into the corium. H&E. X125.

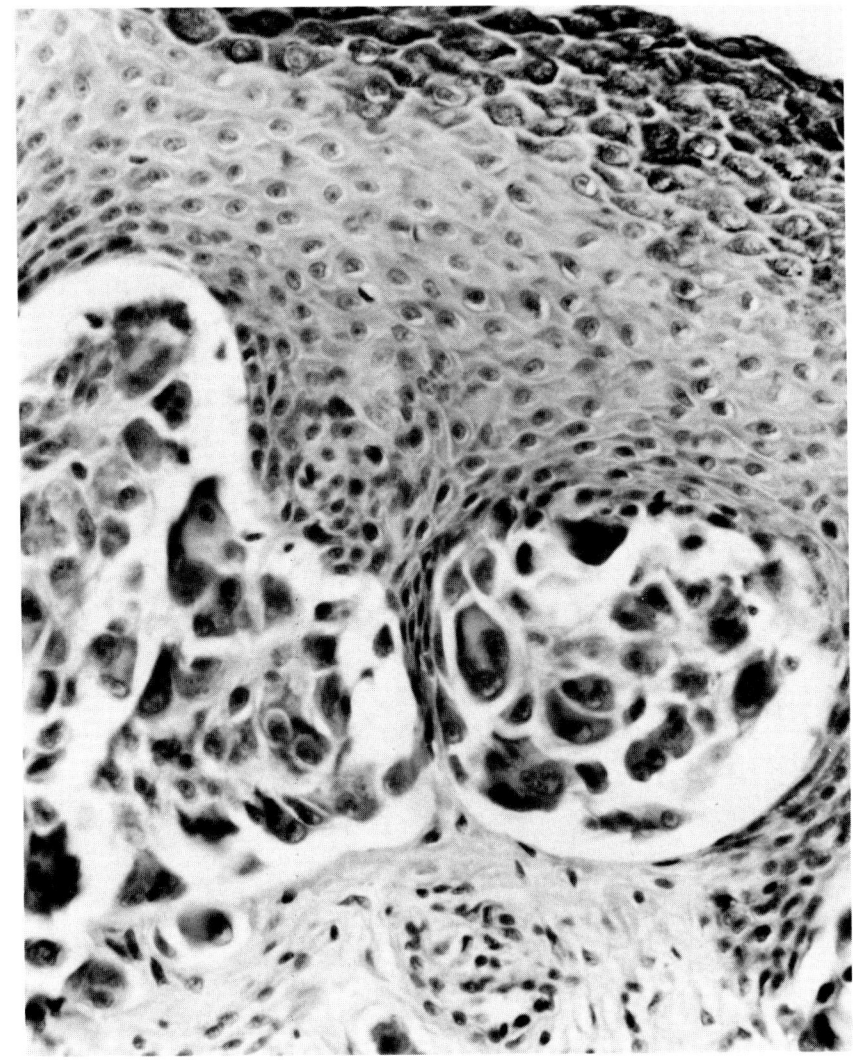

Figure 33–20.
Spitz nevus. Epithelioid junctional nests show several multinucleated giant cells. H&E. X400. (From Kriner and Mehregan. Cutan Pathol 5:90, 1978.)

Recurrence of Nevi after Removal

The desire of many patients to get rid of moles for purely cosmetic reasons has led to the practice of removing only the protruding part either by shaving or by electrodesiccation. With both procedures, intradermal nests of nevus cells and junctional nests connected with the cutaneous appendages are left behind. Occasionally, some weeks or months after surgery, new pigment will become visible in the scar, causing concern to patient and physician alike. On excision of the lesion, a characteristic histologic picture (Fig. 33–23) is found.[70] Often, there are intradermal nests of nevus cells, separated from the epidermis by some scar tissue. The overlying epidermis contains individual and grouped nevus cells forming a new and often deeply pigmented junction nevus. Sometimes these cells are somewhat more irregular than spontaneous junction nevi, but in several fairly large series of cases, no clinical or histologic evidence for development of malignancy was found in this situation.[71] The new nevus probably arises from preexisting junctional cells either at the periphery of the incompletely removed lesion or in the epithelium of hair follicles within the mole. Such new lesions are diagnosed properly as *recurrent junction nevi.*

Regression of Nevus Cell Nevi and Sutton's Halo Nevus

An estimated 20 to 30 percent of nevi disappear through fibrosis or atrophy in old age. In others, the nevus cells seem to be crowded out by development of fat cells (Fig. 33–24). This phenomenon is not atrophy, but rather a new formation of a lipomatous nevus in the mole. Some nevi, however, disappear in a most unusual manner and often

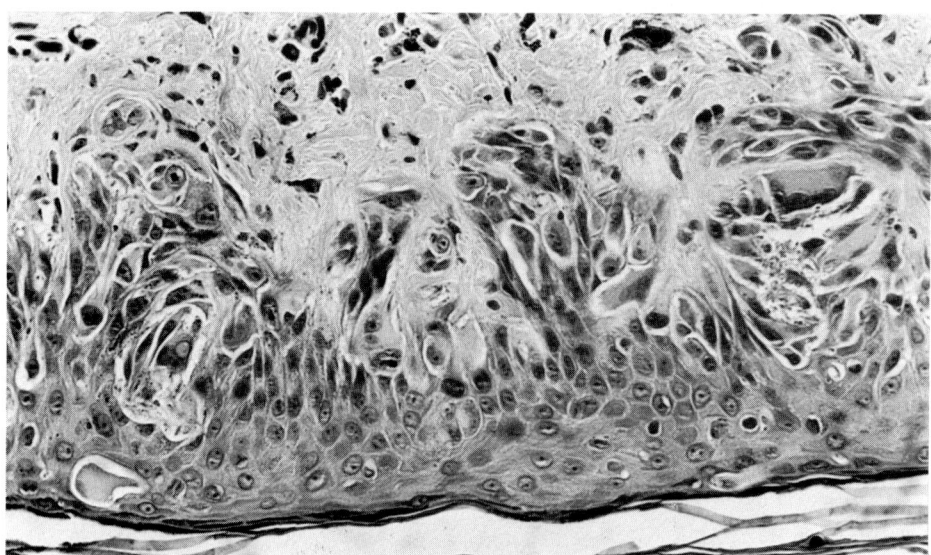

Figure 33–21.
Spitz nevus. Proliferation of spindle-shaped melanocytes forming nests at the dermoepidermal junction. In epidermis are several degenerated cells with homogeneous and eosinophilic cytoplasm. H&E. X250.

early in life.[72] The nevus that is at the center of *leukoderma acquisitum centrifugum* (Fig. 33–25) is most commonly a compound nevus but may be predominantly intradermal. A heavy inflammatory cell infiltrate surrounds the nevus cell nests in the dermis and approaches closely the nests at the dermoepidermal junction. The infiltrate appears immunologically mediated and consists mainly of suppressor/cytotoxic T lymphocytes. A few histiocytes and plasma cells may also be present[73] (Fig. 33–26). At the time the lesion is biopsied, nevus cells may be hard to recognize. The nevus cell nests within heavy inflammatory infiltrate may be identified by immunostaining for S-100 protein.[74] Macrophages with melanin granules are often present. The surrounding epidermis is free of pigment, but nonpigmented melanocytes may be present. There are nevi that undergo the same process of destruction without development of a clinical white halo, and there is an occasional halo nevus without signs of inflammation. It is important to be aware of these lesions in order to avoid mistaking them for malignant melanoma or for infectious granuloma or lymphoma.

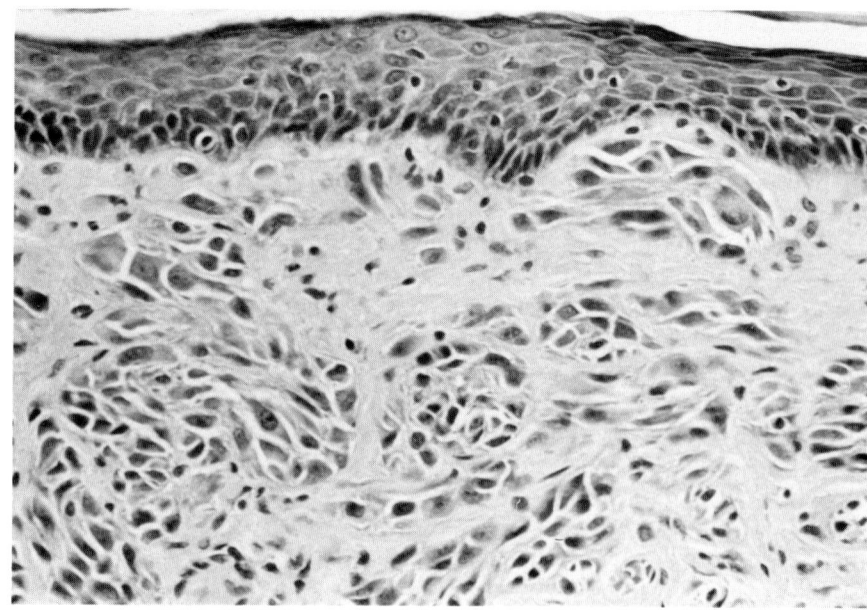

Figure 33–22.
Benign juvenile melanoma (Spitz nevus), intradermal. Plump large cells have predominantly spindle shape and are arranged in ill-defined nests. No melanin. H&E. X250.

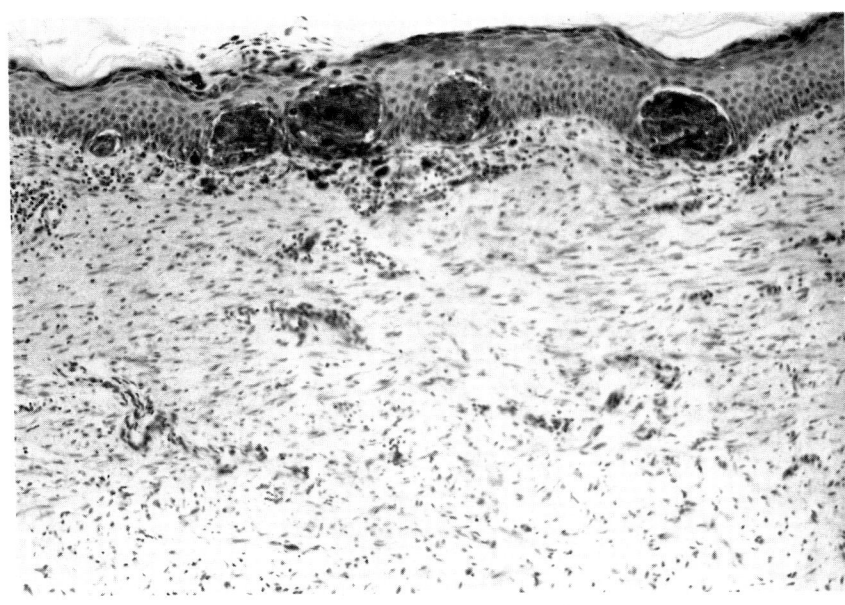

Figure 33-23.
Recurrent junction nevus. Several deeply pigmented nevus cell nests are present at the dermoepidermal junction. Dermis is replaced with scar tissue. H&E. X225.

Congenital Nevi

Approximately 1 percent of newborns may have congenital nevi.[75] These may be small (less than 1.5 cm), medium (1.5 to 20 cm), or large (20 cm or more) in size. An impressive variety involving the entire lower trunk area is known as "bathing trunk nevus." Some congenital nevi develop early in fetal life at the stage at which the dermis and various cutaneous adnexae are organizing. These show nevus cell nests in all layers of dermis at the periphery of the pilosebaceous structures and eccrine glands surrounded in a fine network of collagen, reticulum, and elastic fibers.[76-79] The majority of bathing trunk

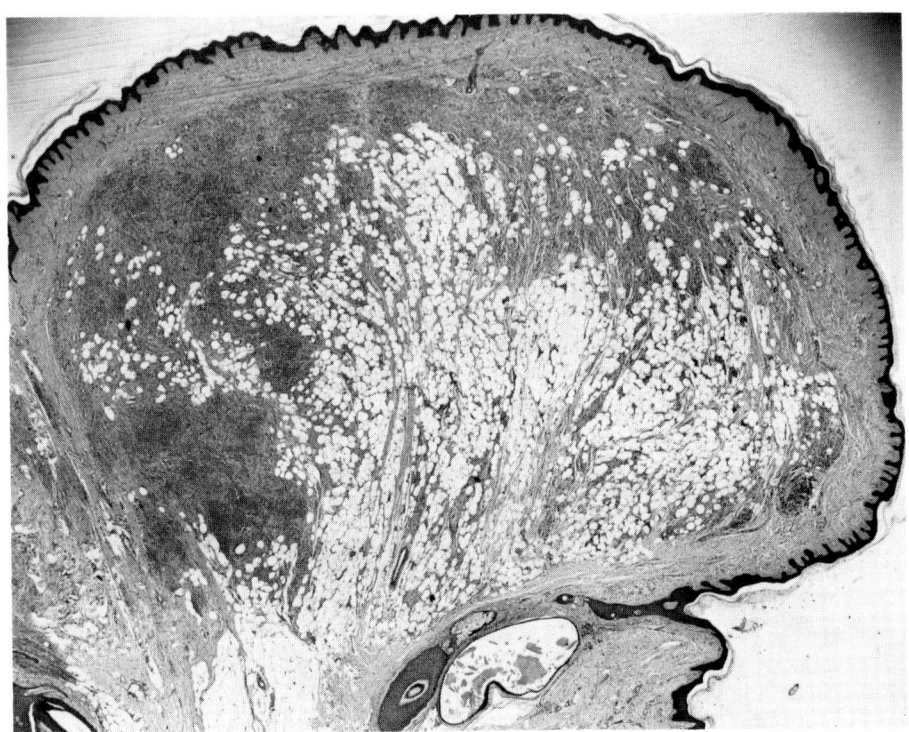

Figure 33-24.
Sessile intradermal nevus with fat tissue. Such pictures may be interpreted as combined nevocellular and lipomatous tumor, or as fat tissue replacing an old cellular nevus. H&E. X30.

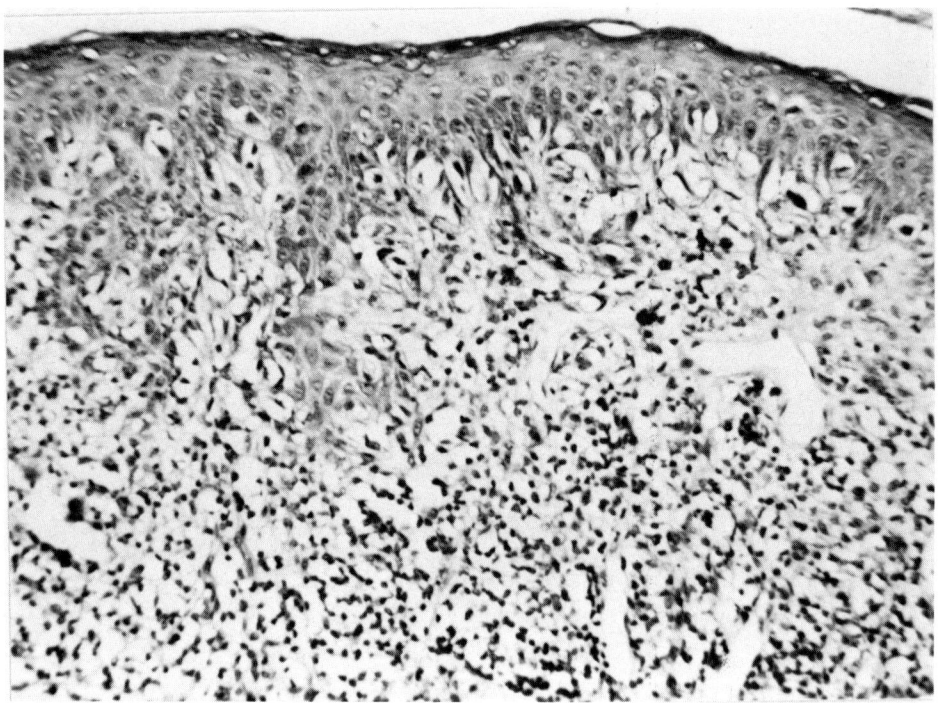

Figure 33–25.
Halo nevus of Sutton. The epidermis shows melanocytic hyperplasia and junctional nests. Dermis contains lymphohistiocytic infiltrate. H&E. X250.

nevi are in this category. Smaller congenital nevi may develop later in the fetal life. These may show only a few nests of nevus cells in the upper dermis with foci of junctional activity involving the epidermis and the cutaneous adnexae and may resemble early acquired melanocytic nevi.[80] Individuals born with *giant* (bathing trunk) nevi may have central nervous system involvement and malignant melanoma may develop in any location involved. Incidence of malignant melanoma developing in small congenital nevi is most likely not significant. A variant of congenital nevus is *cerebriform intradermal nevus* involving the scalp with clinical manifestation of cutis verticis gyrata. Histologically, there is full thickness dermal involvement similar to that of large congenital nevi.[81,82]

Dermal Melanocytes

Dermal melanocytes derive from neuroectoderm but do not reach the epidermis. They stay permanently in the dermis. They are widely distributed in the skin of animals, but in man they are restricted to certain areas except under pathologic circumstances. They are commonly found in the back skin, especially in the sacral area, of newborns of darker skinned races, where they form the so-called "Mongolian spot" (see next section). Dermal melanocytes

are individualistic cells having ameboid appearance. They are dopa positive and contain melanosomes.

Lesions Related to Dermal Melanocytes

Mongolian Spot and Oculomucocutaneous Melanosis

Mongolian spot is a bluish macular lesion located over the sacral area. It occurs in 10 to 25 percent of babies of Southern European stock, 60 percent of newborns in India, and in over 90 percent of American blacks as well as in Orientals.[83] The presence of dermal melanocytes in the skin of the lower back is indeed a universal human attribute but is clinically inapparent in light-skinned children. In very dark-skinned children the spot may be overlooked, or it may not be recognized when it occupies most of the dorsal trunk, a not uncommon occurrence in blacks. The cells are large, ameboid-looking elements which are sparsely scattered in the reticular portion of the dermis and probably cease functioning shortly after birth, except in the relatively few cases of *persistent* Mongolian spot.[84] Because of their small number, they may be overlooked in H&E sections, and one has to search for them even in O&G sections. They also are the substrate of *nevus of Ota* (nevus fuscoceruleus ophthalmomaxillaris, Fig. 33–27) and the

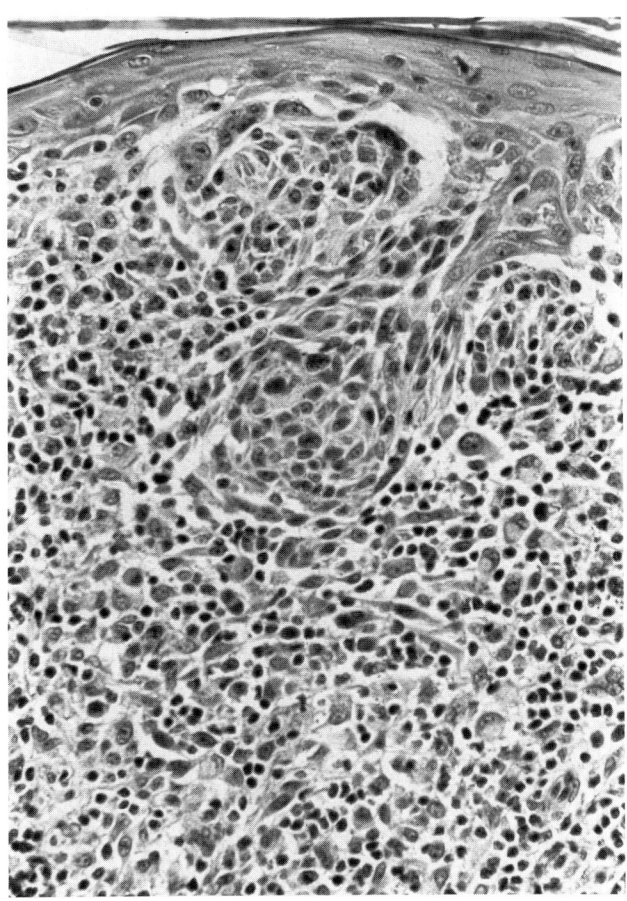

Figure 33–26.
Halo nevus of Sutton. Two nests of nevus cells are recognizable at the dermoepidermal junction. The intradermal nests are surrounded by heavy lymphocytic infiltrate. H&E. X225.

similar *nevus of Ito,* which is situated in the shoulder region.[85] The cells of these lesions are unusually large and present in somewhat greater number in the upper corium. The peculiar powder-stain appearance of these macular melanocytic nevi is due to associated spotty epidermal pigmentation (freckling). Pigmentation of the ectodermal mucous membranes and the sclera of these patients is due to similar cells in the stroma. Nevus of Ota may become complicated with the development of cataract or occular malignant melanoma in the affected side.[86]

Blue Nevus

Localized accumulation of dermal melanocytes forming a papule or small nodule is known as blue nevus of Jadassohn–Tièche.[71] Although it is not usually present at birth, it persists through life once it has formed and thus fulfills the criteria of a true nevus: stable, localized excess of a normal skin constituent. In rare cases, eruptive blue nevi,[72] target lesions,[73] or a large macular hyperpigmented plaque studded with bluish black papules may be found.[87–89] The dermal melanocytes are present as a loose network and are mixed (Fig. 33–28) with a variable number of fibrocytes and melanophages, the latter often containing the bulk of the pigment. The fibrous portion of the dermis also is increased. If one bleaches the melanin in the sections with hydrogen peroxide, the lesion becomes almost indistinguishable from a histiocytoma or dermatofibroma.

Cellular Blue Nevus and Malignant Blue Nevus

In contrast, the cellular blue nevus (Fig. 33–29) consists of densely packed and intersecting bundles of relatively large elongated dermal melanocytes that usually contain little pigment but are interspersed with many melanophages.[90] The tumor may grow deep or reach large size (giant blue nevus, Fig. 33–30).[91] The tendency to grow and occasional instances of malignant transformation speak for a neoplastic nature (Fig. 33–31). Malignant lesions show cells with hyperchromatic and irregularly shaped nuclei and scattered mitotic figures (Fig. 33–32).[92–94] The histologic and cytologic characteristics of cellular blue nevus have given rise to the suggestion that these lesions are pigmented schwannomas. Electron microscopic studies, however, have shown that the tumor cells are melanogenic and are similar to dermal melanocytes.[95]

MALIGNANT MELANOMA

Biology

The incidence of malignant melanoma is increasing and approximately 27,000 new cases are diagnosed in the United States each year. There are multiple etiologic factors in development of malignant melanoma. Carcinogenic properties of ultraviolet light in enhancing progression of precursor melanocytic lesions in the white population discussed recently by Elder[96] does not seem to apply to the acral lentiginous melanomas of blacks and orientals. Histologic review of a large series of early developing malignant melanomas has demonstrated cytologic evidence of pre-existing melanocytic nevi in approximately 25–32 percent of the cases.[97,98] Development

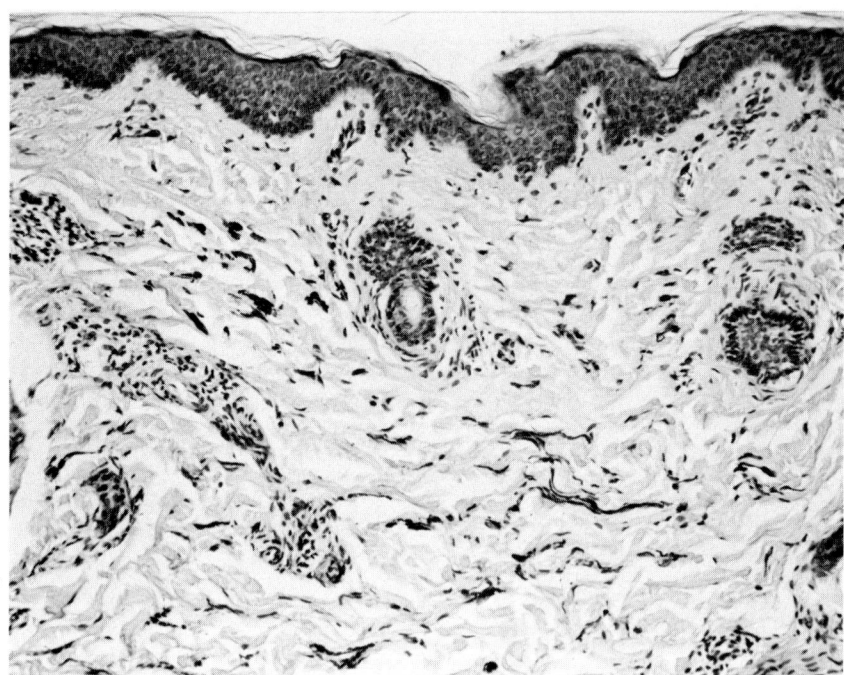

Figure 33–27.
Nevus of Ota. Pigmented dendritic melanocytes are scattered between dermal collagen bundles. H&E. X250.

of malignant melanoma in giant congenital nevi is well documented. It has been suggested that 3–5 percent of malignant melanomas develop in this fashion.[99,100] The relationship between the number of pigmented nevi present and the development of malignant melanoma has been investigated. Individuals with malignant melanoma seem to have a larger number of pigmented nevi than control subjects do.[101] Variation in distribution of pigmented nevi was found among white children in Vancouver.[102] Male children had more pigmented nevi located over the head, neck, and trunk; females had nevi predominantly over the upper and lower extremities. These distribution patterns parallel those of cutaneous melanomas in males and females in adults.

Familial melanoma is transmitted by an autosomal dominant trait.[103,104] One to 6 percent of all malignant melanomas and as much as 44 percent of those with multiple melanomas can be identified as familial. These occur in somewhat younger individuals and are characterized by smaller lesions and a lower Clark level.

Clark's division of malignant melanomas into four categories—lentigo maligna, acral lentiginous melanoma (including mucosal lesions), superficial spreading malignant melanoma, and nodular

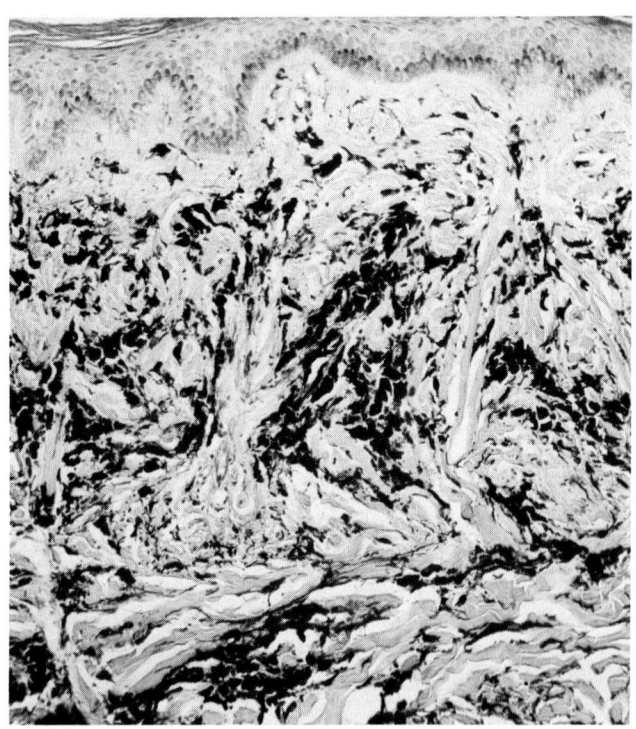

Figure 33–28.
Blue nevus. Strands of lightly pigmented tumor cells are accentuated by massively melanized macrophages. H&E. X135.

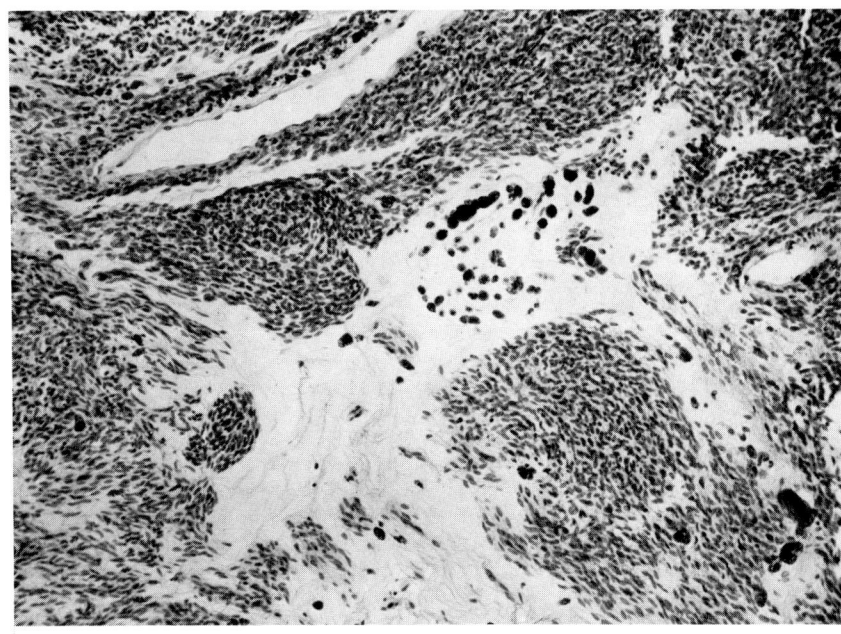

Figure 33–29.
Cellular blue nevus. Most of melanin is in macrophages, while nests of crowded tumor cells contain little pigment. H&E. X135.

melanoma—is based on identification of histologic features of the radial and vertical growth phase. Radial growth phase is defined as a net clinical enlargement of a primary malignant melanoma along radii of an imperfect circle.[105] At this stage, the lesion seems to be flat, round, or oval with irregular border. Histologic details of the radial growth phase is different in lentigo maligna, acral lentiginous melanoma, or superficial spreading malignant melanoma. In a clinical sense, the vertical growth phase

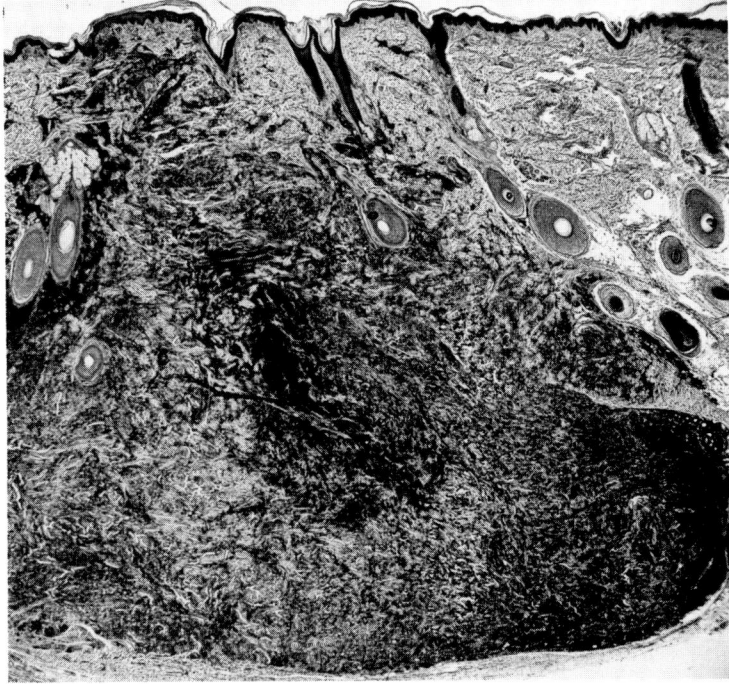

Figure 33–30.
Giant blue nevus. These lesions, which occur most commonly in the sacral area, on the backs of hands and feet, and on the scalp, may reach a size of 2 cm or more and may extend deep into the subcutaneous tissue. Most of the melanin is contained in macrophages, which obscure the fusiform neoplastic, but usually benign, dermal melanocytes. H&E. X14.

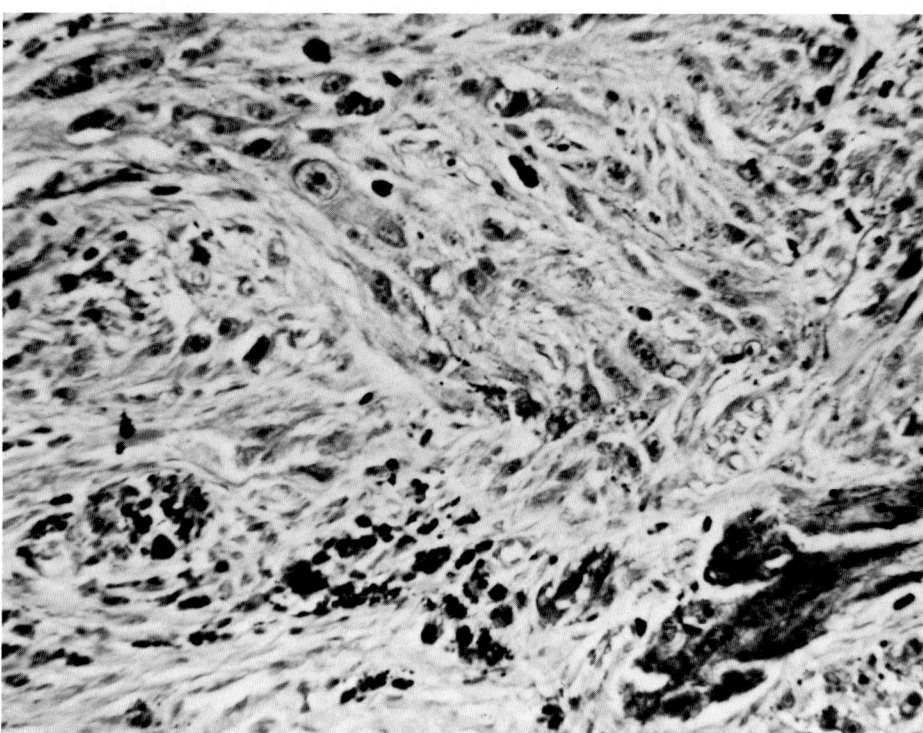

Figure 33–31.
Malignant blue nevus. Atypical, mainly fusiform tumor cells contain only a few small melanin granules. Melanized macrophages attest to the melanogenic nature of the tumor. H&E. X225.

is characterized by focal appearance within a radial growth phase of a new population of cells that tend to expand into a space-taking spherical nodule in a fashion similar to a metastatic lesion.[106]

Lentigo Maligna

Before the turn of the century, Hutchinson described as "infective melanotic freckle" a slowly spreading, macular pigmentation on the faces of elderly individuals, which was later referred to by Dubreuilh as "preblastomatous melanosis." Unfortunately, in a subsequent paper Dubreuilh[107] widened and diluted his concept to include somewhat similar lesions occurring in younger people and on covered surfaces, lesions that we now separate as superficial spreading malignant melanomas. We elected to follow Clark's lead and replaced the older terms with lentigo maligna, which emphasizes the entirely macular nature of the lesion. Lentigo maligna is a distinct type of preinvasive melanoma (malignant melanoma in situ), amounting to about 5 percent of all melanomas. The earliest stage (Fig. 33–33), clinically manifested as a light brown spot, and histologically characterized by the presence of somewhat larger melanocytes may be taken as an early sign of loss of normal territorial behavior and, therefore, of neoplastic derangement of the cells. Yet, for a long time, the melanocytes remain dendritic individuals with small dark nuclei. They do not acquire the cytologic characteristics of nevus cells and do not form theques.[108,109] The epidermis thus has a peculiar, moth-eaten appearance in routine sections (Fig. 33–34).

Gradually, there occurs more pronounced focal crowding of cells, some of which may be carried into the higher epidermal strata and be shed with the horny layer. The number of such cells is relatively small, and the elements remain single and look shrunken and dying in contrast to the pagetoid picture we shall encounter in superficial spreading malignant melanoma. The junctional nests are unevenly spaced and show cells with irregularly shaped nuclei and clear cytoplasm. Melanocytic hyperplasia and nest formation also occur in connection with the infundibular portion of the pilosebaceous structures and less often with the eccrine sweat ducts. The upper dermis shows patchy chronic inflammatory cell infiltrate and macrophages containing melanin pigment granules.

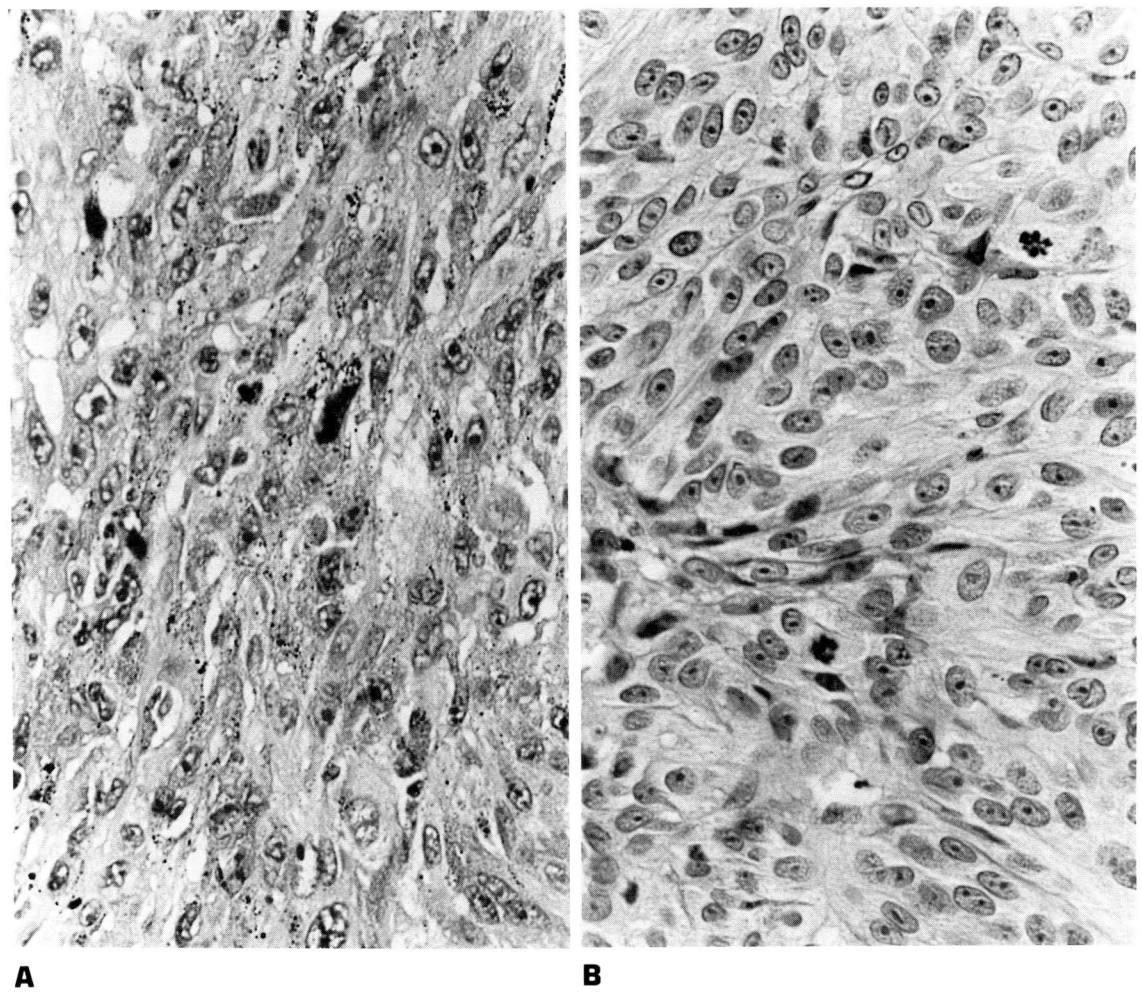

Figure 33–32.
Malignant cellular blue nevus. Pigmented **(A)** and non-pigmented **(B)** areas show cells with large nuclei and scattered mitotic figures. H&E. X400.

Lentigo Maligna Melanoma

As a lentigo maligna progresses, the melanocytic cells become more atypical, show increased tendency to migrate downward within the basement membrane surrounding the hair follicles, and begin to form nests at the junction. Eventually there is disruption of basement membrane and dermal invasion (Fig. 33–35). Detection of early dermal invasion may be facilitated by immunostaining for S-100 protein or HMB-45.[110] When cell nests are present in the dermis, an invasive lentigo maligna melanoma has developed.[111,112] Invasive melanoma developing in lentigo maligna is often of the spindle-celled or desmoplastic variety. An invasive lesion should be graded according to Clark's levels and Breslow's tumor thickness, as will be discussed later.

It is well recognized by dermatologists that malignant melanomas arising in lentigo maligna metastasize late and therefore can often be controlled by local excision. It has also been shown that the radiosensitivity that distinguishes normal melanocytes from benign nevus cells is preserved to some degree in these malignant cells. The biologic basis for these oncologic differences of lentigo maligna melanoma from nodular malignant melanoma, as indicated in Figure 33–36, seems to reside in their origin from melanocytes rather than nevus cells. Histologic differential diagnosis between lentigo

464 MALFORMATION AND NEOPLASIA

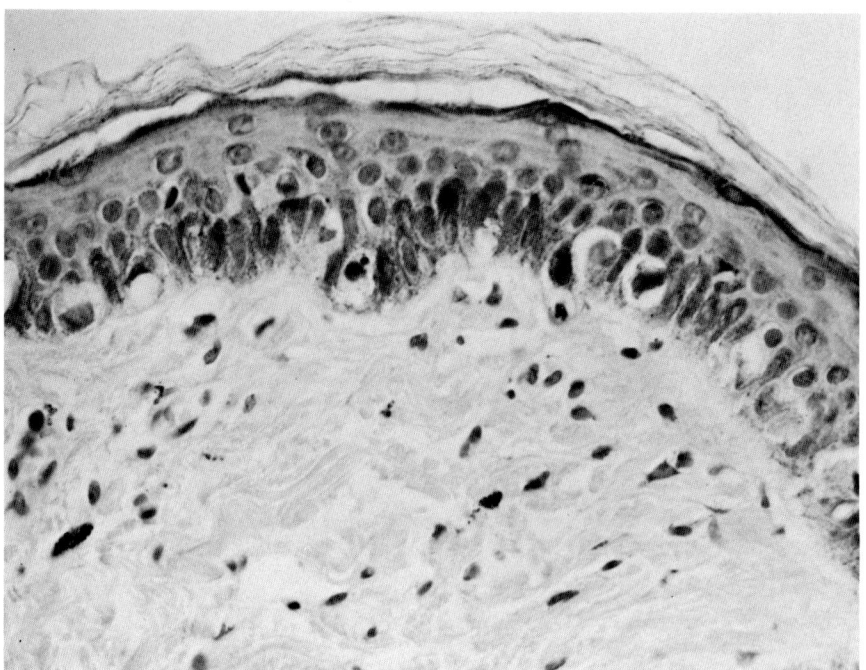

Figure 33—33.
Lentigo maligna, early stage. Epidermis thin without ridges. Increased number of atypical melanocytes in the basal layer. No tendency to nest formation or migration into higher layers. H&E. X600.

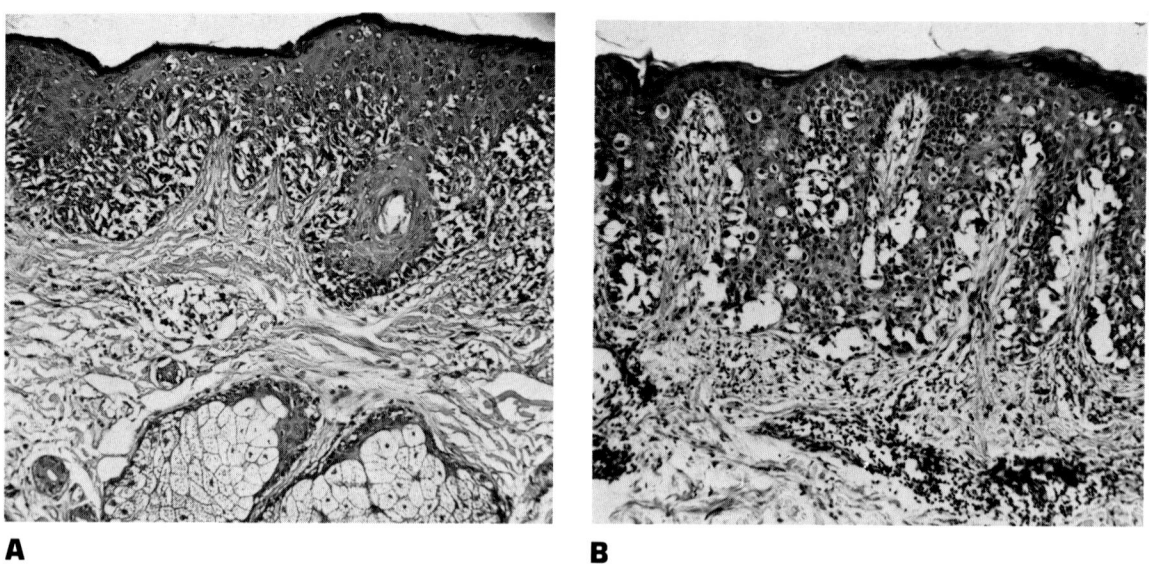

A B

Figure 33—34.
Lentigo maligna. Some degree of epidermal hyperplasia. Crowding of atypical melanocytes in the basal layer produces a moth-eaten appearance while only a few dying cells are present in higher layers. Note atypical melanocytes in basal layer of hair follicle and sebaceous gland in **A.** Both features contrast with the picture of pagetoid melanoma shown in Figure 33—41, where nests of malignant melanoma cells are present in the basal layer and viable tumor cells are disseminated through the prickle cell layers. **A** & **B.** H&E. X90.

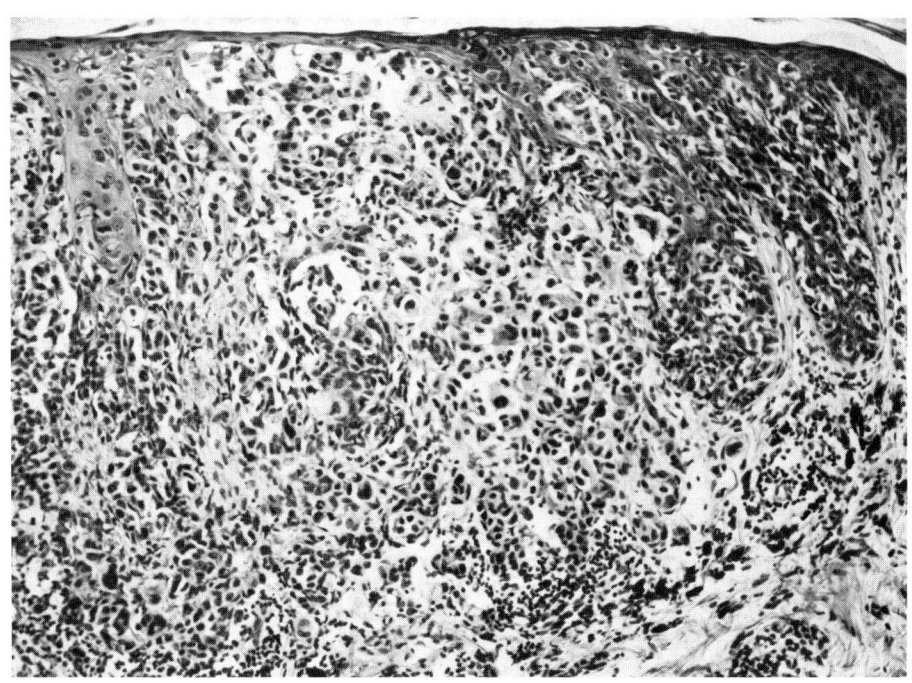

Figure 33–35.
Malignant melanoma developing in lentigo maligna. Persistence of individualized atypical melanocytes in edge of lesion permits diagnosis. H&E. X135.

maligna, lentigo maligna melanoma, and other melanomas is listed in Table 33–4).

Acral Lentiginous Melanoma

Pigmented macular lesions involving palms, soles, and subungual[113,114] areas are separated under the term acral lentiginous melanoma for two reasons. They are not situated in normally light-damaged areas, and the progression to invasion and metastasis is accelerated. The term emphasizes the lentiginous macular character of the lesions.[115] The radial or lentiginous growth phase may evolve over months or years, eventuating into the vertical growth phase

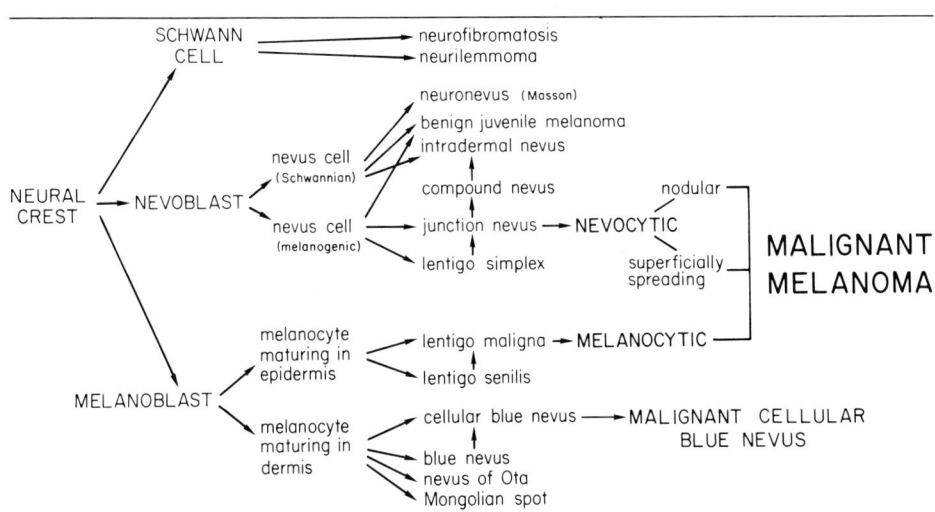

Figure 33–36.
Diagram of neural crest derivation of melanotic tumors. (Adapted from Mishima. Cancer 20:632, 1967.)

TABLE 33–4. DIFFERENTIAL DIAGNOSIS OF MALIGNANT MELANOMAS

Diagnosis	Histologic Features
Lentigo maligna	Crowding of atypical (usually dendritic) pigmented melanocytes in the basal layer. Only minor degree of transepidermal elimination. Later formation of cells nests at the junction. Lymphocytic and plasmacytic infiltrate with pigmented macrophages in upper dermis
Lentigo maligna melanoma	Similar. Nests of atypical melanocytes (dendritic or spindle shaped) at the junction and in dermis. Often downgrowth of melanocytes in outer root sheath and eccrine ducts
Acral lentiginous melanoma	Proliferation of atypical (usually dendritic) pigmented melanocytes in the basal layer. Junctional nests populated with large spindle-shaped or pleomorphic epithelioid cells. Later, dermal invasion with atypical spindle or epithelioid cells and desmoplasia
Superficial spreading malignant melanoma	Large, more or less pigmented (usually round) melanocytic cells in basal layer with strong tendency to nest formation. Invasion of upper epidermal layers in pagetoid fashion and extensive transepidermal elimination. Moderately heavy lymphocytic and plasmacytic dermal infiltrate with pigmented macrophages. Later, nests of malignant melanocytic cells also in dermis, extending to variable depth.
Nodular malignant melanoma	Nests of malignant cells at the junction and in dermis, forming a more or less spherical tumor without appreciable peripheral spread in the epidermis. Variable amount of inflammatory infiltrate in dermis
Malignant blue nevus	Atypical fusiform cells with large nuclei and mitotic figures mixed with deeply pigmented macrophages in the dermis. No epidermal involvement. Variable amount of inflammatory infiltrate.
Metastatic malignant melanoma	Malignant cell nests in dermis, usually without involvement of the junction and often without much inflammatory infiltrate

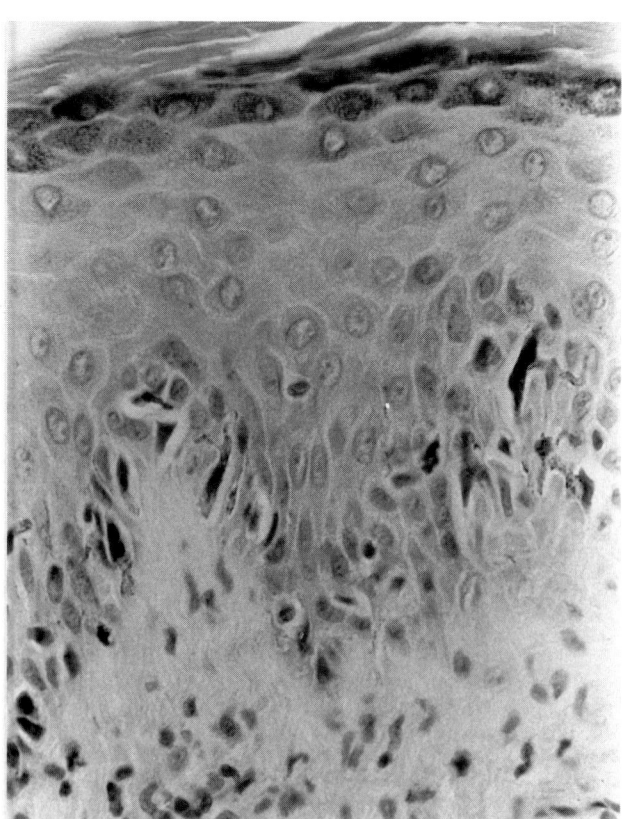

Figure 33–37.
Acral lentiginous melanoma. An early lesion shows atypically large melanocytic cells at the dermoepidermal junction. H&E. X400.

with dermal invasion. The lesion is more common in blacks and orientals and occurs in the sixth to eighth decades of life.[116,117] Weight-bearing areas of soles and subungual areas of thumbs or great toes are common locations.[118]

Acral lentiginous melanoma (Fig. 33–37) in its radial growth phase is characterized histologically by junctional melanocytic hyperplasia (Fig. 33–38). The junctional melanocytes are large, atypical, and show hyperchromatic nuclei[119] and prominent complexes of dendrites (Fig. 33–39).[120] The epidermis shows elongation of the rete ridges and is invaded by upward transmigrating melanocytes (Fig. 33–40). Pagetoid features may be encountered. Junctional nests are irregular, variable in size, and bulge into the dermis. Junctional nests are populated by either elongated, spindle-shaped, or large pleomorphic epithelioid-type cells.

In the vertical growth phase, dermal invasion occurs with poorly defined periphery. The growth is populated with spindle or polygonal epithelioid cells. Desmoplasia may be prominent and neurotropism is present in 14 percent of the cases. Nuclear atypia and mitotic figures are frequent. The growth may be deeply pigmented, or the pigment can be demonstrated by Masson's silver stain. Chronic inflammatory cell infiltrate is always present.

Superficial Spreading Malignant Melanoma

Superficial spreading malignant melanoma appears as a plaque of 1 to several centimeters in diameter,

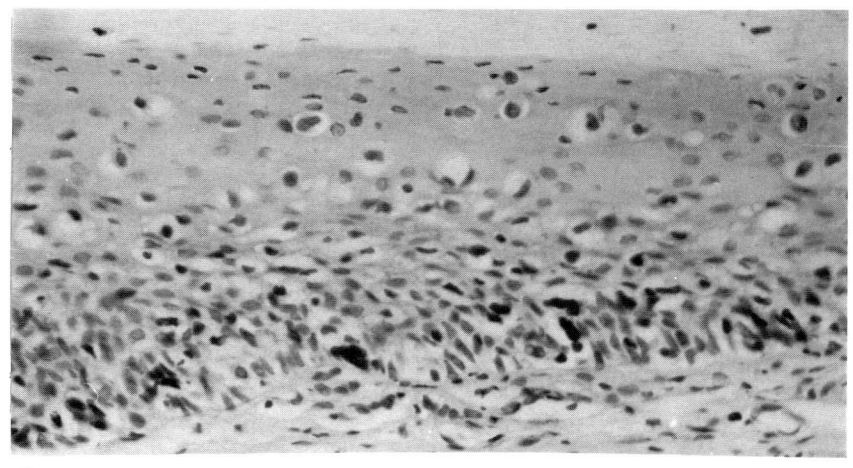

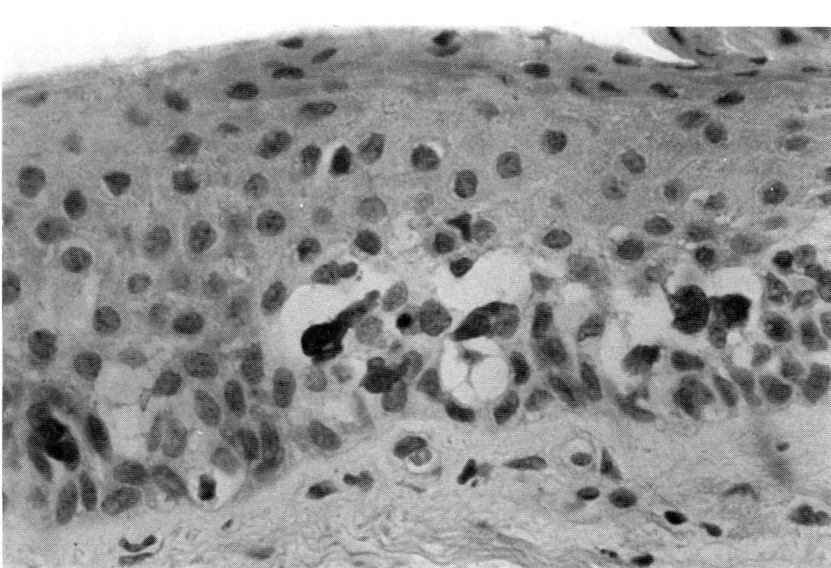

Figure 33–38.
Acral lentiginous melanoma. **A.** Nailbed shows crowing of atypical melanocytic cells at the dermoepidermal junction and upward transmigration into the surface epithelium. H&E. X250. **B.** Details of atypical junctional melanocytes involving the nailbed. H&E. X400.

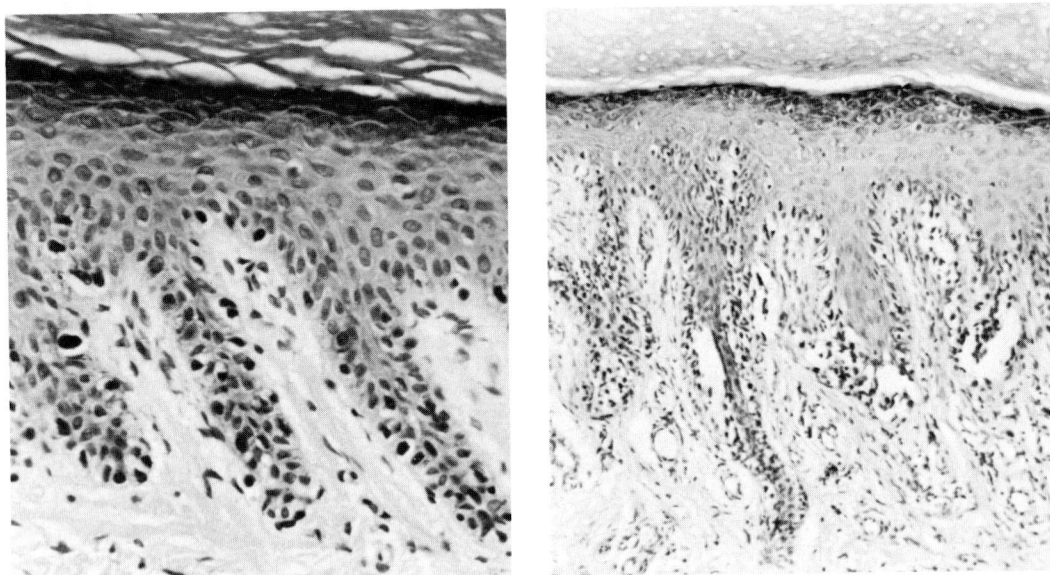

Figure 33–39.
Acral lentiginous melanoma. Shows atypical melanocytic proliferation at the junction and extending downward around a sweat duct. Nests of atypical melanocytes project into the dermis. A few effete melanocytes are eliminated transepidermally. Very little reactive inflammatory infiltrate. H&E. X250. (From Lupulescu et al. Arch Dermatol 107:717, 1973.)

which may be round or arciform with irregular border and angular indentations. The surface may be smooth, slightly elevated, or hyperkeratotic, exhibiting a variety of colors from light brown to black with orange or gray areas. Areas of white depigmentation are indicative of regression.

Histologic features in the early, or radial, phase consist of extensive proliferation of large melanocytic cells with abundant and dusty cytoplasms at the dermoepidermal junction (Fig. 33–41). There is a great tendency for junctional nest formation.[121] Mitotic figures are present and upward transmigra-

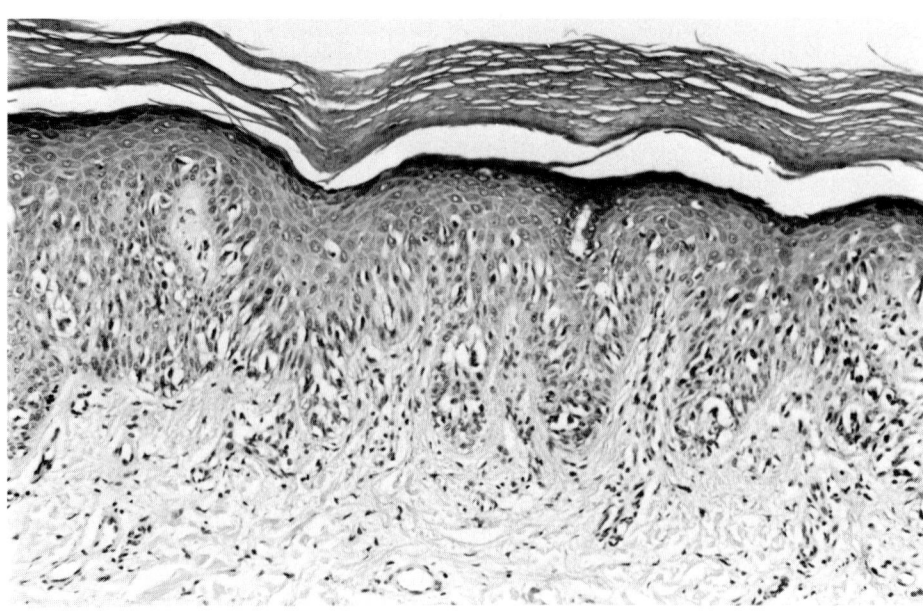

Figure 33–40.
Acral lentiginous melanoma. Diffuse hyperplasia of atypical melanocytes at the dermoepidermal junction and upward transmigration. H&E. X250.

tion of small nests or individual atypical melanocytes within the epidermis is common.[122] Extensive transepidermal elimination of large melanocytic cells is characteristic of the *pagetoid* variety.[123] A lichenoid tissue reaction with basal cell damage associated with lymphohistiocytic infiltrate is observed in the clinically white, regressive areas. The upper dermis shows fibroplasia, macrophages containing melanin, and patchy lymphocytic and plasma cell infiltrate.

The vertical phase is manifested by some increase in thickness of the lesion and development of surface nodularity (Fig. 33–42). Nests of large melanocytic cells extend from the junction down into various levels of the dermis. Desmoplasia and neurotropism is present in approximately 2 percent of the cases.

Nodular Malignant Melanoma

Nodular malignant melanomas are raised hemispherical growths with smooth surfaces that may be red, gray, or deeply pigmented. Some lesions appear richly vascular and resemble granuloma pyogenicum. A few others are completely amelanotic and difficult to recognize clinically. Erythema, ulceration, and pigment spread at the periphery of the nodular lesions are indications of malignancy. Another indication of malignancy in an advanced lesion is peripheral satellitosis. Approximately 30 per-

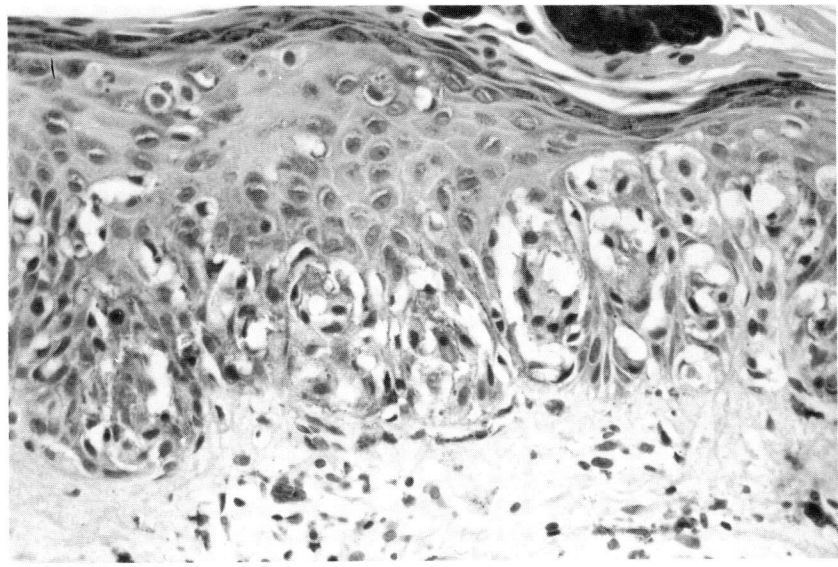

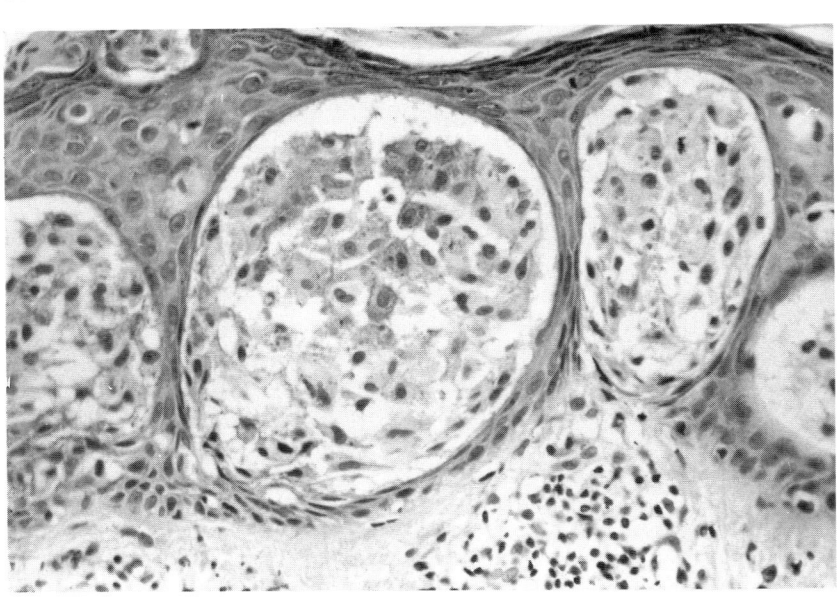

Figure 33–41.
Superficial spreading malignant melanoma. **A.** Nests of malignant melanoma cells at the dermoepidermal junction and pagetoid involvement of the epidermis. H&E. X250. **B.** Large junctional nests populated with cells having abundant cytoplasm and dust-like pigment granules. H&E. X250.

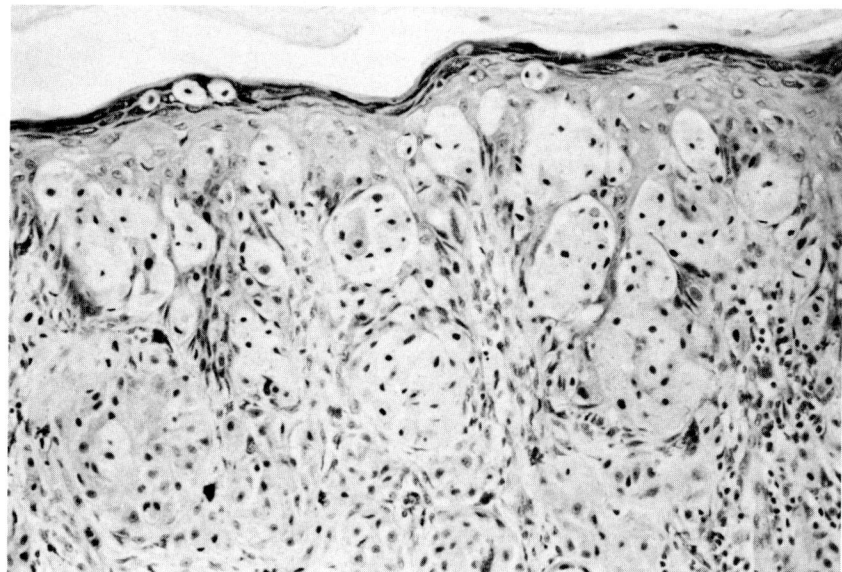

Figure 33–42.
Superficially spreading malignant melanoma producing pagetoid picture in its radial growth phase. Note that there is already vertical growth downward into the dermis. H&E. X250.

cent of patients with malignant melanoma give a history of a previously existing pigmented lesion in the area. The incidence of this association is higher in younger patients.[124]

CRITERIA FOR MALIGNANCY

There are several criteria for malignancy of a melanocytic tumor, some more significant than others.

With the exception of malignant blue nevus, all types of malignant melanomas start at the dermoepidermal junction. The junctional nests are populated with atypically large cells showing variable degrees of melanogenesis. From the junction, tumor cells are carried into the higher epidermal layers and are eliminated (Fig. 33–43). The radial growth phase and dermal invasion is marked by the appearance of a new population of cells that tend to grow in spherical nodules. The cell size has considerable significance. The cells of malignant melanoma usually

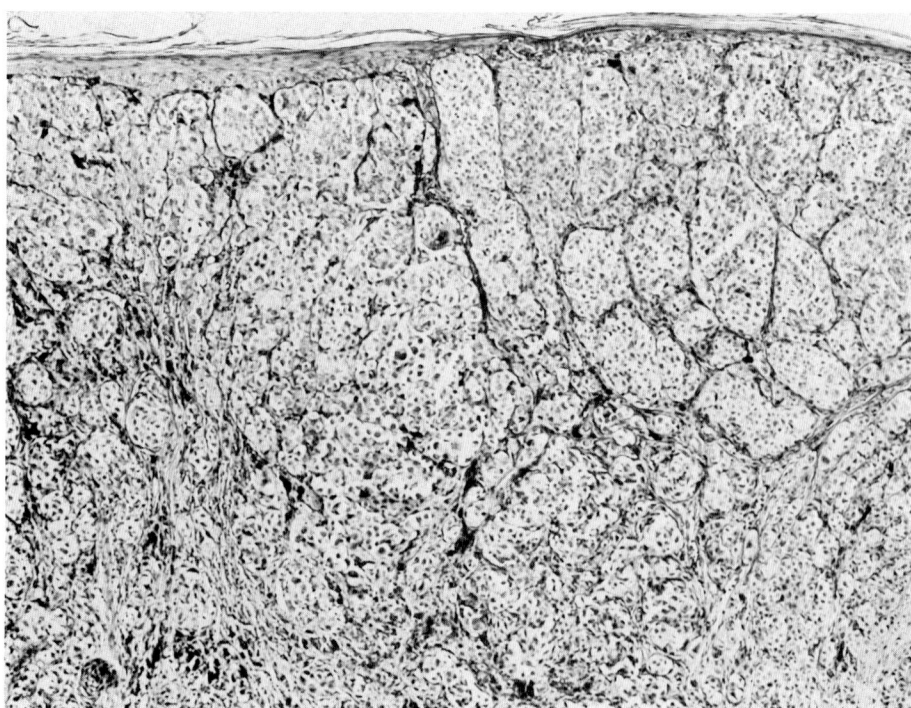

Figure 33–43.
Nodular malignant melanoma. This general view of a bulky and relatively amelanotic tumor illustrates the variability of the tumor cells, which are gathered into unevenly sized nests by scanty stroma. While there is a thin layer of stroma between epidermis and tumor in the left half of the picture, tumor cells replace the lower half of the epidermis in the right half. H&E. X60.

are large and unevenly pigmented. Some cells contain plenty of cytoplasm and dust-like pigment granules. Multiple cell populations may be present, with different clones of cells showing morphologic variations. One important feature of malignant melanoma is the tendency of cells to nest formation, which is retained even in undifferentiated amelanotic lesions. The connective tissue stroma present in benign cellular nevi is no longer appreciated. The elastic fibers are destroyed and the reticulum fibers are few, present only at the periphery of the large tumor nests (Fig. 33–44).[125] This feature is well recognized when a nodular malignant melanoma has developed within a preexisting congenital nevus (Fig. 33–44). The presence of and number of mitoses is of primary importance.[126] Mitotic figures, especially when in dermal nests away from the junction, are an indication of malignancy.

Another important feature is inflammatory reaction composed of lymphocytes and possibly plasma cells. It is practically always present, but may be absent in rapid-growing tumors. On the other hand, it may be found in Spitz nevus, nevus incipiens, and Sutton's halo nevus. Microscopic satellites are another indication of malignancy.[127] These are defined as the presence of tumor nests over 0.05 mm in diameter within the reticular dermis, fat tissue, blood vessels, or lymphatics beneath the principal invasive tumor mass, but separated from it by normal connective tissue in serial sections. Several varieties of malignant melanomas are worthy of special recognition. Malignant melanomas developing in association with the acquired melanocytic nevi appear to have a more favorable prognosis.[128] On the other hand, *amelanotic malignant melanomas* are considered poorly differentiated and usually signify a higher degree of malignant potentiality and poor prognosis.[129] Desmoplastic and neurotropic malignant melanomas are rare, and often develop within preexisting lentigo maligna, acral lentiginous melanoma, and occasionally superficial spreading lesions (Fig. 33–46). Histologically, bundles of elongated and spindle-shaped cells extend from the lower surface of the epidermis into the underlying dermis in fascicles and exhibit variable degrees of desmoplastic stroma.[130–132] Desmoplasia is spotty in the neurotropic variety where a neuromalike infiltrate shows predilection for perineural invasion.[133–136] Mitotic figures are usually plentiful. A completely amelanotic lesion should be histologically differentiated from spindle-cell squamous cell carcinoma and fibrosarcoma. Electron microscopy[137] will dem-

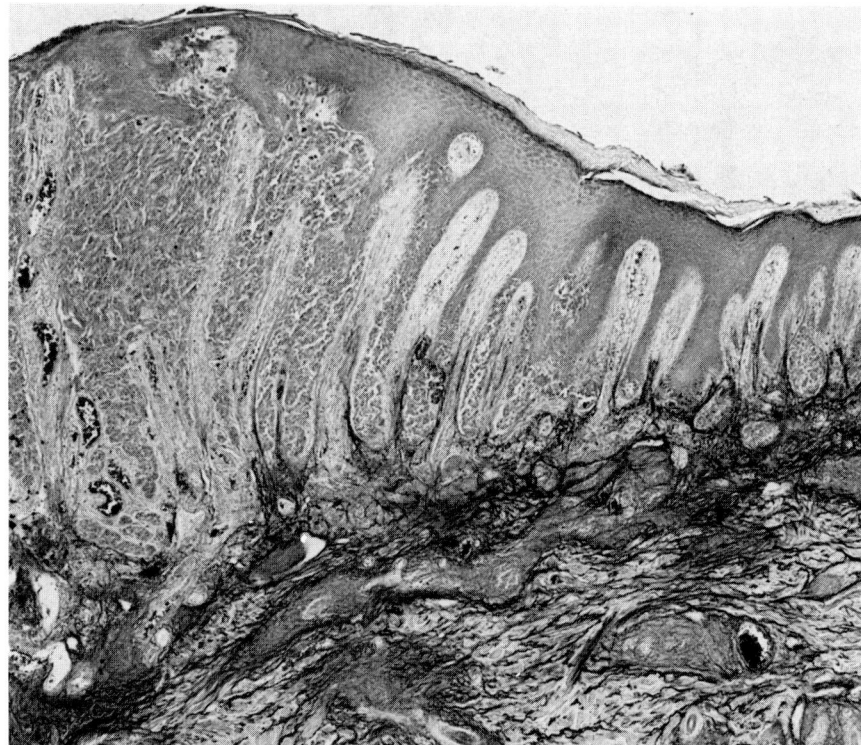

Figure 33–44.
Malignant melanoma developing above a benign intradermal nevus. Presence of elastic fibers in benign part (lower right) and absence in malignant portion (upper left) emphasize difference. O&G. X45.

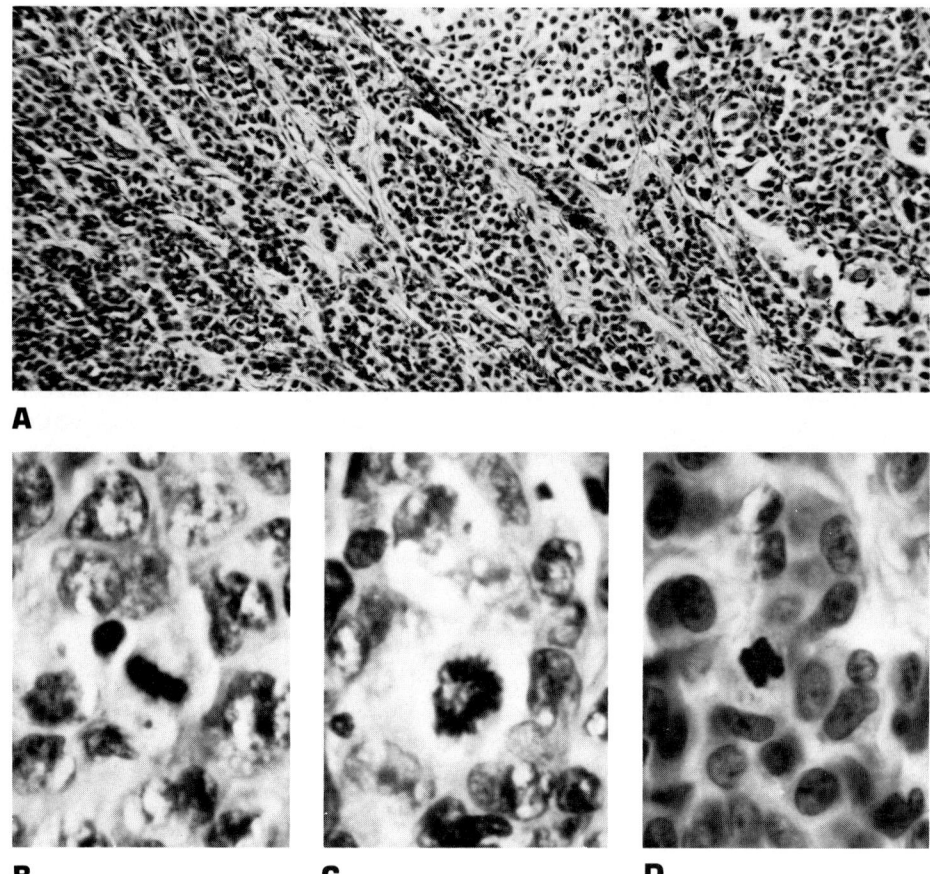

Figure 33–45.
Malignant melanoma. **A.** At higher magnification, relatively large size of cells is evident, when compared with Figure 33–6. There is some indication of nest formation, cells form diffuse masses in other areas, and there is a minimum of stroma. H&E. X125. **B, C,** and **D.** Characteristics of nuclei and mitotic figures. Cell in **C** has more than normal complement of chromosomes. H&E. X1000.

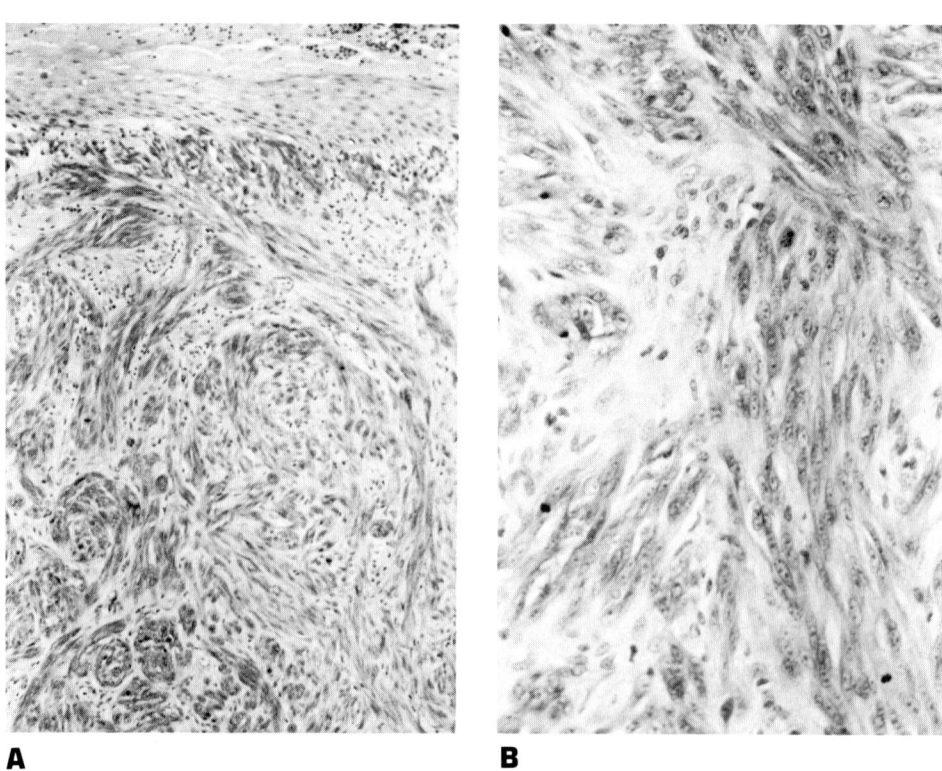

Figure 33–46.
Desmoplastic malignant melanoma. **A.** Bundles of spindle-shaped melanocytes extending from the dermoepidermal junction into the corium. H&E. X250. **B.** Scattered mitotic figures. H&E. X400.

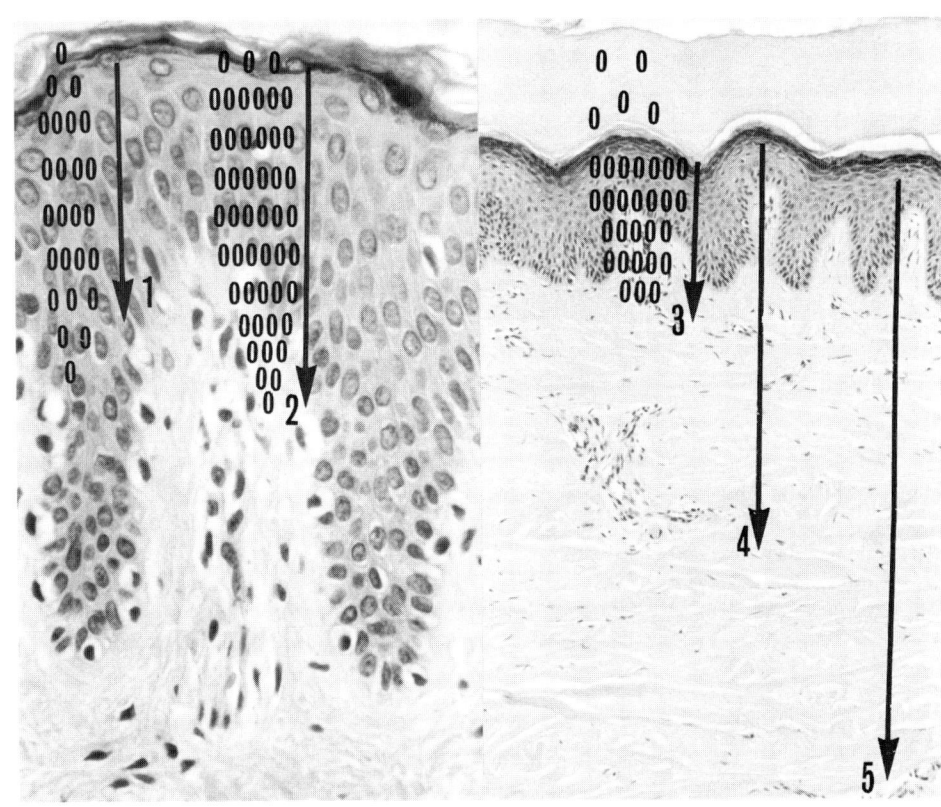

Figure 33–47.
The levels of dermal invasion according to Clark are indicated: level 1, intraepidermal; level 2, invasion of papillae; level 3, involvement of superficial vascular plexus; level 4, invasion of reticular dermis; level 5, involvement of subcutaneous tissue.

onstrate melanin and melanosomes and the tumor cells will stain positive for S-100 protein, HMB-45, and neuron-specific enolase.[138,139]

HISTOLOGIC GRADING OF MALIGNANT MELANOMA AND PROGNOSIS

A major responsibility of the pathologist in the field of malignant melanoma is the prognostication of malignant potentiality and metastatic spread. Clark pioneered in this field and demonstrated that not every malignant melanoma carries the expectation of metastasis.[140] In statistical terms, the depth of penetration is important, and Clark's grading of dermal invasion into levels 2, 3, 4, and 5 is very helpful in predicting which tumors have a high chance of having already seeded themselves in the lymph stream (Fig. 33–47). Clark's level 1 means in situ melanoma with proliferation of malignant melanocytic cells in the confines of the epidermis. Level 2 is characterized by involvement of the papillary layer. Level 3 shows invasion of the superficial vascular plexus; level 4, invasion of pars reticularis; and level 5, involvement of the subcutaneous fat tissue.[141]

Another rule advanced by Breslow advocates actual measurement of maximum tumor thickness under microscope.[142,143] This is achieved by measuring the lesion from the surface of granular layer of the epidermis down to a point that limits the lower border of the growth. Tumors less than 0.75 mm in thickness are apt to behave localized; tumors more than 1.7 mm are most likely to have a high tendency for metastasis.[144–147] To these two indices one may also add other indications of higher degrees of malignancy, such as the index of mitotic figures more than one per high power field, the presence of surface ulceration, microscopic satellites, and absence of immunologic host reaction.[148–150]

REFERENCES

1. Mishima Y: Macromolecular changes in pigmentary disorders. III. Cellular nevi: Subcellular and cytochemical characteristics with reference to their origin. Arch Dermatol 91:536, 1965
2. Nakajima T, Watanabe S, Sato Y, et al: Immunohistochemical demonstration of S100 protein in malignant melanoma and pigmented nevus, and its diagnostic application. Cancer 50:912, 1982
3. Penneys NS, Mogollon R, Kowalczyk A, et al: A survey of cutaneous neural lesions for the presence of myelin basic protein: An immunohistochemical study. Arch Dermatol 120:210, 1984
4. Spann CR, Owen LG, Hodge SJ: The labial melanotic macule. Arch Dermatol 123:1029, 1987
5. Revus J, Clerici T: Penile melanosis. J Am Acad Dermatol 20:567, 1989
6. Leicht S, Youngberg G, Diaz-Miranda C: Atypical pigmented penile macules. Arch Dermatol 124:1267, 1988
7. Barnhill RL, Albert LS, Shama SK, et al: Genital lentiginosis: A clinical and histopathologic study. J Am Acad Dermatol 22:453, 1990
8. Chapel TA, Taylor RM, Pinkus H: Volar melanotic macules. Int J Dermatol 18:222, 1979
9. Narisawa Y, Kohda H: Clinical characteristics of pigmented macules on palms and/or soles appearing after middle age in Japan. J Dermatol 14:430, 1987
10. Vasquez M, Maldonado H, Benmaman C, Sanchez JL: Melasma in men: A clinical and histologic study. Int J Dermatol 27:25, 1988
11. Jimbow K, Szabo G, Fitzpatrick TB: Ultrastructure of giant pigment granules (macromelanosomes) in the cutaneous pigmented macules of neurofibromatosis. J Invest Dermatol 61:300, 1973
12. Frenk E: Étude ultrastructurale des tâches pigmentaires du syndrome d'Albright. Dermatologica 143:12, 1971
13. Grupper C, Pruniéras M, Hincky M, et al: Albinisme partial familiale (piebaldisme): Étude ultrastructurale. Ann Dermatol Syphiligr 97:267, 1970
14. Jimbow K, Fitzpatrick TB, Szabo G, et al: Congenital circumscribed hypomelanosis: A characterization based on electron microscopic study of tuberous sclerosis, nevus depigmentosus, and piebaldism. J Invest Dermatol 64:50, 1975
15. Bisighini G, Moroni P, Davalli R, Lo Scocco G: Su di un caso di LEOPARD syndrome. Chron Dermatol 18:395, 1987
16. Barros MA, Norton Mexedo MF, Mesquita-Guimaraes J: Nunes da ponte A: Sindrome de Peutz-Jeghers. Dois Casos. Med Cutan ILA 14:255, 1986
17. Reed OM, Mellette RJ Jr, Fitzpatrick JE: Cutaneous lentiginosis with atrial myxomas. J Am Acad Dermatol 15:398, 1986
18. Andre P, Janin-Mercier A, Souteyrand P, et al: Lentiginose cutanéo-muqueuse, éphélides et myxome cardiaque. Ann Dermatol Venereol 115:151, 1988
19. O'Neill JF, James WD: Inherited patterned lentiginosis in blacks. Arch Dermatol 125:1231, 1989
20. Abel EA, Reid H, Wood C, Hu C-H: PUVA-induced melanocytic atypia: Is it confined to PUVA lentigines? J Am Acad Dermatol 13:761, 1985
21. Bruce DR, Berger TG: PUVA-induced pigmented macules: A case involving palmoplantar skin. J Am Acad Dermatol 16:1087, 1987
22. Williams HC, Salisbury J, Brett J, DuVivier A: Sunbed lentigines. Brit Med J 296:1097, 1988
23. Mehregan AH: Lentigo senilis and its evolutions. J Invest Dermatol 65:429, 1975
24. Eng AM: Solitary small active junctional nevi in juvenile patients. Arch Dermatol 119:35, 1983
25. Schmoeckel C, Stolz W, Sakai LY, et al: Structure of basement membranes in malignant melanoma and nevocytic nevi. J Invest Dermatol 92:663, 1989
26. Stenback F, Wasenius V-M: Occurrence of basement membranes in pigment cell tumors of the skin, relation to cell type and clinical behavior. J Cutan Pathol 13:175, 1986
27. Bentley-Phillips CB, Marks R: Cell division and metabolic activity of nevus cells: The relationships between anatomy and behaviour in moles. Br J Dermatol 94:559, 1976
28. Miescher G, Albertini A: Histologie de 100 cas de naevi pigmentaires d'après les méthodes de Masson. Bull Soc Fr Dermatol Syphiligr 42:1265, 1935
29. Sagebiel RW: Histologic artifacts of benign pigmented nevi. Arch Dermatol 106:691, 1972
30. Weedon D: Unusual features of nevocellular nevi. J Cutan Pathol 9:284, 1982
31. Soltani K, Pepper MC, Simjee S, Apatoff BR: Large acquired nevocytic nevi induced by the Koebner phenomenon. J Cutan Pathol 11:296, 1984
32. Hughes BR, Cunliffe WJ, Bailey CC: The development of excess numbers of benign melanocytic naevi in children after chemotherapy for malignancy. Br J Dermatol 119 (Suppl 33):30, 1988
33. Stewart DM, Altman J, Mehregan AH: Speckled lentiginous nevus. Arch Dermatol 114:895, 1978
34. Simoes G: Speckled zosteriform lentiginous nevus. J Am Acad Dermatol 4:236, 1981
35. Vion B, Belaich S, Grossin M, Preaux J: Les aspects evolutifs du naevus sur naevus: Revue de la litterature à propos de 7 observations. Ann Dermatol Venereol 112:813, 1985
36. Stern JB, Haupt HM, Aaronson CM: Malignant melanoma in a speckled zosteriform lentiginous nevus. Int J Dermatol 29:583, 1990
37. Kelly JW, Crutcher WA, Sagebiel RW: Clinical diagnosis of dysplastic melanocytic nevi. A clinicopathologic correlation. J Am Acad Dermatol 14:1044, 1986
38. Roush GC, Barnhill RL, Duray PH, et al: Diagnosis of the dysplastic nevus in different populations. J Am Acad Dermatol 14:419, 1986
39. Vignon-Pennamen M-D: Le syndrome du naevus dysplasique. Ann Dermatol Venereol 112:269, 1985

40. Soyer PH, Smolle J. Hödl S, et al: Surface microscopy. A new approach to the diagnosis of cutaneous pigmented tumors. Am J Dermatopathol 11:1, 1989
41. Rahbari H, Mehregan AH: Sporadic atypical mole syndrome: A report of five nonfamilial B-K mole syndrome-like cases and histopathologic findings. Arch Dermatol 117:329, 1981
42. Mehregan AH: Dysplastic nevi: A histopathologic investigation. J Cutan Pathol 15:276, 1988
43. Balkau D, Gartmann H, Wischer W, et al: Architectural features in melanocytic lesions with cellular atypia. Dermatologica 177:129, 1988
44. Ahmed I, Piepkorn MW, Rabkin MS, et al: Histopathologic characteristics of dysplastic nevi. Limited association of conventional histologic criteria with melanoma risk group. J Am Acad Dermatol 22:727, 1990
45. Takahashi H, Yamana K, Maeda K, et al: Dysplastic melanocytic nevus. Electron-microscopic observation as a diagnostic tool. Am J Dermatopathol 9:189, 1987
46. Jimbow K, Horikoshi T, Takahashi H, et al: Fine structural and immunohistochemical properties of dysplastic melanocytic nevi: Comparison with malignant melanoma. J Invest Dermatol 92:304S, 1989
47. Kraemer KH, Greene MH: Dysplastic nevus syndrome, familial and sporadic precursors of cutaneous melanoma. Dermatol Clin 3:225, 1985
48. Rhodes AR, Harrist TJ, Day CL, et al: Dysplastic melanocytic nevi in histologic association with 234 primary cutaneous melanomas. J Am Acad Dermatol 9:563, 1983
49. Duray PH, Ernstoff MS: Dysplastic nevus in histologic contiguity with acquired nonfamilial melanoma. Clinicopathologic experience in a 100-bed hospital. Arch Dermatol 123:80, 1987
50. Rigel DS, Rivers JK, Kopf AW, et al: Dysplastic nevi. Markers for increased risk of melanoma. Cancer 63: 386, 1989
51. Albert LS, Rhodes AK, Sober AJ: Dysplastic melanocytic nevi and cutaneous melanoma: Markers of increased melanoma risk for affected persons and blood relatives. J Am Acad Dermatol 22:69, 1990
52. Aso M, Hashimoto K, Eto H, et al: Expression of Schwann cell characteristics in pigmented nevus. Immunohistochemical study using monoclonal antibody to Schwann cell associated antigen. Cancer 62: 938, 1988
53. Winkelmann RK: Cholinesterase nevus: Cholinesterases in pigmented tumors of the skin. Arch Dermatol 82:17, 1960
54. Schrader WA, Helwig EB: Balloon cell nevi. Am J Pathol 48:60, 1966
55. Goette DK, Doty RD: Balloon cell nevus: Summary of the clinical and histologic characteristics. Arch Dermatol 114:109, 1978
56. Hashimoto K, Bale G: An electron microscopic study of balloon cell nevus. Cancer 30:530, 1972
57. Aloi FG, Coverlizza S, Pippione M: Balloon cell melanoma: A report of two cases. J Cutan Pathol 15:230, 1988
58. Peters MS, Su DWP: Balloon cell malignant melanoma. J Am Acad Dermatol 13:351, 1985
59. Spitz S: Melanomas of childhood. Am J Pathol 24: 591, 1948
60. Allen AC: Juvenile melanomas of children and adults and melanocarcinomas of children. Arch Dermatol 82:325, 1960
61. Smith SA, Day CL, Vander Ploeg DE: Eruptive widespread Spitz nevi. J Am Acad Dermatol 15:1155, 1986
62. Guillot B, Barneon G: Naevomatose juvenile de Spitz. Forme profuse Linéaire. Ann Dermatol Venereol 115:345, 1988
63. Renfro L, Grant-Kels JM, Brown SA: Multiple agminate Spitz nevi. Pediatr Dermatol 6:114, 1989
64. Peters MS, Goellner JR:Spitz naevi and malignant melanomas of childhood and adolescence. Histopathology 10:1289, 1986
65. Paniago-Pereira C, Maize JC, Ackermann AB: Nevus of large spindle and/or epithelioid cells (Spitz nevus). Arch Dermatol 114:1811, 1978
66. Scott G, Chen KTK, Rosai J: Pseudoepitheliomatous hyperplasia in Spitz nevi. A possible source of confusion with squamous cell carcinoma. Arch Pathol Lab Med 113:61, 1989
67. Kamino H, Misheloff E, Ackermann AB, et al: Eosinophilic globules in Spitz's nevi: New findings and a diagnostic sign. Am J Dermatopathol 1:319, 1979
68. Arbuckle S, Weedon D: Eosinophilic globules in the Spitz nevus. J Am Acad Dermatol 7:324, 1982
69. Barr R, Morales RV, Graham JH: Desmoplastic nevus: A distinct histologic variant of mixed spindle cell and epithelioid cell nevus. Cancer 46:557, 1980
70. Schoenfeld RJ, Pinkus H: The recurrence of nevi after incomplete removal. Arch Dermatol 78:30, 1958
71. Park KH, Leonard DD, Arrington JH III, Lund HZ: Recurrent melanocytic nevi: Clinical and histologic review of 175 cases. J Am Acad Dermatol 17:285, 1987
72. Litous P: Halo naevus. Ann Dermatol Venereol 116: 567, 1989
73. Vignale RA, Paciel J, Bruno J, et al: Halo nevus: In situ study with monoclonal antibodies. Med Cutan ILA 14:13, 1986
74. Penneys NS, Mayoral F, Barnhill R, et al: Delineation of nevus cell nests in inflammatory infiltrates by immunohistochemical staining for the presence of S-100 protein. J Cutan Pathol 12:28, 1985
75. Kroon S, Clemmensen OJ, Hastrup N: Incidence of congenital melanocytic nevi in newborn babies in Denmark. J Am Acad Dermatol 17:422, 1987
76. Fenton DA, Mayou B, Atherton D, Black MM: Histopathology of giant congenital melanocytic naevi: Implications for treatment. Br J Dermatol 117 (Suppl 32):40, 1987
77. Stenn KS, Arons M, Hurwitz S: Pattern of Congeni-

tal nevocellular nevi: A histologic study of thirty-eight cases. J Am Acad Dermatol 9:388, 1983
78. Silvers DN, Helwig EB: Melanocytic nevi in neonates. J Am Acad Dermatol 4:166, 1981
79. Nickoloff BJ, Walton R, Pregerson-Rodan K, et al: Immunohistologic patterns of congenital nevocellular nevi. Arch Dermatol 122:1263, 1986
80. Clemmensen OJ, Kroon S: The histology of "congenital features" in early acquired melanocytic nevi. J Am Acad Dermatol 19:742, 1988
81. Orkin M, Frichot BC III, Zelickson AS: Cerebriform intradermal nevus. A case of cutis verticis gyrata. Arch Dermatol 110:575, 1974
82. Berbis Ph, Dor AM, Niel-Bourrelly RM, et al: Naevus cerebriforme intradermique. Ann Dermatol Venereol 114:369, 1987
83. Nanda A, Kaur S, Bhakoo OM, Dhall K: Survey of cutaneous lesions in Indian newborns. Pediatr Dermatol 6:39, 1989
84. Hidano A: Persistent Mongolian spot in the adult. Arch Dermatol 103:680, 1971
85. Dekio S, Koike S, Jidoi J: Nevus of Ota with nevus of Ito. J Dermatol (Tokyo) 16:164, 1989
86. Hartmann LC, Oliver FG, Winkelmann RK, et al: Blue nevus and nevus of Ota associated with dural melanoma. Cancer 64:182, 1989
87. Bondi EE, Elder D, Guerry D, Clark WH Jr: Target blue nevus. Arch Dermatol 119:919, 1983
88. Pittman JL, Fisher BK: Plaque-type blue nevus. Arch Dermatol 112:1127, 1976
89. Toppe F, Haas N: Naevus spilus géant avec naevus bleus. A propos d'un cas. Ann Dermatol Venereol 115:703, 1988
90. Temple-Camp CRE, Saxe N, King H: Benign and malignant cellular blue nevus: A clinicopathological study of 30 cases. Am J Dermatopathol 10:289, 1988
91. Marano SR, Brooks RA, Spetzler RF, Rekate HL: Giant congenital cellular blue nevus of the scalp of a newborn with an underlying scalp defect and invasion of the dura mater. Neurosurgery 18:85, 1986
92. Simon CA, von Overbeck J, Polla L: Naevus bleu malin. Dermatologica 171:183, 1985
93. Kuhn A, Groth W, Gartmann H, Steigleder GK: Malignant blue nevus with metastases to the lung. Am J Dermatopathol 10:436, 1988
94. Goldenhersh MA, Savin RC, Barnhill RL, Stenn KS: Malignant blue nevus. J Am Acad Dermatol 19:712, 1988
95. Bhawan J, Chang WH, Edelstein LM: Cellular blue nevus: An untrastructural study. J Cutan Pathol 7:109, 1980
96. Elder DE: Human melanocytic neoplasms and their etiologic relationship with sunlight. J Invest Dermatol 92:297S, 1989
97. Stolz W, Schmoeckel C, Landthaler M, Braun-Falco O: Association of early malignant melanoma with nevocytic nevi. Cancer 63:550, 1989
98. Gruber SB, Barnhill RL, Stenn KS, Roush GC: Nevomelanocytic proliferations in association with cutaneous malignant melanoma: A multivariate analysis. J Am Acad Dermatol 21:773, 1989
99. Padilla SR, McConnell TS, Gribble JT, Smoot C: Malignant melanoma arising in a giant congenital melanocytic nevus. Cancer 62:2589, 1988
100. Hori Y, Nakayama J, Okamoto M, et al: Giant congenital nevus and malignant melanoma. J Invest Dermatol 92:310S, 1989
101. Grob JJ, Gouvernet J, Aymar D, et al: Count of benign melanocytic nevi as a major indicator of risk for nonfamilial nodular and superficial spreading melanoma. Cancer 66:387, 1990
102. Gallagher RP, McLean DI, Yang PC, et al: Anatomic distribution of acquired melanocytic nevi in white children. A comparison with melanoma: The Vancouver male study. Arch Dermatol 126:466, 1990
103. Kopf AW, Hellman LJ, Rogers GS, et al: Familial malignant melanoma. JAMA 256:1915, 1986
104. Greene MH, Fraumeni JJ Jr: The hereditary variant of malignant melanoma. In: Clark WH, Goldman LI, Mastrangelo MJ (eds): Human Malignant Melanoma. New York: Grune and Stratton, p 139, 1979
105. Clark WH Jr, Elder DE, Van Horn M: The biologic forms of malignant melanoma. Human Pathol 17:443, 1986
106. Kopf AW, Welkovich B, Frankel PE, et al: Thickness of malignant melanoma: Global analysis of related factors. J Dermatol Surg Oncol 13:345, 1987
107. Dubreuilh MW: De La mélanose circonscrite précancereuse. Ann Dermatol Syphiligr 3:129, 1912
108. Mishima Y: Malanosis circumscripta praecancerosa (Dubreuilh): A non-nevoid premelanoma distinct from junction nevus. J Invest Dermatol 34:361, 1960
109. Paul E, Illig L: Fluorescence-microscopic investigation of pigment cells of lentigo maligna (melanosis circumscripta praeblastomatosa Dubreuilh) and lentigo maligna melanoma. Arch Dermatol Res 256:179, 1976
110. Penneys NS: Microinvasive lentigo maligna melanoma. J Am Acad Dermatol 17:675, 1987
111. Michalik EE, Fitzpatrick TB, Sober AJ: Rapid progression of lentigo maligna to deeply invasive lentigo maligna melanoma: Report of two cases. Arch Dermatol 119:831, 1983
112. MacKie RM: Malignant melanocytic tumors. J Cutan Pathol 12:251, 1985
113. Feibleman CE, Stall H, Maize JC: Melanomas of the palm, sole and nailbed: A clinicopathologic study. Cancer 46:2492, 1980
114. Paladugu RR, Winberg CD, Yonemoto RH: Acral lentiginous melanoma: A clinicopathologic study of 36 patients. Cancer 52:161, 1983
115. Bonerandi J-J, Collet-Villette AM, Grob J-J: Melanome acrolentigineux. Ann Dermatol Venereol 114:1141, 1987

116. Margolis RJ, Tong AKF, Byers HR, Mihm MC Jr: Comparison of acral nevomelanocytic proliferations in Japanese and whites. J Invest Dermatol 92:225S, 1989
117. Scrivner D, Oxenhandler RW, Lopez M, Perez-Mesa C: Plantar lentiginous melanoma. A clinicopathologic study. Cancer 60:2502, 1987
118. Saida T: Malignant melanoma in situ on the sole of the foot. Its clinical and histopathologic characteristics. Am J Dermatopathol 11:124, 1989
119. Saida T, Yoshida N: Guidelines for histopathologic diagnosis of plantar malignant melanoma. Two-dimensional coordination of maximum diameters of lesions and degrees of intraepidermal proliferation of melanocytes. Dermatologica 181:112, 1990
120. Saida T, Ohshima Y: Clinical and histopathologic characteristics of early lesions of subungual malignant melanoma. Cancer 63:556,1989
121. Wade TR, White CR: The histology of malignant melanoma. Med Clin North Am 70:57, 1986
122. Stolz W, Schmoeckel C, Welkovich B, Braun-Falco O: Semiquantitative analysis of histologic criteria in thin malignant melanomas. J Am Acad Dermatol 20:1115, 1989
123. Glasgow BJ, Wen DR, Al-Jitawi S, Cochran AJ: Antibody to S-100 protein aids the separation of pagetoid melanoma from mammary and extramammary Paget's disease. J Cutan Pathol 14:223, 1987
124. Rivers JK, Kelly MC, Kopf AW, et al: Age and malignant melanoma: Comparison of variables in different age-groups. J Am Acad Dermatol 21:717, 1989
125. Mehregan AH, Staricco RG: Elastic fibers in pigmented nevi. J Invest Dermatol 38:271, 1962
126. Kühni-Petzoldt C, Keil H, Schöpf E: Prognostic significance of the mitotic rate for patients with thin (< 1.5 mm) melanoma. Z Hautkr 61:15, 1986
127. Harrist TJ, Rigel DS, Day CL, et al: "Microscopic satellites" are more associated with regional lymph node metastases than is primary melanoma thickness. Cancer 53:2183, 1984
128. Friedman RJ, Rigel DS, Kopf AW, et al: Favorable prognosis for malignant melanomas associated with acquired melanocytic nevi. Arch Dermatol 119:455, 1983
129. Bhawan J: Amelanotic melanoma or poorly differentiated melanoma? J Cutan Pathol 7:55, 1980
130. Egbert B, Kempson R, Sagebiel R: Desmoplastic malignant melanoma. A clinicohistopathologic study of 25 cases. Cancer 62:2033, 1988
131. Walsh NMG, Roberts JT, Orr W, Simon GT: Desmoplastic malignant melanoma. A clinicopathologic study of 14 cases. Arch Pathol Lab Med 112:922, 1988
132. Reiman HM, Goellner JR, Woods JE, Mixter RC: Desmoplastic melanoma of the head and neck. Cancer 60:2269, 1987
133. Kossard S, Doherty E, Murray E: Neurotropic melanoma: A variant of desmoplastic melanoma. Arch Dermatol 123:907, 1987
134. Kossard S, Doherty E, Murray E: Neurotropic melanoma. A variant of desmoplastic melanoma. Arch Dermatol 123:907, 1987
135. Warner TFCS, Ford CN, Hafez GR: Neurotropic melanoma of the face invading the maxillary nerve. J Cutan Pathol 12:520, 1985
136. Reed RJ, Leonard DD: Neurotropic melanoma: A varient of desmoplastic melanoma. Am J Surg Pathol 3:301, 1979
137. Nakagawa H, Lee YA, Kikuchi K, et al: Desmoplastic malignant melanoma—An electron microscopic and immunohistochemical study of a case. J Dermatol Tokyo 15:161, 1988
138. Paul E, Cochran AJ, Wen DR: Immunohistochemical demonstration of S-100 protein and melanoma-associated antigens in melanocytic nevi. J Cutan Pathol 15:161, 1988
139. Wick MR, Swanson PE, Rocamora A: Recognition of malignant melanoma by monoclonal antibody HMB-45. An immunohistochemical study of 200 paraffin-embedded cutaneous tumors. J Cutan Pathol 15:201, 1988
140. Mihm MC Jr, Clark WH Jr, From L: The clinical diagnosis, classification, and histogenic concepts of the early stages of cutaneous malignant melanomas. N Engl J Med 284:1078, 1971
141. Cascinelli N: Melanoma today. J Dermatol Tokyo 15: 355, 1988
142. Breslow A: Tumor thickness, level of invasion and node dissection in stage I cutaneous melanoma. Ann Surg 182:572, 1975
143. Breslow A: Prognostic factors in the treatment of cutaneous melanoma. J Cutan Pathol 6:208, 1979
144. Kopf AW, Welkovich B, Frankel R, et al: Thickness of malignant melanoma: Global analysis of related factors. J Dermatol Surg Oncol 13:4, 1987
145. Karakousis CP, Emrich LJ, Rao U: Tumor thickness and prognosis in clinical stage 1 malignant melanoma. Cancer 64:1432, 1989
146. Berdeaux DH, Meyskens FL, Parks B, et al: Cutaneous malignant melanoma. II. The natural history and prognostic factors influencing the development of stage II disease. Cancer 63:1430, 1989
147. Reed KM, Bronstein BR, Mihm MC Jr, Sober AJ: Prognosis for polypoidal melanoma is determined by primary tumor thickness. Cancer 57:1201, 1986
148. Prade M, Bognel C, Charpentier P, et al: Malignant melanoma of the skin: Prognostic factors derived from a multifactorial analysis of 239 cases. Am J Dermatopathol 4:411, 1982
149. Maize JC: Primary cutaneous malignant melanoma: An analysis of the prognostic value of histologic characteristics. J Am Acad Dermatol 8:857, 1983
150. Day CL, Lew RA, Harrist TJ: Malignant melanoma prognostic factors: 4. Ulceration width. J Dermatol Surg Oncol 10:23, 1984

34

EPIDERMAL NEVI AND BENIGN EPIDERMOID TUMORS

Circumscribed areas of skin exhibiting hyperplasia of the epidermis, without appreciable alteration of the normal structure or maturation process and without external cause, may be called "epidermal nevi" regardless of their becoming manifest before or after birth. If circumscribed hyperplasia is associated with retarded but relatively normal maturation of cells and with some alteration of structure, the lesion is then a "benign epidermoid tumor" (see Table VII–1). Considerable disruption of normal epidermal organization, dysplasia of cells, and atypical keratinization are the marks of "malignant epidermoid tumors," which may be precancerous, carcinoma in situ, or invasive carcinoma. The term "epidermoid" is used because such tumors may take their origin not only from epidermal but also from adnexal keratinocytes. Site of origin is not important, and direction of maturation of the tumor cells in an epidermoid manner is the diagnostic feature. Malignant epidermoid tumors are discussed in Chapter 35. Here we deal with epidermal nevi and benign epidermoid tumors, both of which manifest their relatively high level of organization through associated characteristic dermal changes. In fact, most benign epidermoid tumors are fibroepithelial in character. Just as inflammatory epidermal hyperplasia is practically always associated with increase of papillary tissue and just as viral warts have a papillomatous pattern, so do most epidermal nevi and benign epidermoid tumors exhibit papillary hyperplasia.

EPIDERMAL NEVI

Verrucous Epidermal Nevus

Verrucous epidermal nevi (Fig. 34–1) are flesh colored or brown lesions with a smooth or hyperkeratotic surface. They may be present at birth or appear during childhood or adolescence.[1] The lesion is either localized or is arranged in linear fashion (linear verrucous epidermal nevus). Extensive involvement of one extremity or one side of the trunk is known as *nevus unius lateris*. Unilateral or bilateral involvement may show swirled or parallel band following Blashko's lines (Fig. 34–2).[2] Histologically, these lesions show hyperplasia of the epidermis and papillary connective tissue in varying degrees, which is responsible for the hyperkeratotic warty appearance or soft pedunculated lesions. A special form is the *hard nevus of Unna* (Fig. 34–1A) in which all dermal papillae in the area are evenly elongated and produce a serrated configuration of the epidermis which itself is moderately acanthotic and hyperkeratotic.[3]

Verrucous epidermal nevi are differentiated from the organoid nevi by lack of adnexal participation in the nevoid lesion and by the absence of secondary development of nevoid tumors.

Ichthyosis Hystrix

This histologically distinctive lesion may be considered as a variant of verrucous epidermal nevus or a

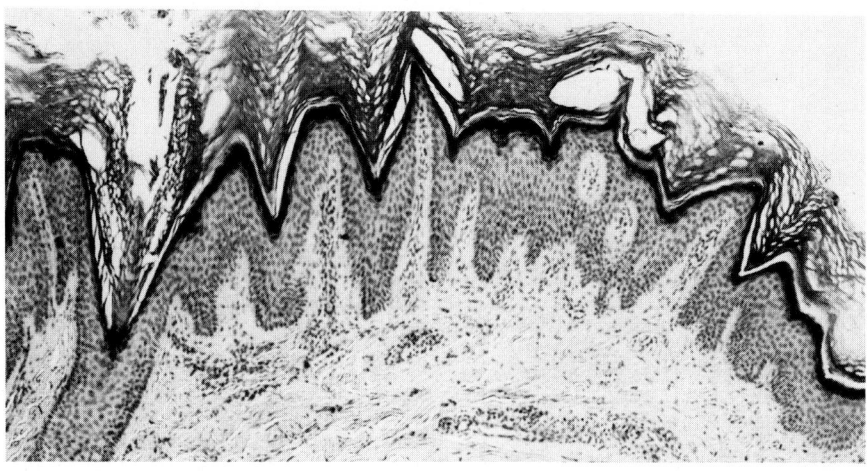

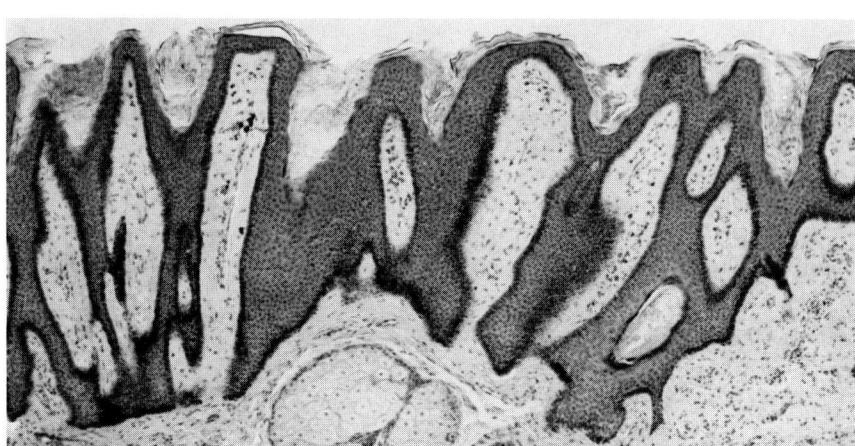

Figure 34–1.
Epidermal nevus. Both lesions are papillomatous. **A.** Hard epidermal nevus with hyperkeratosis and relatively minor connective tissue component. **B.** Soft epidermal nevus which is also pigmented. There is little keratin, and papillae are large. H&E. X70.

form fruste of epidermolytic hyperkeratosis (Chapter 30). Clinically, brown, verrucous, hyperkeratotic lesions appear in linear bands or may involve one segment of the body. Histologically (see Fig. 30–4), the verrucous hyperplastic epidermis shows marked hypergranulosis, with large keratohyalin granules, and vacuolization of the epidermal cells with basketweave-type hyperkeratosis.[4,5]

Inflammatory Linear Verrucous Epidermal Nevus (ILVEN)

ILVEN is characterized by the appearance of scaling, erythematous, and dermatitic lesions in linear unilateral or bilateral distribution.[6–11] The lesion is persistent and is refractory to treatment. Histologically, the acanthotic epidermis shows well-defined areas of hypergranulosis and hyperkeratosis alternating with foci of loss of granular layer and parakeratosis[12,13] (Fig. 34–3). Telangiectasia and mild lymphocytic infiltrate may be present in the underlying dermis.

Pigmented Hairy Epidermal Nevus

Nevus of Becker becomes manifest usually during adolescence over one side of the upper back and shoulder.[14,15] Familial cases are rare.[16,17] In the early stage, velvety macular areas of hyperpigmentation appear in this location and later show hypertrichosis. Smaller macular, hyperpigmented lesions with or without hypertrichosis may also occur in other parts of the body. Histologic sections (Fig. 34–4) show mild epidermal thickening and uniform epidermal hyperpigmentation. Hyperpigmentation results from an overload of melanin in the kera-

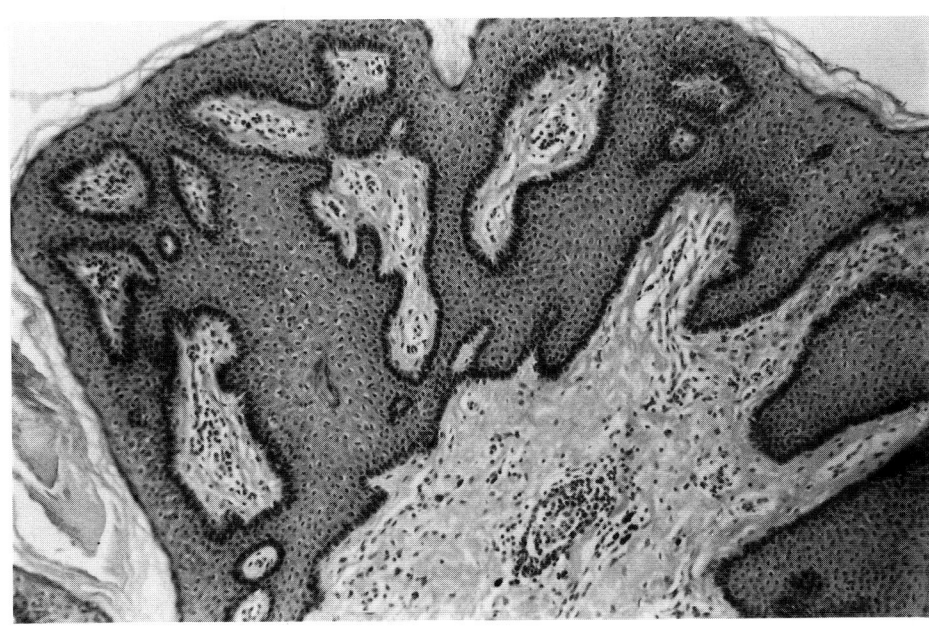

Figure 34–2.
Linear verrucous epidermal nevus. In this case with soft papillomatous lesions epidermal hyperplasia is associated with corresponding papillary connective tissue participation. H&E. X100.

tinocytes.[18,19] There is an increase in the number and size of the pilosebaceous structures and arrector pili muscles.[20,21] Lesions with extensive hyperplasia of hair muscle bundles are classified as "arrector pili or pilar smooth muscle hamartoma."[22–24] Becker's nevus may occur in association with hypoplasia of breast and pectoralis major muscle.[25,26]

White Sponge Nevus

In oral mucosa, white sponge nevus appears as small white plaques or elevated wartlike lesions.[27–29] Histologically, there is thickening of the surface epithelium, which appears edematous and populated with clear cells, and is covered by a thin layer of parakeratosis.

Epidermal Nevus Syndrome

Epidermal nevus syndrome is characterized by an association of linear verrucous epidermal nevus with a variety of congenital developmental abnormalities including the connective tissue, blood vessel, central nervous, and musculoskeletal systems.[30–34] The ma-

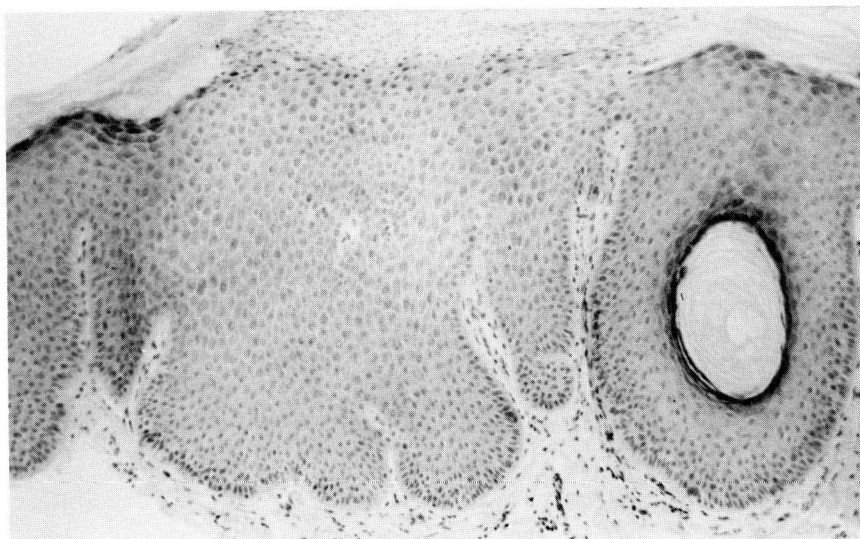

Figure 34–3.
Inflammatory linear verrucous epidermal nevus. Sharply limited blocks of pale-staining parakeratotic epidermis alternate with dark-staining, normally keratinizing blocks, only some of which are associated with follicular openings (right). H&E. X135.

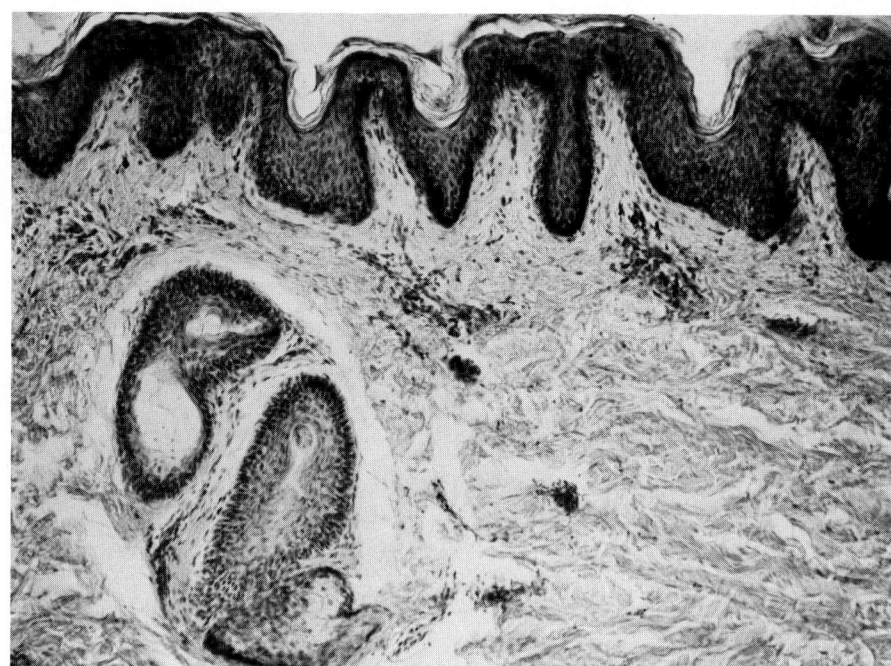

Figure 34–4.
Pigmented hairy epidermal nevus of Becker. Papillomatous, hyperpigmented epidermis associated with hyperplastic pilar complexes. H&E. X135.

jority of cases show histologic changes of hyperkeratotic linear verrucous epidermal nevus, but cases with features of ichthyosis hystrix and inflammatory linear verrucous epidermal nevus also have been reported.[35,36] In another group of cases, inflammatory linear verrucous epidermal nevi have occurred in association with the ipsilateral hypoplasia of trunk and extremities of females, suggesting an x-linked dominant mode of inheritance.[37,38]

Nevoid Hyperkeratosis of Nipples and Areolae

Velvety hyperkeratotic and hyperpigmented lesions occur bilaterally over the nipples and areolae of young women.[39,40] Similar lesions may be present in individuals with ichthyosis or unilaterally as an extension of a linear verrucous epidermal nevus.[41] Histologically (Fig. 34–5A), there is a marked papillomatous configuration of the epidermis and hyperkeratosis with minimal epidermal acanthosis.

Acrokeratosis Verruciformis of Hopf

Acrokeratosis verruciformis of Hopf appears to be a manifestation of Darier's disease in some cases, but it is questionable if one should consider it a form fruste of that disease when it occurs without other manifestations. Histologically (Fig. 34–5B), there is marked papillomatous of the epidermis, with acanthosis and hyperkeratosis resembling church spires.[42]

Acanthosis Nigricans

Velvety hyperkeratotic and hyperpigmented plaques that occur in axillae and in other flexural areas show histologic changes (Fig. 34–6) very similar to those of a verrucous epidermal nevus. Papillomatous hyperplasia of the epidermis and hyperpigmentation occur with minimal epidermal thickening. There are no histologic differences between the benign and malignant varieties.[43]

Reticulated and Confluent Papillomatosis (Gougerot and Carteaud)

The papillomatosis of Gougerot and Carteaud often is found heavily colonized by *Pityrosporum orbiculare* and there is an indication that the papillomatosis is a peculiar tissue reaction to this organism.[44] Histologically (Fig. 34–7), there is mild hyperkeratosis, epidermal acanthosis, and hyperpigmentation.[45]

Multiple Minute Digitate Hyperkeratoses

Minute digitate hyperkeratotic lesions that occur over the chest wall and shoulder show areas of hyperkeratosis with elongation of the epidermal rete

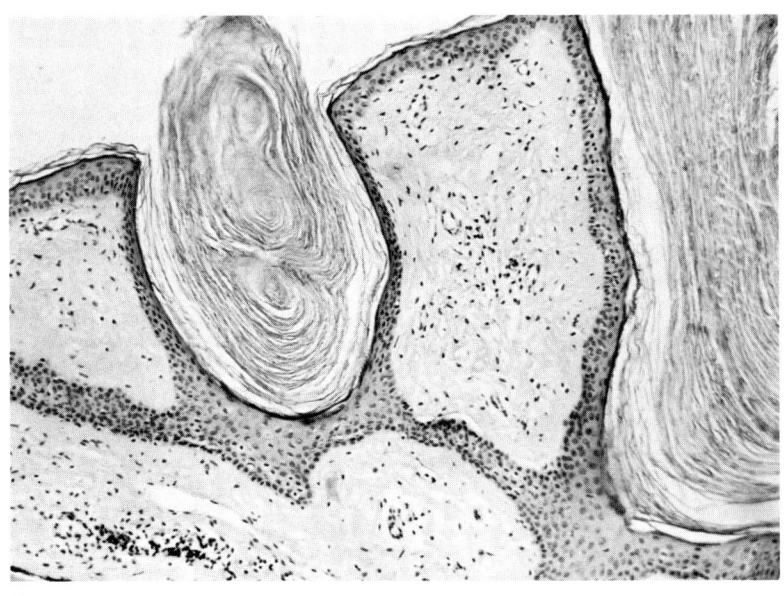

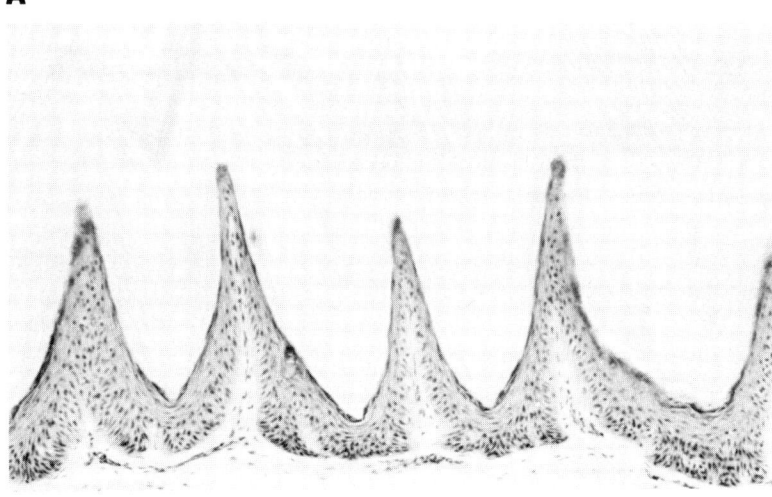

Figure 34–5.
A. Nevoid hyperkeratosis of nipple. Papillomatosis and lamellated hyperkeratosis in association with rather thin epidermis. H&E. X135. (From Mehregan and Rahbari: Arch Dermatol 113:1691, 1977. **B.** Acrokeratosis verruciformis of Hopf. Church spire appearance of long papillae covered by unremarkable heavily keratinized epidermis. H&E. X125.

ridges and hypergranulosis (Fig. 34–8). Minimal lymphocytic infiltrate is present in the underlying dermis.[46–48] One familial incidence, with a father and son affected, has been reported.[49]

Stucco Keratosis

Small grayish white keratotic lesions occur over the distal portions of the lower extremities.[50] Histologically, there is papillomatous hyperplasia of the epidermis with hyperkeratosis in church spire fashion.[51]

SEBORRHEIC VERRUCA

Seborrheic verruca is the prototype of a benign epidermoid neoplasm corresponding in its structural organization and degree of maturity to an adenoma in the spectrum of glandular tumors[52] (see Table VII–1). Structure is mildly distorted, and maturation is retarded but proceeds along normal channels. The tumors, therefore, show an increased proportion of basaloid cells, while typical light-staining prickle cells often are restricted to a few layers below the stratum granulosum. All three major patterns of seborrheic verruca—the solid, the papillomatous, and the reticulated types—basically are combined hyperplasia of epidermis and papillary dermis. The latter is minimal in the solid type (Fig. 34–9), which also shows little or no hyperkeratosis. Ectodermal and mesodermal components are fairly well balanced in the common papillomatous types (Fig. 34–10), characterized by an onionlike lamellation of horny material in recesses and intralesional cysts (Fig. 34–

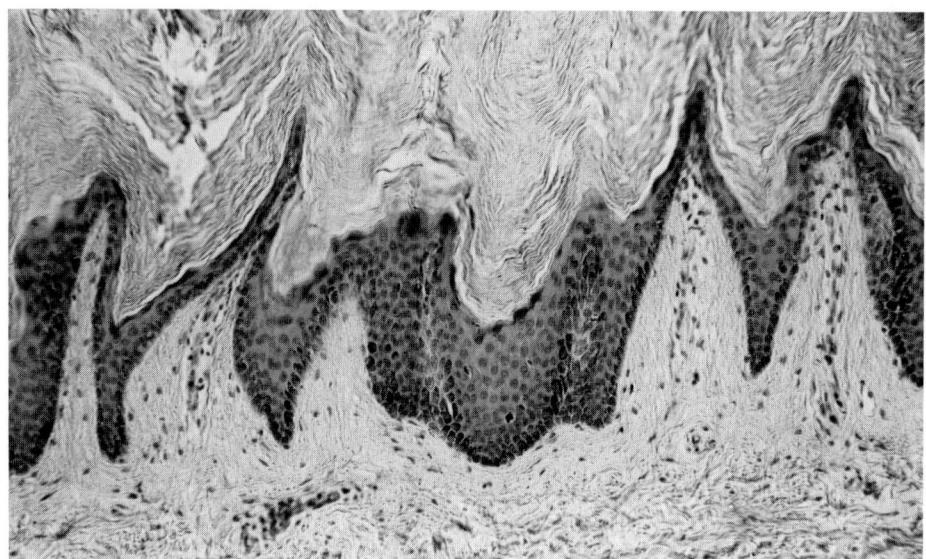

Figure 34–6.
Acanthosis nigricans. The epidermis is neither significantly acanthotic nor hyperpigmented. The clinical picture is due mainly to elongation and increased bulk of papillae and to hyperkeratosis. The dark color has its seat in the horny layer. H&E. X135.

11). The latter are due to "endokeratinization." They originate in deep portions of the thick epithelium and are gradually pushed upward and outward as they enlarge until they merge with the surface keratin. The hypothesis of invagination of the horny layer is ill-conceived, inasmuch as all movement in the epidermis is outward, and examination of suitable lesions in serial sections leaves no doubt about the intraepidermal origin and truly cystic nature of many of these horny pearls. Other cornified cysts and cystlike structures are due to retention of keratin in hair follicles and sweat ducts traversing the verruca. Sweat ducts can be recognized in O&G sections by the eosinophilic staining of their keratin.

The *reticulated* type of seborrheic verruca (Fig. 34–12) is fairly rare and has structural relations to *lentigo senilis*.[53] The typical histologic picture of lentigo senilis shows peculiar club-shaped downward projections of the epidermis, which seem to be true buds of the basal layer and usually are deeply pigmented, especially at the bulbous tips (Chapter 33). They do not penetrate the papillary layer but often are embedded in dense, eosinophilic connective tissue. From this simple pattern, one can find transitions to the complicated lacy appearance of the reticulated type of seborrheic verruca (Fig. 34–13).

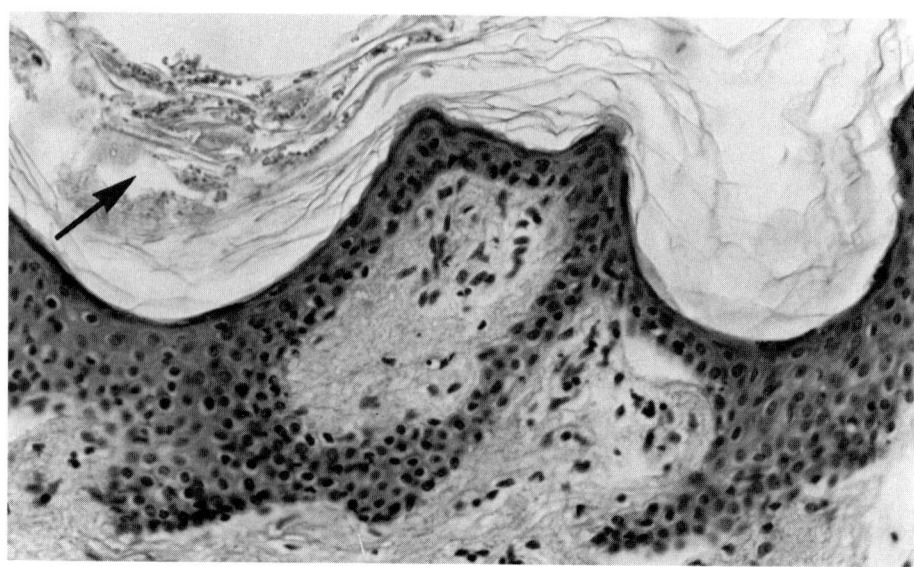

Figure 34–7.
Reticulated and confluent papillomatosis (Gougerot and Carteaud). Papillomatous hyperplasia of the epidermis, with the arrow pointed to the colonies of pityrosporum in the keratin layer. H&E. X125.

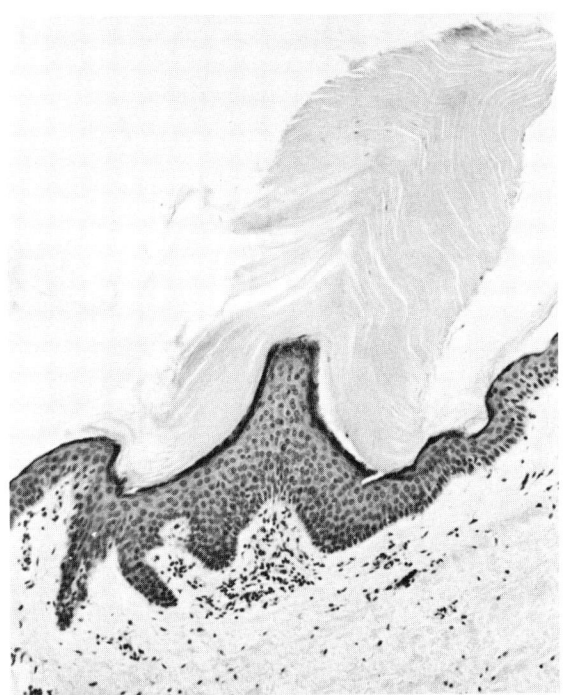

Figure 34–8.
Minute digitate hyperkeratosis. One papilla contains some inflammatory cells. The overlying epidermis has a thick granular layer and is covered by a minute cutaneous horn. H&E. X125.

Seborrheic verrucae have a normal complement of inconspicuous melanocytes and often contain moderate amounts of melanin in their keratinocytes. Some are deeply pigmented (Fig. 34–14). The amount of melanin has no clinical significance.

Not all seborrheic verrucae are populated with small basaloid cells or are pigmented (Fig. 34–15). The "acanthotic" variety shows simple papillomatous epidermal hyperplasia with hypergranulosis and lamellar hyperkeratosis. The histologic pattern of this variety resembles a verrucous epidermal nevus. A "flat" type of seborrheic verruca occurs predominantly over the lower extremities. Histologically shows low-grade papillomatous acanthosis of the epidermis and is often nonpigmented.

Activated Seborrheic Verruca

Seborrheic verrucae have clinical and histologic aspects of sluggishness. They grow very slowly, and the accumulation of large amounts of stagnating keratin and often of pigment supports the impression of slow turnover. Under certain conditions, however, the lesions may increase rather suddenly in size and change their histologic character. Some elderly people suffering from widespread eczematous

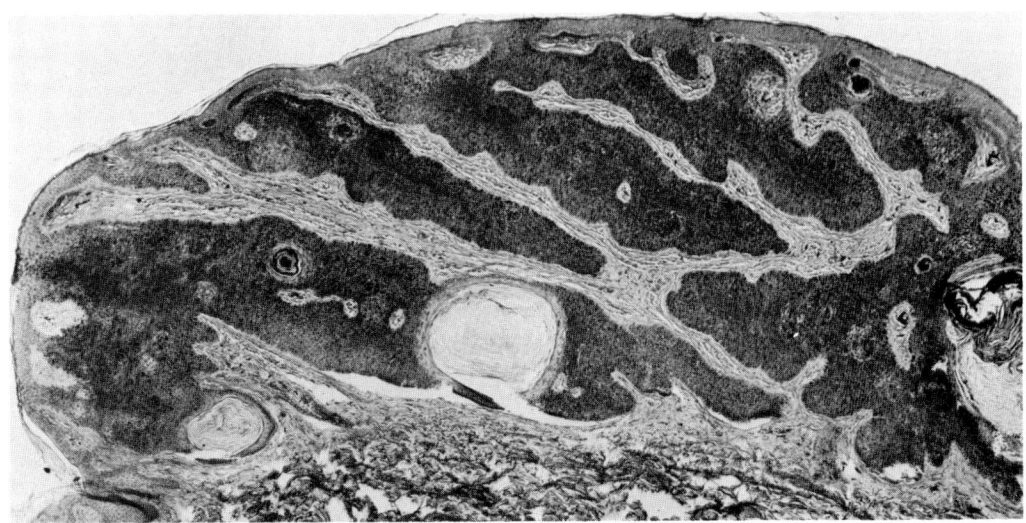

Figure 34–9.
Seborrheic verruca, solid type. This sessile, protruding lesion consists of masses of deeply pigmented basaloid cells changing rather abruptly into a relatively thin stratified layer of larger prickle cells. There is no surface hyperkeratosis and only few keratinizing foci in the substance of the tumor. O&G. X30.

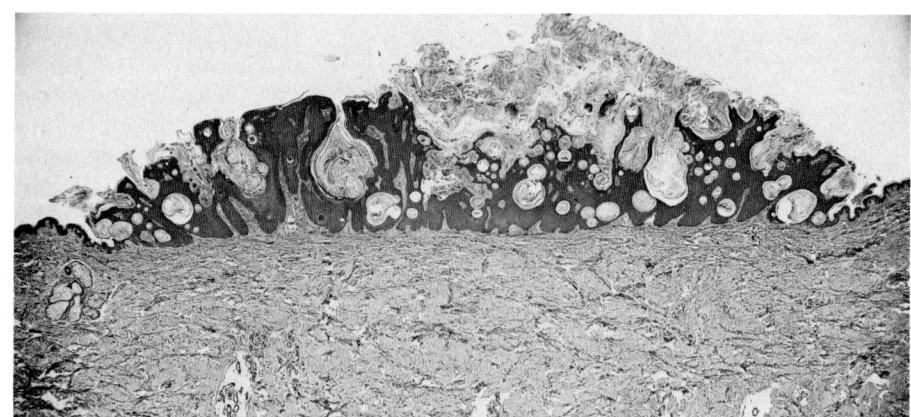

Figure 34–10.
Common type of seborrheic verruca in which many horny cysts move upward to become incorporated in surface hyperkeratosis. Note superficial stuck-on nature of papillomatous lesion. H&E. X14.

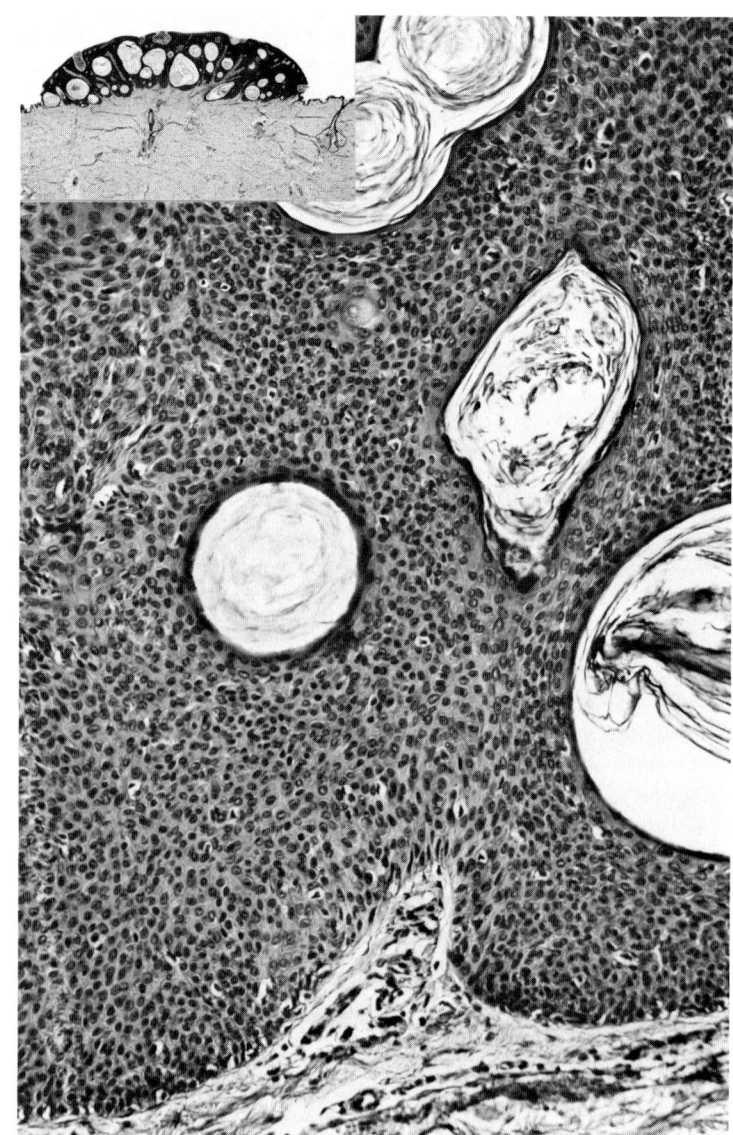

Figure 34–11.
Seborrheic verruca showing development of horny cysts deep in the body of the lesion (endokeratinization) and moving upward to join the surface stratum corneum. In between is another cyst that is a dilated hair follicle containing a few tiny hairs. H&E. X225.

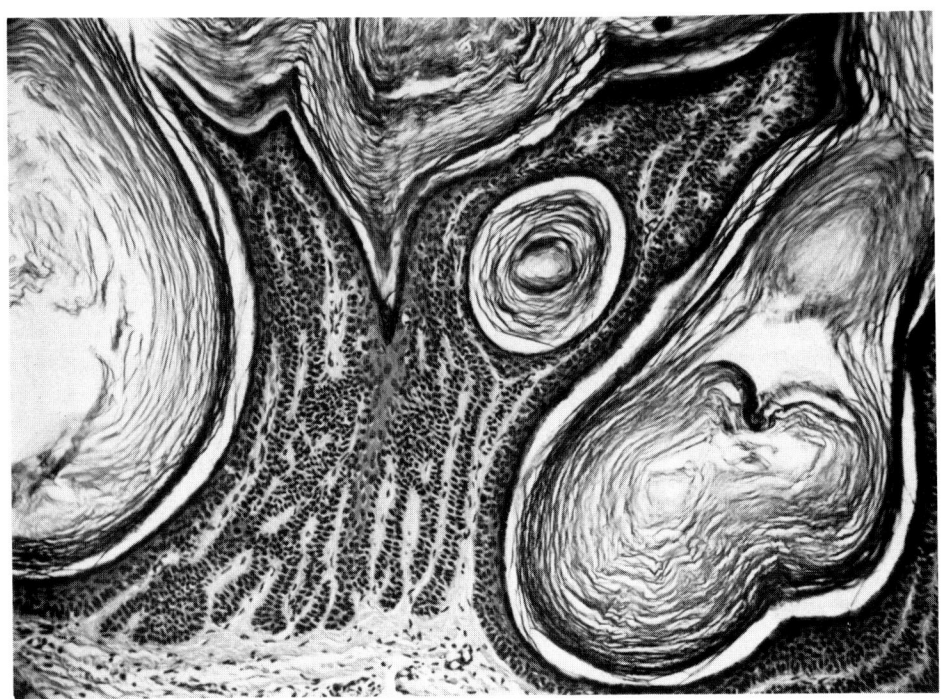

Figure 34–12.
Seborrheic verruca, reticulated type. H&E. X135.

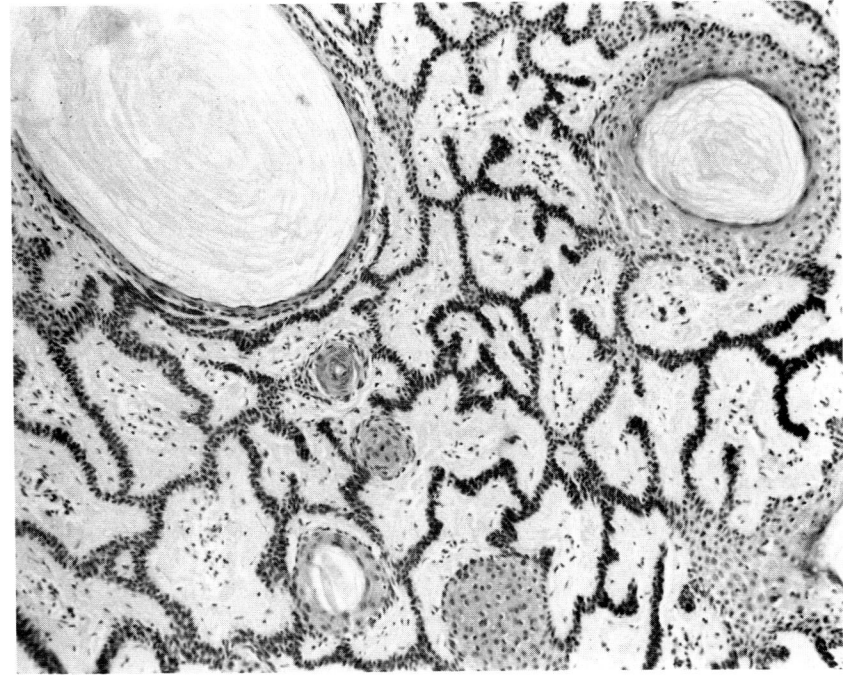

Figure 34–13.
Reticulated and hyperpigmented seborrheic verruca. This lesion is often superimposed on a lentigo senilis. H&E. X125.

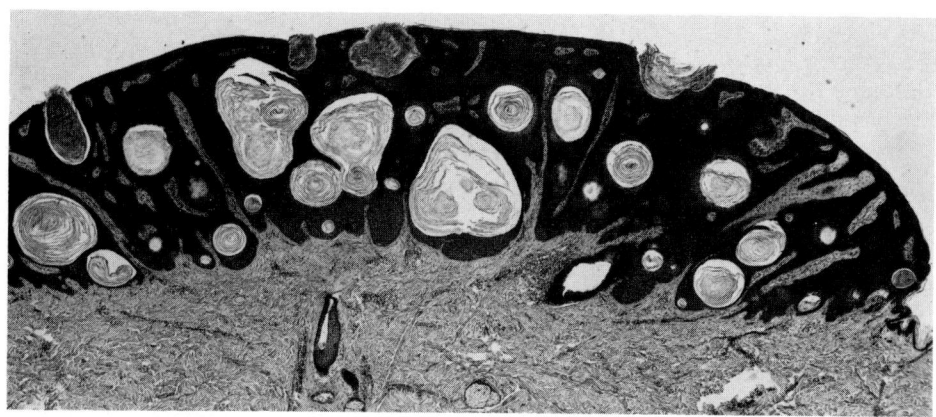

Figure 34-14.
Deeply pigmented seborrheic verruca. Practically every basaloid keratinocyte composing the lesion contains melanin. Melanocytes are few and small. Note papillomatous features of lesion, which lacks any surface hyperkeratosis but contains characteristic horny cysts. H&E. X8.

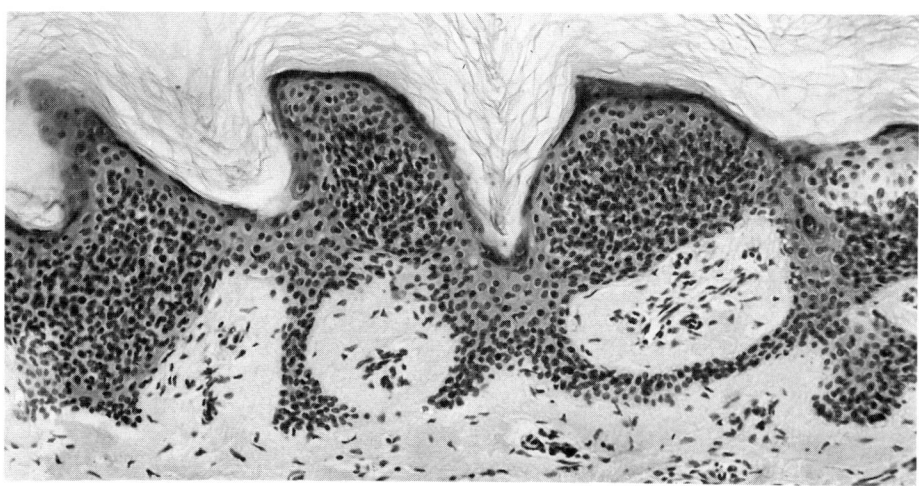

Figure 34-15.
Seborrheic verruca, flat type. **A.** Clonal islands of small basaloid cells within a moderately acanthotic epidermis. H&E. X125. **B.** An acanthotic and hyperkeratotic variety. H&E. X125.

dermatitis or psoriatic erythroderma may develop many small papular lesions, which become manifest when the dermatitis subsides—and then subside gradually themselves. Histologically, they are papillomatous acanthomas[54] in the sense that they have layers of prickle cells above a single basal layer. Biologically, they are tiny seborrheic verrucae, temporarily stimulated into proliferation and precipitous maturation along with the surrounding acanthotic and exfoliating epidermis.

If one irritates a seborrheic verruca, for instance by the application of croton oil, conversion of basal cells into prickle cells also is accelerated, and the proportion of the latter increases.[55] This experience supports the view that the keratinocytes of this benign tumor are not materially deranged in their metabolism but are retarded in their maturation, which is one of the essential criteria of neoplasia. Occasionally, one encounters lesions that present the characteristic structure of the benign epidermoid neoplasm in one part, while another part presents a most unusual architecture (Fig. 34–16) consisting of numerous tiny or larger spheres of prickle cells in concentric arrangement, the larger ones undergoing central keratinization. The spheres, or "squamous eddies," are embedded in a mass of basaloid cells. This picture, to which the name *basosquamous acanthoma* was given by Lund[56] when it was found as the sole substrate of lesions, suggests that a seborrheic verruca has been activated by some inflammatory stimulus, perhaps by infection, and that basaloid cells have been explosively converted into maturing prickle cells in numerous foci. One has to be acquainted with this picture of the activated seborrheic verruca, which otherwise may be misdiagnosed as squamous cell carcinoma.

Clonal Seborrheic Verruca and Intraepidermal Nests

While intralesional nests of prickle cells (squamous eddies) are found in activated seborrheic verrucae and inverted follicular keratosis, other types of seborrheic verruca are characterized by sharply defined nests of basaloid cells.[57] These lesions usually are flat clinically and occur most commonly on the lower extremities. While the histologic picture (Fig. 34–17) closely resembles certain types of intraepidermal epithelioma (Chapter 40), it is identified by finding of a gradual transition zone between the outer cells of the basaloid nests and the surrounding epidermal keratinocytes. Clonal nests of basaloid cells may be deeply pigmented or have an associated increase in the number of dendritic melanocytes (see Melanoacanthoma).

Seborrheic verrucae are benign tumors and are not precancerous. All cases in which development of basal cell epithelioma in seborrheic verruca has been reported are most likely instances of coincidental association of two common tumors of senile

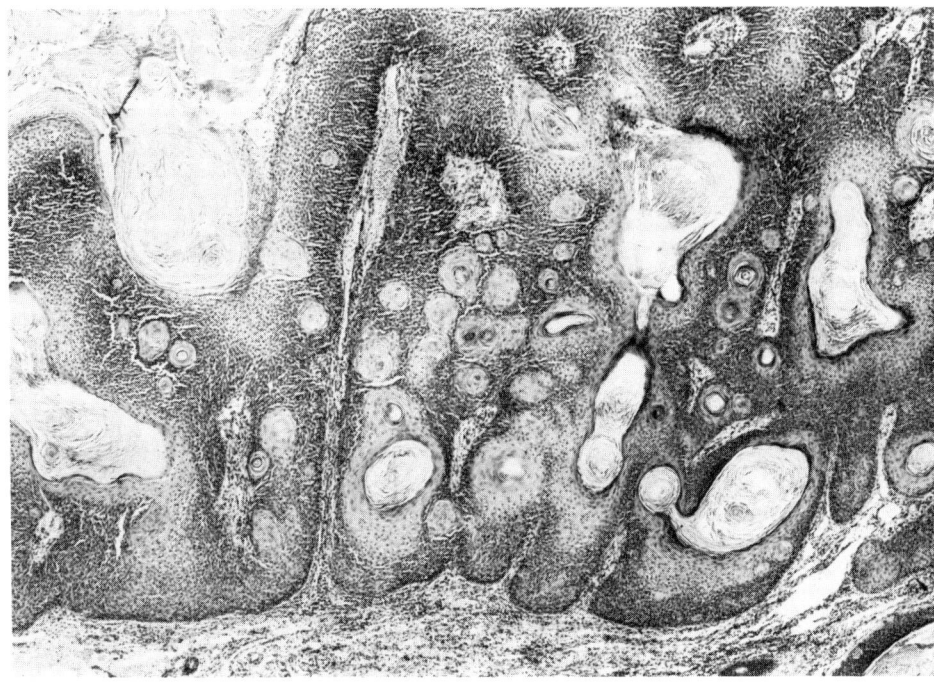

Figure 34–16.
Activated seborrheic verruca with numerous keratinizing centers. This is the pattern of Lund's basosquamous acanthoma and is encountered also in Helwig's inverted follicular keratosis. H&E. ×45.

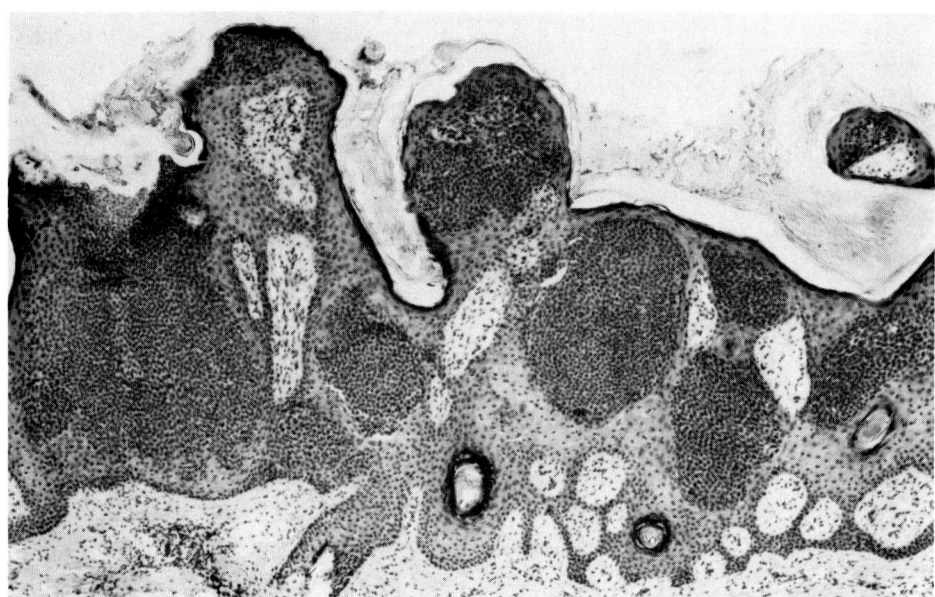

Figure 34–17.
Seborrheic verruca with basaloid nests resembling intraepidermal epithelioma of Jadassohn type. H&E. X45.

skin.[58] The same may be true for development of squamous cell carcinoma. Bowenoid dysplastic cellular changes, however, can occur in seborrheic verruca in rare instances and in long-standing lesions.[59,60] Sudden appearance and rapid increase in size and number of seborrheic verrucae in association with pruritus and internal malignancy is known as the sign of Lesser–Trélat.[61–64] The internal malignancy is often an adenocarcinoma of gastrointestinal tract and occasionally of the lung or a lymphocytic lymphoma.[65]

Melanoacanthoma

Rare but of considerable biologic interest, melanoacanthoma is a lesion, originally described by Bloch as nonnevoid melanoepithelioma, which represents combined benign neoplasia of epidermal keratinocytes and large dendritic melanocytes (Fig. 34–18).[66] The lesion may resemble a seborrheic verruca or may form a large plaque of several centimeters in diameter with a sharply defined periphery.[67] It may consist in full thickness of a mixture of pigmented basaloid cells and dendritic melanocytes. In another histologic form, well-defined islands of small basaloid cells and dendritic melanocytes are present within a generally acanthotic epidermis.

Dermatosis Papulosa Nigra

Closely related to seborrheic verruca, dermatosis papulosa nigra is a hereditable condition involving facial skin of blacks in the form of numerous small deeply pigmented or hyperkeratotic papillomas. Histologically, each lesion shows a central core of fibrovascular tissue and is covered with papillomatous acanthotic and hyperpigmented epidermis.[68]

CLEAR CELL ACANTHOMA (DEGOS)

A striking appearance, both clinically and histologically, is presented by the rare tumor described as *acanthome à cellules claires* by Degos.[69] Solitary or, rarely, multiple tumors,[70,71] often localized on the leg, resemble an exuberant granuloma pyogenicum clinically and consist of a greatly thickened epidermis composed of unusually large keratinocytes, which stain pale in routine sections (Fig. 34–19) because they contain much glycogen.[72] The altered epithelium has cell-sharp margins against normal surrounding epidermis and adnexal units traversing the tumor. Long papillae with blood-filled capillaries characterize Degos' acanthoma as a papilloma and, together with incomplete keratinization, account for the clinical aspect of an angiomatous lesion.

Clear cell acanthoma represents a circumscribed derangement of epidermal metabolism leading to intracellular storage of glycogen granules. Its pattern of reactivity to epithelial membrane antigen (EMA), differences in cytokeratin expression, and lack of reactivity to carcinoembryonic antigen (CEA) rules out relationship with seborrheic verruca or with the intraepidermal sweat duct units.[73–75]

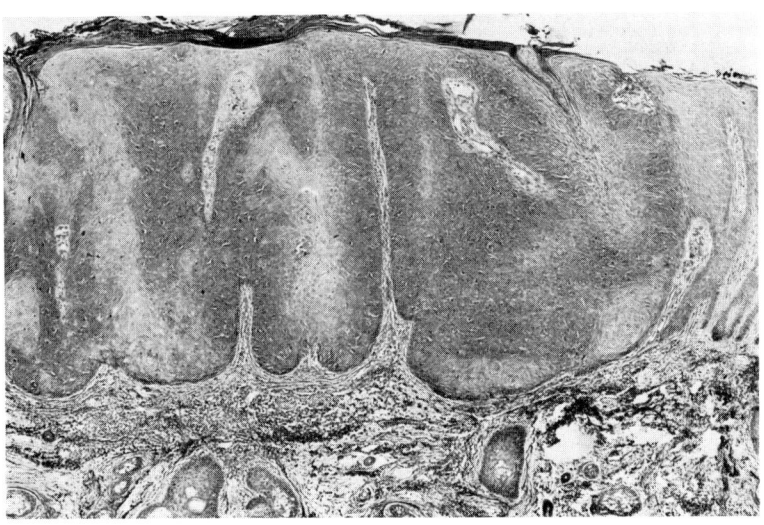
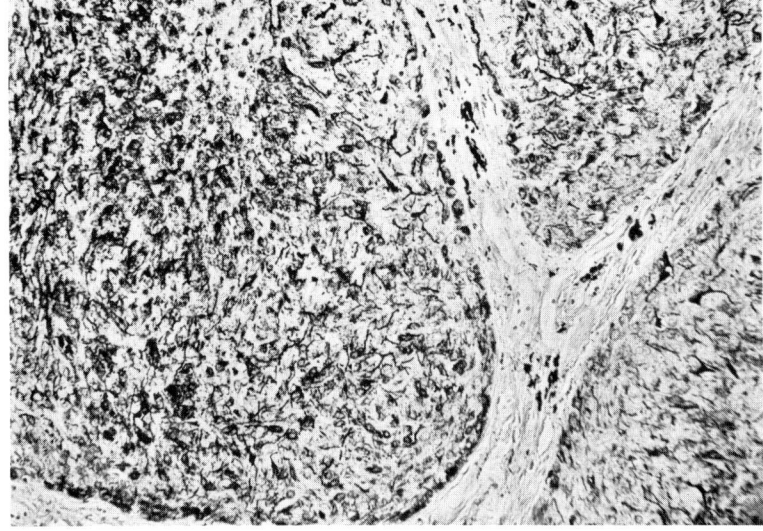

Figure 34-18.
Melanoacanthoma. **A.** Massive papillomatous epidermis is composed of dark and light portions, the latter representing nonpigmented areas of prickle cells. O&G. X30. **B.** Most of melanin is contained in dendritic melanocytes, which are present in profusion between basaloid keratinocytes. Masson silver. X135.
(From Mishima and Pinkus. Arch Dermatol 81: 539, 1966.)

PALMAR PITS

Another instance of localized retarded maturation of epidermis, but with a quite different and peculiar connotation, is palmar pits, which are a marker of the nevoid basal cell epithelioma syndrome.[76,77] They exhibit an increase of basaloid cells within the epidermal rete ridges, poor development of prickle cells, and diminished coherence of keratinocytes (Fig. 34-20), which leads to premature shedding of horny cells and a localized defect in the keratin layer. Disturbances of the papillary dermis indicate that they are, in fact, tiny fibroepithelial neoplasms.[78] In several cases, they progressed to basal cell epithelioma formation.[79]

POROKERATOSIS

Porokeratosis of Mibelli is a misnomer based on the failure to view the skin in three dimensions. The sweat pore is a dot, and the cornoid lamella that encircles the lesion of porokeratosis is a ring that slowly moves eccentrically, crossing the fixed ostia of sweat ducts and hair follicles as it travels (Fig. 34-21). In cutting biopsy sections, we try to orient the tissue so that the lamella is shown in cross section. It then appears as a funnel-shaped depression in the epidermis (Fig. 34-22) usually not associated with a sweat pore. The granular layer is missing in the depth of the depression, and a column of parakeratotic cells rises obliquely from it. It must be em-

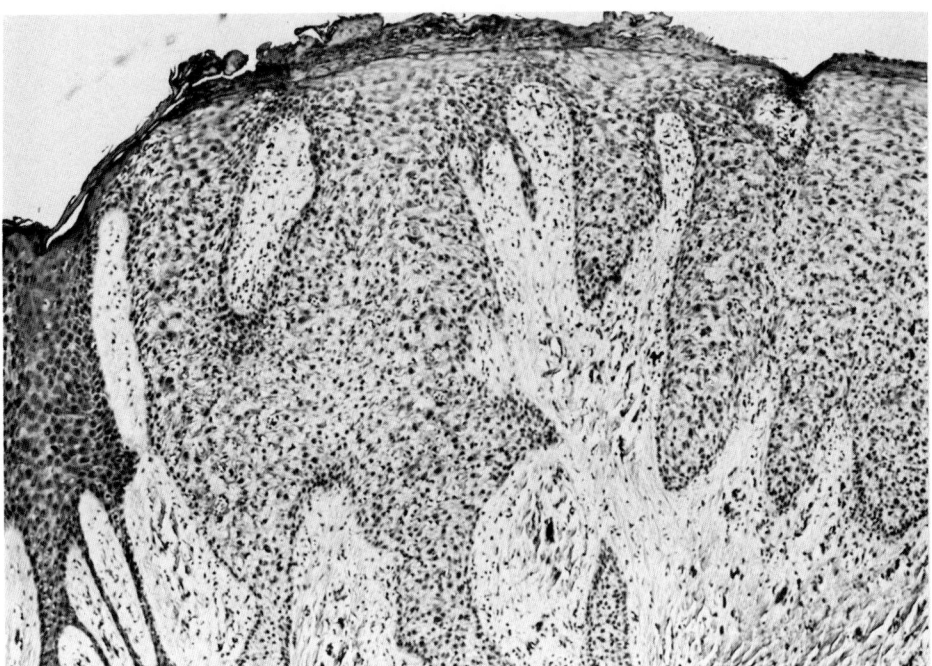

Figure 34–19.
Pale cell acanthoma. Sharp delineation between the dark-staining epidermis at left and the light-staining tumor cells. Both types of epithelium are similarly acanthotic. Nuclei of tumor cells are not enlarged. H&E. X75.

phasized once more that the column is but a cross section of the ring-shaped cornoid lamella. The nature of the lesion is puzzling if we concentrate attention on the ring. Closer examination shows that the entire disk of epidermis inside the ring is abnormal, often hypoplastic, sometimes verrucous. While keratinization usually is normal, parakeratotic plugs resembling the cornoid lamella may be found in follicular and eccrine ostia within the lesion. We pointed out in the previous editions that one might consider porokeratosis as a benign heritable derangement of the metabolism of some epidermal cells. These form a slowly enlarging disk, in which only the active rim expresses the disturbance in the form of parakeratosis. A similar hypothesis has been independently voiced and documented by Reed and Leone,[80] and we, therefore, feel safe in listing Mibelli's disease as a benign epidermal neoplasm. Clinically in the classic form, single or multiple circular lesions show an elevated, hyperkeratotic, and ridged border. Other morphologic forms include the superficial disseminated type[81] and the linear nevoid[82] and punctate varieties.[83,84] Facial plaques[85] and lesions of lips or buccal mucosa may be present. Solitary lesions involving the plantar surface of the foot are known as porokeratosis plantaris discreta.[86] Porokeratosis may occur in individuals with immunosuppression.[87] Long-standing lesions of porokeratosis may become complicated by Bowen's disease, squamous cell carcinoma, and rarely basal cell epithelioma.[88–91]

POROKERATOTIC ECCRINE OSTIAL AND DERMAL DUCT NEVUS

Small keratotic papules arranged into bands or with linear configuration involve the upper and lower extremities and extend into palms and soles.[92–94] Histologically, within a papillomatous acanthotic epidermis are tall parakeratotic columns (cornoid lamellae) in irregular intervals some originating from the underlying hair follicles or eccrine sweat ducts.[95]

LARGE CELL ACANTHOMA

Not exceedingly rare, but rarely diagnosed, is another benign epidermal neoplasm that produces slightly scaling discolored spots and barely infiltrated plaques in the sun-exposed skin of elderly persons, most often female. Biopsies are usually submitted to rule out actinic keratosis, or the le-

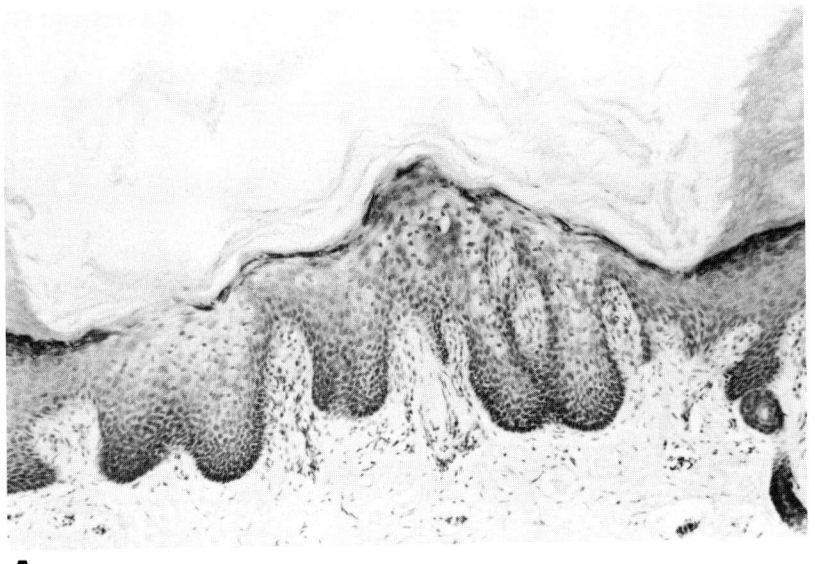

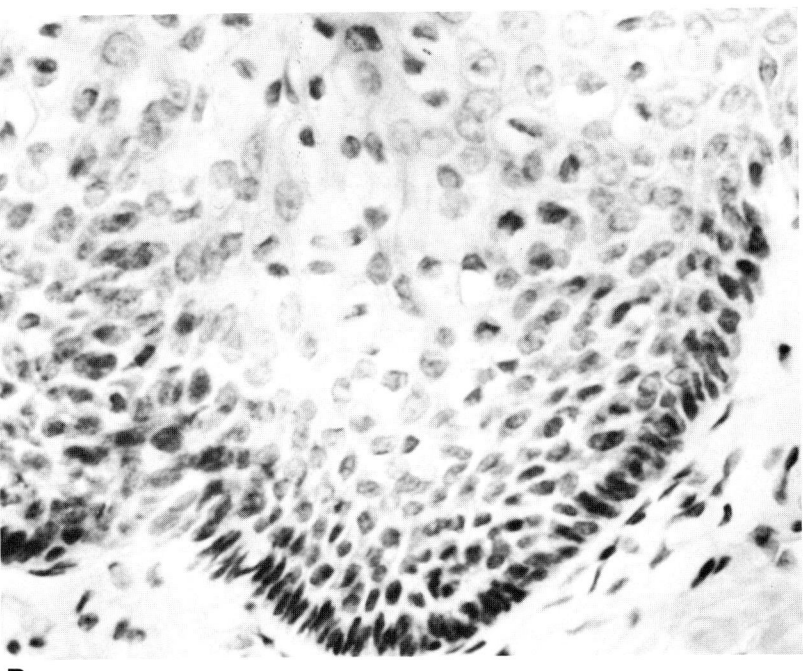

Figure 34–20.
Palmar pit in nevoid basal cell epithelioma syndrome. **A.** Sharply limited area of epidermis with decreased keratinization. Increased cellularity of papillary dermis. H&E. X125. **B.** Palisading basal layer beneath disordered prickle cells resembles somewhat a basal cell epithelioma. H&E. X400.

sions are removed for cosmetic reasons.[96] The histologic picture at first suggests normal skin or a flat papilloma until one becomes aware of the unusually large size not only of the cytoplasm but of the nuclei of keratinocytes as well. There may be slight anisocytosis but never enough to confuse the lesion with Bowen's disease. The granular and keratin layers are thickened, and the epidermis often is hyperpigmented. Mild inflammatory infiltrate may be present in the upper dermis. Closer examination reveals that the nuclei are larger, but not paler staining, than the nuclei of normal epidermis and adnexa and that mitoses, when present, also are bulkier but do not seem to contain a larger number of chromosomes. Photocytometry[97] confirmed that the nuclei are hyperploid. The lesions, which were described as large cell acanthoma (Fig. 34–23), appear to be entirely benign.

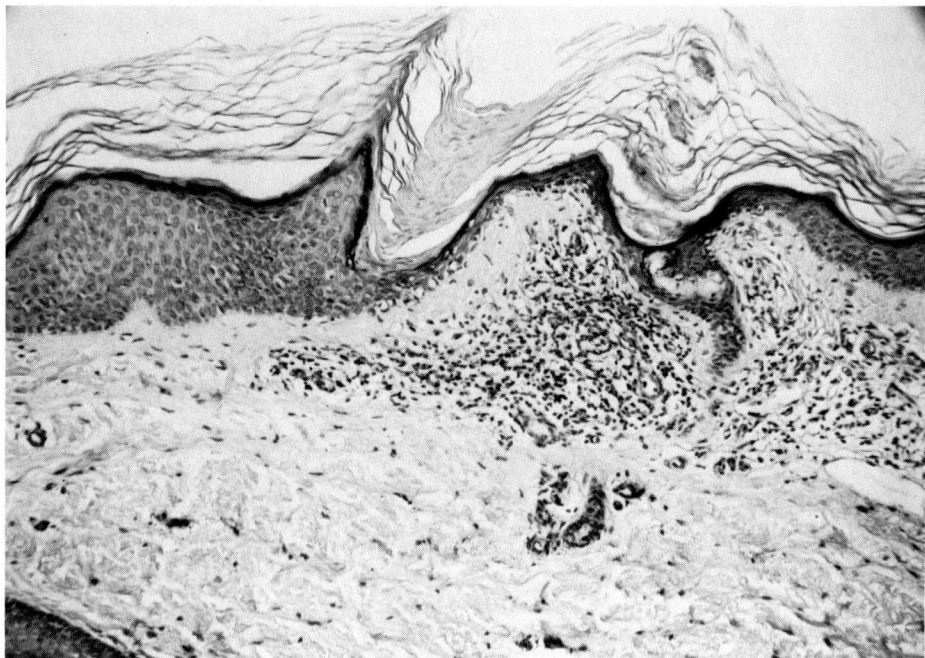

Figure 34–21.
Porokeratosis of Mibelli. Border of lesion is characterized by break in granular layer and oblique parakeratotic plug representing cross section of cornoid lamella. Note that this lesion has no relation to sweat duct, epidermis does not return to normal inside ring, and sweat duct in this area is dilated and hyperkeratotic. Note also inflammatory infiltrate. H&E. X135.

ACANTHOLYTIC ACANTHOMA

The solitary hyperkeratotic papule or nodule is located predominantly over the trunk and occasionally extremities.[98] Histologically, there is epidermal acanthosis, papillomatosis, and hyperkeratosis. Acantholysis is a prominent histologic feature occurring in various levels of the acanthotic epidermis from the suprabasal to granular.

KERATODERMA PALMARE ET PLANTARE

The various heritable forms of diffuse keratoderma of palms and soles represent peculiar intermediates between generalized nevoid disturbances of the integument, which we discussed in Chapter 30, and the localized malformations, with which we deal in this chapter. This ambivalence is accentuated by

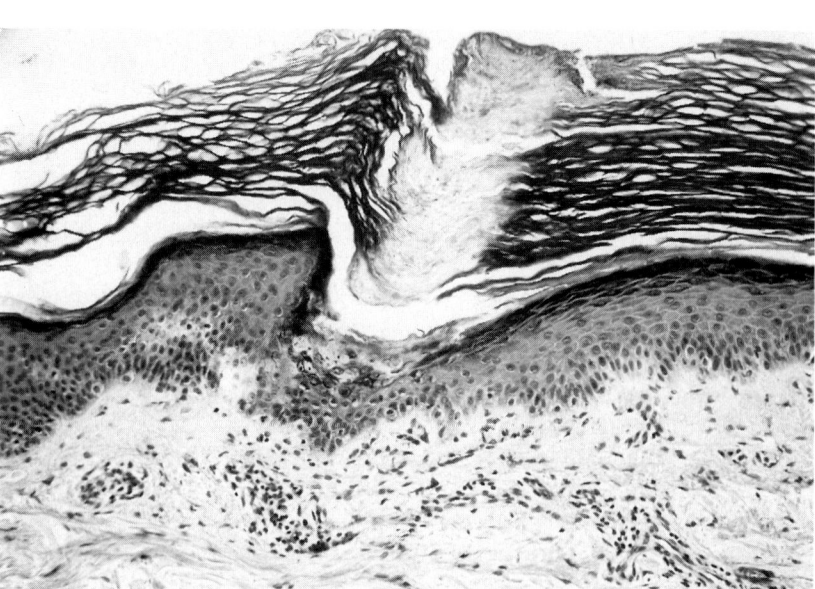

Figure 34–22.
Porokeratosis of Mibelli. Parakeratotic cornoid lamella is originating within a cup-shaped area of epidermal depression. H&E. X185.

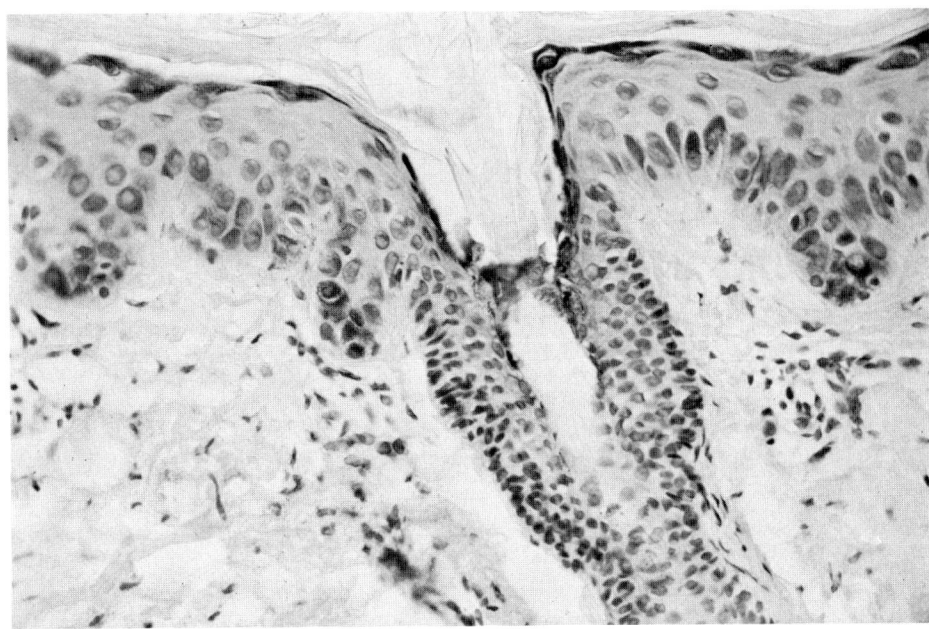

Figure 34–23.
Large cell acanthoma. Sharp contrast between the normal sized cells of a hair follicle and abnormally large cells forming an epidermis-like surface epithelium with normal keratinization. Nuclei and cytoplasm are large, and the nuclei are sufficiently variable to arouse suspicion of Bowen's dermatosis. There are no dyskeratotic cells, however, and mitoses, if present, are restricted to the basal layer. H&E. X225.

rare cases in which diffuse volar keratoderma has the histologic features of epidermolytic hyperkeratosis (Chapter 30). Keratodermas of palms and soles, whether occurring in families or as isolated cases, show pure epidermal hypergranulosis and hyperkeratosis (Fig. 34–24). Clinical manifestation may be localized or diffuse or may show linear configuration (striate keratoderma). Reed and Porter[99] listed 25 different types of volar keratoderma, and at least three more have been added since.[100–102] Keratoderma punctatum palmare et plantare refers to discrete lenticular lesions histologically characterized by a small cup-shaped area of epidermal depression containing dense orthokeratotic material (Fig. 34–25A). At the base of the lesion, the epidermis shows mild thickening and hypergranulosis.

CALLOSITIES AND CLAVUS

Callosities are localized areas of hyperkeratosis in response to chronic irritation and can occur in any location. Clavus refers to lesions appearing most commonly over the weight-bearing areas of the sole. They are histologically characterized by a central parakeratotic horny plug situated within a funnel-shaped area of epidermal depression (Fig. 34–25B). The epidermis may become very thin under the center of the lesion.

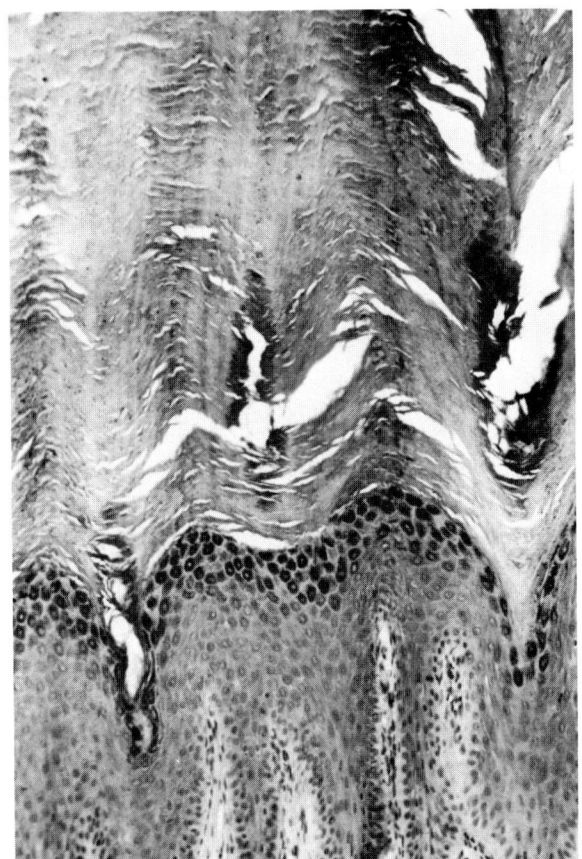

Figure 34–24.
Keratoderma palmare. Diffuse acanthosis, hypergranulosis, and hyperkeratosis. Sweat ducts normal (compare with Fig. 2–40). H&E. X125.

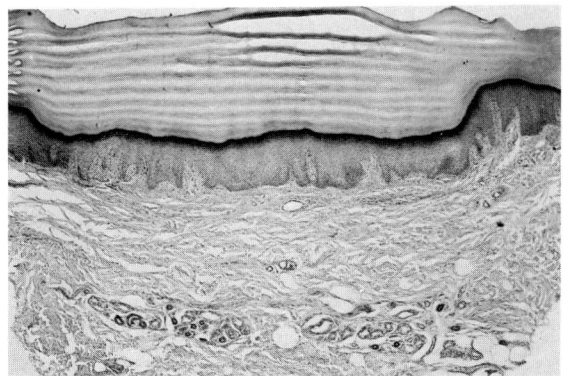

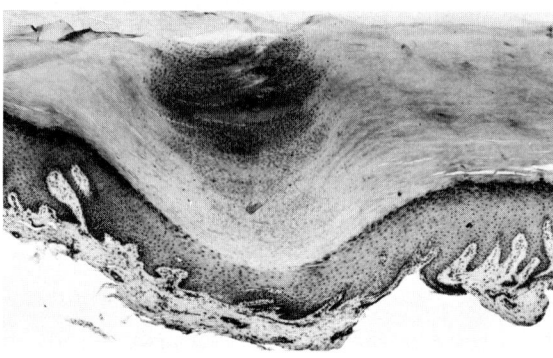

Figure 34–25.
A. Keratoderma palmare punctatum. Sharp-edged depression of epidermis. Striated appearance of the keratotic plug is shattering artifact caused by its brittleness. Epidermis has normal structure; dermis is slightly compressed. H&E. X45. *B.* Clavus. Relatively small lesion shows cup-shaped depression and thinning of epidermis, loss of granular layer, and parakeratosis of center of horny plug, all of which characterize the clavus. H&E. X45.

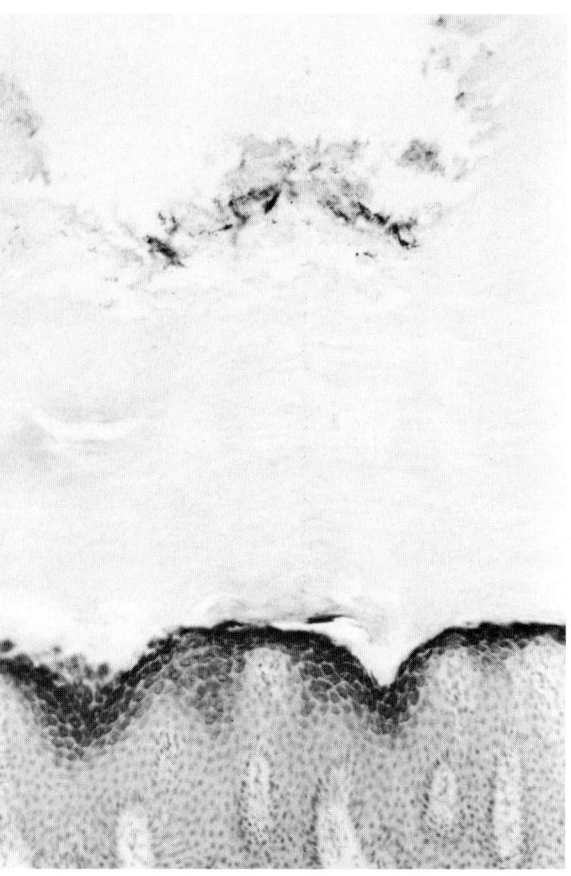

Figure 34–26.
Pitted keratolysis. Keratin layer partly destroyed by Corynebacterium growing in the upper layers of entirely normal stratum corneum. H&E. X125.

PITTED KERATOLYSIS

Superficial dissolution of the plantar keratin layer by species of *Corynebacterium*[103] produces shallow circular or circinate erosions. Filamentous and coccoid microorganisms are present within the keratin layer in eroded areas (Fig. 34–26). In a recent case reported from the Middle-East *dermatophilus congolensis* has been identified as causative agent.[104]

RETICULATED PIGMENTED ANOMALY OF THE FLEXURES

Dowling–Degos disease[105–107] is a rare genodermatosis transmitted by an autosomal dominant trait.[85] It is characterized by appearance of reticulated and dark brown macular pigmentation of face, trunk, and extremities, more pronounced over the flexural areas. Histologically (Fig. 34–27), there are areas of hyperpigmentation and downward budding of basaloid cells in connection with the lower surface of the epidermis, resembling a lentigo senilis or reticulated form of seborrheic verruca. Similar budding of basaloid cells occurs in connection with the infundibular portion of the hair follicles.

RETICULATE ACROPIGMENTATION

Kitamura's reticulate acropigmentation is inherited as an autosomal dominant trait.[108–110] It is manifested by networks of freckle-like pigmented areas

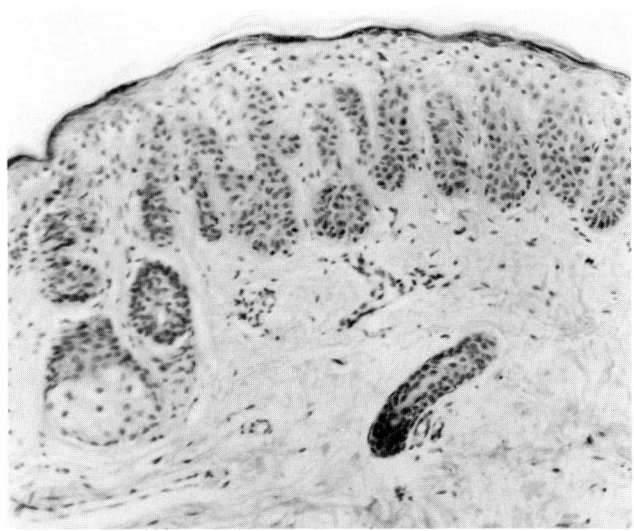

Figure 34–27.
Reticulated pigmented anomaly of the flexures. Picture resembles lentigo senilis or reticulated seborrheic verruca. H&E. X250.

over the extremities and later in other skin areas. Histologic findings include mild epidermal atrophy and an increase in the number of dopa-positive junctional melanocytes.

REFERENCES

1. Rogers M, McCrossin I, Commens C: Epidermal nevi and the epidermal nevus syndrome. A review of 131 cases. J Am Acad Dermatol 20:476, 1989
2. Jackson R: The lines of Blaschko: A review and reconsideration. Observations of the cause of certain unusual linear conditions of the skin. Br J Dermatol 95:349, 1976
3. Su DWP: Histopathologic varieties of epidermal nevus. Am J Dermatopathol 4:161, 1982
4. Zeligman I, Pomeranz J: Variations of congenital ichthyosiform erythroderma: Report of cases of ichthyosis hystrix and nevus unius lateris. Arch Dermatol 91:120, 1965
5. Adam JE, Richards R: Ichthyosis hystrix: Epidermolytic hyperkeratosis; discordant in monozygotic twins. Arch Dermatol 107:278, 1973
6. Kaidbey KH, Kurban AK: Dermatitic epidermal nevus. Arch Dermatol 104:166, 1971
7. Pegum JS, Darley CR: Inflammatory linear verrucous naevus. Br J Dermatol (Suppl 19) 105:78, 1981
8. Landwehr AJ, Starink TM: Inflammatory linear verrucous epidermal naevus: Report of a case with bilateral distribution and nail involvement. Dermatologica 166:107, 1983
9. Valdez RP, Balina LM, Kien MC: Nevo epidermico verrugoso inflamatorio (NEVIL) de disposicion bilateral. Rev Argent Dermatol 64:276, 1983
10. Morag C, Metzker A: Inflammatory linear verrucous epidermal nevus: Report of seven new cases and review of the literature. Pediatr Dermatol 3:15, 1985
11. Wood WH, Pellegrini AE: Inflammatory linear verrucous epidermal nevus. J Assoc Mil Dermatol 14:7, 1988
12. Altman J, Mehregan AH: Inflammatory linear verrucous epidermal nevus. Arch Dermatol 104:385, 1971
13. Dupré A, Christol B: Inflammatory linear verrucous epidermal nevus: A pathologic study. Arch Dermatol 113:767, 1977
14. Becker SW: Concurrent melanosis and hypertrichosis in distribution of nevus unius lateris. Arch Dermatol 60:155, 1949
15. Tymen R, Forestier JF, Boutet B, Colomb D: Naevus tardif de Becker: A propos d'une serie de 100 observations. Ann Dermatol Venereol 108:41, 1981
16. Fretzin DF, Whitney D: Familial Becker's nevus. J Am Acad Dermatol 12:589, 1985
17. Jain HC, Fisher BK: Familial Becker's nevus. Int J Dermatol 28:263, 1989
18. Boiron G, Surlève-Bazeille JE, Maleville J: Ultrastructure of Becker's melanosis. J Cutan Pathol 5:299, 1978
19. Panizzon R, Brungger H, Vogel A: Problems of the Becker's nevus: A clinical-histological-electron microscopic examination of 39 patients. Hautarzt 35:578, 1984
20. Haneke E: The dermal component in melanosis naeviformis Becker. J Cutan Pathol 6:53, 1979
21. Chapel TA, Tavafoghi V, Mehregan AH, Gagliardi C: Becker's melanosis: An organoid hamartoma. Cutis 27:410, 1981
22. Johnson MD, Jacobs AH: Congenital smooth muscle hamartoma. A report of six cases and a review of the literature. Arch Dermatol 125:820, 1989
23. Banafe JL, Ghrenassia-Canal S, Vancina S: Nevus musculaire lisse. Ann Dermatol Venereol 107:929, 1980
24. Slifman NR, Harrist TJ, Rhodes AR: Congenital arrector pili hamartoma: A case report and review of the spectrum of Becker's melanosis and pilar smooth muscle hamartoma. Arch Dermatol 121:1034, 1985
25. Blanc F, Jeanmougin M, Civatte J: Naevus de Becker et hypoplasie mammaire. Ann Dermatol Venereol 115:1127, 1988
26. Moore JA, Schosser RH: Becker's melanosis and hypoplasia of the breast and pectoralis major muscle. Pediatr Dermatol 3:34, 1985
27. Frithiof L, Banoczy J: White sponge nevus (leukoedema exfoliativum mucosae oris): Ultrastructural observations. Oral Surg 41:607, 1976
28. Jorgenson RJ, Levin LS: White sponge nevus. Arch Dermatol 117:73, 1981
29. Alinovi A, Benaldi D, Pezzarossa E: White sponge

nevus: Successful treatment with penicillin. Acta Derm Venereol 63:83, 1983
30. Camacho Martinez F, Moreno Gimenez JC: Syndrome du naevus épidermique (de Solomon, Fretzin et DeWald). Ann Dermatol Venereol 112:143, 1985
31. Golitz LE, Weston WL: Inflammatory linear verrucous epidermal nevus: Association with epidermal nevus syndrome. Arch Dermatol 115:1208, 1979
32. Haustein UF, Süss E: Inflammatorischer lineärer verruköser epidermaler naevus (ILVEN). Dermatol Monatsschr 164:120, 1978
33. Goldberg LH, Collins SAB, Siegel DM: The epidermal nevus syndrome: Case report and review. Pediatr Dermatol 4:27, 1987
34. Hornstein L, Bove KE, Towbin RB: Linear nevi, hemihypertrophy, connective tissue hamartomas, and unusual neoplasms in children. J Pediatr 110:404, 1987
35. Raynaud F, Saurat J H: Le syndrome de Solomon (syndrome du naevus épidermique) sa place en pédiatrie générale. Ann Pediatr 29:46, 1982
36. Mehregan AH: Epithelial nevi and benign tumors of the skin and their associated systemic conditions. J Dermatol (Tokyo) 12:10, 1985
37. Laplanche G, Grosshans E, Gabriel-Robez O, Happle R, Enjolras O: Hyperplasie épidermique et hémidysplasie corporelle hypoplasique congénitales homolaterales (Démembremeut du syndrome de Solomon). Ann Dermatol Venereol 107:729–739, 1980
38. Moulin G, Barrut D, Franc MP, Fauchet R: C.H.I.L.D. syndrome: Naevus épidermique et hémidysplasie corporelle hypoplasique homolatérale. Ann Dermatol Venereol 109:793, 1982
39. Ferrando J, Navarra E, Torres MJ: Hiperqueratosis neviforme de la areola mamaria. Med Cutan ILA 9:285, 1981
40. Kuhlman DS, Hodges SJ, Owen LG: Hyperkeratosis of the nipple and areola. J Am Acad Dermatol 13:596, 1985
41. Mehregan AH, Rahbari H: Nevoid hyperkeratosis of nipples and areolae. Arch Dermatol 113:1691, 1977
42. Schneller WA: Acrokeratosis verruciformis of Hopf. Arch Dermatol 106:81, 1972
43. Jeanmougin M: Les acanthosis nigricans. Ann Dermatol Venereol 112:531, 1985
44. Roberts SOB, Lachapelle JM: Confluent and reticulate papillomatosis (Gougerot-Carteaud) and *Pityrosporum orbiculare*. Br J Dermatol 81:841, 1969
45. El-Tonsy M H, El-Benhawi M O, Mehregan A H: Confluent and reticulated papillomatosis. J Am Acad Dermatol 16:893, 1987
46. Goldstein N: Multiple minute digitate hyperkeratoses. Arch Dermatol 96:692, 1967
47. Yoon SW, Gibbs RB: Multiple minute digitate hyperkeratoses. Arch Dermatol 111:1176, 1975
48. Goodfield M, Rowell NR: Disseminated minute keratoses. Br J Dermatol 117 (Suppl 32):72, 1987
49. Frenk E, Mevorah B Leu F: Disseminated spiked hyperkeratosis: An unusual discrete nonfollicular keratinization disorder. Arch Dermatol 117:412, 1981
50. Willoughby C, Soter NA: Stucco keratosis. Arch Dermatol 105:859, 1972
51. Shall L, Marks R: The pathology and pathogenesis of stucco keratoses. Br J Dermatol 117(Suppl):32, 1987
52. Mehregan AH, Rahbari H: Benign epithelial tumors of the skin: 1. Epidermal tumors. Cutis 19:43, 1977
53. Mehregan AH: Lentigo senilis and its evolutions. J Invest Dermatol 65:429, 1975
54. Horiuchi Y: Multiple seborrheic verrucae following eczema. A case report. J Dermatol (Tokyo) 16:505, 1989
55. Mevorah B, Mishima Y: Cellular response of seborrheic keratosis following croton oil irritation and surgical trauma. Dermatologica 131:452, 1965
56. Lund HZ: Atlas of Tumor Pathology: Tumors of the Skin. Sec. 1. Fascicle 2. Washington DC, Armed Forces Institute of Pathology, 1957
57. Mehregan AH, Pinkus H: Intraepidermal epithelioma. A critical study. Cancer 17:609, 1964
58. Mikhail GR, Mehregan AH: Basal cell carcinoma in seborrheic verruca. J Am Acad Dermatol 6:500, 1982
59. Bloch PH: Transformation of seborrheic keratosis into Bowen's disease. J Cutan Pathol 5:361, 1978
60. Rahbari H: Bowenoid transformation of seborrheic verrucae (keratoses). Br J Dermatol 101:459, 1979
61. Curry SS, King LE: The sign of Leser–Trélat: Report of a case with adenocarcinoma of duodenum. Arch Dermatol 116:1059, 1980
62. Lambert D, Fort M, Legoux A, Chapuis J-L: Le signe de Leser–Trélat. A propos de 2 observations. Ann Dermatol Venereol 107:1035, 1980
63. Hattori A, Umegae Y, Kataki S, et al: Small cell carcinoma of the lung with Leser–Trélat sign. Arch Dermatol 118:1017, 1982
64. Holdiness MR: The sign of Leser–Trélat. Int J Dermatol 25:564, 1986
65. Halevy S, Halevy J, Feuerman EJ: The sign of Leser–Trélat in association with lymphocytic lymphoma. Dermatologica 161:183, 1980
66. Mishima Y, Pinkus H: Benign mixed tumor of melanocytes and malpighian cells. Melanoacanthoma: Its relationship to Bloch's benign non-nevoid melanoepithelioma. Arch Dermatol 81:539, 1960
67. Prince C, Mehregan AH, Hashimoto K, Plotnick H: Large melanoacanthomas: A report of five cases. J Cutan Pathol 11:309, 1984
68. Hairston MA Jr, Reed RJ, Derbes VJ: Dermatosis papulosa nigra. Arch Dermatol 89:655, 1964
69. Degos R, Civatte J: Clear cell acanthoma: Experience of eight years. Br J. Dermatol 83:248, 1970
70. Brownstein MH: The benign acanthomas. J Cutan Pathol 12:172, 1985
71. Trau II, Fisher BK, Schewach-Millet M: Multiple clear cell acanthomas. Arch Dermatol 116:433, 1980
72. Cotton DWK, Mills PM, Stephenson TJ, Underwood JCE: On the nature of clear cell acanthomas. Br J Dermatol 117:569, 1987
73. Baden TJ, Woodley DT, Wheeler CE Jr: Multiple clear cell acanthoma. Case report and delineation of base-

ment membrane zone antigens. J Am Acad Dermatol 16:1075, 1987
74. Hashimoto T, Inamoto N, Nakamura K: Two cases of clear cell acanthoma: An immunohistochemical study. J Cutan Pathol 15:27, 1988
75. Naeyaert JM, Bersaques J, Geerts M-L, Kint A: Multiple clear cell acanthomas. A clinical, histological, and ultrastructural report. Arch Dermatol 123:1670, 1987
76. Howell JB, Mehregan AH: Story of the pits. Arch Dermatol 102:583, 1970
77. Hashimoto K, Howell JB, Yamanishi Y, et al: Electron microscopic studies of palmar and plantar pits of nevoid basal cell epithelioma. J Invest Dermatol 59:380, 1972
78. Covo JA: The pits in the nevoid basal cell carcinoma syndrome. Arch Dermatol 103:568, 1971
79. Holubar K, Matras H, Swalik AV: Multiple palmar basal cell epitheliomas in basal cell nevus syndrome. Arch Dermatol 101:679, 1970
80. Reed RJ, Leone P: Porokeratosis: A mutant clonal keratosis of the epidermis: I. Histogenesis. Arch Dermatol 101:340, 1970
81. Shumack SP, Commens CA: Disseminated superficial actinic porokeratosis: A clinical study. J Am Acad Dermatol 20:1015, 1989
82. Rahbari H, Cordero AA, Mehregan AH: Linear porokeratosis: A distinctive clinical variant of porokeratosis of Mibelli. Arch Dermatol 109:526, 1974
83. Lestringant GG, Berge T: Porokeratosis puctata palmaris et plantaris. Arch Dermatol 125:816, 1989
84. Patrizi A, Passarini B, Minghetti G, Masina M: Porokeratosis palmaris et plantaris disseminata: An unusual clinical presentation. J Am Acad Dermatol 21:415, 1989
85. Mehregan AH, Khalili H, Fazel Z: Mibelli's porokeratosis of the face. J Am Acad Dermatol 3:394, 1980
86. Montgomery RM: Porokeratosis plantaris discreta. Cutis 20:711, 1977
87. Neumann RA, Knobler RM, Metze D, Jurecka W: Disseminated superficial porokeratosis and immunosuppression. Br J Dermatol 199:375, 1988
88. Coskey RJ, Mehregan AH: Bowen disease associated with porokeratosis of Mibelli. Arch Dermatol 111:1480, 1975
89. Otsuka F, Huang J, Sawara K, et al: Disseminated porokeratosis accompanying multicentric Bowen's disease. Characterization of porokeratotic lesions progressing to Bowen's disease. J Am Acad Dermatol 23:355, 1990
90. Chernosky ME, Rapini RP: Squamous cell carcinoma in lesions of disseminated superficial actinic porokeratosis. A report of two cases. Arch Dermatol 122:853, 1986
91. Sarkany I: Porokeratosis of Mibelli with basal cell epithelioma. Proc R Soc Med 66:435, 1973
92. Driban NE, Cavicchia JC: Prokeratotic eccrine ostial and dermal duct nevus. J Cutan Pathol 14:118, 1987
93. Aloi FG, Pippione M: Porokeratotic eccrine ostial and dermal duct nevus. Arch Dermatol 122:892, 1986
94. Fernandez-Redondo V, Toribio J: Porokeratotic ostial and dermal duct nevus. J Cutan Pathol 15:393, 1988
95. Coskey RJ, Mehregan AH, Hashimoto K: Porokeratotic eccrine duct and hair follicle nevus. J Am Acad Dermatol 6:940, 1982
96. Rahbari H, Pinkus H: Large cell acanthoma: One of the actinic keratoses. Arch Dermatol 114:49, 1978
97. Fand SB, Pinkus H: Polyploidy in benign epidermal neoplasia. J Cell Biol 47:2, pt 2, 1970, p 52a
98. Brownstein MH: Acantholytic acanthoma. J Am Acad Dermatol 19:783, 1988
99. Reed WB, Porter PS: Keratosis. Arch Dermatol 104:99, 1971
100. Brown FC: Punctate keratoderma. Arch Dermatol 104:682, 1971
101. Onwukwe F, Mihm MC, Toda K: Hereditary papulotranslucent acrokeratoderma: A new variant of familial punctate keratoderma? Arch Dermatol 108:108, 1973
102. Herman PS: Punctate keratoderma. Arch Dermatol 109:910, 1974
103. Tilgen W: Pitted keratolysis (keratolysis plantare sulcatum). J Cutan Pathol 6:18, 1979
104. Gillum RL, Qadri HSM, Al-Ahal MN, et al: Pitted keratolysis: A manifestation of human dermatophilosis. Dermatologica 177:305, 1988
105. Wilson-Jones E, Grice K: Reticulated pigmented anomaly of the flexures. Arch Dermatol 114:1150, 1978
106. Howell JB, Freeman RG: Reticular pigmented anomaly of the flexures. Arch Dermatol 114:400, 1978
107. Kikuchi I, Inoue S, Narita H, et al: The broad spectrum of Dowling Degos disease, including Haber's syndrome: A hereditary abnormal reactivity to stimulation, increasing with age? Case reports and management. J Dermatol (Tokyo) 10:361, 1983
108. Crovato F, Nazzari G, Rebora A: Dowling-Degos disease (reticulate pigmented anomaly of the flexures) is an autosomal dominant condition. Br J Dermatol 108:473, 1983
109. Woodley DT, Caro I, Wheeler CE Jr: Reticulate acropigmentation of Kitamura. Arch Dermatol 115:760, 1979
110. Bajaj AK, Gupta SC: Reticulate acropigmentation of Kitamura: A report of two families. Dermatologica 168:247, 1984

35

EPIDERMAL PRECANCER, SQUAMOUS CELL CARCINOMA, AND PSEUDOCARCINOMA

In this chapter we discuss purely epithelial neoplasias in contrast to the organoid fibroepithelial lesions dealt with in the previous chapter. Whether and to what extent the mesoderm is involved in the causation of human cutaneous precanceroses and carcinomas is a question irrelevant to diagnostic interpretation of characteristic histologic changes. We can diagnose a dysplastic precancerous stretch of epidermis regardless of the presence of actinic elastosis and other dermal changes, and their presence or absence should not influence our judgment. The significant features are cytologic alteration of keratinocytes in a manner leading to an abnormal end product. This change involves a limited number of cells that are distinctly different from their normal neighbors, on which they abut with a sharp border. From this no-mixing, no-transition feature we deduct that the neoplastic cells are a clone or stock, heritably deranged and not just temporarily altered through external influences emanating from the body in general (e.g., hormones) or from supporting connective tissue.

A clone of irreversibly altered neoplastic cells may replace a stretch of epidermis, yet remain in the boundaries of a basement membrane. Alternately, it may form distinct nests within a framework of persistent epidermis, or it may grow invasively down into the dermis. In the latter case, the basement membrane, which is evidence of epithelial-mesenchymal interrelations, usually is lost, and all trace of fibroepithelial coordination has disappeared. In any of the three situations, the mesoderm does not participate in forming the tumor. At most it exhibits an inflammatory reaction and other secondary changes found commonly in cancer of any organ.

PRECANCEROUS KERATOSES

"Keratosis" is a clinical term and has been applied rather loosely to many lesions exhibiting increased and usually adherent keratin formation thought not to be due to an inflammatory process. Histopathologic study cannot really accept keratosis as a diagnostic term, and it was pointed out that seborrheic keratosis is a papilloma and is better designated a seborrheic verruca (disregarding that seborrheic is also inappropriate). One might say that all neoplasms of keratinocytes are "acanthomas,"[1] and this term has been applied to some recently delineated lesions (clear cell acanthoma, large cell acanthoma, acantholytic acanthoma, Chapter 34). The name keratosis, however, is ingrained, and we shall continue using it for actinic and other precancerous keratoses. Objections have frequently been raised against the use of "precancerous" in histologic diagnosis because it includes prophecy. It is, however, one of the principal tasks of the pathologist to imply prognosis in his diagnostic interpretation. The con-

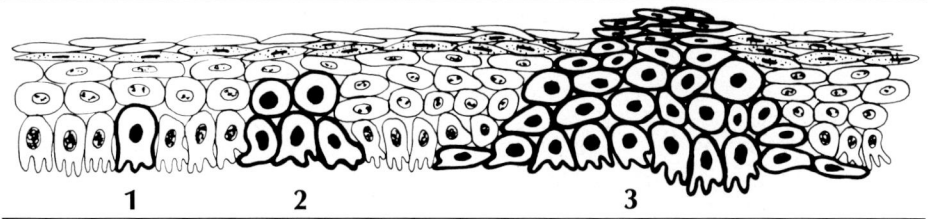

Figure 35–1.
Diagram illustrates three stages of development of a solar keratosis as prototype of epidermal malignant transformation. (1) Heritable perversion of a single basal germinal cell which by multiplication (2) produces more abnormal basal cells and keratinizing cells. (3) When abnormal products reach surface, clinical keratosis results. Meanwhile, abnormal germinal cells undermine normal epidermis, thus producing a slanting cell-sharp border. (From Pinkus. In Kopf and Andrade (eds): Year Book of Dermatology, 1967. Courtesy of Year Book Medical Publishers.)

cept of *precancerosis* is based essentially on statistical data which show the more or less frequent association of a certain type of lesion with cancer developing in it.[2–4] Similarly, we can diagnose a precancerous lesion by certain histologic and cytologic criteria without waiting for it to progress to invasive carcinoma. On the other hand, if we accept the thesis that the cells composing the keratosis are irreversibly altered and have acquired some of the properties characteristic of malignant neoplasia (Fig. 35–1), we can apply the term "carcinoma in situ." Which term we prefer to use depends on personal choice and extraneous circumstances.

The two principal lesions in this group are actinic keratoses and the precancerous dermatosis of Bowen. Certain variants, like erythroplasia of Queyrat, cutaneous horns and xeroderma pigmentosum will be mentioned. The outstanding differential feature between a typical actinic keratosis (keratosis senilis) and a typical Bowen's disease is that the former consists of fairly even squamous cells ending in parakeratosis without a granular layer, whereas the latter consists of uneven cells exhibiting dyskeratosis, but may have a granular layer and orthokeratosis. We shall see that transitions exist.

Actinic Keratosis
Keratosis Senilis (Freudenthal)

Although the diagnosis keratosis senilis has been supplanted in clinical usage by actinic keratosis, it remains a useful histologic diagnostic term if we define it by the features originally delineated by Freudenthal and reemphasized and biologically interpreted by Pinkus.[5] The diagram (Fig. 35–2) illustrates that actinic keratosis consists of deranged epi-

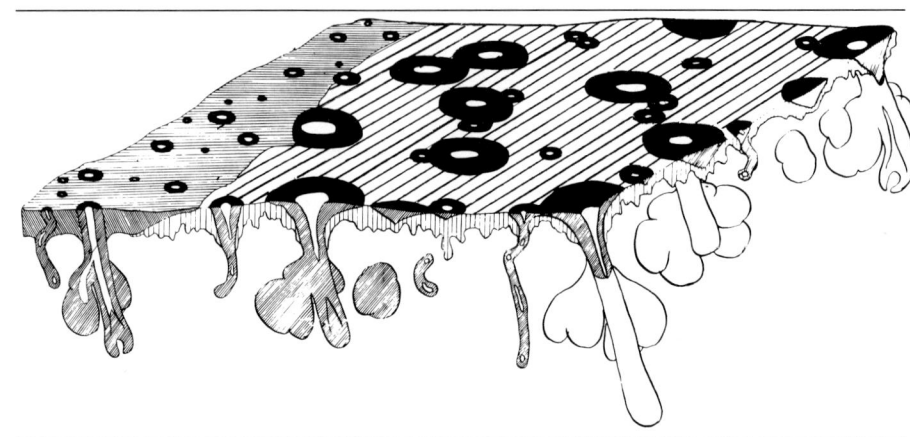

Figure 35–2.
Diagram illustrating three-dimensional architecture of actinic keratosis. Cut borders of epidermal plate show what is seen in two-dimensional vertical sections. Dysplastic epidermis borders on and creeps under normal epidermis and adnexal epithelium. The latter forms hyperplastic umbrellas which may merge on surface, thus submerging dysplastic epithelium. (From Pinkus. Am J Clin Pathol 29:193, 1958.)

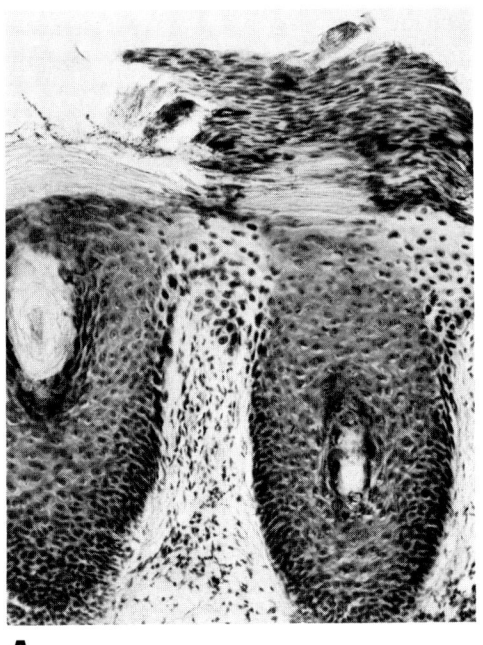
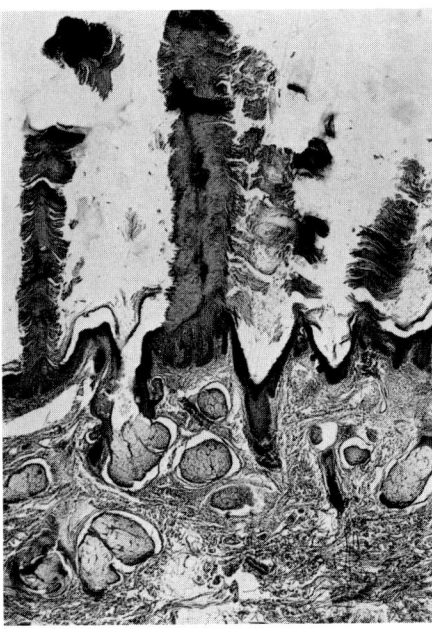

Figure 35–3.
Keratosis senilis type of actinic keratosis. Illustrated are sharp borders of dysplastic epidermis and hyperplastic adnexal epithelium with production of alternating stretches or columns of parakeratotic and orthokeratotic horny material. **A.** H&E. X135. **B.** H&E. X35.

dermal keratinocytes that are demarcated sharply from hyperplastic but otherwise normal adnexal keratinocytes and from the normal surrounding epidermis. In a histologic section (corresponding to the cut edges of the three-dimensional diagram), we see (Figs. 35–3 and 35–4) lighter staining, more eosinophilic epidermal prickle cells arising from an often irregular basal layer and ending as nucleated (parakeratotic) flakes without the formation of a granular layer. In between, there are follicular and eccrine ostia lined with multiple layers of darker staining cells that form a hyperplastic granular

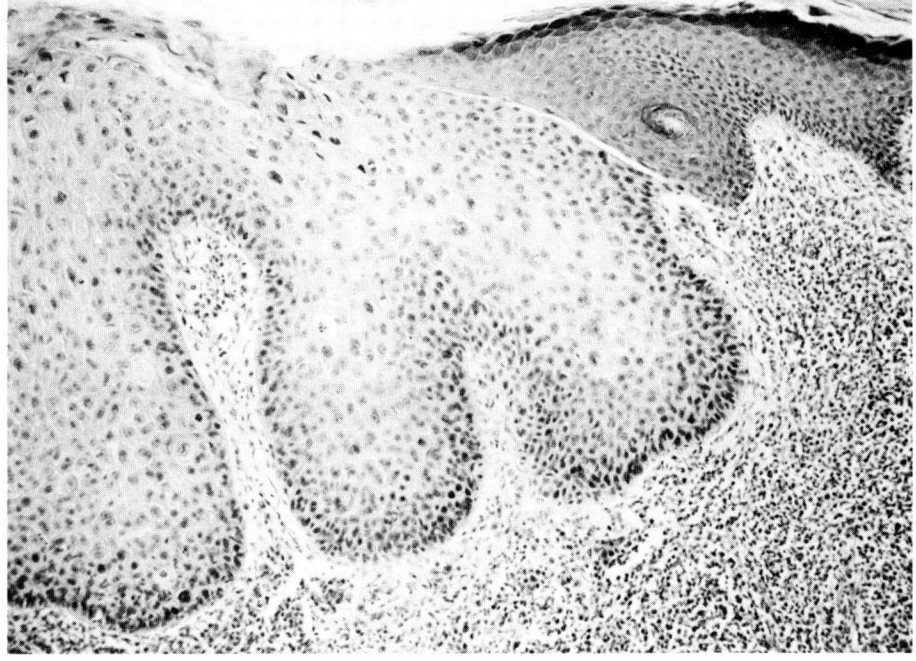

Figure 35–4.
Actinic keratosis, lateral edge. Sharp slanting border of bowenoid epithelium and normal epidermis, including a sweat duct. Lack of cohesion between the two types of epithelium. Strong reactive inflammatory infiltrate in dermis. H&E. X135.

layer and orthokeratotic horny material.[6] It is characteristic that the border between the two types of epithelium is sharp and that it usually does not run vertically but forms a slant or slanting curve (Fig. 35–4).[7] Most often, the adnexal keratinocytes cover more surface, whereas epidermal keratinocytes cover more dermal junction and often extend like a collar downward around adnexal ostia (Fig. 35–5).[8] In some spots (Fig. 35–5B), however, adnexal epithelium barely reaches the surface, a sign that the balance in the struggle between the competing keratinocytes is being tipped. Occasionally, adnexal epithelium is completely submerged by dysplastic epidermis (Fig. 35–6). In other areas, the umbrella-like spreading of adnexal keratinocytes from adjacent ostia may merge on the surface (Figs. 35–3A and 35–5A) and submerge the dysplastic epidermal cells. Such pictures falsely suggest that only the lower part of the epidermis is deranged, the upper being normal. Examination of the diagram and biologic interpretation of the events explain the situation. There is over- and undersliding of normal and dysplastic keratinocytes of different provenience, not maturation of atypical basal strata into normal upper strata. The basal layer of the keratosis may be straight or may show mild or pronounced atypical budding. Ultrastructural changes in actinic keratosis are similar to those of Bowen's disease.[9] These include widened intercellular spaces with microvilli formation, a decrease in the number of desmosomes, a decrease in the amount of tonofilaments, aggregation of tonofibrils, binucleated keratinocytes, mitotic figures, and discontinuity of the basal lamina, with cytoplasmic projections of the basal cells into the upper dermis.

These matters are discussed in detail because biologic insight into the mechanics of actinic keratosis helps the student to grasp the concepts of cutaneous carcinogenesis and also assists in the diagnosis of unusual lesions and in the interpretation of small fragments of tissue obtained from curettings of this type of lesion.

If we retrace theoretically the development of actinic keratosis to its beginning, we arrive at the one deranged stem cell of the carcinoma in situ, as illustrated in Figure 35–1. A clinical lesion is not apparent until the third stage has been reached, and histologic diagnosis is possible only slightly earlier. The diagram illustrates that actinically damaged skin can carry many more foci of deranged epidermis than are clinically visible, a fact nicely demonstrated by the effects of local application or systemic administration of 5-fluorouracil, which brings out all the subclinical lesions, and supported by findings that the epidermis surrounding a keratosis is not normal.[10] Some clinically apparent lesions may regress spontaneously.[11]

Any actinic keratosis, whether keratosis senilis or other type, is of course associated with actinic changes in the dermis, especially with elastotic alteration. In addition, there is an infiltrate of round cells, which may be mild or heavy and which often includes plasma cells and, occasionally, eosinophils.[12,13] This type of infiltrate is associated with practially all malignant neoplastic skin lesions, whether they are invasive or not, and is of considerable diagnostic significance even though it may be absent in rare cases. It should alert the pathologist to look for the diagnostic epidermal changes, as in the atrophic form of actinic keratosis (Fig. 35–7).

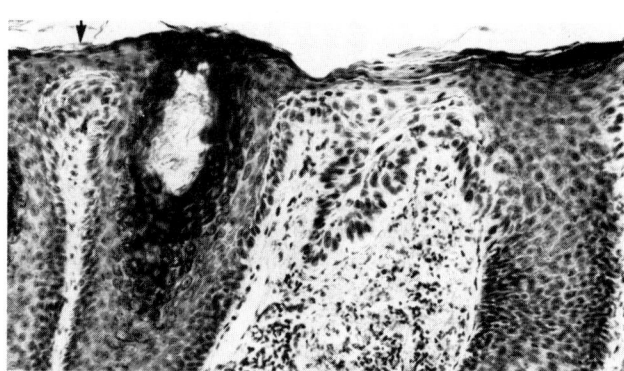

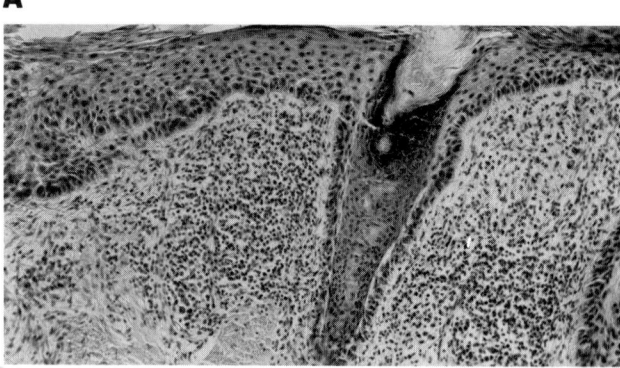

Figure 35–5.
Actinic keratosis. **A.** Atypical budding of dysplastic epidermis between hair follicles. Dysplastic epithelium also creeps down around the follicles, which form umbrellas on the surface. Adnexal epithelium has joined at left side of picture (arrow), cutting dysplastic epithelium off from access to the surface. H&E. X135. **B.** Dysplastic epidermis has crept far down on outside of sweat duct and begins to overpower it. While ductal keratinocytes still spread on surface to left and form keratohyalin layer, they do not reach surface on right. Note reactive inflammatory infiltrate in **A** and **B**. H&E. X70.

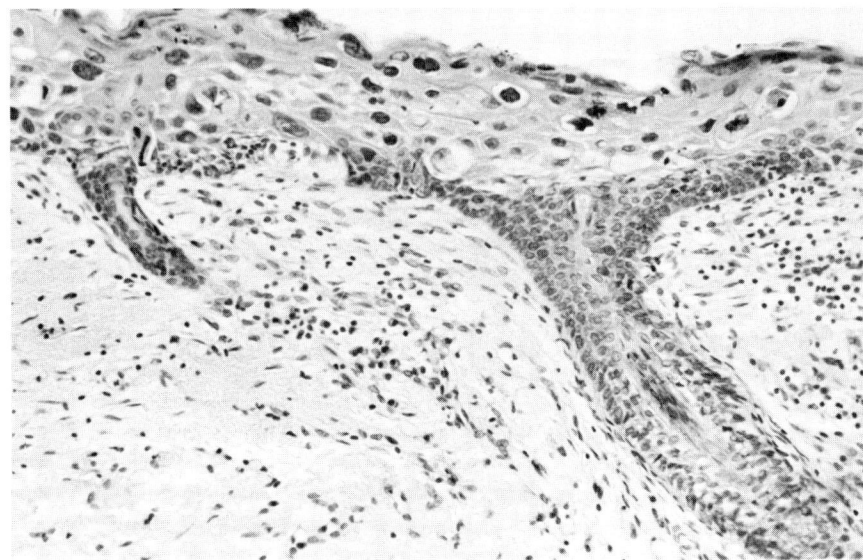

Figure 35-6.
Unusual picture of actinic keratosis in which a solid layer of dysplastic epidermis covers the surface, while a sweat duct and a hair follicle spread below it. H&E. X125.

Our early hypothesis that it is a tissue immune reaction to the neoplastic cells that the organism recognizes as nonself long before they become invasive has become more acceptable. A similar interpretation has been advanced for the inflammatory infiltrate in basal cell epithelioma and squamous cell carcinoma.[14]

Variants of Actinic Keratosis

One of the more common variants of classic actinic keratosis is the *Darierlike form* (Fig. 35-8), in which a section will show a single layer of dysplastic cells at the dermoepidermal junction separated by a cleft from fairly normal upper layers of epidermis. Acantholytic degenerating or dyskeratotic cells may float in the fluid-filled cleft.[15] This picture is explained as an extreme case of the biologic process. If the dysplastic cells become more vigorous and invasive, they then form *acantholytic squamous cell carcinoma* (Fig. 35-21).

Occasionally dysplastic epidermal epithelium has been completely submerged by a new epidermis (Fig. 35-8B) originating from the cutaneous adnexa. A confusing picture then results, in which the

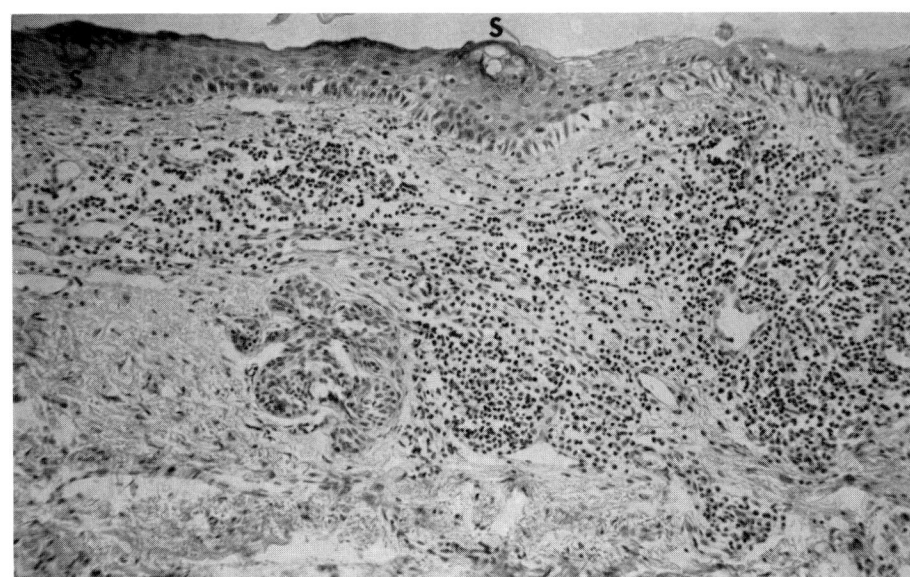

Figure 35-7.
Atrophic actinic keratosis. Dysplastic basal cells form quickly degenerating upper layers without keratohyalin in right half of picture and extend below normally keratinizing epidermis of adnexal provenience almost to left border of picture. Two intraepidermal center(s) are cross sections of sweat duct lumina. Branching epithelial island in dermis is a tangential section of bulge proliferation of a hair follicle (Chap. 2). Note heavy inflammatory reaction. H&E. X135.

lower part of the epidermis appears anaplastic while the upper parts appear normal and keratinize with formation of keratohyalin granules.

Another common variant is produced by the epidermal cells becoming more dyskeratotic in a bowenoid manner. The histologic picture then resembles that of Bowen's disease, and it is difficult to decide in some cases whether one is dealing with true Bowen's disease in a sun-exposed area or with a *bowenoid actinic keratosis* (Fig. 35–9). The significance of differentiation is clinical because an actinic keratosis is more apt to become invasive. In cases of the bowenoid type, but also in some lesions of less dysplastic character, the epidermis may become quite hyperplastic, and, at low power, the picture may resemble a cutaneous papilloma. Attention to cytologic detail will lead to the correct diagnosis of a "hyperplastic variant" of actinic keratosis.

A fourth variant may be called *atrophic actinic keratosis*. These lesions look red and atrophic clinically, have an adherent scale, and are painful on blunt pressure. They resemble discoid lupus erythematosus in all these respects and usually are biopsied for differential diagnosis. Histologically (see Fig. 35–7), the epidermis is atrophic, and the upper corium contains heavy lymphocytic infiltrate associated with some telangiectasia. The zone of actinic elastosis is more or less destroyed. At first glance, the infiltrate may appear to be the most significant feature, and the resemblance to lupus erythematosus may be striking, but closer inspection reveals the distinguishing features. The epidermis has no granular layer and is parakeratotic. It also may show some cellular atypicality and always is sharply delineated against the hyperplastic and hyperkeratotic adnexal ostia. In discoid lupus, ostial and epidermal epithelia are equally atrophic and orthokeratotic. The dermal infiltrate usually contains plasma cells in the keratosis.

A fifth variant is the *spreading pigmented actinic keratosis*[16–18] (Fig. 35–10). Usually, melanocytes do not survive long in the deranged epithelium. If they do, the question of lentigo maligna may arise but is usually ruled out by the dysplastic changes of the keratinocytes. Pigmented lesions often spread beyond the usual dimensions of an actinic keratosis. Another form of pigmented lesion is a combination of actinic keratosis and lentigo senilis in one area (Fig. 35–11).

Other Actinic Keratoses

That exposure to ultraviolet rays causes the formation of pyknotic cells in the epidermis has been

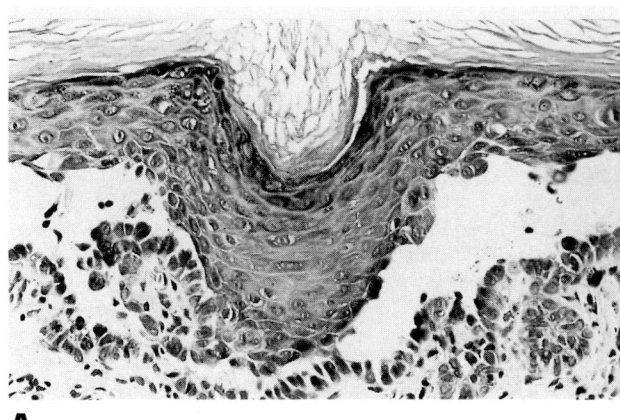

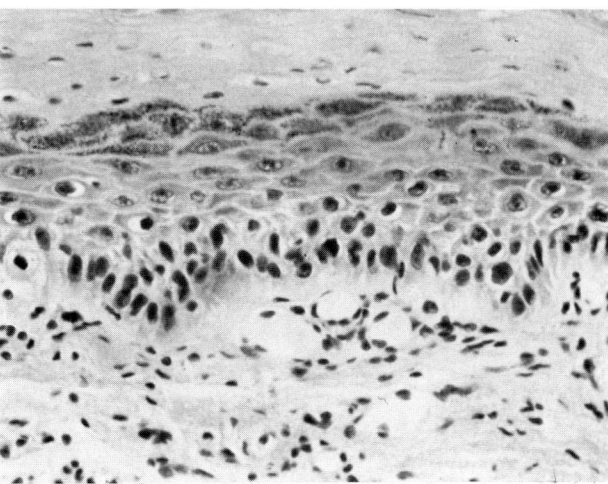

Figure 35–8.
A. Darier-like actinic keratosis shows foci of downward budding of basaloid cells and suprabasal acantholysis. H&E. X225. **B.** In this form of actinic keratosis the lower portion of the epidermis appears dysplastic while the upper part shows keratohyalin granules. H&E. X225.

known for many years (Chapter 3). The recent introduction of combined psoralen and long-wave ultraviolet ray exposure (PUVA) in the treatment of psoriasis and other disorders has caused new interest in the effect of UV on the epidermis.[19] Focal dysplasia was found in about one half of the cases[20] and persisted for 1 year after the start of the therapy. Whether such cells may survive after treatment is discontinued remains to be seen, but clinical experience of larger numbers of actinic keratoses, keratoacanthomas, and squamous cell carcinomas in treated skin leads to that conclusion.[21,22] The effect of PUVA on epidermal melanocytes is responsible

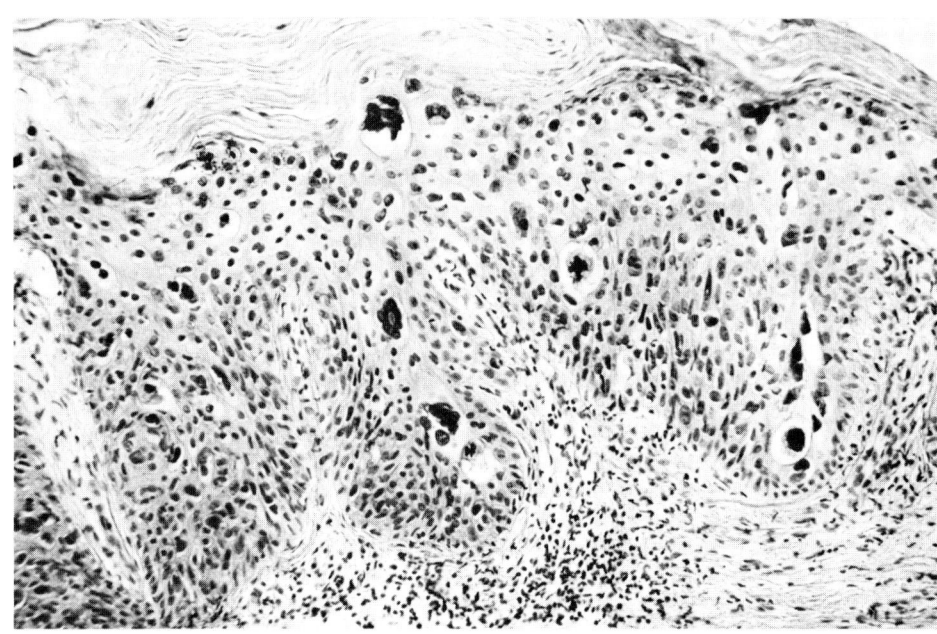

Figure 35–9.
Bowenoid actinic keratosis. Extreme dysplasia of epidermis is indistinguishable from pictures seen in Bowen's dermatosis (Fig. 35–12). Presence of actinic elastosis and information that the lesion is situated in actinic skin influence the judgment. H&E. X135.

for the development of stellate freckles and extensive xeroderma pigmentosum-like changes.[23,24]

Other light-induced epidermal lesions include the lichen planus-like keratosis (lichenoid actinic keratosis)[25] discussed in Chapter 9 and disseminated superficial actinic porokeratosis and large cell acanthoma discussed in Chapter 34.

BOWEN'S PRECANCEROUS DERMATOSIS (CARCINOMA IN SITU) AND ERYTHROPLASIA OF QUEYRAT

The precancerous dermatosis described by Bowen in 1912[26] is the first recognized example of carcinoma in situ. Clinically, it forms flat scaly or elevated crusted plaques, and some lesions may be exuberantly papillomatous and hyperkeratotic. The general histologic features consist of a full thickness loss of epidermal stratification (windblown appearance), great variability of nuclear size and depth of staining (poikilokaryosis), occurrence of mitoses in all layers of the living epidermis, and presence of atypical cells, some with multiple nuclei and dyskeratotic cells (Fig. 35–12). The surface may be parakeratotic or orthokeratotic. There is usually some degree of acanthosis, and the rete ridges are uneven and plump. Papillae may be inconspicuous or elongated. Dermal changes include superficial telangiectasia and chronic inflammatory cell reaction.

The balance between dysplastic epidermis and adnexal epithelium often is disturbed in Bowen's disease to the disadvantage of the adnexa. Instead of forming hyperkeratotic umbrellas (Fig. 35–13), the follicular epithelium often just reaches the skin surface (Fig. 35–13C). In many cases, dyskeratotic epidermis invades ostial territory (Fig. 35–13D) and may replace follicular epithelium all the way down to the sebaceous duct without disturbing the basement membrane. The symbiosis between keratinocytes and melanocytes is disturbed in Bowen's disease, and melanocytes disappear gradually, just as they do in actinic keratoses. Plaques of the anogenital region, however, are often deeply pigmented and may be multiple.[27,28]

Similar changes are found in keratoses due to sunlight, x-rays or other ionizing radiation, and ar-

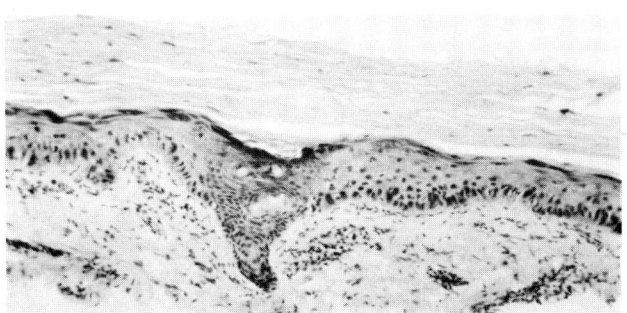

Figure 35–10.
Pigmented actinic keratosis. Melanocytes persist and form melanin in a keratosis of the back of the hand. Melanin is being carried into the horny layer. H&E. X125.

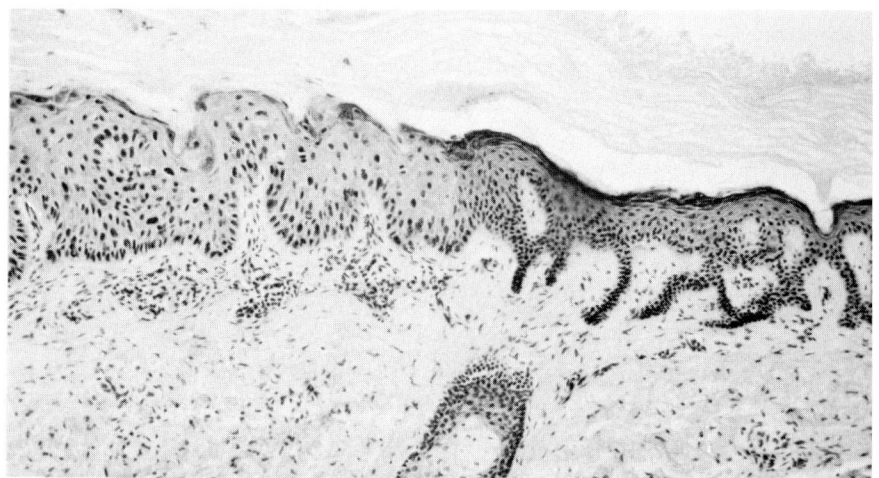

Figure 35-11.
A common association of actinic keratosis (left) and lentigo senilis (right) in chronic actinic exposed skin of forearm. H&E. X125.

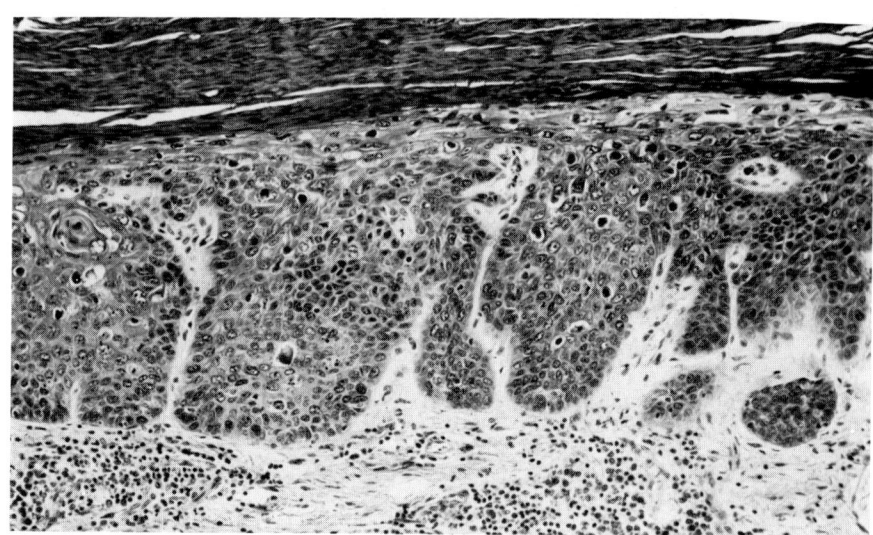

Figure 35-12.
Bowen's precancerous dermatosis. Acanthosis and dyskeratosis are shown in both figures. **A.** Parakeratosis and considerable inflammatory infiltrate. **B.** Horny layer is mainly orthokeratotic and includes some dyskeratotic cells. Inflammatory infiltrate is unusually mild. H&E. X135.

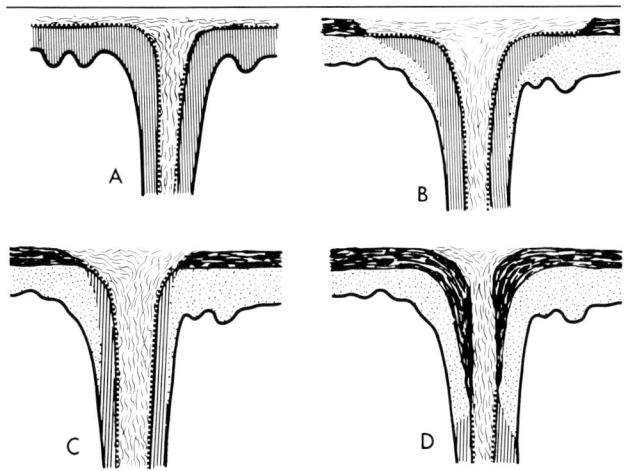

Figure 35-13.
Diagram illustrating shifting balance between adnexal and dysplastic epidermal keratinocytes in Bowen's disease and other precancerous conditions. **A.** In normal skin, epidermal and infundibular keratinocytes are indistinguishable and form orthokeratotic keratin through intermediate stage of a granular layer indicated by dots. **B.** Umbrella-like spread of orthokeratotic adnexal epithelium while parakeratotic epidermis forms a collar around the follicle. (Compare with Figs. 35-2 to 35-5.) **C.** Beginning repression of adnexal epithelium which just reaches skin surface corresponding to situation in Figure 35-5B on right. **D.** Follicular territory taken over by dysplastic epidermis. Adnexal epithelium is present deeper down. Basement membrane (heavy black line) remains intact. Careful examination of tissue sections shows this situation not infrequently in Bowen's disease. (From Pinkus. In McKenna (ed): Modern Trends in Dermatology, 1966. Courtesy of Butterworth & Co., Ltd.)

senic. These lesions are called "bowenoid." The term Bowen's disease may be restricted to the lesions located over the open skin surface. Carcinoma in situ is used for exactly similar changes occurring on mucous membranes, such as conjunctiva, on urethra, and in the nailbed and nail matrix.[29-31]

Epithelial cells of Bowen's disease characteristically have a nucleus that is large in relation to cytoplasm (Fig. 35-14). The number of individually keratinizing cells often is relatively small. In the clonal variety of Bowen's disease, relatively well-defined islands of anaplastic cells are present within a generally acanthotic epidermis (Fig. 35-15). The intraepidermal islands may be populated with small cells having hyperchromatic nuclei or large cells with abundant and light-staining cytoplasms resembling Paget's disease. In Bowen's disease the entire thickness of epidermis is dysplastic; in Paget's disease the epidermal keratinocytes between the Paget cells appear normal. In some lesions, the anaplastic epidermis is populated with small, dark-staining cells (basaloid type). This is commonly found on the semimucous membranes and merges into the full-blown histologic picture of erythroplasia of Queyrat (Fig. 35-16). The latter is usually accompanied by very heavy dermal infiltrates of lymphocytes and plasma cells.

Papillomavirus has been identified in Bowen's disease of extragenital location.[32] The relationship of Bowen's disease with internal malignancy has been ruled out in two recent clinical investigations.[33,34]

CUTANEOUS HORN

Cutaneous horn is a clinical diagnosis.[35,36] The pathologist is compelled to diagnose the underlying condition, which might be an epidermal nevus, ichthyosis hystrix, verruca vulgaris, inverted follicular keratosis, seborrheic verruca, or actinic keratosis. Other lesions may include keratoacanthoma, an open epidermoid cyst, an invasive squamous cell carcinoma (Fig. 35-17), or basal cell epithelioma.[37] Trichilemmal horn is made up of dense keratinous material, at the base of which the epithelium shows trichilemmal type of keratinization.[38] Some of these are open trichilemmal cysts.

XERODERMA PIGMENTOSUM

One precancerous condition is in a class by itself. It has been shown,[39] although there are exceptions, that all the cells of patients afflicted with xeroderma pigmentosum are unable to repair ultraviolet-induced DNA damage properly.[40] A proportion of the defective cells acquire the properties of neoplastic cells early in life and progress from precancer to manifest cancer, usually in the absence of underlying actinic elastosis. Squamous cell carcinomas, basal cell epitheliomas, malignant melanomas, and cutaneous sarcomas may arise. These lesions do not differ histologically from other tumors of their respective types, and no special discussion is needed. Xeroderma pigmentosum, however, is of tremendous biologic and pathogenetic interest because it proves the direct damaging influence of ultraviolet rays on the genetic material of those cells that later become

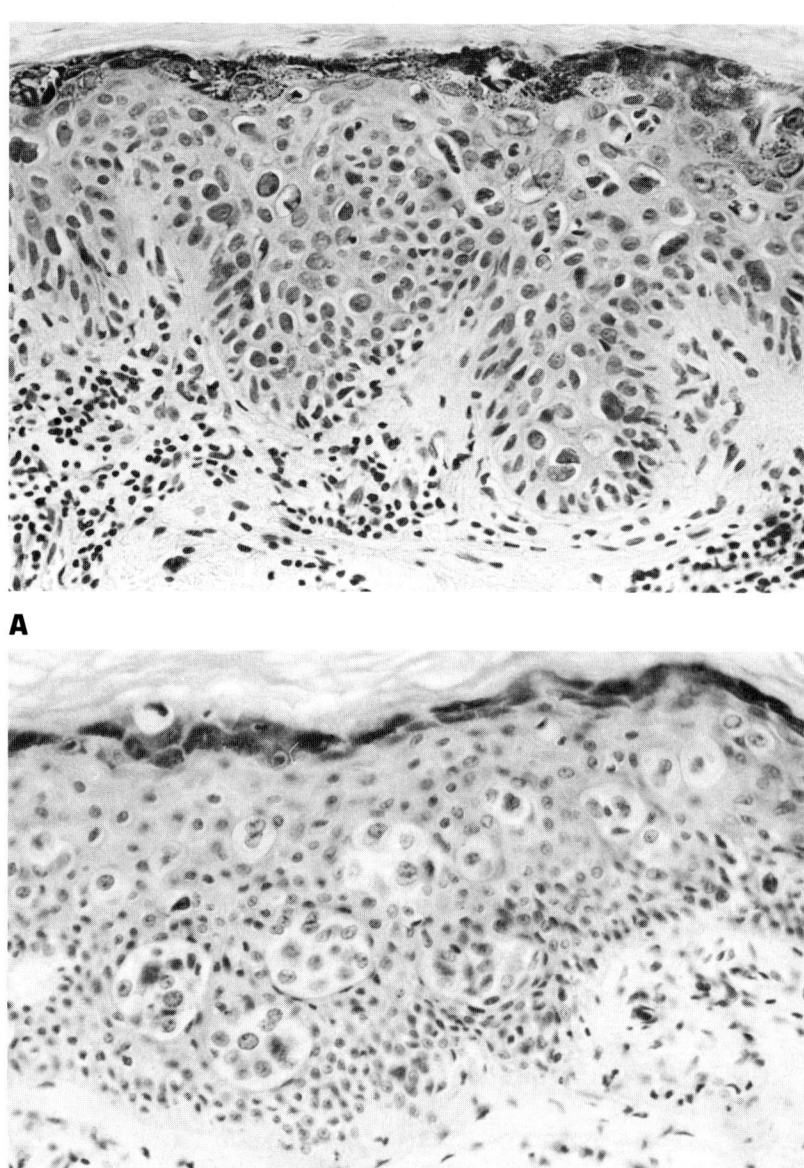

Figure 35–14.
Bowen's disease. **A.** Cell details, especially the relatively large size of many nuclei in relation to cytoplasm. H&E. X250. **B.** Borst phenomenon (Fig. 40–17) lateral to replacement of entire epidermis by dysplastic cells. Such pictures are found occasionally and indicate the mobility of the malignant cells. H&E. X250.

neoplastic. Similar mechanisms may act much more slowly in normal skin.

PROGRESSION FROM PRECANCEROSIS TO CANCER

If we accept the concept that any epidermal precancerous lesion is, in fact, carcinoma in situ, we can rephrase the heading and discuss histomechanisms by which an in situ lesion becomes invasive. Attention has been focused on the basement membrane by old authors and new. Redefinition of the basement membrane (Chapters 2 and 5) as that thin layer between mesoderm and epithelium that can be demonstrated by the PAS method has led to a fairly general agreement that the basement membrane disappears wherever squamous epithelium becomes invasive. This fact should not be interpreted to mean that the neoplastic epithelium has acquired the power to break through the confining barrier or that a hole in the barrier permits the cells to slip through. Basement membrane formation is an expression of ectodermal–mesodermal interaction.[41] Its disappearance indicates cessation of this intertissue coor-

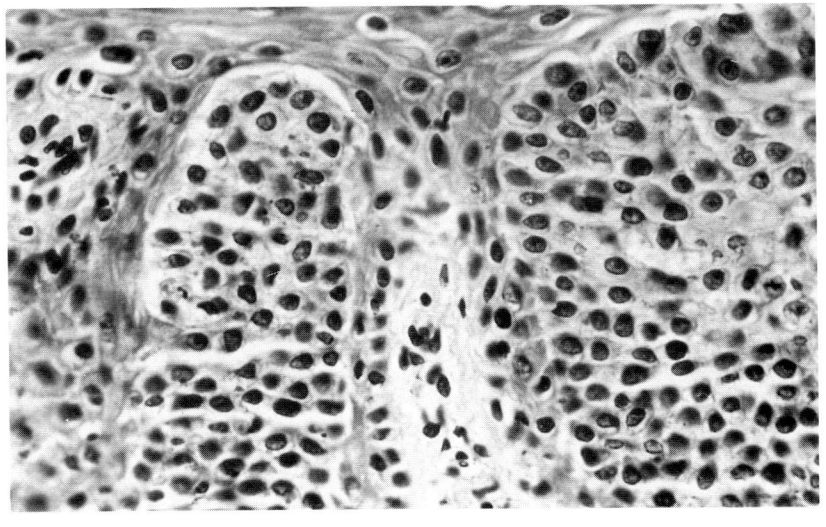

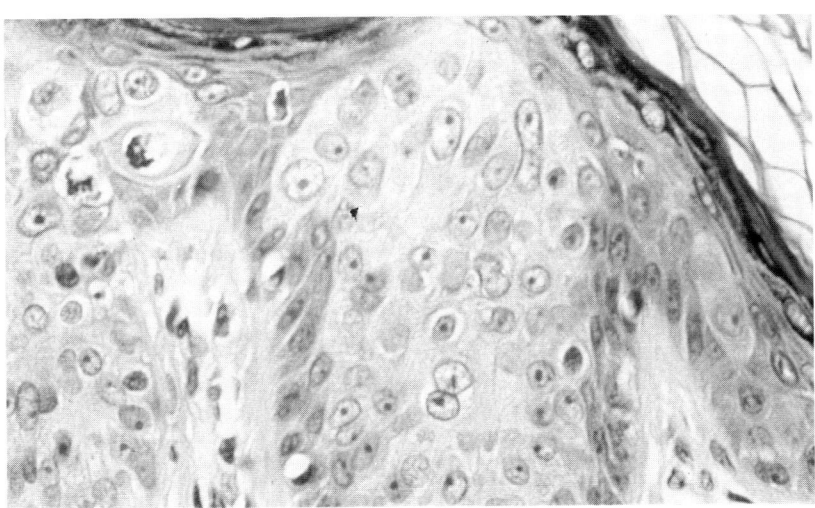

Figure 35–15.
Clonal Bowen's disease. **A.** Well-defined islands of small anaplastic cells with dark staining nuclei. H&E. X400. **B.** Islands of large cells with irregularly shaped nuclei and abundant light staining cytoplasms. H&E. X400.

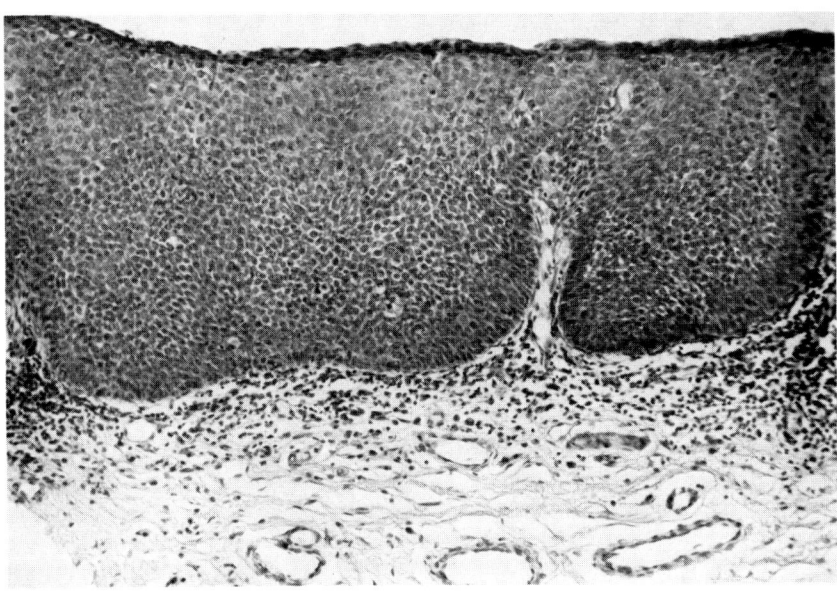

Figure 35–16.
Erythroplasia of Queyrat. Thick epidermis consists almost entirely of nonkeratinizing basaloid cells (épithéliome nu) with only slight indication of dysplasia. Relatively mild inflammatory infiltrate. H&E. X135.

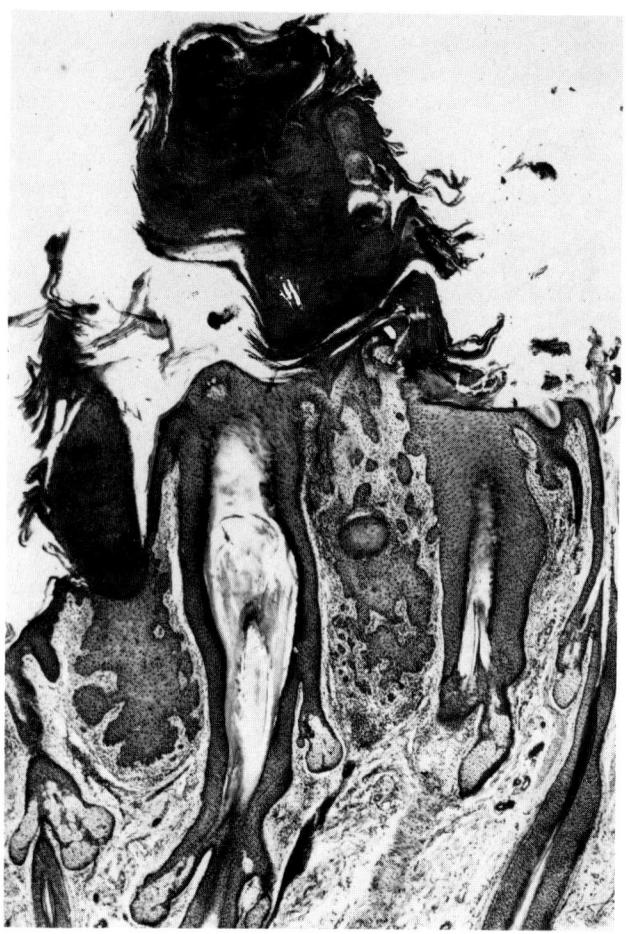

Figure 35–17.
Early squamous cell carcinoma arising in actinic keratosis. Atypical interfollicular budding (Figs. 35–3B and 35–5A) has been replaced by frank invasion of dermis down to level of sebaceous glands. Massive parakeratotic material forms a small cutaneous horn. H&E. X35.

dination and, therefore, is a secondary, although highly valuable, diagnostic feature.

Actinic and other keratoses, including Bowen's disease, can become invasive by three different routes. The most direct and obvious one is increased budding of the neoplastic epithelium into the dermis between the adnexa (Fig. 35–17). A second route is the creeping of epithelium on the outer surface of hair follicles and sweat ducts within the basement membrane. The third one is repression of adnexal epithelium (Fig. 35–13) and occupation of follicular territory (Fig. 35–18), as discussed for Bowen's disease. In all cases, the basement membrane eventually disappears, and the epithelium becomes truly invasive and destructive. It is important to realize that recurrences of keratoses after relatively superficial excision or destruction may have their origin in epithelia that have reached middermis by the last two routes without actually having invaded the corium. It is wise to point this out to the clinician in appropriate cases.

SQUAMOUS CELL CARCINOMA

The diagnosis of squamous cell carcinoma is generally accepted and understood in the United States. Other synonymous terms are "epidermoid carcinoma," "prickle cell cancer," "spinous cell carcinoma," or "spinalioma," the latter being common usage in German. Darier's designation *épithélioma pavimenteux typique* has been replaced by "carcinoma (or épithélioma) spinocellulaire" in French.

Although cutaneous squamous cell carcinoma (Fig. 35–19) most commonly arises in the epidermis, it may arise in adnexal epithelium and in keratinous cysts, most of which are of adnexal origin. Derivation, therefore, is not important for diagnosis. All true carcinomas of the skin are squamous cell carcinomas, with the exception of rare adenocarcinomas of sebaceous and sudoriparous nature. Basal cell carcinomas belong to a different class of tumors. They are members of the tribe of organoid adnexoid tumors and, therefore, are designated as "basal cell epitheliomas." The tumor cell of squamous cell carcinoma is a heritably deranged keratinocyte which has escaped from the regulatory influences of the organism to the extent that it grows invasively and destructively into the mesoderm and may demonstrate its relative autonomy by metastasis, although this event occurs relatively late and is encountered but rarely in modern practice. The squamous cancer cell preserves its ability for maturation in the form of keratinization to a greater or lesser degree and may lose it completely. *Histologic grading* of squamous cell carcinoma was put on this basis by Broders,[42] who devised four classes: grade I, tumors in which more than 75 percent of cells are maturing (differentiating); grade II, 75 to 50 percent differentiating cells; grade III, 50 to 25 percent differentiating cells; and grade IV, fewer than 25 percent differentiating cells. Although this system has many practical and theoretic flaws, it remains a simple means of descriptively expressing degree of maturation. Many pathologists prefer to say well-differentiated, poorly differentiated, and undifferentiated. Histologic grading of squamous cell carcinoma can be further advanced by measurement of tumor thickness, depth of dermal invasion, degree of cellular

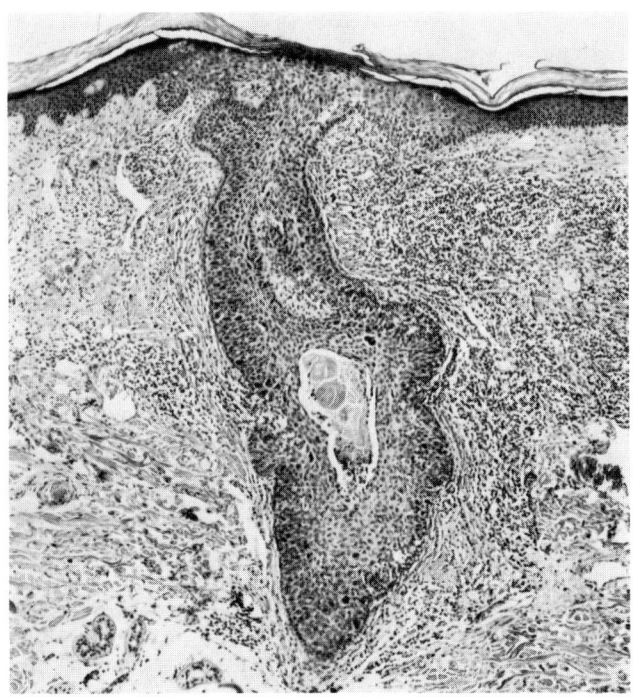

Figure 35–18.
Extensive invasion of a hair follicle by dysplastic epidermis of Bowen's disease. Patient had been treated locally with 5-fluorouracil, and lesion appeared clinically cured. Drug did not destroy cells hidden in follicle, and surviving dyskeratotic epithelium is now secondarily spreading on surface. Clinical history is essential to explain paradoxical picture. H&E. X60.

atypia, and number of mitotic figures per high power field.[43]

The derangement of the epidermoid cancer cell changes its morphology so that no normal basal cells are present (Fig. 35–20). Even the outermost cells of a cancer nest are relatively large and pale-staining elements in most instances and exhibit little tendency to palisading. They are closely applied to the surrounding connective tissue, and the retraction spaces that we shall encounter in basal cell epithelioma are absent. Yet PAS stain reveals the absence of a basement membrane in most instances. Nuclei have large nucleoli. Mitotic figures, sometimes atypical, may be found in all layers of a nodule.[44] Toward the center of larger nests, the cells may undergo fairly normal keratinization with formation of keratohyalin, but, more commonly, they form parakeratotic material.[45] Thus, irregular horn pearls are produced that must be separated from the squamous eddies and horny pearls seen in activated seborrheic verruca (Chapter 34). Individual cell keratinization may occur. If it predominates, the lesion assumes a bowenoid character.

Acantholytic Squamous Cell Carcinoma

Pronounced acantholytic tendency may lead to the formation of irregular cavities lined with atypical cells and filled with dyskeratotic or plainly degen-

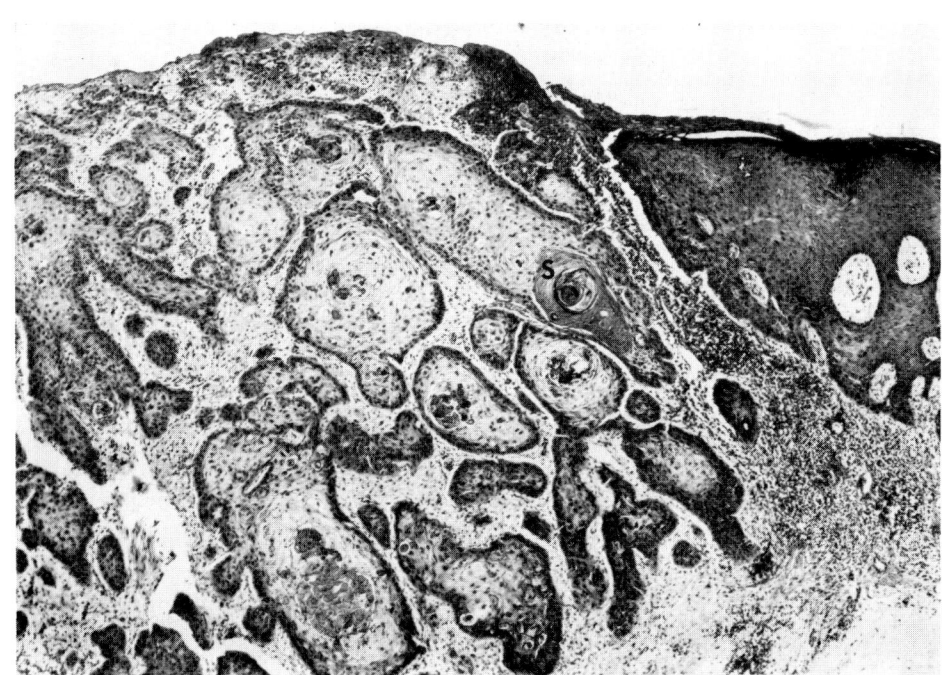

Figure 35–19.
Invasive squamous cell carcinoma, keratinizing. Tumor would be Broders' grade II. Hyperplastic obstructed sweat duct(s) is enveloped by malignant epithelium. H&E. X70.

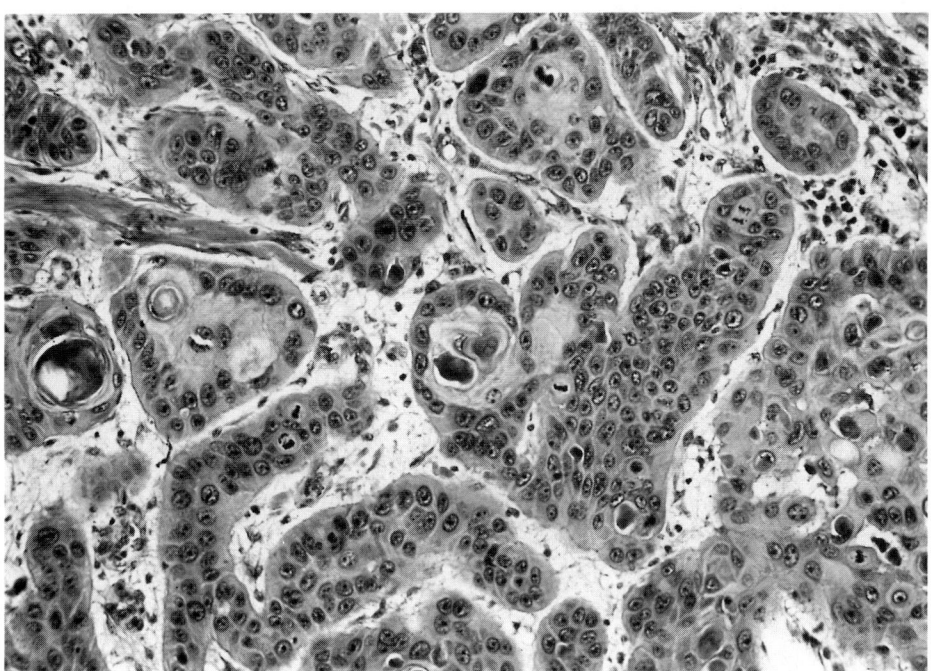

Figure 35–20.
Squamous cell carcinoma, well differentiated. H&E. X225.

erating elements.[46] One part or the entire invasive tumor masses may be involved. Such cancers often are derived from Darier-like actinic keratosis and have been called "adenoacanthomas,"[47] a term that should be abandoned since there is no evidence of true glandular differentiation. Acantholytic squamous cell carcinoma (Fig. 35–21) appears to be the most straightforward and unmistakable designation, but adenoid or pseudoglandular carcinoma and carcinoma segregans also have been used.

Immature Tumors

Even squamous cell carcinomas that have lost all ability to keratinize (Fig. 35–22) do not resemble basal cell epitheliomas. Invasive lesions developing in preexisting Bowen's disease may consist predominantly of atypical basaloid cells with foci of squamous metaplasia, follicular or sebaceous differentiation.[48] If one encounters a completely immature tumor, however, the differential diagnosis between squamous cell carcinoma, adenocarcinoma, and amelanotic melanoma must be weighed carefully. In some cases, it may be impossible without resorting to special histochemical or immunostaining techniques.[49] Silver and dopa reaction and immunostaining for S-100 protein or HMB-45 can be used to identify amelanotic malignant melanomas. Stains for acid mucopolysaccharide and lipids and immunostaining for CEA may be applied for recognition of adenocarcinomas.

Small-Cell Squamous Carcinomas

There are a few actinic keratoses of the keratosis senilis type in which the dysplastic cells are small and basaloid and may give rise to small-celled carcinomas simulating basal cell epithelioma in their early stages. Lack of fibrous stroma, the absence of retraction spaces and PAS-positive basement membrane identifies these lesions as squamous cell cancers.

Spindle Cell Squamous Carcinomas

Spindle cell squamous carcinomas were first described as recurrent tumors after x-ray treatment.[50] It is also observed in severely actinic exposed facial skin in association with actinic keratosis. Histologically, bundles of large spindle-shaped cells extend from the lower surface of the epidermis down, exhibiting hyperchromatic nuclei, multinucleated giant cells, and mitotic figures (Fig. 35–23).[51] There is no tendency for keratinization and no dyskeratotic cells. Differential diagnosis from atypical fibroxanthoma, malignant fibrous histiocytoma, and desmoplastic malignant melanoma may require special studies. Fresh tissue or formalin-fixed material may

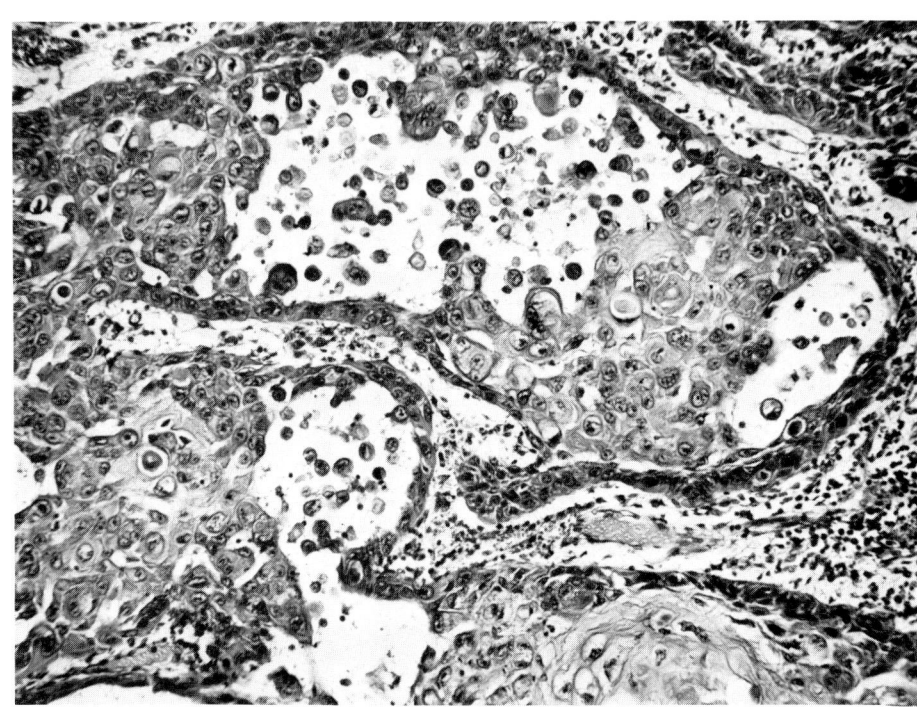

Figure 35–21.
Acantholytic squamous cell carcinoma. Often arises in Darier-like actinic keratosis (Fig. 35–8). H&E. X135.

be suitable for immunostaining for keratin, S-100 protein, and other tissue markers;[52] electron microscopy for demonstration of tonofilament and desmosomes between the tumor cells.

Verrucous Carcinoma of Skin

Under the picturesque name of *epithelioma cuniculatum*,[53] deeply invasive and destructive forms of squamous carcinoma were described, which penetrate the foot from the volar surface and resemble a rabbit warren on cross section.[54,55] These tumors (Fig. 35–24) show slow progressing biologic behavior similar to the verrucous carcinoma of the oral mucosa (Chapter 46) and the destructive lesions of giant condyloma acuminatum. These three varieties of carcinoma do not show much cellular atypicality or tendency to squamous pearl formation. The tumor

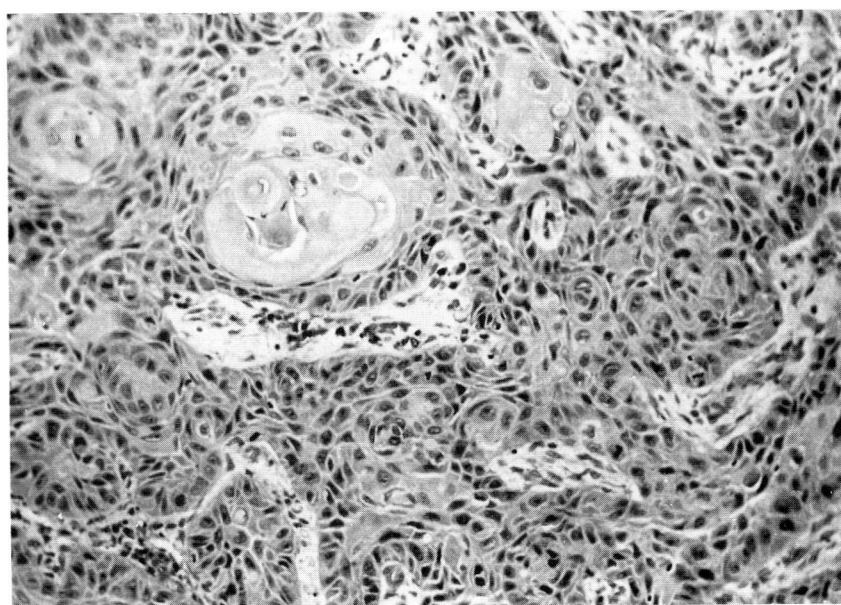

Figure 35–22.
Squamous cell carcinoma exhibiting only a few individually keratinizing cells. Note absence of retraction spaces. H&E. X225

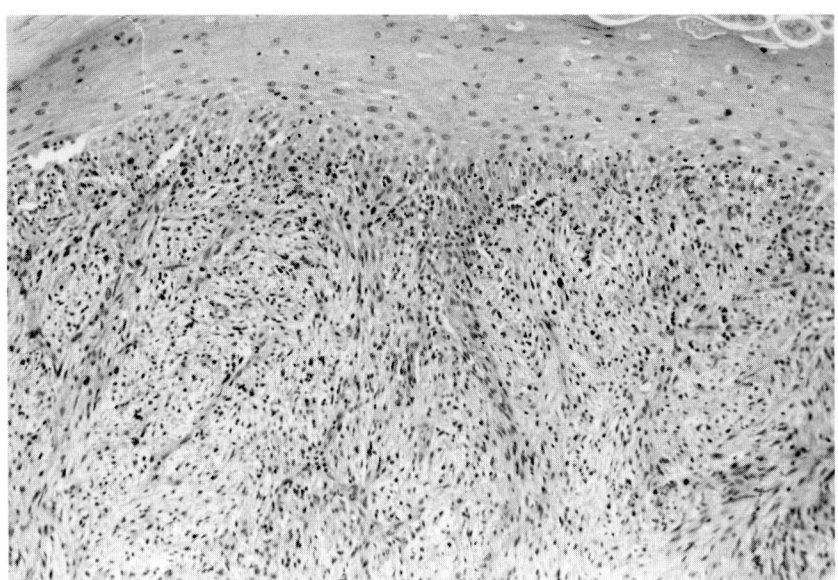

Figure 35—23.
Spindle cell squamous carcinoma. Bundles of anaplastic spindle-shaped cells extend down from the lower surface of the epidermis. H&E. X125.

masses are well differentiated. Their frontal edge advances in a pushing manner, destroying tissue without obvious invasion by individual sprouts and heavy chronic inflammatory cell reaction. Sufficiently large and deep biopsies are needed for diagnosis.

Squamous cell carcinoma of the ectodermal mucous membranes and its precursor lesions have special features and require special differential considerations. They will be discussed in Chapter 46.

PSEUDOCARCINOMA

Under this heading are discussed two separate phenomena: one usually referred to as *pseudoepitheliomatous proliferation* associated with various inflammatory processes, the other known as *keratoacanthoma* or self-healing squamous cell carcinoma.

Pseudoepitheliomatous Proliferation

In ordinary acanthosis and in papillomatosis, the rete ridges and papillae increase in length and bulk and lift the suprapapillary epidermis above the level of the surrounding skin. Although often described in the literature, there is no downgrowth of rete ridges in any of these conditions.[56] The true baseline of the papillae–epidermis unit remains undisturbed, as can be shown simply by staining for elastic fibers (Chapter 2). In some inflammatory diseases, however, usually in the group of granulomatous inflammation, rarely in severe lichen simplex chronicus and hypertropic lichen planus, the nonneoplastic epidermis indeed grows down into the pars reticularis. One cannot always be sure, however, how much of the stratified epithelium found deep in the skin may take its origin from hair roots and eccrine glands.[57] The general configuration of the invasive formations may be indistinguishable from true carcinoma, but pronounced cellular atypy is absent, and nuclei usually are normochromatic and relatively small in relation to cytoplasm. Nucleoli may be as large as in carcinoma, and a basement membrane between epithelium and mesoderm commonly is absent. Central keratinization may occur. It often contains an admixture of inflammatory cells in which infective microorganisms may be found. In most cases, the underlying inflammatory process is sufficiently evident to permit diagnosis, but awareness and careful examination may be needed to avoid mistakes. We shall see that at least one mesodermal tumor, granular cell myoblastoma, also provokes pseudoepitheliomatous epidermal proliferation.

In contrast to neoplastic epithelium, the epidermis returns to normal when the primary condition heals. While this knowledge does not help in the examination of specific specimens, it is one of the best arguments against any concept that development of carcinoma depends only on the opportunity for normal cells to break through the basement membrane.

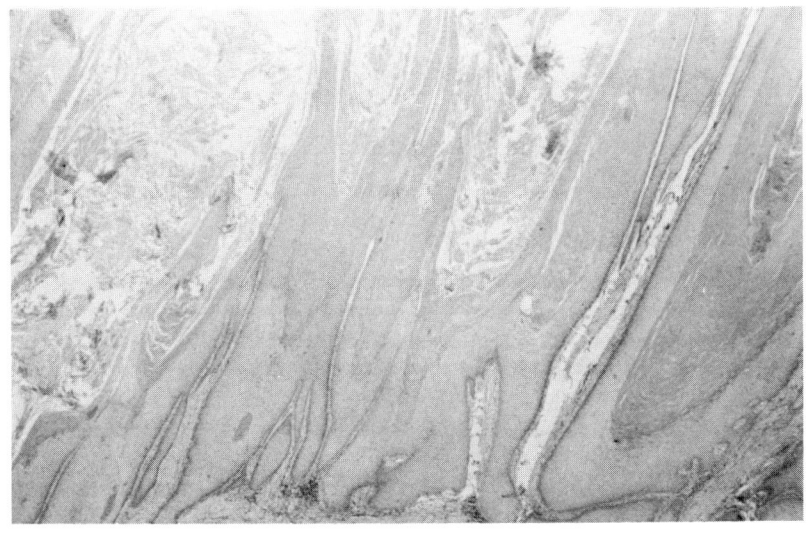

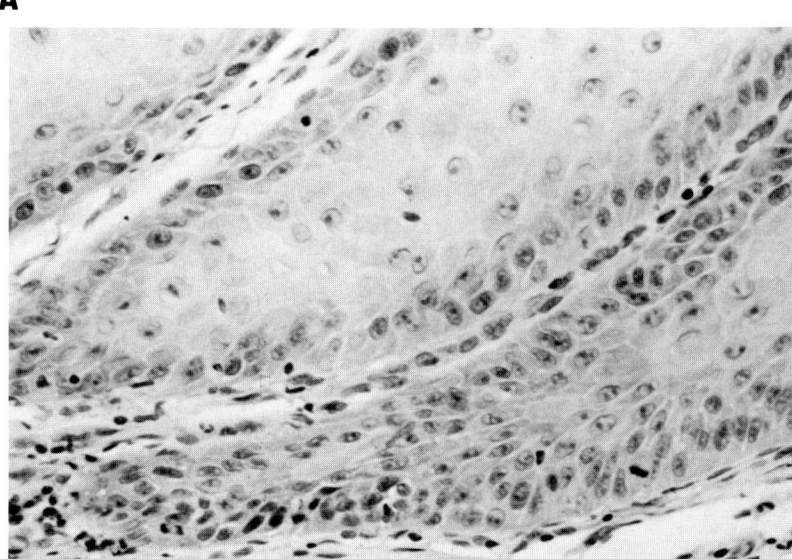

Figure 35-24.
Verrucous carcinoma of skin. **A.** demonstrates the deceptively benign aspect at low power. H&E. X10. **B.** shows absence of a well-formed basal layer and slight atypicality of cells. Mitoses and large nucleoli. H&E. X250.

Papillomatosis Cutis Carcinoides

A special case is Gottron's papillomatosis cutis carcinoides.[58] These broad plaques located on the lower extremities have a clinical resemblance to so-called pyoderma vegetans but are in no way related to verrucous carcinoma of the sole of the foot. Histologically, they show great acanthosis and papillomatosis, often extending downward into the dermis, but the cells are relatively normal prickle cells and keratinize normally in association with a vascular connective tissue stroma.

Keratoacanthoma

The concept of *self-healing squamous cell carcinoma* is only a few decades old and, like the concept of benign juvenile melanoma, was developed on a catamnestic clinical basis. Pathologists then were forced to refine their histologic criteria and, in many cases, to change their diagnoses on specimens previously diagnosed as cancer.

We describe a keratoacanthoma (Fig. 35-25) as a heavily keratinized squamous cell lesion that is definitely destructive and invasive but stops

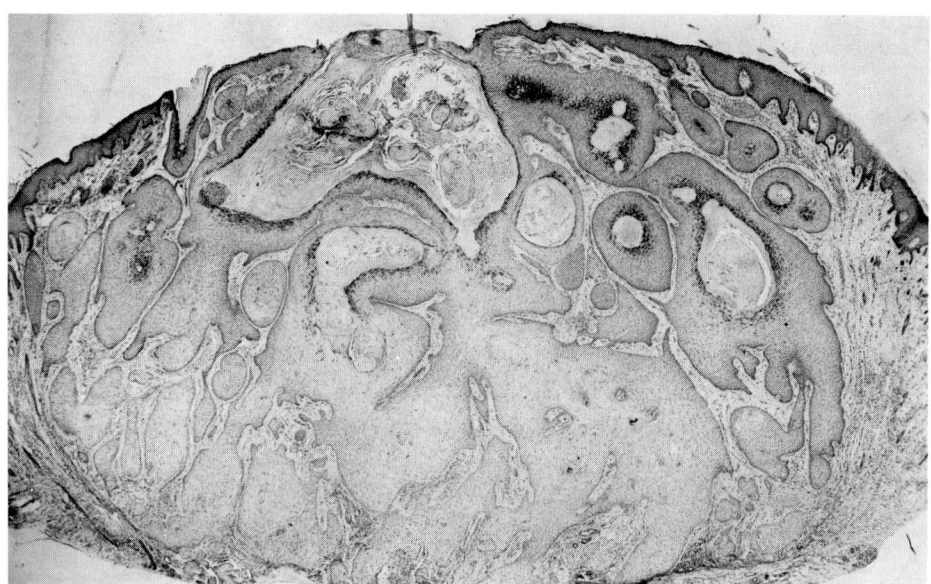

Figure 35–25.
Keratoacanthoma. Note pale-staining nuclei and cytoplasm of invasive epithelium. H&E. X14.

growing spontaneously and subsides, leaving a scar.[59] It spreads laterally below the epidermis, leading to a picture of buttress formation on cross section with a horn-filled, very irregular crater in the center. Histologic criteria include the presence of mitoses only in the outermost layer, growth not deeper than the sweat coils, relatively normal nuclear–cytoplasmic ratio, absence of dyskeratosis, and mainly orthokeratotic maturation of central cells. None of these rules is without exception, however, and invasion of blood vessels and neural sheaths in the subcutaneous tissue may occur.[60,61] The characteristic buttress formation by the surrounding epidermis may also be seen in some slow-growing, well-differentiated squamous cell carcinomas without a tendency to spontaneous involution. Tangential sectioning and convolution of the advancing margin may cause difficulties in exactly locating mitoses. A rarely mentioned but striking and helpful feature in O&G sections (Fig. 35–26) is survival of elastic fiber remnants in the epithelial masses.[62] Collagen fibers may also be demonstrated by specific stains.[63] Although histologic diagnosis usually is possible on an adequate biopsy specimen, which must include the edge and the lower pole of the tumor, there remain cases in which the final decision has to be based on clinicopathologic correlation: a rapidly growing tumor exhibiting histologic features of a well-differentiated squamous cell carcinoma is a keratoacanthoma, while a very slowly growing lesion with similar histology but no self-healing tendency during a year or more is a carcinoma.

Cytologic criteria are important. Most keratoacanthomas do not exhibit cytologic abnormalities, and a highly dysplastic epithelium is not compatible with the diagnosis even if the pattern of the entire tumor is classic. This differentiation is, of course, impossible to prove because total excision of the lesion will lead to cure whether it was a keratoacanthoma or an early squamous cell carcinoma. It is, however, of value to advise the clinician not to neglect a dysplastic tumor because it has the configuration of keratoacanthoma.

We recognize that the histologic differentiation of a well keratinizing squamous cell carcinoma and keratoacanthoma is not always satisfactory and therefore suggest that the lesion is best treated by complete surgical excision.[64]

Two distinctive forms of multiple keratoacanthomas are recognized.[65] The *Ferguson–Smith* type occurs in childhood and adolescence among members of families.[66] Circular lesions with elevated border and crateriform center appear within a 6- to 8-week period and eventually regresses leaving atrophic scars. The *Grzybowski* type appears later in life. Numerous pinhead to bean-size keratotic lesions evolve within 4 to 8 months and gradually disappear leaving many pitted scars.[67,68] The histopathology of the eruptive form may involve a single hair follicle with pseudoepitheliomatous proliferation of the follicular epithelium and may resemble a chronic folliculitis.

Diagnosis of keratoacanthoma is more difficult when the nail bed is involved.[69,70] Subungual keratoacanthoma shows clinically acute manifestations

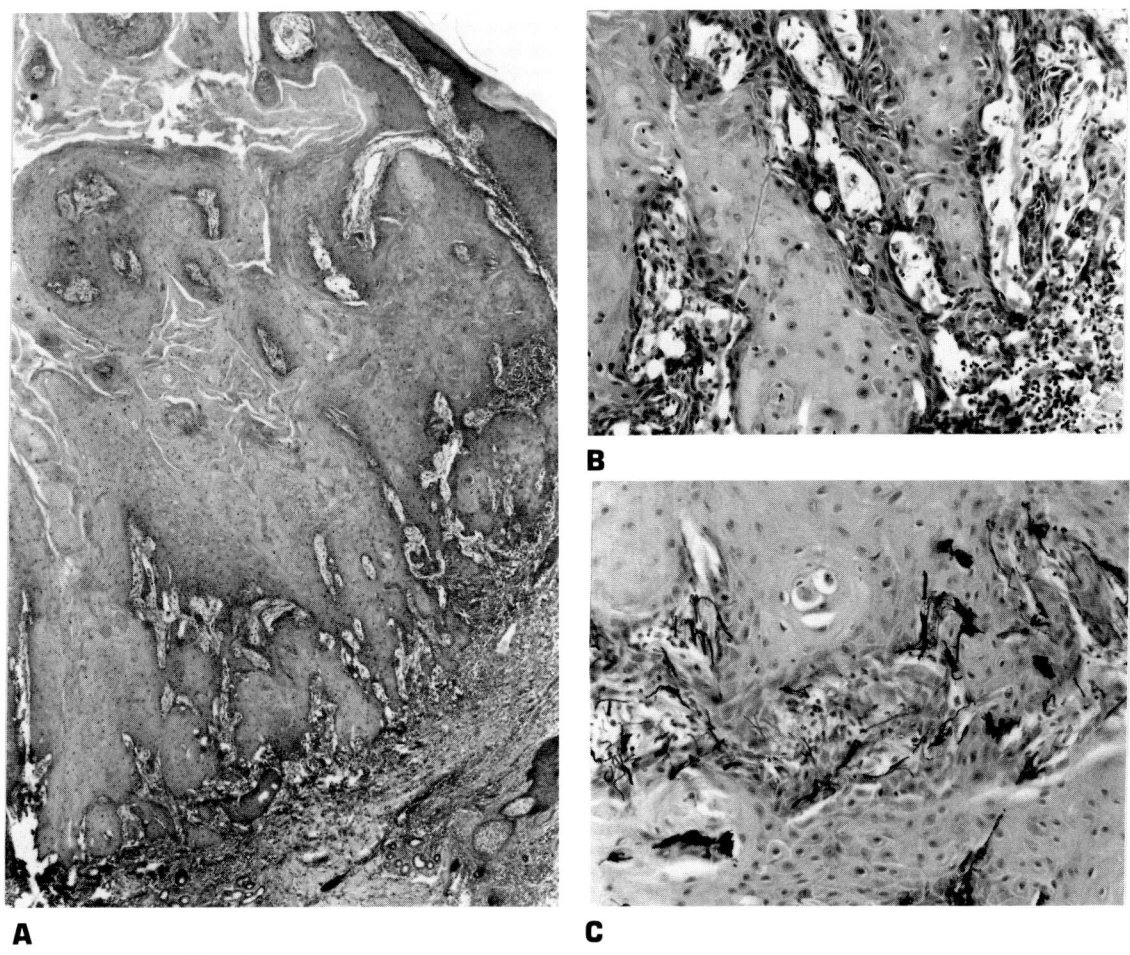

Figure 35–26.
Keratoacanthoma. **A.** Massive proliferation of highly keratinizing squamous epithelium with peripheral marginal buttress formation. H&E. X45. **B.** Well-differentiated tumor epithelium. H&E. X400. **C.** Well-differentiated tumor masses incorporating fragments of elastic fibers. O&G. X400.

with pain and swelling, suggesting an infection. X-ray film will show an underlying bone erosion. Histologically, large masses of well-keratinized epithelium with numerous dyskeratotic cells extend into the subcutaneous tissues.

REFERENCES

1. Brownstein MH: The benign acanthomas. J Cutan Pathol 12:172, 1985
2. Marks R, Rennie G, Selwood TS: Malignant transformation of solar keratoses to squamous cell carcinoma. Lancet 1:795, 1988
3. Marks R, Rennie G, Selwood T: The relationship of basal cell carcinomas and squamous cell carcinomas to solar keratoses. Arch Dermatol 124:1039, 1988
4. Mehregan AH: Actinic keratosis and actinic squamous cell carcinoma. A comparative study of 800 cases observed in 1968 and 1988. J Cutan Aging Cosmet Dermatol 1:47, 1988
5. Pinkus H: Keratosis senilis. Am J Clin Pathol 29:193, 1958
6. Hashimoto K, Mehregan AH: Tumors of the Epidermis. Boston: Butterworths, 1990
7. Balin AR, Lin AN, Pratt L: Actinic keratoses. J Cutan Aging Cosmet Dermatol 1:77, 1988
8. Bhawan J: Histology of epidermal dysplasia. J Cutan Aging Cosmet Dermatol 1:95, 1988
9. Kimura S: Ultrastructure of senile keratosis. J Dermatol Tokyo 7:255, 1980
10. Johnson TM, Rapini RP, Duvic M: Inflammation of actinic keratoses from systemic chemotherapy. J Am Acad Dermatol 17:192, 1987
11. Marks R, Foley P, Goodman G, et al: Spontaneous

remission of solar keratoses: The case for conservative management. Br J Dermatol 115:649, 1986
12. Pinkus H, Jallad MS, Mehregan AH: The inflammatory infiltrate of precancerous skin lesions. J Invest Dermatol 41:247, 1963
13. Avgerinou G, Nicolis G, Vareltzidis A, Stratigos J: The dermal cellular infiltrate and cell-mediated immunity in skin carcinomas. Dermatologica 171:238, 1985
14. Guillen FJ, Day CL Jr., Murphy GF: Expression of activation antigens by T cells infiltrating basal cell carcinomas. J Invest Dermatol 85:203, 1985
15. Carapeto FJ, García-Perez A: Acantholytic keratosis. Dermatologica 148:233, 1974
16. James MP, Wells GC, Whimster IW: Spreading pigmented actinic keratoses. Br J Dermatol 98:373, 1978
17. Subrt P, Jorizzo JL, Apisarnthanarax P, et al: Spreading pigmented actinic keratosis. J Am Acad Dermatol 8:63, 1983
18. Dinehart SM, Sanchez RL: Spreading pigmented actinic keratosis. An electron microscopic study. Arch Dermatol 124:680, 1988
19. Epstein JH: Photocarcinogenesis, skin cancer, and aging. J Am Acad Dermatol 9:487, 1983
20. Cox AJ, Abel EA: Epidermal dystrophy. Occurrence after psoriasis therapy with psoralen and long-wave ultraviolet light. Arch Dermatol 115:567, 1979
21. Abel EA, Cox AJ, Farber EM: Epidermal dystrophy and actinic keratoses in psoriasis patients following oral psoralen photochemotherapy (PUVA): Follow-up study. J Am Acad Dermatol 7:333, 1982
22. Niemi KM, Niemi A, Kanerva L: Morphologic changes in epidermis of PUVA-treated patients with psoriasis with or without a history of arsenic therapy. Arch Dermatol 119:904, 1983
23. Miller RA: Psoralens and UV-A induced stellate hyperpigmentation freckling. Arch Dermatol 118:619, 1982
24. Lorette G, Jafar R, Grojean M-F, et al: Xeroderma pigmentosum-like changes. Arch Dermatol 119:873, 1983
25. Berger TG, Graham JH, Goette DK: Lichenoid benign keratosis. J Am Acad Dermatol 11:635, 1984
26. Degos R, Civatte J, Belaïch S, et al: Maladie de Bowen cutanée ou muceuse. A propos de 243 cas. Ann Dermatol Syphiligr 103:5, 1976
27. Lloyd KM: Multicentric pigmented Bowen's disease of the groin. Arch Dermatol 101:48, 1970
28. King CM, Yates VM, Dave VK: Multicentric pigmented Bowen's disease of the genitalia associated with carcinoma in situ of the cervix. Br J Venereol Dis 60:406, 1984
29. Coskey RJ, Mehregan AH, Fosnaugh R: Bowen's disease of the nail bed. Arch Dermatol 106:79, 1972
30. Dieteman DF: Bowen's disease of the nail bed. Arch Dermatol 108:577, 1973
31. Baran RL, Gormley DE: Polydactylous Bowen's disease of the nail. J Am Acad Dermatol 17:201, 1987
32. Stone MS, Noonan CA, Techen J, Bruce S: Bowen's disease of the feet. Presence of human papilloma virus 16 DNA in tumor tissue. Arch Dermatol 123:1517, 1987
33. Chuang TY, Reizner GT: Bowen's disease and internal malignancy. A matched case-control study. J Am Acad Dermatol 19:47, 1988
34. Reymann F, Ravnborg L, Schou G, et al: Bowen's disease and internal malignant diseases. A study of 581 patients. Arch Dermatol 124:677, 1988
35. Mehregan AH: Cutaneous horn: A clinicopathologic study. Dermatol Digest 4:45, 1965
36. Bart RS, Andrade R, Kopf AW: Cutaneous horn: A clinical and histopathologic study. Acta Derm Venereol 48:507, 1968
37. Sandbank M: Basal cell carcinoma at the base of cutaneous horn. Arch Dermatol 104:97, 1971
38. Kimura S, Trichilemmal keratosis (horn): A light and electron microscopic study. J Cutan Pathol 10:59, 1983
39. Reed WB, Landing B, Sugarman G, et al: Xeroderma pigmentosum: Clinical and laboratory investigation of its basic defect. JAMA 207:2073, 1969
40. Cleaver JE: Xeroderma pigmentosum: Genetic and environmental influences in skin carcinogenesis. Int J Dermatol 17:435, 1978
41. Gay S, Kresina TF, Gay R, et al: Immunohistochemical demonstration of basement membrane collagen in normal human skin and in psoriasis. J Cutan Pathol 6:91, 1979
42. Broders AC: Practical points on the microscopic grading of carcinoma. NY State J Med 32:667, 1932
43. Immerman SC, Scanlon EF, Christ M, Knox KL: Recurrent squamous cell carcinoma of the skin. Cancer 51:1537, 1983
44. McGibbon DH: Malignant epidermal tumors. J Cutan Pathol 12:224, 1985
45. Pinkus H, Mehregan AH: Premalignant skin lesions. Clin Plastic Surg 7: 289, 1980
46. Nappi O, Pettinato G, Wick MR: Adenoid (acantholytic) squamous cell carcinoma of the skin. J Cutan Pathol 16:114, 1989
47. Carapeto FJ, García-Perez A: Adenoacanthoma: A review of twenty cases, compared with the literature. Dermatologica 145:269, 1972
48. Kao GF: Carcinoma arising in Bowen's disease. Arch Dermatol 122:1124, 1986
49. Hashimoto K, Eto H, et al: Anti-keratin monoclonal antibodies: Production, specificities and applications. J Cutan Pathol 10:529, 1983
50. Martin HE, Stewart FW: Spindle cell epidermoid carcinoma. Am J Cancer 24:273, 1935
51. Evans HL, Smith LJ: Spindle cell squamous carcinoma and sarcoma-like tumors of the skin. Cancer 45:2687, 1980
52. Penneys NS, Nadji M, et al: Prekeratin in spindle cell tumors of the skin. Arch Dermatol 119:476, 1983
53. Wilkinson JD, Black MM: Carcinoma cuniculatum: A clinicopathologic study of 21 cases. Arch Dermatol 116:1390, 1980

54. Kao GF, Graham JH, Helwig EB: Carcinoma cuniculatum (verrucous carcinoma of the skin): A clinicopathologic study of 46 cases with ultrastructural observations. Cancer 49:2395, 1982
55. Horn L, Sage R: Verrucous squamous cell carcinoma of the foot: A report of five cases. J Am Podiatr Med Assoc 78:227, 1988
56. Civatte J: Pseudo-carcinomatous hyperplasia. J Cutan Pathol 12:214, 1985
57. Grunwald MH, Lee JY, Ackerman AB: Pseudocarcinomatous hyperplasia. Am J Dermatopathol 10:95, 1988
58. Nikolowski W: Papillomatosis cutis carcinoides, in Braun-Falco O, Petzold D (eds): Fortschritte der praktischen Dermatologie und Venerologie, vol 7. Berlin: Springer-Verlag, 1973, p 36
59. Kingman J, Callen JP: Keratoacanthoma. A clinical study. Arch Dermatol 120:736, 1984
60. Poiares Baptista A, Born M: L'invasion perinerveuse dans le kerato-acanthome. Ann Dermatol Venereol 109:27, 1982
61. Cooper PH, Wolfe JT III: Perioral keratoacanthomas with extensive perineural invasion and intravenous growth. Arch Dermatol 124:1397, 1988
62. Bowers D, Bhawan J, Tsay A: Transepithelial elimination of elastic fibers in keratoacanthoma: An ultrastructural study. J Invst Dermatol 92:407, 1989
63. Bakker PS, Tjon A, Joe SS: Inclusion of elastic and collagen fibers in keratoacanthoma. Ned Tijdschr Geneeskd 112:1358, 1968; 113:371, 1969
64. Piscioli F, Boi S, Zumiani G, Cristofolini M: A gigantic metastasizing keratoacanthoma. Report of a case and discussion on classification. Am J Dermatopathol 6:123, 1984
65. Reid BJ, Cheesbrough MJ: Multiple keratoacanthoma: A unique case and review of the current classification. Acta Derm Venereol 58:169, 1978
66. Belaich S, Escande J-P, Crickx B, et al: Epitheliomatose spontanement curable de Ferguson-Smith. Ann Dermatol Venereol 112:697, 1985
67. Balus I, Fazio M, Carducci M, et al: Une variete rare de kerato-acanthome multiple: Le kerato-acanthome eruptif. Ann Dermatol Venereol 108:995, 1981
68. Lloyd KM, Madsen DK, Lin PY: Grzybowski's eruptive keratoacanthoma. J Am Acad Dermatol 21:1023, 1989
69. Keeney GL, Banks PM, Linscheid RL: Subungual keratoacanthoma. Report of a case and review of the literature. Arch Dermatol 124:1074, 1988
70. Gonzalez-Ensenat A, Vilalta A, Torras H: Keratoacanthome peri et sous-ungueal. Ann Dermatol Venereol 115:329, 1988

36

NEVUS SEBACEOUS AND SEBACEOUS TUMORS

The spectrum of adnexoid neoplasia discussed in the introduction to Section VII (Table VII–1) is most clearly seen in tumors related to sebaceous glands. We use the cautious expression "related" because the possibility exists that tumors of sebaceous structure may arise in nonsebaceous adnexal matrix, although most sebaceous tumors probably have their origin in sebaceous glands.

ORGANOID NEVUS (NEVUS SEBACEUS OF JADASSOHN)

It is not uncommon to find two or more of the adnexa participating in nevus formation, and these lesions often also involve the epidermis and the supporting connective tissue. Such nevi are best diagnosed as organoid nevi (Fig. 36–1), since they involve the entire skin organ. To focus diagnosis on only that structure which happens to be most prominent in the individual lesion leads to confusion, while realization of the true, complicated nature of such organoid nevi (Fig. 36–2) creates a unified concept and leads to proper prognostic and therapeutic conclusions.

Organoid nevi are most commonly located on the scalp, but may be found on the face, neck, and trunk in descending frequency. They have a definite life history in three stages.[1] Usually present at birth and in their most common location on the scalp, they manifest as hairless areas with yellow to orange surface discoloration. In this juvenile stage, the epidermis may be somewhat acanthotic. The pilosebaceous structures are small and incompletely formed (Fig. 36–3). Only a very small minority show apocrine glands. The second stage, during the adolescence, is characterized by a definite increase in the thickness of the lesion, which may show yellow surface nodularity or verrucous hyperkeratosis. The area remains hairless. Histologic findings now may be diagnosed as *nevus sebaceus of Jadassohn* due to the presence of many large sebaceous lobules. The hair follicles remain small, recognizable only by buds of basaloid cells in connection with the lower surface of the epidermis. The epidermis shows verrucous hyperplasia and may be hyperpigmented. One-half of the lesions show ectopic apocrine glands. The third stage, during the adult life, is distinguished by development of a variety of benign and malignant tumors within the area of nevoid malformation (Fig. 36–4). The most common adnexal tumor developing in organoid nevi is syringocystadenoma papilliferum. Others include solid and syringoid hidradenomas, apocrine cystadenoma, trichilemmoma, inverted follicular keratosis, and sebaceous epithelioma.[2–4] The incidence of basal cell epithelioma has been reported as high as 10 to 20 percent. True malignant lesions such as squamous cell carcinoma, eccrine and apocrine adenocarcinomas, and undifferentiated adnexal carcinomas may occur on rare occasions.[5,6] Organoid nevi with exten-

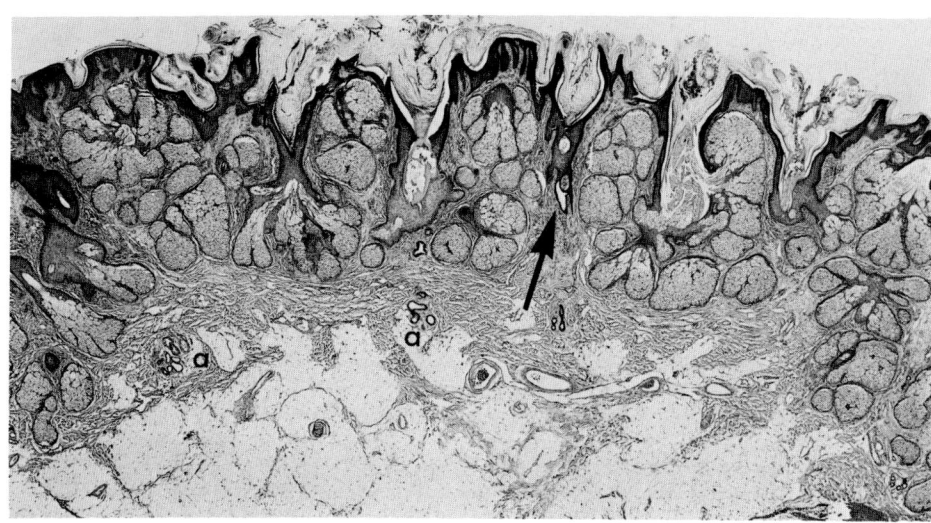

Figure 36–1.
Organoid nevus of scalp in adult life. While in this case preponderance of large sebaceous glands seems to justify diagnosis of nevus sebaceus, one should not overlook papillomatous hyperplasia of epidermis, underdevelopment of hair roots, and presence of apocrine glands (a). Arrow points to dilated apocrine duct. H&E. X30.

sive scalp involvement or with linear lesions in midfacial locations may be associated with mental deficiency, seizures, or hamartomatous lesions in kidneys, eyes, skeletal or central nervous systems as part of a neurocutaneous syndrome (nevus sebaceus syndrome).[7–13]

To diagnose an organoid nevus as an aplastic birth defect or nevus verrucosus in childhood and overlook its potential to develop as nevus sebaceus later does a disservice to the patient because it prevents corrective prophylactic treatment, which ideally consists of complete excision deep enough to remove apocrine coils. Furthermore, failure to be cognizant of the broad concept of organoid nevus results in confusion of a field that can be understood clearly by synthesis of biologic and pathologic facts.[14]

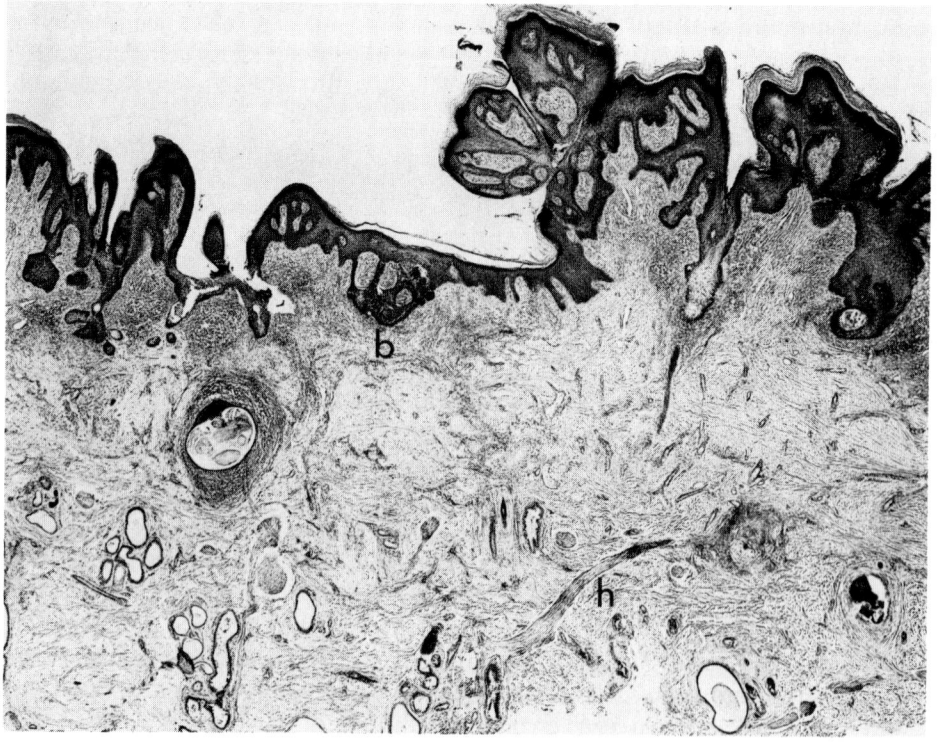

Figure 36–2.
Organoid nevus of scalp in adult life. In this case, not only hair roots but also sebaceous glands are underdeveloped. Epidermis is papillomatous, apocrine glands are present, and mesodermal portion of skin is obviously abnormal. h, hair muscle; b, atypical basaloid proliferation which may be a malformed hair root or a tiny basal cell epithelioma. H&E. X28. (From Mehregan and Pinkus. Arch Dermatol 91: 574, 1965.)

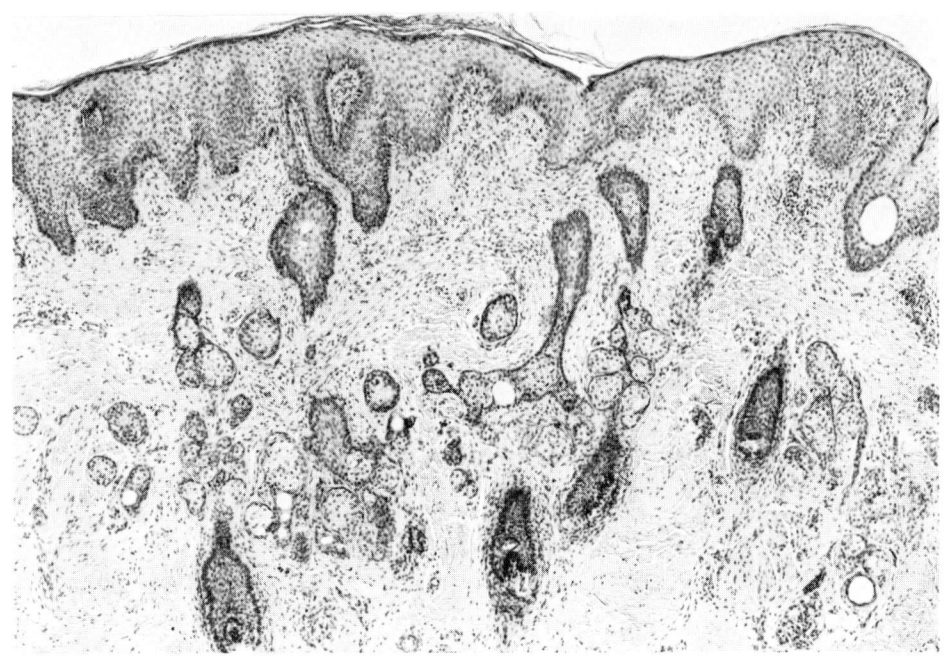

Figure 36–3.
Infantile form of organoid nevus of scalp (Wolters' nevus epitheliomatosus capitis). Acanthotic, somewhat papillomatous epidermis, malformed and underdeveloped pilosebaceous complexes, abnormal connective tissue. H&E. X75. (From Mehregan and Pinkus. Arch Dermatol 91:574, 1965.)

SENILE SEBACEOUS HYPERPLASIA

Senile sebaceous hyperplasias are small yellowish nodular lesions occurring on the faces of middle-aged or older individuals. They consist of excessively large and crowded lobes of sebaceous glands[15] (Fig. 36–5). There is some accentuation of the basal layer, which exhibits a low labeling index when injected with tritiated thymidine. The process of maturation proceeds in the normal fashion. Labeled cells are retained in acini much longer, and the sebocytes are smaller.[16] Sebaceous hyperplasia may also occur in a large nodular form resembling an epithelial cyst,[17] involving the areola following pregnancy,[18] in a linear pattern,[19] or in a diffuse form giving a facial impression of cutis verticis gyrata.[20]

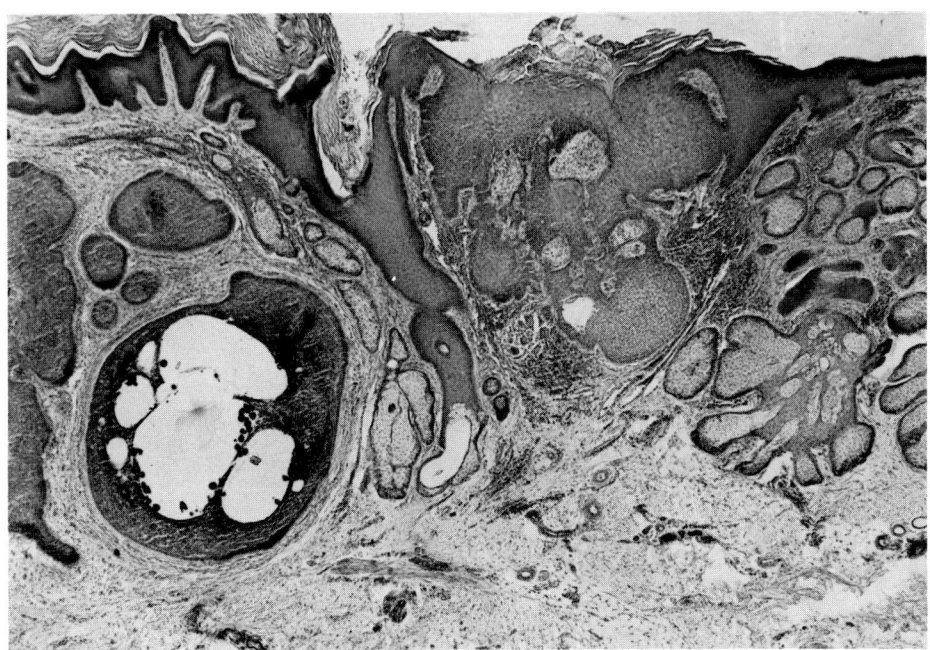

Figure 36–4.
Third phase in life history of organoid nevus of scalp. In this case, pigmented basal cell epithelioma (left) and solid hidradenoma of clear cell type (center) have developed in nevus sebaceus which persists in right third of picture. H&E. X21. (From Mehregan and Pinkus. Arch Dermatol 91:574, 1965.)

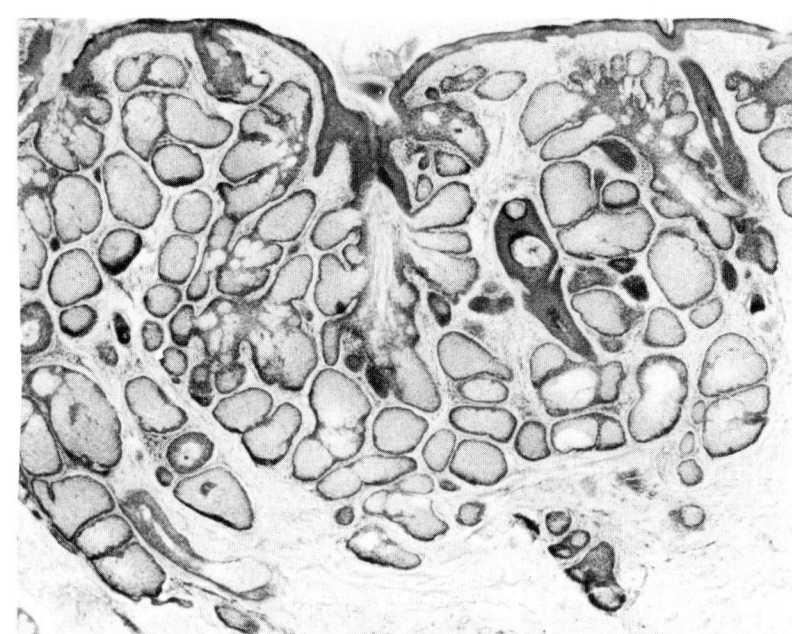

Figure 36–5.
Senile sebaceous hyperplasia. A nodular growth consists of numerous well-differentiated lobules of sebaceous glands, some in connection with a central follicle. H&E. X25.

SEBACEOUS TRICHOFOLLICULOMA

Solitary nodular lesions with a central depressed area from which multiple hairs are extruded, occurring over the nose, have been described as sebaceous trichofolliculoma[21] (Fig. 36–6). Many large sebaceous follicles, terminals, and vellus hair follicles are found in connection with a central epithelial-lined sinus, which may show surface opening.[22]

SEBACEOUS ADENOMA

Sebaceous adenomas are rare. These are yellow nodular lesions, often present on the face, chest, or back. Lesions are made up of massive aggregations of sebaceous lobules with multiple layers of small basaloid cells in their periphery and relatively small sebocytes (Fig. 36–7). The lobular structure of the glands, however, is well preserved (Fig. 36–8).

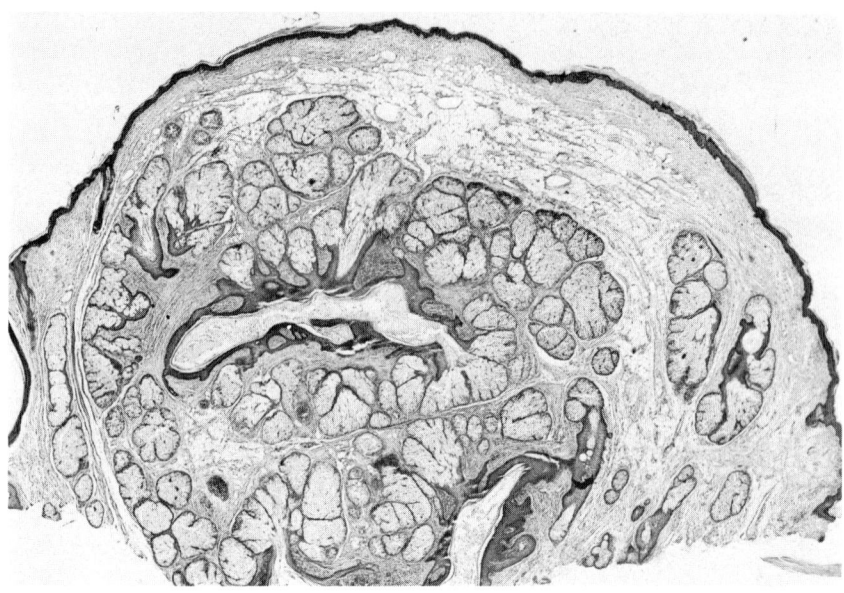

Figure 36–6.
Sebaceous trichofolliculoma. Numerous sebaceous lobules and small hair follicles in association with a central cystic follicular pore. H&E. X10.

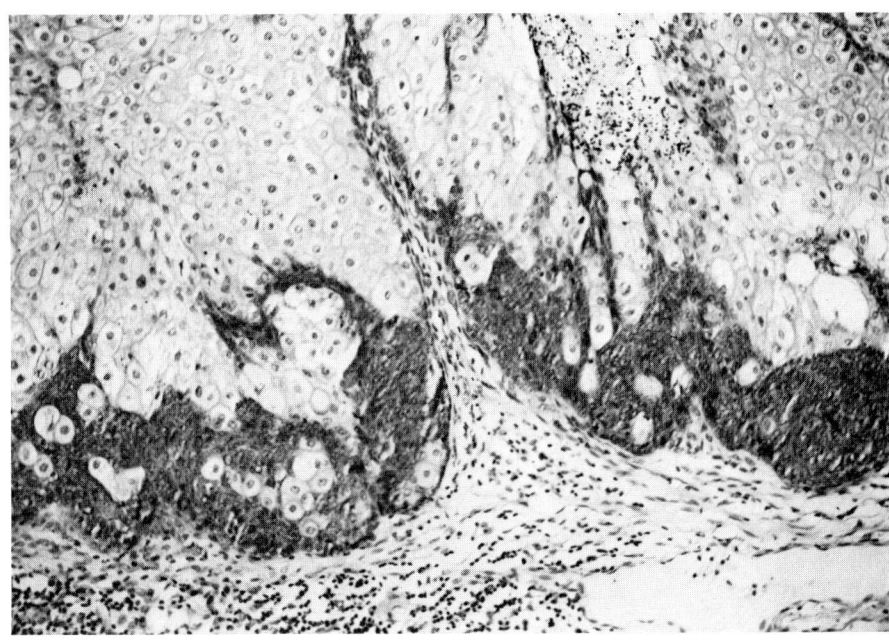

Figure 36–7.
Sebaceous adenoma. H&E. X135.

SEBACEOUS EPITHELIOMA

In sebaceous epithelioma, the architecture of the gland is more or less completely obliterated, and the tumors consist mainly of solid masses of basaloid cells displaying focal ability for sebaceous maturation (Fig. 36–9). Central cystic spaces may contain sebaceous and degenerated cellular material. Scattered mitotic figures and chronic inflammatory cell reaction are also present. Below this type of tumor on the ladder of maturity are lesions that we may call basal cell epitheliomas with sebaceous differentiation, because the growth consists predominantly of basaloid cells and only small groups or single cells show this tendency.

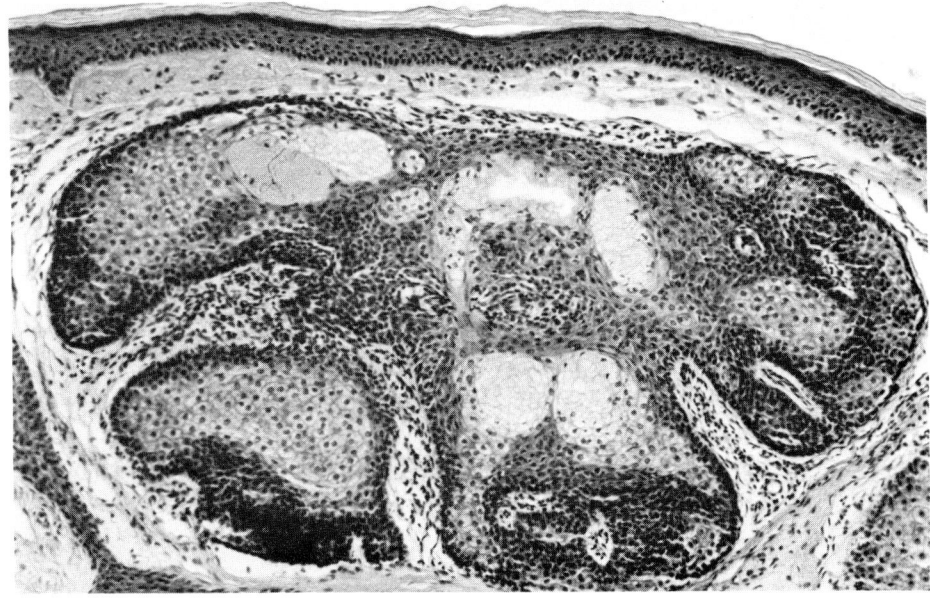

Figure 36–8.
Sebaceous adenoma. Multiple sebaceous lobules with several rows of basaloid cells in their periphery and small sebocytes. H&E. X125.

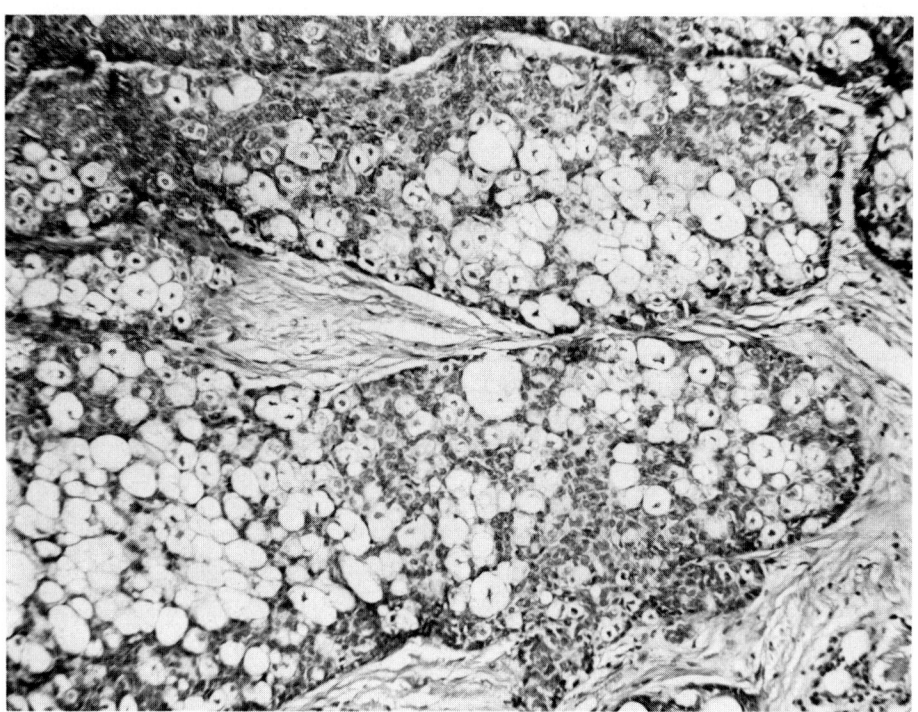

Figure 36–9.
Sebaceous epithelioma. H&E. X135.

MUIR–TORRE SYNDROME

Multiple sebaceous tumors in association with low grade and often multiple malignant neoplasms of the digestive tract are known as Muir–Torre syndrome.[23–30] Histologically, the sebaceous tumors are sebaceous adenomas, sebaceous epitheliomas, basal cell epitheliomas with sebaceous differentiation, and sebaceous carcinomas. Keratoacanthoma-like lesions consist of massive proliferation of follicular sheath epithelium and may exhibit foci of sebaceous differentiation (Fig. 36–10). Muir–Torre syndrome is closely related to the cancer family syndrome.[31,32]

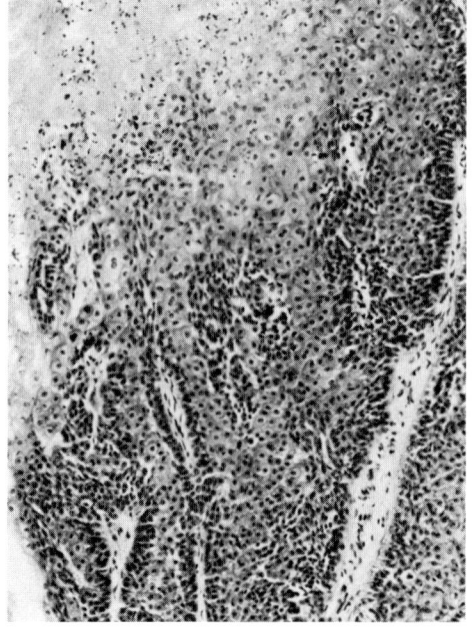 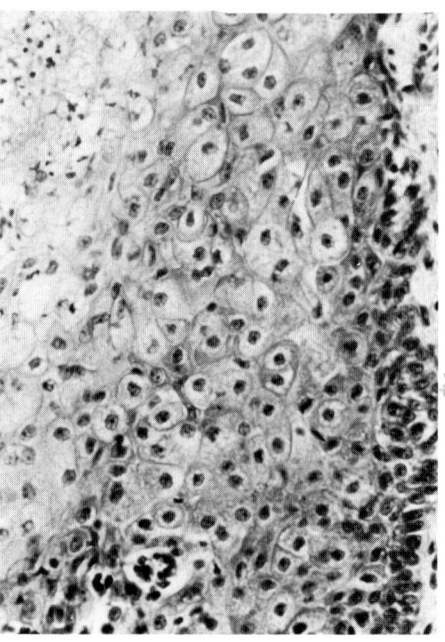

Figure 36–10.
Muir–Torre syndrome. A keratoacanthoma-like lesion of leg shows massive proliferation of follicular sheath epithelium and foci of sebaceous differentiation. H&E. X125.

REFERENCES

1. Mehregan AH, Pinkus H: Life history of organoid nevi: Special reference to nevus sebaceus of Jadassohn. Arch Dermatol 91:574, 1965
2. Wilson-Jones E, Heyl T: Naevus sebaceus: A report of 140 cases with special regard to the development of secondary malignant tumors. Br J Dermatol 82:99, 1970
3. Bonvalet D, Barrandon Y, Foix Ch, Civatte J: Tumeurs annexielles benignes de survenue tardive sur naevus verruco-sebace (Jadassohn): A propos de 7 cas. Ann Dermatol Venereol 110:337, 1983
4. Alessi E, Wong SN, Advani HH, Ackerman AB: Nevus sebaceus is associated with unusual neoplasms. An atlas. Am J Dermatopathol 10:116, 1988
5. Domingo J. Helwig EB: Malignant neoplasms associated with nevus sebaceus of Jadassohn. J Am Acad Dermatol 1:545, 1979
6. Tarkhan II, Domingo J: Metastasizing eccrine porocarcinoma developing in a sebaceous nevus of Jadassohn. Report of a case. Arch Dermatol 121:413, 1985
7. Lovejoy FH Jr, Boyle WE Jr: Linear nevus sebaceous syndrome: Report of two cases and a review of the literature. Pediatrics 52:382–387, 1973
8. Chalub EG, Volpe JJ, Gado MH: Linear nevus sebaceous syndrome associated with porencephaly and nonfunctioning major cerebral venous sinuses. Neurology 25:857, 1975
9. Moskowitz R, Honig PJ: Nevus sebaceus in association with an intracranial mass. J Am Acad Dermatol 6:1078, 1982
10. Clancy RR, Kurtz MB, Baker D, et al: Neurologic manifestations of the organoid nevus syndrome. Arch Neurol 42:236, 1985
11. Kang WH, Koh YJ, Chun SI: Nevus sebaceus syndrome associated with intracranial arteriovenous malformation. Int J Dermatol 26:382, 1987
12. Pujol RM, Tuneu A, De Moragas JM, et al: Sindrome del nevus sebaceo lineal. Med Cutan ILA 15:280, 1987
13. Diven DG, Solomon AR, McNeely MC, Font RL: Nevus sebaceus associated with major ophthalmologic abnormalities. Arch Dermatol 123:383, 1987
14. Mehregan AH: Epithelial nevi and benign tumors of the skin and their associated systemic conditions. J Dermatol Tokyo 12:10, 1985
15. Mehregan AH: Sebaceous tumors of the skin. J Cutan Pathol 12:196, 1985
16. Lunderschmidt C, Plewig G: Circumscribed sebaceous gland hyperplasia: Autoradiographic and histoplanometric studies. J Invest Dermatol 70:207, 1978
17. Kudoh K, Hosokawa M, Miyazawa T, Tagami H: Giant solitary sebaceous gland hyperplasia clinically simulating epidermoid cyst. J Cutan Pathol 15:396, 1988
18. Catalano PM, Ioannides G: Areolar sebaceous hyperplasia. J Am Acad Dermatol 13:867, 1985
19. Fernandez N, Torres A: Hyperplasia of sebaceous glands in a linear pattern of papules: Report of four cases. Am J Dermatopathol 6:237, 1984
20. Blanchet-Barden C, Servant JM, Bao LeTaun, Puissant A: Hyperplasie sebacée acquise à type de cutis verticis gyrata sensible au 13-Cis-Retinoid. Ann Dermatol Venereol 109:749, 1982
21. Plewig G: Sebaceous trichofolliculoma. J Cutan Pathol 7:394, 1980
22. Silva LG: Trichofoliculoma sebaceo. Med Cutan ILA 10:51, 1982
23. Rulon DB, Helwig EB: Multiple sebaceous neoplasms of the skin: An association with multiple visceral carcinomas especially of the colon. Am J Clin Pathol 60:745, 1973
24. Schwartz RA, Flieger DN, Saied NK: The Torre syndrome with gastrointestinal polyposis. Arch Dermatol 116:312, 1980
25. Housholder MS, Zeligman I: Sebaceous neoplasms associated with visceral carcinomas. Arch Dermatol 116:61, 1980
26. Fahmy A, Burgdorf WC, et al: Muir–Torre syndrome: Report of a case and re-evaluation of the dermatopathologic features. Cancer 49:1898, 1983
27. Banse-Kupin L, Morales A, Barlow M: Torre's syndrome: Report of two cases and review of the literature. J Am Acad Dermatol 10:803, 1984
28. Finan MC, Connolly SM: Sebaceous gland tumors and systemic disease: A clinicopathologic analysis. Medicine 63:232, 1984
29. Graham R, McKee P, McGibbon D, Heyderman E: Torre–Muir syndrome. An association with isolated sebaceous carcinoma. Cancer 55:2868, 1985
30. Schwartz RA, Goldberg DJ, Mahmood F, et al: The Muir–Torre syndrome: A disease of sebaceous and colonic neoplasms. Dermatologica 178:23, 1989
31. Lynch HT, Lynch PM, et al: The cancer family syndrome: Rare cutaneous phenotypic linkage of Torre's syndrome. Arch Intern Med 141:607, 1981
32. Lynch HT, Fusaro RM, Roberts L, et al: Muir–Torre syndrome in several members of a family with a variant of the cancer family syndrome. Br J Dermatol 113:295, 1985

37
HAIR NEVI AND HAIR FOLLICLE TUMORS

HAIR NEVI

Hair and hair follicle are involved in several nevi. Localized growth of unusually strong hairs is a hair nevus, while crowding of many tiny mature follicles (Fig. 37–1) constitutes a hair follicle nevus. Circumscribed patches of scalp hair of divergent color or texture may be classified as nevi. The most common form is the *white forelock* (poliosis), which may occur alone or as part of piebaldism (Chapter 31), but patches of red hair in a brown scalp or other abnormalities may be observed (*dichromism*). The *woolly-hair nevus* of Wise[1–3] in a straight-haired scalp has found its counterpart in the *straight-hair nevus* in a negroid scalp.[4,5] The excessive development of hairs in common pigmented moles and in bathing-trunk (animal pelt) nevi can properly be classified as hair nevus (nevus pilosus). Very rare, indeed, are cases in which vellus hair follicles are found within the nevi of sole or family members having circumscribed patches of vellus hairs on their palms.[6–8]

Nevus Comedonicus

In nevus comedonicus a number of cystic dilated hair follicles containing pigmented horny plugs (Fig. 37–2) occur in a localized area or in linear arrangement.[9–11] Occurrence in homozygous twins suggests an autosomal dominant inheritance.[12] Dilated follicles are lined with infundibular epithelium keratinizing with formation of keratohyalin granules. Sebaceous lobules may be observed in connection with the wall of the cystic follicles in early lesions. A histologic variant is characterized by occurrence of epidermolytic hyperkeratosis in dilated follicles.[13] Underlying calcification and extensive inflammation with development of cysts and abscesses may complicate the lesion.[14,15] Secondary benign tumors are rare and malignant changes do not occur.[16] Nevus comedonicus may occur in association with skeletal abnormalities and central nervous system manifestations.[17] Ocular changes may be present in the form of congenital cataract.[18]

HAIR FOLLICLE TUMORS

A number of hair follicle tumors are listed in Table VII–1 in descending order of maturation. The variety of such tumors is greatly increasing, due to more thorough observations of a multiplying number of investigators of dermal pathology. This tendency is welcome, as it seems advisable to organize and subdivide the field for several reasons. The question of benign versus malignant can be answered with more confidence if one is familiar with all varieties of

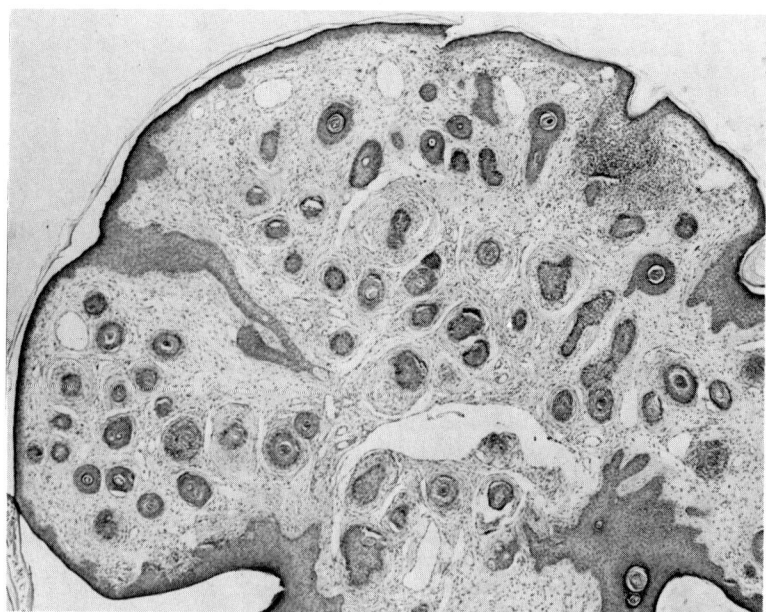

Figure 37–1.
Hair follicle nevus. Numerous tiny but mature hair follicles with thick fibrous root sheath in a pedunculated papillomatous papule. H&E. X60.

tumors.[19] Several variants have unexpected associations with generalized systemic disease, whereas this association is uncommon in others. Finally, we must take into consideration the tendency of the mind of the inquisitive pathologist, who is not satisfied until a definite diagnostic term can be affixed to a particular tumor. On the next pages we describe a fairly long list of tumors, and it will become obvious that hair follicle epithelium can deviate from normal not only in the vertical order of maturity but also in several horizontal directions of organization. How much of this intellectual differentiation between various tumors is of practical significance to the clinician is a question that every pathologist has to answer in considering the circumstances of the individual case.

Trichofolliculoma

The most organized nevoid tumor related to the entire hair follicle has been appropriately called trichofolliculoma. It consists of one or several keratinized sinuses (Fig. 37–3) into which dozens of abortive hair roots enter from all sides. The central keratin-filled sinus and the surrounding hair follicles are embedded in a well-organized fibrous stroma forming a well-defined neoplasm.[20] Some of the newly formed hair follicles produce nothing but a rudimentary matrix, others form an inner root sheath, and some produce tiny colorless filaments (trichoids) that may appear on the skin surface as cottony or silky strands.[21] That many hair roots open into a common sinus and that they may have secondary branches constitutes adenomatous deviation from normal organization. The lower degree of maturation fits this pattern, distinguishing trichofollic-

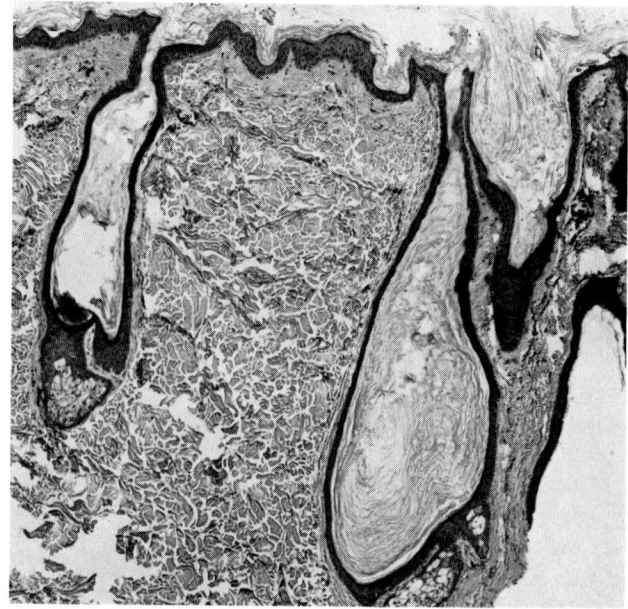

Figure 37–2.
Nevus comedonicus. Saccular dilation of the lengthened pilosebaceous duct. Sebaceous glands situated at an unusually deep level in the dermis. Hair roots atrophic. H&E. X75.

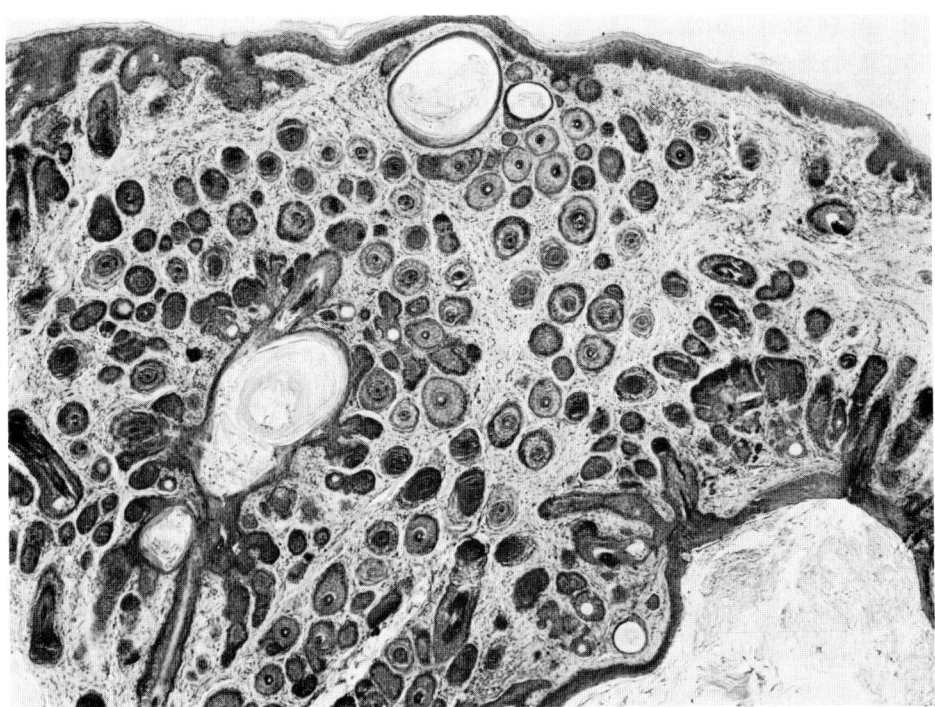

Figure 37–3.
Trichofolliculoma. Branching hair follicles achieve varying degrees of maturation, and some form tiny hairs. H&E. X45. (From Pinkus and Mehregan. In Schnyder (ed.) Haut und Anhangsgebilde, 1973. Courtesy of Springer-Verlag.)

uloma as an adenomatous neoplasm from mature hair follicle nevus.

Trichoadenoma

Solitary intracutaneous nodule of trichoadenoma occurs over the face or on the trunk.[22] This is a moderately well-differentiated tumor (Fig. 37–4) consisting of solid masses of cells and small horny cysts with stratified epithelium of outer root sheath character that keratinizes in both epidermoid and trichilemmal fashions forming soft or dense keratin.[23] No hair roots are formed. It is, therefore, a tumor of the adenomatous level of organization and exhibits differentiation toward the pilosebaceous canal.

Dilated Pore

Dilated pore of Winer[24] may be considered as a simple type of follicular sheath neoplasm (Fig. 37–5). Thick proliferating folds of outer root sheath epithelium line a central cystic space. The dilated follicle may be funnel-shaped, round, multilobulated, or dish-like with a wide opening.[25] The lesion shows a central horny plug and clinically resembles a large blackhead.[26]

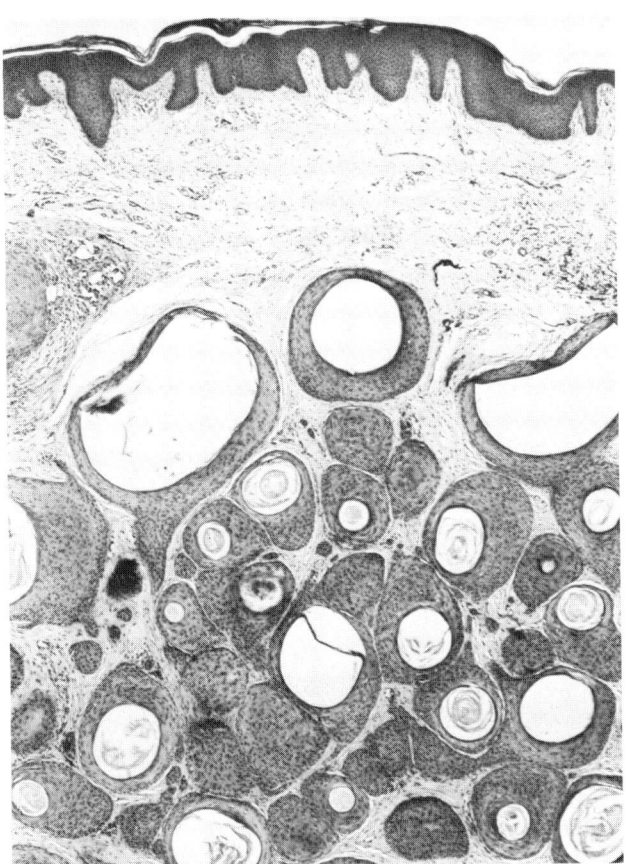

Figure 37–4.
Nikolowski's trichoadenoma. H&E. X70.

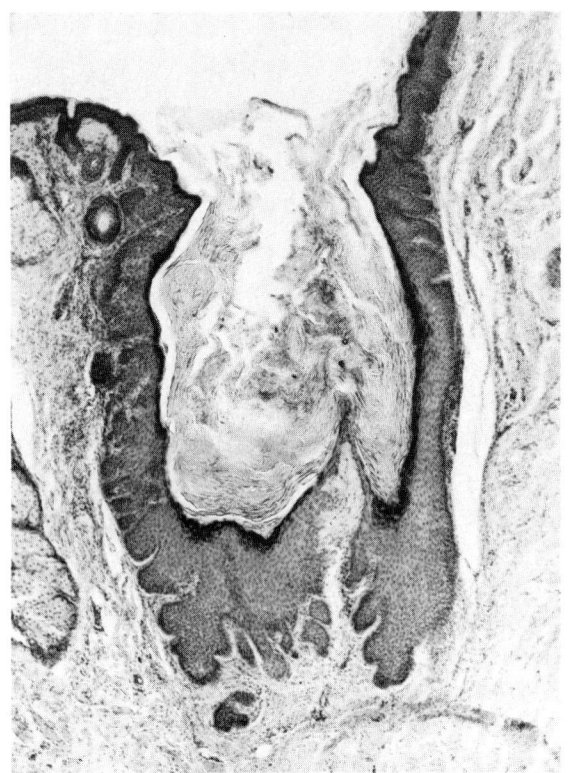

Figure 37–5.
Winer's dilated pore. H&E. X45.

Pilar Sheath Acanthoma

Related to dilated pore, pilar sheath acanthoma lesion appears most commonly over the upper lip area (Fig. 37–6). Massive proliferation of follicular sheath epithelium occurs, extending from the wall of a central cystic cavity into the surrounding dermis in all directions and often down to the level of striated muscles.[27] Keratinization is with formation of keratohyalin granules (Fig. 37–7). Areas populated with clear epithelial cells and occasional abortive hair follicles may be present.[28,29]

Tumor of Follicular Infundibulum

A less mature follicular neoplasm is the tumor of follicular infundibulum,[30,31] in which masses of rather light-staining outer-root-sheath-type cells (Fig. 37–8) form a shelf or fenestrated plate below the epidermis, which they penetrate wherever there is a follicular opening. This tumor resembles, in some respects, the growth pattern of the very superficial type of basal cell epithelioma but seems to be even more benign in its clinical behavior and consists of cells resembling those of follicular infundibulum.[32,33] There is, however, a single case report of a patient with multiple tumors of follicular infundibulum complicated with development of superficial basal cell epithelioma.[34]

Inverted Follicular Keratosis

Also known as *follicular poroma*,[35] inverted follicular keratosis appears as keratotic nodular lesions over the face and occasionally elsewhere.[36,37] Hyperplastic follicular epithelium (Fig. 37–9) extends from the surface into the dermis surrounded by fibrovascular stroma. Maturation is retarded so that the percentage of small basaloid cells is increased at the periphery of the tumor lobules. In the center, numerous foci of keratinization occur forming

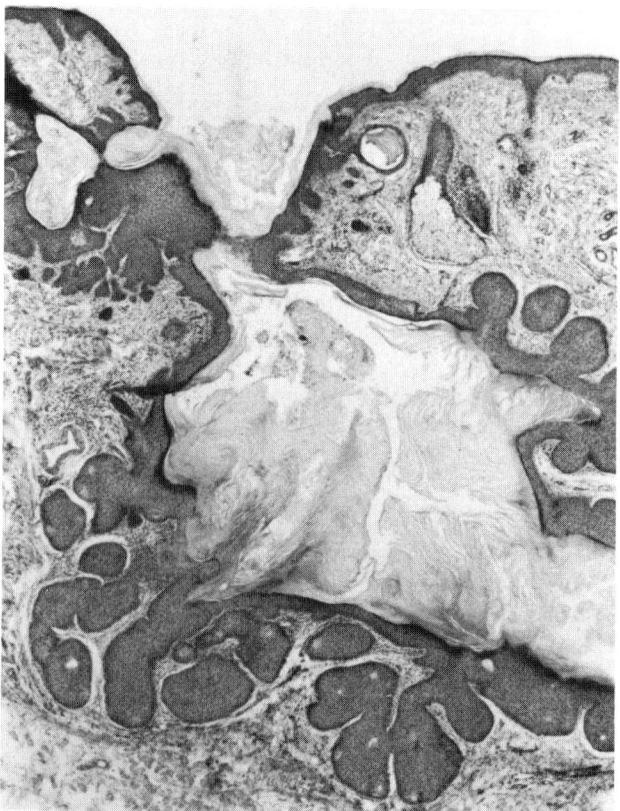

Figure 37–6.
Pilar sheath acanthoma. Similar to dilated pore in formation of a horny plug, it branches out with massive proliferation of follicular sheath epithelium in all directions. H&E. X25.

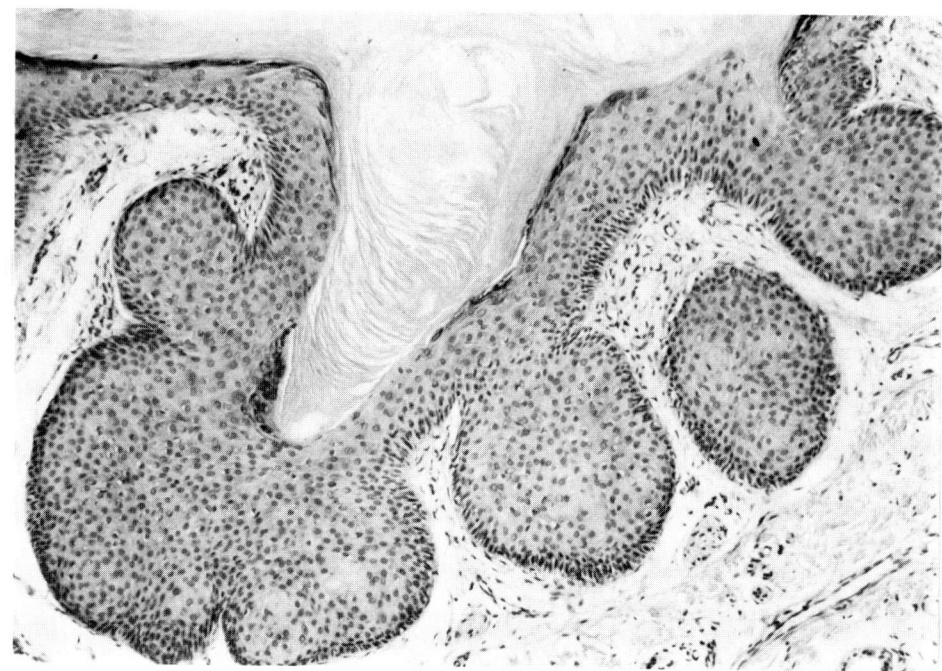

Figure 37–7.
Pilar sheath acanthoma. Massive proliferation of follicular sheath epithelium in connection with a central cystic dilated follicular pore. H&E. X125.

squamous eddies[38] (Fig. 37–10). Early lesions may show a connection with an underlying hair follicle or sebaceous gland. A papillomatous and hyperkeratotic lesion of inverted follicular keratosis may resemble a verruca vulgaris. There are, however, no vacuolated cells and immunostaining for the papilloma virus common antigen have been negative.[39]

Trichilemmoma

Massive proliferation of follicular sheath epithelium (Fig. 37–11) is seen in connection with the lower surface of the epidermis. The tumor epithelium (Fig. 37–12) is made up of light-staining cells with abundant glycogen granules. At the periphery, the tumor cells palisade and rest on a layer of homogeneous basement membrane, thus resembling the outer root sheath of the hair follicle.[40,41] Trichilemmomas are usually superficial. A case with long-standing scalp lesions showing extensive dermal and subcutaneous fat involvement and with benign cytologic features has been reported.[42]

Cowden's Disease "Multiple Hamartoma Syndrome"

This autosomal dominant inherited disease is characterized by skin manifestations and multiple system involvements. The majority of facial lesions are trichilemmomas. Acral lesions are benign or punctate keratoses and oral lesions are fibromas.[43–45] Other system involvements include thyroid adenoma and adenocarcinoma, fibrocystic disease and carcinoma of breast, multiple polyps of the gastrointestinal tract, diverticula of the colon, ovarian cysts, leiomyoma, and carcinoma of the uterus.[46–48]

Pilomatricoma

The single tumor definitely related to hair matrix is *Malherbe's calcifying epithelioma,* which therefore may be properly called pilomatricoma.[49,50] The living portions of this tumor (Fig. 37–13) strongly resemble the nonstratified mass of small, dark-staining cells of the pilar matrix. In an early lesion, the upper part of a hair follicle may be present in almost normal fashion, while the deep portion is occupied by a pilomatricoma (Fig. 37–14). The peripheral masses of small basaloid hair matrix-type cells show transformation into fully keratinized shadow cells toward the center of the lesion.[51] Trichocyte-type cytokeratins have been demonstrated in the keratinizing (transitional) and shadow cells. Shadow cells have a strong tendency for calcification.[52]

Bone formation is observed in a few cases. A foreign-body-type granuloma is often present around

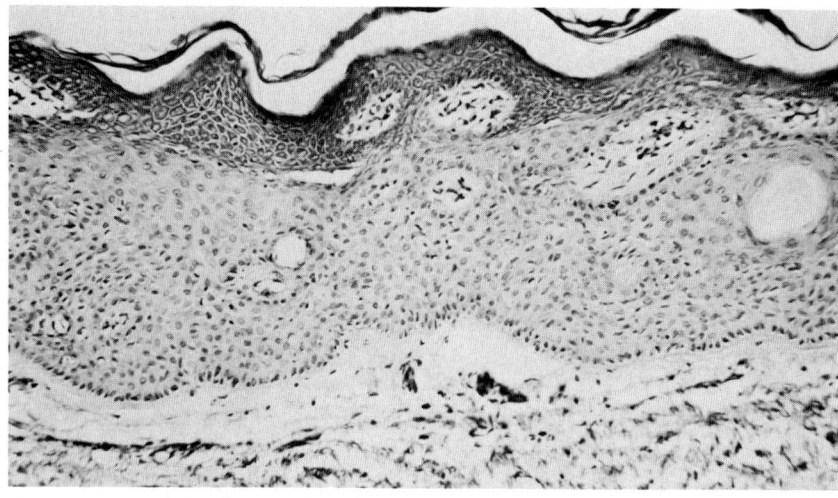
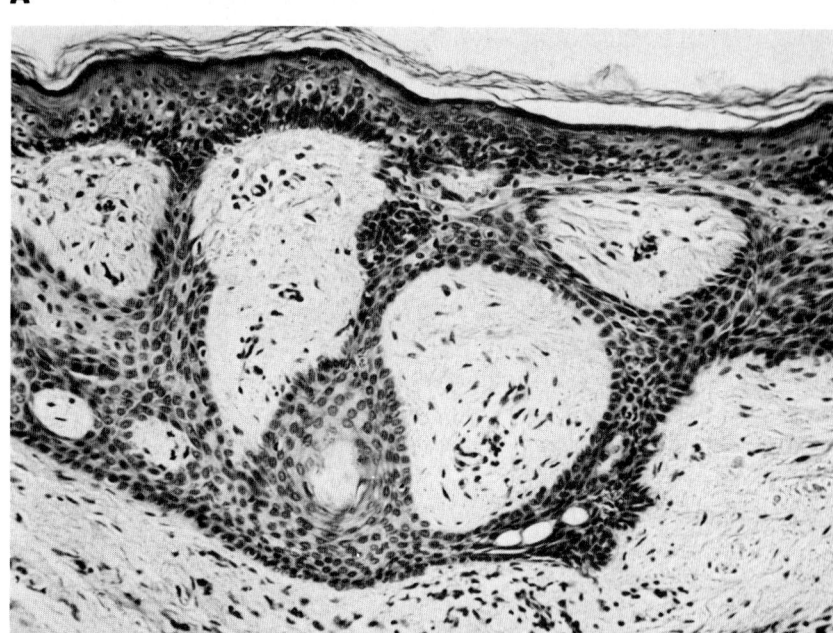

Figure 37–8.
Tumor of follicular infundibulum. Benign neoplastic epithelium forms a plate below the epidermis, with which it is in multiple contact. The tumor stains lighter than the epidermis, is not pigmented, and is embedded in moderately mature stroma. **A.** Van Gieson. X70. **B.** H&E. X180.

the keratinized areas within the fibrous stroma of the lesion. Anetodermic changes due to loss of collagen and elastic fibers may be clinically observed.[53] Unusually large lesions with deep dermal involvement occur. Superficial perforation may lead to elimination of the tumor epithelium and calcified material.[54] Multiple and familial cases have been reported.[55] Another development is the association of pilomatricomas with myotonic muscular dystrophy.[56–59] Several cases with malignant pilomatricoma reported show combined histologic features of pilomatricoma with dysplastic cellular changes, squamous metaplasia, and scattered mitoses (see Chapter 41).

TRICHOEPITHELIOMA

In the systematic spectrum of adnexoid tumors, there is a level of maturity at which much of the tumor may have the characteristics of quite imma-

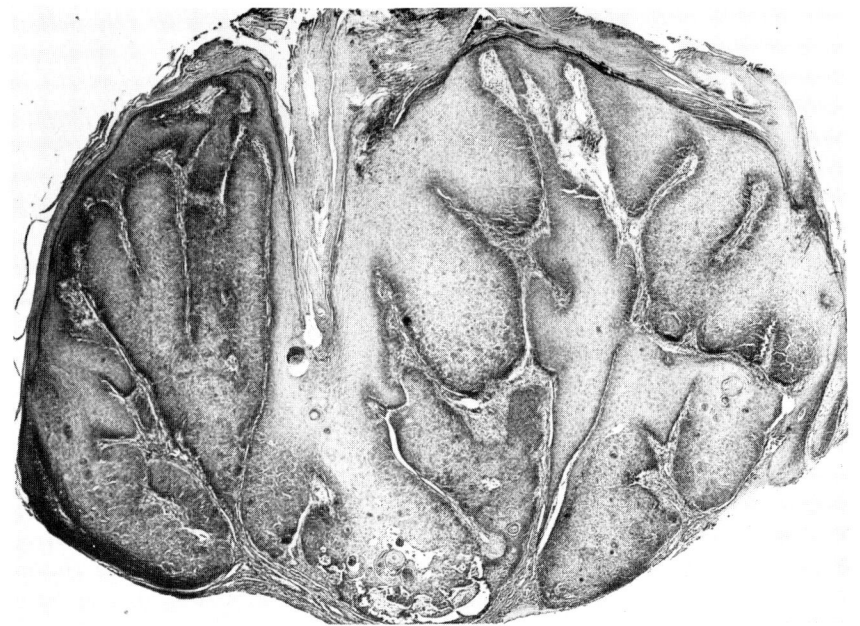

Figure 37–9.
Follicular poroma (inverted follicular keratosis) contains recognizable remnant of involved hair follicle in center and is characterized by smooth outline of the proliferating epithelium that contains numerous squamous eddies (see Fig. 37–10). Compare with Figure 35–25 (keratoacanthoma) consisting of large, light-staining prickle cells. H&E. X23. (From Mehregan. Arch Dermatol 89:229, 1964.)

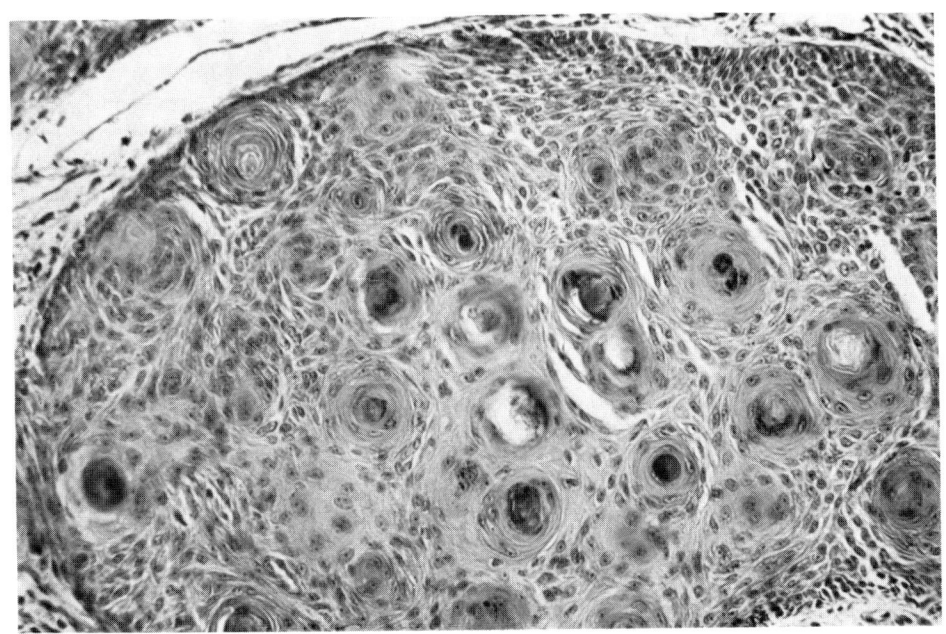

Figure 37–10.
Squamous eddies in inverted follicular keratosis (follicular poroma). H&E. X185. (From Mehregan. Arch Dermatol 89: 229, 1964.)

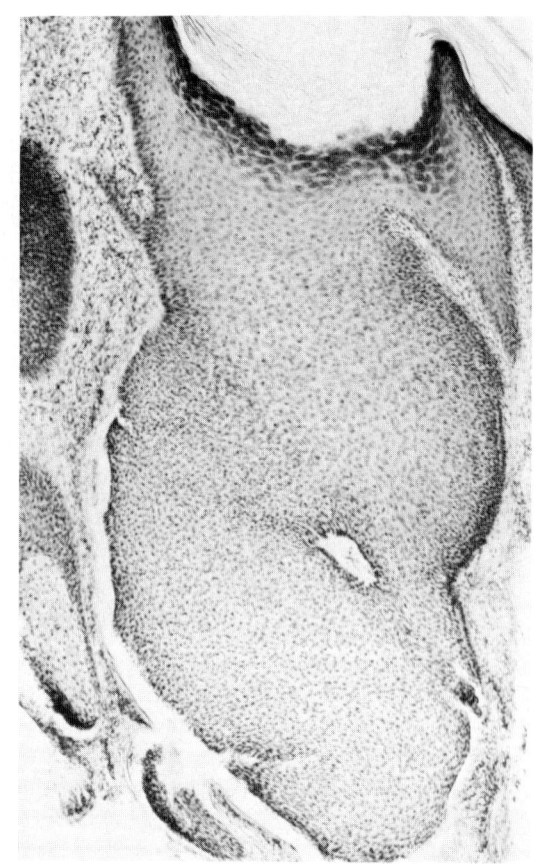

Figure 37-11.
Trichilemmoma. Solid plug of follicular sheath epithelium extends into the dermis. The cells are fairly small but light-staining because they contain glycogen. H&E. X125.

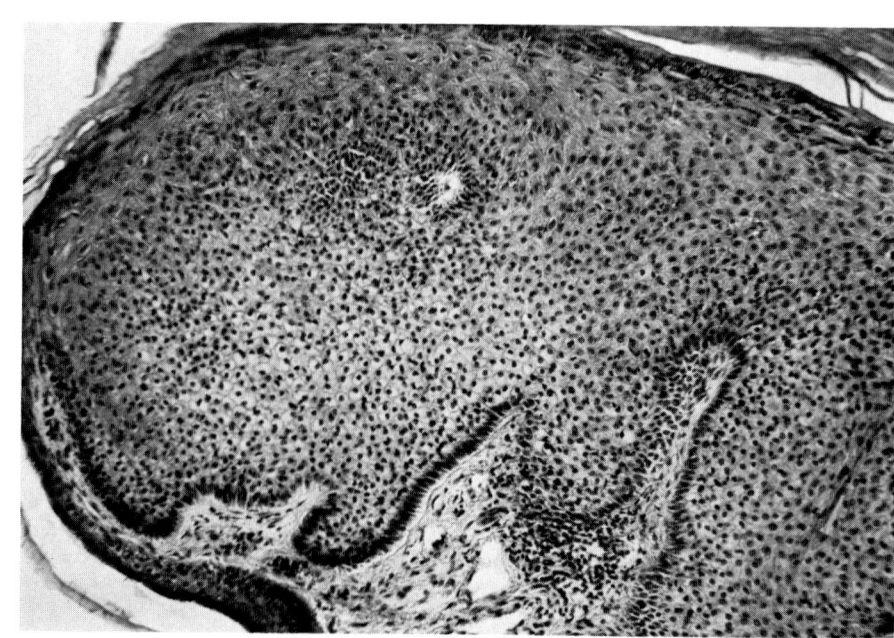

Figure 37-12.
Trichilemmoma. Small portion of lesion to show clear cell character of epithelium and palisading basal layer which rests on a well-defined basement membrane. Tumor cells keratinize in epidermoid fashion on surface. H&E. X135.

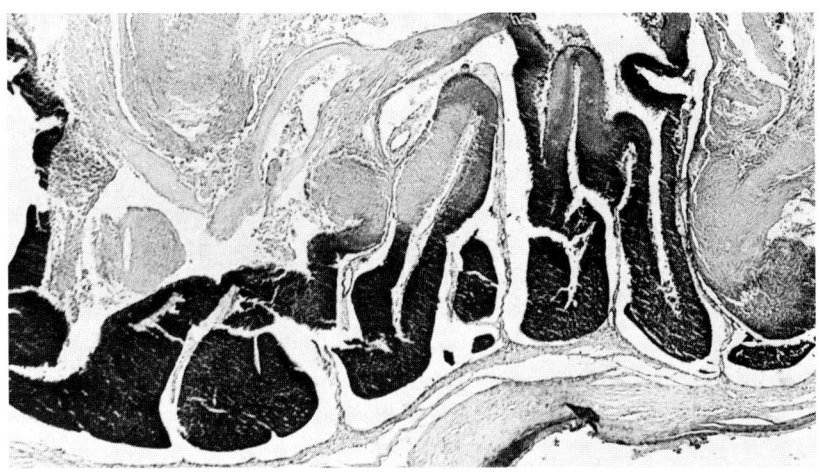
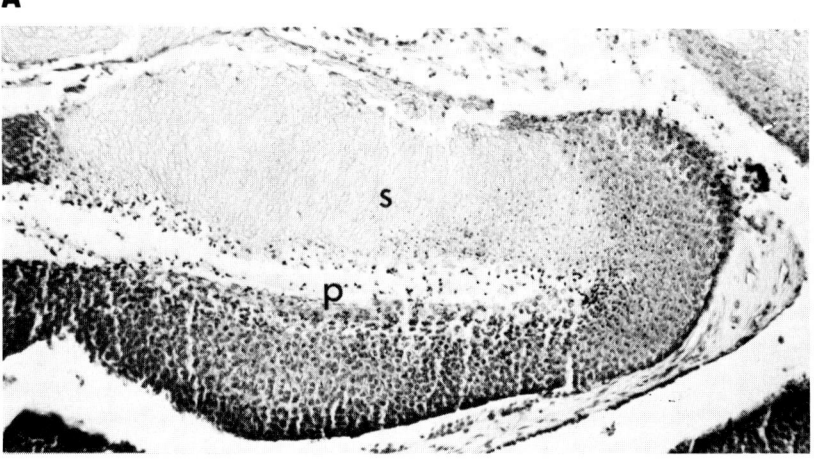

Figure 37–13.
Pilomatricoma. Calcification was not present in this case. **A.** Masses of small dark-staining cells contrast with lighter-staining squamous cells and shadow cells. H&E. X60. **B.** Details of three cellular components: basaloid (b), prickle (p), and shadow (s) cells. H&E. X135.

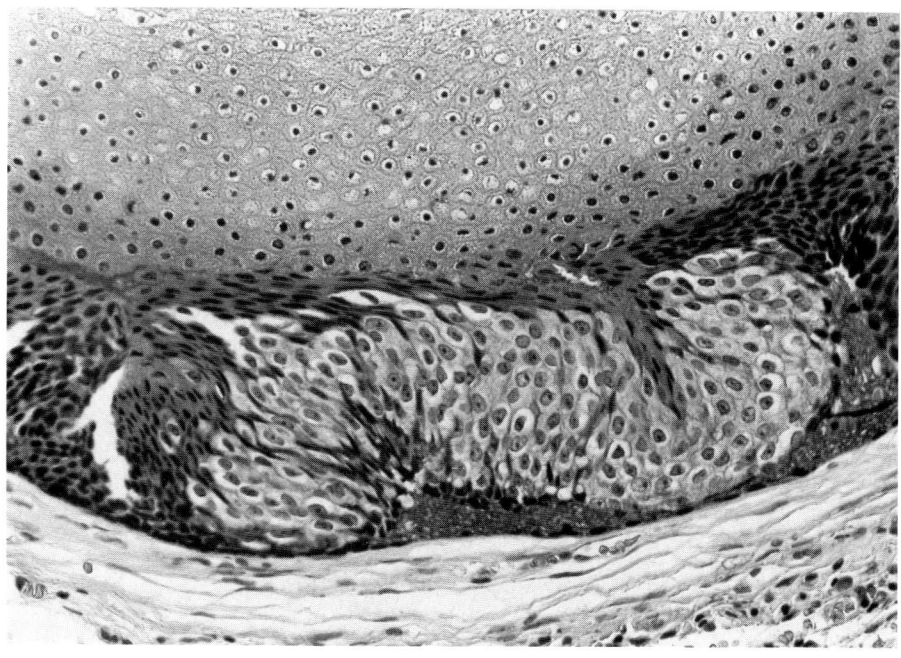

Figure 37–14.
Pilomatricoma shows transformation of small hair matrix-type cells to the fully keratinized shadow cells. H&E. X400.

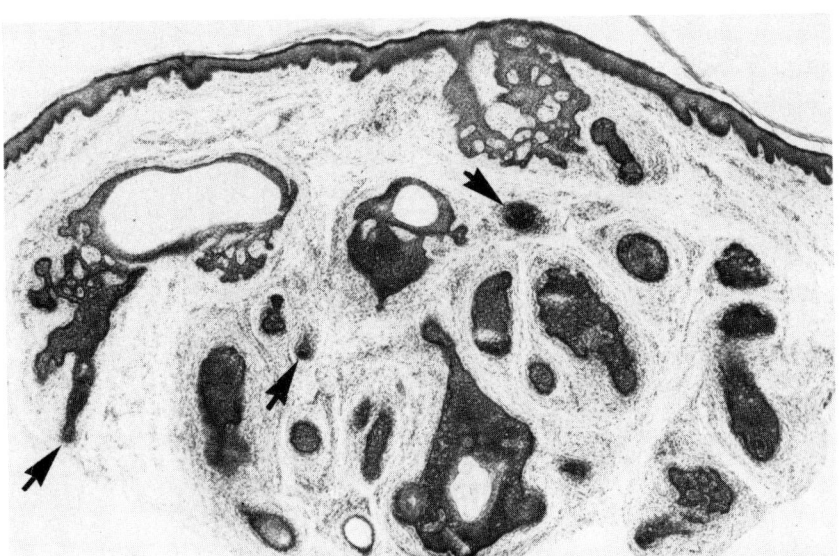

Figure 37–15.
Trichoepithelioma. Rudimentary hair papilla-matrix configurations indicated by arrows. H&E. X45.

ture basal cell epithelioma, while small foci or larger parts show maturation in the direction of sebaceous gland, hair root, or other recognizable adnexal structures. Tumors with features of maturation resembling various parts of the hair follicle are common and vary from basal cell epitheliomas with peculiar antler-like-type of growth (Fig. 37–15), or with occasional rudimentary hairbulb-like structures, to typical trichoepitheliomas.

Trichoepithelioma may be solitary or multiple (*epithelioma adenoides cysticum*). The multiple variety may be familial, transmitted by an autosomal dominant trait.[60]

Histologically, in addition to solid epithelial nests, which often show antler-like branching, there often are tiny keratinizing cysts resembling milia and rudimentary hair papillae, consisting of small areas of crowding of palisaded basal cells surrounded by aggregation of elongated fibroblasts.[61] (Fig. 37–16). Formation of an organized hair is extremely

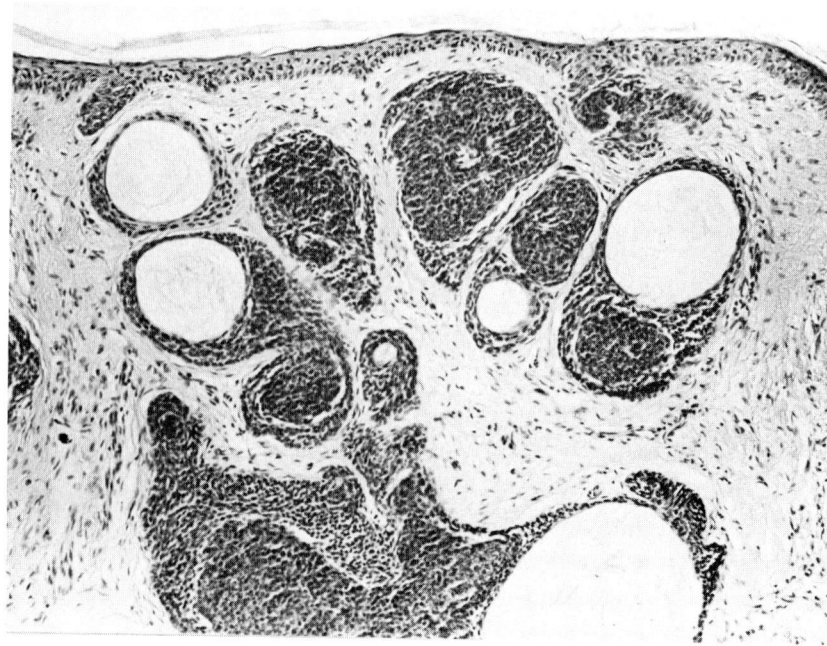

Figure 37–16.
Trichoepithelioma. Solid masses of basaloid cells and small keratin cysts in a well-organized fibrous stroma. H&E. X125.

rare. The nests usually show peripheral palisading, and the central cells may be lighter staining and larger, like those of premalignant fibroepithelial tumors (Chapter 40). The stroma also shows a relatively high degree of maturity and may form sulfated mucopolysaccharides and elastic fibers. Retraction spaces formed between the tumor epithelium and fibrous stroma in basal cell epithelioma are not common in trichoepitheliomas. Separation occurs between the fibrous tumor stroma and the surrounding dermal connective tissue (Fig. 37–17). Large solitary and histologically immature trichoepitheliomas occur in perianal area or on extremities and may consist predominantly of small solid nests or branching cords of basaloid cells with no tendency for keratinization or horn cyst formation.[62,63]

In routine diagnosis, it is not always simple to classify one or the other tumor as either trichoepithelioma or basal cell epithelioma. The absence or presence of inflammatory infiltrate, characteristic of basalioma, is a helpful clue. For practical purposes, one should keep in mind that the individual tumor of cases with multiple epithelioma adenoides cysticum tends to remain small, while solitary trichoepitheliomas of similar histologic appearance grow progressively larger and should be treated like basal cell epitheliomas. Trichoepitheliomas may occur in association with lupus erythematosus and dystrophia unguis congenita or as part of "Rombo" syndrome.[64–66]

Desmoplastic Trichoepithelioma

Desmoplastic trichoepithelioma is usually a solitary, firm nodule with a central depressed area appearing over the facial skin in all ages. Histologically (Fig. 37–18), there is marked resemblance to a morphealike type of basal cell epithelioma consisting of small nests and thin strands of basaloid cells embedded in dense fibrotic stroma.[67,68] They also show, however, multiple foci of keratin cyst formation, areas of calcification, and foreign-body granuloma. Lesions with this histologic pattern have been reported in association with melanocytic nevi as a combined malformation.[69,70]

Basaloid Follicular Hamartoma

Basaloid follicular hamartoma may occur as a single plaque of alopecia, in linear unilateral distribution resembling a systematized epidermal nevus, or in the generalized form with diffuse alopecia and fine papular lesions.[71,72] Histologically, all three types show transformation of individual hair follicles into small basaloid hamartomas that may resemble miniature premalignant fibroepithelial tumors, small trichoepitheliomas, or basal cell epitheliomas (Fig.

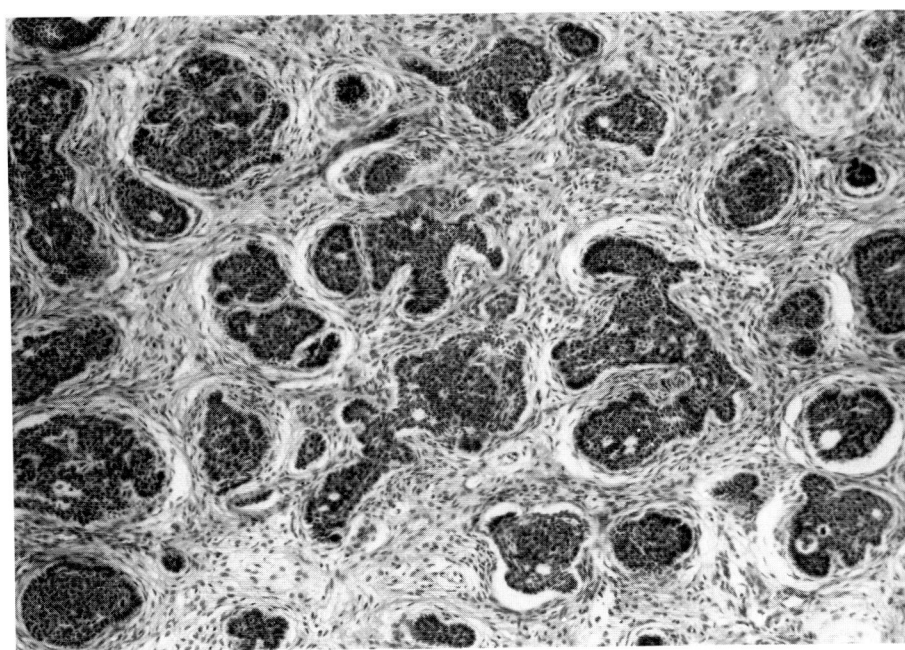

Figure 37–17.
Poorly differentiated trichoepithelioma consists of small solid masses and branching nests of basaloid cells and abortive hair follicles embedded in a well-organized fibrovascular stroma. H&E. X125.

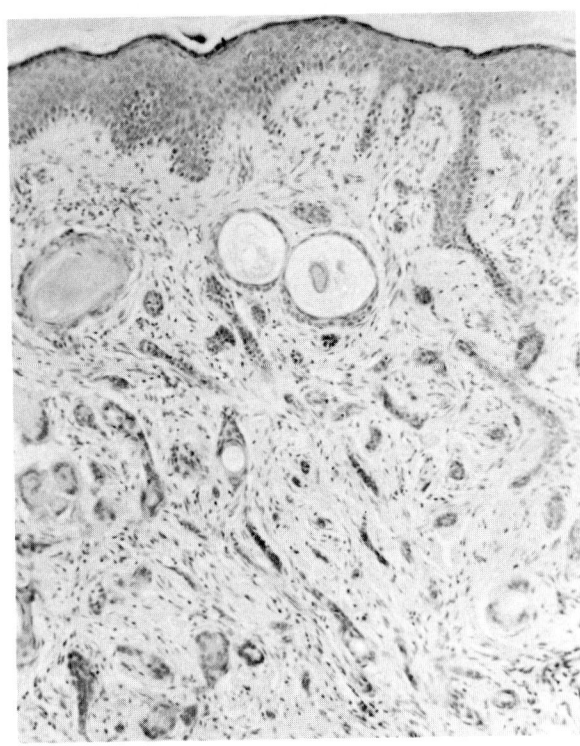

Figure 37-18.
Desmoplastic trichoepithelioma. Compare with Figure 40-21. H&E. X125.

37-19). Women with the generalized form had associated myasthenia gravis.[73-77]

Atrophodermia Vermicularis and Other Follicular Hamartomas

Long known as a clinical curiosity, atrophodermia vermicularis, which produces a worm-eaten appearance of the skin of the cheeks, has been shown to be due to malformation of all portions of the skin (Fig. 37-20) and may be considered another form of peculiarly localized organoid nevus. Small sebaceous glands, incompletely formed hair follicles, and abnormal connective tissue characterize the histologic findings in this condition.[78] *Haber syndrome* is a rare familial condition characterized by rosacea-like facial dermatosis, keratotic plaques, and pitted scars. Follicular atrophy and budding of basaloid cells in connection with comedo-like follicles are seen in the facial lesions.[79-80]

TUMORS OF PERIFOLLICULAR CONNECTIVE TISSUE

The connective tissue component of the pilar apparatus gives rise to three different forms of neoplasms (Chapter 42), including perifollicular fibroma, fibrofolliculoma, and trichodiscoma.

Perifollicular Fibroma

Single or multiple firm papulonodular lesions of perifollicular fibroma appear most commonly over the face, head, and neck regions (see Fig. 42-5). Histologically, there is concentric proliferation of fibrous connective tissue surrounding small vellus-type follicles.[81-83]

Fibrofolliculoma

Fibrofolliculomas are usually multiple, firm papules 2 to 4 mm in diameter, some of which show a central hair. Histologically, in the center of each lesion is a cystic follicle containing keratinous material. The infundibular epithelium shows outward epithelial projections surrounded by proliferation of connective tissue fibers (Fig. 37-21).[84]

Trichodiscoma

The hair disk (haarscheibe) is a slowly adapting touch receptor in mammalian skin occurring in close vicinity to the hair follicles (see Fig. 2-37). It con-

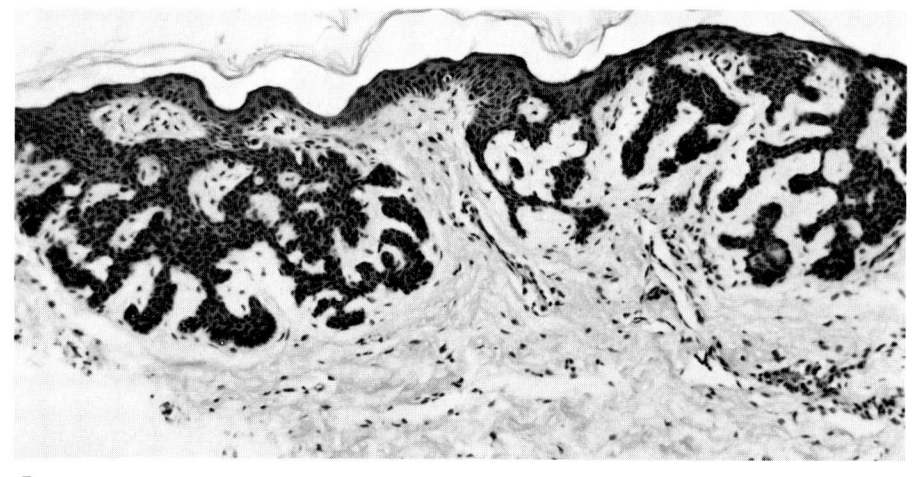
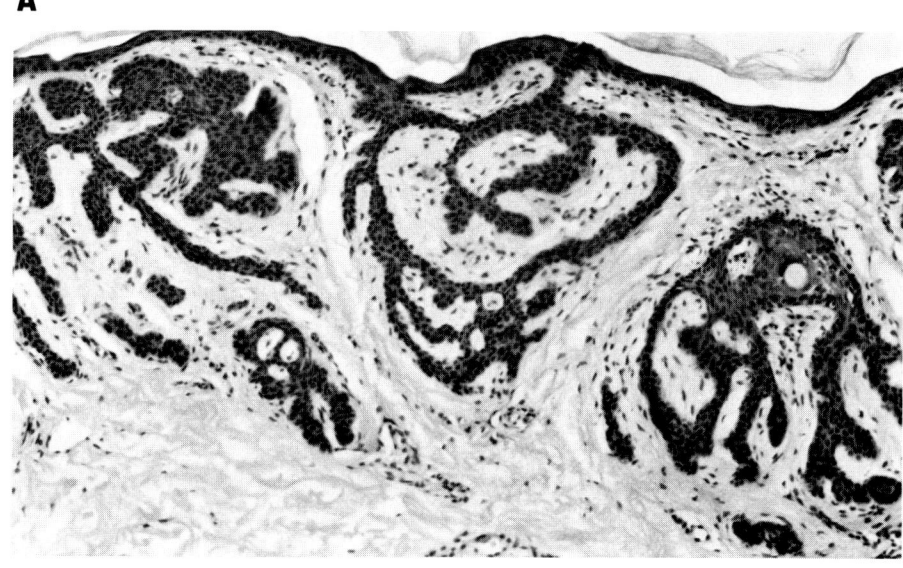

Figure 37–19.
Basaloid follicular hamartoma. **A** and **B.** Hair follicles are transformed into strands and thin septae of basaloid cells surrounded by fibrous stroma. H&E. X125.

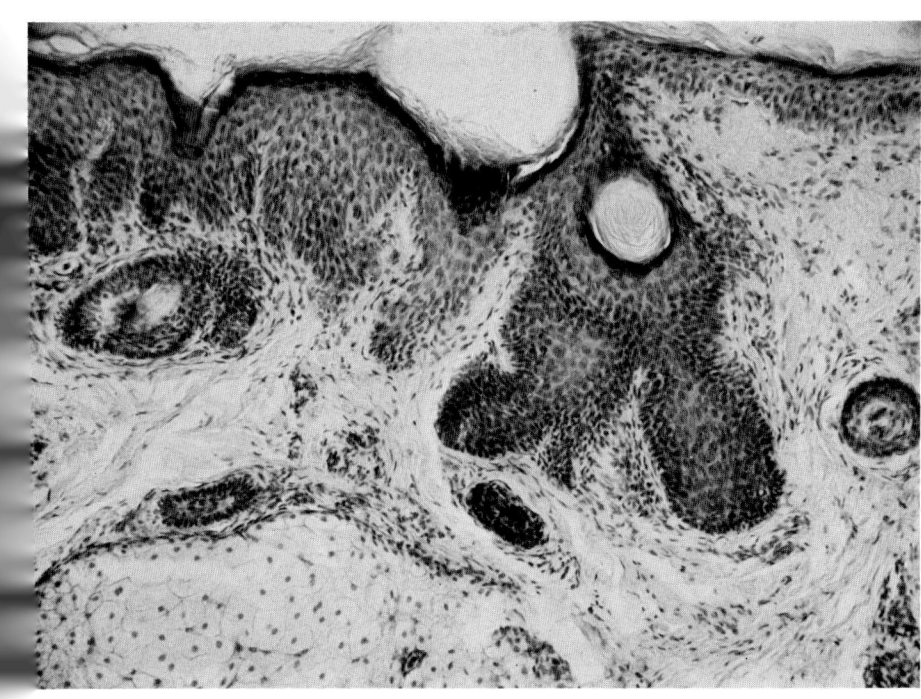

Figure 37–20.
Atrophodermia vermiculata. Minor malformation of epidermis, pilar apparatus, and dermis. H&E. X180.

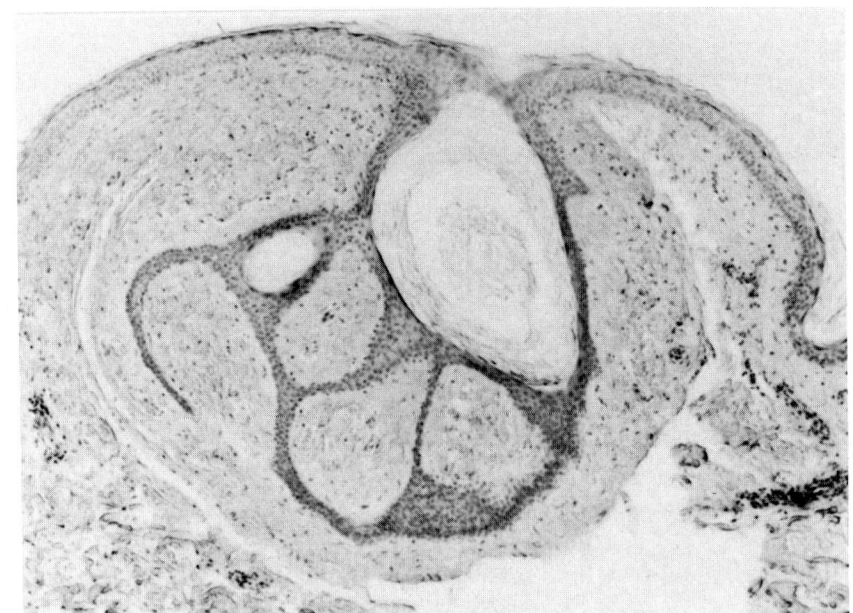

Figure 37–21.
Fibrofolliculoma (Birt–Hogg–Dubé). The upper part of the follicle is surrounded by a well-defined fibrous sheath tumor supporting a net-like proliferation of the upper outer root sheath. Follicle plugged with keratin. The sebaceous gland (not shown in this section) is displaced downward. H&E. X125. (From Weintraub and Pinkus. J Cutan Pathol 4:289, 1977.)

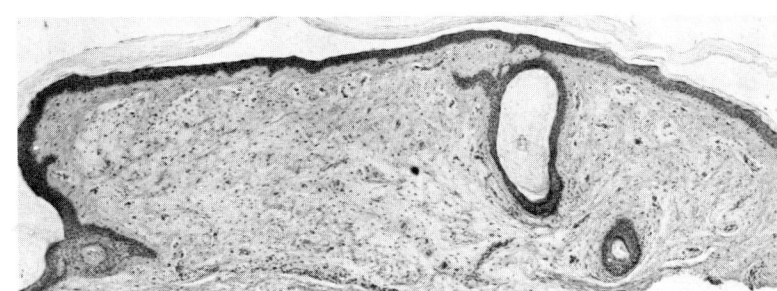

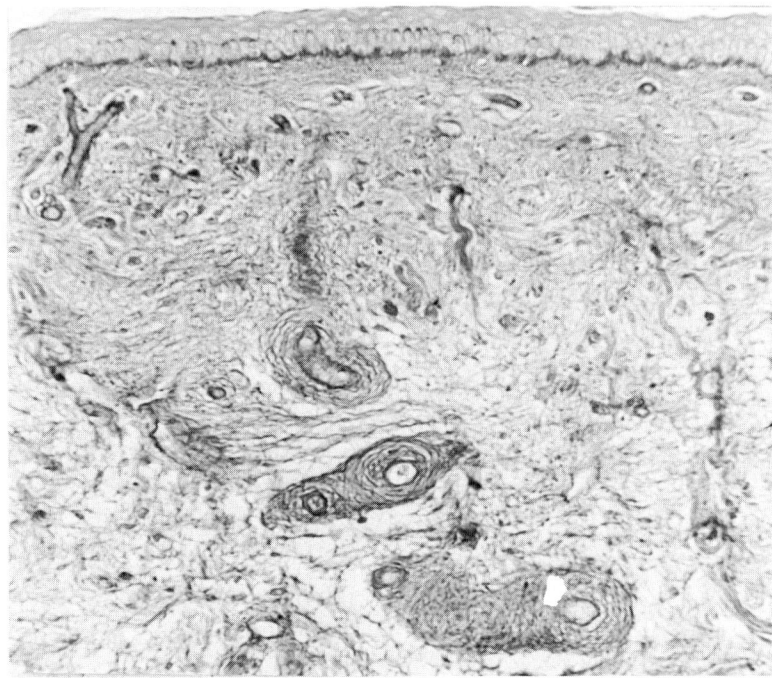

Figure 37–22.
Trichodiscoma. **A.** Picture includes the greater portion of a flat sessile papule. Oblique sections of two hair follicles, which open near the rim of the tumor. H&E. X30. **B.** Blood vessels enveloped in PAS-positive lamellae are embedded in ground-substance-rich connective tissue. Alcian blue–PAS. X180.

sists of a well-vascularized dermal connective tissue and thick myelinated nerves in contact with Merkel cells in the basal layer of epidermis. Neoplasia of the dermal pad of this organ is manifest as numerous, small, 1- to 3-mm papular lesions. Histologically (Fig. 37–22), the dome-shaped parafollicular lesion is made up of richly vascular connective tissue with abundant alcian-blue-reactive material.[85–87] Multiple fibrofolliculomas with trichodiscomas and acrochordons occur as Birt–Hogg–Dube syndrome.[88–94]

REFERENCES

1. Domonkos A: Wooly hair nevus. Arch Dermatol 85:568, 1962
2. Hutchinson PE: Woolly hair. Trans St Johns Hosp Dermatol Soc 60:160, 1974
3. Lantis SDH, Pepper MC: Woolly hair nevus: Two case reports and a discussion of unruly hair forms. Arch Dermatol 114:233, 1978
4. Gibbs RC, Berger RA: The straight hair nevus. Int J Dermatol 9:47, 1970
5. Downham TF, Chapel TA, Lupulescu AP: Straight hair nevus syndrome: A case report with scanning electron microscopic findings of hair morphology. Int J Dermatol 15:438, 1976
6. Mehregan AH, Coskey RJ: Pigmented nevi of sole: Report of two cases with histologic evidence of hair follicle formation. Arch Dermatol 106:886, 1972
7. Schnitzler ML: Dysembryoplasie pilaire circonscrite des paumes. Un cas familial. Bull Soc Fr Dermatol Syphiligr 80:323, 1973
8. Jackson CE, Callies OC, Krull EA, Mehregan AH: Hereditary hairy cutaneous malformation of palms and soles. Arch Dermatol 111:1146, 1975
9. Leppard B, Marks R: Comedone nevus: A report of nine cases. Trans St Johns Hosp Dermatol Soc 59:45, 1973
10. Nabai H, Mehregan AH: Nevus comedonicus: A review of the literature and report of twelve cases. Acta Dermatol Venereol 53:71, 1973
11. Beck MH, Dave VK: Extensive nevus comedonicus. Arch Dermatol 116:1048, 1980
12. Giam YC, Ong BH, Rajan VS: Nevus comedonicus in homozygous twins. Dermatologica 162:249, 1981
13. Aloi FG, Molinero A: Nevus comedonicus with epidermolytic hyperkeratosis. Dermatologica 174:140, 1987
14. Urry LE, Mellette JR Jr, Fitzpatrick JE: Nevus comedonicus with associated cutaneous calcification. J Assoc Mil Dermatol 14:30, 1988
15. Milton GP, DiGiovanna JJ, Peck GL: Treatment of nevus comedonicus with ammonium lactate lotion. J Am Acad Dermatol 20:324, 1989
16. Dudley K, Barr WG, Armin A, Massa MC: Nevus comedonicus in association with widespread, well-differentiated follicular tumors. J Am Acad Dermatol 15:1123, 1986
17. Engber PB: The nevus comedonicus syndrome: A case report with emphasis on associated internal manifestations. Int J Dermatol 17:745, 1978
18. Whyte HJ: Unilateral comedo nevus and cataract. Arch Dermatol 97:533, 1968
19. Rosen LB: A review and proposed new classification of benign acquired neoplasms with hair follicle differentiation. Am J Dermatopathol 12:496, 1990
20. Pinkus H, Sutton RL Jr: Trichofolliculoma. Arch Dermatol 91:46, 1965
21. Mehregan AH: Hair follicle tumors of the skin. J Cutan Pathol 12:189, 1985
22. Rahbari H, Mehregan AH, Pinkus H: Trichoadenoma of Nikolowski. J Cutan Pathol 4:90, 1977
23. Bonvalet D, Duterque M, Ducret J-P: Tricho-adenome de Nikolowski. Ann Dermatol Venereol 115:1186, 1988
24. Winer LH: The dilated pore, a trichoepithelioma. J Invest Dermatol 23:181, 1954
25. Klövekorn G, Klövekorn W, Plewig G, Pinkus H: Riesenpore und Haarscheidenakanthom: Klinische und histologische Diagnose. Hautarzt 34:209, 1983
26. Mehregan AH: Infundibular tumors of the skin. J Cutan Pathol 11:387, 1984
27. Mehregan AH, Brownstein MH: Pilar sheath acanthoma. Arch Dermatol 114:1495, 1978
28. Bhawan J: Pilar sheath acanthoma: A new benign follicular tumor. J Cutan Pathol 6:438, 1979
29. Smolle J, Kerl H: Das "pilar sheath acanthoma"—ein gutartiges follikuläres hamartom. Dermatologica 167:335, 1983
30. Mehregan AH, Butler JD: Tumor of follicular infundibulum. Arch Dermatol 83:924, 1961
31. Mehregan AH: Tumor of follicular infundibulum. Dermatologica 142:177, 1971
32. Casas JG, Palacios AM, Schroh RG, et al: Tumor del infundibulo folicular. Rev Argent Dermatol 62:223, 1981
33. Kossard S, Finley AG, Poyzer K, Kocsard E: Eruptive infundibulomas. A distinctive presentation of the tumor of follicular infundibulum. J Am Acad Dermatol 21:361, 1989
34. Schnitzler L, Civatte J, Robin F, DeMay CL: Tumeurs multiples de l'infundibulum pilaire avec degenerescence baso-cellulaire. A propos d'un cas. Ann Dermatol Venereol 114:551, 1987
35. Duperrat B, Mascaro JM: Une tumeur bénigne développée aux depens de l'acrotrichium ou partie intraépidermique du follicule pilaire: Porome folliculaire (acanthome folliculaire intraépidermique; acrotrichoma). Dermatologica 126:291, 1963
36. Mehregan AH: Inverted follicular keratosis. Arch Dermatol 89:229, 1964
37. Helwig EB: Inverted follicular keratosis. In Seminar on the Skin: Neoplasms and Dermatoses. American Society of Clinical Pathology, International Congress of Clinical Pathology, Washington, DC, Sept 1954.

Chicago, American Society of Clinical Pathology, 1955
38. Mehregan AH: Inverted follicular keratosis is a distinct follicular tumor. Am J Dermatopathol 5:467, 1983
39. Mehregan AH, Nadji M: Inverted follicular keratosis and verruca vulgaris: An investigation for the papilloma virus common antigen. J Cutan Pathol 11:99, 1984
40. Ackerman AB, Wade TR: Tricholemmoma. Am J Dermatopathol 2:207, 1980
41. Headington JT: Tricholemmoma: To be or not to be? Am J Dermatopathol 2:225, 1980
42. Mehregan AH, Medenica M, Whitney D, Kato I: A clear cell pilar sheath tumor of scalp: Case report. J Cutan Pathol 15:380, 1988
43. Starink TM, Meijer CJLM, Brownstein MH: The cutaneous pathology of Cowden's disease: New findings. J Cutan Pathol 12:83, 1985
44. Starink TM, Hausman R: The cutaneous pathology of facial lesions in Cowden's disease. J Cutan Pathol 11:331, 1984
45. Johnson BL, Kramer EM, Lavker RM: The keratotic tumors of Cowden's disease: An electromicroscopic study. J Cutan Pathol 14:291, 1987
46. Barax CN, Lebwohl M, Phelps RG: Multiple hamartoma syndrome. J Am Acad Dermatol 17:342, 1987
47. Shapiro SD, Lambert CW, Schwartz RA: Cowden's disease. A marker for malignancy. Int J Dermatol 27:232, 1988
48. Pujol RM, Ravella A, Noguera X, et al: Sindrome de hamartomas multiples. Med Cutan ILA 16:322, 1988
49. Ni C, Kimball GP, Craft JL, et al: Calcifying epithelioma: A clinicopathologic analysis of 67 cases with ultrastructural study of 2 cases. Int Ophthalmol Clin 22:63, 1982
50. Taaffe A, Wyatt EH, Bury HPR: Pilomatricoma (Malherbe). A clinical and histological survey of 78 cases. Int J Dermatol 27:477, 1988
51. Jacobson M, Ackerman AB: "Shadow" cells as clues to follicular differentiation. Am J Dermatopathol 9:51, 1987
52. Moll I, Heid H, Moll R: Cytokeratin analysis of pilomatrixoma: Changes in cytokeratin-type expression during differentiation. J Invest Dermatol 91:251, 1988
53. Moulin G, Bouchet B, DosSantos G: Les modifications anétodermiques du tégument au-dessus de tumeurs de Malherbe. Ann Derm Venereol 105:43, 1978
54. TarPorten HJ, Sharbaugh AH: Extruding pilomatricoma. Report of a case. Cutis 22:47, 1978
55. Wong WK, Somburanasin R, Wood MG: Eruptive multicentric pilomatricoma (calcifying epithelioma). Arch Dermatol 106:76, 1972
56. Harper PS: Calcifying epithelioma of Malherbe: Association with myotonic muscular dystrophy. Arch Dermatol 106:41, 1972
57. Chiaramonti A, Gilgore RS: Pilomatricomas associated with myotonic dystrophy. Arch Dermatol 114:1363, 1978
58. Aso M, Shimao S, Takahashi K: Pilomatricomas: Association with myotonic dystrophy. Dermatologica 162:197, 1981
59. Delfino M, Monfrecola G, Ayala F, et al: Multiple familiar pilomatricomas: A cutaneous marker for myotonic dystrophy. Dermatologica 170:128, 1985
60. Brownstein MH: The genodermatopathology of adnexal tumors. J Cutan Pathol 11:457, 1984
61. Brooke JD, Fitzpatrick JE, Golitz LE: Papillary mesenchymal bodies: A histologic finding useful in differentiating trichoepitheliomas from basal cell carcinomas. J Am Acad Dermatol 21:523, 1989
62. Long SA, Hurt MA, Santa Cruz DJ: Immature trichoepithelioma: Report of six cases. J Cutan Pathol 15:353, 1988
63. Tatnall FM, Wilson Jones E: Giant solitary trichoepitheliomas located in the perianal area: a report of three cases. Br J Dermatol 115:91, 1986
64. Winkelmann RK: Hair follicle tumors. In Orfanos CE, Montagna W, Stüttgen G (eds): Hair Research. Berlin: Springer-Verlag, 1981
65. Michaelsson G, Olsson E, Westermark P: The Rombo syndrome. A familial disorder with vermiculate atrophoderma, milia, hypotrichosis, trichoepitheliomas, basal cell carcinomas and peripheral vasodilation with cyanosis. Acta Derm Venereol 61:497, 1981
66. Cramer M: Trichoepithelioma multiplex and dystrophia unguis congenita: A new syndrome. Acta Derm Venereol 61:364, 1981
67. Brownstein MH, Shapiro L: Desmoplastic trichoepithelioma. Cancer 40:2979, 1977
68. MacDonald DM, Wilson-Jones E, Marks R: Sclerosing epithelial hamartoma. Clin Exp Dermatol 2:153, 1977
69. Brownstein MH, Starink TM: Desmoplastic trichoepithelioma and intradermal nevus: A combined malformation. J Am Acad Dermatol 17:489, 1987
70. Fukui Y, Ono H, Umemura T, Hasegawa M: A combined case of desmoplastic trichoepithelioma and nevus cell nevus. J Dermatol (Tokyo) 17:506, 1990
71. Mehregan AH, Baker S: Basaloid follicular hamartoma. Report of three cases with localized and systematized unilateral lesions. J Cutan Pathol 12:55, 1985
72. Geffner RE, Goslen JB, Santa Cruz DJ: Linear and dermatomal trichoepitheliomas. J Am Acad Dermatol 14:927, 1986
73. Brown AC, Crounse RG, Winkelmann RK: Generalized hair follicle hamartoma. Associated with alopecia, aminoaciduria and myasthenia gravis. Arch Dermatol 99:478, 1969
74. Ridley CM, Smith N: Generalized hair follicle hamartoma associated with alopecia and myasthenia gravis: Report of a second case. Clin Exp Dermatol 6:283, 1981
75. Starink TM, Lane EB, Meijer CJL: Generalized trichoepitheliomas with alopecia and myasthenia gravis: Clinicopathologic and immunohistochemical study and comparison with classic desmoplastic trichoepithelioma. J Am Acad Dermatol 15:1104, 1986
76. Weltfriend S, David M, Ginzburg A, Sandbank M:

Generalized hair follicle hamartoma: The third case report in association with myasthenia gravis. Am J Dermatopathol 9:428, 1987
77. Miyakawa S, Araki Y, Sugawara M: Generalized trichoepitheliomas with alopecia and myasthenia gravis. J Am Acad Dermatol 19:361, 1988
78. Rozum TL, Mehregan AH, Johnson SAM: Folliculitis ulerythematosa reticulata. Arch Dermatol 106:388, 1972
79. Sanderson KV, Wilson HTH: Haber's syndrome: Familial rosacea-like eruption with intraepidermal epithelioma. Br J Dermatol 77:1, 1965
80. Seiji M, Otaki N: Haber's syndrome. Familial rosacea-like dermatosis with keratotic plaques and pitted scars. Arch Dermatol 103:452, 1971
81. Zackheim HS, Pinkus H: Perifollicular fibromas. Arch Dermatol 82:913, 1960
82. Cramer HJ: Multiple perifollikuläre Fibrome. Hautarzt 19:228, 1968
83. Freeman RG, Chernosky ME: Perifollicular fibroma. Arch Dermatol 100:66, 1969
84. Starink TM, Brownstein MH: Fibrofolliculoma: Solitary and multiple types. J Am Acad Dermatol 17:493, 1987
85. Pinkus H, Coskey R, Burgess GH: Trichodiscoma. Benign tumor related to haarscheibe (hair disk). J Invest Dermatol 63:212, 1974
86. Starink TM, Kisch LS, Meijer CJLM: Familial multiple trichodiscomas. A clinicopathologic study. Arch Dermatol 121:888, 1985
87. Balus L, Crovato F, Breathnach AS: Familial multiple trichodiscomas. J Am Acad Dermatol 15:603, 1986
88. Fujita WH, Barr RJ, Headley JI: Multiple fibrofolliculomas with trichodiscomas and acrochordons. Arch Dermatol 117:32, 1981
89. Balus L, Fazio M, Sacerdoti G, et al: Fibrofolliculomes, trichodiscomes et acrochordons. Syndrome de Birt–Hogg–Dubé. Ann Dermatol Venereol 110:601, 1983
90. Iranzo P, Martin E, Del Olmo JA, Mascaro JM: El sindrome de Birt–Hogg–Dube como forma de expresion de la esclerosis tuberosa. A proposito de dos observaciones personales en dos hermanas. Med Cutan ILA 13:145, 1985
91. Moreno A, Puig L, De Moragas JM: Multiple fibrofolliculomas and trichodiscomas. Dermatologica 171:338, 1985
92. Ubogy-Rainey Z, James WD, Lupton GP, Rodman OG: Fibrofolliculomas, trichodiscomas, and acrochordons: The Birt–Hogg–Dube syndrome J Am Acad Dermatol 16:452, 1987
93. Curley RK, Mortimer PS, Marsden RA: Hereditary multiple fibrofolliculomas: Syndrome of Birt, Hogg and Dube. Br J Dermatol 119 (Suppl 33):67, 1988
94. Bayrou O, Blanc F, Moulonguet I, et al: Syndrome de Birt–Hogg–Dube. Fibrofolliculomes, trichodiscomes et acrochordons. Ann Dermatol Venereol 117:37, 1990

38

CYSTS RELATED TO THE ADNEXA

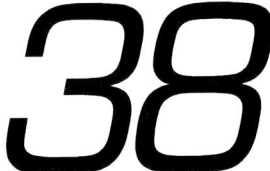

Cysts are properly considered simple benign neoplasms, even though they increase in size more through accumulation of keratinous or fluid contents than through proliferation of the cells in their walls and may be morphologically indistinguishable from retention cysts in some cases. One may introduce a classification (Fig. 38–1) based, as we have done in most of this section, on histologic resemblance rather than on origin.[1] There are two principle types of cutaneous cysts, each with two subdivisions. One type has glandular epithelium in its wall; the other has keratinizing lining. A few cysts are combinations of the two types.

GLANDULAR CYSTS

Hidrocystomas

Cysts having two concentric layers of nonkeratinizing epithelium and containing fluid (Fig. 38–2) can be assumed to be related to sweat glands. When the wall is very thin, one may have to examine it closely at high power in order to recognize the double row of flat nuclei. Tangential sectioning, on the other hand, may produce the false impression of multilayered stratification.[2] Classification as eccrine or apocrine may be arbitrary or impossible in some cases. The presence of columnar, or at least bulging, luminal cells speaks for apocrine derivation, which is made certain if intracellular lipid or pigmented granules can be demonstrated.[3,4] Similarly, Moll's gland cyst of the eyelid consists mainly of two rows of small cuboidal ductal cells. Electron microscopy, however, shows secretory cells that contain large lamellar inclusions that are PAS positive and diastase resistant.[5]

Mucinous Syringometaplasia

The clinical manifestation is a keratotic nodule resembling plantar verruca vulgaris. Histologically, there is a central sinuslike dilated eccrine duct lined in the superficial portion by a layer of stratified squamous epithelium. Deeper parts are branching and the glandular epithelium shows marked mucinous metaplasia with many goblet cells (Fig. 38–3).[6–8]

Steatocystoma Multiplex

Sebaceous cysts, in spite of the widespread use of the name, are exceedingly rare. The only type of cyst that definitely has sebaceous cells and lobules in its wall is steatocystoma multiplex (Fig. 38–4).[9] This is characterized by the appearance of single (*steatocystoma simplex*)[10] or numerous small intracutaneous cystic lesions usually over the trunk and occasionally elsewhere. Familial occurrences in several gen-

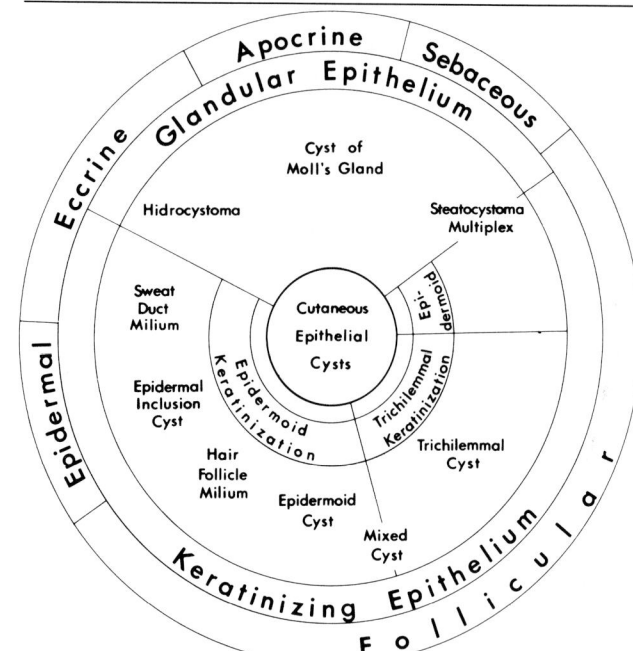

Figure 38–1.
Diagram showing diagnostic names of cutaneous epithelial cysts in relation to type of maturation of their epithelium. There is overlap between glandular and keratinizing maturation in eccrine and pilosebaceous cysts. In keratinizing group, epidermoid and trichilemmal types of maturation occur.

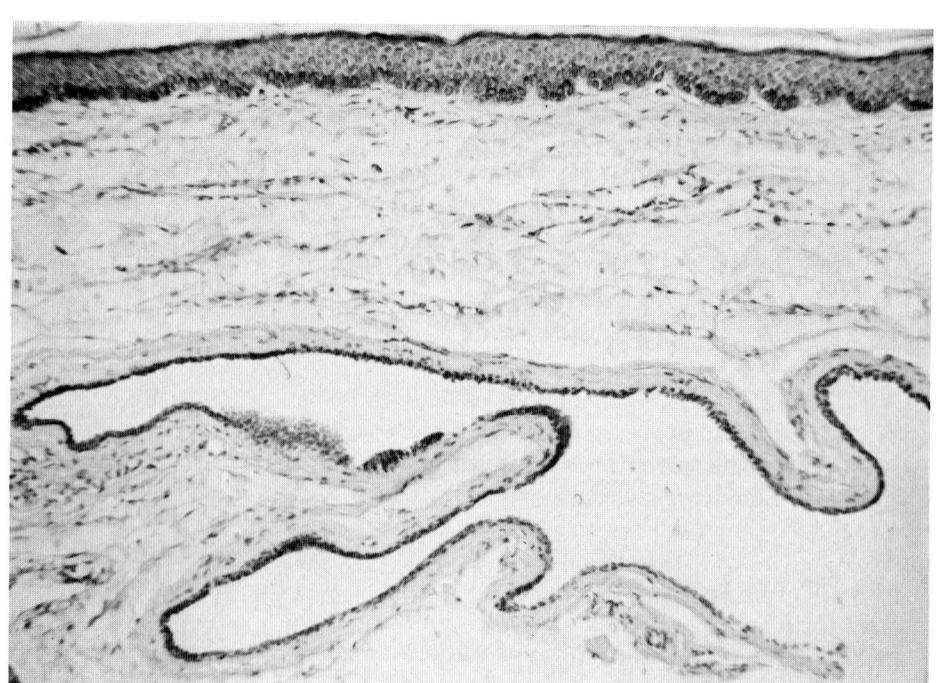

Figure 38–2.
Eccrine hidrocystoma. Collapse of the ruptured cyst gives the false impression of papilliferous projection of the wall, which is lined by two rows of flat or cuboid cells. H&E. X135.

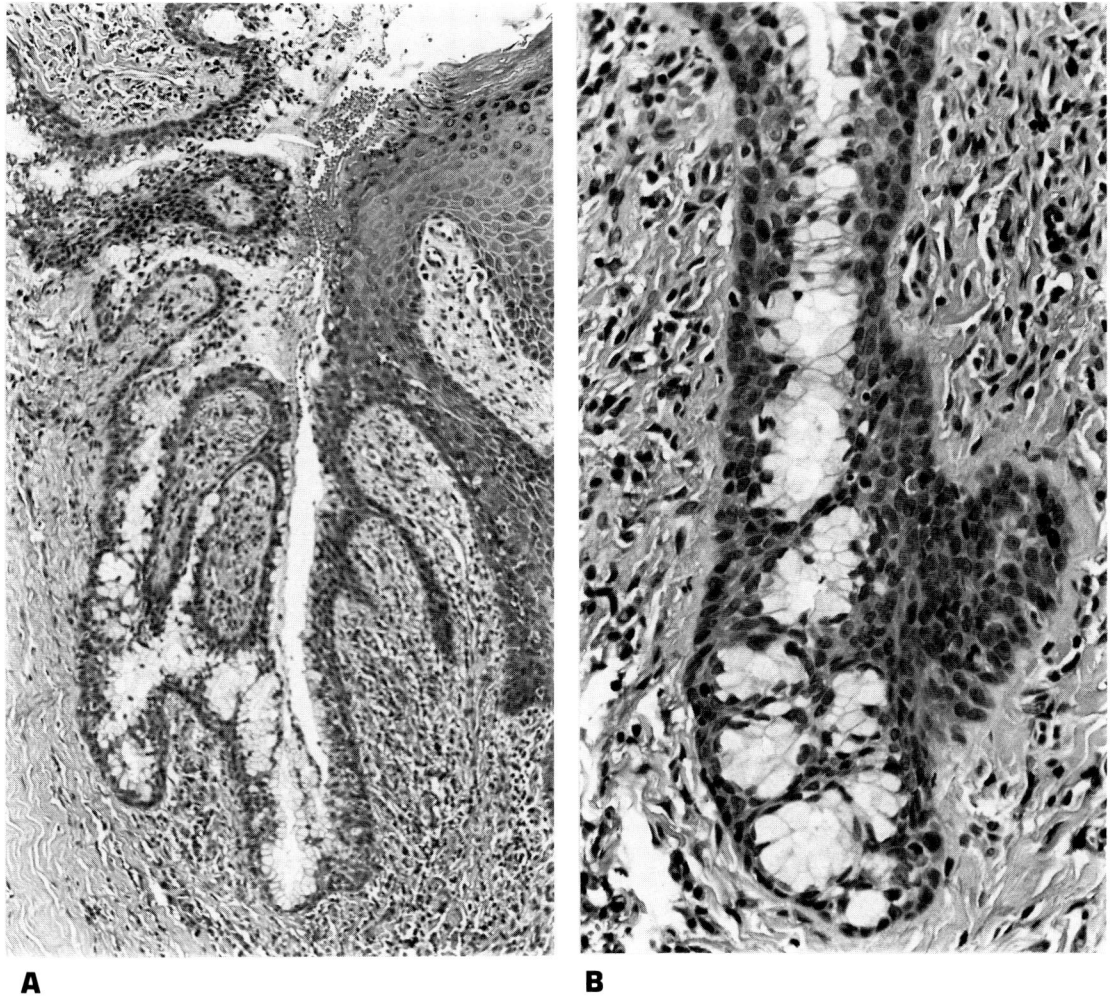

Figure 38–3.
Mucinous syringometaplasia. **A.** *A sinuslike dilated eccrine duct in part lined with mucin containing cells. H&E, X125.* **B.** *Proliferation and mucinous metaplasia of eccrine ductal epithelium. H&E. X400.*

erations suggest an autosomal dominant mode of inheritance.[11] In these lesions, large portions of the cyst lining consist of thin, stratified, and partly keratinizing epithelium, perhaps related to the sebaceous duct.[12] Sebaceous lobules are present in connection or form a portion of the cyst wall. Since, however, these cysts often contain hairs and must, therefore, have hair roots in their makeup, they are actually pilosebaceous cysts, and perhaps simple dermoids.

KERATINOUS CYSTS

All keratinous cysts are lined by stratified epithelium, which may be thin or thick. They keratinize either with formation of keratohyalin, forming a relatively loosely lamellated horny material resembling that of epidermis, or without keratohyalin, in which case the contents are dense and may look amorphous in H&E sections but can be shown to

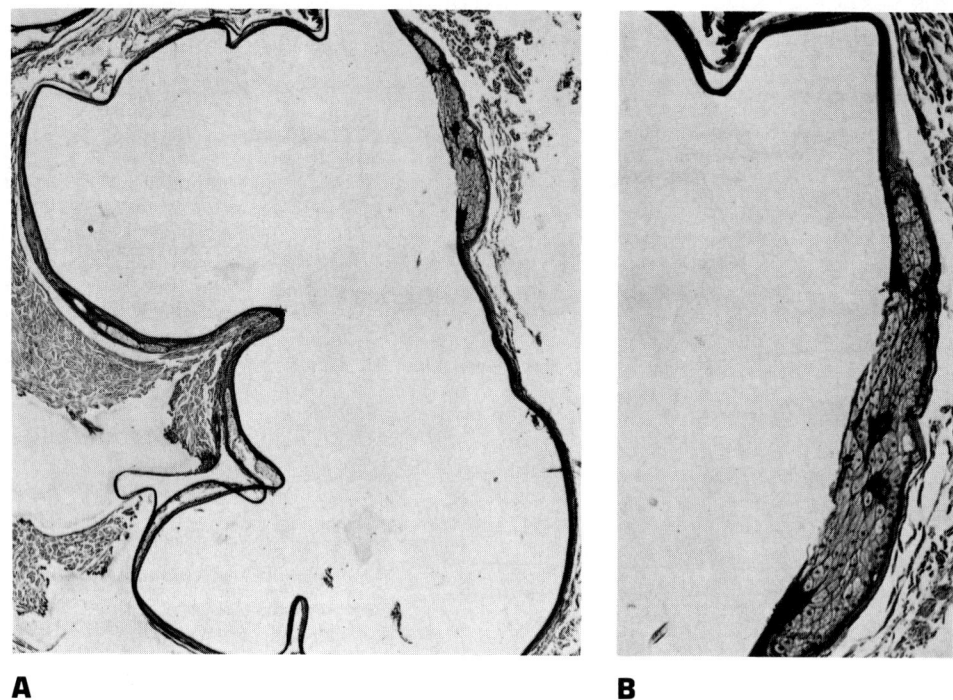

Figure 38—4.
Steatocystoma multiplex. The contents of the cyst consisting of a soft mixture of keratinous flakes and sebum have disappeared during preparation of the paraffin sections. **A.** H&E. X27. **B.** Detail of part of wall in which sebaceous cells border lumen. Rest of cyst wall consists of stratified epithelium. H&E. X73.

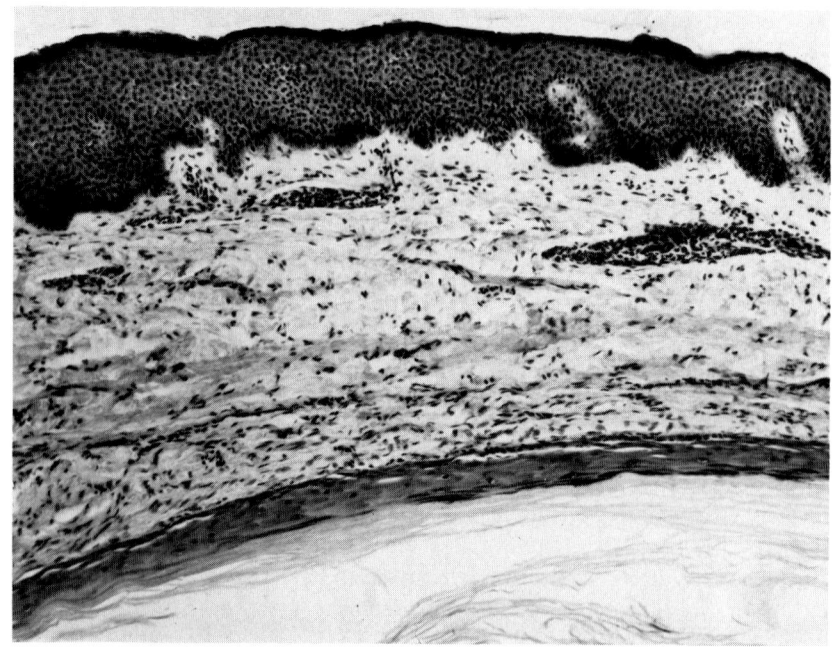

Figure 38—5.
Part of wall of an epidermoid cyst in comparison with epidermis. Cyst consists of flat basal and squamous cells with thin granular layer and flaky epidermoid keratin. H&E. X135.

resemble trichilemmal keratin by a variety of other staining procedures.

Epidermoid Cysts

Because the epidermal type of keratinization is encountered in several extraepidermal tissues in the skin (acrosyringium, follicular infundibulum, sebaceous duct) and outside the skin (esophagus, cervix uteri), and can be induced in many other epithelia (squamous metaplasia), it appears wise not to speculate about the origin of cysts containing this type of maturation and to call them epidermoid cysts rather than epidermal cysts.[13] Actually cysts of this type may originate in occluded hair follicles, in outer root sheath epithelium (facial milia), in obstructed eccrine ducts (retention milia in blistering dermatoses). A few perhaps are secondary to trauma and implantation of epidermis (epidermoid inclusion cyst). Epidermoid cysts of sole or of subungual location may be of this variety.[14-16]

The only basis for diagnosing an epidermoid cyst (Fig. 38–5) is the presence of stratified epithelium with a well-developed and (at least almost) continuous layer of flattened cells containing keratohyalin granules and transforming into soft epidermal-type horny material. Epidermoid cysts may contain considerable melanin in heavily pigmented individuals. Progressive darkening of cysts without increase of general skin color has been reported as a sign of hemochromatosis.[17]

Eruptive Vellus Hair Cysts

Hyperpigmented papular eruption over the chest wall or extremities of children and young adults is the clinical manifestation of eruptive vellus hair cysts.[18-22] Congenital and familial cases have also been reported.[23-25] Cystic dilated and thin-walled vellus hair follicles are present in middermis containing keratinous material and thin hair shafts. Breakdown of the cyst wall gives rise to foreign-body granuloma. Some lesions regress spontaneously (Fig. 38–6).

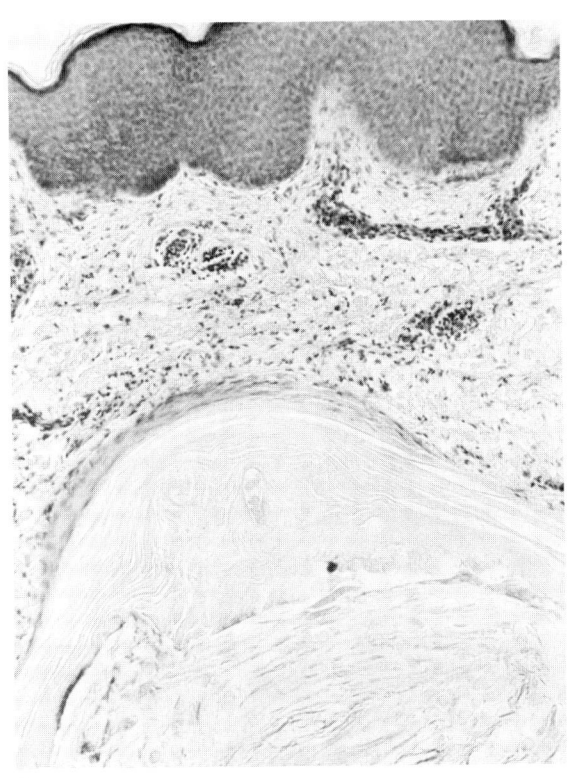

A

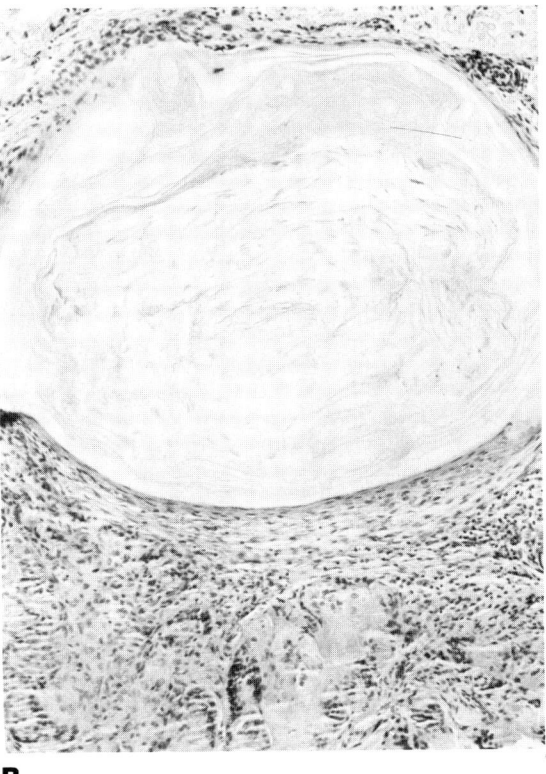

B

Figure 38–6.
Eruptive vellus hair cyst is a follicular retention cyst. **A.** Cross section of coiled-up vellus hair in cyst. **B.** Foreign-body granuloma below cyst. H&E. X125.

Pigmented Follicular Cyst

The pigmented follicular cyst is usually a single lesion often diagnosed as a pigmented nevus.[26] The cyst wall is made up of infundibular epithelium. The content is soft keratin and many coarse and pigmented hair shafts. One or more growing hair follicles may be associated with the cyst wall (Fig. 38–7).[27]

Trichilemmal Cysts

The other type of keratinous cyst has been recognized as having its prototype in the outer root sheath (trichilemma) at the level of the follicular isthmus and in the sac surrounding the lower end of the catagen and telogen hair (see Fig. 2–32) that produces the hair club.[28] Thus, trichilemmal cyst is the new term to replace the misnomer "sebaceous cyst." Trichilemmal cysts (Fig. 38–8) are common, most frequently encountered on the scalp, and have a tough stratified lining resting on a well-developed, but usually not thick, basement membrane that permits one to shell them out without breaking the wall. Histologically, in young cysts, the epithelium consists of large, rather pale-staining cells that do not flatten but become more bulky toward the inside. The large vesicular nucleus fades, and the cell joins

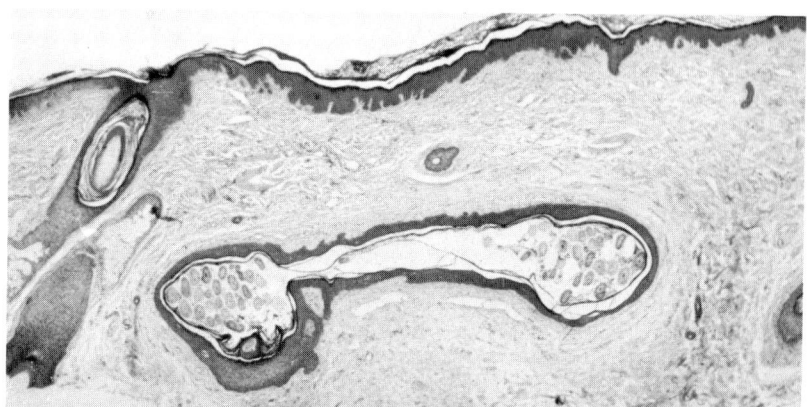

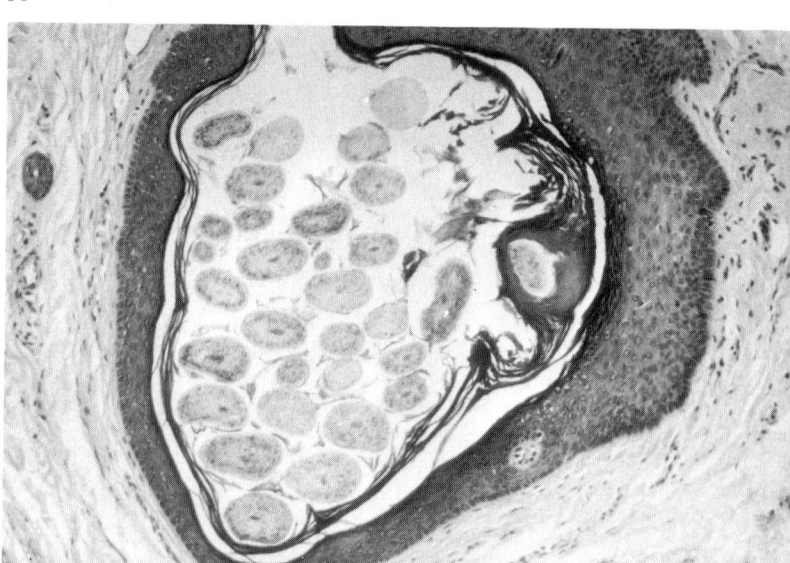

Figure 38–7.
Pigmented follicular cyst. Cyst lined with follicular epithelium contains many pigmented hairs. **A.** H&E. X60. **B.** H&E. X135. (From Mehregan and Medenica. J Cutan Pathol 9:423, 1982.)

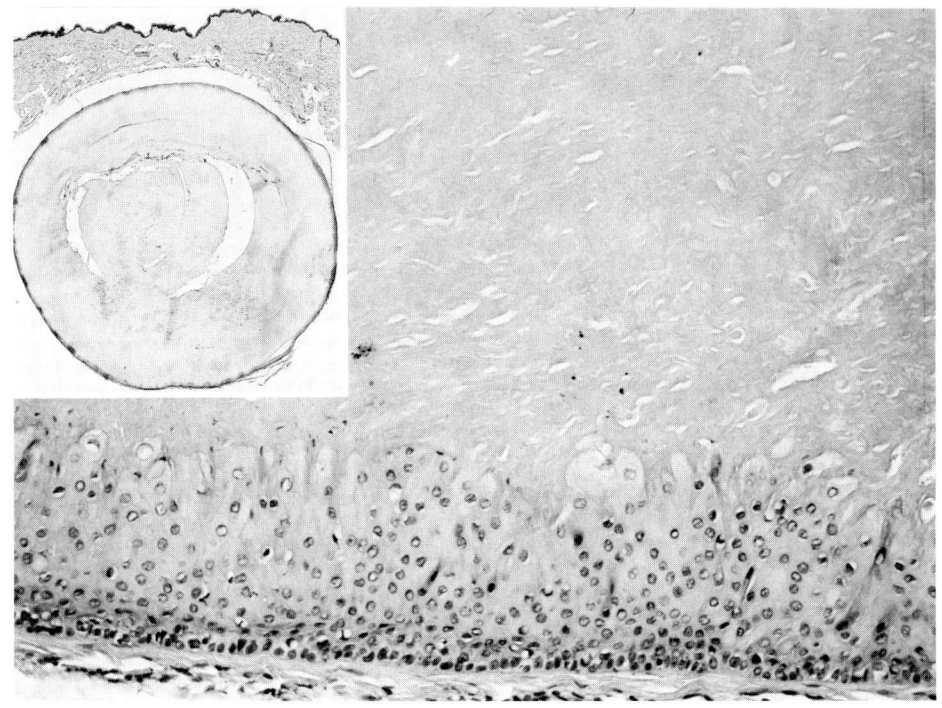

Figure 38–8.
Trichilemmal cyst. Inset shows the entire cyst in typical location in the deep dermis and below. The main picture shows part of the thick wall consisting of stratified epithelium. The cells get larger toward the lumen and fade individually into the dense keratinized mass without formation of keratohyalin. A few remnants of nuclei survive. Compare with Figure 2–32, cross section of catagen hair club. H&E. X250. Inset H&E. X5.

the dense central mass of keratin. Keratohyalin usually is absent but may occur in occasional cells. There is a characteristic interlocking of nucleated and keratinized cells similar to that seen in the formation of the club hair. Cell boundaries of complicated pattern can be demonstrated by PAS stain. In older cysts, the epithelium may be flattened and the boundary between wall and contents more smooth. The dense keratin often breaks down into granular masses and may calcify. If the wall ruptures, a foreign-body-type granuloma may replace it partly or completely. Cutaneous horn that is made up of dense keratotic material with the base showing trichilemmal keratinization (trichilemmal horn) may represent a trichilemmal cyst that has opened to the surface and should be differentiated from a horn developing over a trichilemmoma.[29,30] A cyst with a surface opening lined with infundibular epithelium that changes abruptly to trichilemmal keratinization is reported as *hybrid cyst*[31] (Fig. 38–9).

Proliferating Trichilemmal Cyst (Pilar Tumor)

Although we have listed the proliferating trichilemmal cyst in the follicular neoplasms classification, we have elected to discuss it in this chapter. We have observed histologic indication that inflammation due to rupture of the wall of a trichilemmal cyst sets into motion a new proliferative cycle leading to the formation of a multilobulated lesion. Proliferating trichilemmal lesions may also develop in the skin of individuals with multiple and hereditary trichilemmal cysts.[32,33]

Proliferating trichilemmal cysts or pilar tumors are usually large intracutaneous multilobulated nodules or exophytic lesions located over the head and neck areas.[34] Large infiltrative lesions may show hair loss, superficial ulceration, and crusting. Histologically (Fig. 38–10), massive proliferation of follicular sheath epithelium occupies a major portion of the dermis and extends into the subcutaneous fat tissue. There are many central areas of trichilemmal keratinization and keratin cyst formation.[35,36] Some areas may consist of proliferating, glycogen-laden clear cells resembling the outer root sheath epithelium. Abnormally large cells with hyperchromatic nuclei may give the impression of dysplasia.[37] PAS-positive basement membrane is preserved in many areas. Fibrovascular proliferation and foci of foreign-body granuloma are present. While the majority of cases follow a benign course, a

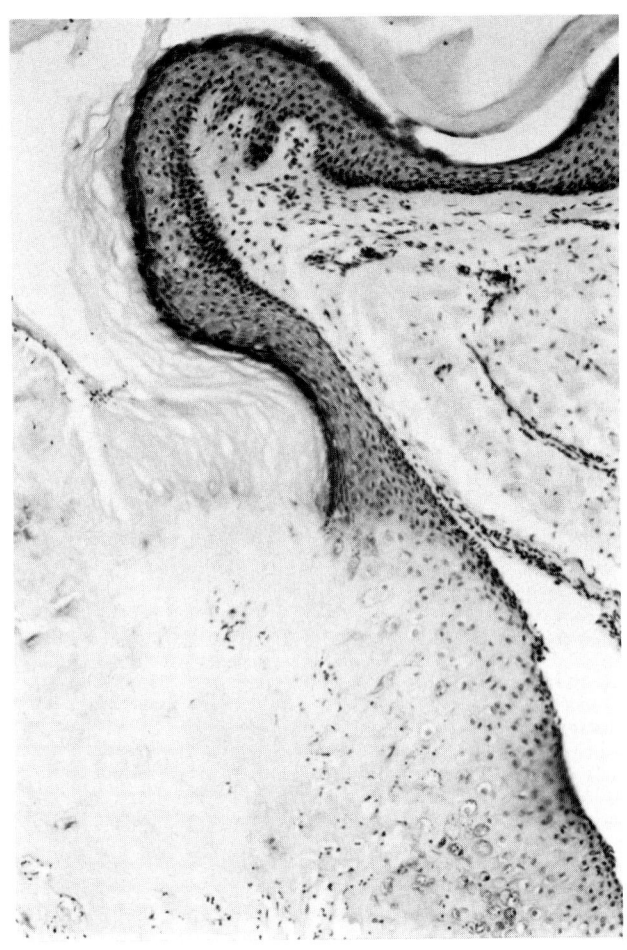

Figure 38-9.
Hybrid cyst. Abrupt transformation from the infundibular to trichilemmal keratinization. H&E. X125.

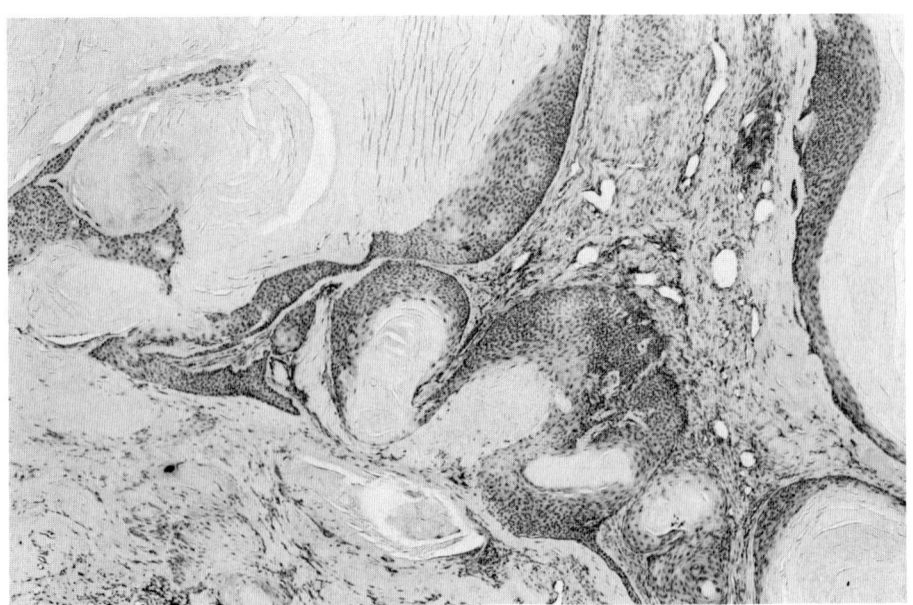

Figure 38-10.
Proliferating trichilemmal cyst. Part of large tumor is shown. Secondary cysts form in wall of larger ones, break down, and disappear with foreign-body reaction. H&E. X54.

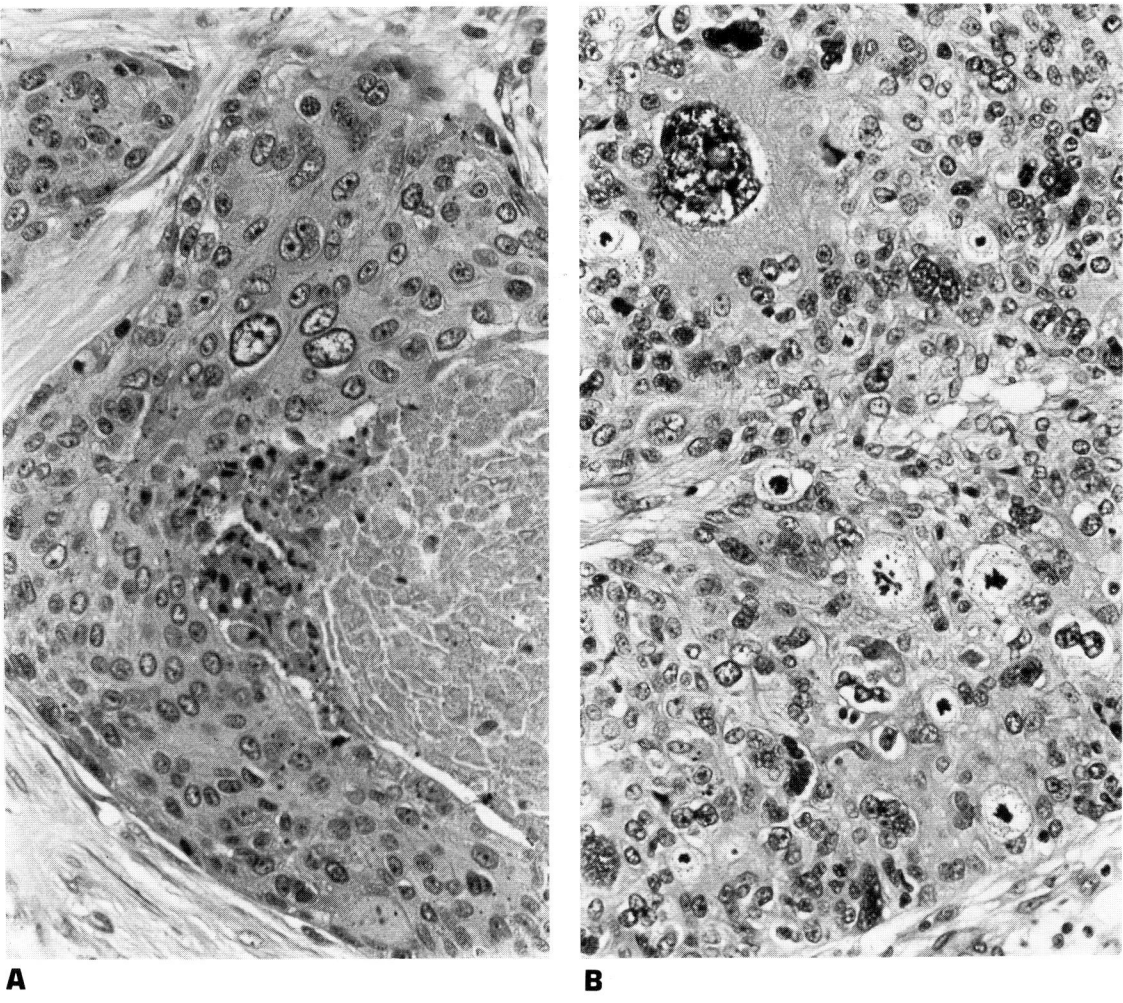

Figure 38–11.
Malignant proliferating trichilemmal cyst (pilar tumor). H&E. X400.

limited number of cases with malignant pilar tumors have been reported (Fig. 38–11).[38,39]

Other Types

True *dermoid cysts* (Fig. 38–12) usually localized in the subcutis[40] are rarely encountered in dermatologic practice. We mentioned that steatocystoma multiplex may be of this type. Whether the formation of a well-developed papillary body with epithelial ridges and vascular papillae constitutes evidence of dermoid remains questionable. Small hair follicles, sebaceous lobules, and, occasionally, sweat ducts may be present in the cyst wall.

Solitary and multilobulated cystic lesions in the lower extremities of women in their second or third decades of life occur in deep dermis of subcutaneous fat tissue lined by a simple columnar ciliated epithelium and have been described as *cutaneous ciliated cysts* (Fig. 38–13).[41–45] An embryonal developmental defect of the male genitalia is *median raphe cysts* near the glans penis. The cystic spaces are lined by pseudostratified columnar epithelium of one to-four cells in thickness.[46,47] Sinuses containing intes-

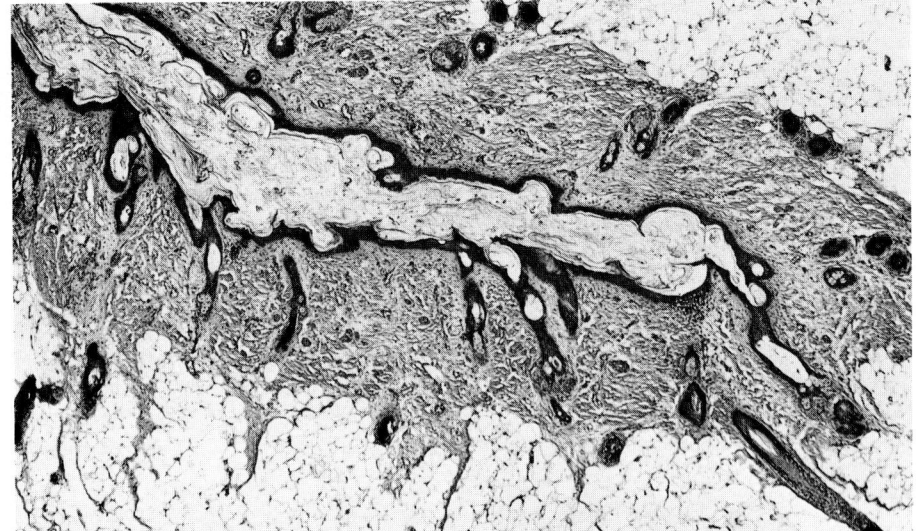

Figure 38–12.
Small dermoid cyst of ovary. The lining of the cyst consists of epidermis-like epithelium from which cutaneous adnexa grow into the surrounding dermis and fat tissue. H&E. X5.

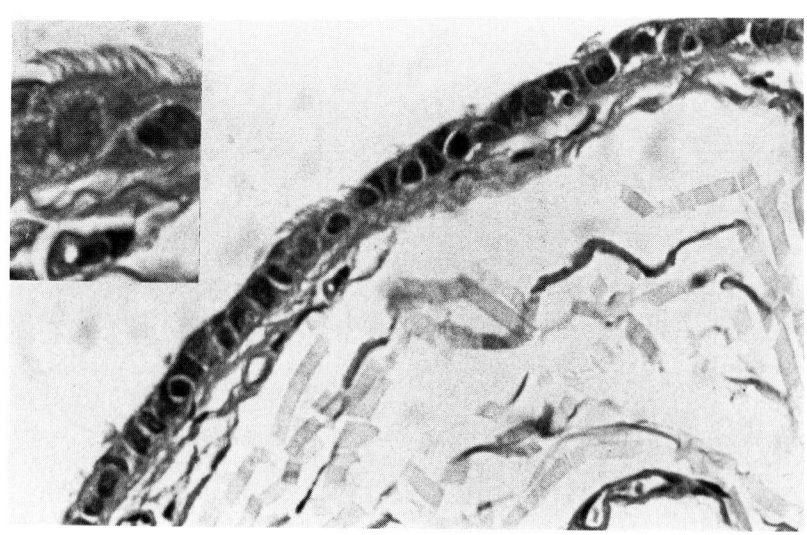

Figure 38–13.
Cutaneous ciliated cyst. A cyst lined with a simple layer of columnar ciliated epithelium. H&E. X400. Inset H&E. X1100.

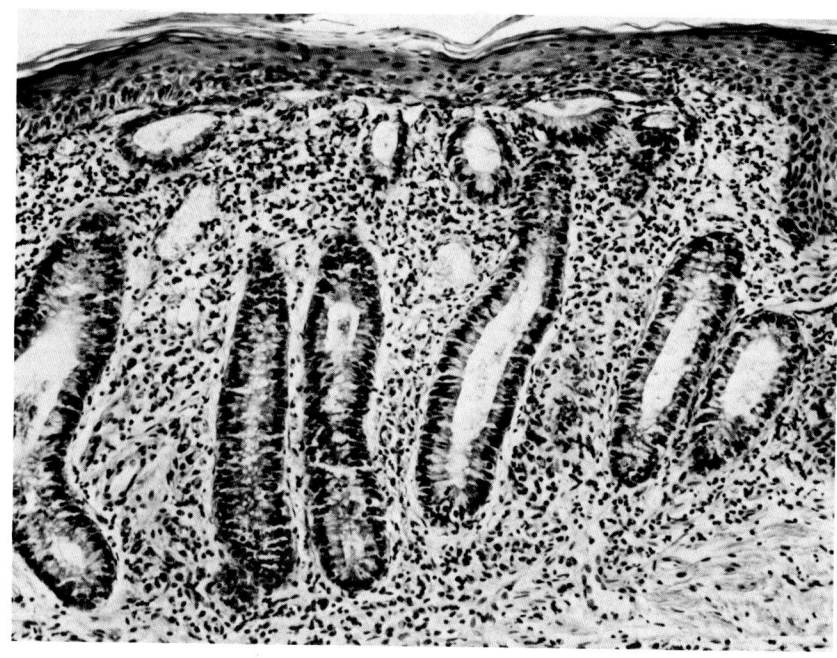

Figure 38–14.
Omphaloenteric polyp. Glandlike structures lined with intestinal crypt epithelium beneath epidermoid surface in an umbilical polyp. H&E. X150.

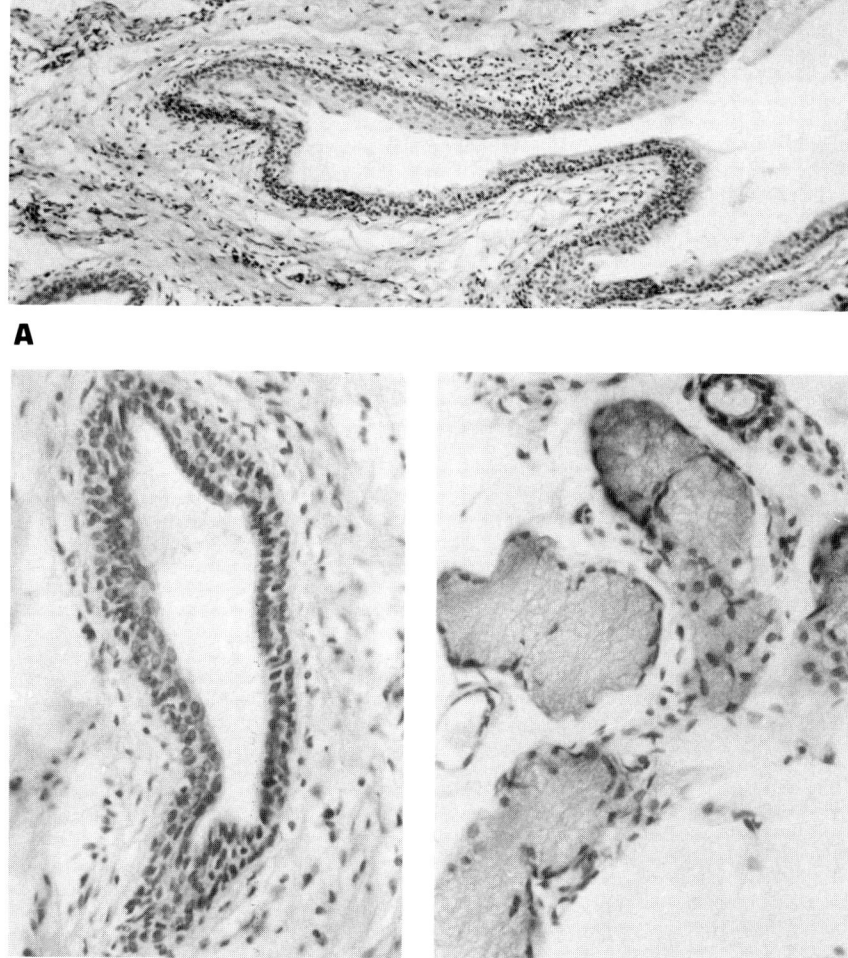

Figure 38–15.
Bronchogenic cyst. Pseudostratified epithelium and mucous cells. H&E. **A.** X125. **B.** and **C.** X250.

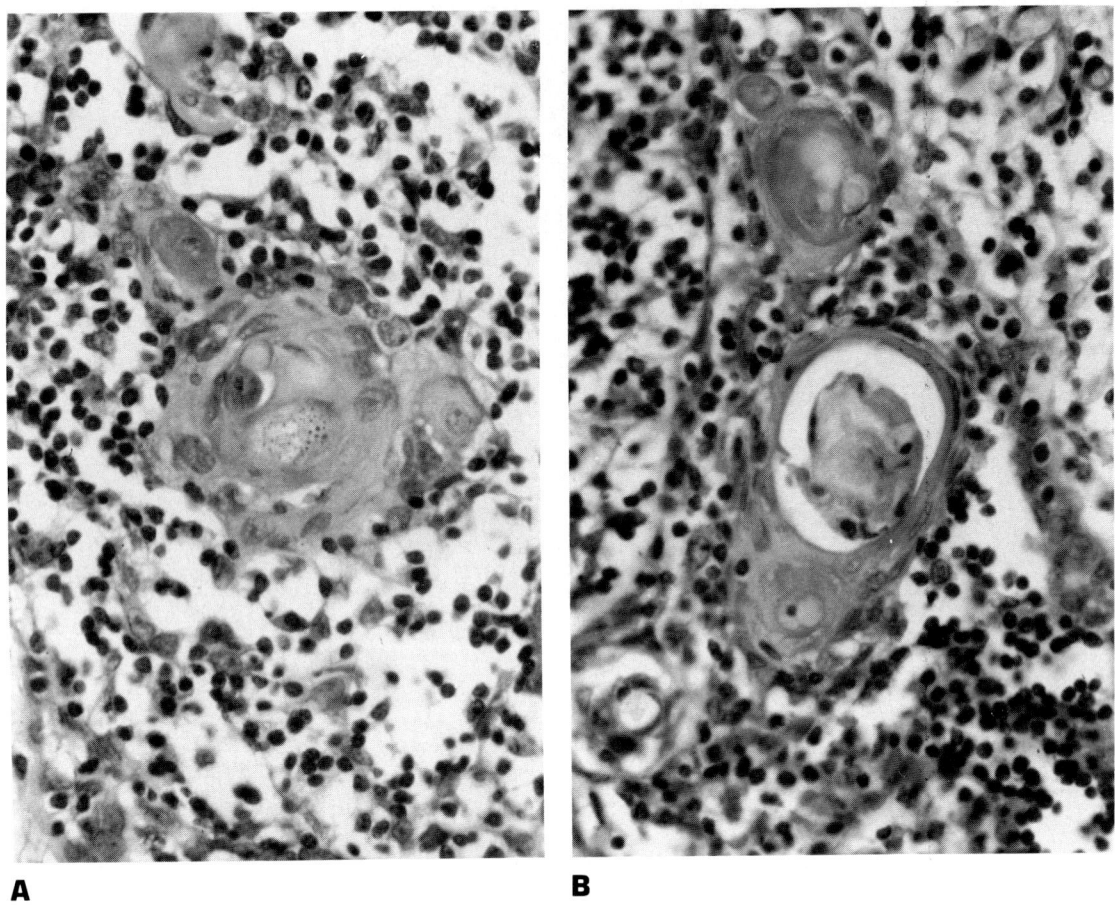

Figure 38—16.
Thymic cyst is made up of thymic tissue and Hassall's corpuscles. H&E. X400.

tinal mucosa (Fig. 38–14) occur in the umbilicus as remnants of the omphaloenteric canal. Over the manubrium, one encounters occasional *bronchogenic cysts* (Fig. 38–15), which are lined with pseudostratified, ciliated epithelium containing goblet cells.[48,49] Smooth muscle, seromucous glands and, rarely, lymphoid nodules and cartilage may be present. Branchial cleft cyst shows a lining of stratified squamous epithelium and often lymphoid structures.[50–52] *Thymic cysts* are rare and are histologically characterized by the presence of thymic tissue with Hassall's corpuscles in the cyst wall (Fig. 38–16).[53,54] The occurrence of endometriosis in the skin should also be mentioned.[55]

REFERENCES

1. Bode U, Plewig G: Klassifikation follikularer Zysten: Epidermalzysten einschliesslich Sebocystomatosis Gunther, Steatocystoma multiplex und Trichilemmalzysten. Hautarzt 31:1, 1980
2. Smith JD, Chernosky ME: Hidrocystomas. Arch Dermatol 108:676, 1973
3. Mehregan AH: Apocrine cystadenoma. Arch Dermatol 90:274, 1964
4. Fukuda M, Kato H, Hamada T: Apocrine hidrocystoma. A report of five cases and review of the Japanese literature. J Dermatol Tokyo 16:315, 1989
5. Hashimoto K, Zagula-Mally ZW, Youngberg G, Leicht S: Electron microscopic studies of Moll's gland cyst. J Cutan Pathol 14:23, 1987
6. King DT, Barr RJ: Syringometaplasia:Mucinous and squamous variants. J Cutan Pathol 6:284, 1979
7. Mehregan AH: Mucinous syringometaplasia. Arch Dermatol 116:988, 1980
8. Scully K, Assaad D: Mucinous syringometaplasia. J Am Acad Dermatol 11:503, 1984
9. Holmes R, Black MM: Steatocystoma multiplex with unusually prominent cysts on the face. Br J Dermatol 102:711, 1980

10. Brownstein MH: Steatocystoma simplex: A solitary steatocystoma. Arch Dermatol 118:409, 1982
11. Feinstein A, Trau H, Movshovitz M, Schewach-Millet M: Steatocystoma multiplex. Cutis 31:425, 1983
12. Taniguchi S, Hirone T: Light and electron microscopic studies of steatocystoma multiplex. In Orfanos CE, Montagna W, Stüttgen G (eds): Hair Research. Berlin: Springer-Verlag, 1981
13. Pinkus H: Epidermoid cysts or epidermal inclusion cysts? Arch Dermatol 111:130, 1975
14. Lemont H: Keratinous cysts of the foot: A histologic review of 120 cases. J Am Podiatr Assoc 65:103, 1975
15. Fisher BK, Macpherson M: Epidermoid cyst of the sole. J Am Acad Dermatol 15:1127, 1986
16. Fanti PA, Tosti A: Subungual epidermoid inclusions: Report of 8 cases. Dermatologica 178:209, 1989
17. Leyden JJ, Lockshin NA, Kriebel S: The black keratinous cyst: A sign of hemochromatosis. Arch Dermatol 106:379, 1972
18. Easterly NB, Fretzin DF, Pinkus H: Eruptive vellus hair cysts. Arch Dermatol 113:500, 1977
19. Burns DA, Calnan CD: Eruptive vellus hair cysts. Clin Exp Dermatol 6:209–213, 1981
20. Watson A: Eruptive vellus hair cysts. Int J Dermatol 21:273, 1982
21. Pepin R, Robin J, et al: Kystes eruptifs à duvets. Ann Dermatol Venereol 109:799, 1982
22. Barnadas M, Moreno A, DeMoragas JM: Quiste velloso eruptivo. Med Cutan ILA 11:117, 1983
23. Piepkorn MW, Clark L, Lombardi DL: A kindred with congenital vellus hair cyst. J Am Acad Dermatol 5:661, 1981
24. Benoldi D, Allegra F: Congenital eruptive vellus hair cysts. Int J Dermatol 28:340, 1989
25. Mayron R, Grimwood RE: Familial occurrence of eruptive vellus hair cysts. Pediatr Dermatol 5:94, 1988
26. Mehregan AH, Medenica M: Pigmented follicular cysts. J Cutan Pathol 9:423, 1982
27. Caballero LR, Yus ES: Pigmented follicular cyst. J Am Acad Dermatol 21:1073, 1989
28. Pinkus H: "Sebaceous cysts" are trichilemmal cysts. Arch Dermatol 99:554, 1969
29. Brownstein MH: Trichilemmal horn: Cutaneous horn showing trichilemmal keratinization. Arch Dermatol 114:1831, 1978
30. Nakamura K: Two cases of trichilemmal-like horn. Arch Dermatol 120:386, 1984
31. Brownstein MH: Hybrid cyst: A combined epidermoid and trichilemmal cyst. J Am Acad Dermatol 9:872, 1983
32. Mehregan AH, Hardin I: Generalized follicular hamartoma, complicated by multiple proliferating trichilemmal cysts and palmar pits. Arch Dermatol 107:435, 1973
33. Stranc MF, Bennet MH, Mehmed EP: Pilar tumour of the scalp developing in hereditary sebaceous cysts. Br J Plast Surg 24:82, 1971
34. Janitz J, Wiedersberg H: Trichilemmal pilar tumors. Cancer 45:1594, 1980
35. Miyairi H, Takahashi S, Morohashi M: Proliferating trichilemmal cyst: An ultrastructural study. J Cutan Pathol 11:274, 1984
36. Poiares Baptista A, Garcia E, Silva L, Born MC: Proliferating trichilemmal cyst. J Cutan Pathol 10:178, 1983
37. Brownstein MH, Arluk DJ: Proliferating trichilemmal cyst: A simulant of squamous cell carcinoma. Cancer 48:1207, 1981
38. Saida T, Oohara K, Hori Y, Tsuchiya S: Development of a malignant proliferating trichilemmal cyst in a patient with multiple trichilemmal cysts. Dermatologica 166:203, 1983
39. Mehregan AH, Lee KC: Malignant proliferating trichilemmal tumors: Report of three cases. J Dermatol Surg Oncol 13:1339, 1987
40. Brownstein MH, Helwig EB: Subcutaneous dermoid cysts. Arch Dermatol 107:237, 1973
41. Farmer ER, Helwig EB: Cutaneous ciliated cysts. Arch Dermatol 114:70, 1978
42. Clark JV: Cutaneous ciliated cysts. Arch Dermatol 114:1246, 1978
43. True L, Golitz LE: Ciliated plantar cyst. Arch Dermatol 116:1066, 1980
44. Leonforte JF: Cutaneous ciliated cystadenoma in man. Arch Dermatol 118:1010, 1982
45. Patterson JW, Pittman DL, Rich JD: Presternal ciliated cyst. Arch Dermatol 120:240, 1984
46. Asarch RG, Golitz LE, Sausker WF, Kraye SM: Median raphe cysts of the penis. Arch Dermatol 115:1084, 1979
47. Golitz LE, Robin M: Median Raphe canals of the penis. Cutis 27:170, 1981
48. Van Der Putte SCJ, Toonstra J: Cutaneous "bronchogenic" cyst. J Cutan Pathol 12:404, 1985
49. Muramatsu T, Shirai T, Sakamoto K: Cutaneous bronchogenic cyst. Int J Dermatol 29:143, 1990
50. Finn D, Buchlater I, Sarti E, et al: First branchial cleft cysts: Clinical update. Laryngoscope 97:136, 1987
51. Jaworsky C, Murphy GF: Cystic tumors of the neck. J Dermatol Surg Oncol 15:21, 1989
52. Hogan D. Wilkinson RD, Williams A: Congenital anomalies of the head and neck. Int J Dermatol 19:479, 1980
53. Sanusi D, Carrington PR, Adams DN: Cervical thymic cyst. Arch Dermatol 118:122, 1982
54. Barr RJ, Santa Cruz DJ, Pearl RM: Dermal thymus. A light microscopic and immunohistochemical study. Arch Dermatol 125:1681, 1989
55. Verret J-L, Leclech C: Aspects dermatologiques de la pathologie ombilicale. Ann Dermatol Venereol 115:621, 1988

SWEAT APPARATUS TUMORS

Our ability to diagnose and classify those tumors that are related to sweat glands has increased in recent years with the development of enzyme histochemical patterns and ultrastructural and immunostaining characteristics. Immunostaining directed against various epithelial antigens including cytokeratins, S-100 protein, carcinoembryonic antigen (CEA), epithelial membrane antigen, and gross cystic disease fluid protein-15 (GCDFP-15) have been applied to fresh-frozen or paraffin-fixed tissue sections for identification of sweat gland tumors.[1–6]

In trying to organize the field on a biologic basis according to modern standards, we are using the term "sweat apparatus" for all parts of the gland: secretory, ductal, and poral. This is necessary because the old classification of tumors of the duct (syringadenomas) and of the coil (spiradenomas) does not take into consideration that a good portion of the eccrine coil also consists of duct and does not make allowance for the specific properties of the intraepithelial duct. Next, it is undeniable for anyone acquainted with principles of terminology that *hidradenoma* means sweat adenoma and therefore stands for benign sweat apparatus tumor in a general sense. Hidradenoma cannot be used for any particular tumor without adding a qualifying adjective, be it in the classic Latin form or in modern French or English, for example, hidradenoma papilliferum, *hidradénome éruptif,* nodular hidradenoma. Other names that have been generally accepted, for example, syringoma, eccrine spiradenoma, and eccrine poroma, may well be continued in use if their meaning is clearly understood as designating certain types of hidradenoma and not being outside the limits of that general term. We discourage, however, the growing tendency to describe and name every new hidradenoma because of minor variation and will attempt a classification on sound general principles.

We use the same two principles we outlined for sebaceous tumors: degree of maturation and morphologic resemblance to normal parts of the sweat apparatus, after first sorting out eccrine from apocrine tumors, inasmuch as these two types of glands are distinct in embryologic origin, anatomic structure, and secretory function (see Table VII–1).[7]

SWEAT GLAND NEVI

Hyperplasia of mature eccrine or apocrine glands in a localized area constitutes a sweat gland nevus. *Eccrine nevus*[8–10] is rare and can manifest itself as an area of hyperhidrosis with or without surface epidermal changes (Fig. 39–1). Eccrine angiomatous nevus refers to a usually singular tender nodular lesion (Fig. 39–2) characterized histologically by localized hyperplasia of mature eccrine glands, an increased number of dilated capillary blood vessels, and sometimes small hair follicles.[11,12] Very rare is

564 MALFORMATION AND NEOPLASIA

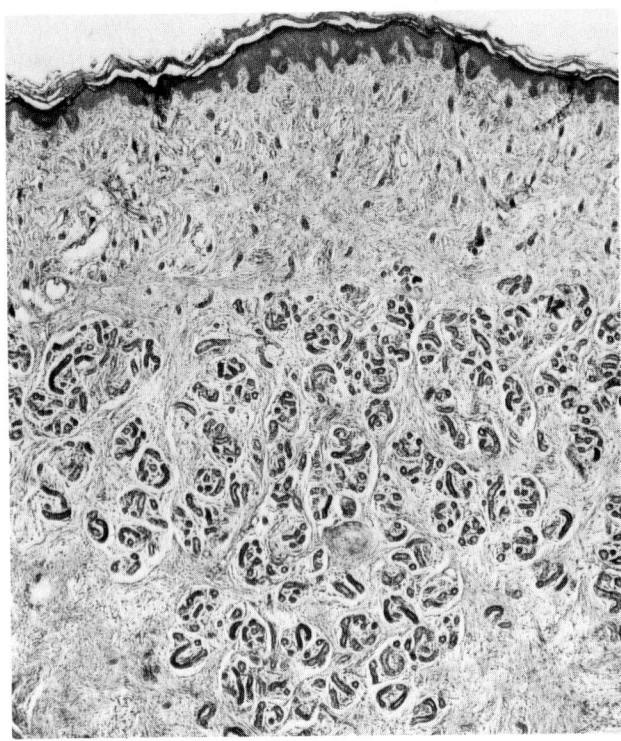

Figure 39–1.
Eccrine nevus (nevus sudoriparus). Increased number and size of structurally normal eccrine apparatuses. Epidermis slightly papillomatous. H&E. X60.

pure *apocrine nevus* in the form of a localized lesion exhibiting an increase in the number of mature apocrine glands.[13] Apocrine hyperplasia also occurs within an organoid nevus, and lesions of this type have been reported as apocrine nevus.[14,15]

Supernumerary Nipple

Supernumerary nipple (polythelia) usually appears along the embryonic milk lines which run from the anterior axillary fold to the inner thighs. It may be single or multiple and can occasionally occur in other locations. The lesion usually is a light brown nodule often associated with hairs. Histologically (Fig. 39–3), it shows a corrugated pattern of epidermis over a central pilosebaceous structure. In the dermis are a number of smooth muscles and mammary glands.[16]

APOCRINE TUMORS

Apocrine Cystadenoma

The cystic nodular lesion of apocrine cystadenoma appears most commonly over the face and occasionally elsewhere.[17–19] The growth may be skin color or

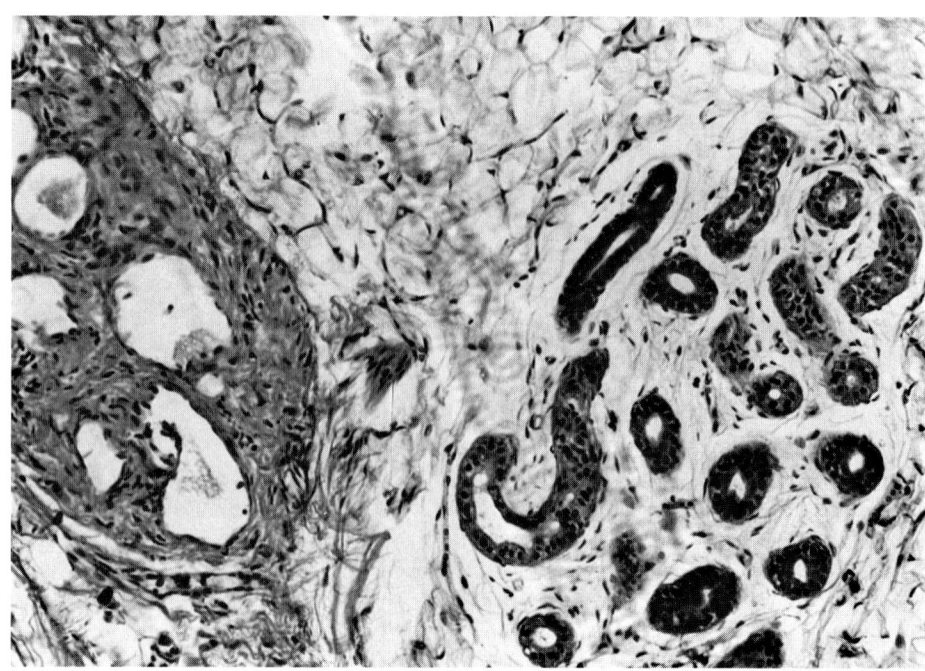

Figure 39–2.
Eccrine angiomatous nevus. A combination of hemangioma and eccrine hyperplasia. H&E. X125.

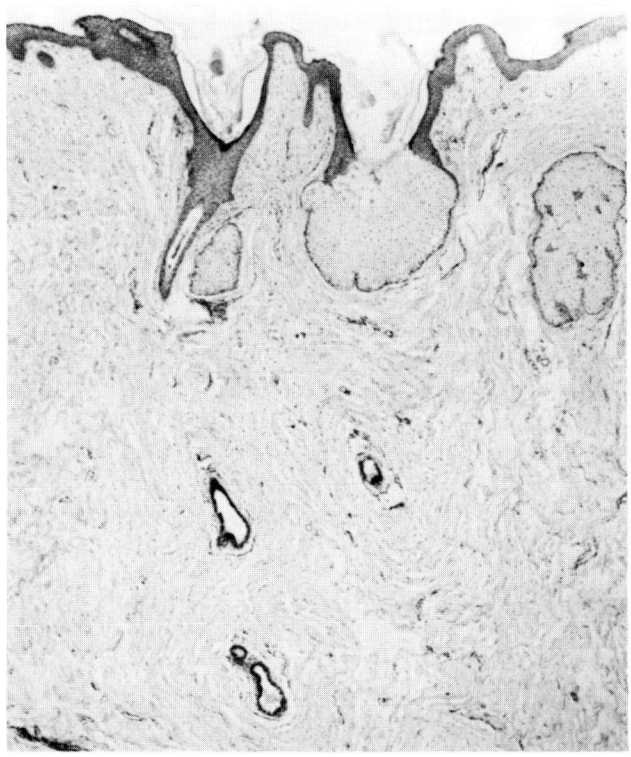

Figure 39–3.
Supernumerary nipple. Hair follicles, free sebaceous glands, and milk ducts in the dermis, which contains multiple strands of smooth muscle. H&E. X25.

deeply pigmented, resembling a blue nevus or a pigmented basal cell epithelioma. Histologically (Fig. 39–4), multiple cystic spaces containing secretory material are present in the dermis. Deep cystic cavities are lined with apocrine-type secretory epithelium of high columnar cells with basilar nuclei resting over an outer layer of elongated myoepithelial cells. Small papillomatous projections of secretory epithelium extend into the central cavity indicating an adenomatous lesion. Superficial cysts are lined by a thin layer of ductal epithelium. Lipochrome granules present in the cytoplasm of high columnar cells and in the secretory material inside the cysts are most likely responsible for the deep pigmentation of some lesions.[20]

Syringadenoma Papilliferum

Syringadenoma papilliferum occurs most commonly on the scalp over a preexisting organoid nevus but may also appear by itself and elsewhere.[21] Papilliferous and tubular structures (Fig. 39–5) extend from the surface into the dermis surrounded by fibrovascular stroma that contains an unusually large number of plasma cells.[22,23] The epithelial lining usually consists of high columnar luminal cells resting on a row of flat or cuboidal cells (Fig. 39–6).

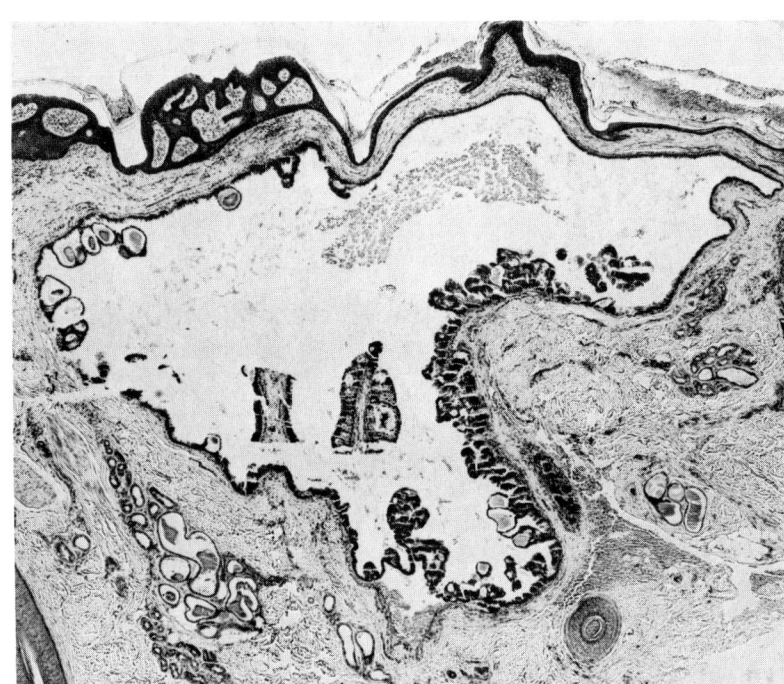

Figure 39–4.
Apocrine cystadenoma developed in organoid nevus. Apocrine and eccrine coils are present near tumor, which consists mainly of two-layered epithelium lining a large cyst and papilliferous projections into lumen. Papillomatous epidermal lesion is part of the preexistent nevus. H&E. X30. (From Mehregan. Arch Dermatol 90:274, 1964.)

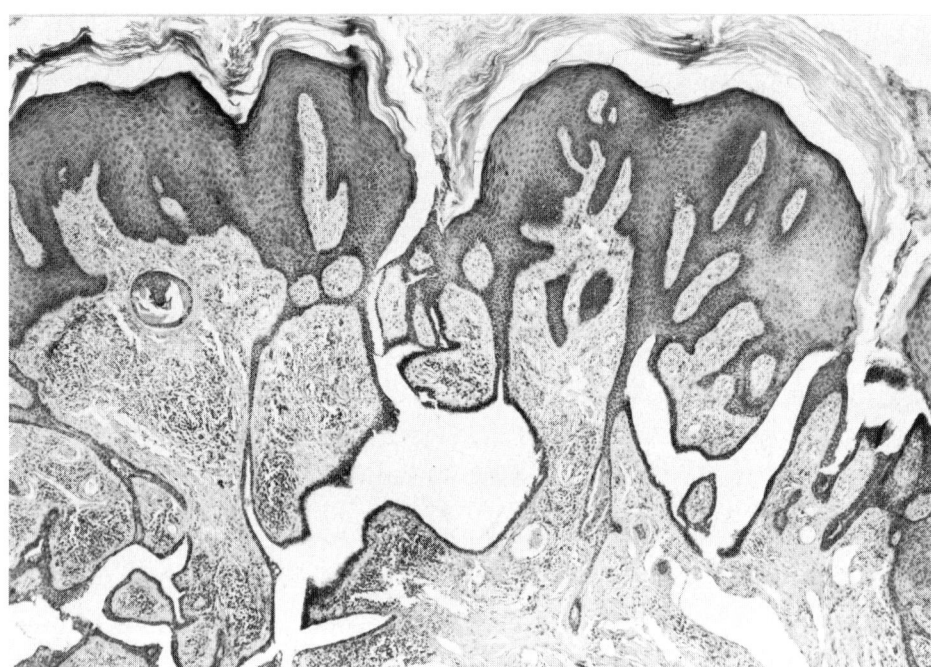

Figure 39–5.
Syringocystadenoma papilliferum. Multiple papilliferous sinuses lined with ductal epithelium and open to the surface epidermis. H&E. X70.

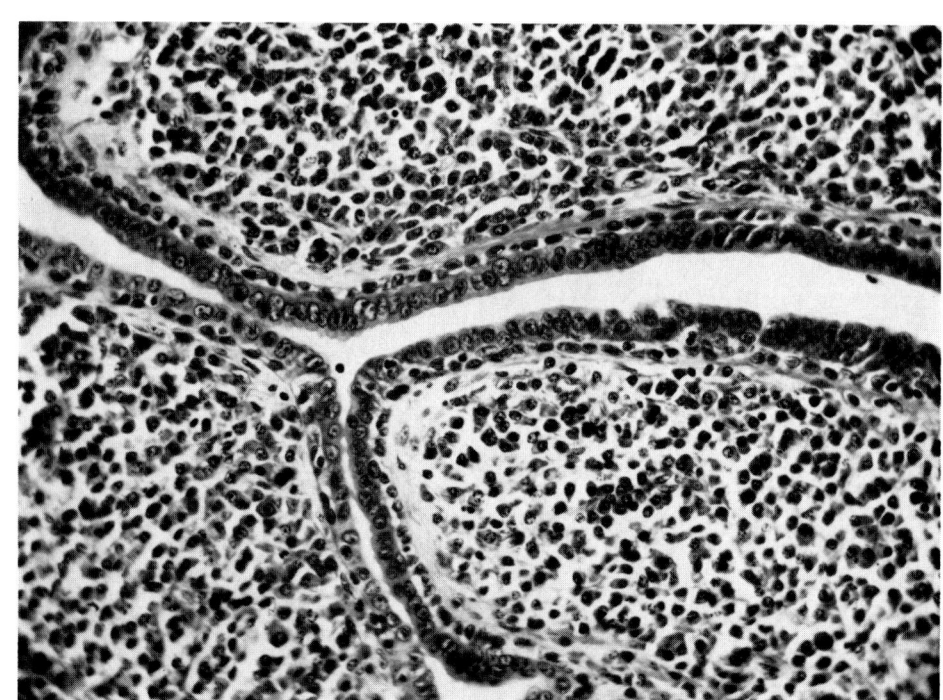

Figure 39–6.
Cellular details of papilliferous syringocystadenoma. Lumen-lining columnar or cuboidal cells rest on outer layer of flat epithelial cells. Stroma contains many plasma cells. H&E. X280.

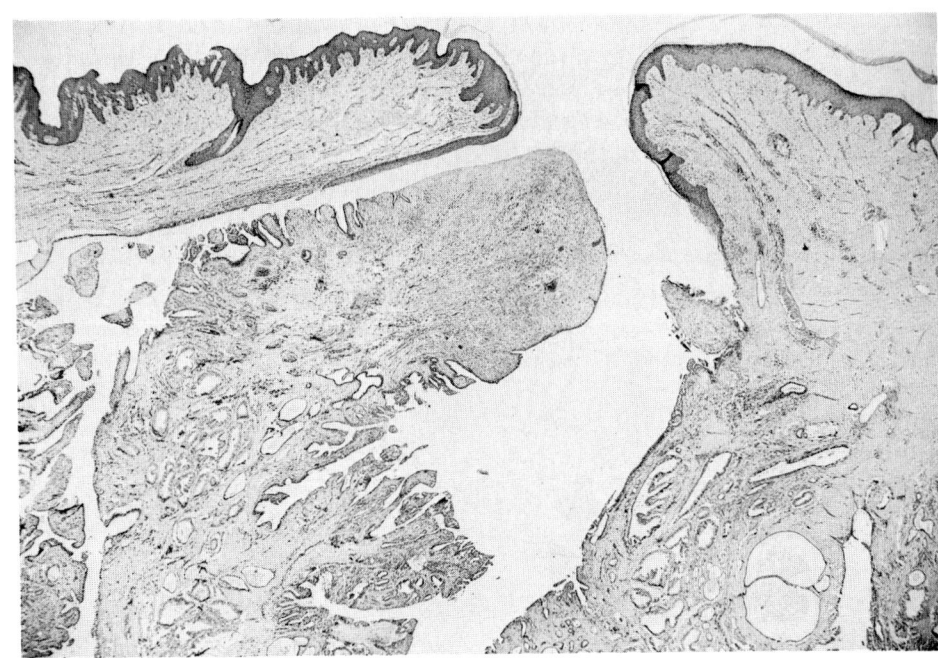

Figure 39–7.
Hidradenoma papilliferum of vulva. Large sinus filled with, and surrounded by, adenomatous tissue. Epithelial cells appear light because they have eosinophilic cytoplasm. H&E. X30.

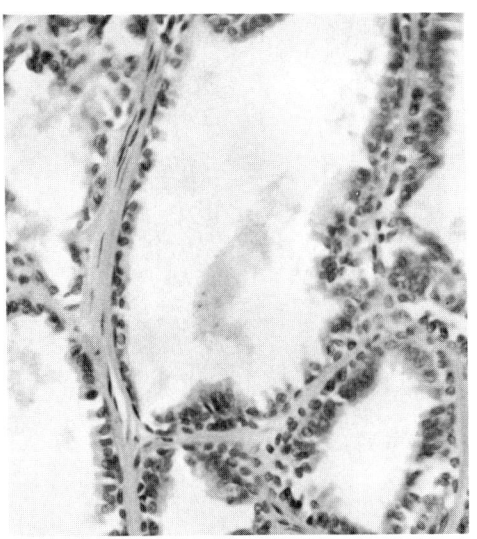

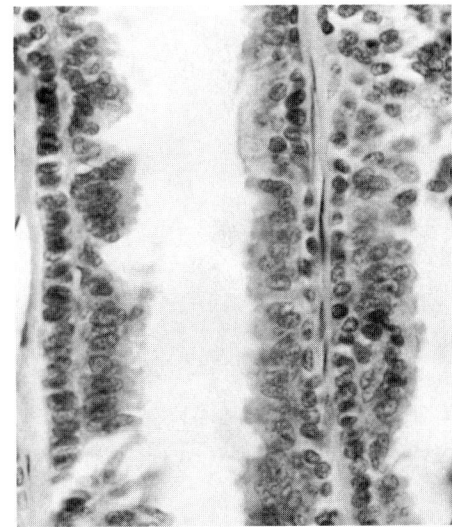

Figure 39–8.
Tubular apocrine adenoma. Inner layer of high columnar cells resting over a layer of cuboidal or flattened cells and basement membrane. H&E. **A** and **B.** X250.

A **B**

Hidradenoma of Vulva (Hidradenoma Papilliferum)

This freely movable nodular lesion of vulva may show superficial erosion and moisture, suggesting active secretion.[24,25] Microscopically (Fig. 39–7), numerous papilliferous projections lined by high columnar apocrine-type secretory epithelium extend from the wall of the cyst into the central cavity.[26]

Tubular Apocrine Adenoma

A well-defined, solitary, intracutaneous, nodular growth is histologically distinctive by the presence of cystic dilated and branching tubular structures surrounded by fibrovascular stroma.[27–30] In the lining of the tubular structures is an inner layer of high columnar cells resting over an outer layer of flattened or cuboidal cells and a basement membrane (Fig. 39–8). The enzyme pattern and electron microscopic findings confirm apocrine differentiation.[27]

Erosive Adenomatosis of the Nipple

This lesion, also called *florid papillomatosis of the nipple ducts,* shows nodular enlargement of the nip-

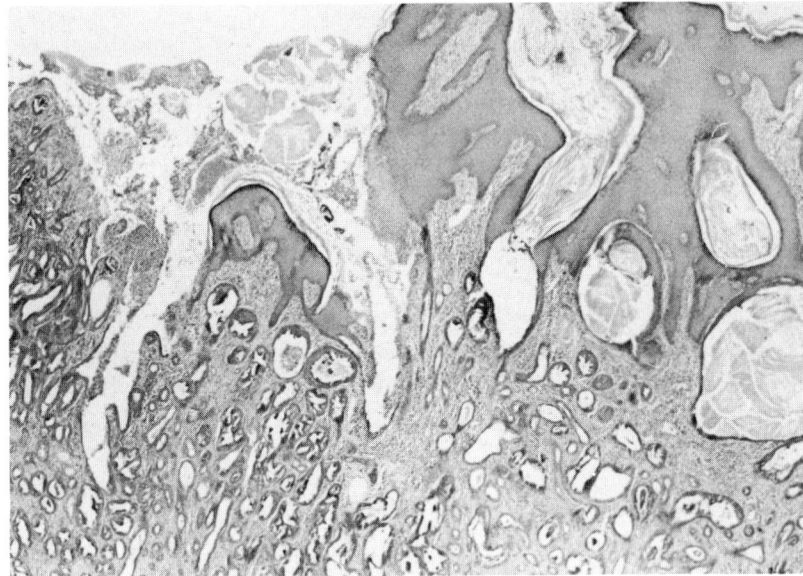

A

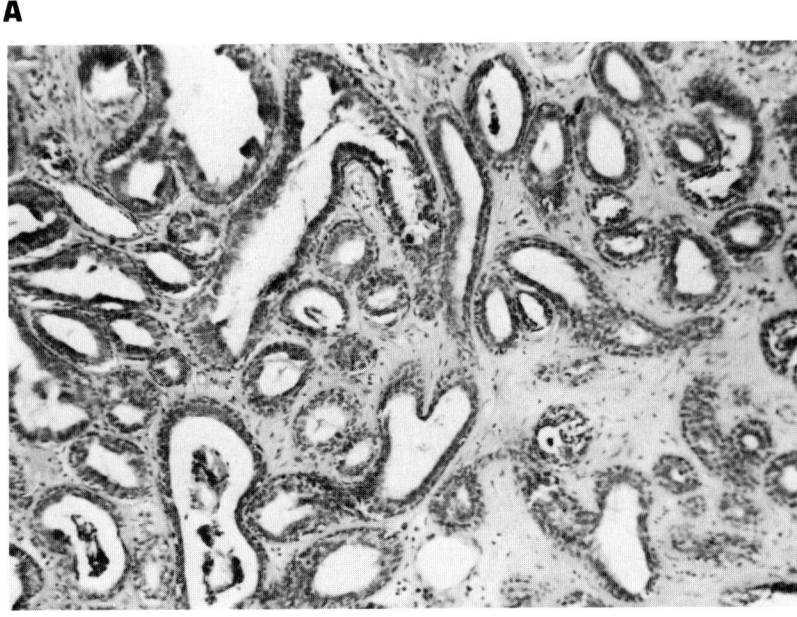

B

Figure 39–9.
Erosive adenomatosis of nipple. Similar to Figure 39–5, but no plasma cell infiltrate. H&E. **A.** X45. **B.** X125.

ple with superficial erosions and blood-stained or serous discharge.[31] The growth is well defined and shows numerous branching ducts and tubular structures extending from the surface deep into the dermis (Fig. 39–9).[32] The papillary structures are lined by an inner layer of columnar cells and an outer layer of flattened or cuboidal cells resting on the basement membrane.[33]

Cutaneous Cylindroma

We discuss here with deliberation the cutaneous cylindroma, as the epitheliomatous representative of the pilary complex including the apocrine glands. Cylindroma is often located over the hair-bearing areas such as face and scalp; it never appears on the palms or soles and and rarely involves the trunk or extremities. The growth is undifferentiated and therefore its enzyme pattern has not been established for either eccrine or apocrine derivation. There are two clinical manifestations. The *solitary* type occurs over the face and scalp during adulthood. The *multiple* variety appears earlier in life forming exophytic nodules involving the forehead and scalp in turban areas called "turban tumors."[34–36] Histologically (Fig. 39–10), cylindroma is a dermal lesion but occasionally may extend into the subcutaneous fat tissue. Solid masses of basaloid cells are closely applied to one another like pieces of a jigsaw puzzle. Tumor lobules are well defined and are surrounded by a layer of PAS-positive hyaline sheath and show small hyalin globes among the basaloid cells. There are occasional sweat glandular lumen formations. Multiple cylindromas can occur with multiple trichoepitheliomas as a dominantly inherited trait.[43,44] Dermal cylindromas may be associated with eccrine spiradenomas and membranous basal cell adenoma of the parotid gland.[37,38] Malignant degeneration of cylindroma may lead to invasion of subcutaneous tissues or distant metastasis (see Chapter 41).

ECCRINE TUMORS

Hidroacanthoma Simplex (Syringoacanthoma)

Hidroacanthoma simplex is a superficial eccrine neoplasm clinically resembling a flat type of seborrheic verruca or a plaque of Bowen's disease.[39] Histologically (Fig. 39–11), there are circumscribed islands of small and uniform basaloid cells in the confines of an acanthotic epidermis. The tumor cells contain glycogen granules and are well defined from the surrounding epidermal keratinocytes.[40,41] Eccrine sweat ducts may enter and disappear within the tumor islands. Occasionally, there are areas of sweat-duct-like lumina formation.[42]

Eccrine Poroma and Dermal Duct Tumor

Eccrine poromas are benign tumors (Fig. 39–12) that manifest ductal as well as keratinizing epidermoid maturation similar to the epithelium of the sweat pore (acrosyringium, eccrine epidermal sweat duct unit).[43] Although they are most common on the nonhairy parts of the foot, they have been found in most other regions of the body surface. They are almost always single. Multiple and diffuse lesions may be associated with hidrotic ectodermal dysplasia.[44–46] Typically, eccrine poromas are superficial, often protruding or sessile, but occasionally they may project down into the dermis or form the superficial portion of a nodular hidradenoma.

The degree of organization of eccrine poroma is usually on the epitheliomatous rather than the adenomatous or acanthomatous level. The tumor consists mainly of peculiar small and uniform epithelial cells with only occasional slit-like or cystic lumina.[47,48] PAS stain shows abundant glycogen granules in the tumor cells and a sharp line of demarcation between the tumor epithelium and the surrounding epidermis (Fig. 39–13). The tumor masses are embedded in a richly vascular stroma that often produces the clinical appearance of a vascular neoplasm. Tumors of similar structure situated entirely in the dermis (Fig. 39–14) have been described as *dermal duct tumor*.[49] The vascular stroma is not prominent and the histochemical and electron microscopic findings suggest differentiation toward the dermal portion of the eccrine sweat duct unit.[50] Occasionally, these tumors may show melanin pigmentation.

Eccrine Syringofibroadenoma

Linear eccrine poroma and acrosyringeal nevus occur in multiple papular form with linear distribution and appear to be closely related to the often single nodular lesion described by Mascaro as eccrine syringofibroadenoma.[51,52] Histologically, spongelike tumor masses show in cross sections thin strands and septae of small cuboidal acrosyringeal cells with plenty of fibrovascular stroma in between (Fig. 39–15).[53,54]

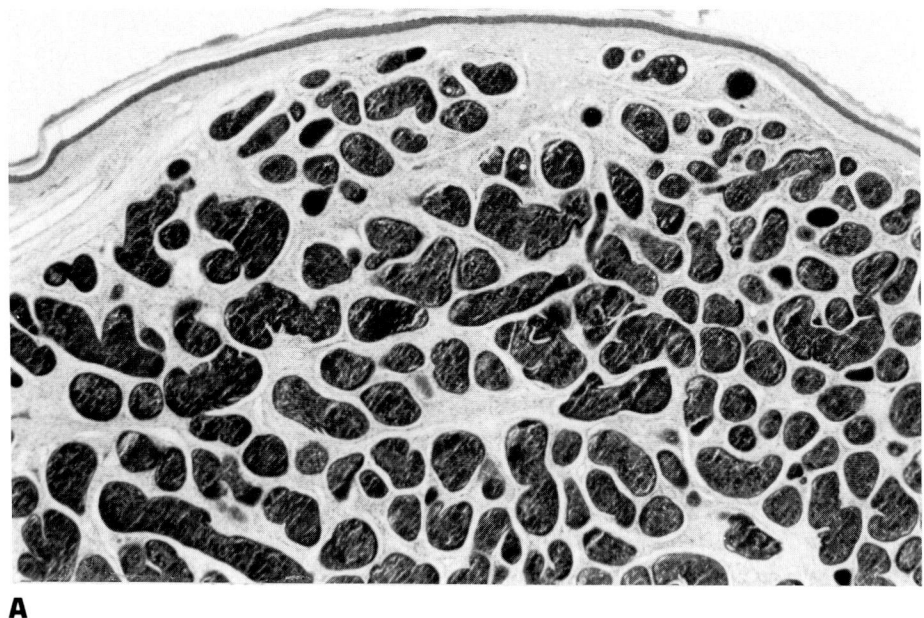

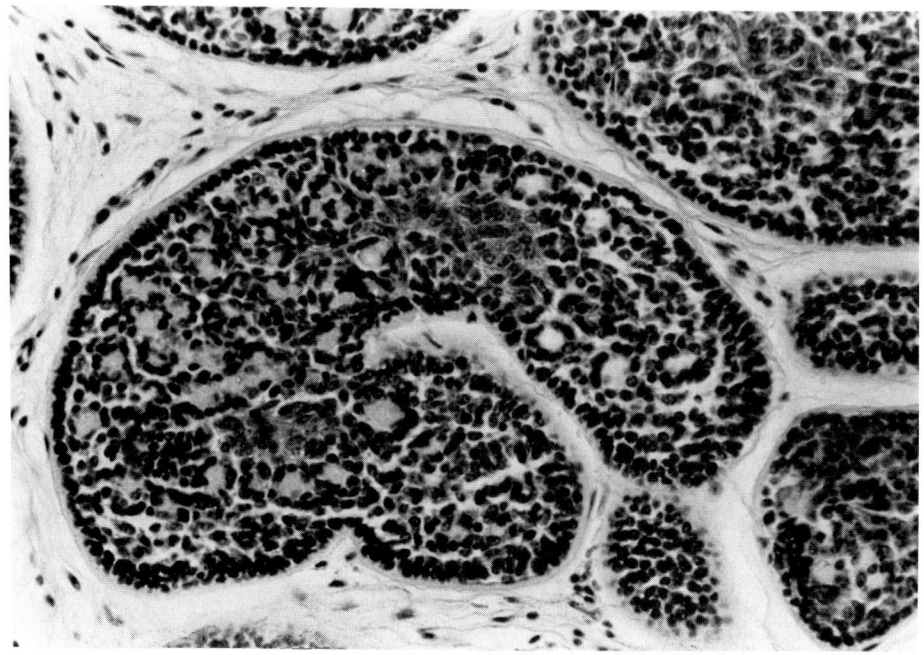

Figure 39–10.
Cutaneous cylindroma. **A.** The characteristic jigsaw puzzle arrangement of the tumor masses. H&E. X25. **B.** Masses of basaloid cells surrounded by hyaline sheath. H&E. X250.

Papillary Eccrine Adenoma

Papillary eccrine adenoma is a counterpart of the tubular apocrine adenoma occurring as a solitary nodular lesion over the extremities.[55,56] Histologically (Fig. 39–16), it is characterized by the presence of cystic dilated and branching ductal structures with areas of papillary projections into the central lumen. Ductal structures are lined by an outer layer of flattened or cuboidal cells. The inner cells may be flattened, cuboidal, or columnar. The central cystic lumen contains an amorphous eosinophilic secretory material.[57–60]

Syringoma

Syringoma was formerly favored to be apocrine but is now considered to be eccrine. The apocrine nature was proposed because the papular lesions appear

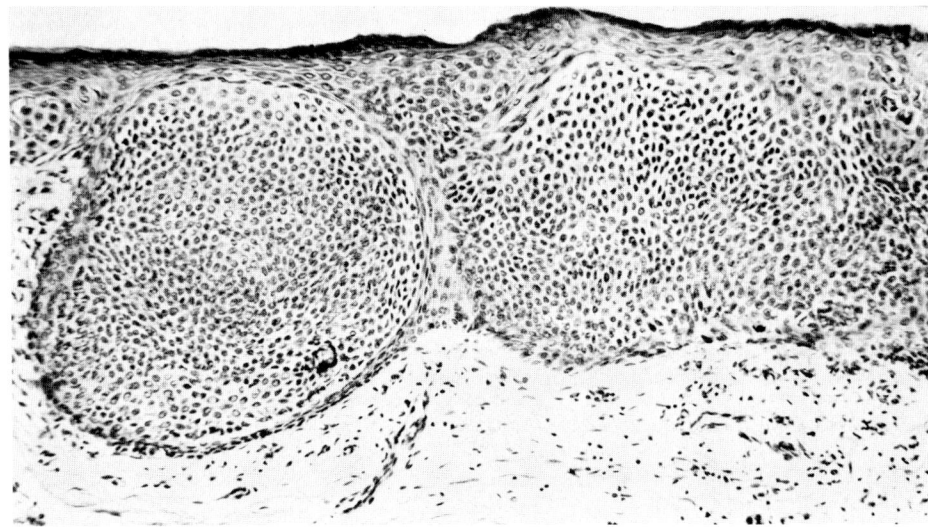

Figure 39–11.
Hidroacanthoma simplex. Intraepidermal nests of poroma-like cells (Fig. 39–12) are sharply delineated around their entire periphery and are in cytoplasmic (desmosomal) contact with surrounding epidermal keratinocytes in many places. H&E. X180.

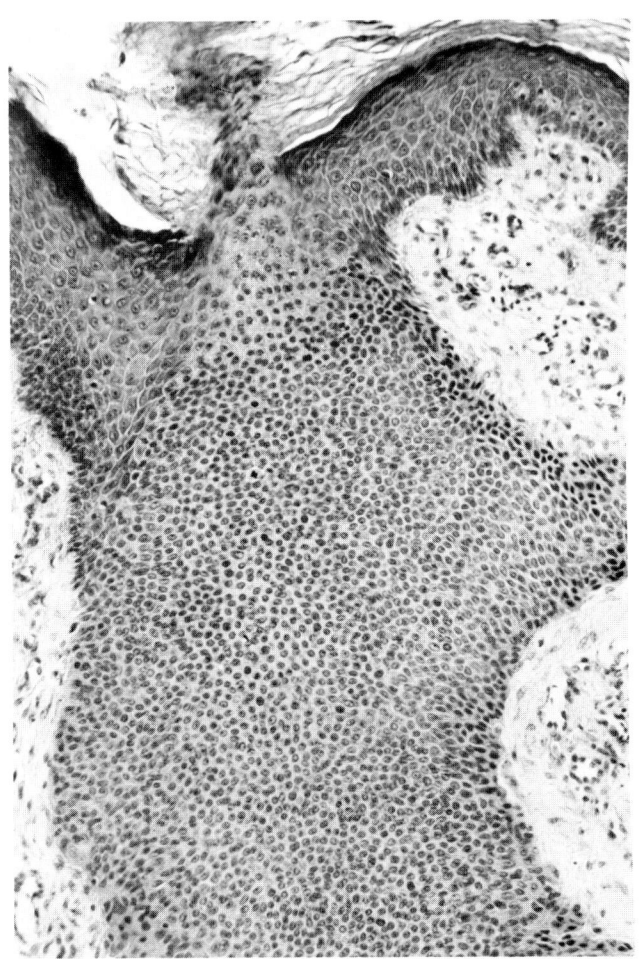

Figure 39–12.
Eccrine poroma. Part of a tumor shows even, small epithelial cells without a palisading outer layer. Sharp dividing line between tumor and normal epidermis which it penetrates. Near the skin surface, tumor cells become larger, prickle cell-like and show incomplete keratinization. In other areas, keratohyalin may be formed. H&E. X135.

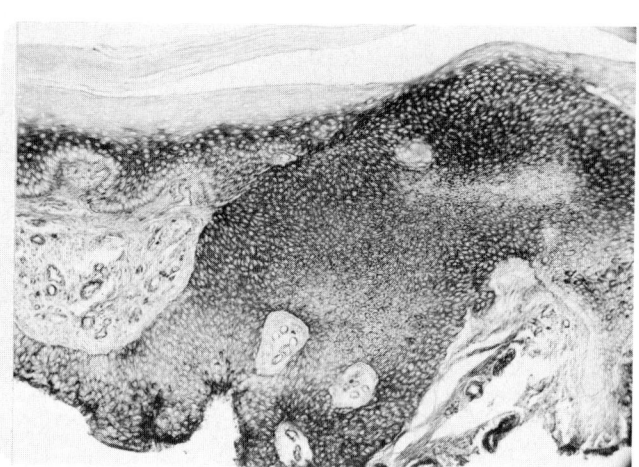

Figure 39–13.
Eccrine poroma stained for glycogen shows sharp division between epidermis (no glycogen in basal layer, considerable glycogen in lower prickle cells) and tumor (glycogen in every cell, including peripheral cells). Where tumor reaches the skin surface, it begins to keratinize, and the cells lose their glycogen. PAS–light green. X90. (From Pinkus, Rogin, and Goldman. Arch Dermatol 74:511, 1956.)

most commonly within the orbital skin in an area in which well-developed Moll's glands and rudimentary apocrine glands are present. When the lesions are widespread they are found within the apocrine triangle between axillae and pubes including vulva.[61,62] Lesions of back or extremities are relatively rare.[63] The eccrine origin, however, is supported by the enzyme pattern and electron microscopic findings of eccrine acrosyringeal differentiation (Fig. 39–17).[64] Syringomas are tumors exhibiting variable organizations of their epithelial portion, which is capable of producing horny material, foamy (clear) cells (clear cell syringoma), and fairly good ductal structures.[65] The small solid epithelial nests and cystic ductal structures, some with comma-like tails, are embedded in a specific connective tissue stroma that constitutes a major portion of the lesion (Fig. 39–18). Eruptive syrin-

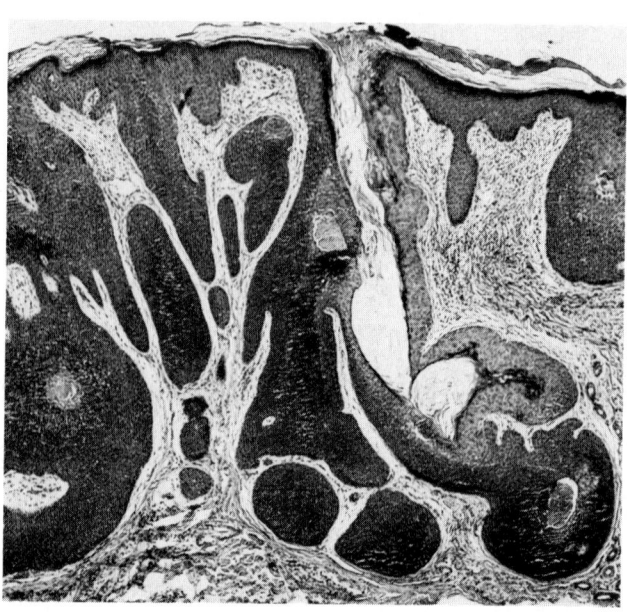

Figure 39–14.
Nodular hidradenoma combining features of eccrine poroma and Winkelmann's dermal duct tumor. Tumor masses are in multiple broad contact with epidermis and a deformed hyperplastic eccrine duct. H&E. X30.

SWEAT APPARATUS TUMORS   573

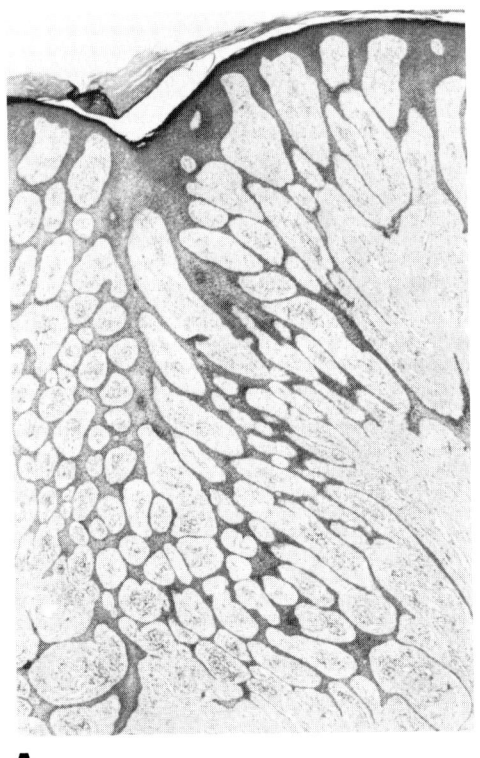
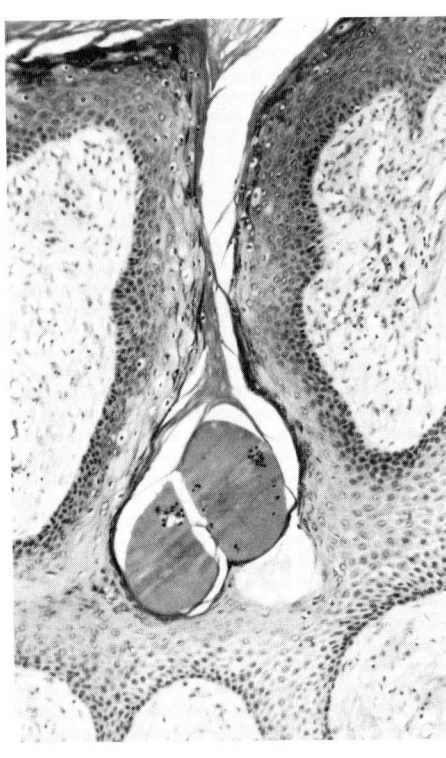

Figure 39–15.
Eccrine syringofibroadenoma. Spongelike masses of acrosyringeal cells are filled in between with a well-organized fibrous stroma. H&E. **A.** X25. **B.** X125.

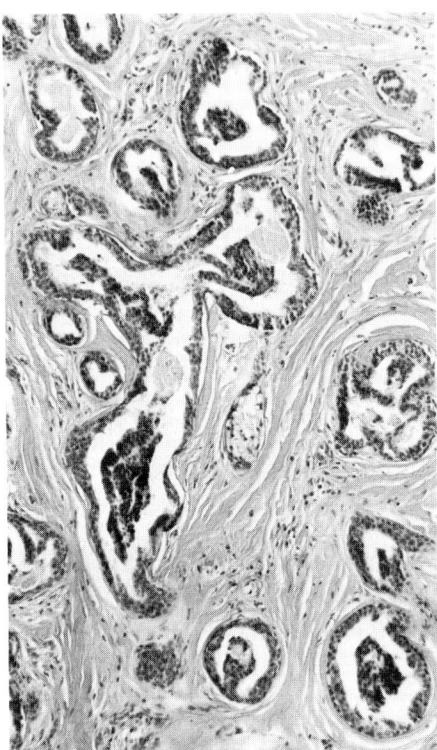
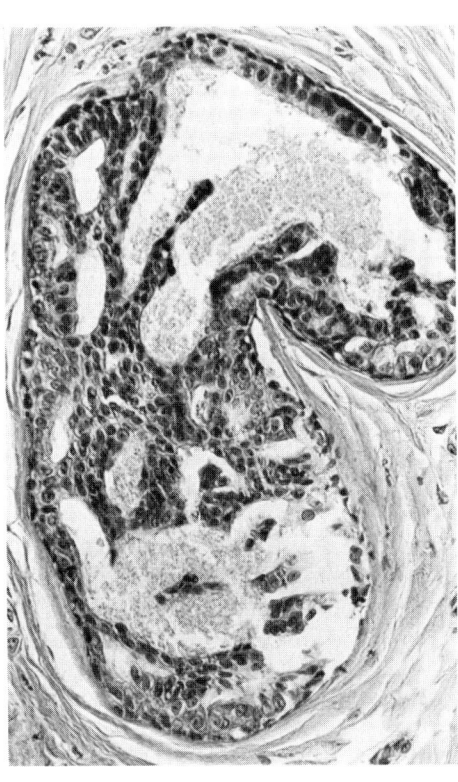

Figure 39–16.
Papillary eccrine adenoma. Tubular structures lined with two or more rows of cuboidal cells. H&E. **A.** X125. **B.** X250.

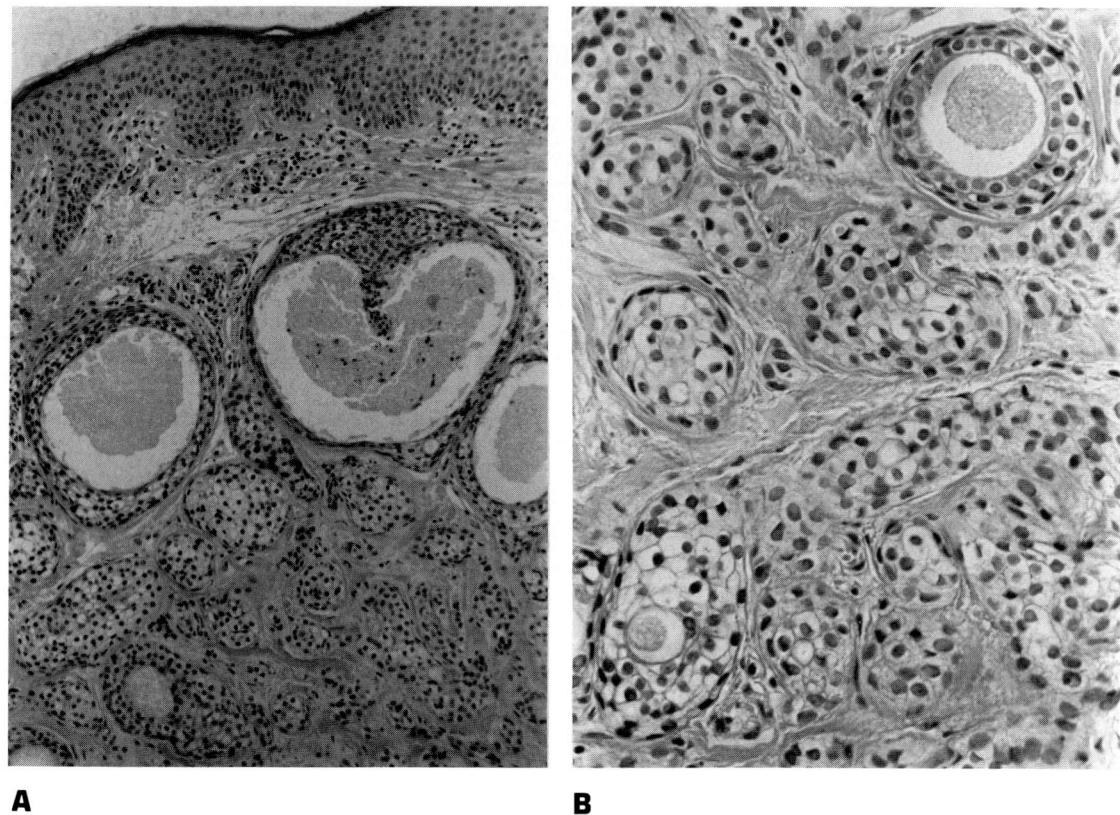

Figure 39–17.
Clear cell syringoma. **A.** Solid nests and dilated sweat ductal structures lined with cells having clear cytoplasms. H&E. X125. **B.** Solid nests of clear cells and ductal structures. H&E. X250.

gomas may be diffuse, linear, or show unilateral distribution.[66–68] Diffuse familial type is dominantly inherited.[69] Syringomas may occur in association with Down syndrome in a significant number of cases.[70,71] They are also found in association with Marfan and Ehlers–Danlos syndromes.[72]

Eccrine Spiradenoma

Eccrine spiradenoma provides a good example of a well-defined entity, some variants of which preserve enough tubular structure to impress as adenomas, while most of them have so low an organization that they are on the level of epitheliomas. In some tumors, the stroma is so prominent and vascular that they may be mistaken for hemangiomas or glomangiomas.[73] The term "spiradenoma," based on Unna's old classification, does not specify ductal or secretory maturation, and the wisdom of this restraint has been shown by electron microscopic investigation.[74] That eccrine spiradenoma usually is situated deep in the skin or in the hypoderm may be taken as additional evidence for its relation to the sweat coil. Eccrine spiradenoma may be solitary, multiple, or show linear distribution.[75–78] The growth is made up of solid masses surrounded by a richly vascular stroma (Fig. 39–19). The tumor masses are made up of proliferation of two types of cells forming thin cords with an interconnected pattern. The inner cells are large, light staining, and often surround central lumen. Peripheral cells are small with compact nuclei and a small amount of

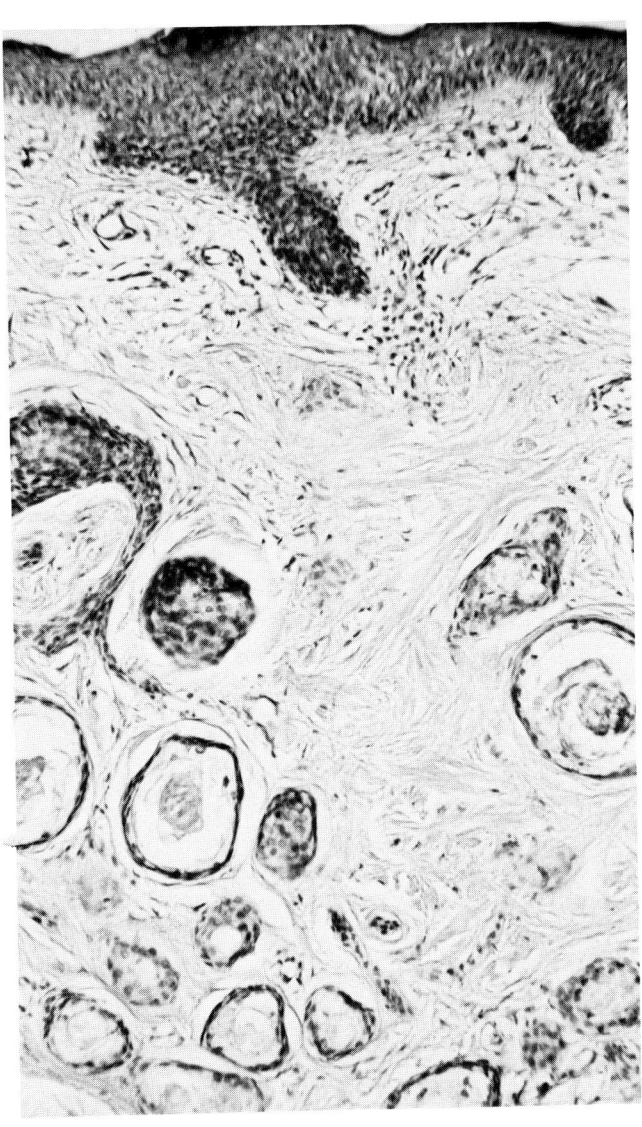

Figure 39–18.
Syringoma. Cystic sweat ductal structures contain secretory material and are embedded in fibrous stroma. H&E. X125.

cytoplasm. Malignant transformation of eccrine spiradenoma is rare (see Chapter 41).

Clear Cell Hidradenoma
Eccrine Acrospiroma

In this category are nodular hidradenomas consisting of cells arranged into solid masses with only occasional organization into lumen-lining order (Fig. 39–20). The tumor cells are either small (epidermoid) or large with abundant and clear cytoplasm containing glycogen granules (clear cells).[79] Connection with the surface epidermis and cystic areas containing secretory material may be present.[80] Stroma can be scant or copious but does not usually exhibit the maturation encountered in other hidradenomas. Electron microscopy has demonstrated cells with ductal and secretory features.[81]

Chondroid Syringoma
(Mixed Tumor of the Skin)

This cutaneous neoplasm has many structural resemblances to the mixed tumor of salivary glands. The clinical manifestation is a solitary intradermal or subcutaneous firm nodule.[82,83] Histologically

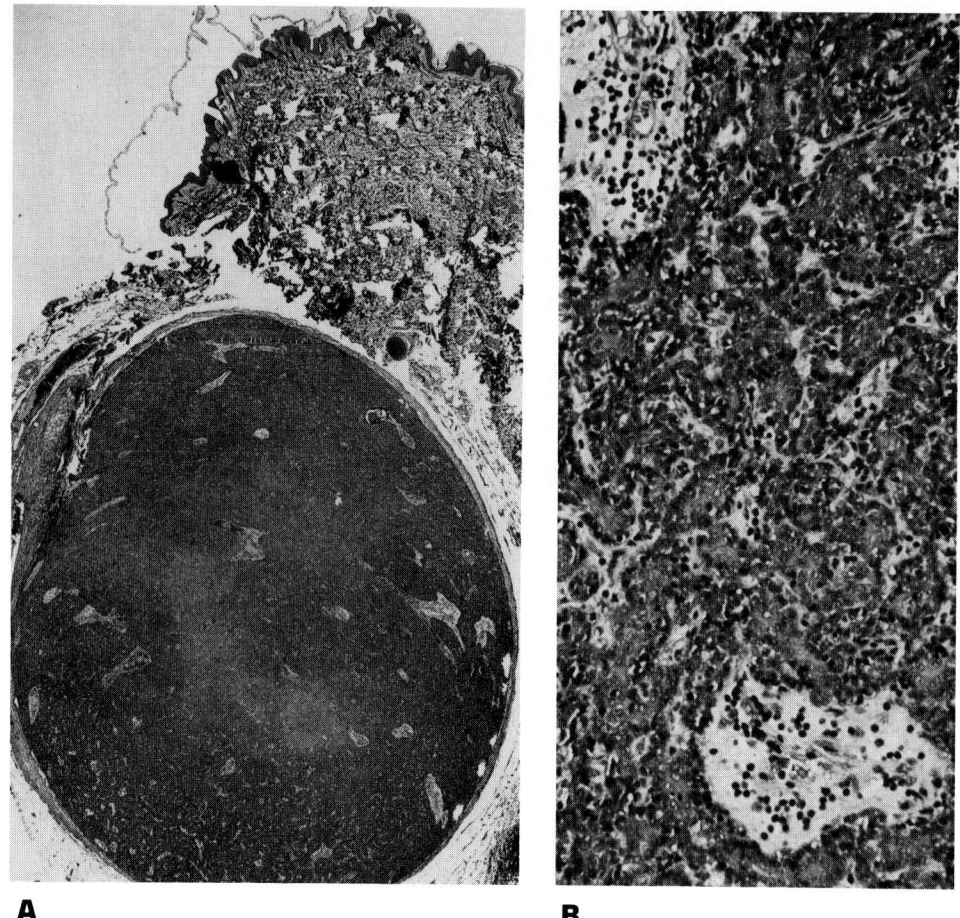

Figure 39–19.
Eccrine spiradenoma. **A.** Typical picture of a well-demarcated tumor, in deep dermis and subcutaneous tissue. Note vascular stroma in interior and a few ductlike lumina in periphery of epithelial nodule. H&E. X14. **B.** Two types of epithelial cells form interconnected cords closely interwoven with stroma. H&E. X225.

(Fig. 39–21), the growth is made up of branching tubules, closely packed ductal structures and, individual epithelial cells embedded in a distinctively myxomatous stroma that often shows chondroid areas. The papillary structures are lined with an inner layer of dark staining cells that give positive reaction for keratin and CEA, suggesting eccrine differentiation. The outer, light-staining cells show faint keratin and no CEA staining and appear to be less differentiated.[84,85]

In another study utilizing immunologic markers, occurrence of both apocrine and eccrine forms of mixed tumor has been suggested (Fig. 39–22).[86]

Occasionally one encounters a solitary lesion combining the histologic features of a mixed tumor of the skin with foci of sebaceous and follicular differentiation.[87] Malignant mixed tumors of the skin are rare. Histologic features indicating malignancy include nuclear pleomorphism, scattered mitotic figures, squamous metaplasia, and stromal or vascular invasion.[88,89]

Aggressive Digital Papillary Adenoma

A single painless mass that occurs over the fingers and toes or the adjacent palmoplantar areas shows

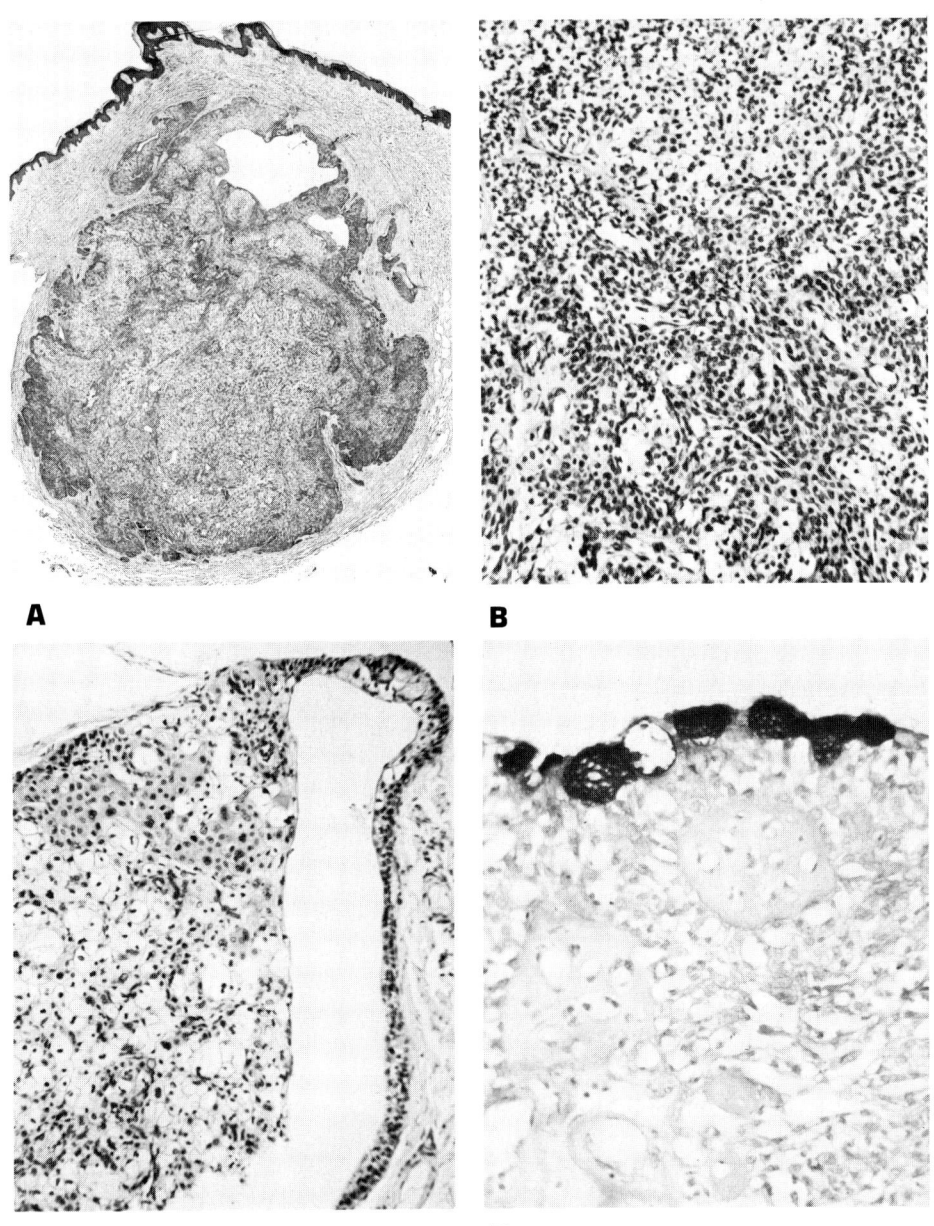

Figure 39–20.
Nodular hidradenoma, clear cell type. **A.** Solid tumor which was connected to epidermis in other parts of block consists of lighter- and darker-staining areas, contains several ductlike lumina, and a few larger cystic spaces (solid-cystic hidradenoma). H&E. X8. **B** and **C.** Cellular patterns indicating that large clear cells are modifications of smaller cells with more solid cytoplasm. Tumor cells border lumen without arranging themselves into a definite lining; note appearance of goblet cells in right upper corner. H&E. X90. **D.** Goblet cells containing PAS-positive material which was found to stain with aldehyde fuchsin and alcian blue, an indication that it is sialomucin. Diastase-digested PAS–hematoxylin. X185.

histologically an aggressive growth pattern (Fig. 39–23). Branching tubular and cystic dilated ductal structures show areas of papillary projections into the central lumina.[90] The fibrous stroma may be thin or dense and may show hyalinized collagen bundles. Some lesions show cellular atypia, nuclear pleomorphism, mitotic figures, and invasion of the surrounding soft tissues indicating malignancy.[91,92]

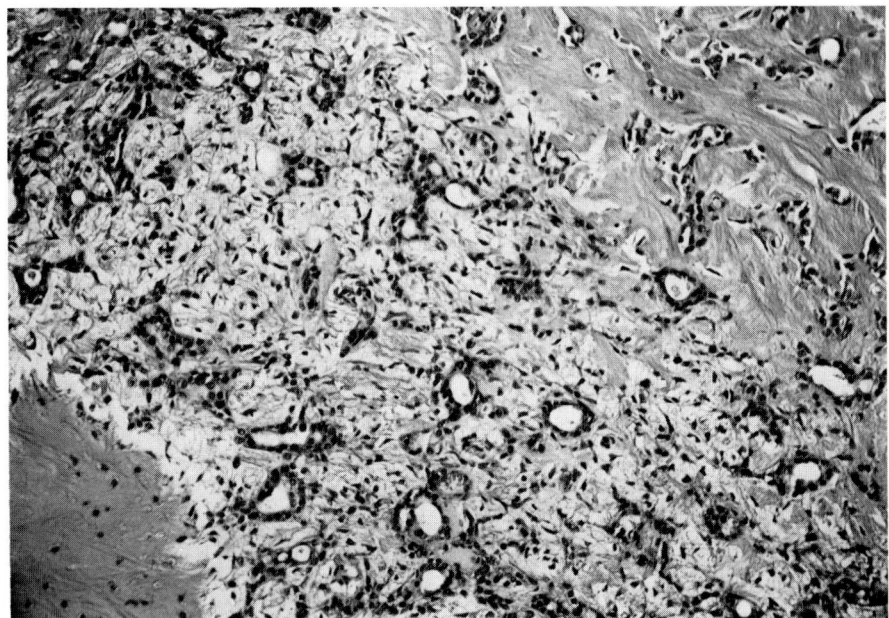

Figure 39–21.
Chondroid syringoma (mixed tumor of skin). In this type of tumor, tubular epithelial structures seem to dissolve into individual cells, which eventually are embedded in amorphous metachromatic matrix resembling cartilage, a process also seen in mixed tumors of salivary glands. H&E. X135.

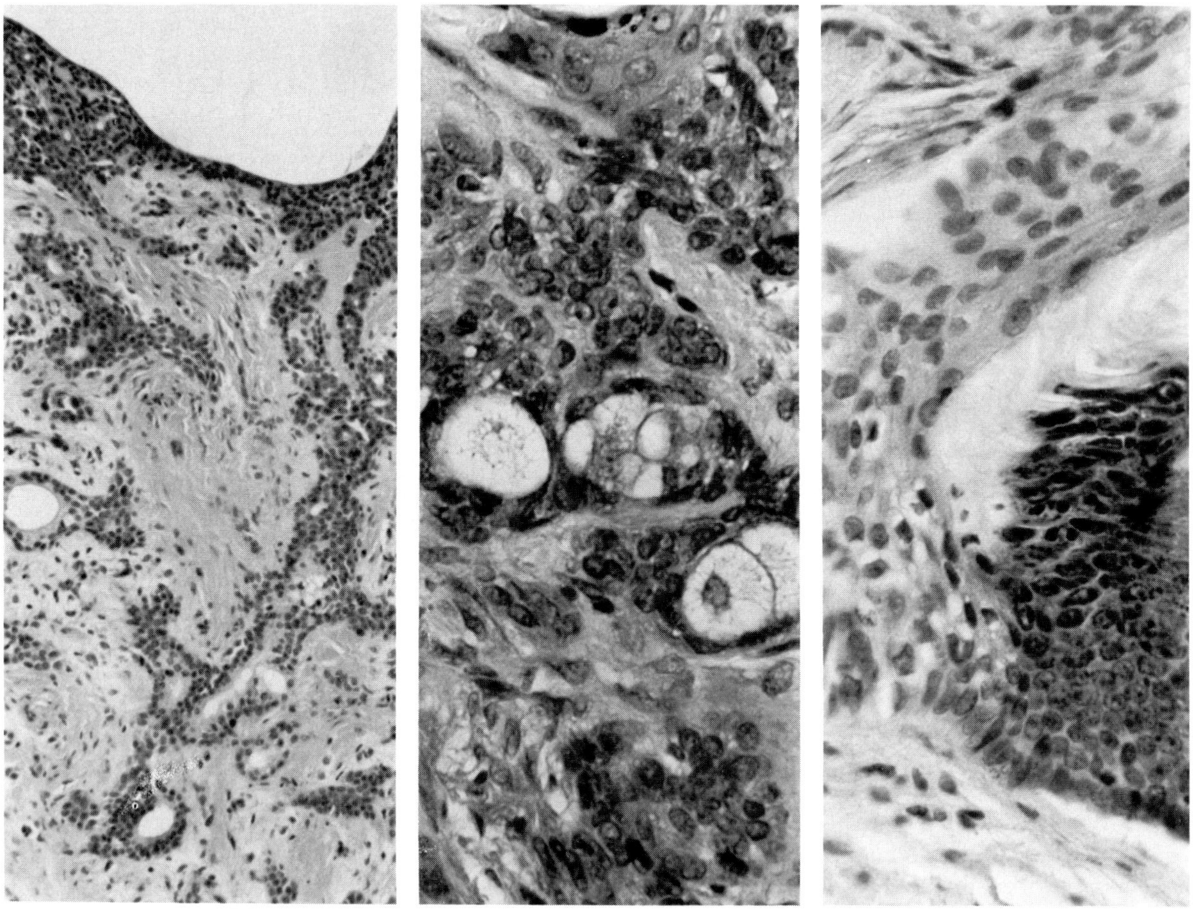

Figure 39–22.
Mixed tumor of the skin. **A.** Branching sweat ductal structures embedded in a mixomatous stroma. H&E. X250. **B.** Focus of sebaceous differentiation. H&E. X400. **C.** An area of hair matrixlike structure formation. H&E. X400.

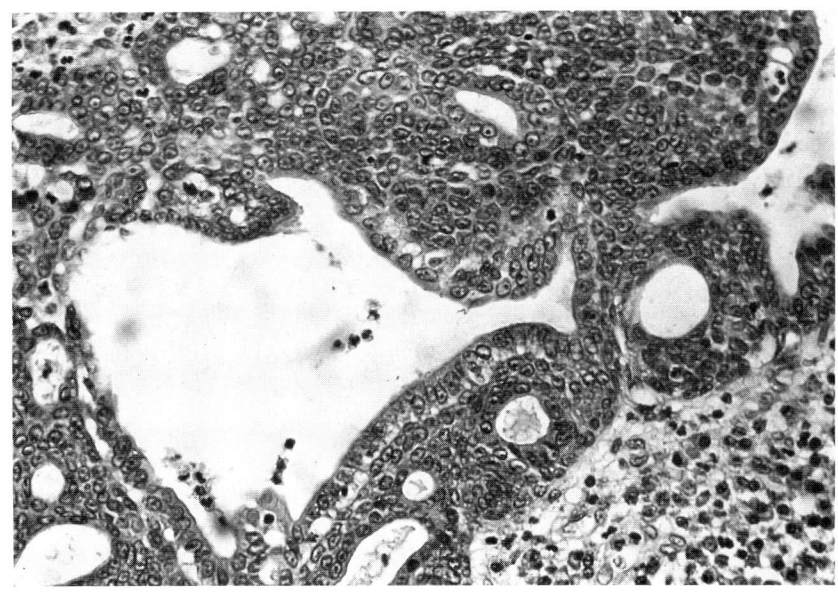

Figure 39-23.
Aggressive digital papillary adenoma. There are solid areas and cystic dilated ductal structures. Note also some chronic inflammatory cell reaction at right-lower portion. H&E. X250.

REFERENCES

1. Johnson WC: Histochemistry of cutaneous adnexa and selected adnexal neoplasms. J Cutan Pathol 11:352, 1984
2. Penneys NS: Immunohistochemistry of adnexal neoplasms. J Cutan Pathol 11:357, 1984
3. Hashimoto K, Kanzaki T: Appendage tumors of the skin: Histogenesis and ultrastructure. J Cutan Pathol 11:365, 1984
4. Maiorana A, Nigrisoli E, Papotti M: Immunohistochemical markers of sweat gland tumors. J Cutan Pathol 13:187, 1986
5. Mazoujian G, Margolis R: Immunohistochemistry of gross cystic disease fluid protein (GCDFP-15) in 65 benign sweat gland tumors of the skin. Am J Dermatopathol 10:28, 1988
6. Suzuki Y, Hashimoto K, Kato I, et al: A monoclonal antibody, SKH1, reacts with 40 Kd sweat gland-associated antigen. J Cutan Pathol 16:66, 1989
7. Hashimoto K, Mehregan AH, Kumakiri M: Tumors of skin appendages. Boston: Butterworths, 1987
8. Donati P, Amantea A, Balus L: Eccrine angiomatous hamartoma: A lipomatous variant. J Cutan Pathol 16:227, 1989
9. Imai S, Nitto H: Eccrine nevus with epidermal changes. Dermatologica 166:84, 1983
10. Kikuchi I, Kuroki Y, Inoue S: Painful eccrine angiomatous nevus on the sole. J Dermatol Tokyo 9:329, 1982
11. Avril MF, Duvillard P, Lebbe C, et al: Naevus eccrine comedinien et angiomateux avec spiradenomes et cylindromes multiples. Ann Dermatol Venereol 114:1326, 1987
12. Velasco JA, Almeida V: Eccrine-pilar angiomatous nevus. Dermatologica 177:317, 1988
13. Kim JH, Hur H, Lee CW, Kim YT: Apocrine nevus. J Am Acad Dermatol 18:579, 1988
14. Rabens SF, Naness JI, Gottlieb BF: Apocrine gland organic hamartoma (apocrine nevus). Arch Dermatol 112:520, 1976
15. Civatte J, Tsoïtis G, Préaux J: Le naevus apocrine. Étude de deux cas. Ann Dermatol Syphiligr 101:251, 1974
16. Mehregan AH: Supernumerary nipple: A histologic study. J Cutan Pathol 8:96, 1981
17. Langer K, Konrad K, Smolle J: Multiple apocrine hidrocystomas on the eyelids. Am J Dermatopathol 11:570, 1989
18. Cramer HJ: Das schwarze hidrocystom (Monfort). Dermatol Monatsschr 166:114, 1980
19. Malhotra R, Bhawan J: The nature of pigment in pigmented apocrine hidrocystoma. J Cutan Pathol 12:106, 1985
20. Mehregan AH: Apocrine cystadenoma. Arch Dermatol 90:274, 1964
21. Helwig EB, Hackney VC: Syringadenoma papilliferum lesions with and without naevus sebaceous and basal cell carcinoma. Arch Dermatol 71:361, 1955
22. Pinkus H: Life history of naevus syringadenomatosus papilliferus. Arch Dermatol Syphiligr 69:305, 1954
23. Niizuma K: Syringocystadenoma papilliferum. Light and electron microscopic studies. Acta Derm Venereol 56:327, 1976
24. Meeker JH, Neubecker RD, Helwig EB: Hidradenoma papilliferum. Am J Clin Pathol 37:182, 1962
25. Woodworth H Jr, Dockerty MB, Wilson RB, et al: Papillary hidradenoma of the vulva: A clinicopathologic study of sixty-nine cases. Am J Obstet Gynecol 110:501, 1971
26. Mehregan AH, Rahbari H: Benign epithelial tumors

of the skin: IV. Benign apocrine gland tumors. Cutis 21:53, 1978
27. Umbert P, Winkelmann RK: Tubular apocrine adenoma. J Cutan Pathol 3:75, 1976
28. Civatte J, Belaïch S, Lauret P: Adénome tubulaire apocrine (quatre cas). Ann Dermatol Venereol 106:665, 1979
29. Warkel RL: Selected apocrine neoplasms. J Cutan Pathol 11:437, 1984
30. Toribio J, Zulaica A, Peteiro C: Tubular apocrine adenoma. J Cutan Pathol 14:114, 1987
31. Rosen PP, Caicco JA: Florid papillomatosis of the nipple. A study of 51 patients, including nine with mammary carcinoma. Am J Surg Pathol 10:87, 1986
32. Brownstein MH, Phelps RG, Magnin PH: Papillary adenoma of the nipple: Analysis of fifteen new cases. J Am Acad Dermatol 12:707, 1985
33. Moulin G, Darbon P, Balme B, Frappart L: Adenomatose erosive du mamelon. A propos de 10 cas avec etude immunohistochimique. Ann Dermatol Venereol 117:537, 1990
34. Vernon HJ, Olsen EA, Vollmer RT: Autosomal dominant multiple cylindromas associated with solitary lung cylindroma. J Am Acad Dermatol 19:397, 1988
35. Crain RC, Helwig EB: Dermal cylindroma (dermal eccrine cylindroma). Am J Clin Pathol 35:504, 1961
36. Munger BL, Graham JH, Helwig EB: Ultrastructure and histochemical characteristics of dermal eccrine cylindroma (turban tumor). J Invest Dermatol 39:577, 1962
37. Ferrandiz C, Campo E, Baumann E: Dermal cylindromas (Turban tumour) and eccrine spiradenomas in a patient with membranous basal cell adenoma of the parotid gland. J Cutan Pathol 12:72, 1985
38. Rockerbie N, Solomon AR, Woo TY, et al: Malignant dermal cylindroma in a patient with multiple dermal cylindromas, trichoepitheliomas, and bilateral dermal analogue tumors of the parotid gland. Am J Dermatopathol 11:353, 1989
39. Warner TFCS, Goell WS, Cripps DJJ: Hidroacanthoma simplex: An ultrastructural study. J Cutan Pathol 9:189, 1982
40. Rahbari H: Hidroacanthoma simplex—A review of 15 cases. Br J Dermatol 109:219, 1983
41. Myskow MW, Gawkrodger DJ, O'Doherty CSJ, McLaren KM: Syringoacanthoma: An acrosyringeal tumour. Dermatologica 181:62, 1990
42. Rahbari H: Syringoacanthoma. Acanthotic lesion of the acrosyringium. Arch Dermatol 120:751, 1984
43. Pinkus H: The discovery of eccrine poroma. J Dermatol Tokyo 2:26, 1979
44. Goldner R: Eccrine poromatosis. Arch Dermatol 101:606, 1970
45. Wilkinson RD, Schopflocher P, Rozenfeld M: Hidrotic ectodermal dysplasia with diffuse eccrine poromatosis. Arch Dermatol 113:472, 1977
46. Mehregan AH: The origin of the adnexal tumors of the skin. A viewpoint. J Cutan Pathol 12:459, 1985
47. Hyman AB, Brownstein MH: Eccrine poroma. An analysis of forty-five new cases. Dermatologica 138:29, 1969
48. Tokura Y, Yoshikuni K, Taraki Y, et al: Immunohistochemically detectable duct-like structures in benign and malignant eccrine poromas: CEA and involucrin immunostaining. J Dermatol Tokyo 16:133, 1989
49. Winkelmann RK, McLeod WA: The dermal duct tumor. Arch Dermatol 94:50, 1966
50. Hu C-H, Marques AS, Winkelmann RK: Dermal duct tumor. A histochemical and electron microscopic study. Arch Dermatol 114:1659, 1978
51. Mascaro JM: Considerations sur les tumeurs fibroepitheliales. Le syringofibroadenome eccrine. Ann Derm Syphiligr 90:146, 1963
52. Civatte J, Jeanmougin M, Barrandon Y, Jimenez de Franch: Siringofibroadenoma ecrino de Mascaro. Discusion de un Caso. Med Cutan ILA 9:193, 1981
53. Mehregan AH, Marufi M, Medenica M: Eccrine syringofibroadenoma (Mascaro). Report of two cases. J Am Acad Dermatol 13:433, 1985
54. Kanitakis J, Zambruno G, Euvrard S, et al: Eccrine syringofibroadenoma. Immunohistological study of a new case. Am J Dermatopathol 9:37, 1987
55. Weedon D: Eccrine tumors: A selective review. J Cutan Pathol 11:421, 1984
56. Falck VG, Jordaan MF: Papillary eccrine adenoma. Am J Dermatopathol 8:64, 1986
57. Oka K, Katsumata M: Eccrine tubular adenoma—A histopathological, histochemical, and ultrastructural study. J Dermatol Tokyo 13:285, 1986
58. Urmacher C, Lieberman PH: Papillary eccrine adenoma. Light-microscopic, histochemical, and immunohistochemical studies. Am J Dermatopathol 9:243, 1987
59. Sexton M, Maize JC: Papillary eccrine adenoma. A light microscopic and immunohistochemical study. J Am Acad Dermatol 18:1114, 1988
60. Tellechea O, Truchetet F, Grosshans E: Adenoma papillar ecrino. Med Cutan ILA 17:85, 1989
61. Carneiro SJC, Gardner HL, Knox JM: Syringomas: Three cases with vulvar involvement. Obstet Gynecol 39:93, 1972
62. Thomas J, Majumdar B, Gorelkin L: Syringoma localized to the vulva. Arch Dermatol 115:95, 1979
63. Metze D, Jurecka W, Gebhart W: Disseminated syringomas of the upper extremities. Case history and immunohistochemical and ultrastructural study. Dermatologica 180:228, 1990
64. Hashimoto K, Blum D, Fukaya T, et al: Familial Syringoma. Case history and application of monoclonal anti-eccrine gland antibodies. Arch Dermatol 121:756, 1985
65. Ambrojo P, Caballero LR, Martinez AA, et al: Clear cell syringoma. Immunohistochemistry and electron microscopy study. Dermatologica 178:164, 1989
66. Holden CA, MacDonald DM: Syringomata: A bathing trunk distribution. Clin Exp Dermatol 6:555, 1981
67. Yung CW, Soltani K, Bernstein JE, Lorincz AL: Uni-

lateral linear nevoid syringoma. J Am Acad Dermatol 4:412, 1981
68. Wilms NA, Douglass MC: An unusual case of preponderantly right-sided syringomas. Arch Dermatol 117:308, 1981
69. Hashimoto K, Blum D, Fukaya T, Eto H: Familial syringoma. Case history and application of monoclonal anti-eccrine gland antibodies. Arch Dermatol 121:756, 1985
70. Lechner W, Dotzer V: Multiple syringome bei Trisomie 21. Z Hautkr 56:1467, 1981
71. Urban CD, Cannon JR, Cole RD: Eruptive syringomas in Down's syndrome. Arch Dermatol 117:374, 1981
72. Dupré A, Bonafé JL: Syringomes, mongolisme, maladie de Marfan et syndrome D'Ehlers–Danlos. Nouvelle entite posant les rapports des syringomes avec les maladies héréditaires du tissue conjonctif. Ann Dermatol Venereol 104:224, 1977
73. Kersting DW, Helwig EB: Eccrine spiradenoma. Arch Dermatol 73:199, 1956
74. Jitsukawa K, Sueki H, Sato S, Anzai T: Eccrine spiradenoma. An electron microscopic study. Am J Dermatopathol 9:99, 1987
75. Revis P, Chyu J, Medenica M: Multiple eccrine spiradenoma: Case report and review. J Cutan Pathol 15:226, 1988
76. Shelley WB, Wood MG: A zosteriform network of spiradenomas. J Am Acad Dermatol 2:59, 1980
77. Tsur H, Lipskier E, Fisher BK: Multiple linear spiradenomas. Plast Reconstr Surg 68:100, 1981
78. Ikeya T: Multiple linear eccrine spiradenoma associated with multiple trichoepithelioma. J Dermatol Tokyo 14:48, 1987
79. Helwig EB: Eccrine acrospiroma. J Cutan Pathol 11:415, 1984
80. Winkelmann RK, Wolff K: Solid-cystic hidradenoma of the skin. Clinical and histopathologic study. Arch Dermatol 97:651, 1968
81. Hashimoto K, DiBella RJ, Level WF: Clear cell hidradenoma: Histological, histochemical, and electron microscopic studies. Arch Dermatol 96:18, 1967
82. Hirsch P, Helwig EB: Chondroid syringoma: Mixed tumor of skin, salivary gland type. Arch Dermatol 84:835, 1971
83. Mills SE: Mixed tumor of the skin: A model of divergent differentiation. J Cutan Pathol 11:382, 1984
84. Terui T, Obata M, Tagami H: Immunohistochemical studies on epithelial cells in mixed tumor of the skin. J Cutan Pathol 13:197, 1986
85. Argenyi ZB, Balogh K, Goeken JA: Immunohistochemical characterization of chondroid syringoma. Am J Clin Pathol 90:662, 1988
86. Hassab-El-Naby H, Tam S, White WL, Ackerman AB: Mixed tumors of the skin. A histological and immunohistochemical study. Am J Dermatopathol 11:413, 1989
87. Apisarnthanarax P, Bovenmyer DA, Mehregan AH: Combined adnexal tumor of the skin. Arch Dermatol 120:231, 1984
88. Harrist TJ, Aretz TH, Mihm MC Jr, Evans GW, Rodriguez FL: Cutaneous malignant mixed tumor. Arch Dermatol 117:719, 1981
89. Ishimura E, Iwamoto H, Kobashi Y, Yamabe H, Ichijima K: Malignant chondroid syringoma. Report of a case with widespread metastasis and review of pertinent literature. Cancer 52:1966, 1983
90. Bourlond A, Frankart M, Vanwijck R, et al: Adenome papillaire eccrine digital agressif. Dermatologica 179:170, 1989
91. Kao GF, Helwig EB, Graham JH: Aggressive digital papillary adenoma and adenocarcinoma. A clinicopathologic study of 57 patients, with histochemical, immunopathological, and ultrastructural observations. J Cutan Pathol 14:129, 1987
92. Ceballos PI, Penneys NS, Acosta R: Aggressive digital papillary adenocarcinoma. J Am Acad Dermatol 23:331, 1990

40
BASAL CELL EPITHELIOMA

TERMINOLOGY

Based on histologic investigation, Krompecher[1] introduced the term "basal cell epithelioma" in 1904 to describe the lesion previously known as Jacob's[2] rodent ulcer. Dubreuilh[3] had previously defined cancer as a malignant neoplasm capable of metastasis and had pointed out that rodent ulcer does not metastasize even when the soft tissues, cartilage, or bone are involved. The term introduced by Krompecher was not satisfactory because it implied derivation from basal cells of the epidermis and because it was not truly a carcinoma. Belisario[4] introduced the term "rodent carcinoma," which did not find many followers. The term "basalioma" has been used in Germany and in other European countries. In all other countries the terms *basal cell epithelioma* and *basal cell carcinoma* are used synonymously among dermatologists.

HISTOGENESIS

As indicated in Table VII–I, basal cell epithelioma is the least mature member of the large tribe of organoid adnexal tumors. It is found at the bottom of the tabulation below all the different adnexal maturations and describes all tumors that do not have morphologic differentiating characteristics of one type or other. Like all the other adnexal tumors, basal cell epithelioma is a fibroepithelial neoplasm consisting of epithelial parenchyma interdependent with mesodermal stroma. This intimal epithelial and mesodermal relationship is the outstanding feature that separates basal cell epithelioma from truly malignant epithelial tumors such as squamous cell carcinoma or adnexal carcinomas.[5] Requirement of the specific fibrous stroma in achieving growth of tumor epithelium in basal cell epithelioma has been well established in experimental autotransplantation.[6] The stroma seems to be necessary for continuation of proliferation of tumor cells in the immature state. Removal of the stroma will result in maturation of basaloid cells into prickle cells and foci of keratinization.[7] Stromal dependency is also the most likely reason for the extremely rare incidence of epithelial cell metastasis.

The point of origin of basal cell epithelioma is not always detectable in histologic sections. In rat skin, Zackheim[8] noted development of basal cell epitheliomas from the lower surface of the epidermis and the infundibular portion of the hair follicles (Fig. 40–1). In early lesions of human superficial basal cell epitheliomas tumor nests were found connected with the lower surface of the epidermis independent of the cutaneous adnexae.[9] Development from the lower surface of the epidermis, however, does not explain some deep seated lesions and those

Figure 40-1.
An early developing basal cell epithelioma. A single tumor nest is connected with the epidermis and is surrounded by retraction space and elongated fibroblasts. H&E. X600.

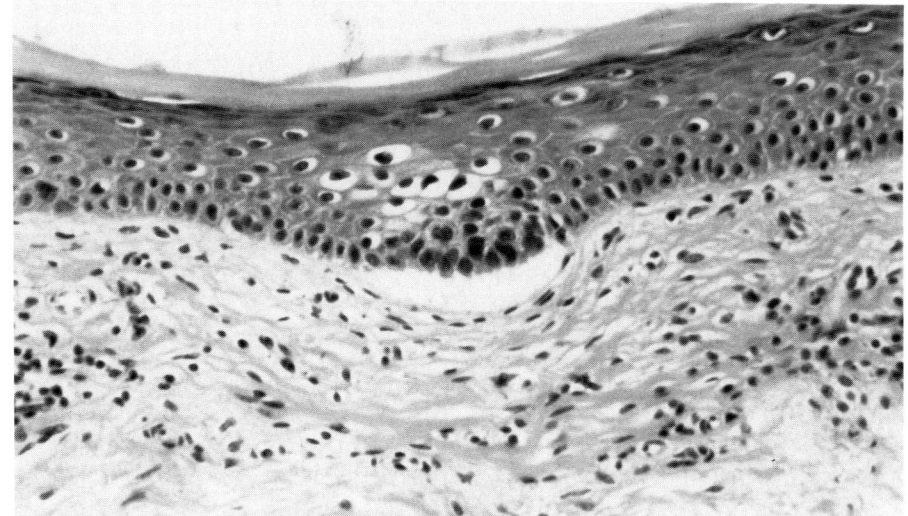

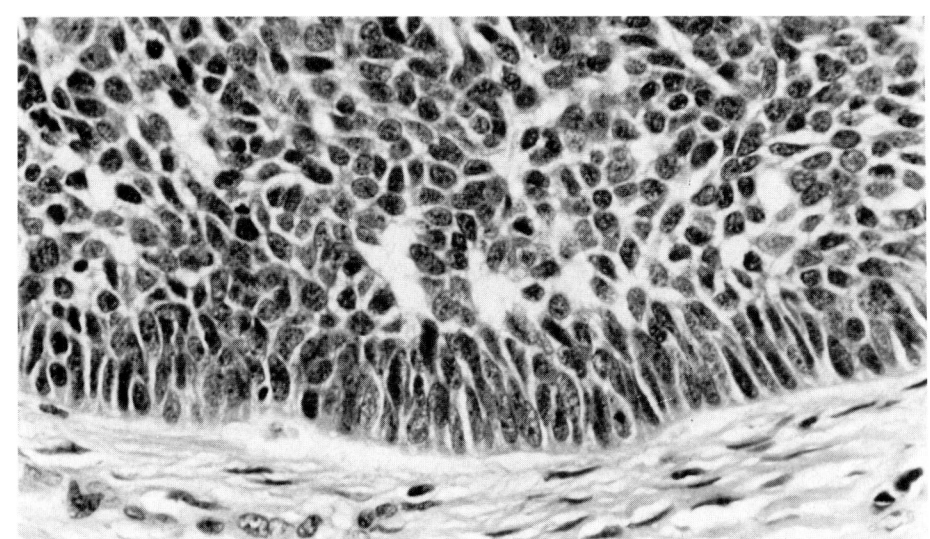

Figure 40-2.
Basal cell epithelioma. **A.** A solid tumor mass surrounded by a layer of cells with palisaded nuclei. H&E. X400. **B.** A solid tumor mass surrounded by a row of cells with palisaded nuclei and inflammatory cell infiltrate within the tumor stroma. H&E. X400.

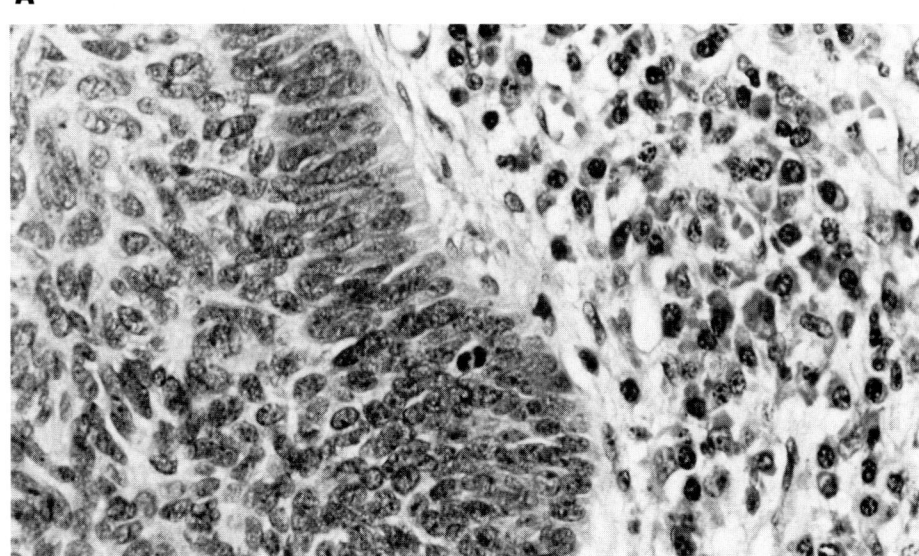

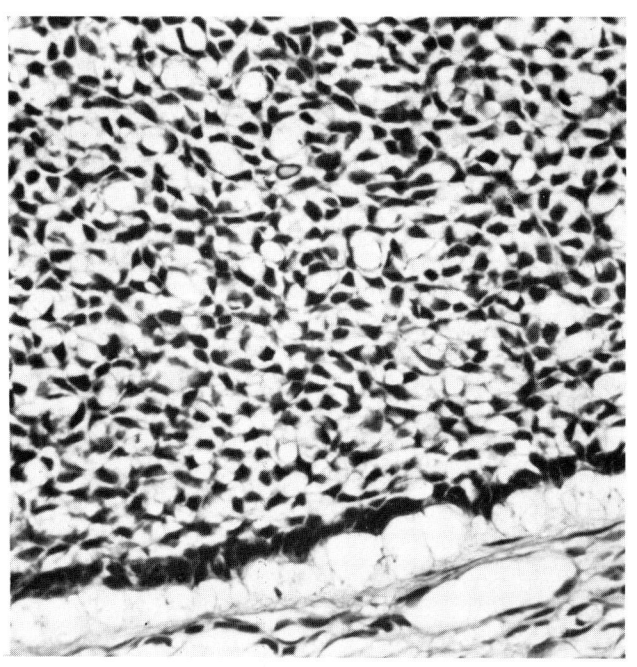

Figure 40–3.
Adamantinoid pattern in basal cell epithelioma. H&E. X370.

of the morphea-like variety that often have no epidermal connection. Pinkus suggested that basal cell epithelioma is a monstrous attempt in adnexogenesis in which both ectodermal and mesodermal components participate just as trichogenesis occurs in the fetus with cooperation of the epithelial germ and the underlying mesynchymal cells. Relation to pilar apparatus is also suggested by others in terms such as "trichoma" and "adnexal carcinoma."[10,11] In support of a relationship of basal cell epithelioma with the pilary complex are histologic observations of follicular differentiation,[12] similarity between the electrophoretic patterns of the fibrous protein extracted from the human basal cell epithelioma and that of the epithelia of the pilary complex, and the similarity of keratin expressions between basal cell epithelioma and the follicular epithelium below the level of isthmus.[13]

EPITHELIAL PORTION

While resembling epidermal or pilar basal cells, the epithelial cells are at most basaloid (Fig. 40–2), a

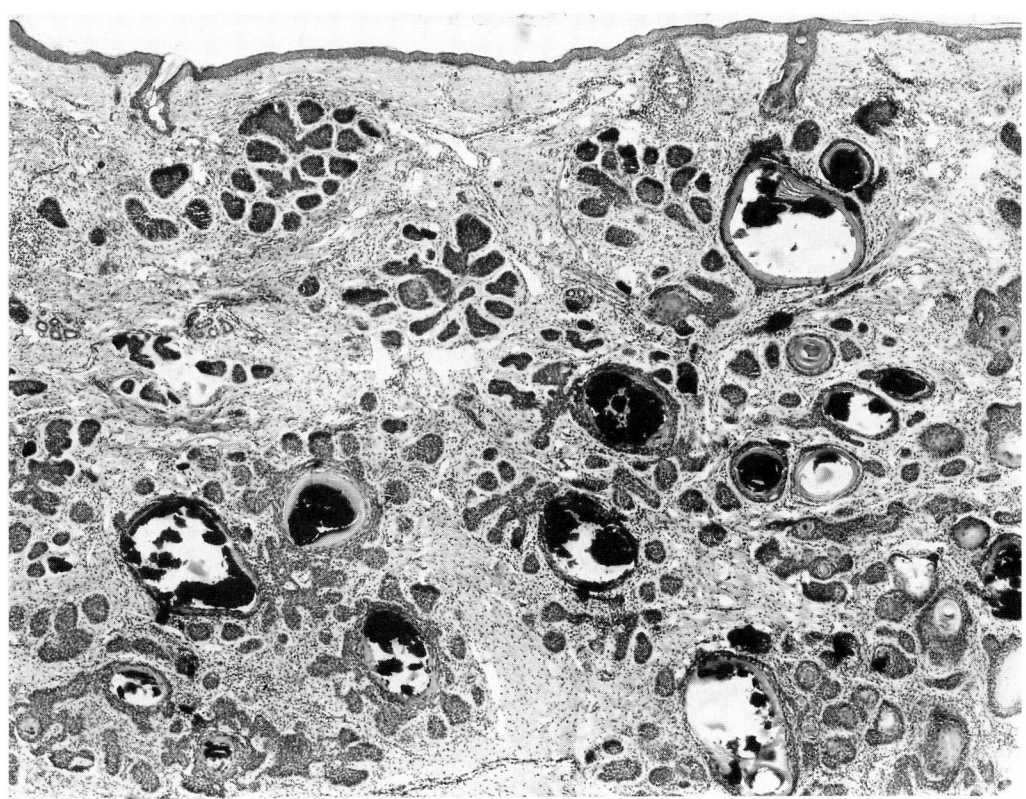

Figure 40–4.
Keratinizing basal cell epithelioma. Some tumor masses show central keratin cyst and areas of calcification. H&E. X75.

fact confirmed by electron microscopy.[14-16] The peripheral cells often form a continuous layer of columnar cells resting in a palisaded arrangement on a PAS-positive basement membrane. This feature may be absent if the tumor cells occur in small clusters or cords. More centrally situated cells may show no particular arrangement or may be more or less fusiform. They often have a larger amount of somewhat lighter staining cytoplasm.

Routine stains usually show no intercellular connections. The cells of basal cell epithelioma usually do not have a well-developed system of tonofibrils. The absence of tonofibrils may account for their relatively small size, for the softness of their cell bodies, which are apt to shrink during histologic processing, and for the inability to keratinize. On the other hand, intercellular bridges (desmosomes) are present, and, in some tumors in which the intercellular spaces contain mucin, a peculiar picture of stellate interconnected cells results (Fig. 40–3). Because of histologic similarity to adamantinoma (an adnexoid epithelioma related to the tooth organ) the term "adamantinoid" is applied.[17]

Keratinization with keratohyalin is very rare in basal cell epithelioma. Its occasional occurrence can be related to epidermoid keratinization, in the sebaceous ducts and the follicular infundibulum. Cornification in the so-called *keratotic* basal cell epithelioma (Fig. 40–4) usually is parakeratotic and often incomplete. We do not recognize metatypical carcinoma (basosquamous carcinoma) as an entity linking basal cell epithelioma with squamous cell carcinoma. We are convinced that most cases of this type are keratinizing basal cell epitheliomas. Other possibilities include pseudoepitheliomatous hyperplasia in a basal cell epithelioma and rare instances of basal cell epithelioma and squamous cell carcinoma developing in close approximity so they are found side by side or intermingled in the same sections.

Pilar differentiation (Fig. 40–5) in a basal cell epithelioma is characterized by the presence of foci of keratinization, keratin cysts, and abortive hair follicle-like structures. Differentiation from solitary trichoepithelioma may be difficult (see Chapter 39).

In most lesions, basaloid cells undergoing mitotic division are present within the rows at the periphery of the tumor masses.[18] In the center tumor cells break down and disappear through the process of apoptosis. If breakdown becomes a prominent feature, cystic spaces are formed and the cavities may reach clinically perceptible size (Fig. 40–6). Other

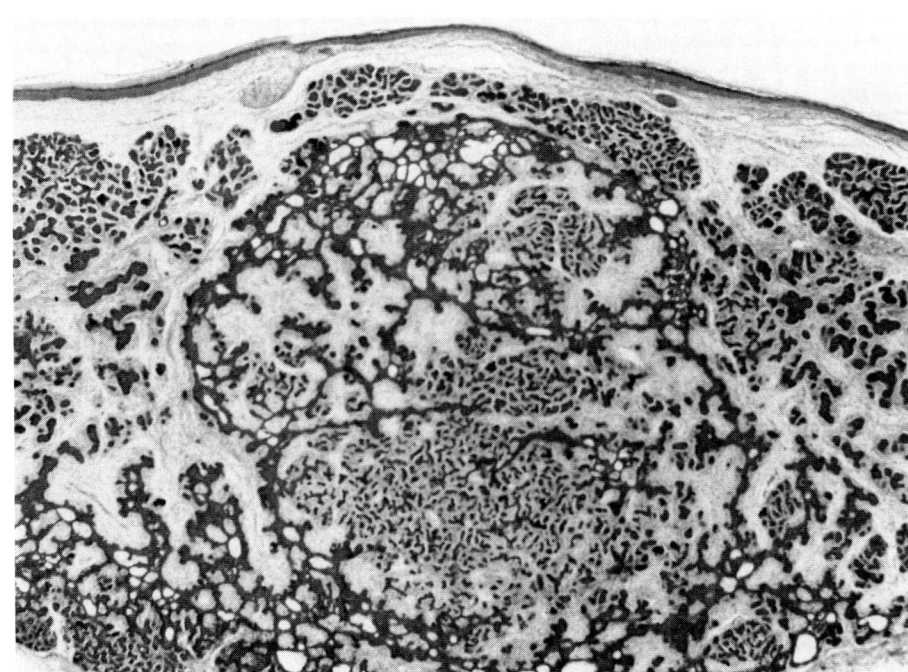

Figure 40–5.
Basal cell epithelioma with follicular differentiation. Note small buds of basaloid cells resembling abortive hair follicles. H&E. X25.

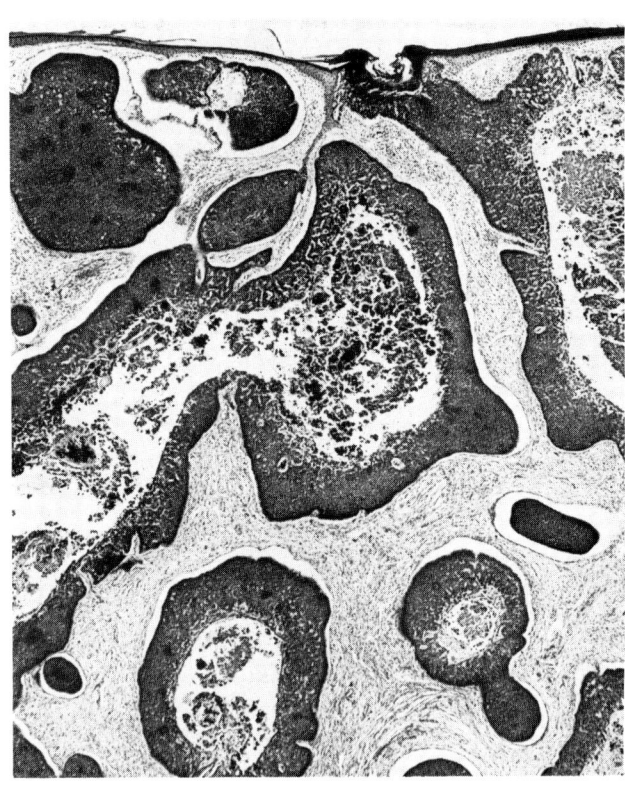

Figure 40-6.
Pseudocystic basal cell epithelioma. Cells degenerate (apoptosis) and disappear in central cavities. Note retraction spaces between epithelial nests and organoid stroma. Tumor approaches and invades epidermis. H&E. X30.

tumors may show cells arranged somewhat regularly around numerous small mucin-filled spaces (Fig. 40–7). The words adenoid or pseudoadenomatous are strictly descriptive when applied to such tumors and do not imply truly glandular nature. Yet another variant is reticulated or plexiform epithelioma (Fig. 40–8) in which two-rowed cords and thin sheets seem to bend around and connect with each other, embedded in a rarefied stroma (Fig. 40–9). In this type, there are no definable epithelial nests, but the entire tumor usually is well circumscribed by a stroma envelope.

Occasionally, all or some of the tumor nests contain multinucleated giant cells or show much variation of cell sizes and shapes that a bowenoid picture results (Fig. 40–10).[19,20] In another rare form, the entire or part of the growth consists of cells with abundant and clear cytoplasm containing glycogen granules (Fig. 40–11).[21–23] A few cases of basal cell epitheliomas with signet-ring cells and with granular cells have also been reported.[24,25]

Yet another variant contains melanin produced by symbiotically present melanocytes (Fig 40–12). The melanin granules may be present mainly within highly dendritic melanocytes or macrophages within the tumor stroma without entering the tumor cells themselves.[26–28] In some instances, however, the basaloid cells retain capacity to accept pigment from dendritic cells and tumor is truly a *pigmented* basal cell epithelioma.

MESODERMAL PORTION

Too little attention has been paid to the stroma of basal cell epitheliomas. Just as stroma is a characteristic feature of benign adnexoid tumors and may constitute the major part of their volume, so it is in basal cell epithelioma. The stroma often is somewhat less mature, more cellular, and less fibrous. A PAS-positive basement membrane usually surrounds the epithelial portions. Mucinous substance, mainly hyaluronic acid, is increased, and

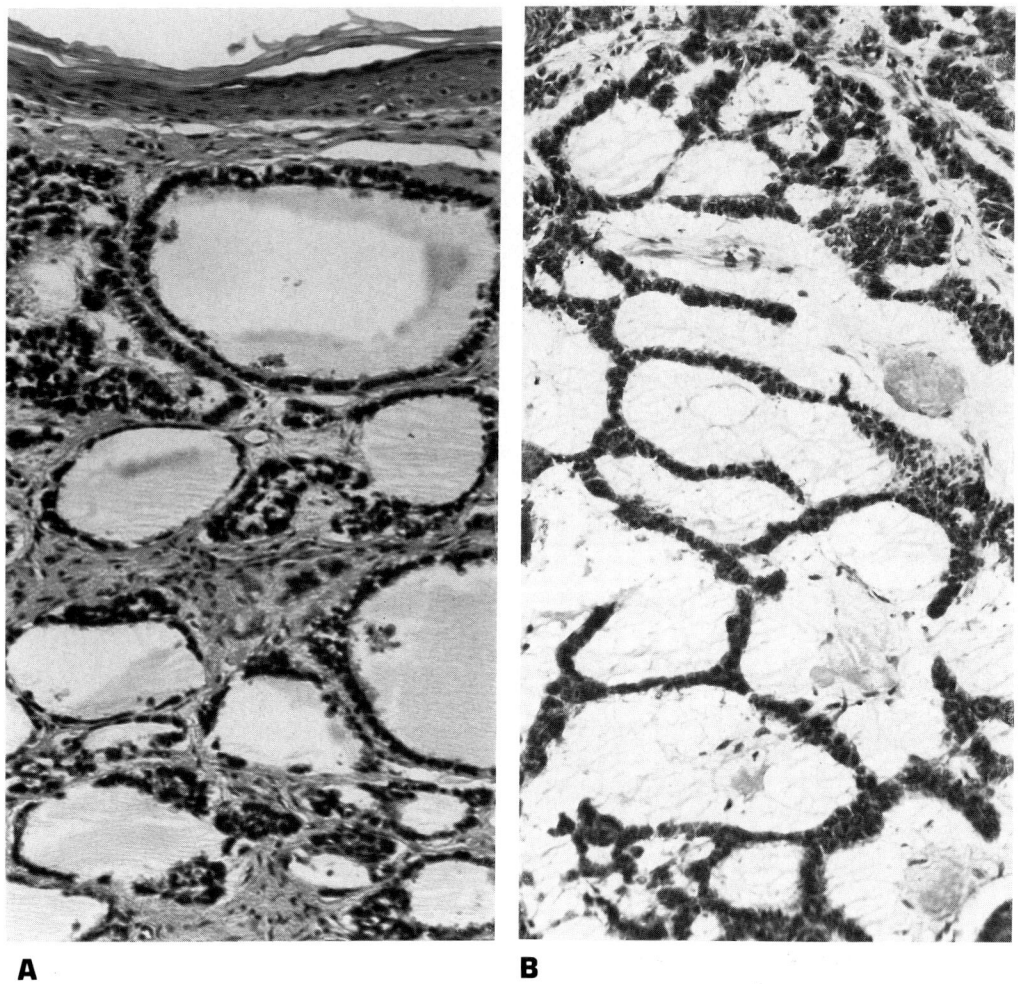

Figure 40–7.
Adenoid basal cell epithelioma. **A.** *Many small mucin-filled cystic spaces. H&E. X125.* **B.** *Extensive mucin deposition between thin septae of basalioma cells. H&E. X125.*

mucin formation may reach considerable proportion around the epithelial nests.[29,30] Sections stained with H&E then show empty halos, so-called retraction spaces (Fig. 40–13). Although some retraction takes place during fixation and dehydration, owing to the softness of the tissues, one can usually show that most of this space is occupied by metachromatic and alcian blue-positive material. There is also evidence of specific synthesis of laminin, fibronectin, and type-IV and type-V collagen.[31,32] The tumor-stromal interface should not be compared to the epidermal–dermal junction of normal skin. The concept of specific constructive metabolic processes in the stroma is supported by the fact that new elastic fibers in typical perifollicular arrangement are found in a small percentage of lesions.[33] In some tumors a dense coat of hyalinized collagenous tissue is formed resembling the hyaline sheaths of cylindromas. Cartilage may rarely develop, but keratin-type amyloid (amyloid K) is not an uncommon deposit in the stroma of basal cell epitheliomas.[34]

Another component of basal cell epithelioma is a cell-mediated inflammatory reaction that consists mainly of T lymphocytes and may include a few plasma cells and eosinophils.[35–37]

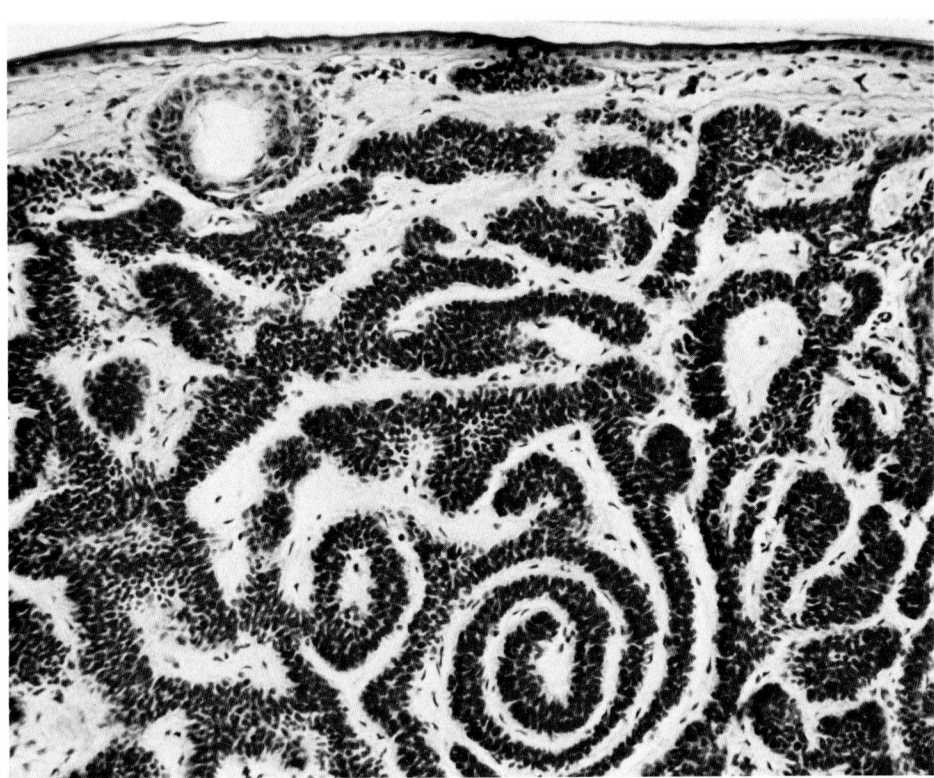

Figure 40–8.
Histologic patterns of basal cell epithelioma. Lacy or plexiform pattern results when myxomatous stroma envelops and separates thin cords and septal sheets of epithelium. H&E. X180.

PREMALIGNANT FIBROEPITHELIAL TUMOR

On the lower part of the trunk or in the groin or thigh region are sometimes found elevated or sessile lesions clinically resembling fibromas but, on microscopic examination, presenting the peculiar picture (Fig. 40–14A) of an epithelial meshwork with hyperplastic mesodermal contents.[38,39] In three-dimensional interpretations we are dealing with an epithelial sponge, the compartments of which are filled with stroma resembling that of benign adnexoid tumors. What look like epithelial cords in paraffin sections actually are cross sections of thin septa. The cells composing them are a little larger and lighter staining than those of basal cell epitheliomas, rather resembling those of trichoepithelioma. In some lesions, solid buds of small dark-staining cells that look like embryonic hair germs or the smallest basaloid nests are found sprouting from the epithelial septa (Fig. 40–14B). These may grow and replace parts or all of the preexisting tumor, a clear case of progression from a benign and balanced fibroepithelial growth to invasive and destructive, yet still organoid, basal cell epithelioma. It was for this reason that Pinkus designated these *premalignant fibroepithelial tumors.*[40]

SUPERFICIAL BASAL CELL EPITHELIOMA

Some varieties of basal cell epithelioma warrant special discussion. A biologically interesting variant is superficial basal cell epithelioma. It occurs most commonly on the trunk, more rarely on the extremities, but may be found on face and scalp as well. Clinically, it is flat, dermatitic, and rarely ulcerated, and may form plaques of several centimeters in diameter. Pigmented lesions may resemble superficial spreading malignant melanoma. Histologically, it consists of a fibroepithelial plate replacing the papillary layer of the skin without invasion into pars reticularis. Its epithelial component is joined to the lower surface of the epidermis in multiple places and may replace short stretches of the epidermis (Fig.

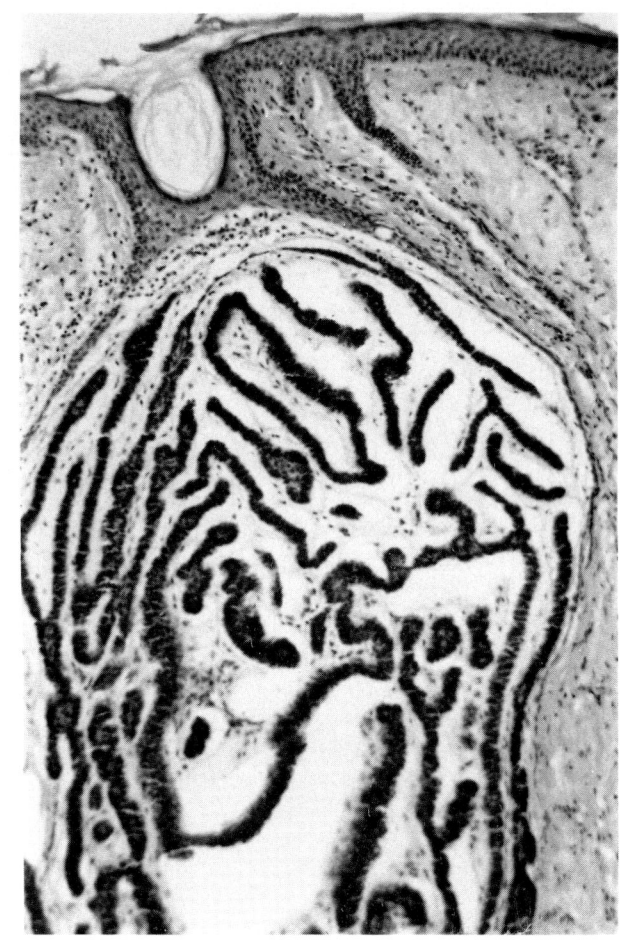

Figure 40-9.
Reticulated basal cell epithelioma shows a myomatous stroma between thin strands and septae of basalioma cells. H&E. X125.

40–15). The lesion advances peripherally as a continuous ring, while in the center are areas of regression.[41] In a majority of lesions, the growth assumes the appearance of a fenestrated plate in which epithelial nests are attached to the lower surface of the epidermis seemingly not connected with each other (Fig. 40–16).[42] Indication of a platelike lesion is easily recognized if one looks at the fibrous tumor stroma that surrounds each epithelial nest and also replaces the papillary dermis continuously within the entire lesion. In a smaller number of lesions, multicentric development of superficial basal cell epithelioma may be proved in serial sections. Whether small or large, superficial basal cell epithelioma can be cured by removing the thin fibroepithelial tumor plate situated above the pars reticularis. Full thickness surgical excision is not necessary.

AGGRESSIVE (INFILTRATING) BASAL CELL EPITHELIOMA

Some facial lesions and occasionally lesions of trunk within the sunlight-protected areas show histologic features indicating an aggressive neoplasm. These include downward extension of the tumor nests in the pathway of the cutaneous adnexa (Fig. 40–17), perivascular and perineural invasion, and involvement of cartilage or bone (Fig. 40–18).[43,44] The advancing border of the growth is made up of small nests or spiky strands of epithelial cells projecting into densely cellular stroma in which many elongated fibroblasts with prominent nuclei extend outward invading the spaces in between the surrounding collagen bundles.[45]

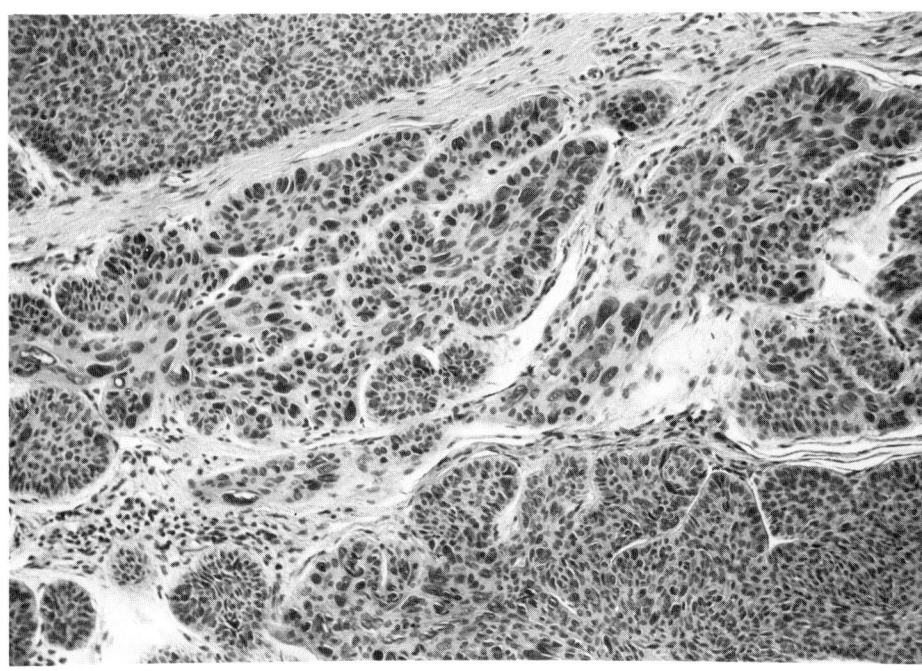

Figure 40–10.
Basal cell epithelioma with bowenoid pattern. Note more conventional appearance in upper left corner. Pattern has no clinical significance and does not denote basosquamous carcinoma. H&E. X135.

SCLEROTIC BASAL CELL EPITHELIOMA

These are often located on the face and neck of relatively older individuals in the form of a solid nodule or infiltrated plaque with or without superficial ulceration (Fig. 40–19). Histologically, small solid tumor nests extend down from the lower surface of the epidermis embedded in a fibrotic stroma. As the growth extends down, the epithelial nests become smaller and the stroma increasingly fibrotic (Fig. 40–20). Marked hyalinization of the fibrous stroma may be present. The inflammatory cell reaction is usually minimal.

MORPHEA-LIKE EPITHELIOMA

Firm, skin-colored, or yellowish white plaques, often having their start at an early age and slowly enlarging for many years before they are detected, constitute another variant of basal cell epithelioma.[46] They should not be confused with relatively superficial lesions on the face that act like brush fire, producing tiny ulcerations in their peripheral advance and leaving behind a somewhat atrophic scar in which residual epitheliomatous nests may be embedded. Morphea-like basal cell epitheliomas grow slowly for 10–20 years before attracting medical attention. The plaquelike lesions show shiny surface

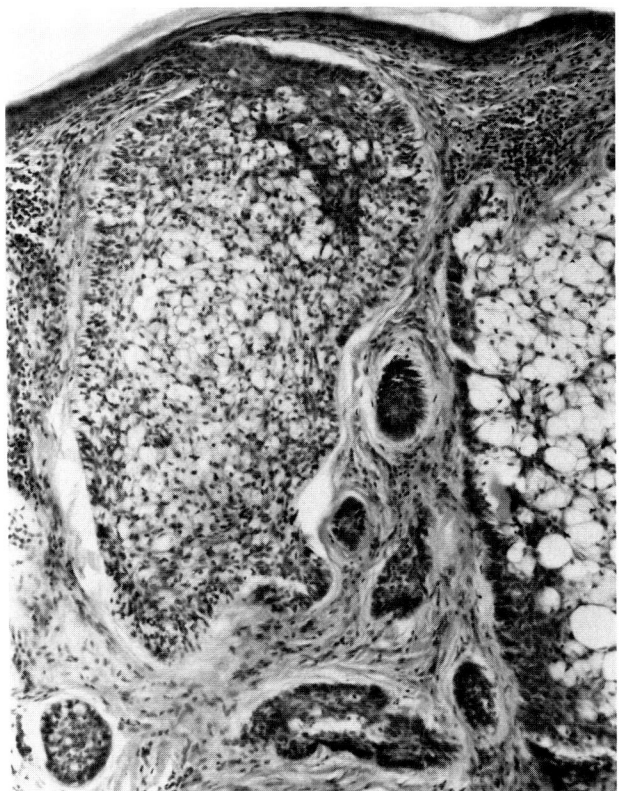

Figure 40–11.
Basal cell epithelioma with clear cells. H&E. X125.

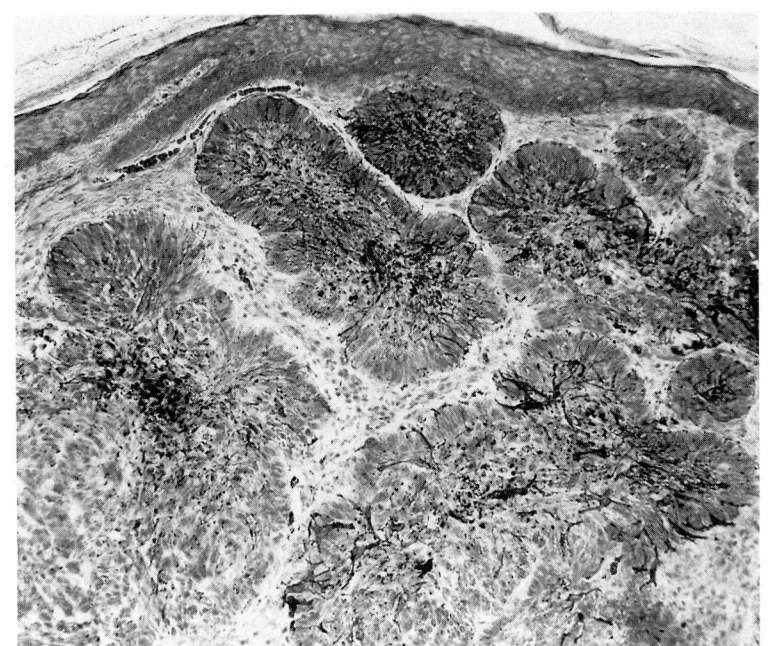

Figure 40–12.
Pigmented basal cell epithelioma. Note numerous dendritic melanocytes among basalioma cells. H&E. X225.

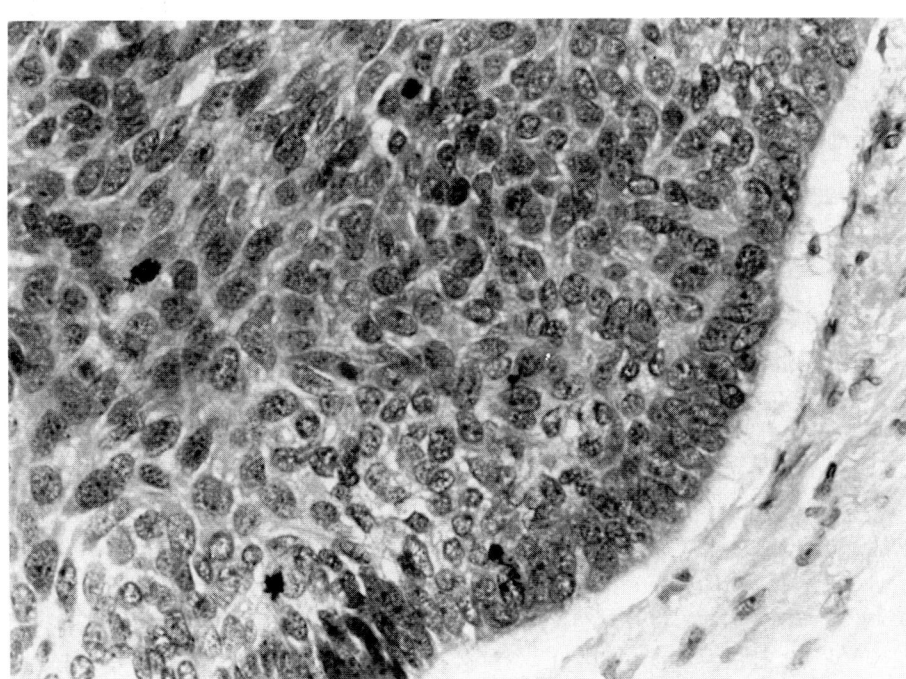

Figure 40–13.
Basal cell epithelioma. A solid mass is surrounded by retraction space and fibrous stroma. H&E. X400.

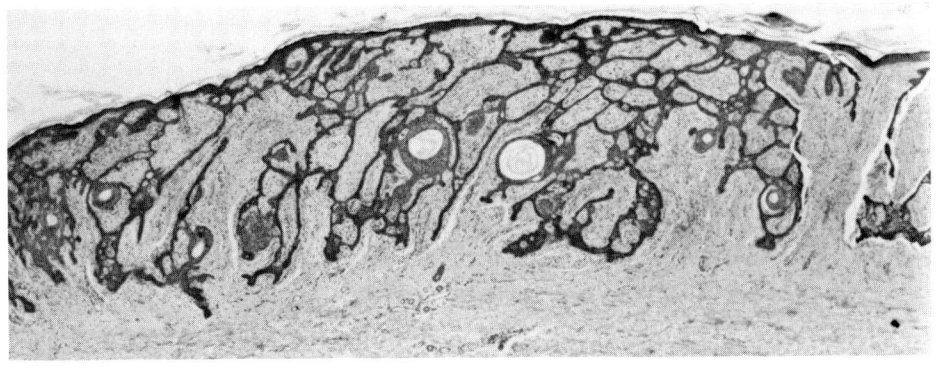

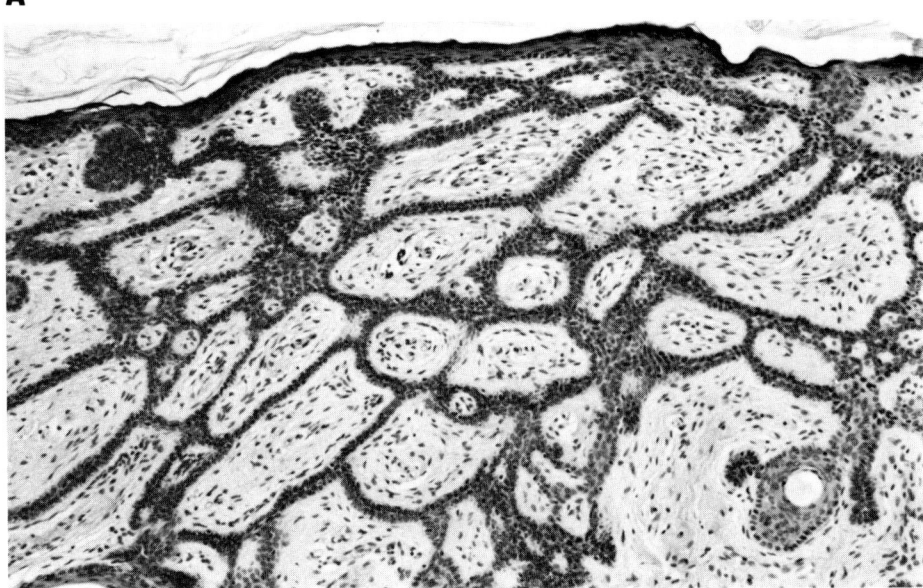

Figure 40–14.
Premalignant fibroepithelial tumor. **A.** An elevated nodular growth with smooth surface. H&E. X25. **B.** Detail of spongelike pattern of epithelial septa between stromal compartments. H&E. X125.

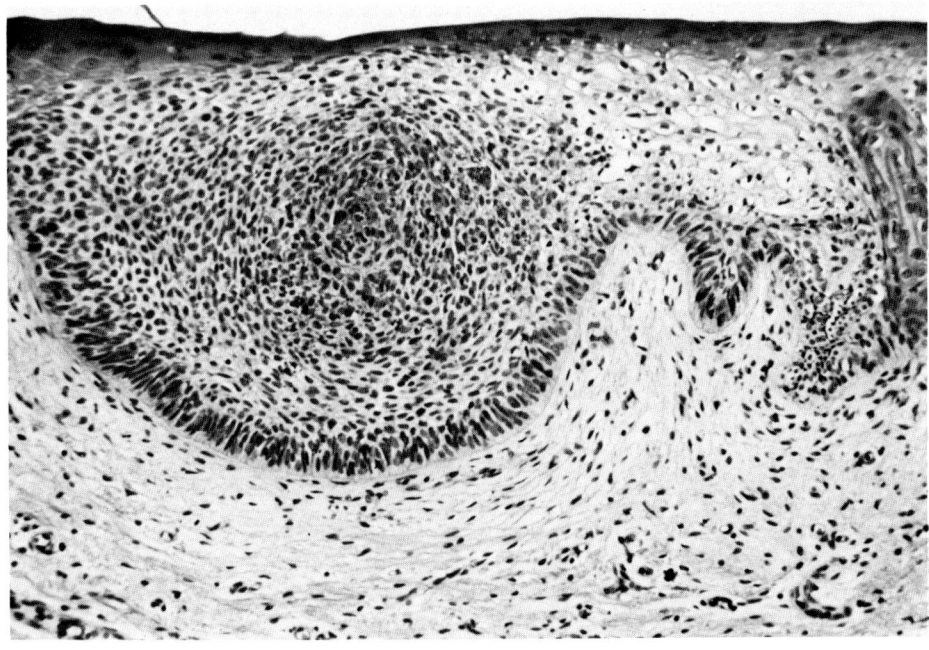

Figure 40–15.
Extremely superficial basal cell epithelioma, which becomes part of the surface epithelium. Keratinizing epidermis at far left is sharply delineated from tumor epithelium, which reaches the surface but does not keratinize. H&E. X185.

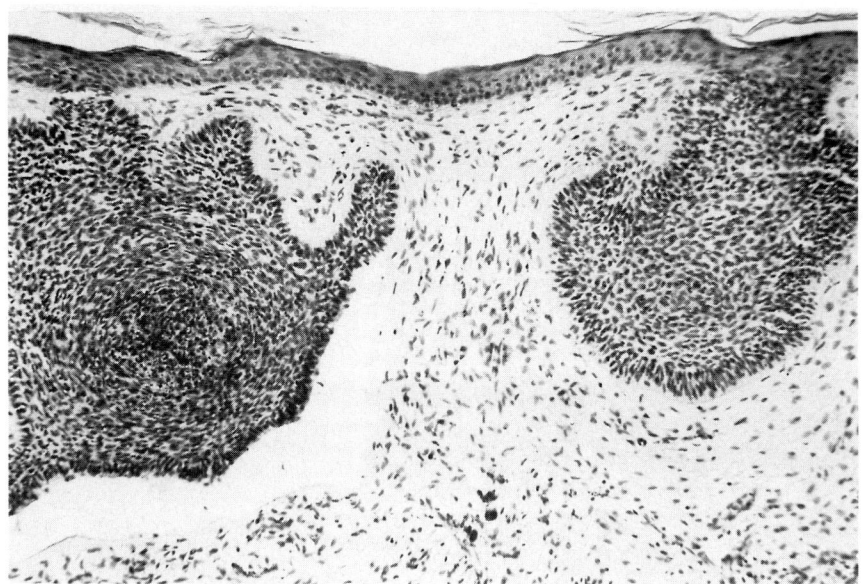

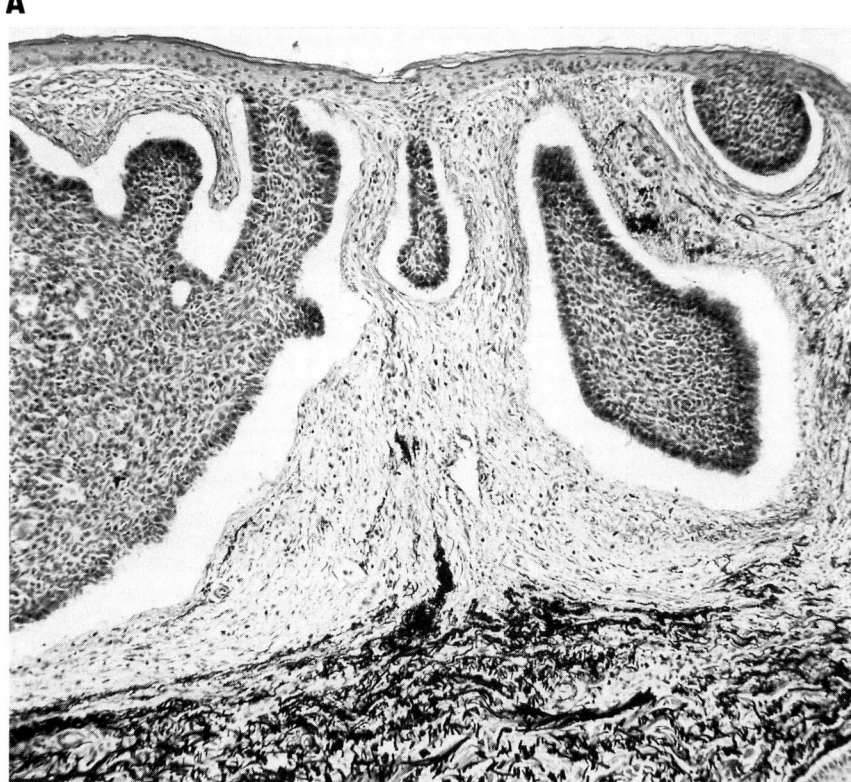

Figure 40–16.
Superficial basal cell epithelioma. **A.** Two solid tumor masses are connected with the lower surface of the epidermis and separated from fibrous stroma by retraction spaces. H&E. X125. **B.** There is a sharp line of definition between the fibrous tumor stroma with no elastic fibers and the underlying normal dermal connective tissue. O&G. X125.

and are rarely ulcerated. On histologic examination, morphea-like basal cell epithelioma (Fig. 40–21) may be mistaken for desmoplastic trichoepithelioma, or for syringoma, owing to the presence of small nests and thin strands of elongated epithelial cells that occasionally widen into keratin-filled whorls or cysts.[47,48] These are embedded in copious and fairly mature connective tissue stroma without much inflammatory reaction. The clinical behavior of these lesions is practically benign, but their eradication is

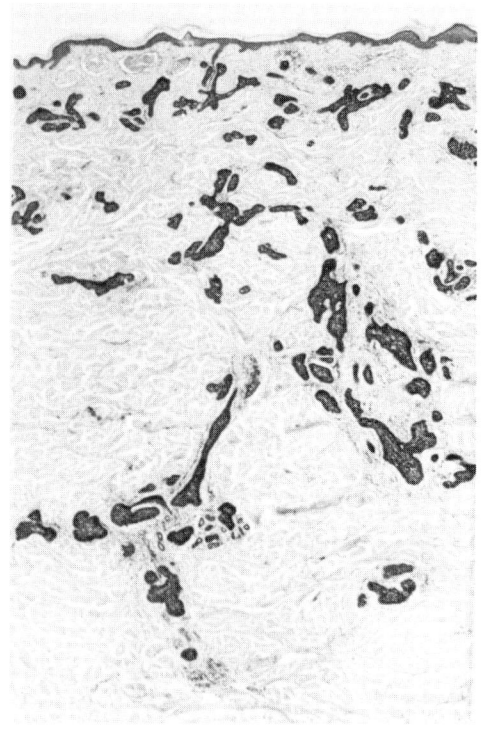
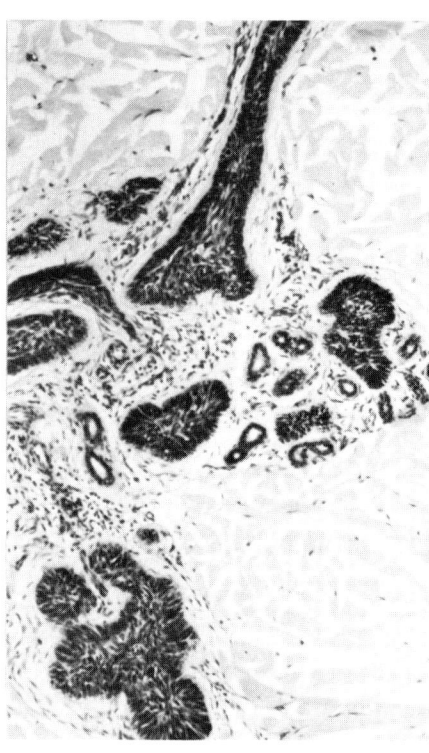

Figure 40–17.
Infiltrating basal cell epithelioma. **A.** Solid tumor masses invading dermis in the path of cutaneous adnexa. H&E. X25. **B.** Solid tumor masses in the level of eccrine sweat coils. H&E. X125.

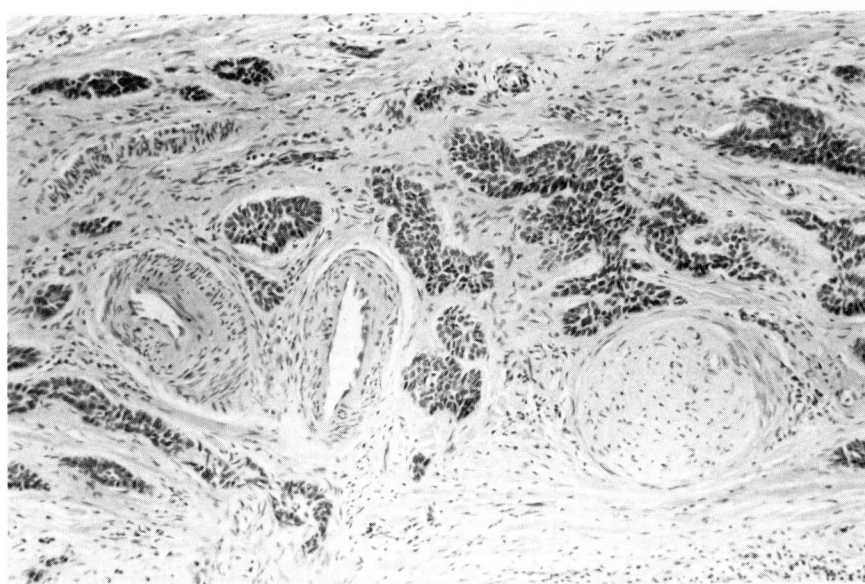

Figure 40–18.
Infiltrating basal cell epithelioma. Tumor masses surrounding deep blood vessels and a nerve trunk. H&E. X125.

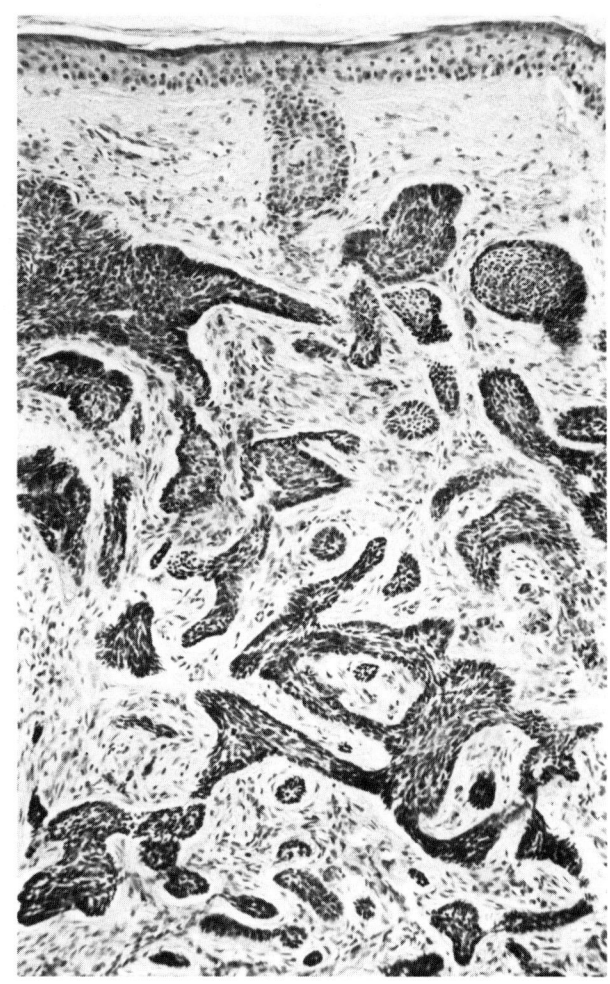

Figure 40-19.
Sclerotic basal cell epithelioma. H&E. X135.

difficult because of an ill-defined periphery, which may require chemosurgery or generous excision, possibly with plastic repair.

NEVOID BASAL CELL EPITHELIOMA SYNDROME

The cutaneous lesions appear early in life and consist of numerous papulonodular lesions over the head and neck areas. Later, in adult life the lesions become large and ulcerated.[49-51] The histopathology of basal cell epitheliomas in the nevoid syndrome is not specific. All epithelial patterns such as solid, adenoid, cystic, and reticulated forms may be encountered.[52]

METASTATIC BASAL CELL EPITHELIOMA

We indicated previously that metastasis in basal cell epithelioma is a rare phenomenon. The incidence in our experience is approximately 0.0005%. Lung, bones, and lymphnodes are common sites of metastatic lesions. There is no specific histologic pattern of basal cell epithelioma that is associated with tendency for metastasis.[53-58] Large aggressively growing and ulcerated lesions, treated inadequately and complicated with recurrences are more likely to metastasize.

INTRAEPIDERMAL EPITHELIOMA

Jadassohn first proposed the concept that basal cell epithelioma may develop and grow within the epi-

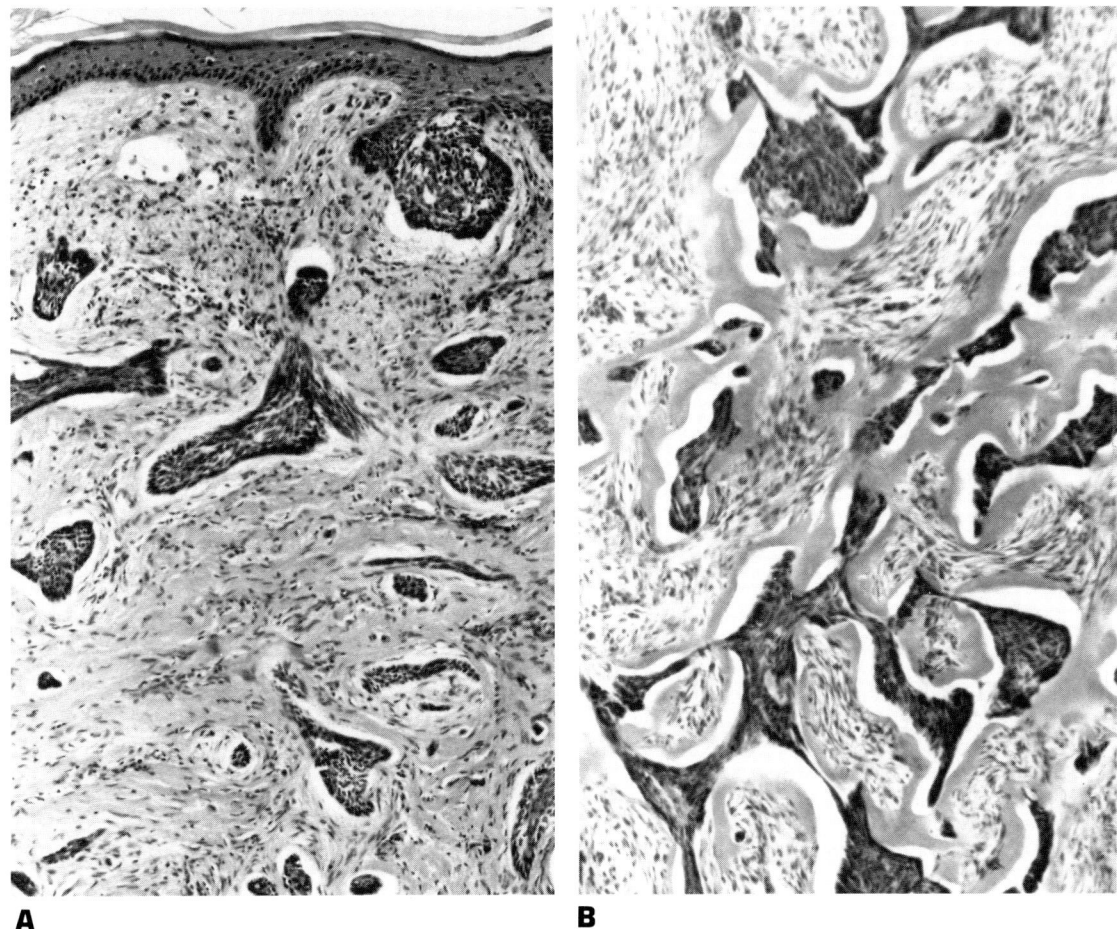

Figure 40–20.
Sclerotic basal cell epithelioma. **A.** Decreasing size of the tumor nests and density of the fibrous stroma. H&E. X125. **B.** Marked hyalinization of the tumor stroma. H&E. X125.

dermis without ever invading the dermis. He reported one case, the true nature of which can no longer be ascertained.[59–60] It may well have been a seborrheic verruca with intraepidermal whorls. The concept was perpetuated, modified, and sometimes confused with other phenomena of intraepidermal malignancy, and one must work with clear definitions in order to untangle the web.

The designation intraepidermal tumor formation should be restricted to the presence of sharply defined nests of neoplastic character surrounded completely by epidermal keratinocytes. This is in contrast to carcinoma in situ, in which a limited area of epidermis is completely replaced by neoplastic cells that extend from the basement membrane to the surface. Examples of the latter are keratosis senilis and Bowen's disease.

Intraepidermal tumor nests may represent three different biologic phenomena that may be designated by the names of Paget, Borst, and Jadassohn. The *Paget* phenomenon consists of adnexal or other nonkeratinocytic tumor cells intruding into the epidermis and forming colonies within it. Examples are Paget's disease, extramammary Paget's, and pagetoid malignant melanoma. The *Borst* phenomenon (Fig. 40–22) was described and clearly defined by that author as the invasion of epidermoid squamous cancer cells into the surrounding epidermis, where they form colonies. Borst observed this phenomenon in a carcinoma of the lip, which also invaded the dermis, and used it as a strong argument for the self-propagation of cancer, as contrasted with the concept of continual conversion of normal cells into cancer cells.[61] The Borst phenomenon may also

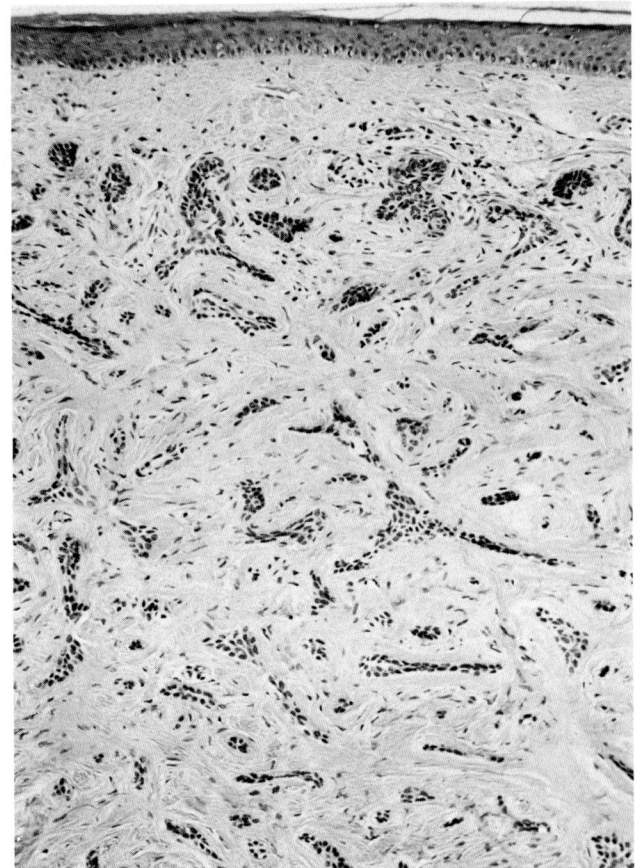

Figure 40–21.
Morphea-like epithelioma. Epithelial cords and occasional lumen-like spaces produce a picture somewhat similar to syringoma and desmoplastic trichoepithelioma. Copious fibrous stroma completely replaces dermis. H&E. X135.

be found in some cases of Bowen disease. The *Jadassohn* phenomenon indicates origin of neoplasia within the epidermis and colony formation of neoplastic cells which remain in the confines of the epidermis. Jadassohn's original observation actually may not have represented this phenomenon but may have been a clonal variety of seborrheic verruca with pseudonests of basaloid cells (see Fig. 34–17). This is indeed the most common type of lesion suggesting intraepidermal neoplasia. Careful study of multiple sections shows that somewhere the border of each nest is not sharp and that the basaloid cells mature into prickle cells. These pseudonests are due to whorling and convolutions (basaloid eddies) within the substance of the seborrheic verruca.

There are, however, true instances of the Jadassohn phenomenon (see Fig. 39–12). They were explained by Smith and Coburn[62] as arising from intraepidermal sweat duct material (hidroacanthoma simplex). This concept has logical appeal and a sound biologic basis in the existence of the acrosyringium as a separate biologic unit. The concept can explain the absence of a demonstrable extraepidermal tumor in some cases of Paget's disease. The principal histologic difference between such cases and hidroacanthoma simplex is that the cells of the latter resemble the intraepidermal eccrine sweat duct unit and are closely connected to each other and surrounding epidermal keratinocytes by desmosomes.[63] Just like the cells of eccrine poroma, they lack an organized system of tonofibrils and are generally incapable of keratinization. Malignant forms of hidroacanthoma simplex are malignant syringoacanthoma and eccrine porocarcinomas, which may combine intraepidermal nests with areas of dermal invasion.[64,65]

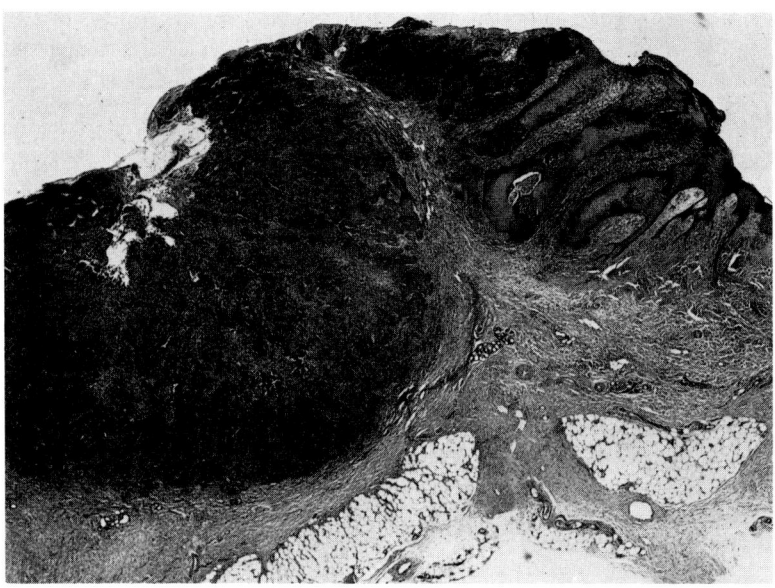

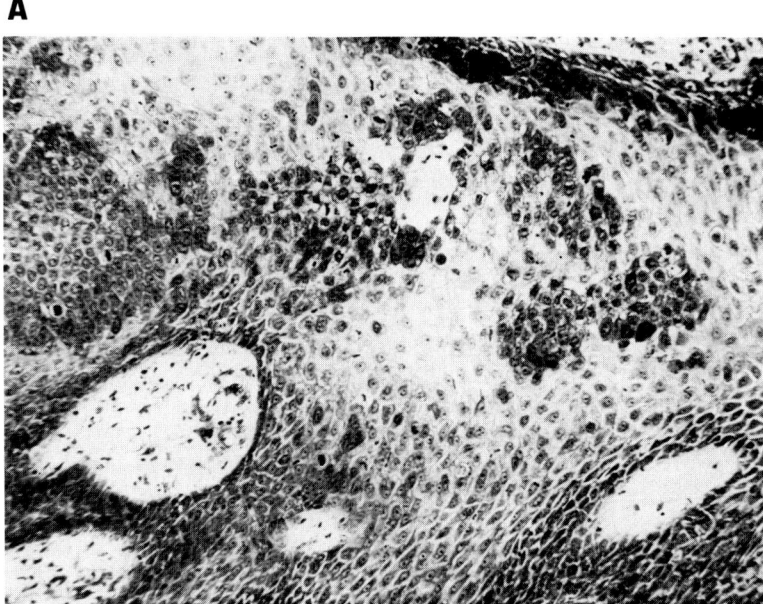

Figure 40–22.
Squamous cell carcinoma of lower lip exhibiting Borst phenomenon. This tumor duplicates almost exactly Borst's original case and is a relatively small-celled, nonkeratinizing carcinoma which has invaded deeply into the dermis and is ulcerated. Nests of squamous carcinoma cells also invade the hyperplastic surrounding epidermis. **A.** H&E. X45. **B.** H&E. X135.

REFERENCES

1. Krompecher E. Der Basalzellenkrebs. Jena: G. Fisher, 1903
2. Jacob A: Observations respecting an ulcer of peculiar character which attacks the eyelids and other parts of the face. Dublin Hosp Rep 4:232, 1827
3. Dubreuihl W: Transactions 2nd International Congress of Dermatology, Vienna, 1892, p 377
4. Belisario JC: Cancer of the Skin. London: Butterworths 1959
5. Pinkus H: Adnexal tumors, benign, not-so-benign, and malignant. In Montagna W, Dobson RL (eds): Carcinogenesis. Advances in Biology of Skin, vol 7. Oxford, New York: Pergamon, 1966, p 255
6. Van Scott EG, Reinertson RP: The modulating influence of the stromal environment on epithelial cells studied in human autotransplants. J Invest Dermatol 36:107, 1961
7. Cooper M, Pinkus H: Intrauterine transplantation of rat basal cell carcinoma as a model for reconversion of malignant to benign growth. Cancer Res 37:2544, 1977
8. Zackheim HS: The origin of experimental basal cell

epitheliomas in the rat. J Invest Dermatol 38:57, 1962
9. Zackheim HS: Origin of the human basal cell epithelioma. J Invest Dermatol 40:283, 1963
10. Wallace SA, Halpert B: Trichoma: Tumor of hair anlage. Arch Pathol 50:199, 1950
11. Foot NC: Adnexal carcinoma of the skin. Am J Pathol 23:1, 1947
12. Tozawa T, Ackerman AB: Basal cell carcinoma with follicular differentiation. Am J Dermatopathol 9:474, 1987
13. Moll R, Franke WW, Volc Platzer B, Krepler R: Different keratin polypeptides in epidermis and other epithelia of human skin, a specific cytokeratin of molecular weight 46,000 in epithelia of the pilosebaceous tract and basal cell epitheliomas. J Cell Biol 95:285, 1982
14. Raidbord HE, Wechsler HL, Fisher ER: Ultrastructural study of basal cell carcinoma and its variants with comments on histogenesis. Arch Dermatol 104:132, 1971
15. Kumakiri M, Hashimoto K: Ultrastructural resemblance of basal cell epithelioma to primary epithelial germ. J Cutan Pathol 5:53, 1978
16. Baden HP, Kubilus J, McGilvray N: Differentiation of basal cell epithelioma in vivo and in culture. J Invest Dermatol 74:246, 1980
17. Lerchin E, Rahbari H: Adamantinoid basal cell epithelioma: A histologic variant. Arch Dermatol 111:586, 1975
18. Grimwood RE, Ferris CF, Mercill DB, Huff JC: The proliferating cells of human basal cell carcinoma are located on the periphery of tumor nodules. J Invest Dermatol 86:191, 1986
19. Tomomichi O, Egawa K, Higo J, Fallas VH: Basal cell epithelioma with giant tumor cells. J Dermatol Tokyo 12:344, 1985
20. Ochiai T, Suzuki T, Morioka S: Basal cell epithelioma with giant cells: Light and electron microscopic study. J Cutan Pathol 14:242, 1987
21. Barr RJ, Williamson C: Clear cell basal cell carcinoma. Arch Dermatol 120:1086, 1984
22. Barnadas MA, Freeman RG: Clear cell basal cell epithelioma: Light and electron microscopic study of an unusual variant. J Cutan Pathol 15:1, 1988
23. Oliver GF, Winkelmann RK: Clear cell basal cell epithelioma: Histopathological, histochemical and electron microscopic findings. J Cutan Pathol 15:404, 1988
24. Cohen RE, Zaim MT: Signet-ring clear-cell basal cell carcinoma. J Cutan Pathol 15:183, 1988
25. Barr RJ, Graham JH: Granular cell basal cell carcinoma. A distinct histopathologic entity. Arch Dermatol 115:1064, 1979
26. Fellner MJ, Katz MJ: Pigmented basal cell cancer masquerading as superficial spreading malignant melanoma. Arch Dermatol 113:946, 1976
27. Deppe R, Pullmann H, Steigleder GK: Dopa-positive Zellen und Melanin im Basaliom. Arch Dermatol Res 256:79, 1976
28. Tezuka T, Ohkuma M, Hirose I: Melanosomes of pigmented basal cell epithelioma. Dermatologica 154:14, 1977
29. McArdle JP, Roff BT, Muller KH: Characterization of retraction spaces in basal cell carcinoma using an antibody to type IV collagen. Histopathology 8:447, 1984
30. Steigleder GK: Besondere Aspekte des Basalioms (Pigmentierung, Stroma, Glucosaminoglycane, Kapillarmuster). Z Hautkr 53–55, 1978
31. Van Cauwenberge D, Pierard GE, Foidart JM, et al: Immunohistochemical localization of laminin, type IV and type V collagen in basal cell carcinoma. Br J Dermatol 108:163, 1983
32. Peltonen J, Jaakkola S, Lask G, et al: Fibronectin gene expression by epithelial tumor cells in basal cell carcinoma: An immunocytochemical and in situ hybridization study. J Invest Dermatol 91:289, 1988
33. Mehregan AH, Staricco RG, Pinkus H: Elastic fibers in basal cell epithelioma. Arch Dermatol 89:33, 1964
34. Satti MB, Azzopardi JG: Amyloid deposits in basal cell carcinoma of the skin. A pathologic study of 199 cases. J Am Acad Dermatol 22:1082, 1990
35. Raffle EJ, MacLeod TM, Hutchinson F: Cell-mediated immune response to basal cell carcinoma. Acta Derm Venereol 61:66, 1981
36. Guillen FJ, Day CL Jr, Murphy GF: Expression of activation antigens by T cells infiltrating basal cell carcinomas. J Invest Dermatol 85:203, 1985
37. Avgerinou G, Nicolis G, Vareltzidis A, Stratigos J: The dermal cellular infiltrate and cell-mediated immunity in skin carcinomas. Dermatologica 171:238, 1985
38. Pasternak F, Civatte J: Les tumeurs fibroepitheliales de Pinkus a localisations extra-dorso-lombo-sacrees. A propos de 31 cas personnals. Ann Dermatol Syphilgr 103:275, 1976
39. Barr RJ, Herter RJ, Stone OJ: Multiple premalignant fibroepitheliomas of Pinkus. A case report and review of the literature. Cutis 21:335, 1978
40. Pinkus H: Premalignant fibroepithelial tumors of skin. Arch Pathol 67:598, 1953
41. Madsen A: Histogenesis of superficial basal cell epitheliomas: Unicentric or multicentric origin. Arch Dermatol 72:29, 1955
42. Lang PG Jr, McKelvey AC, Nicholson JH: Three-dimensional reconstruction of the superficial multicentric basal cell carcinoma using serial sections and a computer. Am J Dermatopathol 9:198, 1987
43. Jacobs GH, Rippey JJ, Altini M: Prediction of aggressive behavior in basal cell carcinoma. Cancer 49:533, 1982
44. Robinson JK, Pollack SV, Robins P: Invasion of cartilage by basal cell carcinoma. J Am Acad Dermatol 2:499, 1980
45. Mehregan AH: Aggressive basal cell epithelioma on sunlight-protected skin. Am J Dermatopathol 5:221, 1983
46. Howell JB, Caro MR: Morphea-like epithelioma. Further observations. Arch Dermatol 75:517, 1956

47. Salasche SJ, Amonette RA: Morpheaform basal cell epitheliomas. A study of subclinical extensions in a series of 51 cases. J Dermatol Surg Oncol 7:387, 1981
48. Richman T, Penneys NS: Analysis of morpheaform basal cell carcinoma. J Cutan Pathol 13:461, 1986
49. Howell JR: The roots of the naevoid basal cell carcinoma syndrome. Clin Exp Dermatol 5:339, 1980
50. Trotten JR: The multiple nevoid basal cell carcinoma syndrome. Report of its occurrence in four generations of a family. Cancer 46:1456, 1980
51. Allison JR Jr: Nevoid basal cell carcinoma syndrome. J Dermatol Surg Oncol 10:200, 1984
52. Pratt MD, Jackson R: Nevoid basal cell carcinoma syndrome. A 15-year follow-up of cases in Ottawa Valley. J Am Acad Dermatol 16:964, 1987
53. Farmer ER, Helwig EB: Metastatic basal cell carcinoma: A clinicopathologic study of seventeen cases. Cancer 46:748, 1980
54. Amonette RA, Salasche SJ, Chesney, TMC, et al: Metastatic basal cell carcinoma. J Dermatol Surg Oncol 7:397, 1981
55. Domarus HV, Stevens PJ: Metastatic basal cell carcinoma. Report of five cases and review of 170 cases in the literature. J Am Acad Dermatol 10:1043, 1984
56. Conley J. Sachs ME, Tomo T, et al: Metastatic basal cell carcinoma of the head and neck. Otolaryngol Head Neck Surg 93:78, 1985
57. Howat AJ, Levick PL: Metastatic basal cell carcinoma. Dermatologica 174:132, 1987
58. Sitz KV, Keppen M, Johnson DF: Metastatic basal cell carcinoma in acquired immunodificiency syndrome-related complex. JAMA 257:340, 1987
59. Rahbari H: Acervate epidermal tumors. Semin Dermatol 3:62, 1984
60. Steffen C, Ackerman AB: Intraepidermal epithelioma of Borst-Jadassohn. Am J Dermatopathol 7:5, 1985
61. Mehregan AH, Pinkus H: Intraepidermal epithelioma: A critical study. Cancer 17:609, 1964
62. Smith JLS, Coburn JG: Hidroacanthoma simplex: Assessment of a selected group of intraepidermal basal cell epitheliomata and of their malignant homologues. Br J Dermatol 68:400, 1956
63. Rahbari H: Hidroacanthoma simplex. A review of 15 cases. Br J Dermatol 109:219, 1983
64. Rahbari H: Syringoacanthoma. Acanthotic lesion of the acrosyringium. Arch Dermatol 120:751, 1984
65. Mehregan AH, Hashimoto K, Rahbari H: Eccrine adenocarcinoma. A clinico-pathologic study of 35 cases. Arch Dermatol 119:104, 1983

41

ADENOCARCINOMA AND METASTATIC CARCINOMA

Adenocarcinomas are rare in the skin. Like benign adnexal tumors, they arise from various skin appendages but are truly malignant and have potentiality for metastasis.

SEBACEOUS ADENOCARCINOMA

The clearest contrast between benign adnexal tumors and adenocarcinomas is provided by neoplasms arising from sebaceous glands.

In Chapter 36, we discussed the spectrum ranging from sebaceous hyperplasia to sebaceous adenoma to sebaceous epithelioma to basal cell epithelioma with sebaceous differentiation. All these are benign fibroepithelial tumors, and the distinction is mainly one of attained or not attained maturity of the cells until the telltale mark of inflammatory infiltrate sets apart the locally malignant but still rather innocuous tumor consisting almost entirely of basaloid cells interacting with supportive stroma.

A sebaceous adenocarcinoma, in contrast, may have many lipid-forming cells, but it has cytologic features of malignancy: large epithelial cells, irregular nuclei with prominent nucleoli, mitotic figures, and no palisading border (Fig. 41–1). It has the appearance of a carcinoma in the sense of general pathology, and it has the ability to metastasize.[1]

Meibomian Carcinoma

Adenocarcinomas of the meibomian glands of the eyelid are relatively more common than those of sebaceous glands of the body surface and are also more dangerous (Fig. 41–2).[2] The growth consists of lobulated masses of basaloid cells, some with irregular and hyperchromatic nuclei and vacuolated cytoplasm containing lipid droplets.[2,3] The tumor cells have propensity to invade the conjunctival epithelium and to cause pagetoid lesions. The pagetoid cells, however, show no PAS-positive or alcian blue-reactive material, and instead stain positive for fat with oil red 0.[4]

ADENOCARCINOMA OF THE SWEAT APPARATUS

In the past decade many published immunohistochemical studies have provided a wealth of new information concerning pathogenesis and differential diagnosis of sweat gland adenocarcinomas.[5–7] Positive staining for carcinoembryonic antigen (CEA), epithelial membrane antigen (EMA), and gross cystic disease fluid protein (GCDFP) have proved useful in differential diagnosis of sweat gland neoplasms from other histologically similar lesions.

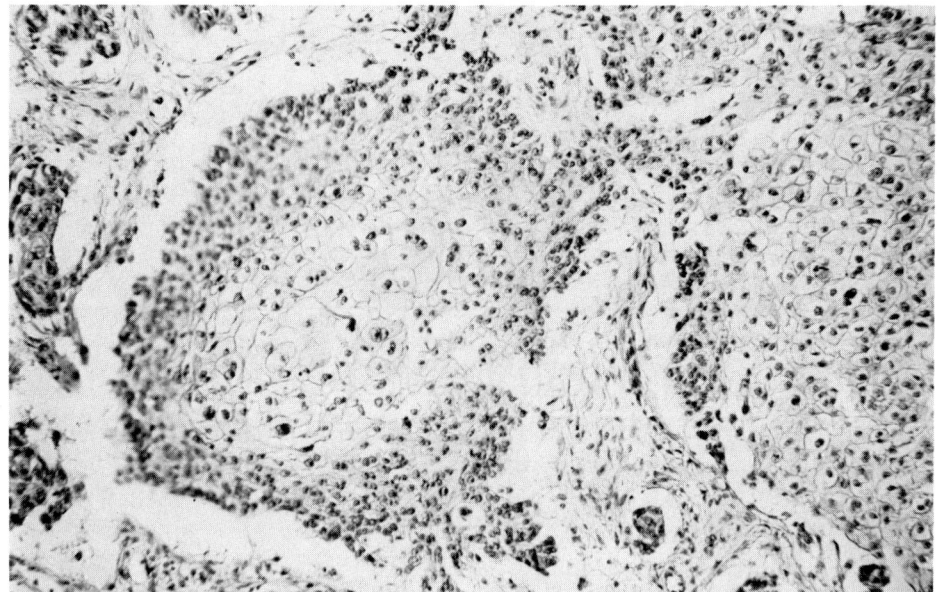

Figure 41–1.
Sebaceous adenocarcinoma. Compare and contrast with sebaceous epithelioma in Figure 36–9. Note cellular atypia and absence of basaloid outer layers. H&E. X135.

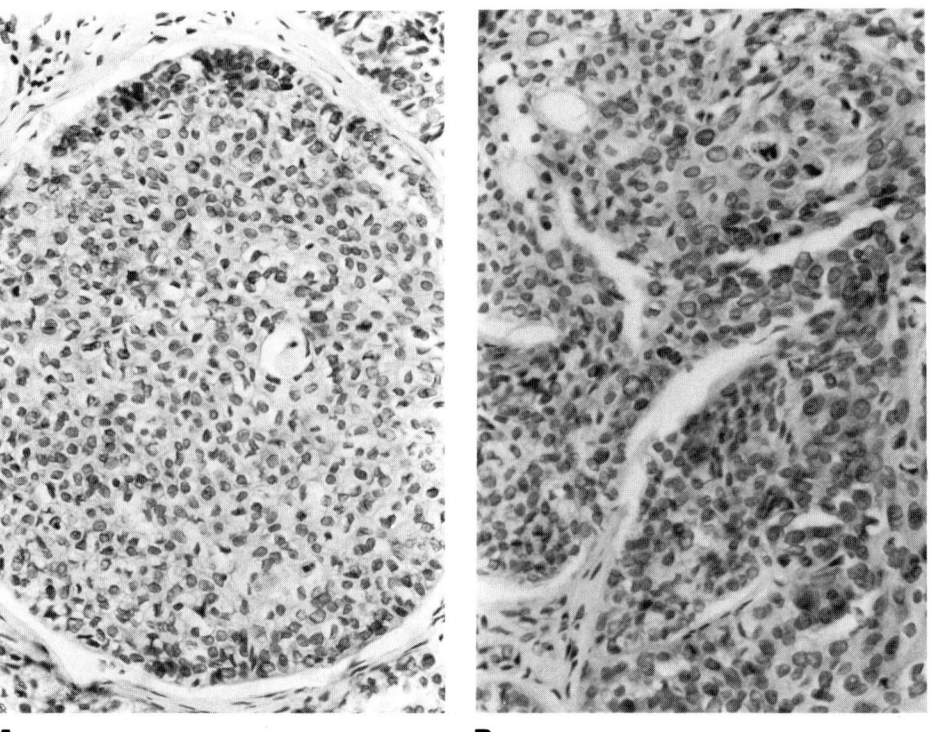

Figure 41–2.
Meibomian carcinoma of eyelid. Solid masses of anaplastic epithelium with foci of sebaceous differentiation. **A** and **B**. H&E. X250.

A B

Eccrine Carcinoma

Primary eccrine carcinomas are relatively rare. At least five different histologic forms have been identified including eccrine porocarcinoma, tubular (adenoid cystic) eccrine carcinoma, microcystic eccrine carcinoma, mucinous eccrine carcinoma, and clear cell eccrine carcinoma.[8]

Eccrine porocarcinoma is biologically instructive in showing that malignant cells of the eccrine apparatus can maintain the ability of their normal progenitors to live within the epidermis and to form pagetoid nests. The lesion is characterized histologically by the presence of well-defined islands of anaplastic cells within an acanthotic epidermis and areas of dermal invasion (Fig. 41–3).[8,9] The tumor epithelium shows cells with irregularly shaped and hyperchromatic nuclei and mitotic figures. The tumor cells contain glycogen and exhibit areas of sweat duct-like lumina formation. Lumina lined with short microvilli are found in electron microscopy. In an interesting case the initial lesion was an ulcerated tumor near the ankle of an elderly woman that metastasized and spread widely in the superficial lymphatics of the skin. In hundreds of places the tumor cells reentered the epidermis from below and produced nodules of intraepidermal nests (Fig. 41–4) along the lower extremity and on the abdomen. A number of similar cases have since been described.[10,11]

Tubular (adenoid cystic) eccrine carcinoma shows numerous cystic dilated and branching tubular structures invading the dermis and the fat tissue surrounding large blood vessels and nerve bundles (Fig. 41–5). Tubular structures are lined by a single layer of luminal cells and one or more rows of cells with hyperchromatic nuclei showing scattered mitotic figures.[12–14] The lumen is filled with PAS-positive and diastase-resistant material. Tubular eccrine carcinoma is notable for its relatively benign

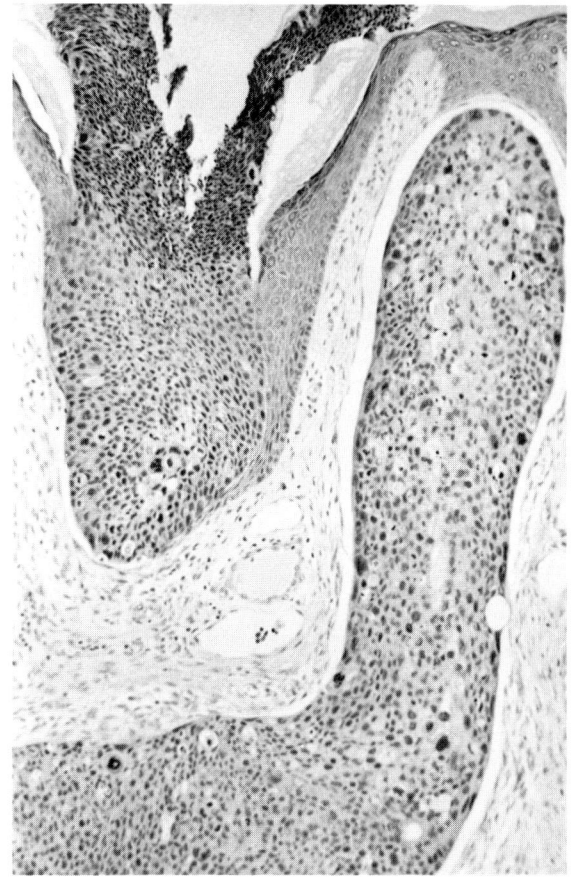

Figure 41–3.
Eccrine porocarcinoma. An intraepidermal island of anaplastic acrosyringeal cells and an area of dermal invasion. H&E. X125.

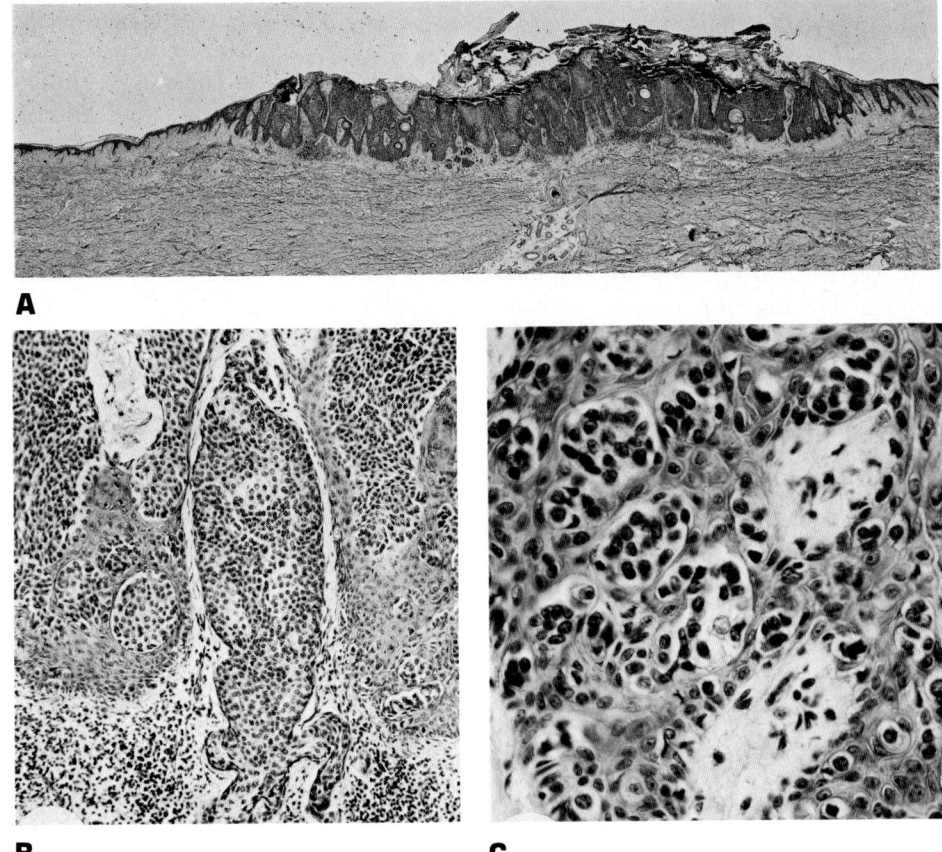

Figure 41–4.
Epidermotropic eccrine carcinoma. **A.** An entire metastatic lesion. H&E. X28. **B.** Tumor nest in a superficial dermal lymph vessel and multiple nests in epidermis. H&E. X90. **C.** Paget-like intraepidermal spread of carcinoma. H&E. X135. (From Pinkus and Mehregan. Arch Dermatol 88: 597, 1963.)

course and rarity of metastasis. Lesions of this type have also been described under basal cell tumors with eccrine differentiation (eccrine epithelioma).[15]

Microcystic eccrine carcinoma[16] is usually a slow-growing nodule located over the upper lip, cheeks or forehead (Fig. 41–6). Histologically, there is extensive dermal involvement by numerous small nests of basaloid or squamous cells, keratin cysts, and areas with sweat-duct-like structure formation. Involvement of the subcutaneous fat tissue with perivascular and perineural invasion may be present.[17–21]

Mucinous (adenocystic) carcinoma is usually intradermal and consists of small groups or thin rows of small basaloid cells floating within pools of acid mucopolysaccharide limited by thin septae of fibrocollagenous tissue (Fig. 41–7). The mucinous stroma gives the color reaction of sialomucin. The epithelial nests may show central sweat-duct-like lumina.[22–25]

Clear cell eccrine carcinoma shows a solid or multilobulated growth made up of cells with round or ovoid nuclei and abundant clear cytoplasms.[26,27] Anaplasia is evident by the presence of large and hyperchromatic nuclei and mitotic figures (Fig. 41–8). Several cases reported in children have been complicated with local recurrences and extensive metastasis unresponsive to chemotherapy.[28]

Malignant Transformation of Eccrine Tumors

Malignant transformation may occur in pre-existing eccrine tumors such as in eccrine spiradenoma, eccrine poroma, papillary eccrine adenoma, and cylindroma.[29–31] These lesions show histologic transformation from benign to malignant areas (Fig. 41–9). Malignant areas show loss of the characteristic histologic pattern, cells with irregularly shaped and hyperchromatic nuclei, and abnormal mitotic

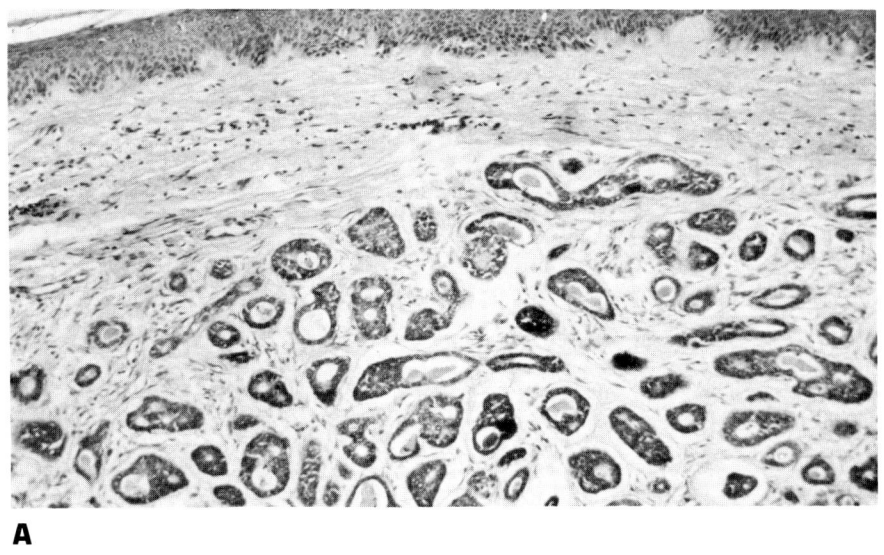
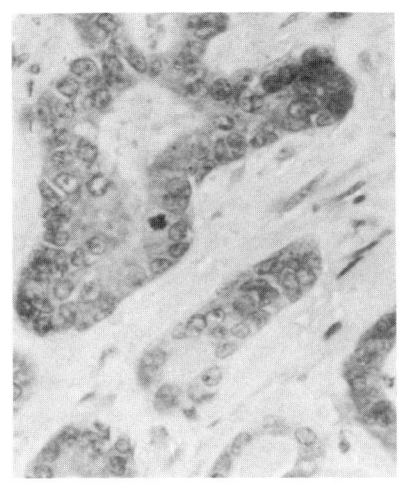
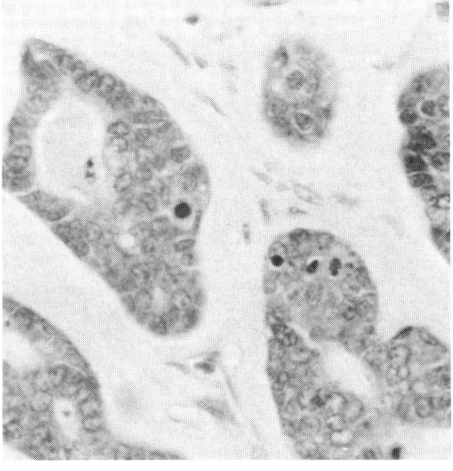

Figure 41–5.
Tubular (adenoid cystic) eccrine carcinoma. **A.** Numerous branching tubular structures. H&E. X125. **B** and **C** show many mitotic figures. H&E. X400.

figures. Other features include foci of squamous metaplasia and surrounding inflammatory cell reaction.[29]

Apocrine Adenocarcinoma and Paget's Disease

Apocrine carcinomas are unusual, and in cases arising in the axilla, relation to aberrant mammary tissue rather than to sweat glands is the preferred interpretation. Special discussion is needed of those lesions known as *extramammary Paget's disease*, which in the majority of cases are of apocrine origin and are occasionally associated with underlying apocrine adenocarcinoma (Fig. 41–10).[32–34]

Paget described the disease of the mammary areola that bears his name and stressed the frequent association with cancer of the breast. His experience has been borne out over the years so regularly that the skin lesion is valid indication for amputation of the breast.[35,36] The question of the origin of Paget cells has been answered satisfactorily in recent years by demonstration of specific glandular cytokeratins and positive immunostaining for CEA and GCDFP indicating that Paget cells are adenocarcinoma cells of glandular origin.[37,38]

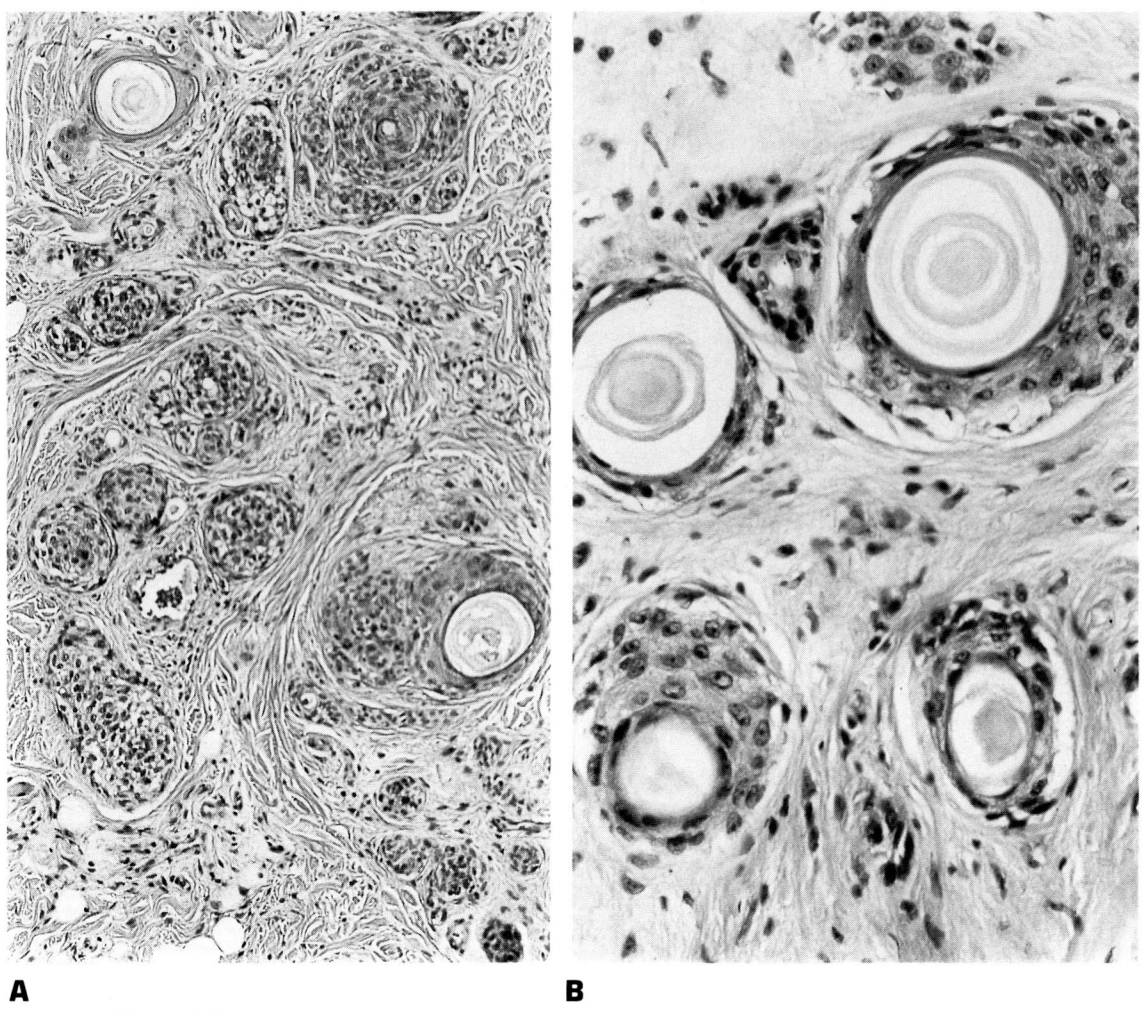

Figure 41–6.
Microcystic eccrine carcinoma. **A.** Small tumor masses infiltrating dermis down to the level of fat tissue. H&E. X125. **B.** Dilated sweat-duct-like structures. H&E. X400.

Extramammary Paget's disease shares many clinical and histologic features with the classic areolar type. Its almost constant location in areas of apocrine gland prevalence, especially axilla and vulva, provides a good basis for the view that it represents *epidermotropic apocrine adenocarcinoma* in most instances.[39,40] In some cases, it was found associated with carcinoma of the rectal mucosa, which is also biologically compatible with the adjoining epidermis.

In Paget's disease of either areolar (Fig. 41–11) or extramammary (Fig. 41–12) type, the epidermis may not be much thickened, but it usually is, and it is covered either by parakeratotic scale or crust. The Paget cells are relatively large and light staining with H&E and are found singly or in smaller and larger groups within the epidermis. Occasionally, they form rosettes, suggesting glandular arrangement, and, in some cases, the epidermis seems to be a bag of keratinocytes filled with masses of the clear nonfibrillar cells. Mitoses are not infrequent and prove that the Paget cells multiply in situ. Paget cells are more prevalent in the lower part of the epidermis but are almost always separated from the dermis by

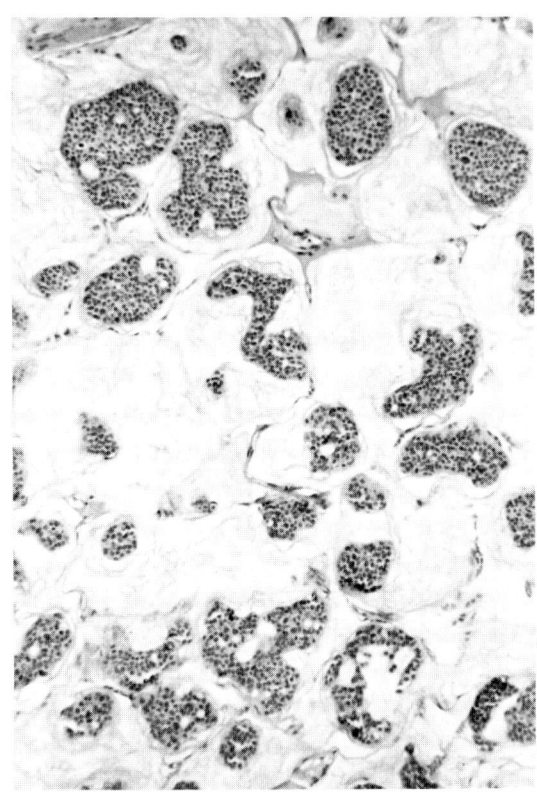

Figure 41–7.
Mucinous carcinoma of skin. A field of moderate expression of the great amount of mucinous stroma that can be associated with small nests of tumor cells. H&E. X250.

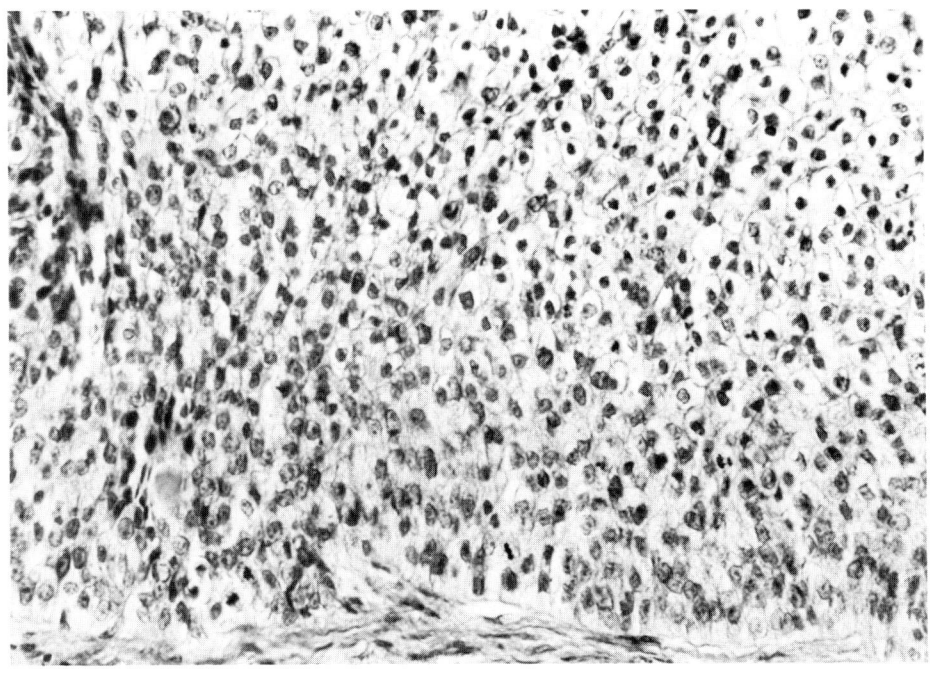

Figure 41–8.
Clear cell eccrine carcinoma. Masses of clear cells with irregular nuclei and scattered mitoses. H&E. X250.

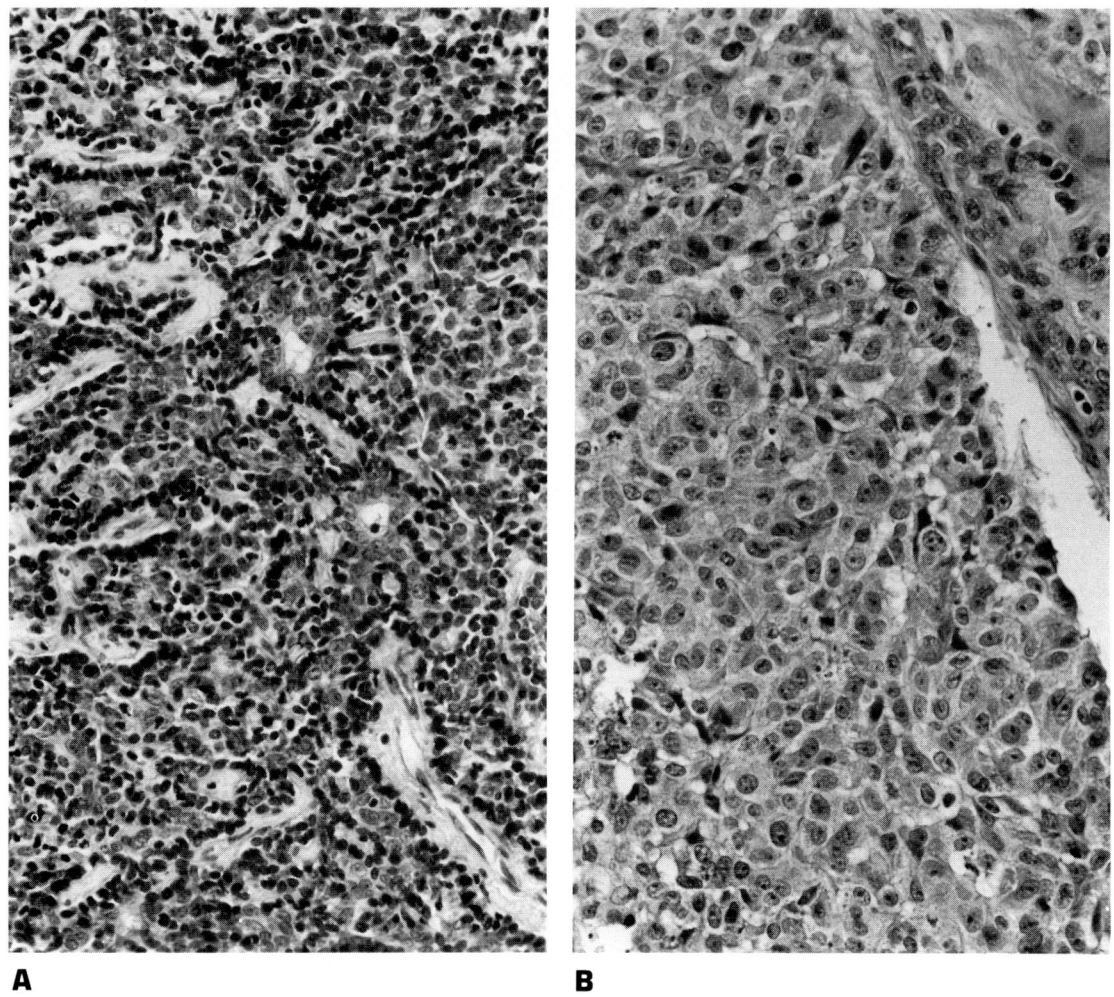

Figure 41–9.
Malignant transformation of eccrine spiradenoma. **A.** The benign portion shows characteristic two types of cell pattern with central luminae. H&E. X125. **B.** Malignant portion shows loss of the tumor pattern and is populated with abnormally large cells. H&E. X125.

a cohesive and fairly intact basal layer. They may invade the dermis, however. They may also be found in the higher epidermal layers, including the stratum corneum, but they do not keratinize themselves. In most cases, the cell is separated from surrounding keratinocytes by a narrow or broader space, not traversed by intercellular bridges. In a few cases, however, intercellular connections are present. This fact does not militate against the adnexal nature of Paget cells, since cells of the intraepidermal adnexal units normally are connected to their neighboring epidermal keratinocytes by bridges. Paget cells of the areolar disease contain glycogen. Those of extramammary cases (Fig. 41–12B) regularly contain PAS-positive and diastase-resistant acid mucopolysaccharides, in most instances, sialomucin, a substance found in hidradenomas. A dense inflammatory infiltrate consisting of small round cells and plasma cells in the upper dermis completes the histologic picture.

In areolar cases, a sufficiently large biopsy often shows the milk ducts affected by a so-called *comedo-type carcinoma,* but other forms of breast cancer may be present. In extramammary cases,

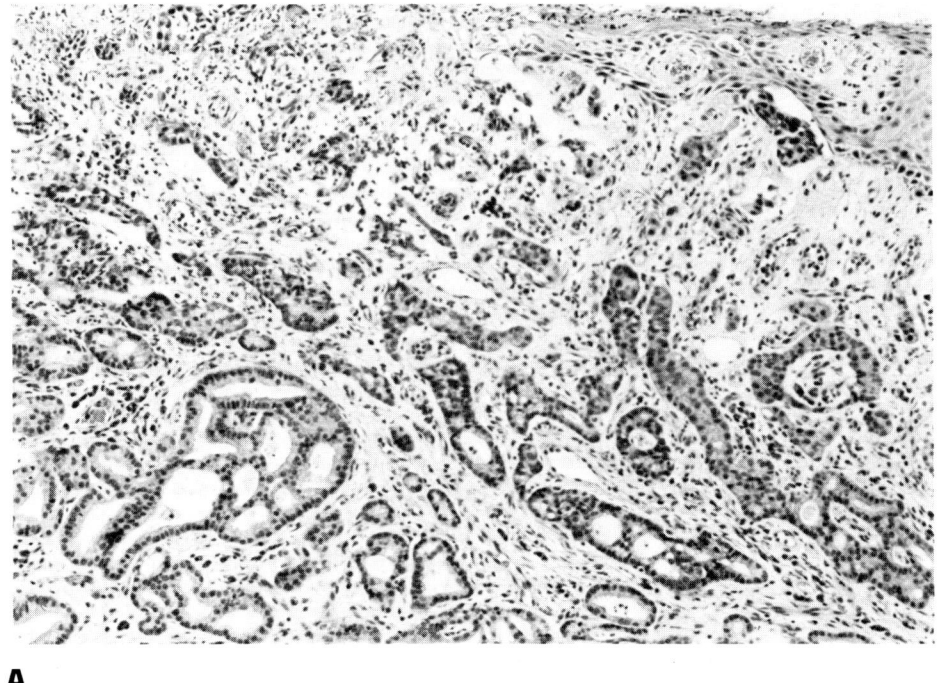

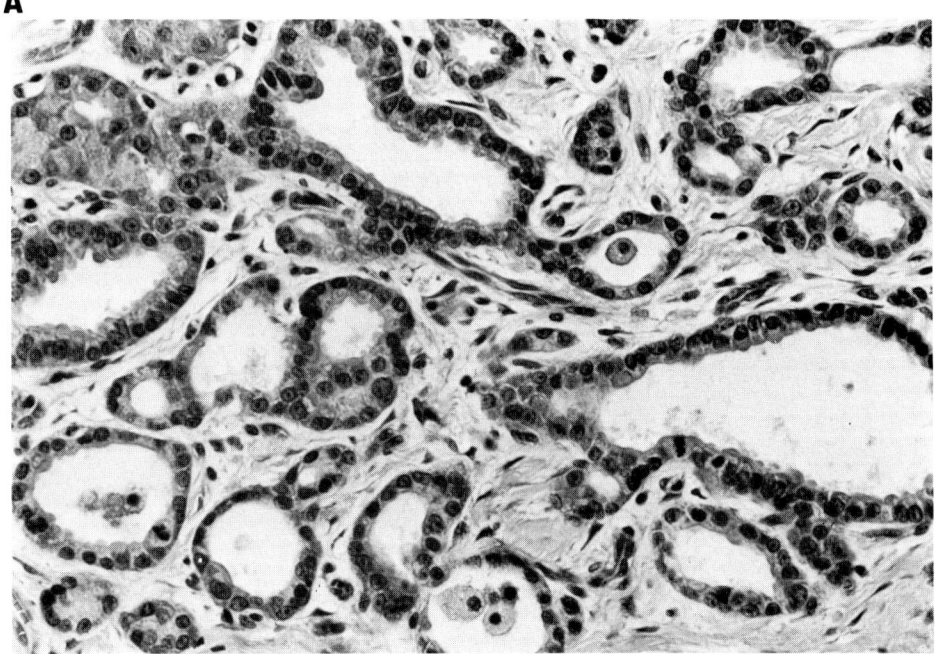

Figure 41—10.
Apocrine adenocarcinoma. Tubular structures lined with high columnar cells and scattered mitoses. **A** also shows pagetoid involvement of the overlying epidermis. **A.** H&E. Original X125. **B.** H&E. Original X250.

Paget cells often are present in the walls of eccrine and apocrine ducts and of hair follicles, presumably as a phenomenon of secondary migration. Careful serial sections may enable one to demonstrate an underlying apocrine gland carcinoma in an axillary lesion. Failure to find such a carcinoma in every case may have two reasons. Usually it proves impractical to examine all tissue in serial or step sections, especially if the superficial lesion is large. Second, the original focus may well be in the poral portion of a gland and may not lead to invasive carcinoma at all.

Beginners may find it difficult to differentiate Paget cells from those of Bowen's disease, on the one hand, and from peculiar large cells of the normal areolar epithelium, on the other. The last

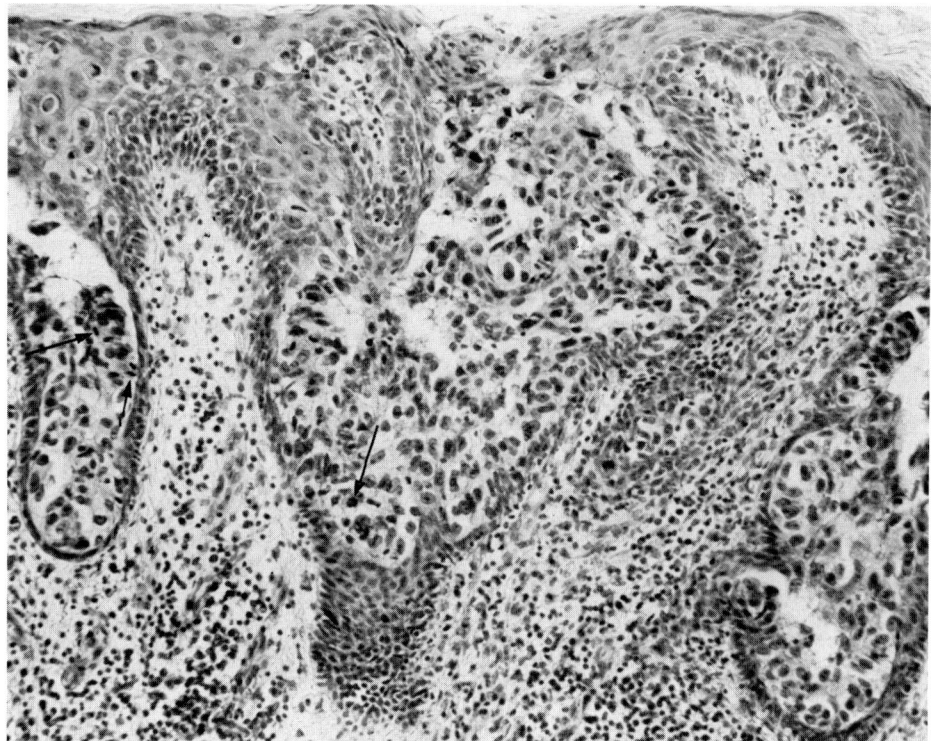

Figure 41–11.
Paget's disease of the nipple. Adenocarcinomatous cells are single or in small and large nests in epidermis. Three mitotic figures in Paget cells indicated by arrows. Epidermal basal layer is intact in most places. H&E. X185. (From Mehregan and Pinkus. Cancer 17:609, 1964.)

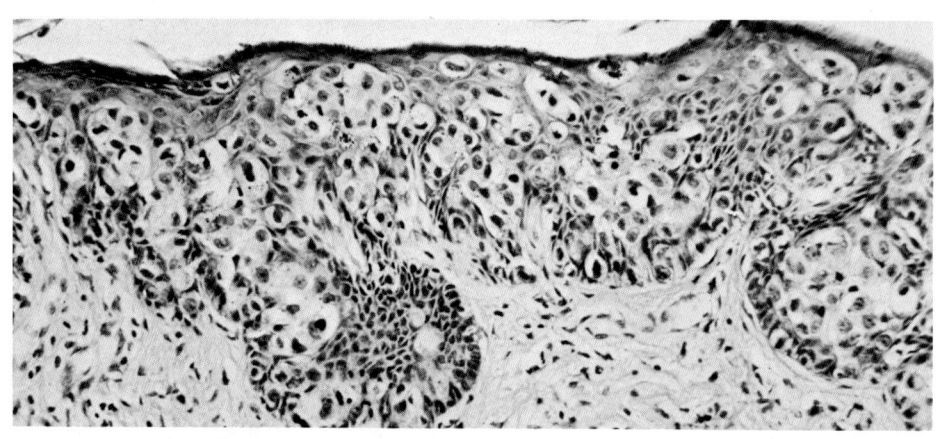

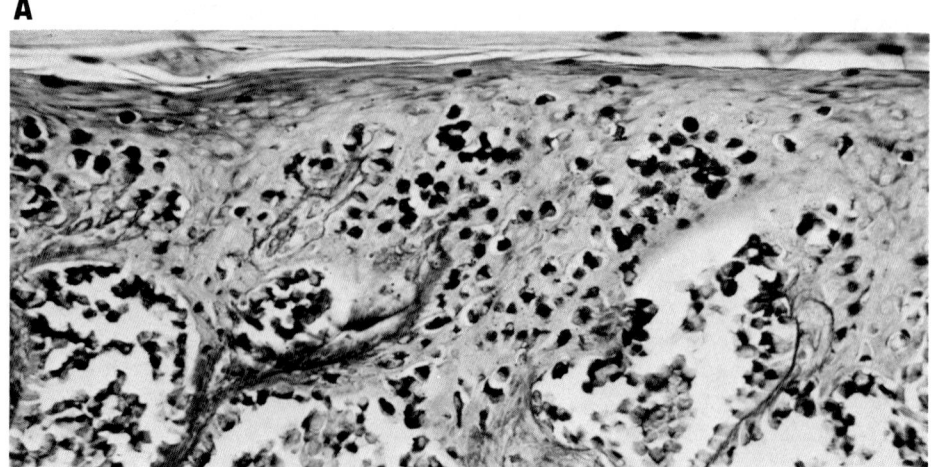

Figure 41–12.
Extramammary Paget's disease. In this case, some nests are not surrounded by basal cells but are confined by basement membrane. **A.** H&E. X180. **B.** Alcian blue–PAS–picric acid stain shows sialomucin in Paget cells not only in living epidermis but also within horny layer. Very dark appearance of mucin is due to its having affinity for alcian blue as well as PAS. X180.

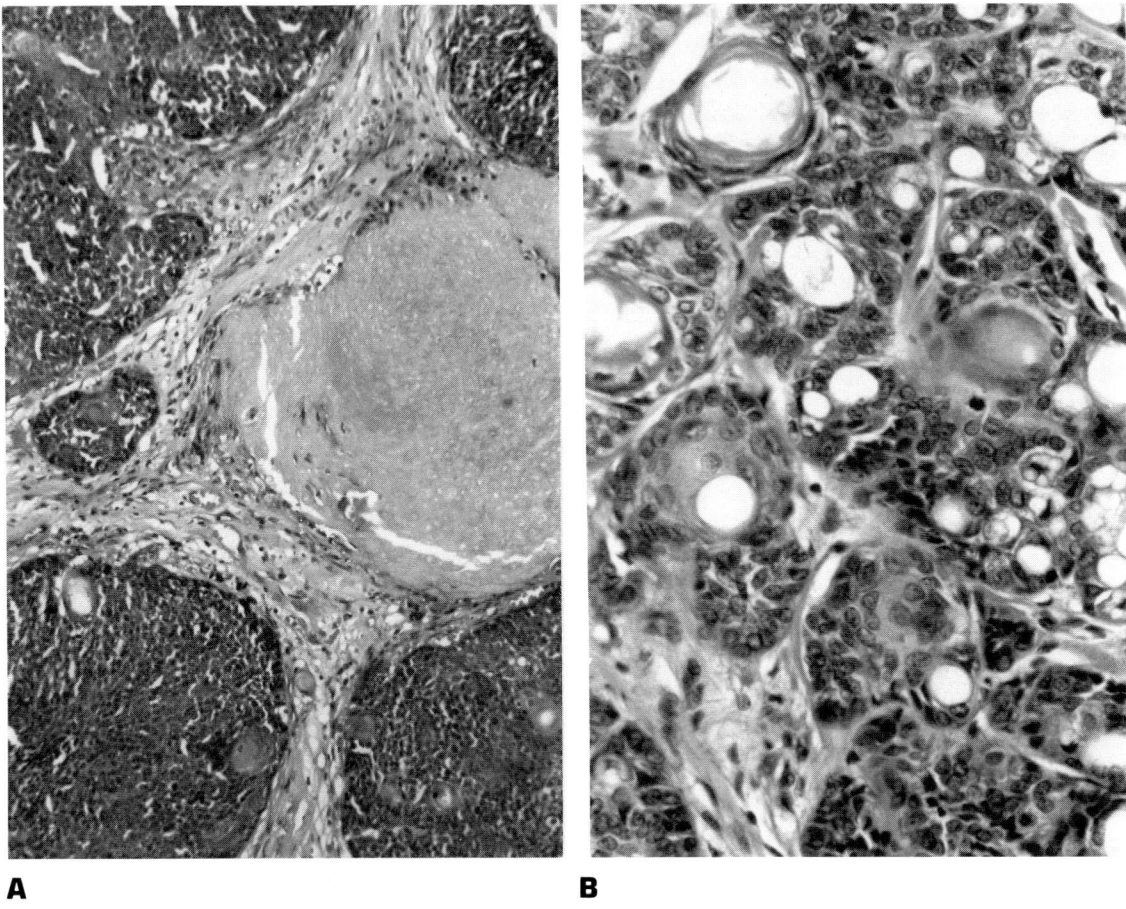

Figure 41-13.
Adnexal (pilary complex) carcinoma. **A.** *Solid masses of basaloid cells and an area of keratinization with formation of shadow cells. H&E. X125.* **B.** *Another area shows foci of sebaceous and sweat-duct-like differentiation. H&E. X225.*

named are prickle cells with a large halo around the nucleus (intracellular edema). Thus, the empty space is between nucleus and cytoplasm, the cell adhering to surrounding cells with numerous desmosomes. In the Paget cell, nucleus and cytoplasm form a unit, and the empty space surrounds the entire cell. In Bowen's disease, some epidermal cells may undergo individual cell keratinization and become separated from their neighbors. This process is only one feature of the general dysplasia exhibited by the epidermis. In Paget's disease epidermal keratinocytes retain fairly normal morphology, although they may be compressed. Paraffin-embedded tissue sections may be stained for CEA antigen, which would give a positive reaction in mammary and extramammary Paget's disease but will be negative in Bowen's disease.[41] Superficially spreading malignant melanoma has pagetoid features but may be differentiated in fresh material by the positive dopa reaction or in paraffin sections by the demonstration of melanin and premelanin (Fontana–Masson method) and also by the absence of acid mucopolysaccharides or glycogen in melanoma cells. Immunostaining for S-100 protein or HMB-45 will result in a positive reaction in pagetoid malignant melanoma. Staining for CEA will be negative.

Pilomatrix Carcinoma

A neoplasm combining histologic features of pilomatricoma with obviously malignant cytologic features is known as pilomatrix carcinoma.[42-46] This tumor shows an aggressive growth pattern and a tendency for distant metastasis. Histologically, there are solid masses of small basaloid cells with central areas of keratinization with formation of shadow cells. The tumor masses show no palisading or fibrous stroma.

There are foci of squamous metaplasia and numerous mitotic figures.

Adnexal (Pilary Complex) Carcinoma

In rare occasions malignant skin lesions consist of solid masses of small basaloid cells with no palisading or retraction space formation and numerous mitotic figures (Fig. 41–13). Areas of squamous metaplasia, trichilemmal type of keratinization, sebaceous differentiation, and rarely sweat-duct-like lumina formation suggest relationship to pilar apparatus.[47] Differentiation from basal cell epithelioma is essential as the undifferentiated adnexal carcinomas have potentiality for local lymphnode involvement and distant metastasis.

Trabecular Carcinoma Neuroendocrine Carcinoma (Merkel Cell Tumor)

Trabecular carcinoma of Toker[48] appears as a solitary erythematous nodule over the sun-exposed areas of head, face, and neck and occasionally elsewhere.[49,50] The growth originates in the dermis and consists of solid sheets of round cells or cells arranged in anastomosing cords and trabecular pattern. Rosette formation is rare.[51] Connection with the surface epidermis or with the cutaneous adnexa is not common (Fig. 41–14). The tumor cells show a narrow rim of amphophylic cytoplasm surrounding a vesicular nucleus that contains multiple nucleoli. Mitotic figures are abundant and angioinvasion, predominantly of lymphatics, is present in one third of

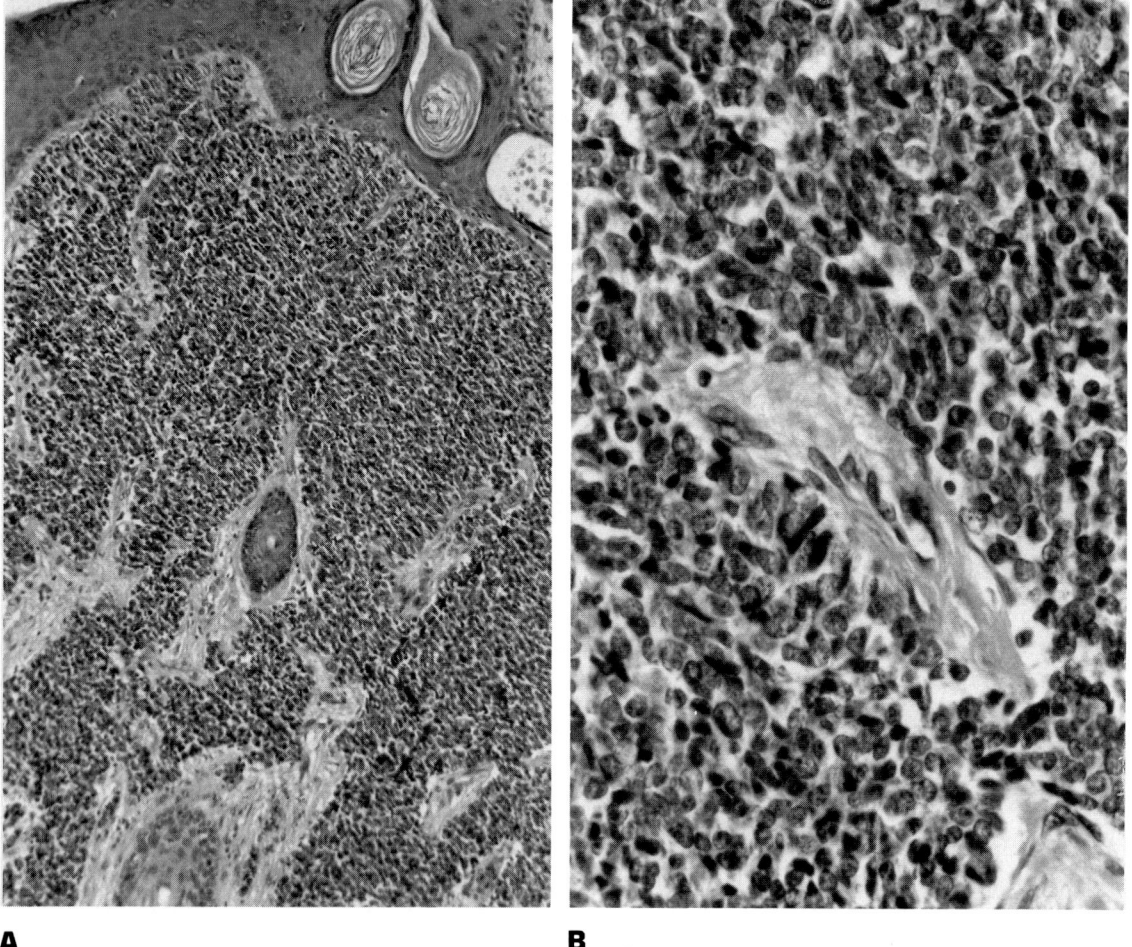

Figure 41–14.
Trabecular (Merkel cell) carcinoma. **A.** Extensive dermal involvement by masses of small basaloid tumor cells. H&E. X125. **B.** The tumor masses show no evidence of adnexal differentiation, no palisading or retraction space formation. H&E. X400.

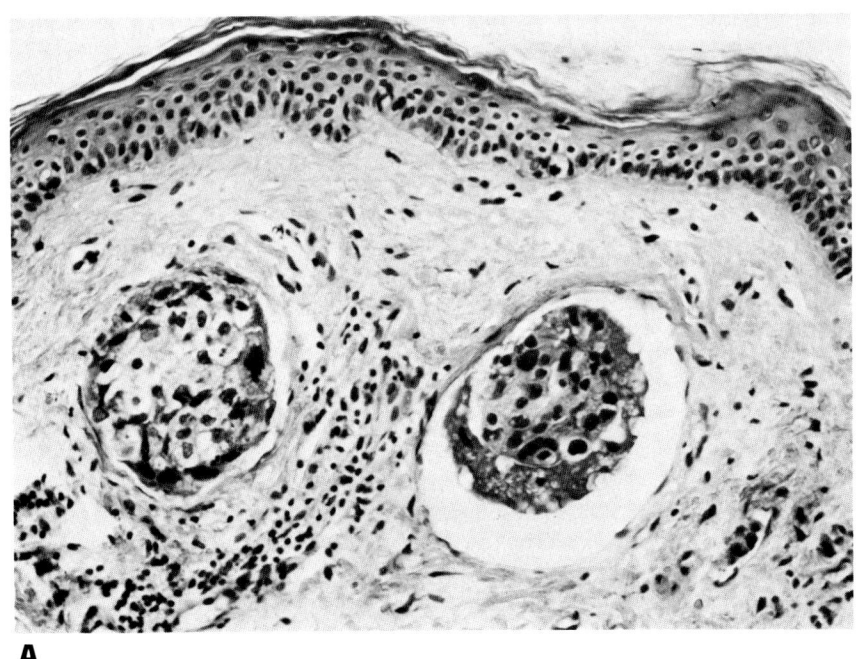

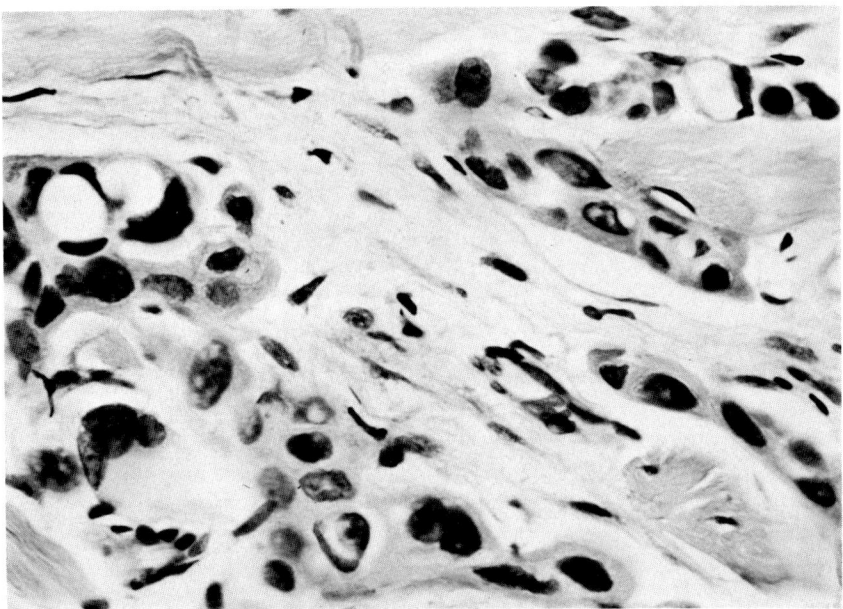

Figure 41–15.
Carcinoma metastatic to skin. **A.** Clinically erysipelas-like lesion produced by obstruction of lymphatics in carcinoma of breast. H&E. X225. **B.** Signet-ring cells in metastatic carcinoma of colon. H&E. X465.

the lesions. Positive identification is made by electron microscopic observation of electron-dense core secretory granules or by positive immunostaining for neuron-specific enolase and synaptophysin.[52–54]

METASTATIC CARCINOMA

Cutaneous metastasis of internal cancer is relatively rare but is of diagnostic importance[55,56] because it may be the first manifestation of metastasis of a supposedly cured malignancy or even the first manifestation of an undiscovered carcinoma.[57,58]

With the exception of hypernephroma and a few other tumors,[59] the histologic features of cutaneous metastases do not permit identification of the primary site. The most common histologic form of growth is the formation of solid cords and thin strands of anaplastic cells infiltrating the interfascicular spaces of the dermis. Presence of signet-ring cells, which contain mucin (Fig. 41–15B), suggests a primary focus in the gastrointestinal tract. Involvement of the superficial dermal lymphatics produces inflammatory (erysipelatoid)[60] lesions (Fig. 41-15A). Rarely, carcinomatous cords approach and even invade the epidermis. Paget-like pictures may be encountered.

The scalp is a site of predilection for metastatic cancer, especially of the breast. Any nodule arising on the scalp of an elderly person should be suspect. In rare cases, a patch of alopecia without tumor formation may be the site of a scirrhous carcinoma, with thin strands and small nests of large cells embedded within a fibrotic stroma that chokes off hair roots.[61] Another clinical form is Sister Marie-Joseph nodule of umbilicus secondary to the adenocarcinoma of the digestive tract.[62]

REFERENCES

1. Wick MR, Goellner JR, Wolfe JT, et al: Adnexal carcinomas of the skin. 11. Extraocular sebaceous carcinomas. Cancer 56:1163, 1985
2. Rao NA, Hidayat AA, McLean IW, et al: Sebaceous carcinoma of the ocular adnexa: A clinicopathologic study of 104 cases with five-year follow up data. Hum Pathol 13:113, 1982.
3. Nakamura S, Nakayama K, Nishihara K, Imai T: Sebaceous carcinoma—with special reference to histopathologic differential diagnosis. J Dermatol Tokyo 15:55, 1988
4. Lee SC, Roth LM: Sebaceous carcinoma of the eyelid with pagetoid involvement of the bulbar and palpebral conjunctiva. J Cutan Pathol 4:134, 1977
5. Wick MR, Goellner JR, Wolfe JT III, Su DWP: Adnexal carcinomas of the skin. I. Eccrine carcinomas. Cancer 56:1147, 1985
6. Swanson PE, Cherwitz DL, Neumann MP, Wick MR: Eccrine sweat gland carcinoma: An histologic and immunohistochemical study of 32 cases. J Cutan Pathol 14:65, 1987
7. Mita H, Takigawa M, Iwatsuki K, et al: An immunohistologic study on eccrine gland carcinoma. J Am Acad Dermatol 20:693, 1989
8. Mehregan HA, Hashimoto K, Rahbari H: Eccrine adenocarcinoma. A clinicopathologic study of 35 cases. Arch Dermatol 119:104, 1983
9. Bottles K, Sagebiel RW, McNutt NS, et al: Malignant eccrine poroma. Case report and review of the literature. Cancer 53:1579, 1984
10. Pinkus H, Mehregan AH: Epidermotropic eccrine carcinoma. A case combining features of eccrine poroma and Paget's dermatosis. Arch Dermatol 88:597, 1963
11. Landa NG, Winkelmann RK: Epidermotropic eccrine porocarcinoma. J Am Acad Dermatol 24:27, 1991
12. Cooper PH, Adelson GL, Holthaus WH: Primary cutaneous adenoid cystic carcinoma. Arch Dermatol 120:774, 1984
13. Wick MR, Swanson PE: Primary adenoid cystic carcinoma of the skin. A clinical, histological and immunocytochemical comparison with adenoid cystic carcinoma of salivary glands and adenoid basal cell carcinoma. Am J Dermatopathol 8:2, 1986
14. Seab JA, Graham JH: Primary cutaneous adenoid cystic carcinoma. J Am Acad Dermatol 17:113, 1987
15. Sanchez NP, Winkelmann RK: Basal cell tumor with eccrine differentiation (eccrine epithelioma). J Am Acad Dermatol 6:514, 1982
16. Goldstein DJ, Barr RJ, Santa Cruz DJ: Microcystic adnexal carcinoma. A distinct clinicopathologic entity. Cancer 50:566, 1982
17. Miyamoto T, Kambe N, Nishiura S, et al: Microcystic adnexal carcinoma. Electron microscopic and immunohistochemical study. Dermatologica 180:40, 1990
18. Birkby CS, Argenyi ZB, Whitaker DC: Microcystic adnexal carcinoma with mandibular invasion and bone marrow replacement. J Dermatol Surg Oncol 15:308, 1989
19. Lupton GP, McMarlin SL: Microcystic adnexal carcinoma. Report of a case with 30 year follow-up. Arch Dermatol 122:286, 1986
20. Wick MR, Cooper PH, Swanson PE, et al: Microcystic adnexal carcinoma. An immunohistochemical comparison with other cutaneous appendage tumors. Arch Dermatol 126:189, 1990
21. Takamiya M, Shiraishi S, Saeki N, et al: Microcystic adnexal carcinoma with Langerhans cells. J Dermatol Tokyo 15:428, 1988
22. Verola O, Rybojad M, Fegueux S, et al: Adenocarcinome mucineux eccrine cutane. Ann Dermatol Venereol 116:853, 1989
23. Perzin KH, Gullane P, Conley J: Adenoid cystic carcinoma involving the external auditory canal. A clinicopathologic study of 16 cases. Cancer 50:2873, 1982
24. Gardner TW, O'Grady RB: Mucinous adenocarcinoma of the eyelid. A case report. Arch Ophthalmol 102:912, 1984
25. Weber PJ, Hevia O, Gretzula JC, Rabinovitz HC: Primary mucinous carcinoma. J Dermatol Surg Oncol 14:170, 1988
26. Chung CK, Heffernan AH: Clear cell hidradenoma with metastasis: Case report with a review of the literature. Plast Reconstr Surg 48:177, 1971
27. Hernández-Pérez E, Cruz TA: Clear cell hidradenocarcinoma. Report of an unusual case. Dermatologica 153:249, 1976
28. Chow CW, Campbell PE, Burry AF: Sweat gland carcinoma in children. Cancer 53:1222, 1984
29. Galadari E, Mehregan AH, Lee KC: Malignant transformation of eccrine tumors. J Cutan Pathol 14:15, 1987
30. Cooper PH, Frierson HF, Morrison GA: Malignant transformation of eccrine spiradenoma. Arch Dermatol 121:1445, 1985
31. Wick MR, Swanson PE, Kaye VN, Pittelkow MR: Sweat gland carcinoma execcrine spiradenoma. Am J Dermatopathol 9:90, 1987

32. Mitsudo S, Nakanishi I, Koss LG: Paget's disease of the penis and adjacent skin. Its association with fatal sweat gland carcinoma. Arch Pathol Lab Med 105:518, 1981
33. De Blois GG, Patterson JW, Hunter SB: Extramammary Paget's disease. Arising in knee region in association with sweat gland carcinoma. Arch Pathol Lab Med 108:713, 1984
34. Piura B, Zirkin HJ: Vulvar Paget's disease with an underlying sweat gland adenocarcinoma. J Dermatol Surg Oncol 14:533, 1988
35. Ascensao AC, Marques MSJ, Capitao-Mor M: Paget's disease of the nipple. Clinical and pathological review of 109 female patients. Dermatologica 170:170, 1985
36. Serour F, Birkenfeld S, Amsterdam E, et al: Paget's disease of the male breast. Cancer 62:601, 1988
37. Ordonez NG, Awalt H, Mackay B: Mammary and extramammary Paget's disease. An immunocytochemical and ultrastructural study. Cancer 59:1173, 1987
38. Guarner J, Cohen C, DeRose PB: Histogenesis of extramammary and mammary Paget cells. An immunohistochemical study. Am J Dermatopathol 11:313, 1989
39. Merot Y, Mazoujian G, Pinkus G, et al: Extramammary Paget's disease of the perianal and perineal regions. Evidence of apocrine derivation. Arch Dermatol 121:750, 1985
40. Hashimoto T, Inamoto N, Nakamura K: Triple extramammary Paget's disease. Immunohistochemical studies. Dermatologica 173:174, 1986
41. Hamm H, Vroom TM, Czarnetski BM: Extramammary Paget's cells: Further evidence of sweat gland derivation. J Am Acad Dermatol 15:1275, 1986
42. Wood MG, Parhizgar B, Beerman H: Malignant pilomatricoma. Arch Dermatol 120:770, 1984
43. Mir R, Cortes E, Papantoniou PA, et al: Metastatic trichomatricial carcinoma. Arch Pathol Lab Med 110:660, 1986
44. Manivel C, Wick MR, Mukai K: Pilomatrix carcinoma: An immunohistochemical comparison with benign pilomatrixoma and other benign cutaneous lesions of pilar origin. J Cutan Pathol 13:22, 1986
45. Gould E, Kurzon R, Kowalczyk AP, et al: Pilomatrix carcinoma with pulmonary metastasis. Report of a case. Cancer 54:370, 1984
46. Rabkin MS, Wittwer CT, Soong VY: Flow cytometric content analysis of a case of pilomatrix carcinoma showing multiple recurrences and invasion of the cranial vault. J Am Acad Dermatol 23:104, 1990
47. Nakhleh RE, Swanson PE, Wick MR: Cutaneous adnexal carcinomas with divergent differentiation. Am J Dermatopathol 12:325, 1990
48. Toker C: Trabecular carcinoma of the skin. Am J Dermatopathol 4:497, 1982
49. Sibley RK, Dehner LP, Rosai J: Primary neuroendocrine (Merkel cell ?) carcinoma of the skin. I. A clinicopathologic and ultrastructural study of 43 cases. Am J Surg Pathol 9:95, 1985
50. Sibley RK, Dahl D: Primary neuroendocrine (Merkel cell ?) carcinoma of the skin. II. An immunocytochemical study of 21 cases. Am J Surg Pathol 9:109, 1985
51. Rocamora A, Badia N, Vives R, et al: Epidermotropic primary neuroendocrine (Merkel cell) carcinoma of the skin with Pautrier-like microabscesses. Report of three cases and review of the literature. J Am Acad Dermatol 16:1163, 1987
52. Warner TFCS, Uno H, Hafez R, et al: Merkel cells and Merkel cell tumors. Ultrastructure, immunocytochemistry and review of the literature. Cancer 52:238, 1983
53. Hanke WC, Conner CA, Temofeew RK, Lingeman RE: Merkel cell carcinoma. Arch Dermatol 125:1096, 1989
54. Layfield L, Ulich T, Liao S, et al: Neuroendocrine carcinoma of the skin: An immunohistochemical study of tumor markers and neuroendocrine products. J Cutan Pathol 13:268, 1986
55. McKee PH, Cutaneous metastases. J Cutan Pathol 12:239, 1985
56. Tharakaram S: Metastases to the skin. Int J Dermatol 27:240, 1988
57. Brownstein MM, Helwig EB: Patterns of cutaneous metastasis. Arch Dermatol 105:862, 1972
58. Brownstein MM, Helwig EB: Spread of tumors to the skin. Arch Dermatol 107:80, 1973
59. Yamanishi K, Kishimoto S, Hosokawa Y, et al: Cutaneous metastasis from hepatocellular carcinoma resembling granuloma telangiectaticum. J Dermatol Tokyo 16:500, 1989
60. Innocenzi D, Todisco F, Carlesimo OA: Carcinome telangiectasique de Parkes-Weber. Ann Dermatol Venereol 115:1190, 1988
61. Baum EM, Omura EF, Payne RR, Little WP: Alopecia neoplastica—A rare form of cutaneous metastasis. J Am Acad Dermatol 4:688, 1981
62. Powell FC, Cooper AJ, Massa MC, et al: Sister Mary Joseph's nodule. A clinical and histologic study. J Am Acad Dermatol 10:610, 1984

42

MESODERMAL NEVI AND TUMORS

Each of the mesodermal components of the skin can be the source of neoplasms, but their incidence and variability are much smaller than those of epithelial and fibroepithelial tumors. The number and variety of malignant mesodermal neoplasms are even smaller. The more important lesions are listed in Table 42–1, with the exception of vascular tumors, which are discussed in Chapter 43. Rather than giving systematic descriptions, we shall discuss differentiating features and points of biologic significance.

In addition to the usual task of identifying the specific cell or tissue of a tumor, we meet two peculiar difficulties in this field. All mesodermal tissues contain blood vessels, and sometimes it is not easy to decide whether a lesion is primarily or secondarily vascular. Furthermore, reactive proliferation of fibrous tissue must be differentiated from nevoid or neoplastic proliferation.

SCAR VERSUS KELOID VERSUS FIBROMA VERSUS CONNECTIVE TISSUE NEVUS

A good starting point with basic significance is the differentiation of the four conditions listed in the heading. As happens so often in dermatopathology, clinical data are important, and we must try to refine our histologic criteria to fit the clinical course. For instance, there has been much discussion on how to differentiate histologically a temporarily hypertrophic scar from a keloid at the time when the clinician is in doubt within the first few months after surgery, this being the most propitious time to institute treatment. Special stains and more intensive investigation have clarified the differences to some degree.

Every young scar is a new growth of connective tissue and has some features of a neoplasm. However, just as atypical proliferation of epithelium in a healing wound or other tissue defect eventually subsides, so is the stage of proliferation of fibrocytes and blood vessels in a scar followed by a stage of maturation and return to relatively normal tissue homeostasis. *Keloid* tissue, on the other hand, remains immature for prolonged periods and has other peculiar characteristics.

Normal Scar

When scar tissue has replaced a defect in the skin, the area is characterized by three major features. Collagen bundles run a fairly straight course parallel to the skin surface. Small blood vessels extend perpendicularly between epidermis and subcutis, and elastic fibers either are absent or are thin and run parallel to the collagen bundles. Moreover, hair follicles and sweat glands are apt to be absent, and the papillae and rete ridges are either absent or poorly developed.

TABLE 42–1. MESODERMAL NEVI AND TUMORS

Fibrocytic
  Connective tissue nevi
    Collagenous
    Elastic
  Fibroma
    Nodulus cutaneus
    Keloid
    Fibroma molle (pendulum) and acrochordon
    Acquired fibrokeratoma
    Perifollicular fibroma
    Trichodiscoma
    Juvenile hyaline fibromatosis
    Juvenile aponeurotic fibroma
    Palmar and plantar fibromatosis
    Myxoma and myxofibroma
    Chondroma
    Osteoma
    Pseudosarcomatous fasciitis
  Sarcoma
    Dermatofibrosarcoma protuberans
    Spindle cell sarcoma
    Epithelioid sarcoma

Histiocytic
  Benign lesions (Chap. 24)
  Langerhans cell granulomas (Chap. 25)
  Giant cell tumor of tendon sheath
  Malignant fibrous histiocytoma

Lipocytic
  Nevus lipomatosus superficialis and nevus angiolipomatosus
  Lipoma, angiolipoma, and spindle cell lipoma
  Liposarcoma

Muscular
  Leiomyoma
  Leiomyosarcoma
  Rhabdomyosarcoma

For a recent general review of mesodermal tumors, see Hajdu SI: Pathology of Soft Tissue Tumors. Philadelphia, Lea & Febiger, 1979 and Enzinger and Weiss: Soft Tissue Tumors. St. Louis, Mosby, 1983.

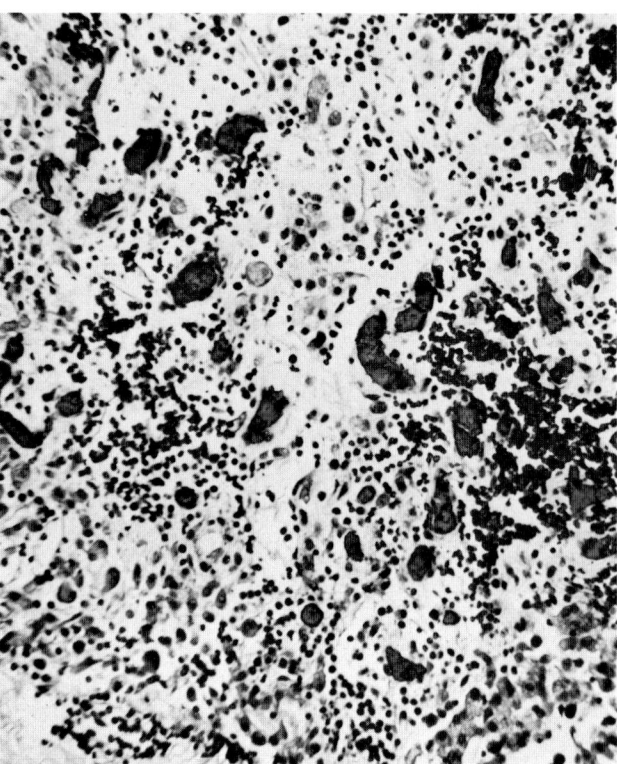

Figure 42–1.
Granulation tissue. Capillary blood vessels and a mixture of inflammatory cells embedded in immature connective tissue. H&E. X180.

This picture comes about because the pars reticularis of the dermis is poorly vascularized, and granulation tissue, the first step in replacement of a tissue defect, arises primarily from the subcutaneous tissue, with some help from adnexal vascular tissue, and from the pars papillaris of the surrounding dermis. We emphasize that we are not dealing here with the healing of an incised and sutured wound but with the restitution of a sizable defect in the skin, such as an ulcer from whatever source. The components of *granulation tissue* (Fig. 42–1), vascular sprouts, and fibrocytes, coming from below, are at first directed vertical to the skin surface. Fibroblastic cells containing myofilaments (myofibroblasts)[1] appear in granulation tissue and contribute to its contraction. Blood vessels later become less numerous, but the persisting ones retain their telltale vertical arrangement. Fibrocytes and the collagen fibers and bundles formed by them are redeployed parallel to the skin surface but never achieve the resilient three-dimensional weave of normal dermis. Elastic fibers often are completely absent. They are regenerated more readily in young individuals but always remain thin. While granulation tissue is rich in ground substance, this soon is reduced, and a maturing scar shows normal staining reactions with mucopolysaccharide and connective tissue stains.

Hypertrophic Scars and Keloids

Hypertrophic scars and keloids, on the other hand, grow in the dermis and produce curvilinear tracts and bundles, several of which form a whorl.[2] The interstitial tissue retains relatively large amounts of mucosaccharides for a longer time, giving H&E sections a bluish tinge. Abnormal cross-linking amino acids have been described as well as the presence of myofibroblasts.[3] In the hypertrophic scar, there is gradual maturation, although the whorled arrangement may persist. In keloids, there is excessive production of extracellular matrix material by dermal fibroblasts leading to the formation of tightly packed nodules of collagen with peripheral blood vessels.[4] The tissue remains rich in cells and ground substance, and the collagen also is abnormal. This is best shown by Luxol fast blue, which stains normal collagen blue and keloid reddish. Later, in old keloids, collagen bundles may become very thick, hyaline, and eosinophilic (Fig. 42–2). There is no new formation of elastic fibers. Keloids that have developed in skin defects (burn keloids, scar keloids) have no normal pars papillaris. So-called *spontaneous keloids*, however, such as those that develop from minor trauma or acne lesions, are separated from the epidermis by fairly normal papillary dermis. Keloids are well circumscribed, often almost encapsulated, in contrast to histiocytomas (fibromas) and papular leiomyomas but similar to angioleiomyomas and neurofibromas.

Connective Tissue Nevi

Under the term *connective tissue nevi* are grouped conditions that are congenital or arise later in life and have a relatively stable excess of mature vascularized connective tissue. It is understood that the sole cell capable of forming connective tissue is the fibroblast, although certain types of basement membrane-related collagens have been attributed to epithelial cells, and formation of elastin to smooth muscle cells. In lesions consisting of an excess of fibers, the fibroblasts usually are inconspicuous. The stimuli that prod them to lay down collagenous fibers, elastic fibers, and ground substance are unknown. We therefore can only describe the lesions we see and group them according to their clinical and histologic correlations, as has been done in Table 42–2.[5] It appears preferable to give such an analysis of various forms of nevoid conditions, rather than to use "connective tissue nevus" as a unifying term. One should remember that blood vessels are an essential part of any connective tissue and may be present in excess (*angiofibromas*).

The *Pringle tumors* of the central face in tuberous sclerosis, for which "adenoma sebaceum" is an unfortunate misnomer, are true angiofibromas and are due to nevoid hyperplasia of vascular connective tissue either between or around hair follicles. *Shagreen plaques* of other regions are larger accumulations of mature connective tissue of the pars reticularis, and periungual fibromas are almost indistinguishable from acquired acral fibrokeratomas. The *Buschke–Ollendorff syndrome*[6] consists of multiple skin papules of mature collagenous and elastic tissue in association with osteopoikilosis (see Chapter 27), which also may be found associated with other types of *collagenoma*[7,8] and elastic tissue nevi. It seems likely that the histologically similar papules of *epidermolysis bullosa et albopapuloidea* of Pasini, which contain degraded chondroitin sulfate,[9] also belong here. Other connective tissue nevi have been described as *nevus elasticus* and *juvenile elastoma*. Nevus elasticus of the Lewandowsky type actually is a minus nevus as far as elastic fibers are concerned and is most likely a collagenous nevus. Lesions described as *juvenile elastoma* (see Fig. 27–1) do consist of circumscribed hyperplasia of elastic tissue. Somewhat similar elastic fiber hyperplasia may be encountered in association with nevus cell nevi.[10]

Fibroma

What constitutes a dermal fibroma is not easy to define. It ought to be a continuing benign proliferation of less than mature connective tissue with deranged architecture. Most fibromas consist of elongated and spindle-shaped fibroblasts and collagen bundles with or without significant increased vascularity. Occasionally, fibromas are poorly cellular and

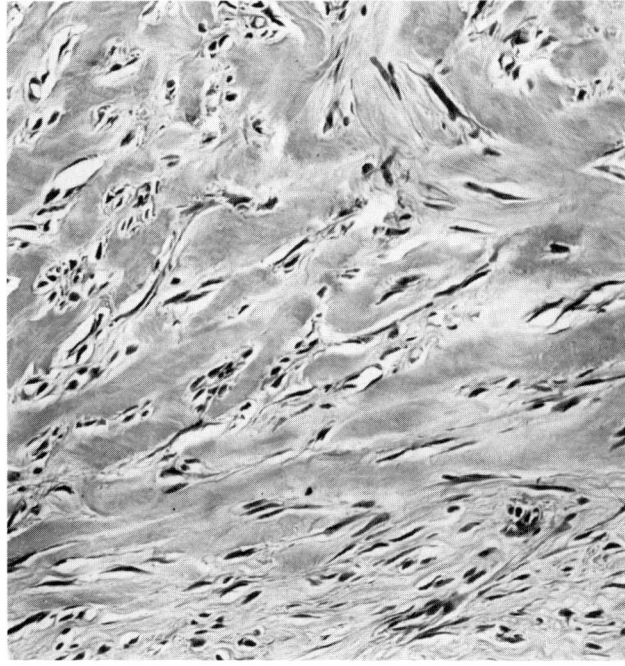

Figure 42–2.
Keloid, central portion exhibiting hyalinized collagen bundles and unusually large fibrocytes. H&E. X225.

TABLE 42–2. CONNECTIVE TISSUE NEVI AND RELATED CONDITIONS

Clinical Diagnosis	Collagen	Elastic Fibers
Pringle tumors	Increased, vascular	Absent
Shagreen patch	Increased	Relatively decreased
Paving stone nevus (Lipschütz)	Hypertrophic, swollen homogeneous	Relatively decreased
Familial cutaneous collagenoma	Increased	Relatively decreased
Dermatofibrosis lenticularis disseminata (Buschke–Ollendorff)	Increased	Decreased
Dermatofibrosis disseminata with microcysts (Verbov)	Increased perifollicular tissue	Decreased
Perifollicular fibroma	Increased perifollicular sheath	Absent
Fibrofolliculoma	Abnormal perifollicular sheath	Absent
Trichodiscoma	Decreased, edematous	Normal
Juvenile elastoma (Weidman)	No significant change	Increased, somewhat abnormal
Nevus elasticus (Lewandowsky)	No significant change	Spottily decreased and abnormal
Zosteriform connective tissue nevus	Abnormal, irregular, fine, short	Reduced, abnormal: shreds, granules
Epidermolysis bullosa et albopapuloidea (Pasini)	Degraded chondroitin sulfate	Absent

Modified from Hegedus and Schor.[5]

consist mainly of markedly sclerotic and hyalinized collagen bundles.[11] The elastic fibers are sparse or completely absent. A common variety is *fibrous papule of the nose*, a small lesion (Fig. 42–3) arising relatively late in life and consisting of fairly cellular fibrous tissue lacking elastic fibers.[12] Its relation with subsiding dermal nevus has been rejected by positive immunostaining for vimentin and negative S-100 protein.[13] Factor XIIIa stain shows positive reaction in 80 percent of cells suggesting development of the lesion from dermal dendrocytes.[14] The tiny papillomatous protrusions on the glans penis and vulva is known as *pearly penile papules* or *hirsutoid papillomas*.[15,16] Each lesion shows a small central core of richly vascular connective tissue covered with a layer of slightly acanthotic epidermis (Fig. 42–4).[17,18]

Perifollicular Fibromas and Trichodiscomas

Other fibromatous lesions are related to the mesodermal portions of the pilar apparatus and have been described as *perifollicular fibromas*[19] and *trichodiscomas*.[20] Both are rare. Their existence, however, emphasizes that the hair follicle has an integral mesodermal component that behaves independently of the interfollicular (skeletal) dermis. This follicle-related mesoderm forms the dermal papilla of the follicle, the perifollicular sheath, the arrector pili muscle, and the dermal pad of the hair disk.

Perifollicular fibromas, which were mentioned in Chapter 37, may be present in three different forms,[21] as small single papules, as larger nodes, and as part of the tuberous sclerosis syndrome (Fig. 42–5). Cases described as multiple perifollicular fi-

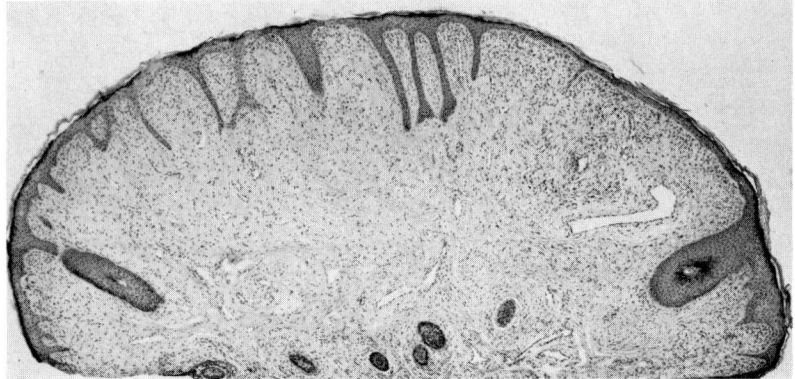

Figure 42–3.
Fibrous papule of nose. This lesion exhibits general, as well as perifollicular, overgrowth of fairly cellular collagenous tissue involving papillae and deeper dermal layers. H&E. X30.

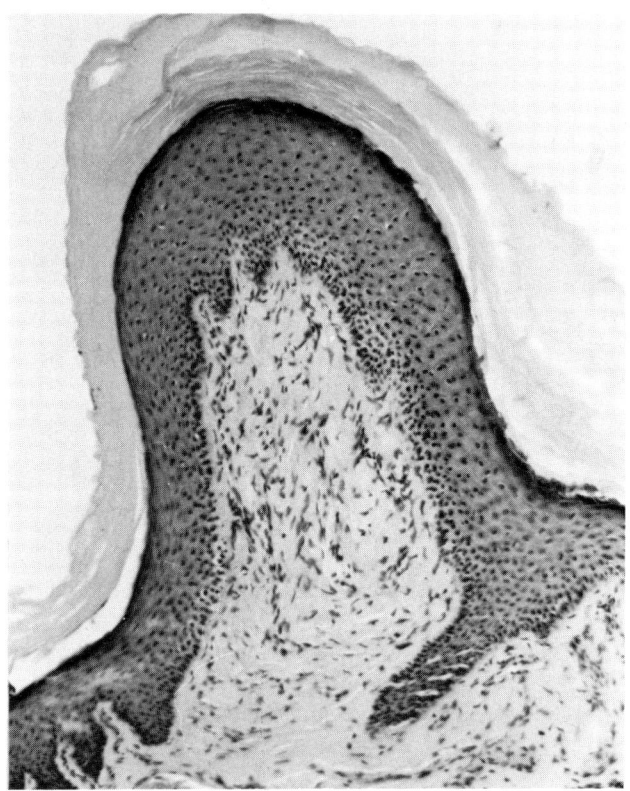

Figure 42–4.
Pearly penile papule. Small digitate lesion shows a central core of fibrous tissue covered with acanthotic epidermis. H&E. X25.

bromas of head and neck[22] seem to belong rather to a closely related entity, the fibrofolliculoma of Birt et al.[23] Histologically perifollicular fibromas are characterized by proliferation of concentric layers of fibrous connective tissue surrounding small pilosebaceous structures.[2]

Acrochordon, Fibroma Pendulum, Acquired Fibrokeratoma, Myxoid Fibroma

In distinction from lesions that are located in the reticular dermis, there are those that project outward from the skin (papillomas) (Fig. 42–6). Most common is the *skin tag* or *acrochordon*. It consists of papillary dermis covered by thin epithelium and, in many cases, seems to be essentially one hyperplastic papilla. In other cases, however, there is more epidermal proliferation, and one wonders whether such a lesion is a papilloma in the sense of a combined new growth of epidermis and mesoderm. This is particularly true in patients who have numerous lesions around the neck which are apt to vary clinically from skin tags to pedunculated seborrheic verrucae.

Fibroma pendulum is the term used for larger and often pedunculated lesions consisting purely of loose connective tissue of papillary type covered by epidermis. Some may contain fat lobules and represent pedunculated lipofibromas. Vascularity varies,

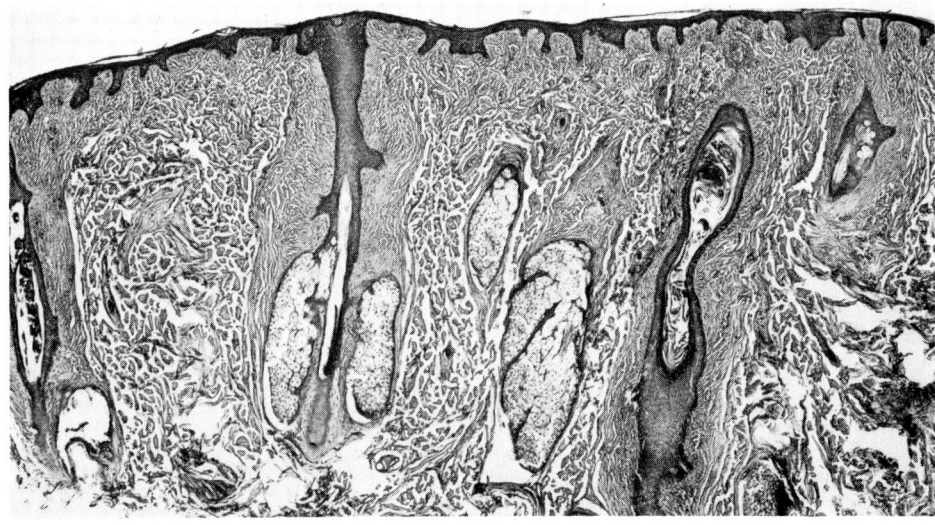

Figure 42–5.
Perifollicular fibromas (nevoid hyperplasia of follicular fibrous sheath) as a manifestation of Pringle's disease (tuberous sclerosis syndrome). H&E. X30.

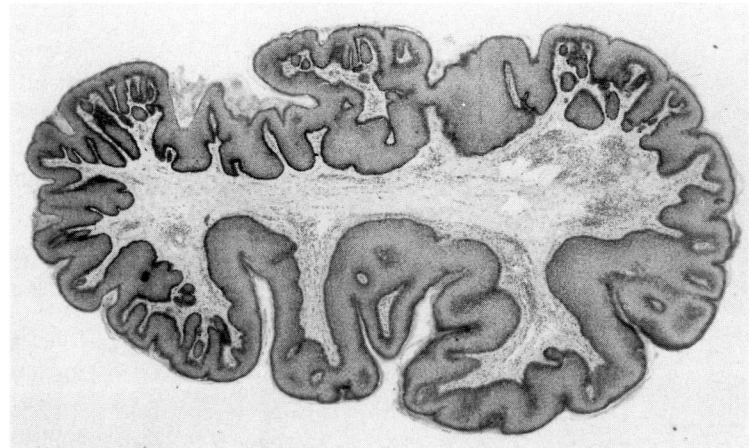

Figure 42–6.
Fibroepithelial polyp (acrochordon). H&E. X25.

and inflammation or torsion of the pedicle may lead to engorgement and hemorrhagic infarction. Fibroma pendulum does not contain hair follicles or sweat glands. If elastic fibers are present, they are of the thin papillary type.

Another not uncommon lesion occurring predominantly on fingers (Fig. 42–7) is *acquired digital fibrokeratoma*.[24,25] Its differentiation from papillomas with hyperkeratotic acanthotic epidermal covering may seem to be a histologic nicety but actually has a biologic basis. The connective tissue core represents the pars reticularis as well as the pars papillaris and may include the two types of elastic fibers found in these layers. Some lesions also contain sweat ducts. Similar lesions occur on acral parts of the limbs other than the digits. The periungual fibromas (Koenen tumors) present in patients with tuberous sclerosis show changes very similar to those of the acquired fibrokeratomas.[26]

Digital *myxoid fibromas* occur in single or multiple familial forms. Warty nodular lesions consist of a central core of richly vascular and markedly myxomatous fibrous connective tissue covered by an acanthotic and often hyperkeratotic epidermis (Fig. 42–8).[27]

LESIONS WITH UNUSUAL DIFFERENTIATION OF CONNECTIVE TISSUE

Myxomas

Cutaneous myxomas or myxoid neurofibromas (Fig. 42–9) occur in association with diffuse pigmented skin lesions (lentigines and nevi), cardiac (atrial) myxomas, and endocrine tumors.[28–30] The skin lesions are either dermal or subcutaneous and show well-defined areas in which elongated fibroblasts are embedded in abundant mucinous stroma.

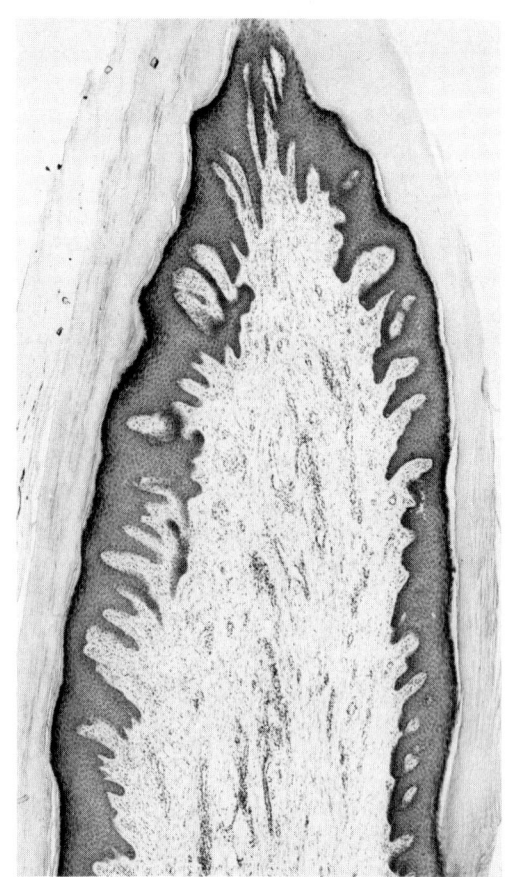

Figure 42–7.
Acquired digital fibrokeratoma. H&E. X30.

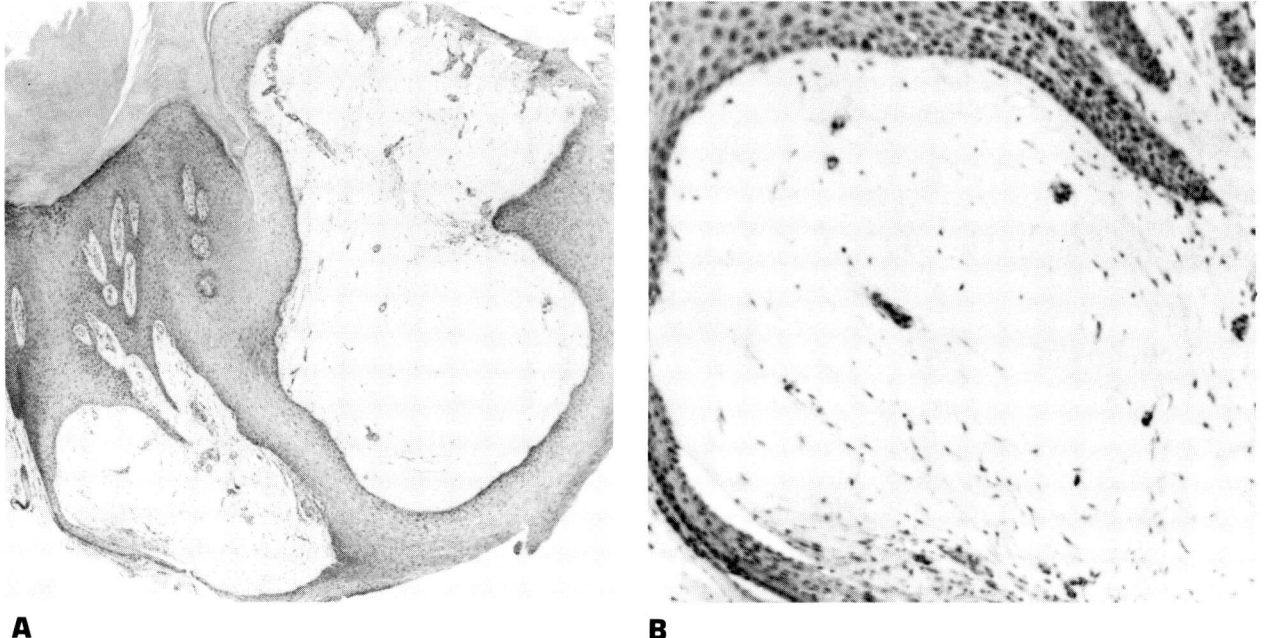

Figure 42–8.
Digital myxofibroma. A hyperkeratotic lesion shows massive proliferation of highly myxomatous fibrous connective tissue covered with acanthotic epidermis. **A.** H&E. × 25. **B.** H&E. × 125.

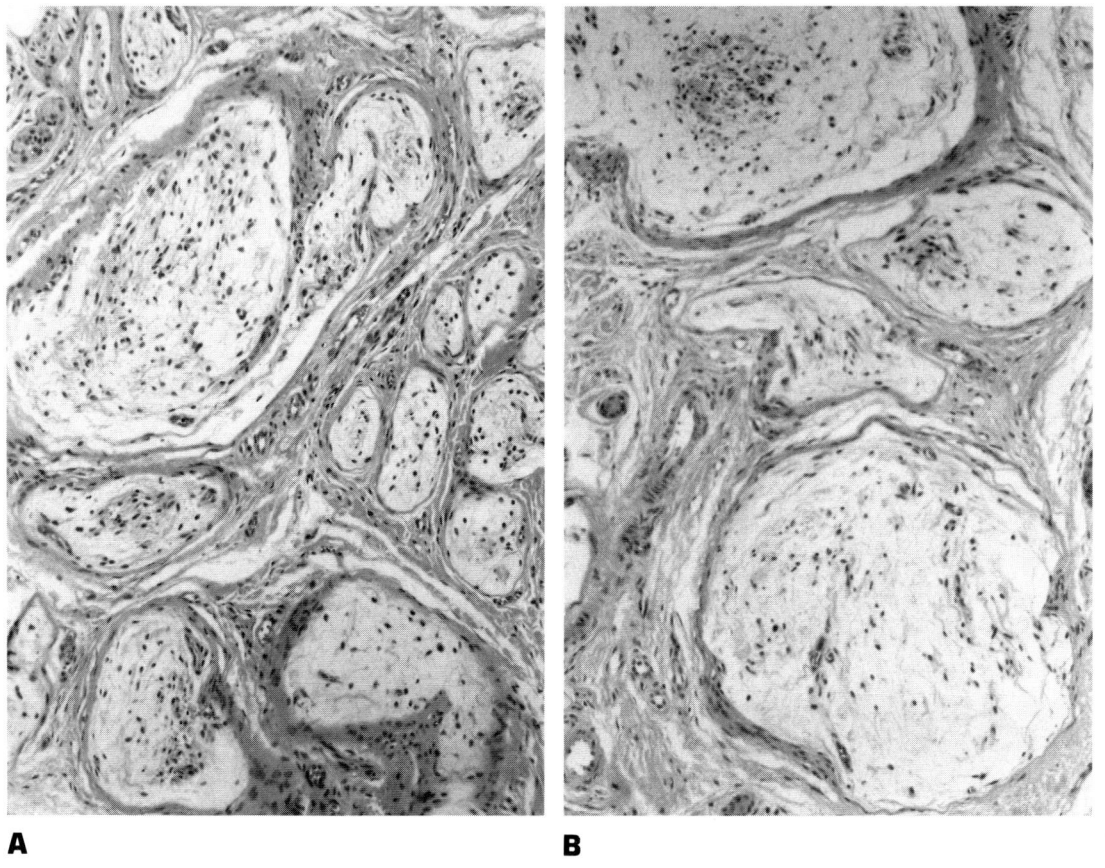

Figure 42–9.
Cutaneous myxoma (nerve sheath myxoma). Lobulated tumor masses are made up of elongated cells with small nuclei embedded in a myxoid stroma. **A** and **B.** H&E. X125.

Giant Cell Tumor of Tendon Sheath (Localized Nodular Tenosynovitis)

Giant cell tumor of tendon sheath is most commonly located on the fingers, forming a deep-seated nodular growth with attachment to the underlying tendon sheath. The growth is solid and lobulated. Densely cellular areas consist of proliferation of histiocytes containing hemosiderin or lipid granules and foreign-body-type multinucleated giant cells (Fig. 42–10).[31] Less cellular areas show proliferation of elongated fibroblasts in a hyalinized collagenous stroma. Electron microscopy shows histiocyte-like cells containing numerous lysosomes, fibroblasts with abundant rough endoplasmic reticulum, and myofibroblasts.[32]

Juvenile Hyaline Fibromatosis

Under the term juvenile hyaline fibromatosis a number of cases have been reported in which large tumors appeared around the head, with small papules elsewhere and destructive lesions in long bones.[33] The tumors consisted of proliferation of fibroblasts and endothelial-lined capillaries (Fig. 42–11) embedded in a homogeneous PAS-positive ground substance.[34] This bizarre manifestation, possibly inherited in an autosomal recessive manner results in extensive tissue destruction and osteolytic bone lesions ending fatally or persisting into the adult life.[35,36]

Juvenile aponeurotic fibroma

This occurs in the palms and soles of young children. It measures from one to several centimeters in diameter and consists of solid proliferation of cells with round or oval nuclei embedded in a matrix of collagenous tissue, showing foci of calcification and chondroid differentiation (Fig. 42–12).[37]

Palmar and plantar fibromatosis

This occurs in childhood in the form of single or rarely multiple nodular growth made up of dense proliferation of elongated fibroblasts and collagenous tissue forming intersecting bundles.[38]

Fibrous Hamartoma of Infancy

This benign soft tissue tumor appears within the first 2 years of life.[39] The growth is made up of three tissue components: fibrous, adipose, and myxoid mesenchymal element. Dense fibrocollagenous areas appear as bands or septae extending in various directions. Mature fatty tissue and areas of moderate to dense cellular proliferation in a myxoid stroma are also present. Electron microscopy shows that a majority of cells are myofibroblasts.[40]

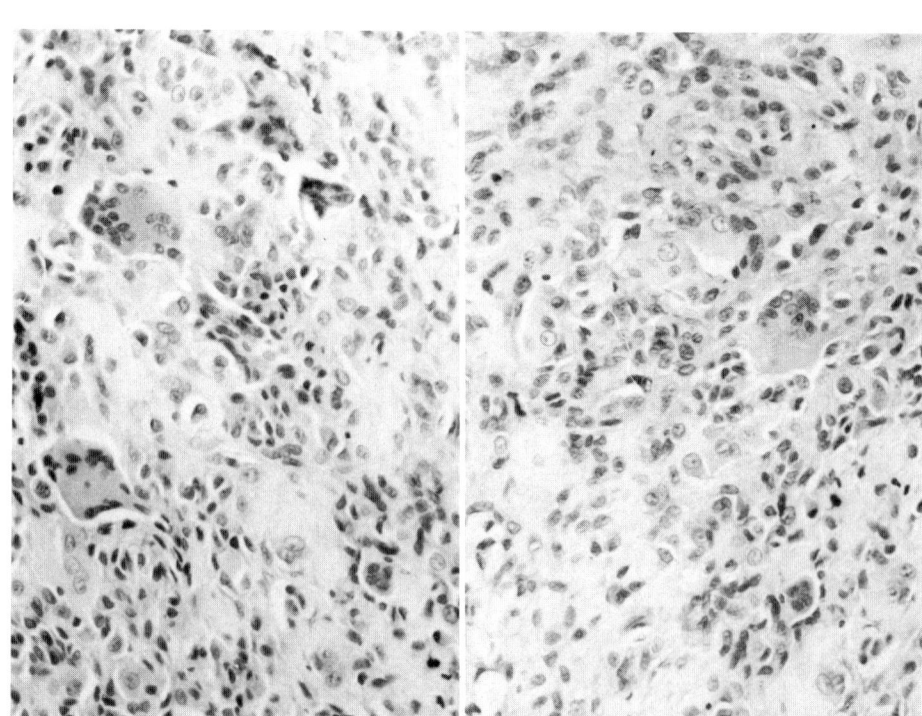

Figure 42–10.
Giant cell tumor of tendon sheath. These accumulations of histiocytes, macrophages, and multinucleated giant cells actually are foreign-body granulomas. H&E. X250.

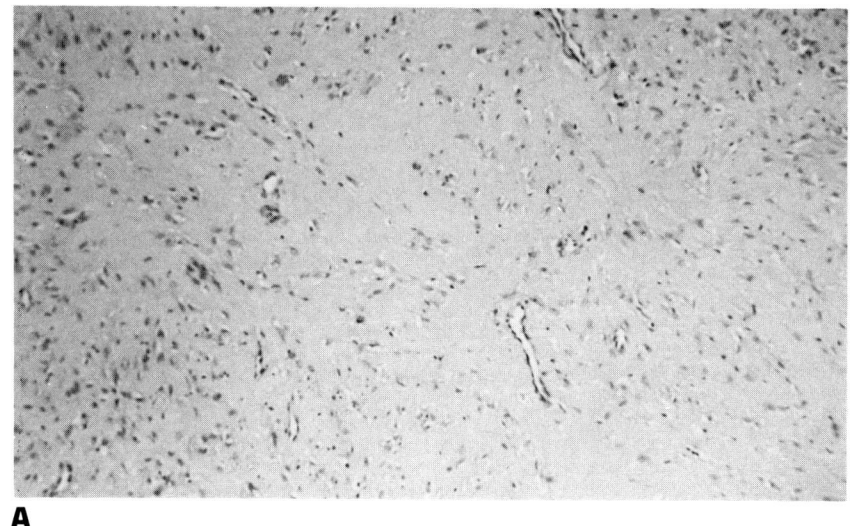
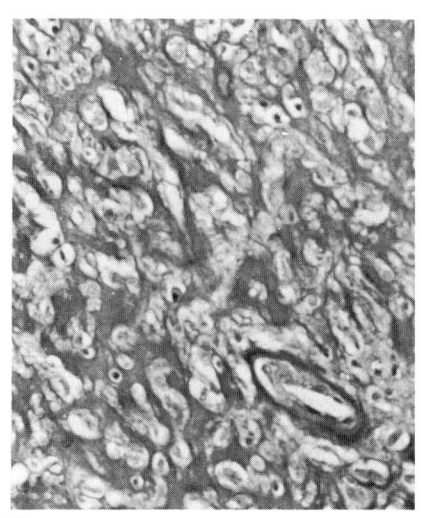
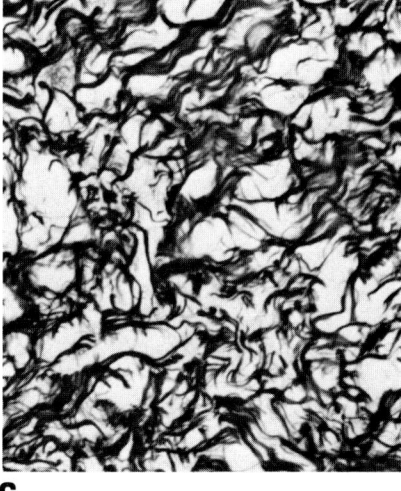

Figure 42–11.
Juvenile hyaline fibromatosis. **A.** *Fibroblasts and endothelial-lined capillaries embedded in a homogeneous ground substance. H&E. X100.* **B.** *PAS stain shows positive reaction of the hyaline material in the ground substance. X275.* **C.** *Reticulum stain demonstrates a rich network of reticulum fibers. X275. (Courtesy of Drs. J.K. Maniar and E. Wilson-Jones.)*

Giant Cell Fibroblastoma

Giant fibroblastoma is another fibrohistiocytic lesion that appears in childhood forming dermal or subcutaneous nodules.[41,42] The growth is richly vascular and consists mainly of massive proliferation of pleomorphic spindle-shaped cells in a paralleled undulating pattern, myxoid areas, and sinusoid spaces lined by multinucleated giant cells.[43] Immunostaining for vimentin is positive. Desmine, S-100 protein, and alpha-l-antichymotrypsin are negative. Factor VIII stains only the endothelial cells of the capillary blood vessels but not the tumor cells.[44]

Osteoma and Chondroma

Bone formation occurs in the skin and subcutaneous tissue under a variety of circumstances and was discussed in Chapter 28. Whether osteoma (Fig. 28–3) in the sense of primary neoplastic bone formation exists is the skin is doubtful. Cases in which multiple tiny spheres of bone have been found on face and neck may follow lesions of acne vulgaris or represent ossification of multiple epithelial milia. A few benign cartilaginous tumors have been found in the skin.[45] We have seen two such lesions over the cartilaginous portion of the nose (Fig. 42–13).

SARCOMA VERSUS HISTIOCYTOMA VERSUS PSEUDOSARCOMA

Tumors consisting predominantly of proliferation of spindle and fusiform cells are difficult to classify

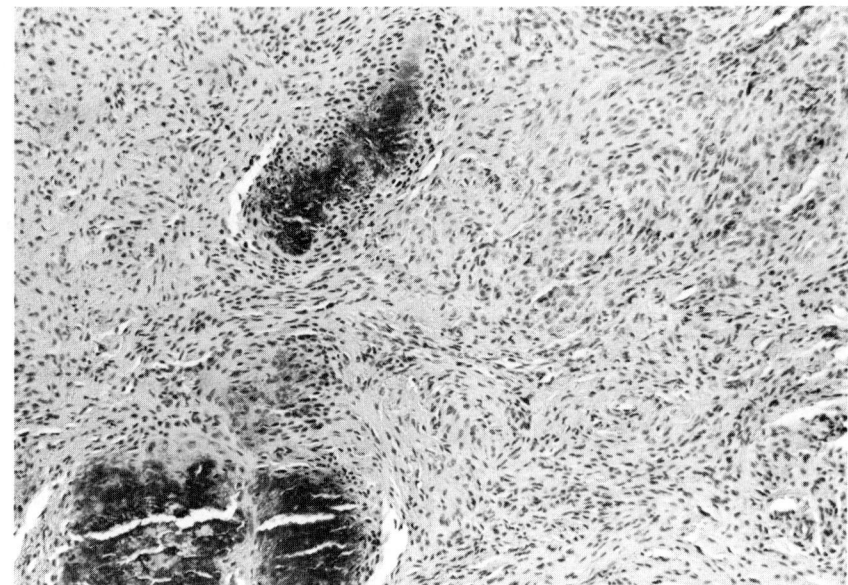

Figure 42–12.
Juvenile aponeurotic fibroma. A solid fibrous tumor with areas of calcification and chondroid differentiation. H&E. X125.

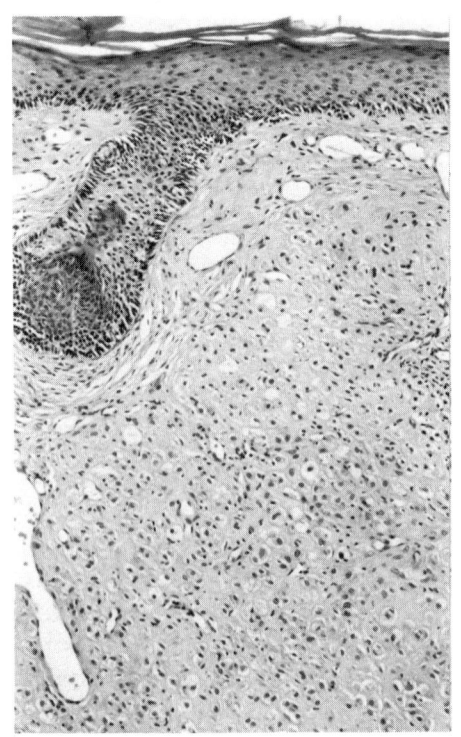 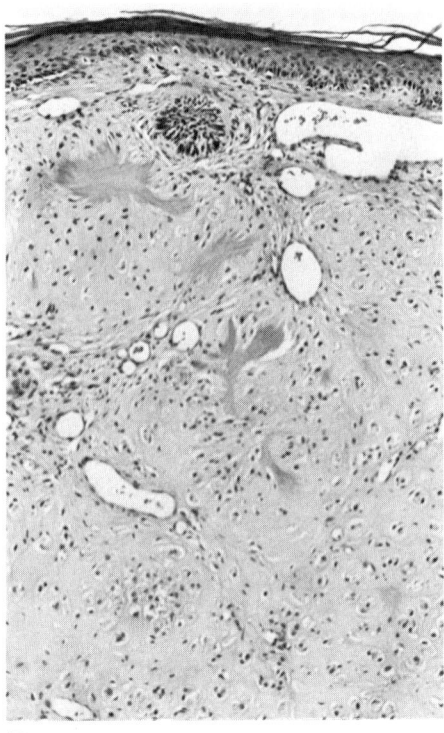

Figure 42–13.
Chondroma. A solid lesion of nose made up of cartilagenous tissue. **A** and **B**. H&E. X125.

because a light microscopic differentiation of fibroblasts and histiocytes is not satisfactory. As pointed out in Chapters 2 and 5, histiocytes are identified by their ability to phagocytose. An inactive (resting) histiocyte is just a fixed-tissue-type cell, although the electron microscope may reveal lysosomes and other differentiating features. It must be kept in mind, however, that fibrocytes and histiocytes most likely can transform one into the other.

In routine sections one sees a spectrum of fibrous tumors ranging from densely cellular histiocytomas to mainly collagenous dermatofibromas. The term "fibrous histiocytoma" is applicable to this entire class of lesions. Malignant lesions consisting predominantly of fusiform cells are discussed in four categories: spindle cell sarcoma, epithelioid sarcoma, malignant fibrous histiocytoma, and dermatofibrosarcoma protuberans. Kaposi's hemorrhagic sarcoma is discussed in Chapter 43.

Spindle Cell Sarcoma

Spindle cell sarcoma consists of streams and bundles of large fusiform cells varying more or less in size of nuclei and cytoplasm and containing numerous mitoses (Fig. 42–14). Interstitial tissue is minimal.[46-49] As a rule the tumor arises in deeper tissues and invades subcutis and dermis. Histologic grading has been proposed based on the tumor size, depth of invasion, degree of tumor cell differentiation, number of mitotic figures, and cell necrosis.[50,51] Lesions with a higher number of mast cells have been associated with better prognosis and longer 5-year survival rate.[52] Fibrosarcomas may occur at any age, during infancy, or may be congenital.[53]

Epithelioid Sarcoma

Epithelioid sarcoma involves predominantly distal extremities of young adults and tends to grow deep along the fascial planes, aponeuroses, and tendon sheaths (Fig. 42–15). The growth is made up of large plump epithelial-appearing cells imitating areas of granuloma formation or invasive squamous cell carcinoma.[54,55] Heavy lymphocytic infiltrate is associated and there are numerous mitotic figures.[56] Positive expression of vimentin and cytokeratins (45 Kd and 54 Kd), specific for simple epithelia, indicates that epithelioid sarcoma masquerades a carcinoma.[57,58]

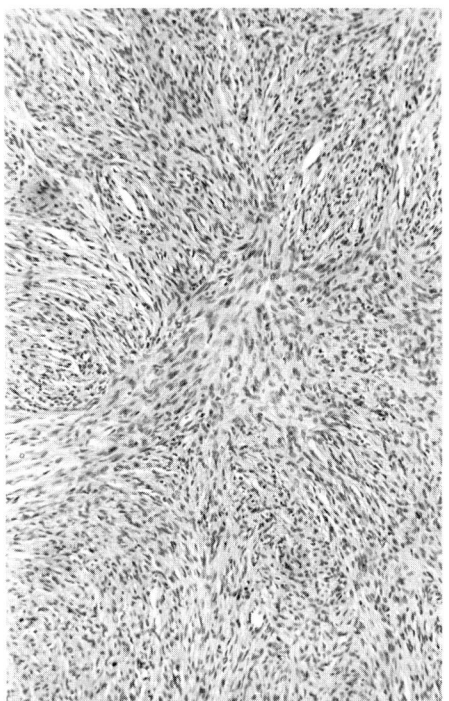
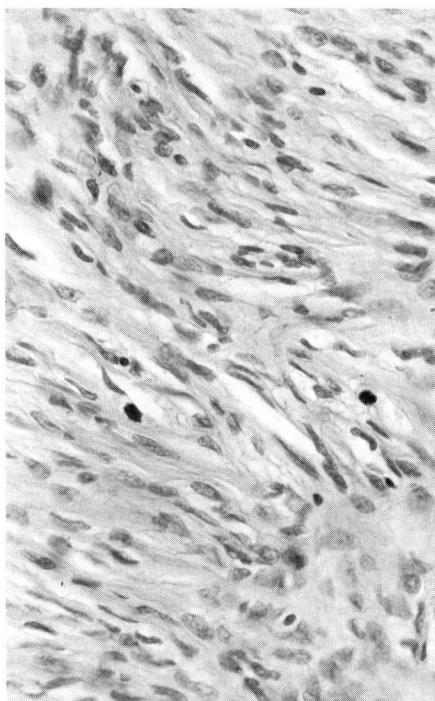

Figure 42–14.
Infantile fibrosarcoma. Marked with dense cellularity, poor collagen formation, and mitotic figures. H&E. **A.** X125. **B.** X600.

A **B**

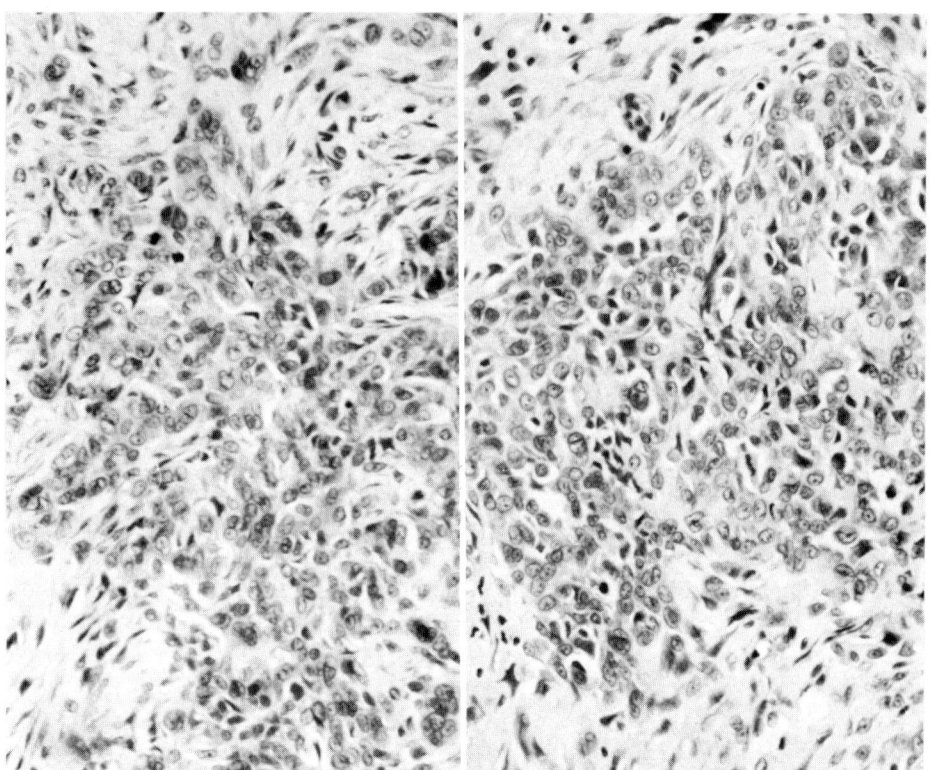

Figure 42–15.
Epithelioid sarcoma. Differentiation of these tumors from spindle cell squamous carcinomas and atypical fibroxanthomas may be difficult. H&E. X225.

Malignant Fibrous Histiocytoma and Atypical Fibroxanthoma

Malignant fibrous histiocytoma (Fig. 42–16) is the most common soft tissue sarcoma of older adults at peak age around the sixth or seventh decade of life. Prognosis is related to the size and depth of the lesion and degree of cytologic malignancy.[59–61] The growth is made up of proliferation of spindle-shaped and elongated fibroblasts in whorled and storiform configuration. Large histiocytes with granular and eosinophilic cytoplasm and multinucleated giant cells are present in addition to a number of mitotic figures.[62,63]

The significance of atypical fibroxanthoma has changed since its introduction as a benign and pseudomalignant neoplasm.[64–66] In a majority of cases, this lesion may be considered to be a superficial form of malignant fibrous histiocytoma. The superficial and often exophytic nature of the growth may be responsible for its benign course.[67]

Atypical fibroxanthomas occur mainly in actinically damaged skin and consist either of dysplastic spindle cells forming poorly developed bundles or of bizarre polygonal cells and multinucleated giant cells or of a mixture of these cell types (Fig. 42–17).[68] They infiltrate the surroundings in irregular fashion but usually do not recur after excision. Some well-documented cases of metastasis indicate that these are true neoplasms.[69,70]

Dermatofibrosarcoma Protuberans

Dermatofibrosarcoma protuberans is a slow growing neoplasm slightly elevated and indurated, red or bluish in color, located predominantly on the trunk and extremities and occasionally on the face and scalp.[71,72] The lesion shows a tendency for local recurrences. Metastasis is rare (Fig. 42–18). Histologically, dermatofibrosarcoma protuberans is charac-terized by involvement of dermis and the subcuta-neous fat tissue by massive proliferation of elongated and spindle-shaped cells forming intersecting bundles with a cartwheel-type arrangement. The tumor bundles are densely cellular and show scattered mitotic figures. The tumor stroma stains blue with Van Gieson suggesting the presence of collagen bundles. The collagen bundles, however, do

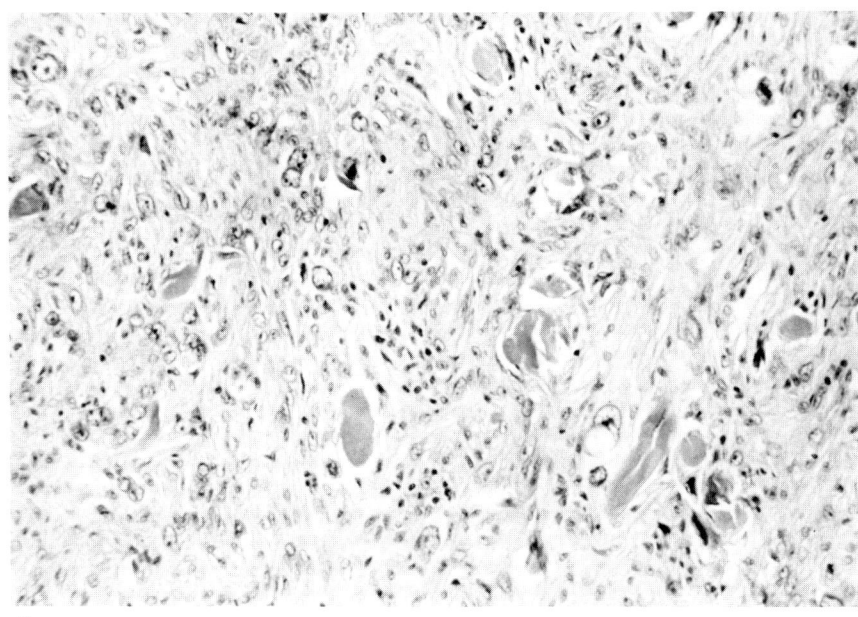

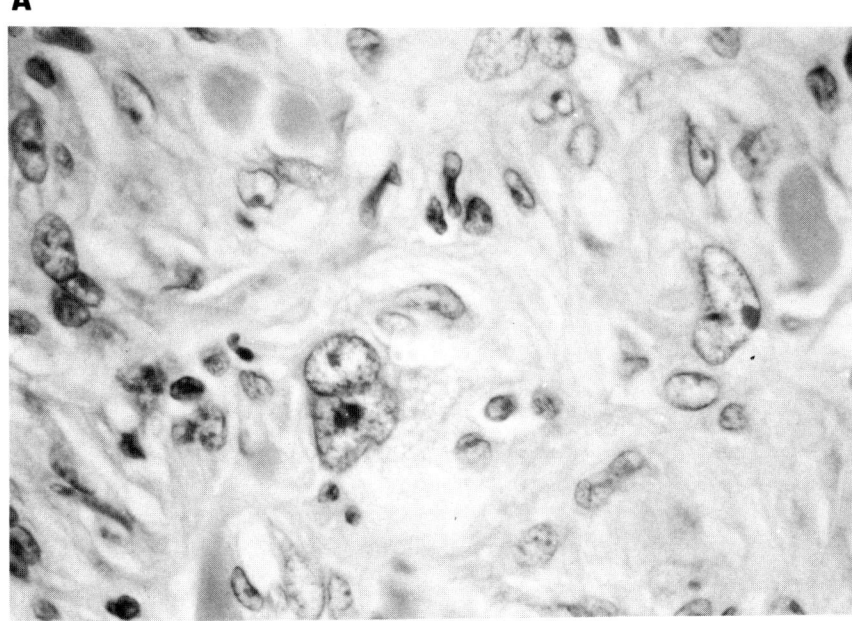

Figure 42-16.
Malignant fibrous histiocytoma. Mixture of small and large atypical cells invading fibrous tissue. H&E. **A.** X125. **B.** X600.

not show birefringence under polarized light.[73] The border of the lesion is ill-defined and fingerlike projections extend into the underlying tissue. At the surface, a shelf of tumor cells extend outward to variable distance at the periphery of the lesion. Electron microscopic findings have suggested fibroblast or modified fibroblast origin.[74] Tissue cultures favor histiocytic derivation.[75]

Pigmented Dermatofibrosarcoma Protuberans (Bodnar Tumor)

Bodnar tumor is a rare usually exophytic and multilobulated neoplasm involving dermis and the subcutaneous tissue (Fig. 42–19). Histologically, it is characterized by massive proliferation of spindle-shaped cells arranged in a tight storiform pattern

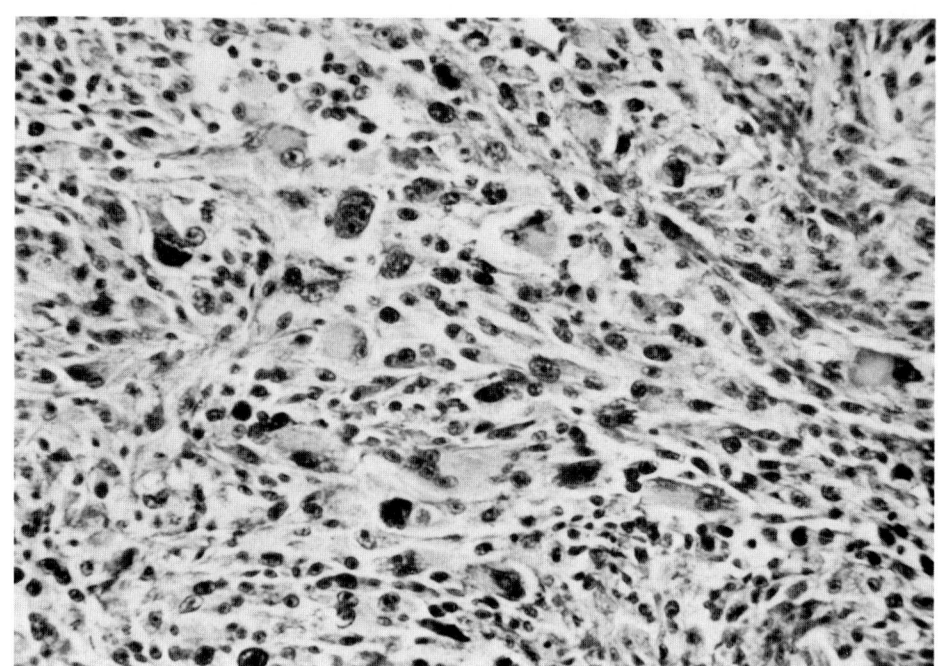

Figure 42–17.
Atypical fibroxanthoma. Greatly variable histiocytes, some multinucleated and foamy. H&E. X225.

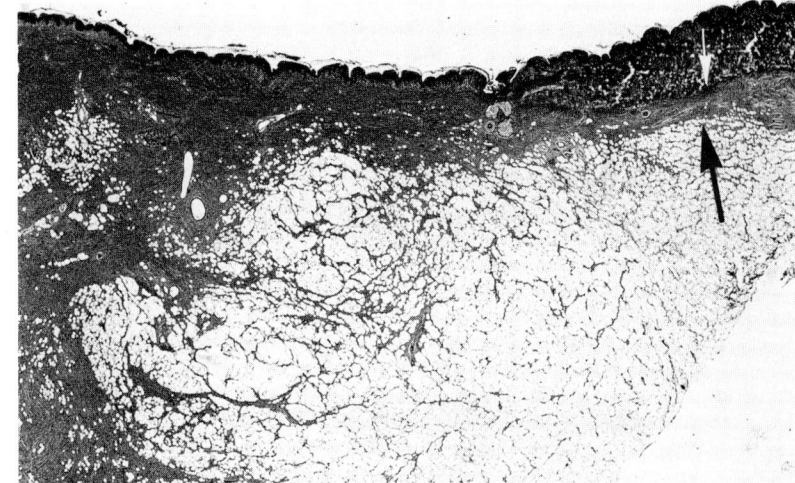

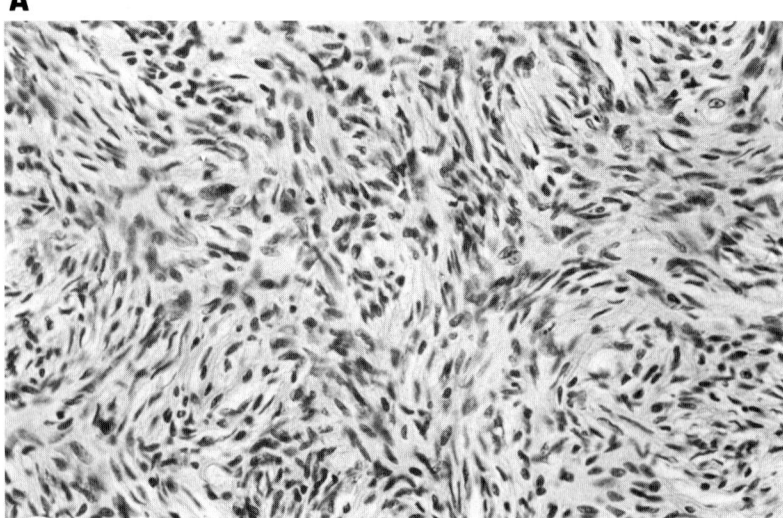

Figure 42–18.
Dermatofibrosarcoma protuberans. **A** shows at left the edge of tumor which infiltrates dermis and subcutaneous tissue. While infiltration of subcutaneous tissue subsides toward right, there is a shelf of tumor tissue at border of dermis and hypoderm extending to edge of specimen at right. Upper and lower borders are indicated by arrows. H&E. X9. **B.** Cartwheel pattern. H&E. X225.

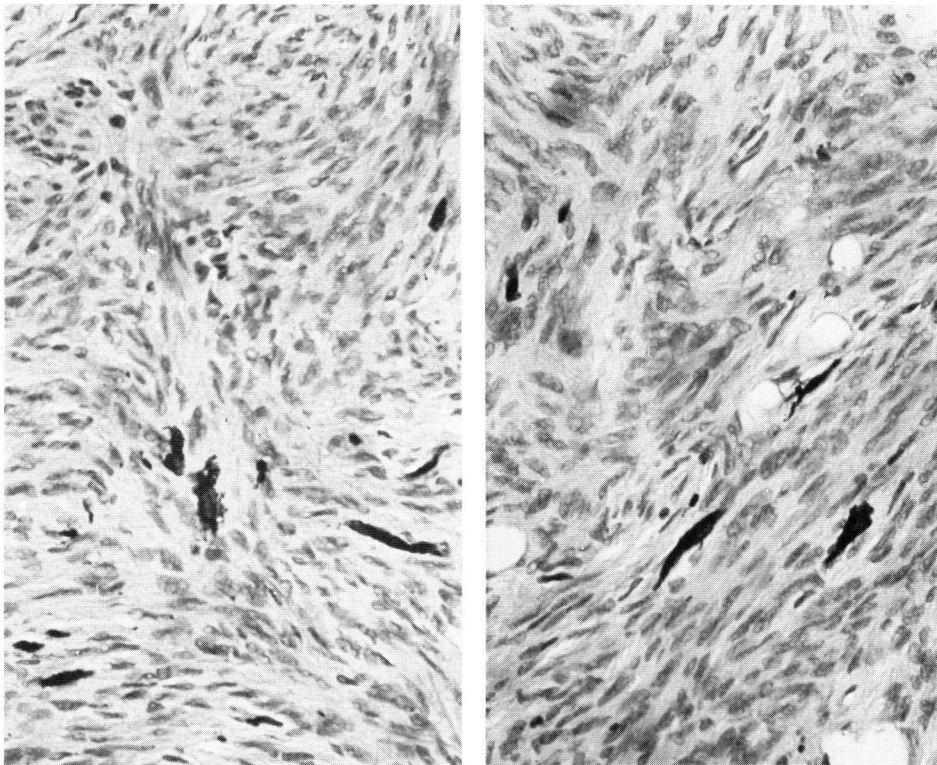

Figure 42–19.
Bodnar tumor shows storiform pattern of dermatofibrosarcoma protuberans and scattered pigmented dendritic melanocytes. H&E. X400.

mixed with a smaller population of melanin-forming dendritic cells.[76,77] Histogenesis is controversial. S-100 protein and neuron specific enolase give positive reaction in dendritic cells. It is most likely that Bodnar tumor is of both histiocytic and neural origin.[78]

Nodular (Pseudosarcomatous) Fasciitis

Nodular fasciitis occurs most commonly over the extremities and within the subcutaneous fat tissue. The overall structure of the growth, with a central solid area and fingerlike projections into the surrounding fat lobules, gives an impression of a highly invasive neoplasm.[79,80] In some areas the growth consists of dense proliferation of elongated and spindle-shaped fibroblasts and small endothelial-lined capillaries. In other areas the elongated fibroblasts are embedded in a mucinous stroma. The lesion is benign and shows no tendency for recurrence. (Fig. 42–20).[78]

Recurrent Digital Fibrous Tumor of Childhood

Mentioned here are fibrous tumors occurring on digits in children and having a strong tendency to recurrence but a relatively benign histologic picture, although they may extend from the lower epidermal surface deep into the subcutaneous tissue. These recurring digital fibrous tumors of childhood[81–82] consist of whorls of spindle cells and fibrous tissue (Fig. 42–21A) and are identified by large cytoplasmic inclusions (Fig. 42–21B), which are visible in H&E sections but are much better demonstrated by phosphotungstic acid hematoxylin. They are not viral bodies (Fig. 42–22). The spindle cells show the features of myofibroblasts on ultrastructural examination.[83,84]

LEIOMYOMA, ANGIOLEIOMYOMA, AND LEIOMYOSARCOMA

Many leiomyomas are so mature that the border between a smooth muscle nevus and a benign neoplasm is difficult to draw histologically. Most leiomyomas (Fig. 42–23) appear to be related to arrector pili muscle in localization and structure. Their frequent occurrence as multiple lesions[85] becomes more plausible if we remember (Chapter 2) that in fetal

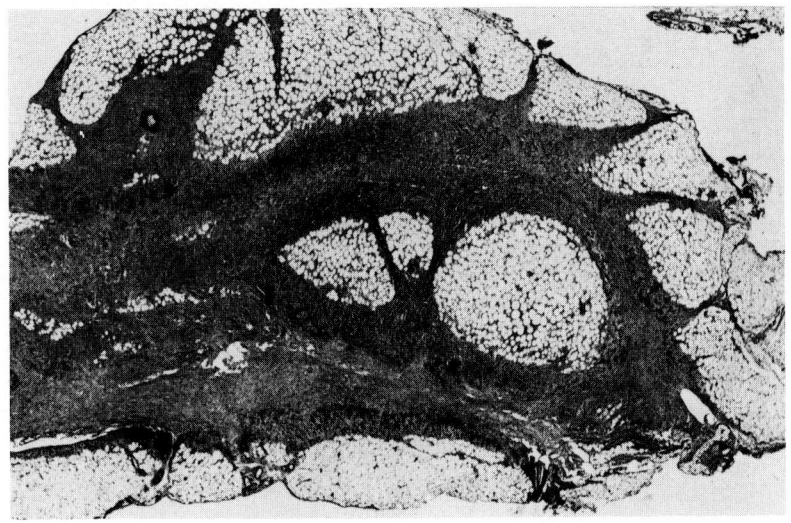

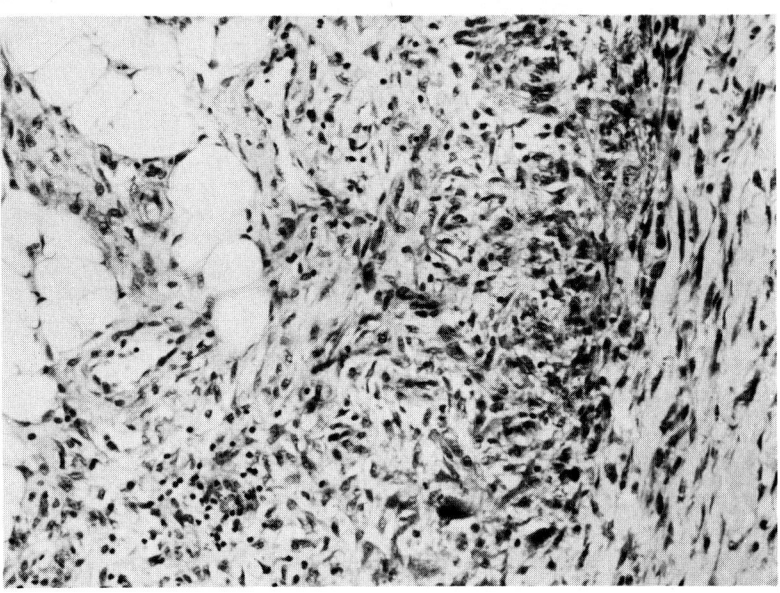

Figure 42–20.
Nodular (pseudosarcomatous) fasciitis. **A.** Subcutaneous nodule consists of densely cellular central area from which processes extend into surrounding fat tissue and suggest invasion. H&E. X14. **B.** In the periphery of the lesion, there is a zone of granulomatous proliferation consisting of newly formed capillary blood vessels, histiocytes, giant cells, and scattered round cells. H&E. X135. (From Mehregan. Arch Dermatol 93: 204, 1966.)

life hair muscles originate in a diffuse metachromatic zone of the mesoderm, in spatial relation to, but not actually as part of, the fibroepithelial hair germ. Excessive production of muscle in these predisposed fields may lead to hamartomatous lesions, which may be stable, mature muscle nevi (congenital arrector pili hamartoma) or less mature, progressively growing neoplasms.[86–88] Other much less common angioleiomyomas are related to vascular muscle.[89,90] These usually are solitary spherical lesions (Fig. 42–24) in the subcutaneous tissue of the legs, predominantly in women, and are easily diagnosed by their sharply defined border and the histologic findings of many dilated endothelial-lined vascular spaces surrounded by bundles of smooth muscles. Trichrome stain will provide sharp contrast between red muscle bundles and the surrounding bluish staining dermal collagenous tissue.

Leiomyomas of a lesser degree of maturity have to be differentiated from histiocytomas and fibromas, and this may not be easy in H&E sections. One should remember that smooth muscle cells are somewhat larger than fibroblasts, and usually form fairly long and straight bundles, which intersect rather than whorl. Formation of much collagen may be disturbing, and in trichrome stains (Van Gieson or Masson–Mallory) the collagen may actually overshadow the cellular element. On the other hand, as

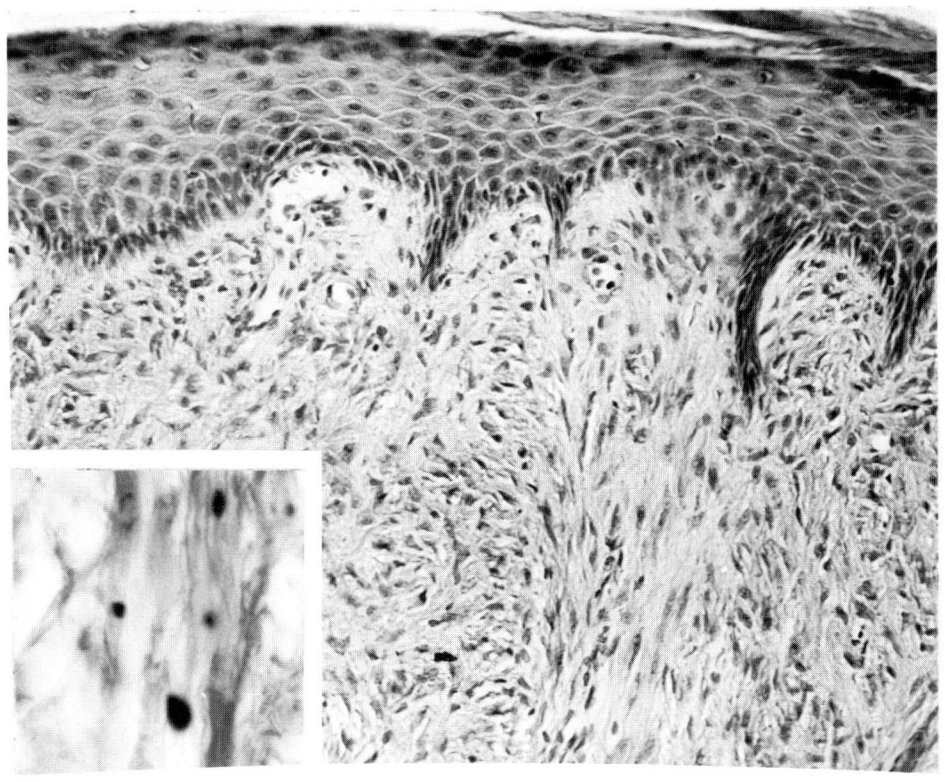

Figure 42–21.
Digital fibrous tumor of childhood. H&E. ×180. Inset shows cytoplasmic inclusions. H&E. ×800.

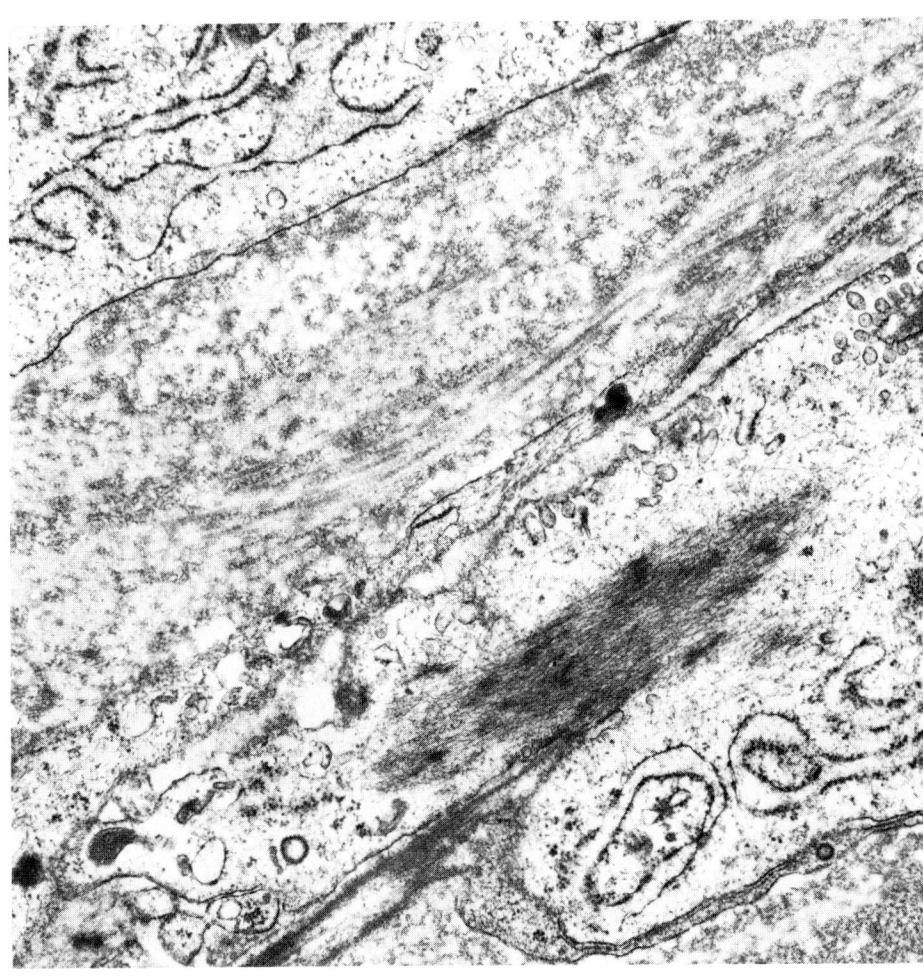

Figure 42–22.
Portion of a myofibroblast shows a bundle of myofilaments running along the cell axis. ×33,670. (Courtesy of Dr. J. Bhawan.)

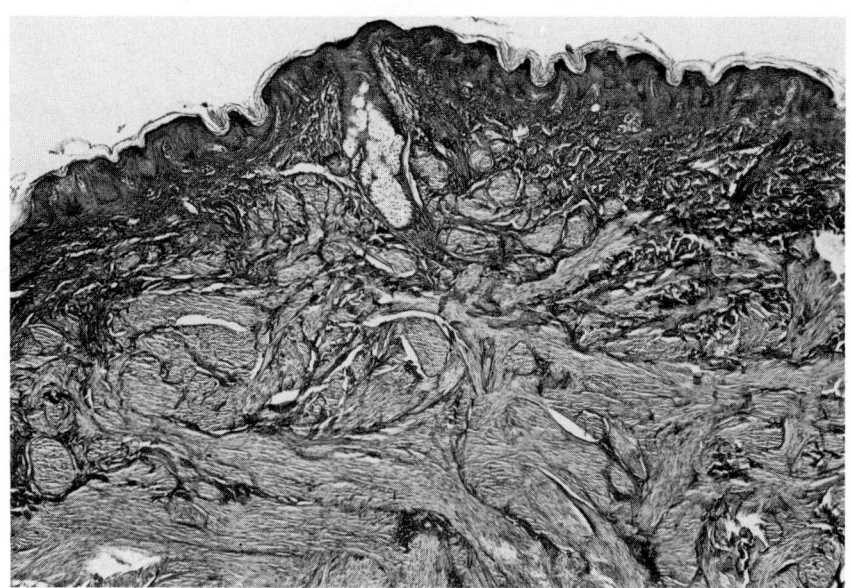

Figure 42–23.
Leiomyoma. Yellow-staining (light) masses of smooth muscle contrast with red-staining (dark) collagen bundles. Van Gieson. X45.

mentioned in Chapter 24, histiocytomas and fibromas contain only disjointed remnants of old elastic fibers, while leiomyomas frequently have newly formed elastic fibers running parallel to the cell bundles.

Leiomyosarcomas involving dermis and the subcutaneous fat tissue are rare.[91-95] The growth consists of massive proliferation of pleomorphic spindle-shaped cells with hyperchromatic nuclei arranged into irregular fascicles and infiltrating the spaces between the collagen bundles (Fig. 42–25). Occasional multinucleated giant cells are present and mitotic figures may exceed one or two per high power field.[95] Immunostaining will be positive for vimentin and desmin. Ninety percent also will express muscle-specific actin.[93]

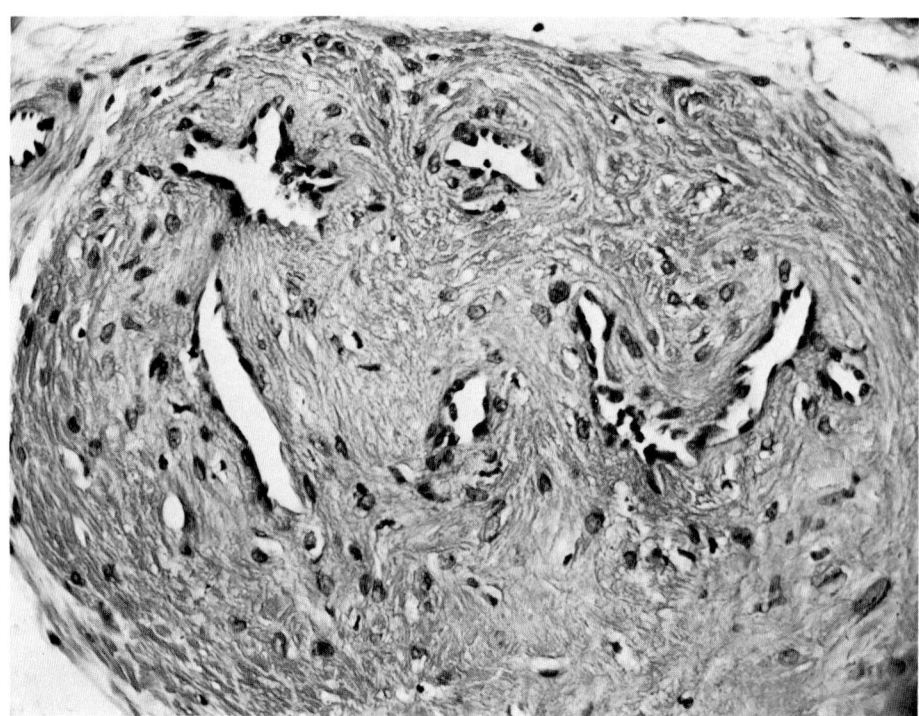

Figure 42–24.
Angioleiomyoma. Vascular channels embedded in a nodule of smooth muscle cells and strongly metachromatic ground substance. H&E. X135.

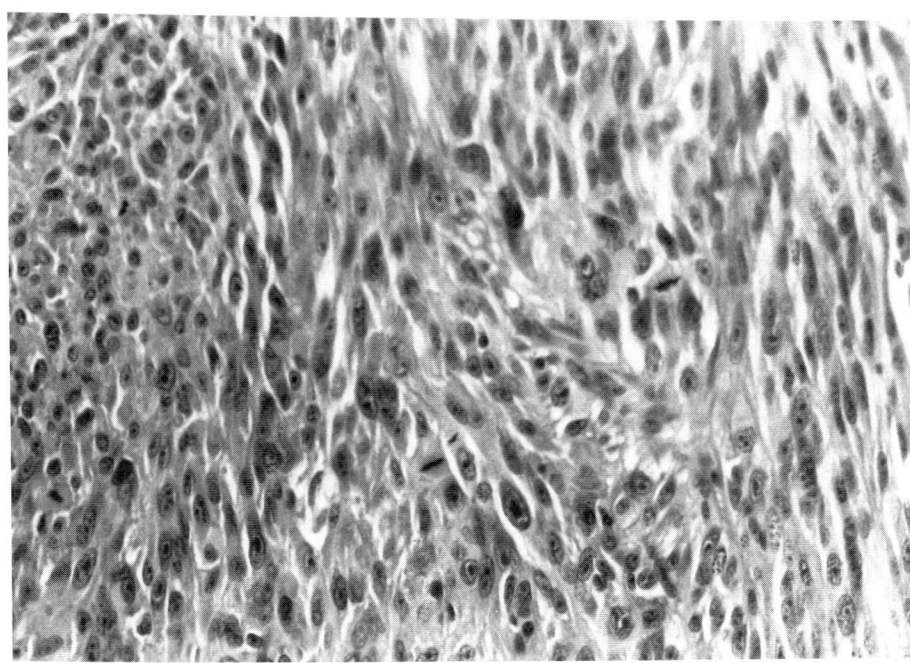

Figure 42–25.
Leiomyosarcoma. Tumor bundles show large cells with irregularly shaped nuclei and mitotic figures. H&E. X400.

Rhabdomyosarcoma occurring in the skin is extremely rare.[96,97] Dermis and the subcutaneous fat tissue show nests and cords of small round to spindle-shaped cells with hyperchromatic nuclei and scanty eosinophilic cytoplasms. The tumor cells are PAS positive due to the presence of intracytoplasmic glycogen granules. Cross striations are not observed. Immunostaining for desmin and antimyoglobin is positive.[96]

LIPOMA, ANGIOLIPOMA, AND LIPOSARCOMA

It is much more common to find normally constituted fat tissue in abnormal location or in abnormal amount than to find histologic aberrations truly classifiable as benign or malignant neoplasms.

Fat tissue develops in the embryo from small vascular foci (primitive fat organs), which by continuous accumulation of specific perivascular cells and their conversion into fat cells form individual fat lobules. *Subcutaneous lipomas* may be solitary, multiple familial, or multiple with symmetric distribution.[98–100] They may vary in size and are not well demarcated. They consist of lobulated masses of mature fat cells separated by thin septae of collagen bundles. *Angiolipomas*, on the other hand, are usually well-defined and are often painful.[101] They consist of proliferation of fat and vascular tissues in different proportions (Fig. 42–26).

Spindle cell lipomas occur over the posterior neck and shoulder of male adults.[102] The growth is often well defined and consists of lobules of mature fat cells and uniform spindle cells and some birefringent collagen fibers (Fig. 42–27). The proportion of lipocytes and spindle cells varies in different portions of the same lesion with the spindle cells dominating in some areas.[103] *Pleomorphic lipoma*, which occurs principally in older men over the neck and shoulder areas, shows in contrast with the uniform histologic pattern of lipomas an admixture of variably sized lipocytes, spindle cells, and bizarre and pleomorphic multinucleated giant cells associated with interlacing bundles of dense birefringent collagen.[104,105] The appearance may suggest liposarcoma. *Liposarcomas* are very rare in dermatologic material. Well-differentiated liposarcomas show normal appearing fat cells interspersed among large anaplastic cells with hyperchromatic nuclei. Less-differentiated lesions may resemble fibrosarcoma, myxosarcoma, or myxomatous neurofibromas.

NEVUS LIPOMATOSUS SUPERFICIALIS AND FOCAL DERMAL HYPOPLASIA

Fat tissue, beyond the small amounts normally present around the deeper parts of hair follicles and

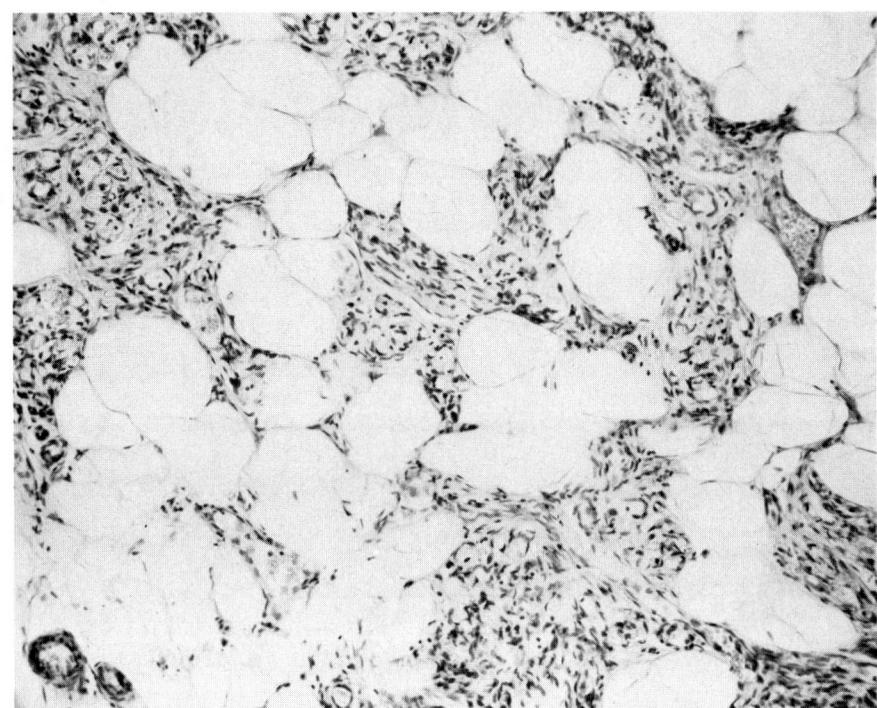

Figure 42–26.
Angiolipoma. Small portion of tumor is shown to demonstrate vascular tissue between normal-appearing fat cells. H&E. X135.

sweat coils, is encountered within the skin in two conditions. The *nevus lipomatosus superficialis* of Hoffman and Zurhelle (Fig. 42–28) usually occurs as grouped yellowish nodular lesions situated over the normal skin around the hip region, mainly of adolescent girls.[106] Histologically, it is characterized by the development of lobules of fat tissue around the capillary blood vessels within the pars reticularis of the dermis.[107,108] There may be associated increased dermal elastic fibers. The other lesion is *focal dermal hypoplasia* (Goltz syndrome), which is present at birth and has atrophic skin lesions and other as-

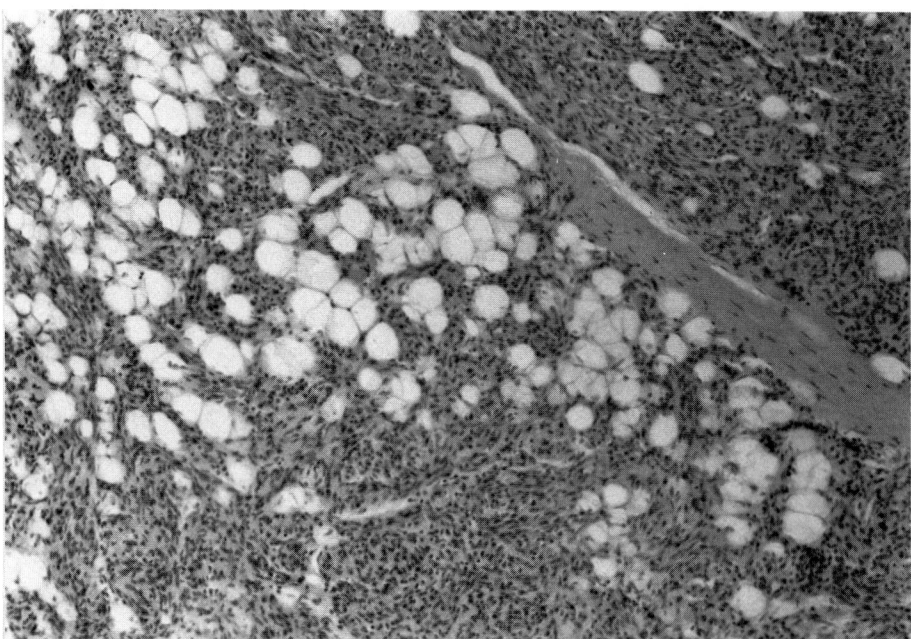

Figure 42–27.
Spindle cell lipoma shows a mixture of lipocytes and spindle-shaped cells in varying proportions. H&E. X125.

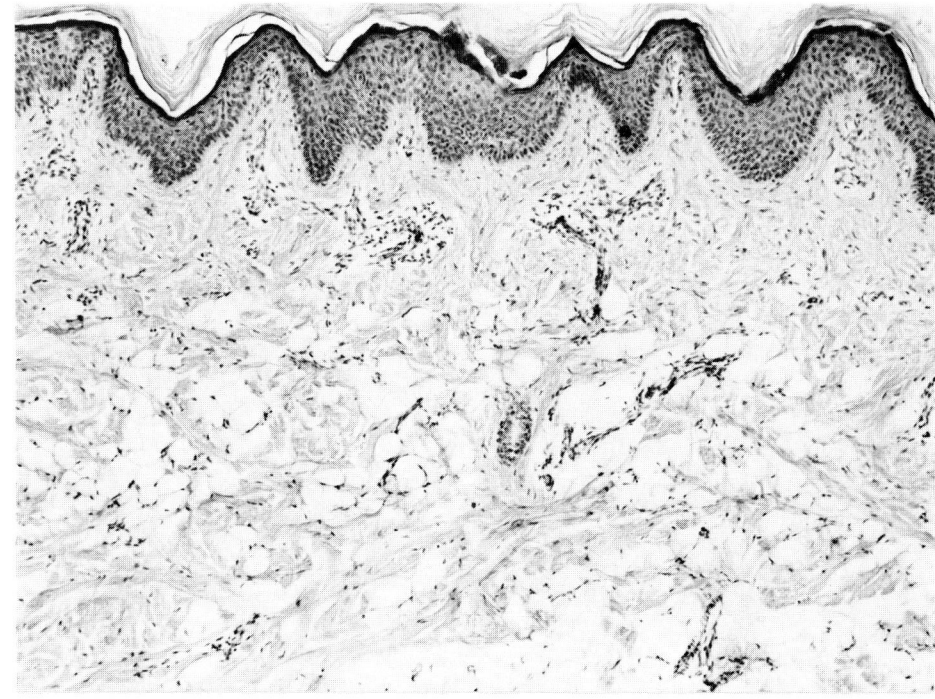

Figure 42–28.
Nevus lipomatosus superficialis. Fat cells of the nevus infiltrate and partly replace the reticular dermis. They remain below the superficial vascular plexus and also are not part of the subcutaneous tissue. H&E. X45. (From Mehregan, Tavafoghi, and Gandtchi. J. Cutan Pathol 2:307, 1975.)

sociated abnormalities (Fig. 42–29).[109] In the early multiform or striate atrophic skin areas the epidermis is thin. The papillary dermis appears edematous and shows some increased vascularity and loss of superficial elastic fibers.[110] The later-appearing striate or papillomatous lesions show multiple lobulated masses of ectopic fat tissue formed within the papillary and reticular dermis evolving into the full picture of Howell's *nevus angiolipomatosus* (Fig. 42–30).[111]

Hibernoma

Yet another rare, and not really cutaneous, nevoid neoplasm has the structure of brown fat tissue, a type of vascular tissue with multivacuolar fat cells,

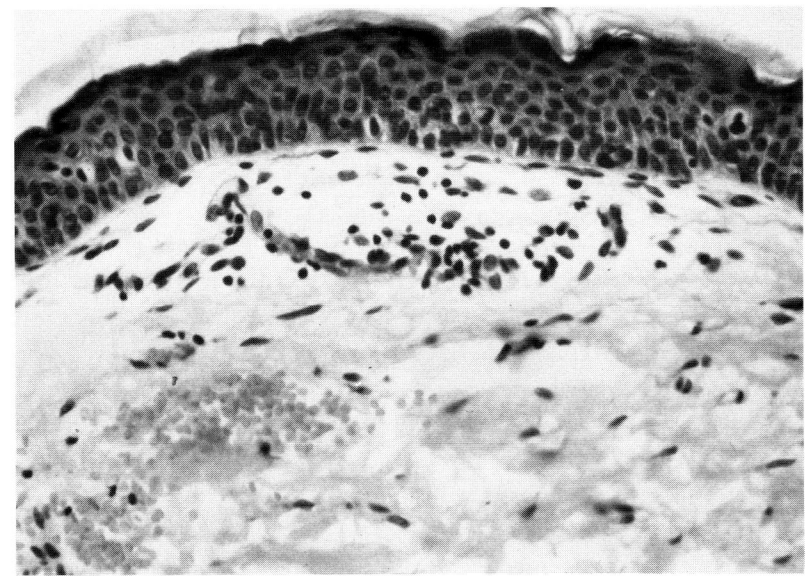

Figure 42–29.
Focal dermal hypoplasia. An early atrophic lesion. H&E. X225.

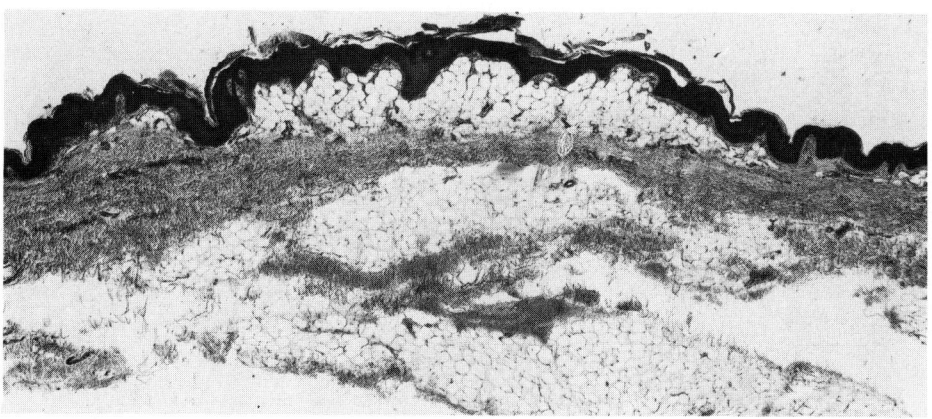

Figure 42–30.
Nevus angiolipomatosus. Nevoid fat tissue occupies pars papillaris of dermis and is separated from subcutaneous fat tissue by pars reticularis, which is being encroached on rather than being hypoplastic. H&E. X21.

which occurs mainly between the shoulder blades and probably is related to heat regulation in babies.[75] Because this tissue is prominently found in hibernating mammals, the tumor was given the name hibernoma.[112] There is, however, the possibility[113] that this rare lesion truly represents neoplasia of fat tissue with retarded maturation.

REFERENCES

1. Majno G, Sabbiani G, Hirschel BJ, et al: Contraction of granulation tissue in vitro: similarity to smooth muscle. Science 173:548, 1971
2. Linares HA, Kirscher CW, Dobrkonsky M, et al: The histiocytic organization of the hypertrophic scar in humans. J Invest Dermatol 59:323, 1972
3. Moriguchi T, Fujimoto D: Crosslink of collagen in hypertrophic scar. J Invest Dermatol 72:143, 1979
4. Abergel PR, Pizzurro D, Meeker CA, et al: Biochemical composition of the connective tissue in keloids and analysis of collagen metabolism in keloid fibroblast cultures. J Invest Dermatol 84:384, 1985
5. Hegedus SI, Schorr WF: Familial cutaneous collagenoma. Cutis 10:283, 1972
6. Schimpf A, Roth W, Kopper J: Dermatofibrosis lenticularis disseminata mit Osteopoikilie (Buschke–Ollendorff Syndrom). Dermatologica 141:409, 1970
7. Schorr WF, Optiz JM, Rayes CN: The connective tissue nevus-osteopoikilosis syndrome. Arch Dermatol 106:208, 1972
8. Smith LR, Bernstein BD: Eruptive collagenoma. Arch Dermatol 114:1710, 1978
9. Sasai Y, Saito N, Seiji M: Epidermolysis bullosa dystrophica et albopapuloidea; report of a case and histochemical study. Arch Dermatol 108:554, 1973
10. Mehregan AH, Staricco RG: Elastic fibers in pigmented nevi. J Invest Dermatol 38:271, 1962
11. Rapini RP, Golitz LE: Sclerotic fibromas of the skin. J Am Acad Dermatol 20:266, 1989
12. Rosen LB, Suster S: Fibrous papules. A light microscopic and immunohistochemical study. Am J Dermatopathol 10:109, 1988
13. Spiegel J, Nadji M, Penneys NS: Fibrous papule. An immunohistochemical study with an antibody to S-100 protein. J Am Acad Dermatol 9:360, 1983
14. Cerio R, Rao BK, Wilson Jones E: An immunohistochemical study of fibrous papule of the nose: 25 cases. J Cutan Pathol 16:194, 1989
15. Magid M, Garden JM: Pearly penile papules: Treatment with the carbon dioxide laser. J Dermatol Surg Oncol 15:552, 1989
16. Ingordo V, Michelini M, Anonide A: Hirsuties papillaris penis: Incidenza nella popolazione giovanile italiana. Chron Dermatol 19:195, 1988
17. Kohda H, Hino Y, Fukuda H: Hirsutoid papillomas of vulvae. J Dermatol Tokyo 13:154, 1986
18. Grob JJ, Collet-Villette AM, Andrac L, Bonerandi JJ: Papillomatose hirsutoide de la vulve. Ann Dermatol Venereol 114:1235, 1987
19. Zackheim HS, Pinkus H: Perifollicular fibromas. Arch Dermatol 82:913, 1960
20. Pinkus H, Coskey RJ, Burgess GA: Trichodiscoma; a benign tumor related to haarscheibe (hair disk). J Invest Dermatol 63:212, 1974
21. Pinkus H: Perifollicular fibromas: Pure periadnexal adventitial tumors. Am J Dermatopathol 1:341, 1979
22. Birt AS, Hogg GR, Dubé WJ: Hereditary multiple fibrofolliculomas with trichodiscomas and acrochordons. Arch Dermatol 113:1674, 1977
23. Weintraub R, Pinkus H: Multiple fibrofolliculomas (Birt-Hogg-Dubé) associated with a large connective tissue nevus. J Cutan Pathol 4:289, 1977
24. Kint A, Baran R, De Keyser H: Acquired (digital) fibrokeratoma. J Am Acad Dermatol 12:816, 1985
25. Cooper PH, Mackel SE: Acquired fibrokeratoma of the heel. Arch Dermatol 121:386, 1985
26. Kint A, Baran R: Histopathologic study of Koenen tumors. Are they different from acquired digital fibrokeratoma? J Am Acad Dermatol 18:369, 1988
27. Coskey RJ, Mehregan AH, Lupulescu AP: Multiple vascular fibromas and myxoid fibromas of the fingers.

A histologic and ultrastructural study. J Am Acad Dermatol 2:425, 1980
28. Ortonne JP: L'association myxomes cardiaques-lesions cutanees pigmentees: Nouveau syndrome cardio-cutane? Ann Dermatol Venereol 113:1279, 1986
29. Carney AJ, Headington JT, Su DWP: Cutaneous myxomas. A major component of the complex of myxomas, spotty pigmentation, and endocrine overactivity. Arch Dermatol 122:790, 1986
30. Vidaillet HJ Jr, Seward JB, Fyke EF III, et al: "Syndrome myxoma": A subset of patients with cardiac myxoma associated with pigmented skin lesions and peripheral and endocrine neoplasms. Br Heart J 57:247, 1987
31. Ushijima M, Hashimoto H, Tsuneyoshi M, Enjoji M: Giant cell tumor of the tendon sheath (Nodular tenosynovitis). A study of 207 cases to compare the large joint group with the common digit group. Cancer 57:875, 1986
32. Sapra S, Prokopetz R, Murray AH: Giant cell tumor of tendon sheath. Int J Dermatol 28:587, 1989
33. Kan AE, Rogers M: Juvenile hyaline fibromatosis: An expanded clinicopathologic spectrum. Pediatr Dermatol 6:68, 1989
34. Mayer-de-Silva A, Poiares-Baptista A, Rodrigo FG, Teresa-Lopes M: Juvenile hyaline fibromatosis. A histologic and histochemical study. Arch Pathol Lab Med 112:928, 1988
35. Quintal D, Jackson R: Juvenile hyaline fibromatosis. A 15-year follow-up Arch Dermatol 121:1062, 1985
36. Camarasa JG, Moreno A: Juvenile hyaline fibromatosis. J Am Acad Dermatol 16:881, 1987
37. Mehregan AH: Superficial fibrous tumors in childhood. J Cutan Pathol 8:321, 1981
38. Dehner LP, Askin EB: Tumors of fibrous tissue origin in childhood. A clinicopathologic study of cutaneous and soft tissue neoplasms in 66 children. Cancer 38:888, 1976
39. Aberer E, Mainitz M, Entacher U, Gebhart W: Fibrous hamartoma of infancy—Infantile subcutaneous myofibroblastoma. Dermatologica 176:46, 1988
40. Paller AS, Gonzalez-Crussi F, Sherman JO: Fibrous hamartoma of infancy. Eight additional cases and a review of the literature. Arch Dermatol 125:88, 1989
41. Chou P, Gonzalez-Crussi F, Mangkornkanok M: Giant cell fibroblastoma. Cancer 63:756, 1989
42. Rosen LB, Amazon K, Weitzner J, Resnick L: Giant cell fibroblastoma. A report of a case and review of the literature. Am J Dermatopathol 11:242, 1989
43. Shmookler BM, Enzinger FM, Weiss SW: Giant cell fibroblastoma. A juvenile form of dermatofibrosarcoma protuberans. Cancer 64:2154, 1989
44. Barr RJ, Young EM, Liao S-Y: Giant cell fibroblastoma: An immunohistochemical study. J Cutan Pathol 13:301, 1986
45. Weinrauch L, Katz M, Pizov G: Primary benign chondroblastoma cutis: Extraskeletal manifestation without bone involvement. Arch Dermatol 123:24, 1987
46. Goette DK, Deffer TA: Postirradiation malignant fibrous histiocytoma. Arch Dermatol 121:535, 1985
47. Laskin WB, Silverman TA, Enzinger FM: Postradiation soft tissue sarcomas. An analysis of 53 cases. Cancer 62:2330, 1988
48. Scott SM, Reiman HM, Pritchard DJ, Ilstrup DM: Soft tissue fibrosarcoma. A clinicopathologic study of 132 cases. Cancer 64:925, 1989
49. Nash AD: Soft Tissue Sarcomas. Histologic Diagnosis. New York: Raven Press, 1989
50. Mandard AM, Petiot JF, Ma MJ, et al: Prognostic factors in soft tissue sarcomas. A multivariate analysis of 109 cases. Cancer 63:1437, 1989
51. Coindre J-M, Bui NB, Bonichon F, et al: Histopathologic grading in spindle cell soft tissue sarcomas. Cancer 61:2305, 1988
52. Ueda T, Aozasa K, Tsujimoto M, et al: Prognostic significance of mast cells in soft tissue sarcoma. Cancer 62:2416, 1988
53. Ninane J, Gosseye S, Panteon E, et al: Congenital fibrosarcoma. Preoperative chemotherapy and conservative surgery. Cancer 58:1400, 1986
54. Carlos Manivel J, Wick MR, Dehner LP, Sibley RK: Epithelioid sarcoma. An immunohistochemical study. Am J Clin Pathol 87:319, 1987
55. Padilla RS, Flynn K, Headington JT: Epithelioid sarcoma. Enzymatic histochemical and electron microscopic evidence of histiocytic differentiation. Arch Dermatol 121:389, 1985
56. Chase DR, Enzinger FM: Epithelioid sarcoma. Diagnosis, prognostic indicators, and treatment. Am J Surg Pathol 9:241, 1985
57. Daimaru Y, Hashimoto H, Tsuneyoshi M, Enjoji M: Epithelial profile of epithelioid sarcoma. An immunohistochemical analysis of eight cases. Cancer 59:134, 1987
58. Wick MR, Manivel JC: Epithelioid sarcoma and isolated necrobiotic granuloma: A comparative immunocytochemical study. J Cutan Pathol 13:253, 1986
59. Kay S: Angiomatoid malignant fibrous histiocytoma. Report of two cases with ultrastructural observations of one case. Arch Pathol Lab Med 109:934, 1985
60. Rooser B, Willen H, Gustafson P, et al: Malignant fibrous histiocytoma of soft tissue. A population-based epidemiologic and prognostic study of 137 patients. Cancer 67:499, 1991
61. Costa C, Schmied E, Saurat J-H: Deux cas d'histiocytome fibreux malin du cuir chevelu. Dermatologica 177:44, 1988
62. Rydholm A, Syk I: Malignant fibrous histiocytoma of soft tissue. Correlation between clinical variables and histologic malignancy grade. Cancer 57:2323, 1986
63. Miettinen M, Soini Y: Malignant fibrous histiocytoma. Heterogeneous patterns of intermediate filament proteins by immunohistochemistry. Arch Pathol Lab Med 113:1363, 1989
64. Fretzin DF, Helwig EB: Atypical fibroxanthoma of skin; clinicopathologic study of 140 cases. Cancer 31:1541, 1973
65. Winkelmann RK, Peters MS: Atypical fibroxanthoma.

A study with antibody to S-100 Protein. Arch Dermatol 121:753, 1985
66. Kuwano H, Hashimoto H, Enjoji M: Atypical fibroxanthoma distinguishable from spindle cell carcinoma in sarcoma-like skin lesions. A clinicopathologic and immunohistochemical study of 21 cases. Cancer 55:172, 1985
67. Enzinger FM, Weiss SW: Soft Tissue Tumors. St. Louis: Mosby, 1983
68. Kuwano H, Hashimoto H, Enjoji M: Atypical fibroxanthoma distinguishable from spindle cell carcinoma in sarcoma-like skin lesions. A clinicopathologic and immunohistochemical study of 21 cases. Cancer 55:172, 1985
69. Glavin FL, Cornwell ML: Atypical fibroxanthoma of the skin metastatic to a lung. Report of a case, features by conventional and electron microscopy, and a review of relevant literature. Am J Dermatopathol 7:57, 1985
70. Helwig EB, May D: Atypical fibroxanthoma of the skin with metastasis. Cancer 57:368, 1986
71. Ding J, Hashimoto H, Enjoji M: Dermatofibrosarcoma protuberans with fibrosarcomatous areas. Clinicopathologic study of nine cases and a comparison with allied tumors. Cancer 64:721, 1989
72. Rockley PF, Robinson JK, Magid M, Goldblatt D: Dermatofibrosarcoma protuberans of the scalp: A series of cases. J Am Acad Dermatol 21:278, 1989
73. Barr RJ, Young EM, King DF: Non-polarizable collagen in dermatofibrosarcoma protuberans: A useful diagnostic aid. J Cutan Pathol 13:339, 1986
74. Lautier R, Wolff HH, Jones RE: An immunohistochemical study of dermatofibrosarcoma protuberans supports its fibroblastic character and contradicts neuroectodermal or histiocytic components. Am J Dermatopathol 12:25, 1990
75. Shindo Y, Akiyama J, Takase Y: Tissue culture study of dermatofibrosarcoma protuberans. J Dermatol Tokyo 15:220, 1988
76. Nakamura T, Ogata H, Katsuyama T: Pigmented dermatofibrosarcoma protuberans. Report of two cases as a variant of dermatofibrosarcoma protuberans with partial neural differentiation. Am J Dermatopathol 9:18, 1987
77. Puig L, De Moragas JM, Matias-Guiu X, Moreno A: Dermatofibrosarcoma protuberans pigmentado (tumor de Bednar). Med Cutan ILA 16:314, 1988
78. Dupree WB, Langloss JM, Weiss SW: Pigmented dermatofibrosarcoma protuberans (Bednar tumor). A pathologic, ultrastructural, and immunohistochemical study. Am J Surg Pathol 9:630, 1985
79. Mehregan AH: Nodular fasciitis. Arch Dermatol 93:204, 1966
80. Bernstein KE, Lattes R: Nodular (pseudosarcomatous) fasciitis. A non-recurrent lesion: Clinicopathologic study of 134 cases. Cancer 49:1668, 1982
81. Iwasaki H, Kikuchi M, Mori R, et al: Infantile digital fibromatosis. Cancer 46:2238, 1980
82. Chung EB, Enzinger FM: Infantile myofibromatosis. Cancer 48:1807, 1981
83. Miyamoto T, Mihara M, Hagari Y, et al: Posttraumatic occurrence of infantile digital fibromatosis. A histologic and electron microscopic study. Arch Dermatol 122:915, 1986
84. Yun K: Infantile digital fibromatosis. Immunohistochemical and ultrastructural observations of cytoplasmic inclusions. Cancer 61:500, 1988
85. Ford GP: Multiple piloleiomyomata. Br J Dermatol 117 (Suppl 32):110, 1987
86. Slifman NR, Harrist TJ, Rhodes AR: Congenital arrector pili hamartoma. A case report and review of the spectrum of Becker's melanosis and pilar smooth muscle hamartoma. Arch Dermal 121:1034, 1985
87. Berberian BJ, Burnett JW: Congenital smooth muscle hamartoma: A case report. Br J Dermatol 115:711, 1986
88. Johnson MD, Jacobs AH: Congenital smooth muscle hamartoma. A report of six cases and a review of the literature. Arch Dermatol 125:820, 1989
89. MacDonald DM, Sanderson KV: Angioleiomyoma of the skin. Br J Dermatol 91:161, 1974
90. Bardach H, Ebner H: Das Angioleiomyom der Haut. Hautarzt 26:638, 1974
91. Jegasothy BV, Gilgor RS, Hull M: Leiomyosarcoma of the skin and subcutaneous tissue. Arch Dermatol 117:478, 1981
92. Flotte TJ, Bell DA, Sidhu GS, Plair CM: Leiomyosarcoma of the Dartos muscle. J Cutan Pathol 8:69, 1981
93. Swanson PE, Stanley MW, Scheithauer BW, Wick MR: Primary cutaneous leiomyosarcoma. A histological and immunohistochemical study of 9 cases, with ultrastructural correlation. J Cutan Pathol 15:129, 1988
94. Moon TD, Sarma DP, Rodriquez FH Jr: Leiomyosarcoma of the scrotum. J Am Acad Dermatol 20:290, 1989
95. Davidson LL, Frost ML, Hanke WC, Epinette WW: Primary leiomyosarcoma of the skin. Case report and review of the literature. J Am Acad Dermatol 21:1156, 1989
96. Perrin C, Lacour J-P, Thyss A, et al: Rhabdomyosarcome sous-cutane de l'enfant. Aspects cliniques, immunologiques et ulstrastructureaux. Ann Dermatol Venereol 115:919, 1988
97. Wiss K, Solomon AR, Reimer SS, et al: Rhabdomyosarcoma presenting as a cutaneous nodule. Arch Dermatol 124:1687, 1988
98. Leffel DJ, Braverman IM: Familial multiple lipomatosis. Report of a case and a review of the literature. J Am Acad Dermatol 15:275, 1986
99. Abensour M, Jeandel C, Heid E: Lipomes et lipomatoses cutanes. Ann Dermatol Venereol 114:873, 1987
100. Ruzicka T, Vieluf D, Landthaler M, Braun-Falco O: Benign symmetric lipomatosis Launois-Bensaude. Report of ten cases and review of the literature. J Am Acad Dermatol 17:663, 1987

101. Howard WR, Helwig EB: Angiolipoma. Arch Dermatol 82:924, 1960
102. Warkel RL, Rehme CG, Thompson WH: Vascular spindle cell lipoma. J Cutan Pathol 9:113, 1982
103. Enzinger FM, Weiss SW: Soft Tissue Tumors. St. Louis: Mosby, 1982, p 313.
104. Shmookler BM, Enzinger FM: Pleomorphic lipoma: A benign tumor simulating liposarcoma. A clinicopathologic analysis of 48 cases. Cancer 47:126, 1981
105. Nigro MA, Chieregato GC, Della Rover GQ: Pleomorphic lipoma of the dermis. Br J Dermatol 116:713, 1987
106. Mehregan AH, Tavafoghi V, Ghandchi A: Nevus lipomatosus cutaneus superficialis (Hoffman-Zurhelle). J Cutan Pathol 2:307, 1975
107. Hann SK, Yang DS, Lee SH: Giant nevus lipomatosus superficialis associated with cavernous hemangioma. J Dermatol Tokyo 15:543, 1988
108. Chanoki M, Sugamoto I, Suzuki S, Hamada T: Nevus lipomatosus cutaneus superficialis of the scalp. Cutis 43:143, 1989
109. Mann M, Weintraub R, Hashimoto K: Focal dermal hypoplasia with an initial inflammatory phase. Pediatr Dermatol 7:278, 1990
110. Howell JB, Freeman RG: Cutaneous defects of focal dermal hypoplasia: an ectomesodermal dysplasia syndrome. J Cutan Pathol 16:237, 1989
111. Howell JB: Nevus angiolipomatosus vs focal dermal hypoplasia. Arch Dermatol 92:238, 1965
112. Bonarandi JJ, Privat Y: Hibernoma. Bull Soc Fr Dermatol Syphiligr 80:72, 1973
113. Angervall L, Nilsson L, Stener B: Microangiographic and histological studies in two cases of hibernoma. Cancer 17:685, 1964

43
VASCULAR NEVI AND TUMORS

Mesodermal neoplasms related to blood and lymph vessels are listed in Table 43–1. A broad practical classification of vascular lesions for clinical purposes might separate lesions that are present at birth or that appear early in childhood from lesions arising later in life. Histologic classification for diagnostic and prognostic purposes might best be based on whether we are dealing with an excess of fully formed vessels, usually blood vessels, or with an excess of vessel-associated cells with or without the formation of vessels. Lesions of the first type are easily recognized and are, with few exceptions, benign. Lesions of the second type may be benign but usually carry implications of malignancy. Their histologic identification may be difficult. "Nevus anemicus," a term that implies local deficiency of blood vessels, is most likely due to hypersensitivity of blood vessels to catecholamines within the localized area.[1]

LESIONS CONSISTING OF VESSELS

Hemangiomas

Objective examination under the microscope without clinical data does not always permit us to say whether an excess of blood vessels in a section is either reactive or nevoid and stable or proliferative in the sense of a benign hemangioma. Hemangiomas[2] generally are subdivided into *capillary* and *cavernous* types. Capillary hemangiomas (Fig. 43–1) are usually an elevated superficial lesion consisting of proliferation of small endothelial lined blood vessels, some containing erythrocytes.[3] Cavernous hemangiomas are deep seated and show larger vascular spaces with thin or thick fibrous walls. Lesions with combined features of capillary and cavernous hemangiomas also occur. *Senile angiomas* are small and show several dilated endothelial lined blood vessels in upper dermis (Fig. 43–2). Venous lake is a bluish lesion often located over the head and neck or lower lip and is characterized by a cystic dilated and thin-walled blood vessel engorged with erythrocytes.

Varicous dilated blood vessels may become occluded by an organized thrombus and give the impression of a nodular hemangioma. Strangulated acrochordon is another lesion that may resemble a traumatized capillary hemangioma. Bartonellosis (verruga peruana) may have so much vascular proliferation that a hemangioma is simulated. The organisms are found in the endothelial cells.[4]

Telangiectasias

A number of vascular lesions are neither congenital (nevoid) and stable nor truly neoplastic. They are

TABLE 43–1. VASCULAR NEVI AND TUMORS

Vascular nevi
  Telangiectatic
  Cavernous

Proliferation of vessels
  Arterial hemangiomas (spiders)
  Acquired hemangiomas, venous lakes, and cirsoid aneurysms
  Angiokeratomas
  Lymphangioma circumscriptum
  Angiosarcoma

Proliferation of cellular elements related to vessels
  Hemangioendothelioma
  Hemangiopericytoma
  Acquired (tufted) angioma
  Granuloma pyogenicum
  Intravascular papillary endothelial hyperplasia
  Aneurysmal (angiomatoid) fibrous histiocytoma
  Epithelioid hemangioma and angiolymphoid hyperplasia with eosinophilia
  Glomangioma
  Malignant angioendothelioma and Stewart–Treves syndrome
  Kaposi sarcoma

---

usually classified as telangiectasias, although vessels larger than capillaries may be affected and some vascular proliferation may be involved. *Nevus flammeus* manifested as a patch of redness is a good example of this type. Another condition is *essential telangiectasia* (Fig. 43–3), appearing as spidery red spots in patchy or unilateral distribution during the adult life.[5] Another is *angioma serpiginosum* that must be separated from pigmented purpuric eruptions (Chapter 13).[6] Similar telangiectasias are found in the CRST syndrome (systemic sclerosis), in thyroid disease,[7] and in Osler's *familial hemorrhagic telangiectasia*. Von Lohuizen's cutis marmorata telangiectatica[8] is another example of widespread livedo-like involvement of the skin in which telangiectatic capillaries and anomalies of larger vessels[9] are combined. Somewhat different are arterial spiders,[10] less appropriately called nevus araneus or spider nevus. They possess a central arteriole with a muscular wall that widens into a subepidermal ampulla and splits up into radiating thin-walled vessels. Yet another eruption bearing the name telangiectasia is related to urticaria pigmentosa (Chapter 45): *telangiectasia macularis eruptiva perstans* presents a combination of more numerous and dilated small vessels in the upper dermis with mild round cell infiltrate and some increase of mast cells. Diagnosis requires staining with toluidine blue or Giemsa solution.

Cirsoid Aneurysm

A peculiar lesion, most commonly encountered as a skin-colored papule on the face or extremities and not usually diagnosed clinically, consists of coiled thick-walled vessels cut in histologic sections in multiple locations and embedded in fibrous stroma. The walls lack normal muscle and elastic fibers and consist mainly of fibrocytes, collagen, and ground substance (Fig. 43–4). Biberstein and Jessner,[11] who first described this lesion, pointed out that these not uncommon lesions are probably not true hemangio-

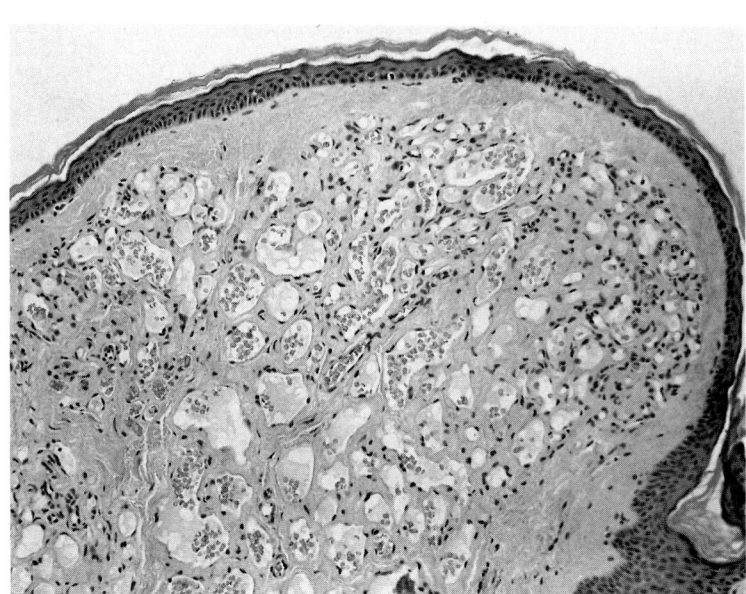

Figure 43–1.
Capillary hemangioma. Nodular vascular growth made up of endothelial-lined capillary blood vessels. H&E. X125.

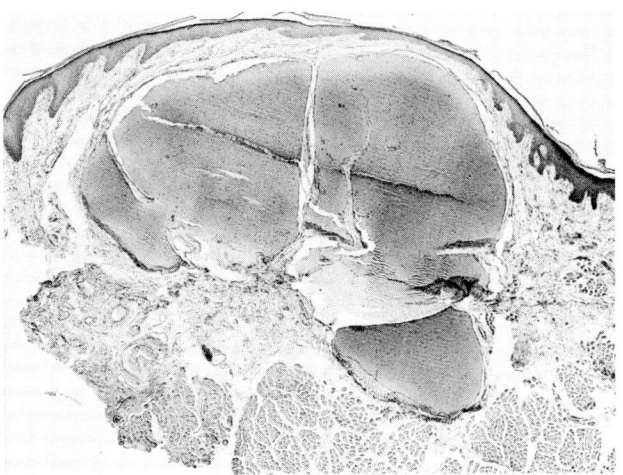

Figure 43–2.
Venous lake (varix) of lip. This is almost a physiologic phenomenon. In many elderly people, the vein near the lateral border of the lower lip between epidermis and skeletal muscle enlarges. It may become thrombosed or cause discomfort due solely to its size, as in the case illustrated. H&E. X45.

mas but cirsoid aneurysms, due to coiling of an abnormal vessel. They have been redescribed as arteriovenous shunts[12,13] or acral arteriovenous tumors.[14] The preferred name is *arteriovenous hemangioma*.

Angiokeratoma

Angiokeratoma is the name given to a superficial hemangioma in which many dilated, endothelial-lined capillaries are present in upper dermis engorged with erythrocytes.[15–17] The overlying epidermis shows reactive hyperplasia, hyperkeratosis, and often intrakeratinous foci of hemorrhages. The lesion is elevated, well-defined, and deep bluish-purple in color. The Mibelli and Fordyce (scrotal or vulvar) types are defined clinically rather than histologically (Fig. 43–5).[18] A localized, nevoid form may be present at birth (*angiokeratoma neviforme*).[17] The Fabry type[19–21] has now been recognized as the expression of metabolic aberration. There is inherited deficiency of alpha-galactosidase leading to the deposition of ceramid trihexosidase. Electron microscopic examination shows dense, laminated inclusions in lysosomes.[19] Under the light microscope, demonstration of lipid droplets in smooth muscle is the diagnostic feature, and these must be looked for in larger vessels and arrector pili muscles. Very similar cutaneous manifestations may be found in *fucosidosis*, an autosomal recessive deficiency of the lysosomal enzyme alpha-L-fucosidase causing accumulation of fucose.[22,23]

Lymphangioma

Lymphangioma, usually encountered in the form of lymphangioma circumscriptum,[24] expresses itself in

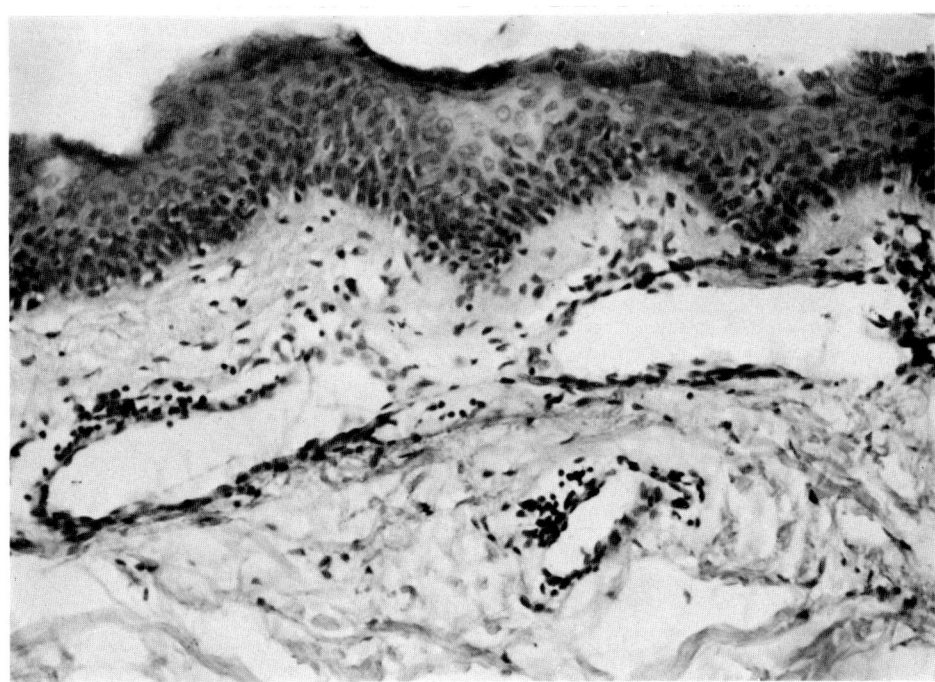

Figure 43–3.
Essential telangiectasia. H&E. X225.

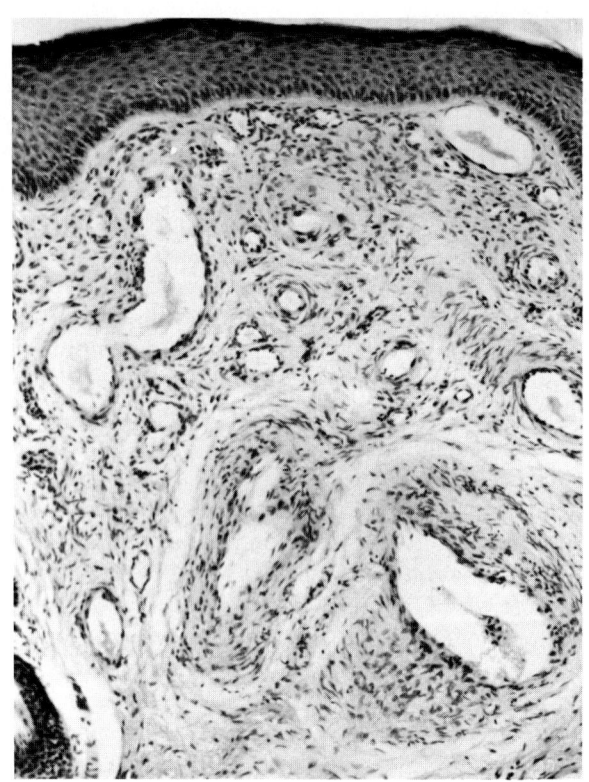

Figure 43–4.
Cirsoid aneurysm, also called arteriovenous hemangioma. Thick-walled coiled-up blood vessels form a papule in facial skin. H&E. X125.

a routine biopsy specimen as multiple endothelium-lined spaces that may be so closely applied to the lower surface of the epidermis as to simulate intraepidermal vesicles (Fig. 43–6). Dilated lymph spaces appear empty or may contain a few lymphocytes or erythrocytes.[25] It is, however, essential to realize that the small superficial angiectasias are in communication with large subcutaneous cisterns consisting of muscle-coated lymphatic vessels and that these must be excised in order to effect cure.[26,27] *Benign lymphangioendothelioma* appears as solitary macular and erythematous plaque over the extremities or trunk. Histologically, delicate, thin-walled endothelial lined clefts and spaces are found in between dermal collagen bundles.[28]

LESIONS DUE TO PROLIFERATION OF VESSEL-ASSOCIATED CELLS

Of the lesions mentioned so far, all consist of well-formed, almost normal vessels in excess. Although the endothelial cells of hemangiomas may be more prominent than those of normal vessels, they are not atypical, and they are not more numerous than needed to line the vascular lumen. If their number exceeds that requirement and if, therefore, they project in papilliferous form into the lumen or form vascular buds and incompletely canalized struc-

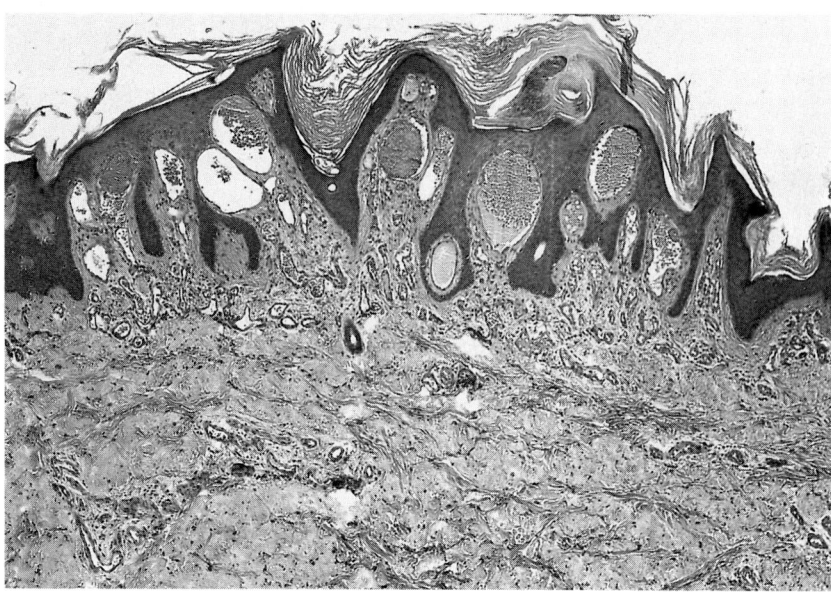

Figure 43–5.
Angiokeratoma. A solitary lesion of lower leg. H&E. X90.

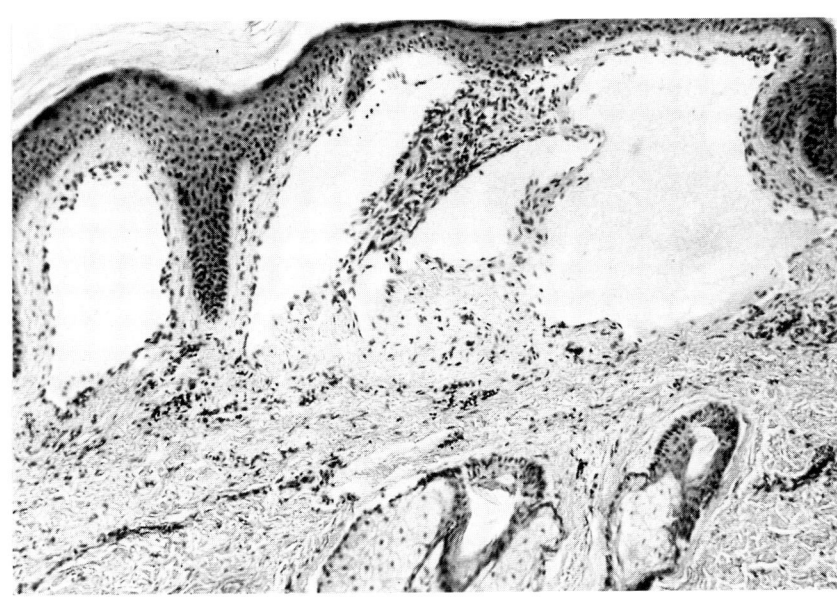

Figure 43–6.
Lymphangioma circumscriptum. H&E. X125.

tures, we are dealing with a tumor consisting of vessel-associated cells, and the differential diagnosis requires much more analysis.

Hemangiopericytoma

Vascular tumors appearing predominantly in childhood and characterized by massive proliferation of endothelial-lined blood spaces surrounded by proliferating rows of elongated pericytes are classified as hemangiopericytomas.[29] Benign and malignant forms may occur. A benign variety occurring soon after birth (Fig. 43–7) is now classified as *cellular angioma of infancy*.[30]

Acquired "Tufted" Angioma (Angioblastoma) (Nakagawa)

Single or multiple patches of angiomatous lesions occur over the upper trunk, neck, or scalp of young

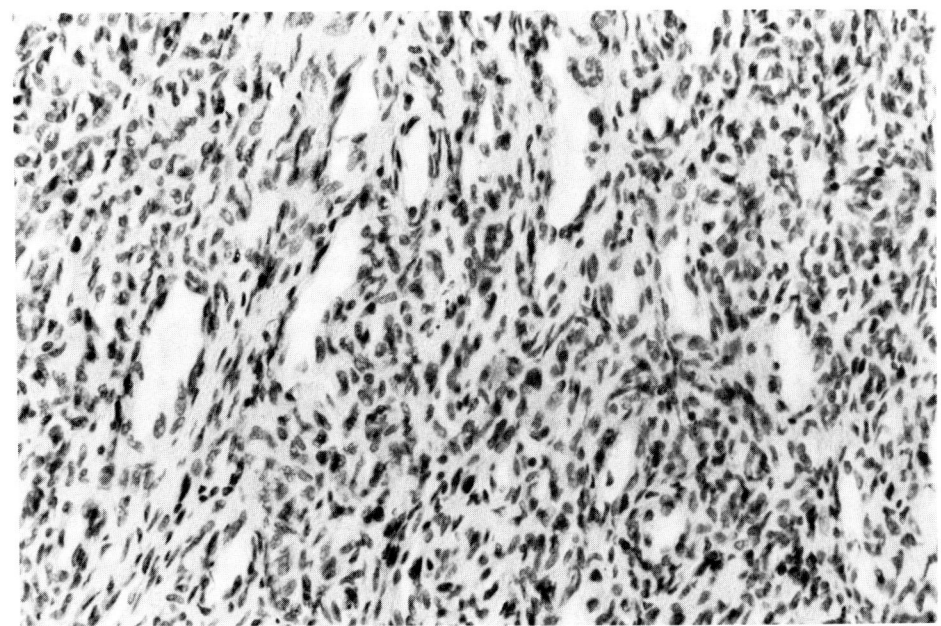

Figure 43–7.
Cellular angioma of infancy. H&E. X125.

individuals. Half of the lesions appear within the first 5 years of life (Fig. 43–8). Histologically, numerous small and circumscribed tufts and lobules of angiomatous tissue are scattered within the dermis. Lobules are composed of small endothelial-lined vessels and solid areas.[31-33] The ultrastructural and immunocytochemical studies suggest that cellular proliferation consists of immature endothelial and perithelial cells with the latter type predominating.[34]

Malignant Proliferating Angioendotheliomatosis

A rare disease characterized by widespread appearance of reddish-brown to blue color lesions is malignant proliferating angioendotheliomatosis (Fig. 43–9). Histologic sections show many dilated dermal blood vessels occluded by colonies of large mononuclear cells showing mitotic figures. Fatal outcome results from extravascular multisystem involvements. Immunohistochemical stains have confirmed these cells as atypical lymphoid tissue.[35-37] The disease is most likely an unusual "angiotropic" manifestation of lymphoma rather than a truly vascular neoplasia.[38]

Granuloma Pyogenicum

Another lesion mimicking a neoplasm but probably exemplifying an inflammatory reactive proliferation is granuloma pyogenicum. It is composed of lobes of incompletely formed vessels (Fig. 43–10) with considerable excess of endothelial and interstitial cells embedded in an edematous stroma. Occasional mitotic figures may be present in a developing lesion. Older lesions may show fibrosis. Characteristically, the lesion is sessile and is fed by a large arterial

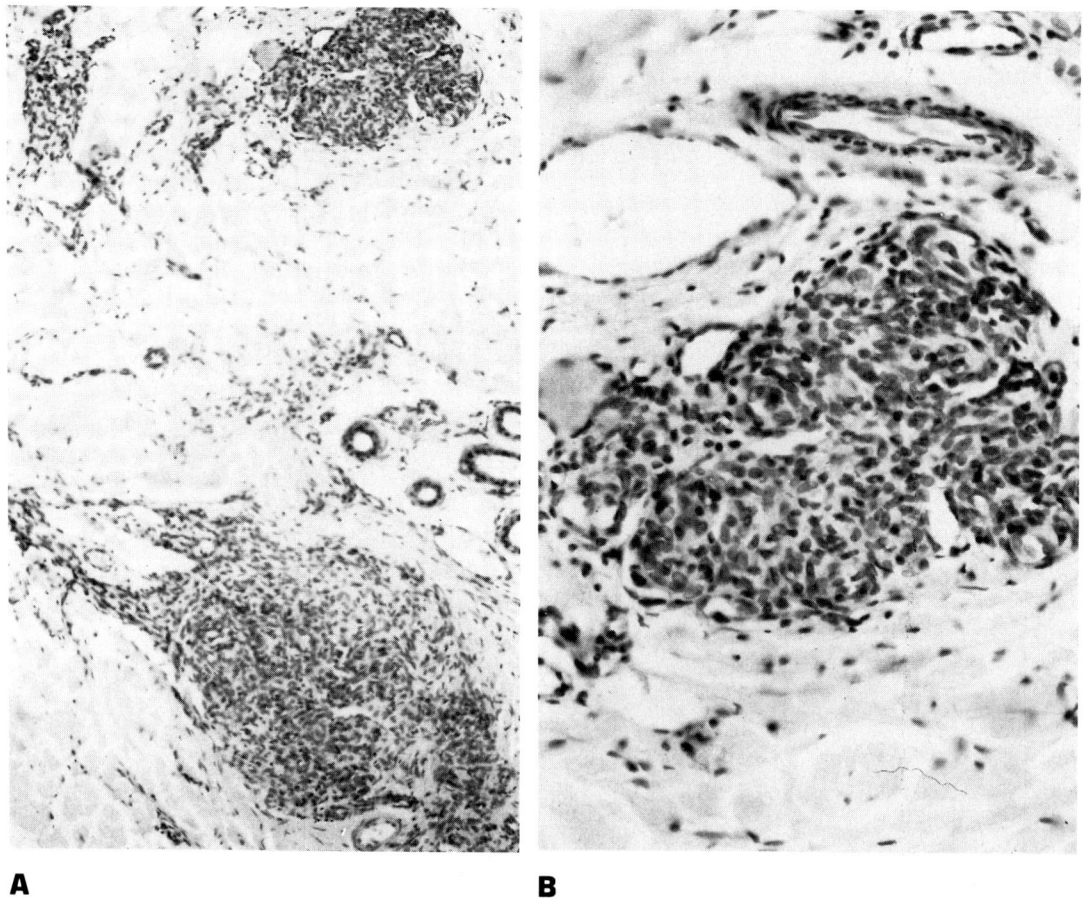

A **B**

Figure 43–8.
*Acquired (tufted) angioma. **A.** Vascular hyperplasia is lobulated. H&E. X125. **B.** Each lobule is made up of proliferation of endothelial cells and pericytes. H&E. X400.*

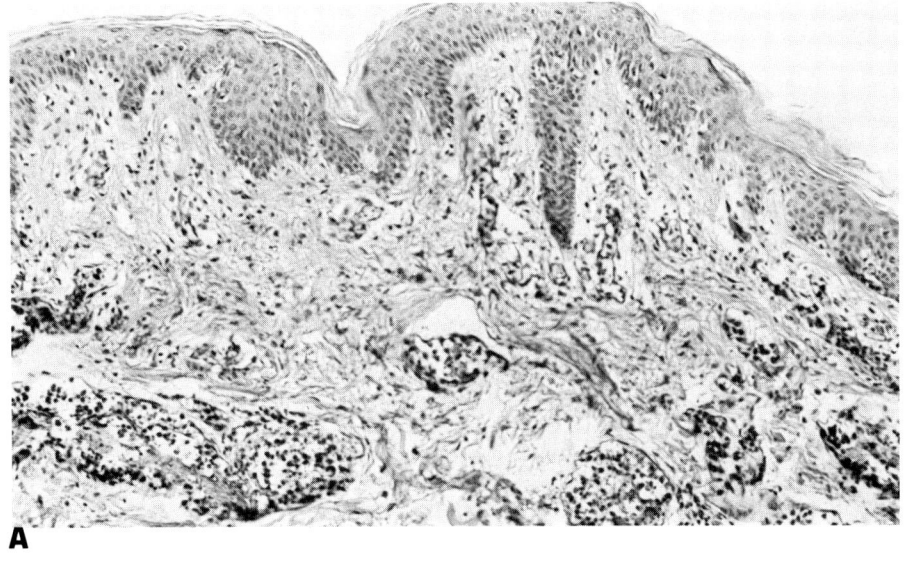
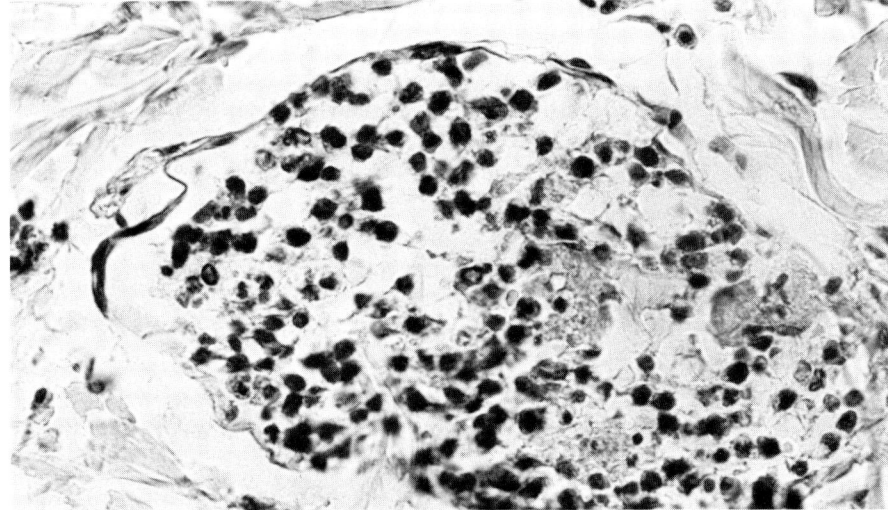

Figure 43–9.
Malignant systematized angioendotheliomatosis. Dermal blood vessels are occluded with small round cells, most likely a lymphomatous process rather than a vascular neoplasia. H&E. **A.** X125. **B.** X400.

vessel entering its base. Therefore, it will recur if this vessel is not excised or destroyed by cauterization. The surface of a granuloma pyogenicum is usually covered by a purulent crust, but that is not essential and is a complication due to mechanical trauma or secondary infection. Protection and mildly antibacterial treatment will cause reepithelization, and many lesions are always covered by thin, smooth epithelium (granuloma telangiectaticum). A frightening but, in fact, harmless experience is the formation of multiple satellites after surgical removal of a granuloma pyogenicum,[39] especially when these secondary lesions develop deep in the skin and thus are histologically indistinguishable from hemangioendothelioma. Cutaneous vascular lesions resembling granuloma pyogenicum have also been reported in Crow–Fukase syndrome.[40]

Bacillary (Epithelioid) Angiomatosis

Multiple cutaneous or mucosal vascular lesions occur in individuals with acquired immunodeficiency syndrome. Up to 1 cm bright red nodular lesions erupt within a few weeks and may disappear spontaneously.[41–43] Histologically, numerous small vascular spaces are lined with plump and cuboidal andothelial cells and are embedded within an edematous stroma and inflammatory cell infiltrate closely resembling granuloma pyogenicum.[44]

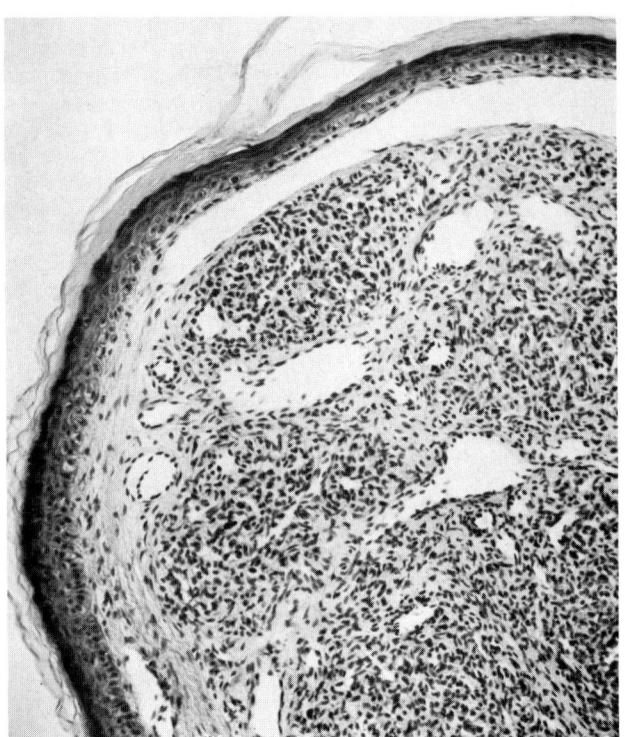

Figure 43–10.
Granuloma pyogenicum. Portion of a well-epithelized sessile lesion is shown. H&E. X135.

Intravascular Papillary Endothelial Hyperplasia (IPEH)

The difficulty of differentiating benign proliferations of vessel-associated cells from neoplasia is exemplified in the lesion first described by Masson in 1923[45,46] as vegetating intravascular hemangioendothelioma (Fig. 43–11). Histologically, there are endothelial-lined papillary projections extending from the wall into vascular lumen. One must remember that in the organization of an intravascular thrombus, there is considerable temporary proliferation of endothelia, perithelia, and other cells. It is generally held now that these processes, if they become excessive, and especially if they take place in preexisting hemangiomas, may mimic "angiosarcoma," another term that has been applied to various malignant forms of vascular proliferation (see Kaposi's sarcoma). It is important in making the diagnosis of IPEH to ascertain the intravascular location of the tumor and to find fibrin, which offers the basis for the florid papillary endothelial proliferation.

Aneurysmal (Angiomatoid) Fibrous Histiocytoma

We elected to discuss this lesion here because of its primary vascular involvement. It occurs as a blue to black nodule in the skin or subcutaneous tissue (Fig. 43–12). Histologically, an aneurysmal vascular space is largely occupied with massive proliferation of histiocytes containing hemosiderin, foam cells, and spindle-shaped fibroblasts.[47] The presence of newly formed blood vessels, extravasated erythrocytes, and the spindle cell stroma may lead to erroneous diagnosis of Kaposi's sarcoma.[48]

EPITHELIOID "HISTIOCYTOID" HEMANGIOMAS ANGIOLYMPHOID HYPERPLASIA WITH EOSINOPHILIA

Angiolymphoid hyperplasia with eosinophilia, atypical granuloma pyogenicum, and some other related vascular lesions occurring over the head, neck, and extremities have been classified under a general term of "epithelioid (histiocytoid) hemangiomas."[49,50]

Angiolymphoid hyperplasia with eosinophilia (Fig. 43–13) occurs most commonly on the face, ears, and scalp in the form of multiple purplish nodules aggregated over an area of dermal infiltration.[51–53] Histologically, thin- and thick-walled dilated vascular spaces are lined with endothelial cells having large and prominent nuclei protruding into the vascular lumina and with eosinophilic and often vacuolated cytoplasm (Fig. 43–14). Thin cords of endothelial cells and incompletely formed blood vessels are present. Cellular atypia and mitotic figures are not observed. The vascular structures are surrounded by an infiltrate of lymphocytes, eosinophils, and scattered mast cells. Lymph follicles are formed within deep dermis or the subcutaneous fat tissue.[54,55]

Recent publications indicate differences between angiolymphoid hyperplasia with eosinophilia and Kimura's disease.[56–59] Kimura's disease occurs in young individuals and shows predilection for involvement of preauricular region in the form of an ill-defined infiltrated plaque without surface angiomatous component. Histologically, many thin-walled blood vessels, lymph follicles, and eosinophils involve deep dermis, the subcutaneous tissues including the salivary glands, lymph nodes, and striated muscles. Histiocytoid or epithelioid endothelial cells are not present.[59]

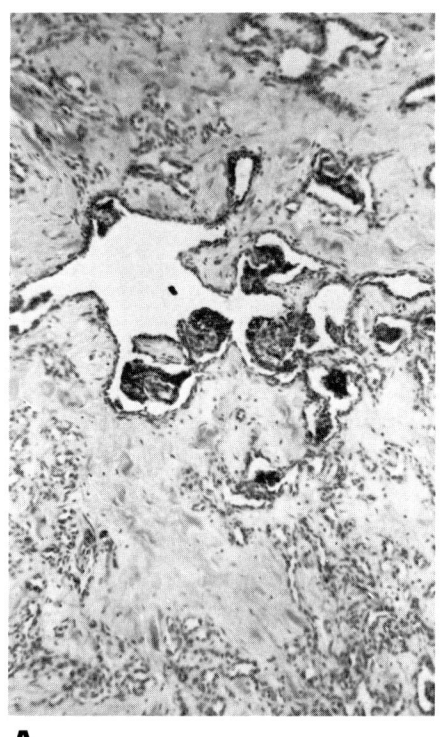 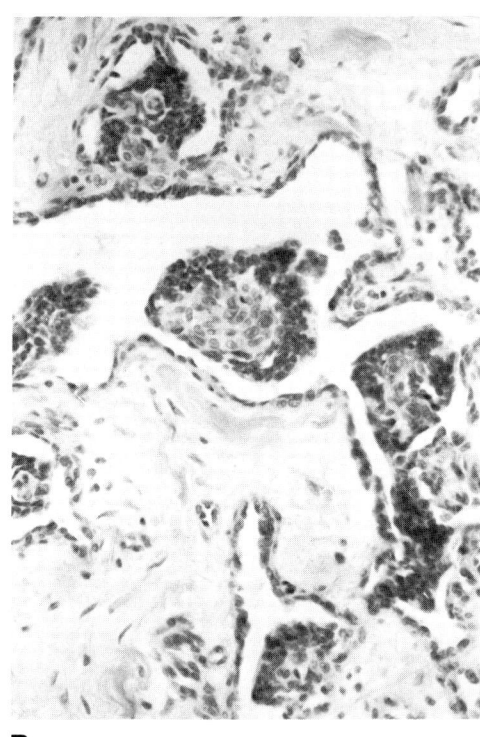

Figure 43–11.
Intravascular papillary endothelial hyperplasia. Endothelial-lined papillary projections into dilated vascular spaces. **A.** H&E. X125. **B.** H&E. X250.

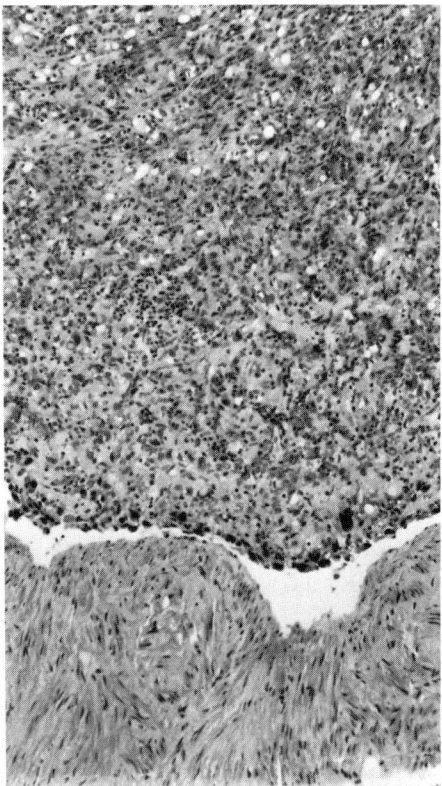 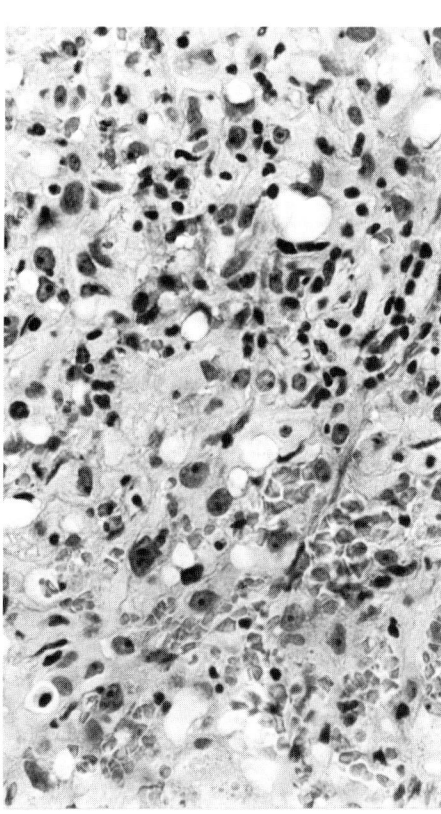

Figure 43–12.
Aneurysmal (angiomatoid) fibrous histiocytoma. **A.** Shows a solid growth within an aneurysmal thick-walled blood vessel. H&E. X125. **B.** The growth is made up of proliferation of histiocytes, foam cells, and scattered lymphocytes. H&E. X600.

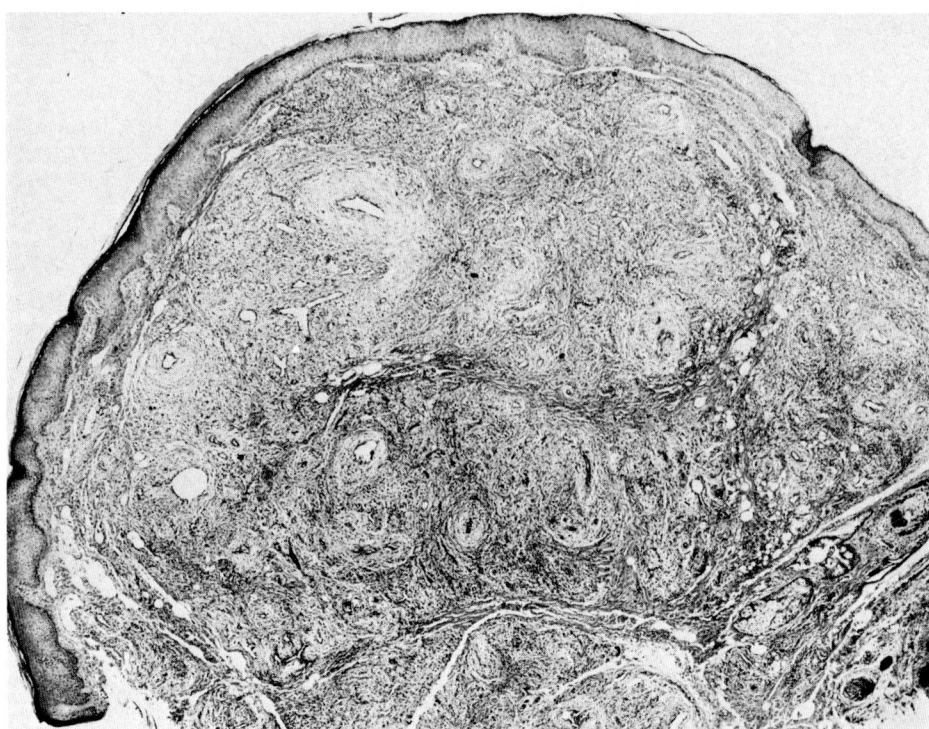

Figure 43–13.
Angiolymphoid hyperplasia with eosinophilia. Nodular lesion consists of unusual blood vessels accompanied by cellular infiltrate rich in lymphocytes and interspersed with eosinophils (see Fig. 43–14). H&E. X14. (From Mehregan and Shapiro. Arch Dermatol 103: 50, 1971.)

Atypical granuloma pyogenicum[60] as well as solitary lesions of epithelioid (histiocytoid) hemangiomas occur in any location and show intradermal proliferation of vascular spaces lined with epithelioid endothelial cells.[61]

Blue Rubber Bleb Nevus

Bean described multiple lesions under this picturesque name. Their relationship to glomangioma was discussed because they also have multiple perivascular layers of epithelioid cells.[62] It seems assured now, however, that blue rubber bleb nevus is clinically and histologically a separate entity. It is clinically associated with systemic cavernous hemangiomas, and fatalities have been reported. Under the electron microscope, the peripheral cells resemble smooth muscle cells.[63,64]

Glomangioma

The neuromyoarterial glomus of Masson gives rise to a tumor called glomangioma or glomus tumor.[65] It may consist of a variable combination of vascular, muscular, and neural components. The most common and most characteristic element is the glomus cell (Fig. 43–15),[66,67] a cuboidal cell with round nucleus and light-staining cytoplasm, which may form solid epithelium-like masses or may be associated with vascular spaces. In the latter case, glomus cells lie outside a lining of flat endothelial cells. While most glomangiomas are single and occur in general on the acral parts of the extremities, a fair number of cases with multiple lesions have been described.[68–70] Locally infiltrating or true glomangiosarcomas are rare.[71]

Malignant Angioendothelioma (Angiosarcoma)

These truly malignant lesions of vascular endothelium are clinically manifested as ill-defined inflammatory plaques or ulcerated nodular lesions located over the scalp or face of elderly individuals.[72–75] Similar lesions may occur following mastectomy, Stewart–Treves syndrome (Fig. 43–16),[76–78] radiation therapy,[79–80] or in chronic leg ulcer.[81] In the skin, one finds numerous dilated vascular spaces lined with large endothelial cells with prominent and hyperchromatic nuclei (Fig. 43–17). Massive en-

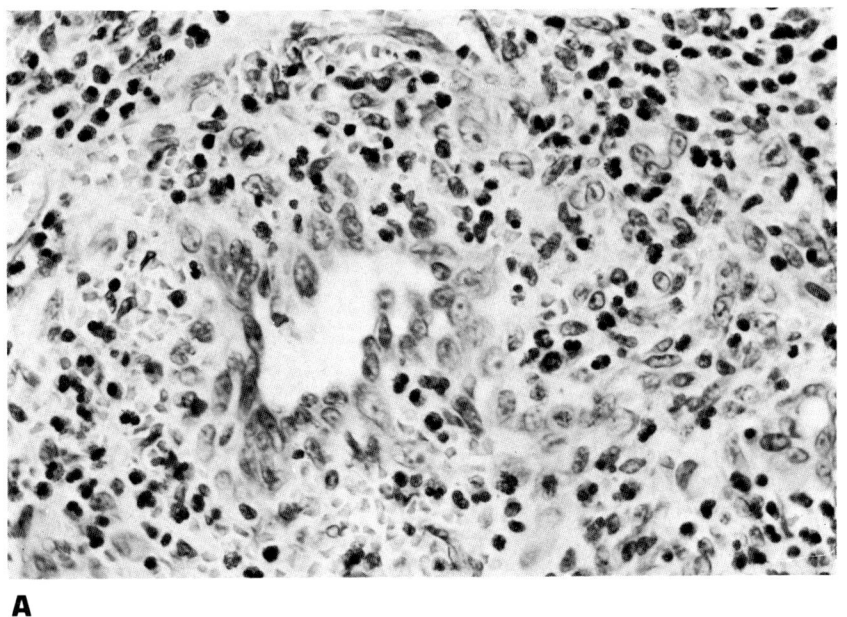

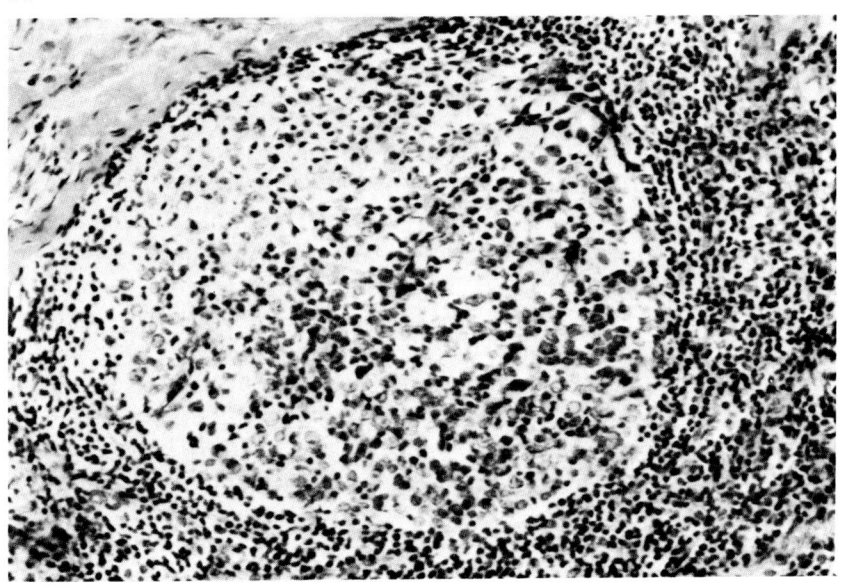

Figure 43–14.
Angiolymphoid hyperplasia with eosinophils. **A.** Small blood vessel surrounded by lymphocytes and fixed-tissue-type cells. Polymorph nuclei belong to eosinophils. H&E. X250. **B.** Lymphoid follicle in deeper portion of lesion. H&E. X250. (From Mehregan and Shapiro. Arch Dermatol 103:50, 1971.)

dothelial cell proliferation may occur in deep dermis, but especially prominent are atypical endothelial cells coating collagen bundles in the reticular dermis (Fig. 43–18).

Kaposi's Sarcoma

To the classic chronic and slowly progressive form of Kaposi's sarcoma that occurs in genetically predisposed individuals in geographic clusters, such as in Africa, Eastern Europe, and North America,[82] a new and more aggressive type has been added in recent years, in immunologically altered individuals affected with AID syndrome, in hemophiliacs receiving factor VIII transfusions, in drug abusers, and in a minority of Haitians. Rapid spread of this form in an epidemic fashion to other sectors of the population suggests an infectious etiology.[83–86]

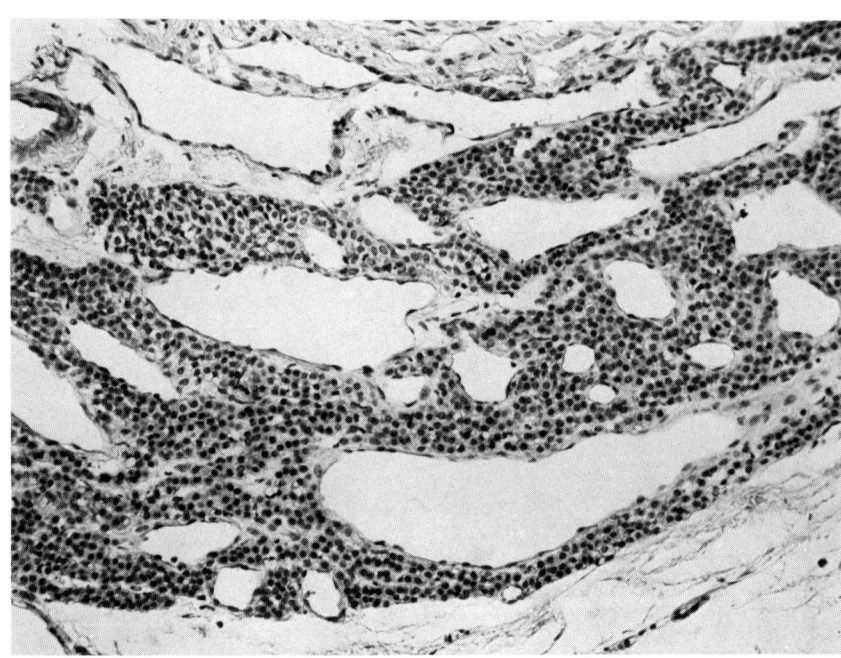

Figure 43–15.
Glomangioma. Cuboidal glomus cells fill spaces between endothelium-lined capillaries. H&E. X180.

Histologically, an early macular or patch stage will show within the upper dermis numerous irregularly shaped vascular spaces lined by endothelial cells having prominent nuclei surrounded by varying degrees of spindle cell proliferation. Scattered lymphocytes and plasma cells may be present.[87] Mitotic figures are not prominent. At this stage immunostaining with polyclonal antibody to type IV collagen will provide a positive reaction (Fig. 43–19).[88] Nodular lesions show massive proliferation of round and spindle-shaped cells forming incomplete blood vessels and slit-like vascular spaces containing erythrocytes. Red cells leaking from the vascular spaces are engulfed by histiocytes with formation of hemosiderin (Fig. 43–20). Scattered mitotic figures and a variable degree of fibrosis are noted. The fusiform cells may prevail over the other cell components and eventually pure spindle cell sarcoma may be observed. Spindle cells are vimentin positive and display laminin and factor VIII RAG reactivity suggesting endothelial derivation.[89] Atypical dermal vessels have also been reported to be present within uninvolved skin areas.[90] The most prominent ultrastructural findings are erythrophagocytosis by the neoplastic spindle cells and endothelial cells and proliferation of primitive vessels.[91] Tubuloreticular structures reported in AIDS-associated form are not observed in the classic variety.[92]

In an early plaque stage, Kaposi's sarcoma may require differential diagnosis from the purplish-pigmented and often hypertrophic plaques of lower legs related to chronic vascular stasis or arteriovenous fistulas.[93] In this condition a plate of newly formed capillary blood vessels is found immediately beneath the epidermis within an edematous and often fibrotic stroma which may also contain a number of macrophages with hemosiderin granules.

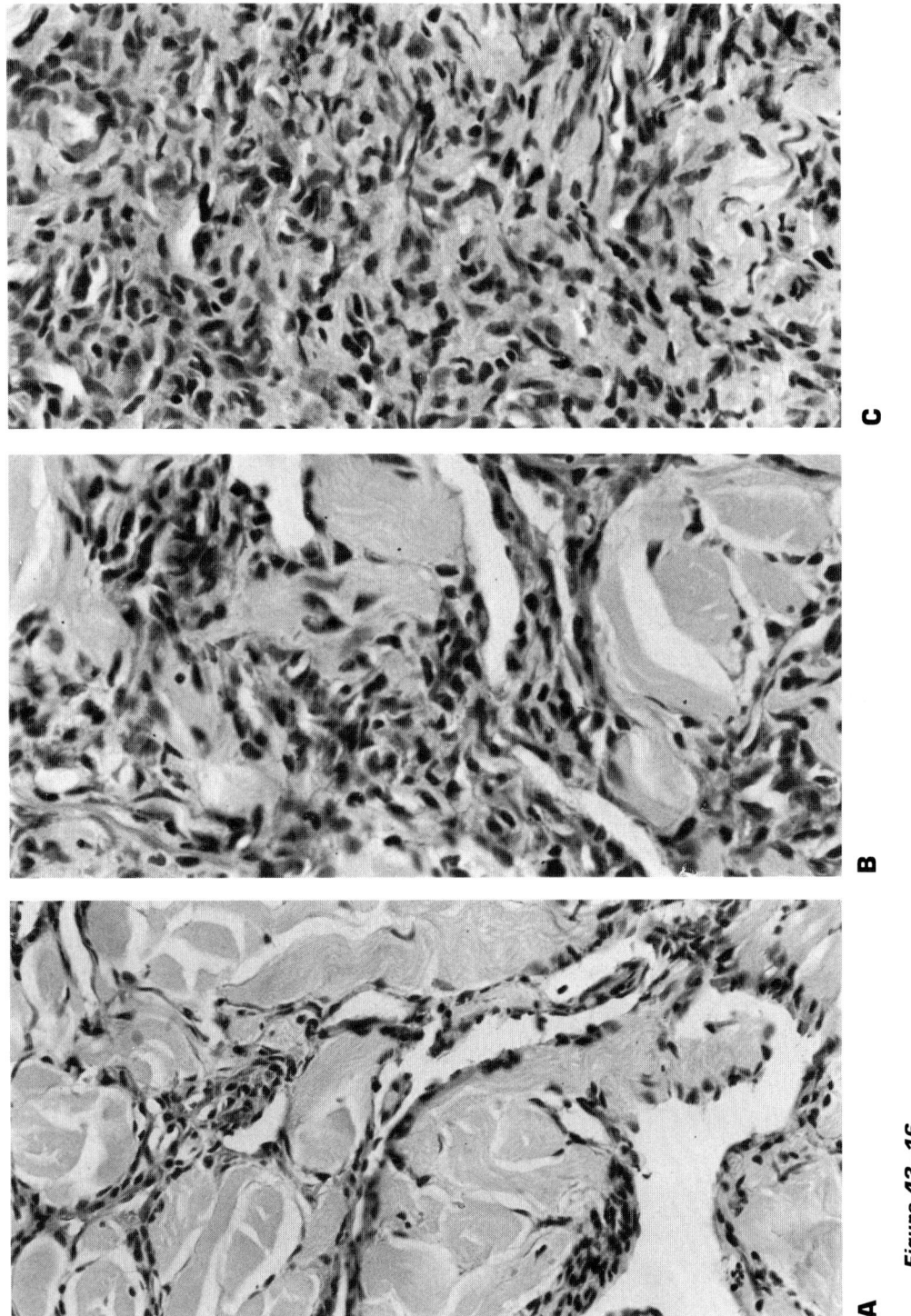

Figure 43–16.
Malignant angioendothelioma of the Stewart–Treves syndrome. **A** and **B.** Malignant endothelial cell proliferation forming vascular spaces in between collagen bundles. H&E. X400. **C.** An area of solid malignant endothelial cell proliferation. H&E. X400.

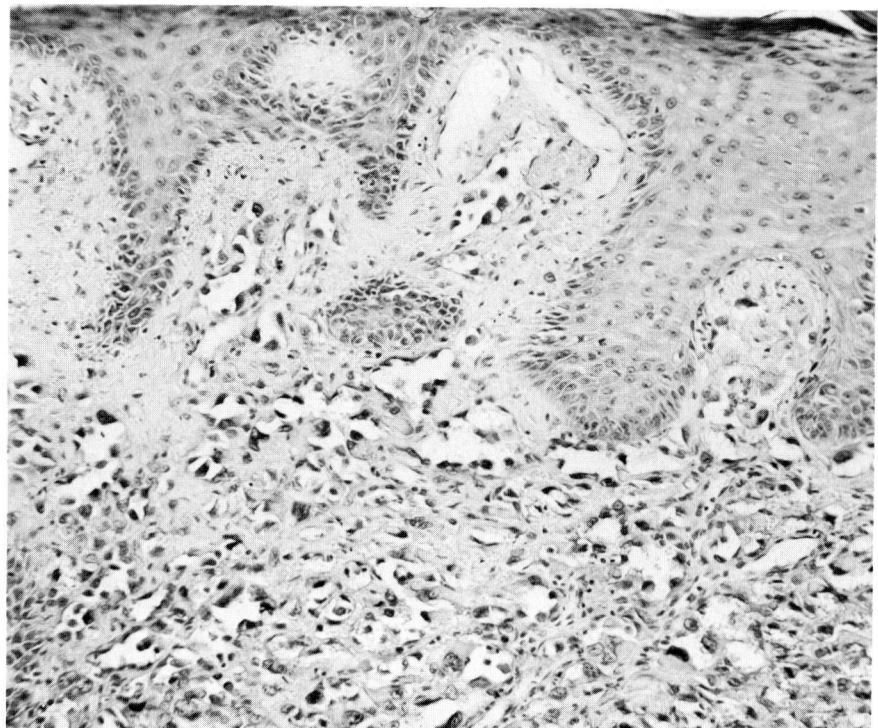

Figure 43–17.
Malignant hemangioendothelioma. Numerous small vascular spaces lined with endothelial cells having large and hyperchromatic nuclei. H&E. X135.

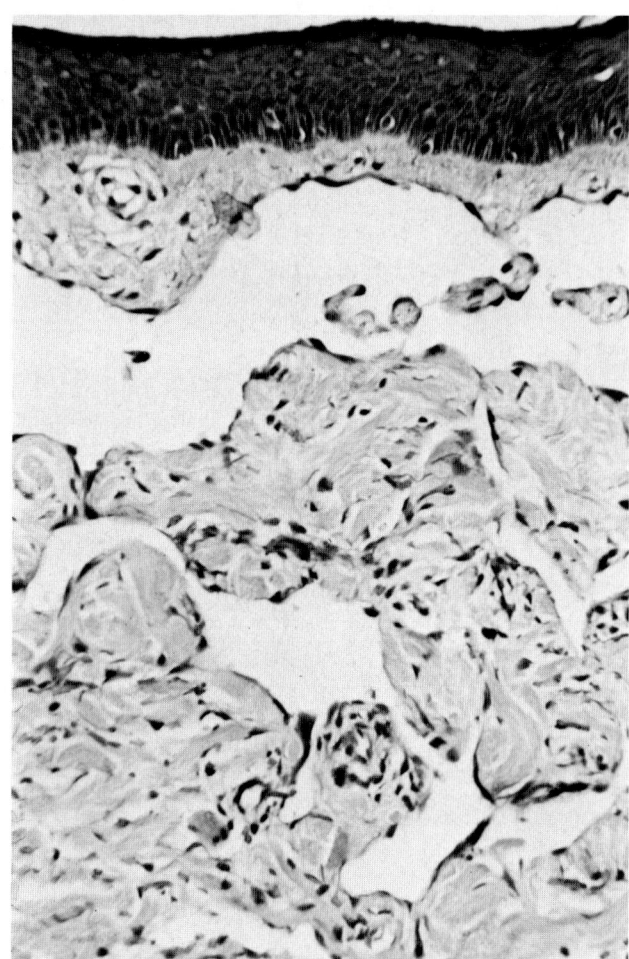

Figure 43–18.
Malignant hemangioendothelioma. Atypical hyperchromatic cells seem to line interfascicular spaces of the dermis rather than form complete blood vessels. H&E. X180.

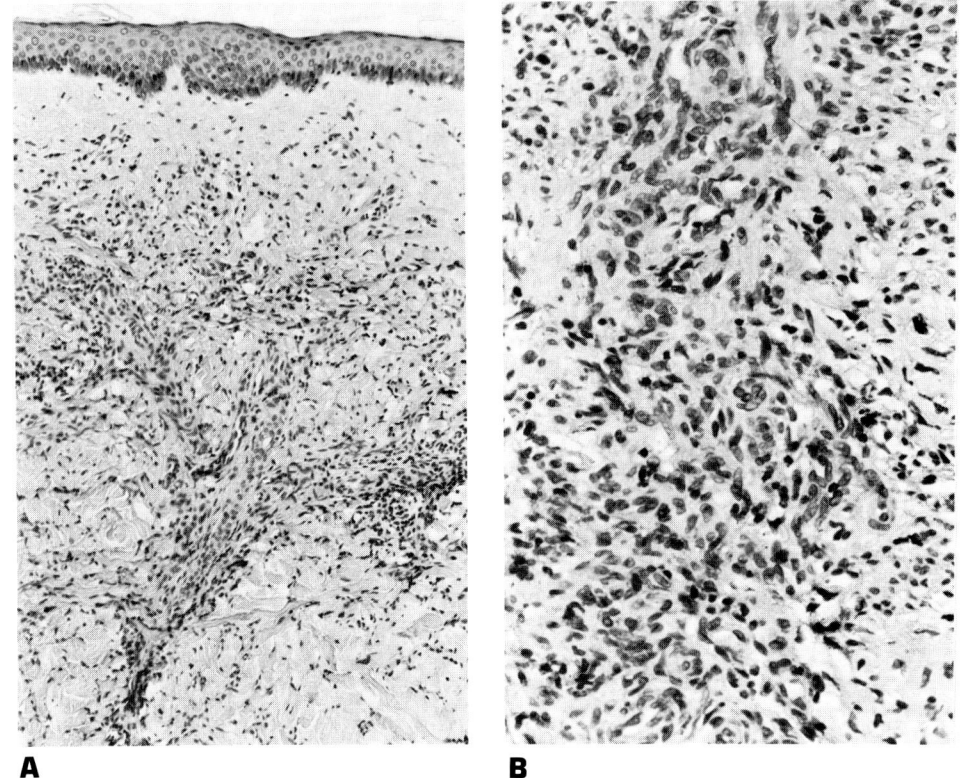

Figure 43-19.
Kaposi's sarcoma in AID syndrome. An early lesion shows perivascular spindle cell proliferation. **A.** H&E. X125. **B.** H&E. X400.

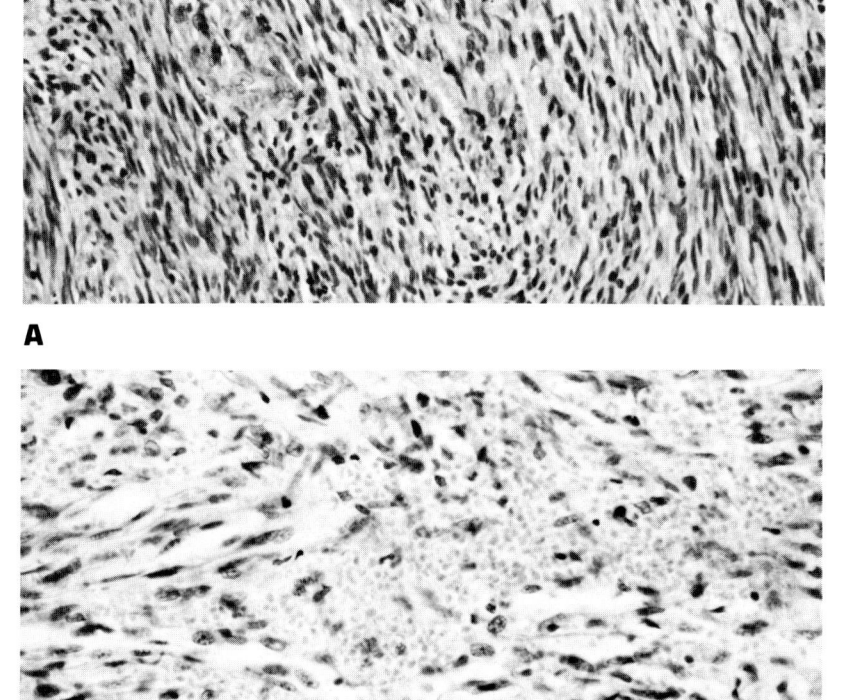

Figure 43-20.
Kaposi's pigmented hemorrhagic sarcoma. **A.** Late stage consisting almost entirely of spindle cells. Many nuclei appear round because they are cross sectioned where the cells streams bend. H&E. X400. **B.** Early phase show vessels and vascular slits lined by endothelial cells. Some round cells, many red blood cells inside and outside of vascular channels. The picture does not show hemosiderin deposits, which are often present. H&E. X400.

REFERENCES

1. Mountcastle AE, Diestelmeier MR, Lupton GP: Nevus anemicus. J Am Acad Dermatol 14:628, 1986
2. Johnson WC: Pathology of cutaneous vascular tumors. Int J Dermatol 15:239, 1976
3. Pesce C, Colacino R: Morphometric analysis of capillary and cavernous hemangioma. J Cutan Pathol 13:216, 1986
4. Arona G, Small O: Verruga peruana o enfermedad de Carrión. Dermatologia, Rev Mexicana 18:20, 1974
5. Okinaga M, Go K, Mizoguchi M: Unilateral dermatolmal superficial telangiectasia. J Dermatol Tokyo 17:638, 1990
6. Marriott PJ, Munro DD, Ryan T: Angioma serpiginosum-familial incidence. Br J Dermatol 93:701, 1975
7. Thomson JA, Mackie RM: Localized secondary telangiectasia in patients with thyroid disease. Br J Dermatol 89:561, 1973
8. Dupont C: Cutis marmorata telangiectatica congenita (Von Lohuizen's syndrome). Br J Dermatol 97:437, 1977
9. Way PH, Herrmann J, Gilbert EF, et al: Cutis marmorata telangiectatica congenita, J Cutan Pathol 1:10, 1974
10. Bean WB: The arterial spider and similar lesions of the skin and mucous membranes. Circulation 8:117, 1953
11. Biberstein HH, Jessner M: A cirsoid aneurysm in the skin. Dermatologica 113:129, 1956
12. Girard C, Graham JH, Johnson WC: Arteriovenous hemangioma (arteriovenous shunt). A clinicopathological and histochemical study. J Cutan Pathol 1:73, 1974
13. Carapeto FJ, Armijo M: Tumeur acrale arterio-veineuse. Ann Dermatol Venereol 105:977, 1978
14. Connelly MG, Winkelmann RK: Acral arteriovenous tumors. Am J Surg Pathol 9:15, 1985
15. Puig L, Llistosella E, Moreno A, DeMorgas JM: Verrucous hemangioma. J Dermatol Surg Oncol 13:1089, 1987
16. Sintes NR, Hernandez PJ, Florencio DV, Solano LJ: Angioqueratoma. A propósito de 93 observaciones. Med Cutan ILA 16:255, 1988
17. Rossi A, Bozzi M, Barra E: Verrucous hemangioma and angiokeratoma circumscriptum: Clinical and histologic differential characteristics. J Dermatol Surg Oncol 15:88, 1989
18. Novick NL: Angiokeratoma vulvae. J Am Acad Dermatol 12:561, 1985
19. Nakumura T, Kaneko H, Nishino I: Angiokeratoma corporis diffusum (Fabry disease) ultrastructural studies of the skin. Acta Derm Venereol 61:37, 1981
20. Carsuzaa F, Rommel A, Bobin P: La maladie de Fabry. Ann Dermatol Venereol 112:643, 1985
21. Frappaz A, Ferrier MC, Hermier C, et al: Angiokeratoma corporis diffusum avec activité enzymatique normale. Ann Dermatol Venereol 114:1383, 1987
22. Smith EB, Graham JL, Ledman JA, et al: Fucosidosis. Cutis 19:195, 1977
23. Dvoretzky I, Fisher BK: Fucosidosis. Int J Dermatol 18:213, 1979
24. Flanagan BP, Helwig EB: Cutaneous lymphangioma. Arch Dermatol 113:24, 1977
25. Whimster IW: The pathology of lymphangioma circumscriptum. Br J Dermatol 94:473, 1976
26. Leshin B, Whitaker DC, Foucar E: Lymphangioma circumscriptum following mastectomy and radiation therapy. J Am Acad Dermatol 15:1117, 1986
27. Eliezri YD, Sklar JA: Lymphangioma circumscriptum: Review and evaluation of carbon dioxide laser vaporization. J Dermatol Surg Oncol 14:357, 1988
28. Wilson-Jones E, Winkelmann RK, Zachary CB, Reda AM: Benign lymphangio-endothelioma. J Am Acad Dermatol 23:229, 1990
29. Maillet PH, Lamesch A, Dawayne PM: L'hémangiopéricytome congénital. A propos de deux cas personels. Chir Pediatr 26:22, 1985
30. Taxy JB, Gray SR: Cellular angiomas of infancy—Ultrastructural study of two cases. Cancer 43:2322, 1979
31. Wilson-Jones E, Orkin M: Tufted angioma (angioblastoma). A benign progressive angioma, not to be confused with Kaposi's sarcoma or low-grade angiosarcoma. J Am Acad Dermatol 20:214, 1989
32. Potts EDA: Tufted angioma. Br J Dermatol 117 (Suppl 32): 54, 1987
33. Padilla SR, Orkin M, Rosai J: Acquired "tufted" angioma (progressive capillary hemangioma). A distinctive clinicopathologic entity related to lobular capillary hemangioma. Am J Dermatopathol 9:292, 1987
34. Kumakiri M, Muramoto F, Tsukinaga I, et al: Crystalline lamellae in the endothelial cells of a type of hemangioma characterized by the proliferation of immature endothelial cells and pericytes-angioblastoma (Nakagawa). J Am Acad Dermatol 8:68, 1983
35. Lim HW, Anderson HM: Angioendotheliomatosis associated with histiocytic lymphoma. J Am Acad Dermatol 13:903, 1985
36. Willemze R, Kruyswijk MRJ, DeBruin CD, et al: Angiotropic (intravascular) large cell lymphoma of the skin previously classified as malignant angioendotheliomatosis. Br J Dermatol 116:393, 1987
37. Wick MR, Rocamora A: Reactive and malignant "angioendotheliomatosis": a discriminant clinicopathological study. J Cutan Pathol 15:260, 1988
38. Petroff N, Koger OW, Fleming MG, et al: Malignant angioendotheliomatosis: An angiotropic lymphoma. J Am Acad Dermatol 21:727, 1989
39. Amerigo J, Gonzalez-Campora R, Galera M, et al: Recurrent pyogenic granuloma with multiple satellites. Clinicopathological and ultrastructural study. Dermatologica 166:117, 1983
40. Jitsukawa K, Hayashi Y, Sato S, Anzai T: Cutaneous angioma in Crow–Fukase syndrome: The nature of globules within the endothelial cells. J Dermatol Tokyo 15:513, 1988

41. Szaniawski WK, Don PC, Bitterman SR, Schachner JR: Epithelioid angiomatosis in patients with AIDS. Report of seven cases and review of the literature. J Am Acad Dermatol 23:41, 1990
42. Axiotis CA, Schwartz R, Jennings TA, Glaser N: AIDS-related angiomatosis. Am J Dermatopathol 11:177, 1989
43. Berger TG, Tappero JW, Kaymen A, LeBoit PE: Bacillary (epithelioid) angiomatosis and concurrent Kaposi's sarcoma in acquired immunodeficiency syndrome. Arch Dermatol 125:1543, 1989
44. Cockerell CJ, LeBoit PE: Bacillary angiomatosis: A newly characterized, pseudoneoplastic, infectious, cutaneous vascular disorder. J Am Acad Dermatol 22:501, 1990
45. Barr RJ, Graham JH, Sherwin LA: Intravascular papillary endothelial hyperplasia. A benign lesion mimicking angiosarcoma. Arch Dermatol 114:723, 1978
46. Hashimoto H, Daimaru Y, Enjoji M: Intravascular papillary endothelial hyperplasia. A clinicopathologic study of 91 cases. Am J Dermatopathol 5:539, 1983
47. Santa Cruz DJ, Kyriakos M: Aneurysmal (angiomatoid) fibrous histiocytoma of the skin. Cancer 47:2053, 1981
48. Sood U, Mehregan AH: Aneurysmal (angiomatoid) fibrous histiocytoma. J Cutan Pathol 12:157, 1985
49. Cavelier-Balloy B, Venencie PY, Lemonnier V, et al: Hémangiome histiocytoide du cuir chevelu. Ann Dermatol Venereol 112:965, 1985
50. Dannaker C, Piacquadio D, Willoughby CB, et al: Histiocytoid hemangioma: A disease spectrum. Report of a case with simultaneous cutaneous and bone involvement limited to one extremity. J Am Acad Dermatol 21:404, 1989
51. Mehregan AH, Shapiro L: Angiolymphoid hyperplasia with eosinophilia. Arch Dermatol 103:50, 1971
52. Dawson J, Mauduit G, Kanitakis J, et al: Unusual vascular tumour of the scalp in association with lymphoid aggregates: A variant of angiolymphoid hyperplasia. J Cutan Pathol 11:506, 1984
53. Olsen TG, Helwig EG: Angiolymphoid hyperplasia with eosinophilia: A clinicopathological study of 116 patients. J Am Acad Dermatol 12:781, 1985
54. Cerio R, Wilson-Jones E: A clinicopathological and immunohistochemical study of angiolymphoid hyperplasia with eosinophilia. Br J Dermatol 119 (Suppl 33):36, 1988
55. Al-Jitawi S, Oumeish OY: Angiolymphoid hyperplasia with tissue eosinophilia. Int J Dermatol 28:114, 1989
56. Kung ITM, Gibson JB, Bannatyne PM: Kimura's disease: A clinicopathological study of 21 cases and its distinction from angiolymphoid hyperplasia with eosinophilia. Pathology 16:39, 1984
57. Maeda K, Jimbow K: Kimura's disease: Immunohistochemistry of infiltrating cells using monoclonal and polyclonal antibodies. J Dermatol Tokyo 13:190, 1986
58. Googe PB, Harris NL, Mihm MC Jr: Kimura's disease and angiolymphoid hyperplasia with eosinophilia: Two distinct histopathological entities. J Cutan Pathol 14:263, 1987
59. Kuo T, Shih L-Y, Chan HL: Kimura's disease: Involvement of regional lymph nodes and distinction from angiolymphoid hyperplasia with eosinophilia. Am J Surg Pathol 12:843, 1988
60. Wilson-Jones E, Bleehen SS: Inflammatory angiomatous nodules with abnormal blood vessels occurring about the ears and scalp (pseudo or atypical pyogenic granuloma). Br J Dermatol 81:804, 1969
61. Ose D, Vollmer R, Shelburne J, et al: Histiocytoid hemangioma of the skin and scapula. A case report with electron microscopy and immunohistochemistry. Cancer 51:1656, 1983
62. Chandon J-P, De Micco C, Lebreuil G, et al: Blue rubber bleb naevus et glomangiomatose: unicité ou dualité? A propos de 2 cas. Ann Dermatol Venereol 105:123, 1978
63. Orange AP: Blue rubber bleb nevus syndrome. Pediatr Dermatol 3:304, 1986
64. Balato N, Montesano M, Lembo G: Blue rubber bleb nevus avec anevrisme arterio-veineux. Ann Dermatol Venereol 113:245, 1986
65. Murata Y, Tsuji M, Tani M: Ultrastructure of multiple glomus tumor. J Cutan Pathol 11:53, 1984
66. Goodman TF, Abele DC: Multiple glomus tumors. A clinical and electron microscopic study. Arch Dermatol 103:11, 1971
67. Reinhard M, Sasse D, Lüders G: Zur Histochemie der Epitheloidzellen in Glomustumoren. Arch Dermatol Forsch 242:165, 1972
68. Landthaler M, Braun-Falco O, Eckert F, et al: Congenital multiple plaquelike glomus tumors. Arch Dermatol 126:1203, 1990
69. McEvoy BF, Waldman PM, Tye MJ: Multiple hamartomatous glomus tumors of the skin. Arch Dermatol 104:188, 1971
70. Tsuneyoshi M, Enjoji M: Glomus tumor. A clinicopathologic and electron microscopic study. Cancer 50:1601, 1982
71. Gould EW, Manivel CJ, Albores-Saavedra J, Monforte H: Locally infiltrative glomus tumors and glomangiosarcomas. A clinical, ultrastructural, and immunohistochemical study. Cancer 65:310, 1990
72. Perrin P, Lemarchand-Venencie F, Bonvalet D, Civatte J: Angiosarcome du cuir chevelu. Ann Dermatol Venereol 112:751, 1985
73. Holden CA, Spittle MF, Wilson-Jones E; Angiosarcoma of the face and scalp, prognosis and treatment. Cancer 59:1046, 1987
74. Blanc D, Quencez E, Billerey C, et al: Angiosarcome de la face de symptomatologie trompeuse. Ann Dermatol Venereol 114:1350, 1987
75. Barttelbort SW, Stahl R, Ariyan S: Cutaneous angiosarcoma of the face and scalp. Plast Reconstr Surg 84:55, 1989
76. Hultberg BM: Angiosarcomas in chronically lymphe-

dematous extremities. Two cases of Stewart–Treves syndrome. Am J Dermatopathol 9:406, 1987
77. Kanitakis J, Bendelac A, Marchand C, et al: Stewart–Treves syndrome: A histogenetic (ultrastructural and immunohistological) study. J Cutan Pathol 13:30, 1986
78. Febre JF, Pourreau-Schneider N, Martin PM, Puissant A: Dosage et modulation des recepteurs steroidiens cutanes sous therapeutique anti-homonale dans le cas d'un syndrome de Stewart–Treves. Ann Dermatol Venereol 115:1035, 1988
79. Handfield-Jones SE, Kennedy CTC, Bradfield JB: Angiosarcoma arising in an angiomatous naevus following irradiation in childhood. Br J Dermatol 118:109, 1988
80. Goette DK, Detlefs RL: Post-irradiation angiosarcoma. J Am Acad Dermatol 12:922, 1985
81. Kofler M, Pichler E, Romani N, et al: Hemangiosarcoma in chronic leg ulcer. Arch Dermatol 124:1080, 1988
82. Friedman-Birnbaum R, Weltfriend S, Katz I: Kaposi's sarcoma: Retrospective study of 67 cases with the classic form. Dermatologica 180:13, 1990
83. Santucci M, Pimpinelli N, Moretti S, Giannotti B: Classic and immunodeficiency-associated Kaposi's sarcoma. Arch Pathol Lab Med 112:1214,1988
84. Lemlich G, Schwam L, Lebwohl M: Kaposi's sarcoma and acquired immunodeficiency syndrome. Postmortem findings in twenty-four cases. J Am Acad Dermatol 16:319, 1987
85. Janier M, Coudere LJ, Morel P, et al: Maladie de Kaposi au cours du SIDA: 31 cases. Ann Dermatol Venereol 114:185, 1987
86. Friedman-Kien AE, Saltzman BR: Clinical manifestations of classical, endemic African, and epidemic AIDS-associated Kaposi's sarcoma. J Am Acad Dermatol 22:1237, 1990
87. Ruszczak ZB, DaSilva AM, Orfanos CE: Kaposi's sarcoma in AIDS. Multicentric angioneoplasia in early skin lesions. Am J Dermatopathol 9:388, 1987
88. Penneys NS, Bernstein M, Leonardi C: Confirmation of early Kaposi's sarcoma by polyclonal antibody to type IV collagen. J Am Acad Dermatol 19:447, 1988
89. Schulze H-J, Rutten A, Mahrle G, Steigleder GK: Initial lesions of HIV-related Kaposi's sarcoma—a histological, immunohistochemical, and ultrastructural study. Arch Dermatol Res 279:499, 1987
90. DeDobbeleer G, Godfrine S, André J, et al: Clinically uninvolved skin in AIDS: Evidence of atypical dermal vessels similar to early lesions observed in Kaposi's sarcoma. J Cutan Pathol 14:154, 1987
91. Kato H, Hamada T, Tsuji T, et al: Kaposi's sarcoma: A light and electron microscopic study. J Dermatol Tokyo 17:414, 1990
92. Konrad K, Schenk P, Rappersberger K: Tuboreticular structures in Kaposi's sarcoma. A comparison of the classical and AIDS-associated forms. Acta Derm Venereol (Stockh) 66:207, 1986
93. Landthaler M, Stolz M, Eckert F, et al: Pseudo-Kaposi's sarcoma occurring after placement of arteriovenous shunt. J Am Acad Dermatol 21:499, 1989

44

NEURAL TUMORS

Tumors arising from the neuroectoderm comprise a limited number of entities in dermal pathology. Their histologic identification and histogenesis has been facilitated in recent years by electron microscopy and by application of various neural-related antigens including S-100 protein, neuron specific enolase (NSE), myelin basic protein (MBP), glial fibrillary acidic protein (GFA), and others.[1,2]

NEUROMA

Proliferation of myelinated nerves (Fig. 44–1), similar to that seen in *amputation neuromas,* may occur in the skin most commonly on the face, as a solitary lesion (palisaded encapsulated neuroma), or in multiple mucosal form, as part of multiple endocrine neoplasia syndrome.[3–6] These are characterized histologically by well-circumscribed intradermal growths of compact and interwoven bundles of nerve fibers without intervening fibrous tissue.[4]

Supernumerary digits in infants contain large nerve trunks and many Meissner's corpuscles in addition to proliferation of blood vessels and fibrous connective tissue (Fig. 44–2). Histologic and electron microscopic features of palisaded encapsulated neuromas as well as supernumerary digits are similar to those seen in peripheral nerve regeneration, suggesting both lesions may be traumatic in origin.[7]

NEUROFIBROMA

The most common cutaneous tumor related to nerves is neurofibroma (Fig. 44–3), which may be solitary and localized, multiple segmental, or diffuse as in *von Recklinghausen's disease.*[8,9] It is differentiated from fibromas and other cutaneous nodules by three features. The cells are relatively small, with short ovoid nuclei, and frequently are not arranged in definite bundles. They often point in all directions. Finely fibrillar interstitial substance does not stain like collagen in trichrome stains and appears light blue rather than pink in O&G sections. The latter also bring out the presence of numerous large mast cells, which are usually roundish rather than ameboid and are scattered throughout the tumor. Large nerve bundles may be encountered (*plexiform neurofibroma*).[10] The neoplasm usually has a sharp border but no capsule. Old lesions may become secondarily fibrotic. Malignant transformation of cutaneous neurofibromas is extremely rare.[11,12]

In relation with neurofibroma, two relatively rare neural neoplasms should be mentioned. *Pacinian neurofibromas* are benign intracutaneous nodular lesions occurring over the acral skin areas and consisting of numerous round neural structures resembling Vater–Pacini corpuscles surrounded by a thin capsule of fibrous connective tissue (Fig. 44–4).[13–15] Dermal *nerve sheath myxomas* or neu-

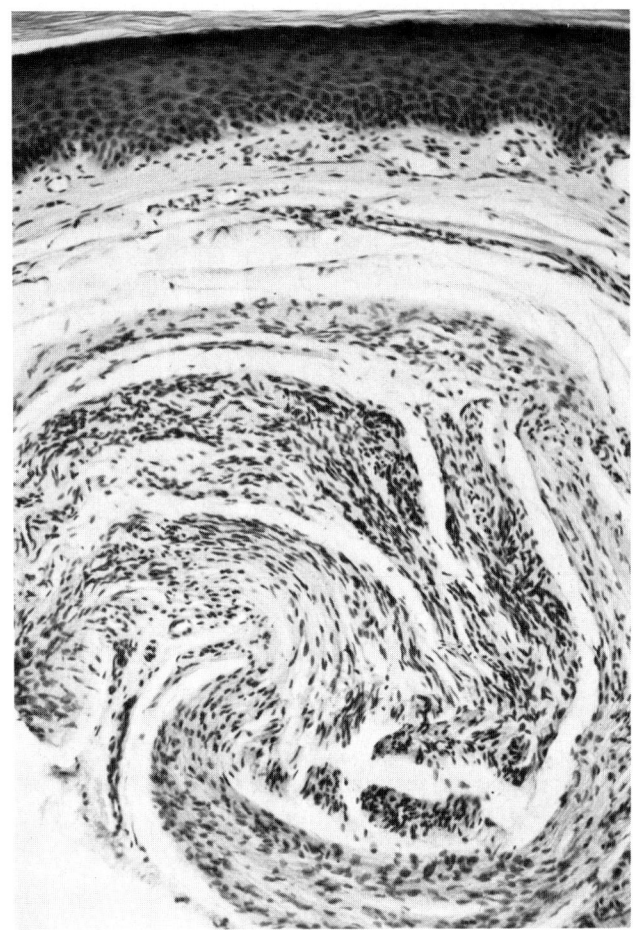

Figure 44–1.
Neuroma in finger skin, probably posttraumatic. H&E. X135.

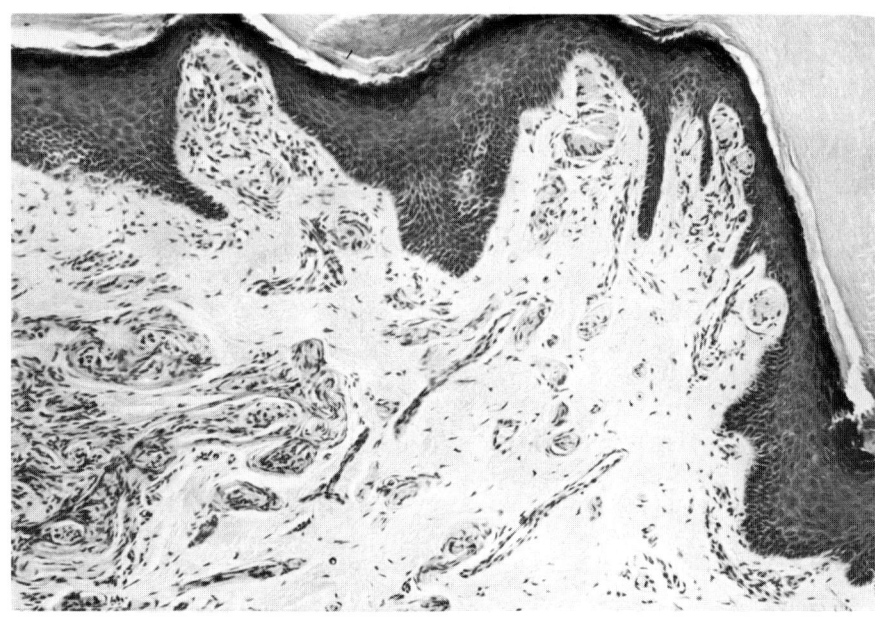

Figure 44–2.
Supernumerary digit—part of a stub-like protrusion in the typical location at the base of the small finger. Large coiled nerve trunks and several deformed Meissner's corpuscles in the sub-epidermal papillae. H&E. X45.

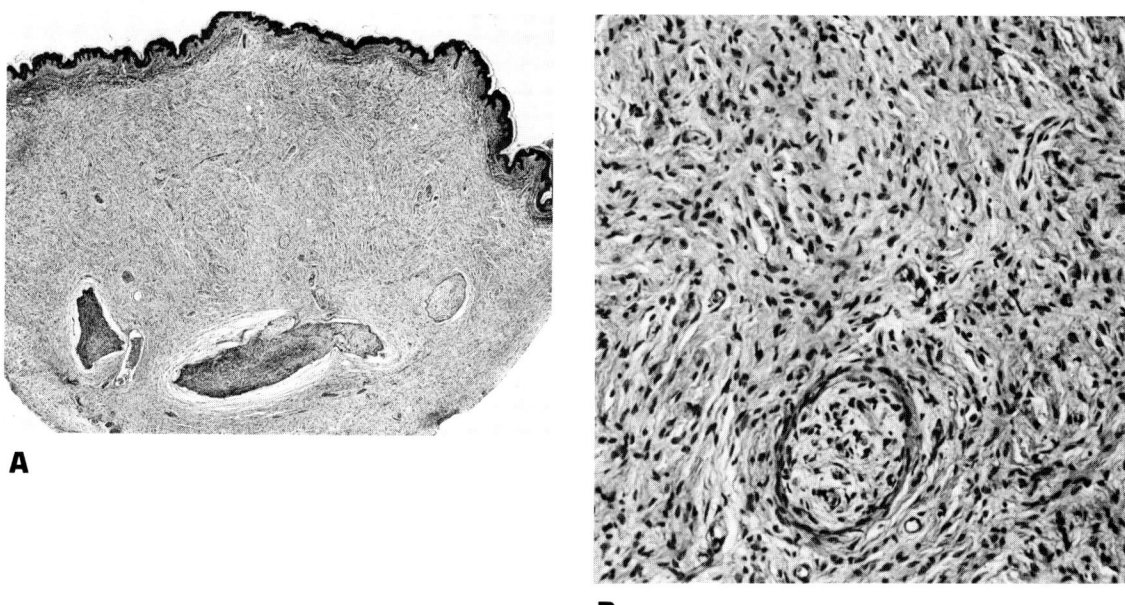

Figure 44–3.
Neurofibroma: Von Recklinghausen type. **A.** Low power shows sharp delineation of tumor without capsule and relative lack of fasciculation. Hypertrophied nerves deep in tumor. H&E. X28. **B.** At higher power, cells are short spindle cells with short nuclei forming convoluted bundles. One deformed nerve near lower border. H&E. X400.

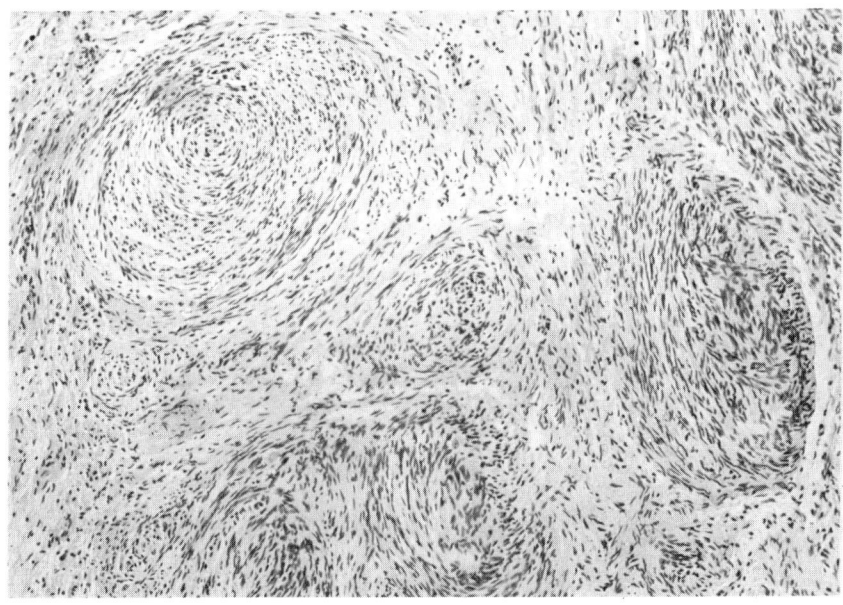

Figure 44–4.
Pacinian neurofibroma. Intracutaneous nodular growth is made up of ovoid neural structures resembling Vater–Pacini corpuscles. H&E. X125.

666 MALFORMATION AND NEOPLASIA

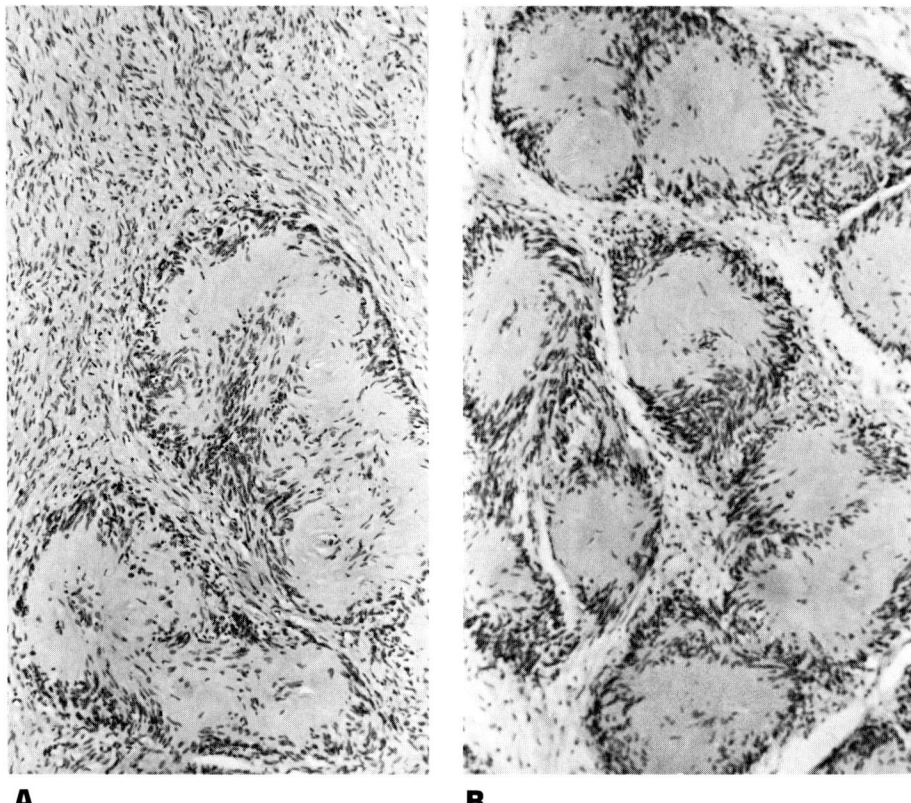

Figure 44–5.
Neurilemmoma. Subcutaneous nodule is made up of cells with elongated and palisaded nuclei and homogenous eosinophilic cytoplasms forming Verocay bodies (Antoni A tissue). **A** and **B**. H&E. X125.

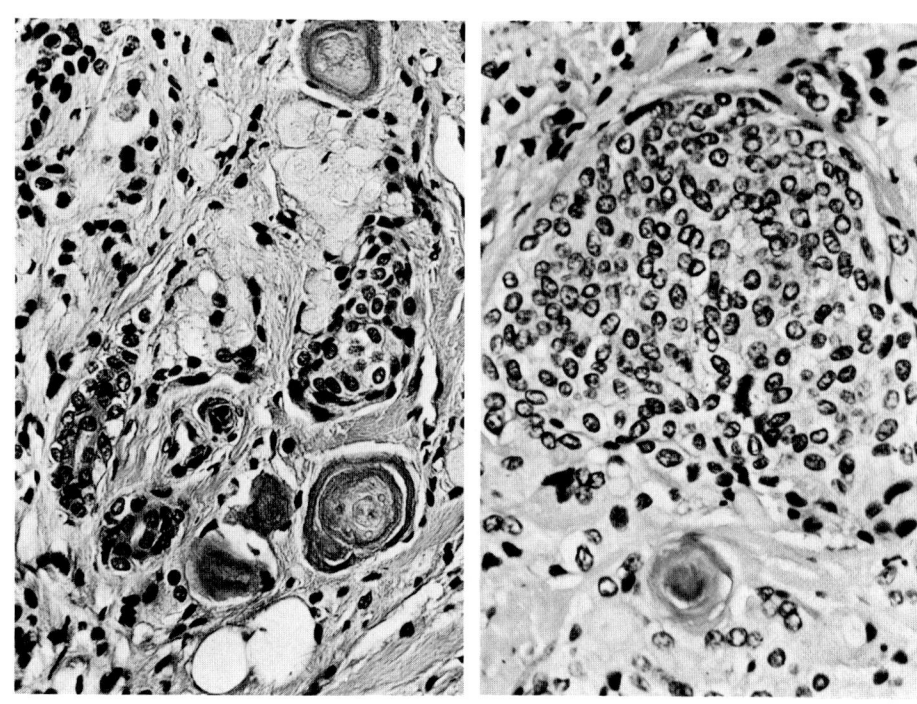

Figure 44–6.
Cutaneous meningioma (psammoma). Nests of meningothelial cells, some of which undergo hyaline degeneration. Lamellated and partly calcified psammoma bodies. H&E. (From Bain and Shnitka Arch Dermatol 74: 590, 1956).

rothekeomas are solitary, well-defined, and often multilobulated intracutaneous neoplasm made up of proliferation of stellate or spindle-shaped cells with small round or ovoid nuclei embedded in a matrix of mucinous material.[16-19] The tumor cells stain positive for S-100 protein.[20]

NEURILEMMOMA

Neurilemmoma (Fig. 44–5) is a benign tumor of Schwann cells, rare in the skin. The characteristic regimentation of nuclei in palisaded fashion and abundant eosinophilic cytoplasms forming Verocay bodies, make it easy to diagnose if this feature is present.[3] Otherwise, neurilemmoma may be suspected if one sees wavy streams of elongated cells resembling the course of nerve bundles. Nerve fibers, however, are usually not demonstrated in routine sections.

OTHER FORMS

Extremely rare are *cutaneous meningiomas*, also called psammomas[21-23] (Fig. 44–6), *gliomas*, usu-

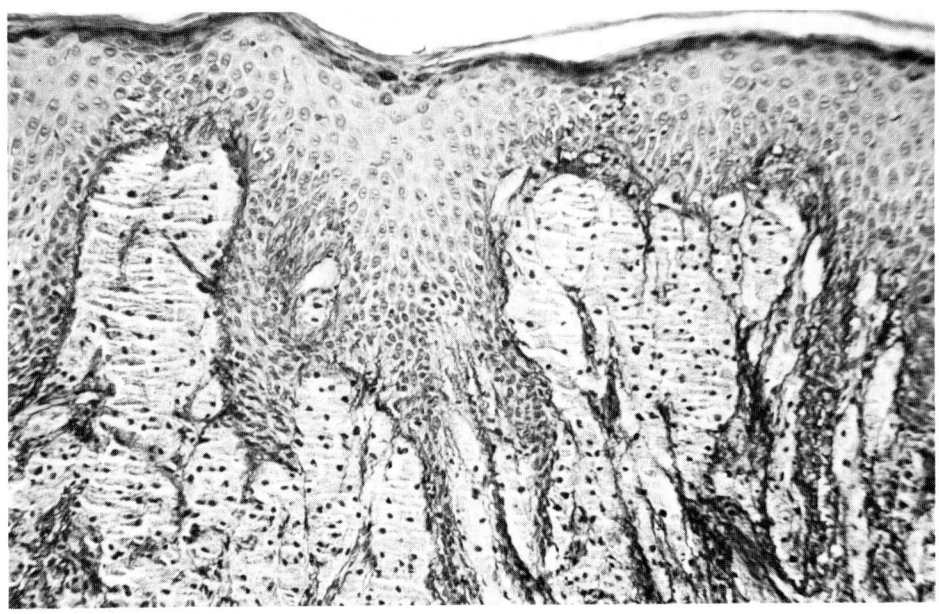

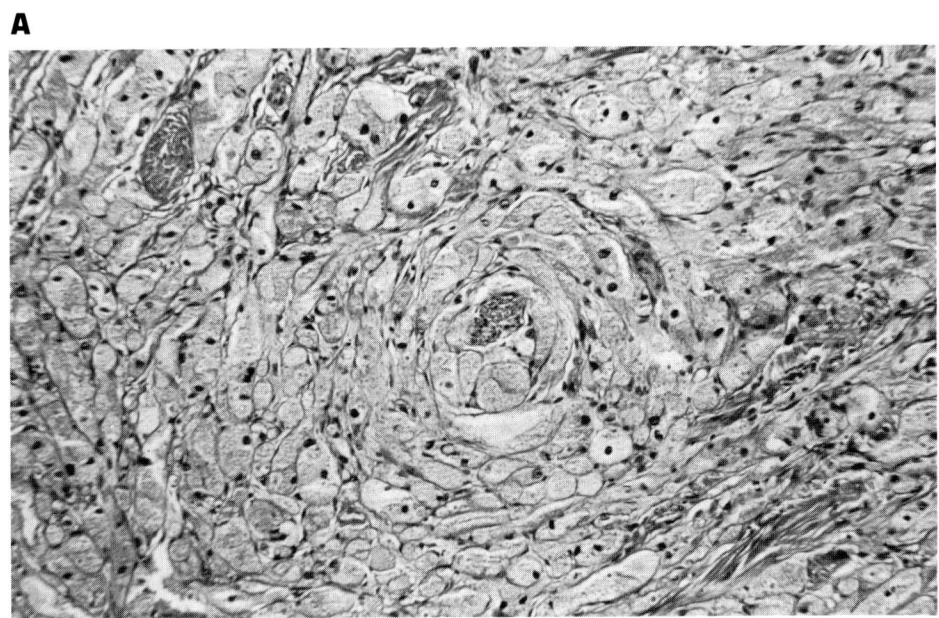

Figure 44–7.
Granular cell myoblastoma (Granular cell tumor). **A.** Pseudoepitheliomatous epidermal hyperplasia overlying a granular cell tumor. H&E. X135. **B.** The growth is made up of large cells with small round nuclei and abundant granular cytoplasms. H&E. X185.

ally developing subcutaneously in the noses of young children[17,18] and having sometimes intracranial connections, and infantile *neuroblastomas,* which may mature into *ganglioneuromas.*

Morton's neuroma is sometimes suspected in painful lesions of the sole, which in many cases are nothing but painful scars resulting from repeated surgical treatment of plantar verrucae or calluses. The true Morton's lesion is local degeneration of an interdigital nerve due to pressure or trauma, and on microscopic examination, it presents degenerating nerve fibers with proliferation of Schwann cells and fibrocytes. Fibrosis may involve the adjacent fat tissue and even adjacent arteries.[24]

Granular Cell Tumor

Granular cell tumor is usually a solitary lesion involving the tongue, skin, or subcutaneous tissue. Dermal lesions appear as raised, firm, well-defined, and non-tender nodules (Fig. 44–7). Histologically, there is extensive dermal involvement with massive proliferation of cells having abundant pale-staining cytoplasm filled with faintly eosinophilic coarse granules. Groups of cells may surround central nerve bundles.[25,26] Ultrastructural observations have eliminated the possibility of myoblastic origin and the recent immunostaining studies utilizing the antiserum to S-100 protein have provided intensepositive staining of the tumor cells suggesting Schwann cell derivation.[27,28]

An intriguing feature of practical importance is the tendency of the overlying epithelium, especially that of mucous membranes, to react with pseudoepitheliomatous proliferation.[29] It may resemble squamous cell carcinoma so much that a superficial biopsy may lead to mistaken diagnosis. In a case of our experience, laryngectomy was barely avoided when a small biopsy from the vocal cord region was first interpreted as carcinoma until a few large granular cells at the lower border of the section led to the correct diagnosis, which was confirmed by conserv-

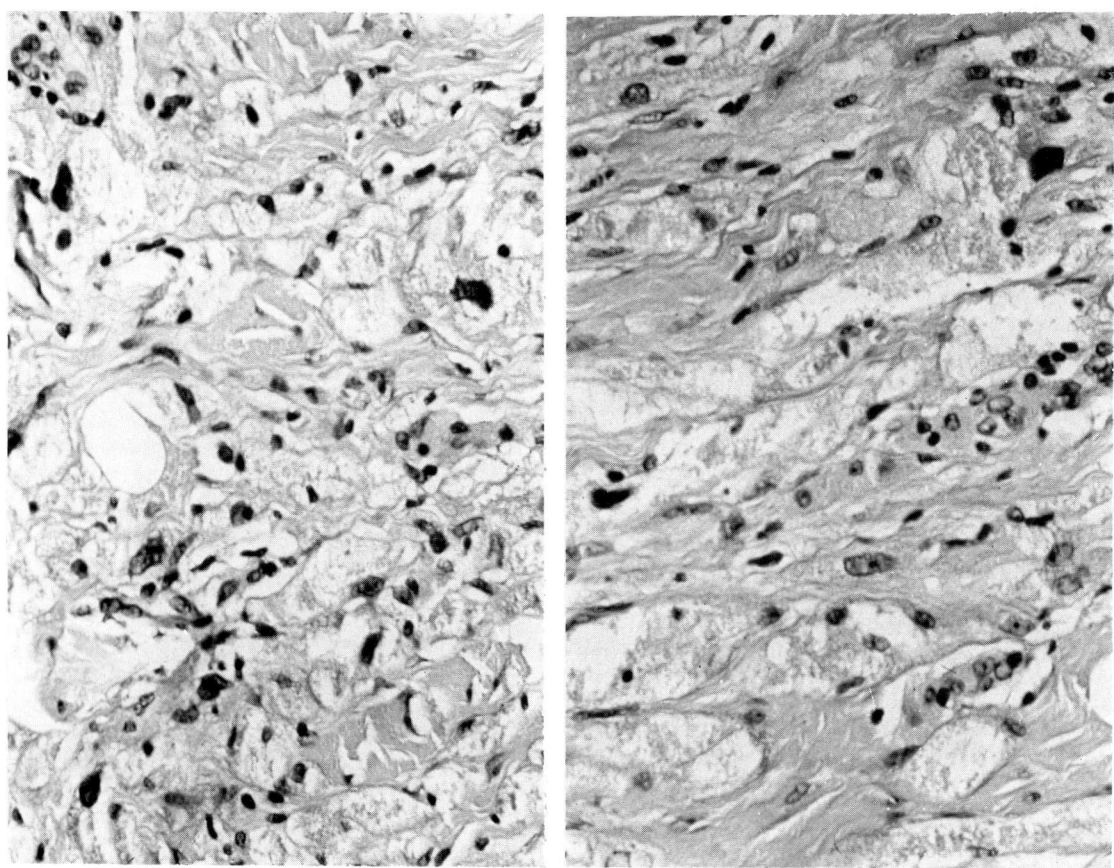

Figure 44–8.
Malignant granular cell myoblastoma. There are many large cells with irregularly shaped nuclei and abundant granular cytoplasms. H&E. X400.

ative surgery (Fig. 44–8). Malignant granular cell tumors occur but rarely.[30] They have the cytologic features of dyplasia with abnormally large cells, irregularly shaped and hyperchromatic nuclei, and mitotic figures.

REFERENCES

1. Aso M, Hashimoto K, Hamzavi A: Immunohistochemical studies of selected skin diseases and tumor using monoclonal antibodies to neurofilament and myelin proteins. J Am Acad Dermatol 13:37, 1985
2. Gray MH, Smoller BR, McNutt S, Hsu A: Immunohistochemical demonstration of Factor XIIIa expression in neurofibromas. Arch Dermatol 126:472, 1990
3. Reed ML, Jacoby RA: Cutaneous neuroanatomy and neuropathology. Normal nerve, neural-crest derivatives, and benign neural neoplasms in the skin. Am J Dermatopathol 5:335, 1983
4. Dover JS, From L, Lewis A: Palisaded encapsulated neuromas. Arch Dermatol 125:386, 1989
5. Winkelmann RK, Aidan-Carney J: Cutaneous neuropathology in multiple endocrine neoplasia. Type 2b. J Invest Dermatol 79:307, 1982
6. Guillet G, Gouthier Y, Tamisier JM, et al: Linear cutaneous neuromas (dermatoneurie en stries): A limited phakomatosis with striated pigmentation corresponding to cutaneous hyperneury (featuring multiple endocrine neoplasia syndrome?). J Cutan Pathol 14:43, 1987
7. Shapiro L, Juhlin EA, Brownstein MH: Rudimentary polydactyly. Arch Dermatol 108:223, 1973
8. Trattner A, David M, Hodak E, et al: Segmental neurofibromatosis. J Am Acad Dermatol 23:866, 1990
9. Jaakkola S, Muona P, James WD, et al: Segmental neurofibromatosis: Immunohistochemical analysis of cutaneous lesions. J Am Acad Dermatol 22:617, 1990
10. Aloi FG, Massobrio R: Solitary plexiform neurofibroma. Dermatologica 179:84, 1989
11. Moulin G, Lombard R: Incidence de la degenerescence des tumeurs nerveuses cutanees dans la maladie de Recklinghausen. Ann Dermatol Venereol 114:807, 1987
12. Dabski C, Reiman HM Jr, Muller SA: Neurofibrosarcoma of skin and subcutaneous tissues. Mayo Clin Proc 65:164, 1990
13. Owen DA: Pacinian neurofibroma. Arch Pathol Lab Med 103:99, 1979
14. McCormack K, Kaplan D, Murray JC, Fetter BF: Multiple hairy Pacinian neurofibromas (nerve-sheath myxomas). J Am Acad Dermatol 18:416, 1988
15. DeKaminsky AR, Glikin I, Torres Cortijo A, et al: Neurofibroma de Vater Paccini. Reporte de tres casos. Med Cutan ILA 17:317, 1989
16. Erlandson RA, Woodruff JM: Peripheral nerve sheath tumors: An electron microscopic study of 43 cases. Cancer 49:273, 1982
17. Nogita T, Someya T, Nakagawa H, et al: Nerve sheath myxoma. An immunohistochemical study of a case. Dermatologica 181:317, 1990
18. Angervall L, Kindblom LG, Haglid K: Dermal nerve sheath myxoma. A light and electron microscopic, histochemical and immunohistochemical study. Cancer 53:1752, 1984
19. Mérot Y, Perrenoud D, Frenk E: Le myxome dermique des gaines nerveuses (neurothecome) de Harkin et Reed: A poropos d'une observations. Ann Dermatol Venereol 116:237, 1989
20. Blumberg AK, Kay S, Adelaar RS: Nerve sheath myxoma of digital nerve. Cancer 63:1215, 1989
21. Nochomovitz LE, Jannotta F, Orenstein JM: Meningioma of the scalp. Light and electron microscopic observations. Arch Pathol Lab Med 109:92, 1985
22. Theaker JM, Fleming KA: Meningioma of the scalp: A case report with immunohistological features. J Cutan Pathol 14:49, 1987
23. Sibley DA, Cooper PH: Rudimentary meningocele: A variant of "primary cutaneous meningioma." J Cutan Pathol 16:72, 1989
24. Asbury AK, Johnson PC (eds): Pathology of Peripheral Nerve. Philadelphia: Saunders, 1978
25. Apisarnthanarax P: Granular cell tumor. An analysis of 16 cases and review of the literature. J Am Acad Dermatol 5:171, 1981
26. Stefansson K, Wollmann RL: S-100 Protein in granular cell tumors (granular cell myoblastoma). Cancer 49:1834, 1982
27. Nakazato Y, Ishizeki J, Takahashi K, Yamaguchi H: Immunohistochemical localization of S-100 protein in granular cell myoblastoma. Cancer 49:1624, 1982
28. Kishimoto S, Arita T, Koishi K, et al: Immunohistochemical and electron microscopic observations in granular cell tumors. J Dermatol Tokyo 13:113, 1986
29. Andreano JM, Tomecki KJ, Bergfeld WF: Huge warty granular cell tumor. Cutis 43:548, 1989
30. Al-Sarraf M, Loud A, Vaitkevicius V: Malignant granular cell tumor. Arch Pathol 91:550, 1971

45
LYMPHOPROLIFERATIVE NEOPLASMS

In approaching histologic and differential diagnosis of lymphoproliferative neoplasms in the skin, one must be aware of several difficulties which make absolute diagnosis hazardous in many cases and impossible in some. The principal difficulties are differentiation between inflammatory and neoplastic infiltrates and identification of cell types. Both difficulties are due in great part to technical factors and to the fact that pathologic classification and diagnostic features described for lymphomas[1] are based on their morphology in lymph nodes. Such criteria as destruction of normal architecture, invasion of capsule, and involvement of peripheral sinuses are not applicable to the skin. Fortunately, the cytologic identification that was unsatisfactory in routine stains is now aided by enzyme histochemistry and by application of various specific monoclonal antibodies in fresh or paraffin-embedded tissue sections.[2-4] A list of various commercially available monoclonal antibodies is given in Table 45–1. For more detailed information we refer our readers to two recent publications on lymphoproliferative disorders of the skin and cutaneous lymphoma.[5-6]

CYTOLOGIC INTERPRETATION

While features of some normal and abnormal cells are mentioned in Chapters 2 and 5, more must be said here about those elements apt to be encountered in lymphoproliferative lesions. A primitive approach to cellular interpretation is this: Cells that are round or roundish without cytoplasmic projections or intercellular connections may be normal or abnormal cells of the lymphoid series, any type of primitive blast form, plasma cells, monocytes, or macrophages, depending on the characteristics of their nuclei and cytoplasm. Cells that are fusiform, stellate, or have obvious intercellular connections are fixed-tissue-type cells and may be fibrocytes, histiocytes, endothelial cells. Specialized cells, such as muscle cells, Schwann cells, or mast cells, are not considered.

Morphology of Cells

T lymphocytes are the most common cells encountered in inflammatory diseases and lymphoproliferative lesions. Development of T lymphocytes involves the following steps: (1) formation of lymphoid stem cells in bone marrow, (2) intrathymic proliferation and differentiation, (3) migration of mature T lymphocytes to T-cell domains in the peripheral lymphoid organs. T lymphocytes are small round cells with round dark-staining nuclei, inconspicuous nucleoli, and scanty cytoplasms. Two subset populations of T lymphocytes are helper–inducer (OKT4 and Leu-3 positive) and cytotoxic–suppressor (OKT8 and Leu-2 positive).

TABLE 45–1. DIFFERENTIATION ANTIBODIES

CD No.	Antibody	Cell type marked	Similar clones
CD1	Leu-6	Thymocytes	OKT6, NA1/34, T6
CD2	Leu-5	Pan-T lymphocytes	OKT11, 9.6, T11
CD3	Leu-4	Mature T lymphocytes	OKT3, T3
CD4	Leu-3	T helper–inducer cells	OKT4, T4
CD5	Leu-1	Pan T lymphocytes	OKT1, T101, T10.2, T1
CD7	Leu-9	T lymphocytes and NK cells	3A1
CD8	Leu-2a,b	T cytotoxic–suppressor cells	OKT8, OKT5, T8
CD10	CALLA	Common acute lymphoblastic leukemia antigen	J5, BA3
CD11b	Leu-15	T suppressor cells, NK cells, monocytes, and granulocytes	CR3, M1, Mo1, Mac1
CD15	Leu-M1	Monocytes, granulocytes	My-1
CD16	Leu-11a,b,c	Fc receptor on neutrophils and NK cells	VEP13, 3G8, L23
CD19	Leu-12	B lymphocytes	B4
CD20	Leu-16	B lymphocytes	B1
CD21	CR2	Mature B lymphocytes	B2
CD22	Leu-14	B lymphocytes	TO15
CD25	IL2	Activated T lymphocytes	Tac, B149.9

Contributed by David Mehregan.

B lymphocytes are lymphocytes differentiated in human bursa equivalent. *Plasma cells* are B lymphocytes that produce immunoglobulins. Plasma cells have round nuclei with cartwheel pattern and basophilic cytoplasms. Lymphoplasmocytic cells are intermediate cells between B lymphocytes and plasma cells. They show nuclei with cartwheel pattern and scanty cytoplasms.[7]

Monocytes-macrophages are round cells having a fair amount of light-staining cytoplasms and indented or kidney-shaped nuclei. In tissue, histiocytes show round nuclei and irregularly shaped cytoplasms with pseudopod-like processes. Histiocytes and macrophages are distinguished by their content of lysosomal enzymes.

Mast cells are difficult to recognize in H&E sections, although their cytoplasms may be slightly basophilic. Giemsa or toluidine blue stain is needed for identification by demonstration of metachromatic intracytoplasmic granules.

Fixed-tissue cells include mainly fibroblasts and endothelial cells. Endothelial cells are identified by their location in the walls of blood vessels and lymphatics. Resting fibrocytes and histiocytes are practically indistinguishable. Fibrocytes are more easily recognized under pathologic conditions such as in the giant form in chronic radiodermatitis, in scar, or in keloid.

Involvement of Dermal Strata

We pointed out in Section III that sparing of the pars reticularis separates most simple inflammatory dermatoses from the lupus erythematosus group and granulomatous inflammation. We now add that involvement of the reticular dermis should make one suspicious also of lymphoproliferative disorders. Again, this rule applies only with reservations to the epidermotropic form of cutaneous T-cell lymphoma especially mycosis fungoides, which may be quite superficial in early stages (see Fig. 45–6). For all other neoplastic diseases of the lymphoreticular system, whether they take the form of leukemia or lymphoma, deep involvement of skin and subcutaneous tissue is characteristic. Figure 45–1 illustrates the most typical distribution, which outlines the entire vasculature of the skin, including superficial and deep plexus and the perforating vessels that usually accompany the adnexa. In leukemia cutis, the cells usually form sharply defined nodular infiltrates around the vessels, while they infiltrate the interfascicular spaces in aggressively growing lymphomas. In lymphomas the Indian-file arrangement of columns of single cells is often seen. A rule of considerable value in differentiating lymphocytic lymphomas from inflammatory diseases, and especially from chronic lupus erythematosus, is that in

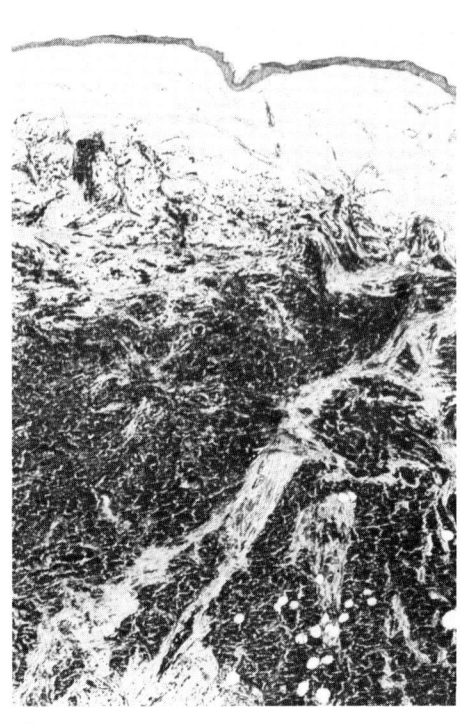
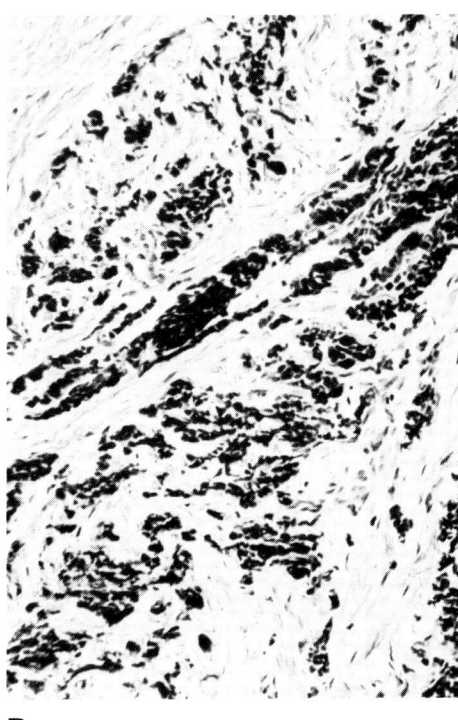

Figure 45–1.
Lymphatic leukemia. **A.** Massive infiltrate does not approach epidermis. H&E. X21.
B. Monomorphic cells in clumps and Indian-file columns between collagen bundles. H&E. X185.

the latter the cells are spaced by edema so that they can easily be scrutinized individually. In a lymphoma, the cells are so tightly packed that their features are obscured except in very thin sections.

STRUCTURAL INTERPRETATION

Since cytologic identification is unsatisfactory in diagnosing non-Hodgkin's lymphomas and pseudolymphomas, we must seek help from the distribution, arrangement, and other structural features of the infiltrate. The important criteria are quantity, polymorphism versus monomorphism, involvement of the various dermal layers, involvement of the epidermis and adnexal structures, and destructiveness.

Quantity of Infiltrate

Heavy cellular infiltrate makes one suspect neoplasia, whereas a minimal number of cells tends to rule it out. This, however, is not an infallible criterion because many granulomas may have just as heavy or heavier infiltrate, and cellularity may be surprisingly small in some lymphomas, especially of the epidermotropic type.

Polymorphism Versus Monomorphism

With the exception of the cutaneous T-cell lymphomas and Hodgkin's disease, most other malignant lymphomas and skin lesions of leukemias show a monomorphous infiltrate or at least one cell type predominating heavily.

Involvement of Epidermis and Adnexa

Leukemic infiltrates do not usually invade the epidermis. They are separated from it by a grenz zone of compressed connective tissue. Lymphomas, on the other hand, may destroy the epidermis and lead to ulceration. It was mentioned in Chapter 25 that Langerhans cell granuloma, which often comes into differential diagnosis, has a strong tendency to invade and even destroy the epidermis. In mycosis fungoides we meet the paradoxical situation that the infiltrate often involves the subpapillary zone more than the papillae, while on the other hand, epidermal invasion in the form of Pautrier abscesses (see Fig. 45–4) is a diagnostic feature. Both phenomena may be found in the same section.

The condition of hair follicles and sweat glands may serve as an indication of the relative benignity or destructiveness of the process. The adnexa may be fairly normal in benign lymphoplasia, although they

TABLE 45–2. A WORKING FORMULATION OF NON-HODGKIN'S LYMPHOMAS FOR CLINICAL USAGE

Low grade malignant lymphoma	Small lymphocytic (consistent with CLL, plasmocytoid) Follicular predominantly small cleaved cell (diffuse areas, sclerosis) Follicular mixed, small cleaved and large cell (diffuse areas, sclerosis)
Intermediate grade malignant lymphoma	Follicular predominantly large cell (diffuse areas, sclerosis) Diffuse small cleaved cell (sclerosis) Diffuse mixed, small and large cell (sclerosis, epithelioid cell component) Diffuse large cell (cleaved cell, noncleaved cell, sclerosis)
High grade malignant lymphoma	Large cell immunoblastic (plasmocytoid, clear cell, polymorphous, epithelioid cell component) Lymphoblastic (convoluted cell, nonconvoluted cell) Small nonconvoluted cell (Burkitt's, follicular areas) Miscellaneous (composite, mycosis fungoides, histiocytic, extramedullary plasmacytoma, others)

Proposed by the Non-Hodgkin's Lymphoma Pathologic Classification Project. Cancer 49:2112, 1982.

are embarrassed by massive infiltrate. They become atrophic in leukemia and are invaded and destroyed by lymphomas. Sebaceous glands usually suffer first, hair follicles next, but eccrine glands are surprisingly resistant.

TERMINOLOGY AND CLASSIFICATION

Concepts and nomenclature of cutaneous lymphoreticular proliferation have grown and changed over the years, just as in other fields of dermatology, but have been influenced much more by parallel developments in general pathology and immunology. Rappaport's classification was morphologic and had to be changed when modern immunologic methods brought new views of histogenesis and function. Five other classifications have been proposed by Lukes and Collins,[8] Dorfman,[9] a British group,[10] the World Health Organization,[11] and a group of German authors (the so-called Kiel classification).[12–13] These systems were re-evaluated and a working formulation for clinical usage was proposed by the non-Hodgkin's lymphoma pathologic classification project in 1982 (see Table 45–2).[14] Leukemia cutis and other rare lesions are discussed only briefly (Table 45–3).

SPECIFIC DISORDERS

Leukemia Cutis

Leukemias are malignant neoplasias of white blood cells characterized by extensive involvement of bone marrow, the presence of abnormal leukocytes in bloodstream, and widespread infiltration of liver, spleen, and lymph nodes. Cutaneous involvement of leukemia may take various morphologic forms and distribution patterns.[15] Multiple soft nodules, infiltrated plaques, and lesions with hemorrhagic tendency may be observed. Specific cutaneous lesions may occur in 20 percent of patients with chronic lymphocytic leukemia (Fig. 45–1). Dermal infiltrate is made up of small mature lymphocytes exhibiting scattered mitoses. Acute lymphocytic leukemia rarely shows skin involvement. The infiltrate consists of medium-sized or large lymphoblasts. Acute and chronic granulocytic leukemias occasionally show skin lesions.[16] In addition to mature neutrophils with lobulated nuclei, myeloblasts with round, oval indented nuclei are also present.

TABLE 45–3. LYMPHOPROLIFERATIVE AFFECTIONS OF THE SKIN

Benign or possibly premalignant
  Parapsoriasis en plaque
  Lymphomatoid papulosis
  Woringer–Kolopp's disease
  Crosti's reticulohistiocytoma of the back
Malignant
  Mycosis fungoides
  Sézary's syndrome
  Primary Hodgkin's disease of the skin
  Primary lymphomas of the skin
  Leukemia cells
Pseudolymphoma
  Arthropod bites
  Actinic reticuloid
  Benign cutaneous lymphoplasia

Extramedullary Plasmacytoma and Multiple Myeloma

Cutaneous lesions characterized by massive plasma cells infiltrate (cutaneous plasmacytoma) may occur as a primary lesion in extramedullary plasmacytoma or as a cutaneous manifestation of multiple myeloma.[17-19] Widespread nodular lesions may involve face, trunk, extremities, or oral mucosa. Dermal infiltrate consists mainly of well differentiated plasma cells (Fig. 45–2).[20,21]

Hodgkin's Disease

Primary cutaneous Hodgkin's disease is very rare. It may appear as eczematous plaques, nodules, and tumors most likely secondary to retrograde lymphatic spread from the involved lymph nodes and is usually associated with poor prognosis.[22,23]

Histopathology of cutaneous Hodgkin's disease is very similar to those of the involved lymph nodes (Fig. 45–3). The most common histologic types are lymphocyte-depleted or the mixed cell variety. One may observe a polymorphous granulomatous infiltrate consisting of epithelioid cells, lymphocytes, plasma cells, neutrophils, eosinophils, and the characteristic Reed–Sternberg cells.[24,25]

Malignant Lymphoma

Malignant lymphomas are by definition locally destructive lesions in contrast to space-occupying leukemic infiltrates or benign cutaneous lymphoplasias (Fig. 45–4).[26-29] Histologically, one finds interfascicular spread of atypical lymphoid cells in pars reticularis in addition to patchy perivascular accumulations. The epidermis often invaded in T-cell lymphomas is usually intact in other cell varieties. Adnexal structures may be involved or completely destroyed. Classification is based on cytologic differentiation, which may be aided by immunohistochemical studies.[30,31]

Small lymphocytic lymphoma (well-differentiated lymphocytic lymphoma) is the most common variety and shows a massive dermal infiltrate made up of cells with small round nuclei and coarsely clumped chromatins with practically no visible cytoplasms. The cells are indistinguishable from normal lymphocytes. *Small cleaved cell lymphoma* (poorly differentiated lymphocytic lymphoma) shows cells with cleaved, indented nuclei, and a small amount of cytoplasms. The cell nuclei are larger and lighter staining than those of the well-differentiated variety. *Large cell lymphoma* (histiocytic lymphoma) shows massive infiltrate of cells with large vesicular nuclei, well-defined nuclear membrane, a few chromatin particles, and one or two nucleoli. The tumor cells show abundant but poorly stained cytoplasms. In *small and large (mixed) type lymphoma* the infiltrate consists of a mixture of small cells with irregular nuclei and large epithelioid type cells. *Lymphoplasmocytic lymphoma* shows a patchy dermal infiltrate of lympho-

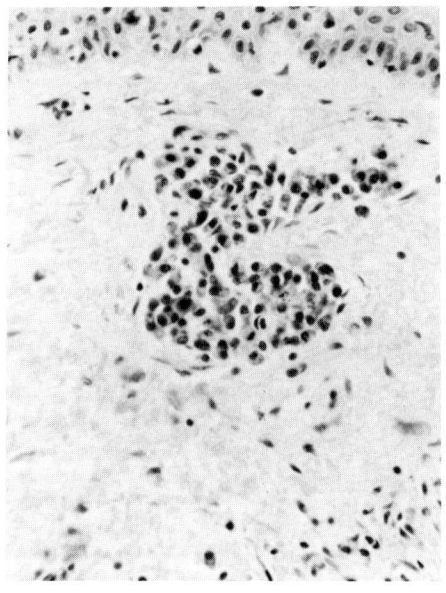
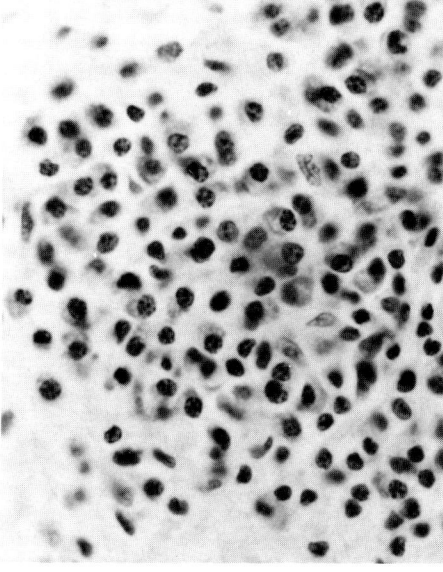

Figure 45–2.
Plasma cell leukemia. Plasma cells in dermis. H&E. **A.** X250. **B.** X800.

A
B

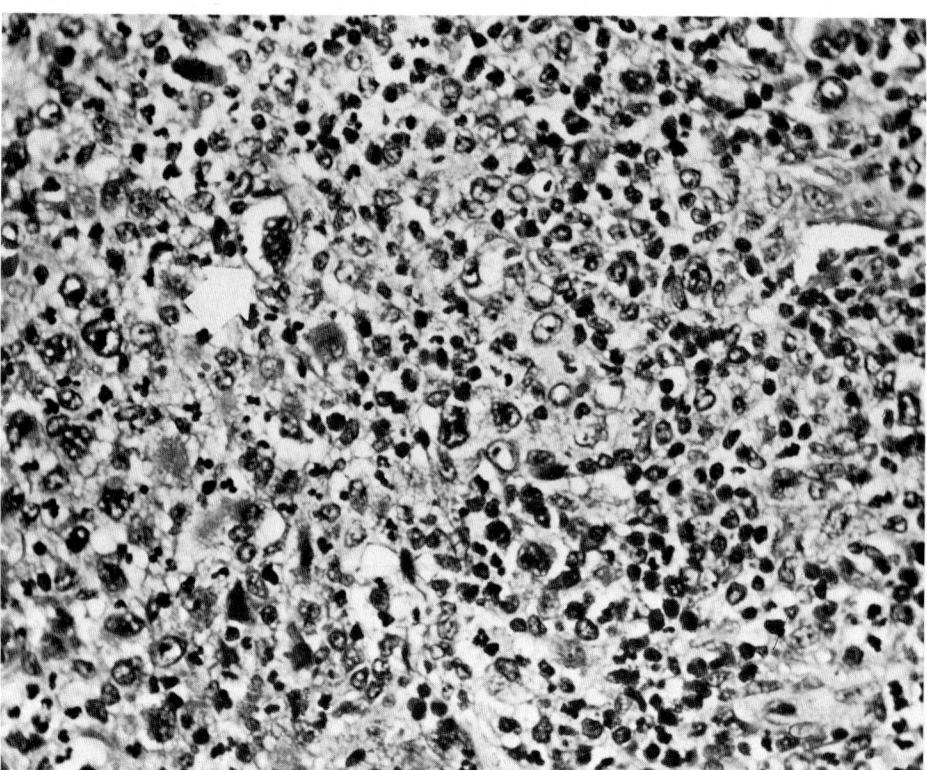

Figure 45–3.
Hodgkin's disease. Mixed infiltrate of atypical mononuclear cells interspersed with a few eosinophils. Reed–Sternberg cells have commonly several nuclei containing very large nucleoli. H&E. X370.

plasmocytoid cells with varying degrees of nuclear pleomorphism.

Mycosis Fungoides

Definition

Mycosis fungoides is the principal form of T-cell lymphoma originating in the skin and often remaining confined to the skin for many years.[32] Lymph node and internal involvement will develop eventually. Mycosis fungoides is a neoplastic, or at least proliferative, process from the beginning, rather than an inflammatory condition. This statement includes parapsoriasis en plaques, erythroderma, or poikiloderma atrophicans as obligatory precursor lesions. On the other hand, mycosis fungoides may superimpose itself on inflammatory diseases such as psoriasis or alopecia mucinosa.

Clinically, mycosis fungoides is characterized by progression from the eczematoid, parapsoriatic, or erythrodermic stage through the plaque stage and into tumor.[33] The course of disease is variable and the stages may occur in reverse order.

The histologic picture may show progression from mixed infiltrate to the predominantly monomorphous infiltrate in the early or late stages. The most reasonable explanation for this seems to be that given by Van Scott et al.[34]: the neoplastic cells may be relatively few in earlier stages and are overshadowed by inflammatory infiltrate, a situation similar to that in Hodgkin's disease. It is assumed that the infiltrate is a reaction to the malignant cells and keeps them in check until, in later stages, the immunologic status of the patient deteriorates. In addition, as in other neoplasms, the neoplastic cell may show progression and change in character. Leukemia, lymphosarcoma, or Hodgkin's disease may develop secondarily in mycosis fungoides.

Histologic Features

In attempting the histologic diagnosis of mycosis fungoides, one must pay attention to the epidermis as well as the dermis. The epidermis often is acanthotic. The rete ridges are long and rounded and often bulbous in cross section (Fig. 45–5). Papillae are correspondingly prominent and often bulbous, the combination producing a festoon-like contour of the dermoepidermal junction in a single section. The epidermis usually shows some intracellular and intercellular edema and also parakeratosis. It often is invaded by mononuclear cells that may lie singly surrounded by a halo or groups within small cav-

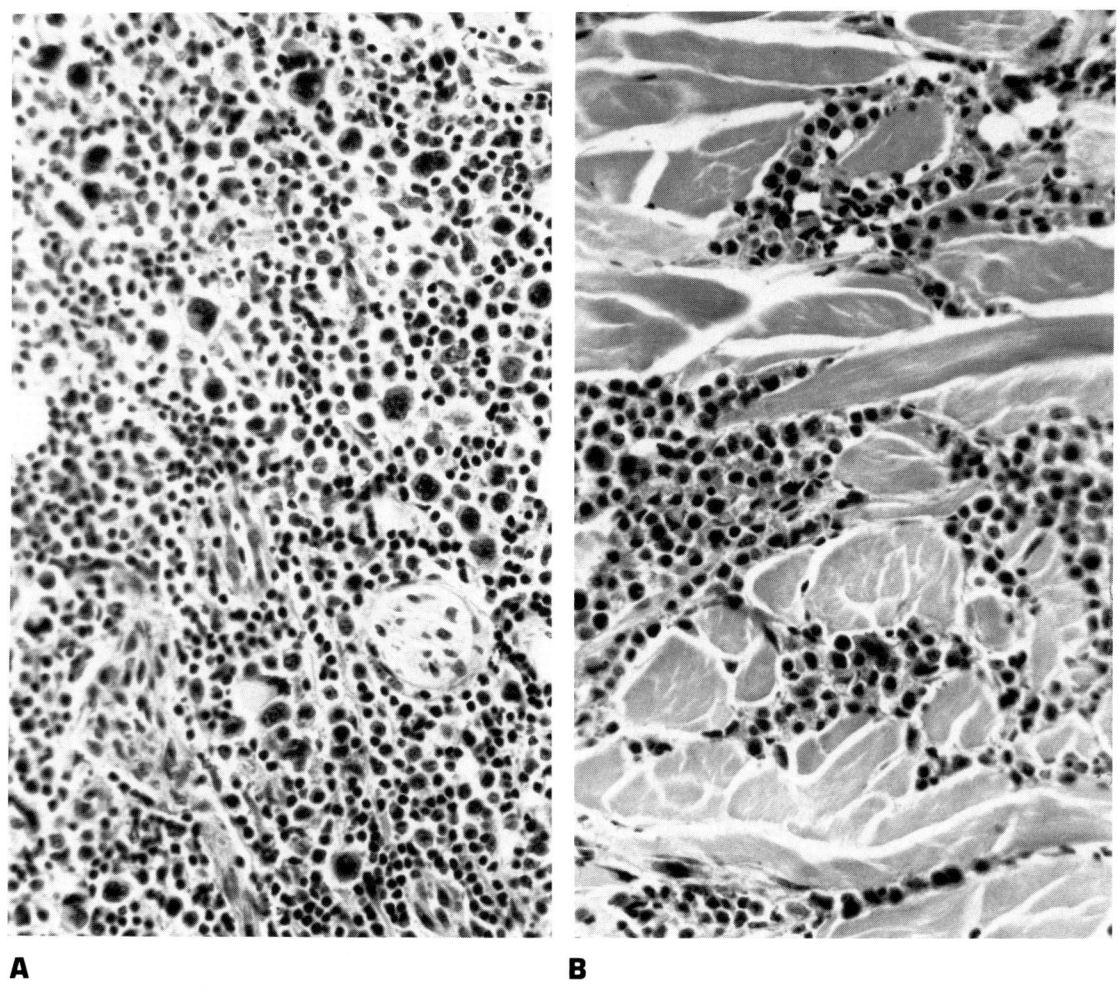

Figure 45–4.
Malignant lymphoma, large cell type. **A.** Massive dermal infiltrate with many abnormal cells having large and irregularly shaped nuclei. H&E. X400. **B.** Involvement of interfascicular spaces. H&E. X400.

ities called Pautrier abscesses (Fig. 45–6). The cells may be simply small round cells but often are larger mononuclears, sometimes possessing atypical nuclei. These are apt to invade the epidermis singly[35,36] in parapsoriasis en plaques. Well-developed Pautrier abscesses are almost pathognomonic for mycosis fungoides, but their absence does not rule out the diagnosis (Fig. 45–7). The number of cells invading the epidermis varies greatly from case to case. In some instances it becomes so great that the epidermis appears honeycombed, and Paget's disease is simulated if the invading cells are large and hyperchromatic (Fig. 45–8). Edelson[37] has pointed out that cutaneous T-cell lymphoma (CTCL) progresses often from the epidermotropic form to a nonepidermotropic form and that this transition carries a poor prognosis, especially if associated with lymph node and other system involvement.

In its classic expression, the dermal infiltrate of mycosis fungoides spares the papillae in spite of its epidermotropism. In the earlier, pretumor stages, infiltrate may form a relatively dense and broad zone in the subpapillary layer and involve the pars reticularis in variable depth. It consists of a mixture of cells in which T lymphocytes of various sizes predominate. Immunostaining suggests predominance of helper–inducer T cells over the suppressor–cytotoxic cells.[38] Plasma cells, eosinophils, and neutrophilic polymorphonuclear cells may be present in descending order of frequency.[39] Mast cells play no significant role. Fixed-tissue-type cells are usually

678 MALFORMATION AND NEOPLASIA

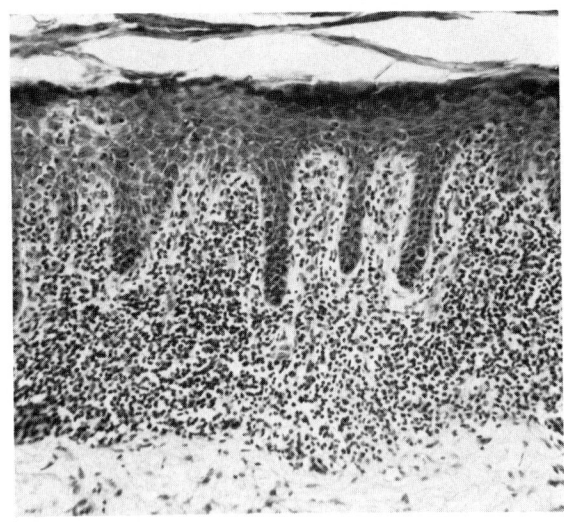

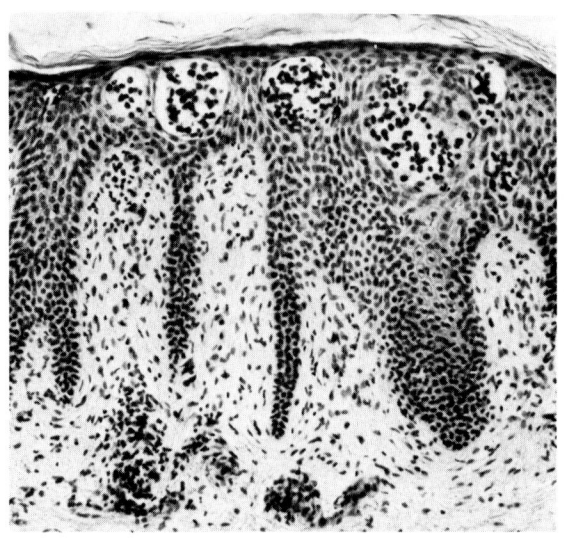

Figure 45–5.
Mycosis fungoides, plaque stage. **A.** Rather diffuse and fairly monomorphous infiltrate, which is heavier in subpapillary layer than in some papillae and does not involve pars reticularis. Acanthotic epidermis is invaded in only a few places. H&E. X135. **B.** Higher degree of acanthosis and crowded Pautrier abscesses in lesion which exhibits relatively mild dermal infiltrate. Many of epidermotropic cells, and some in dermis, are hyperchromatic. H&E. X135.

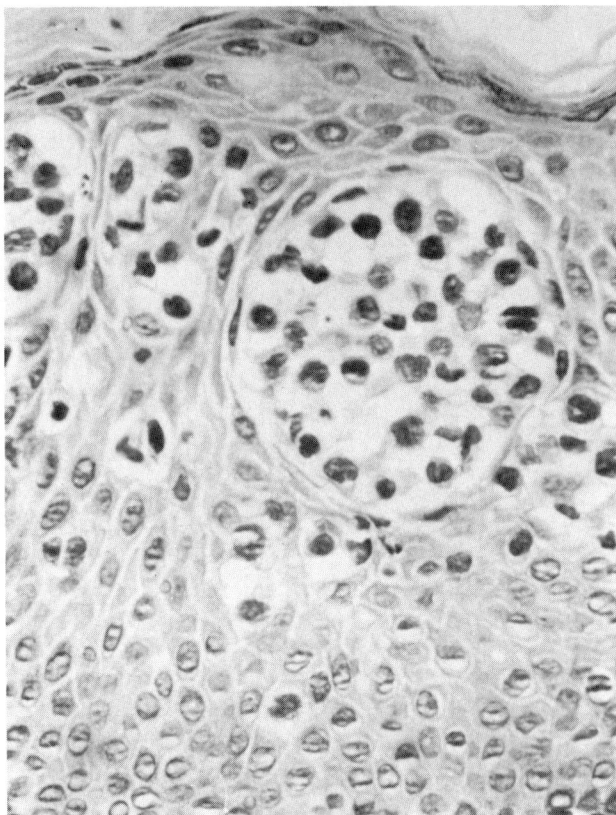

Figure 45–6.
Mycosis fungoides. Pautrier microabscesses. H&E. Original X400.

increased in number, and there may be a diffuse increase of fibrocytes and/or histiocytes throughout the dermis. The characteristic Lutzner or mycosis cells are neoplastic T lymphocytes with hyperchromatic, irregularly shaped, and hyperconvoluted nuclei (Fig. 45–9). Their presence in a significant number within the dermal infiltrate and inside the Pautrier abscess is diagnostic. A few cells with hyperconvoluted nuclei may be observed in various dermatitis and psoriasis. The degree of nuclear hyperconvolution as measured by the nuclear contour index (NCI) is significant.[40] This is achieved by tracing the nuclear contour of 100 T cells in electron micrographs. NCI greater than 6.5 is an indication of T-cell lymphoma.[41,42]

The population of mycosis cells increases in the infiltrated plaques or tumors of mycosis fungoides. Numerous large cells with multilobulated nuclei and atypical mitotic figures are frequently observed (Fig. 45–10).[43]

Differential Diagnosis

Commonly, the pathologist is requested to rule out or to confirm the diagnosis of mycosis fungoides in a patient having long-standing eczema, parapsoriasis, or other ill-defined skin eruptions. Mycosis fungoides has a chronic and slowly progressive course during which its clinical manifestations and histo-

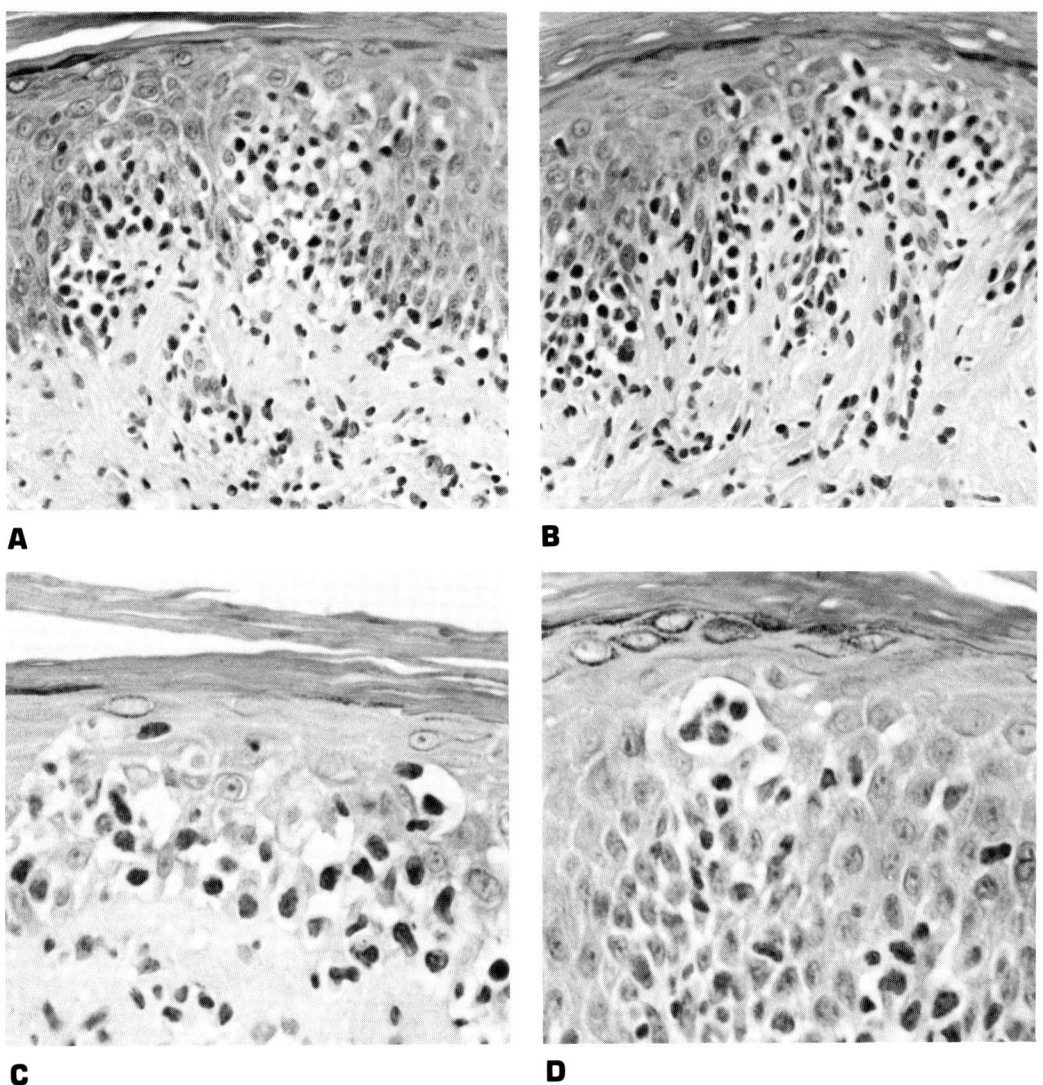

Figure 45–7.
Epidermotropic lymphoma. Hyperchromatic cells invade the epidermis diffusely, forming Pautrier abscesses occasionally. Relatively few of these cells are present in the dermis. H&E. **A** and **B**. X400. **C** and **D**. X600.

logic features become increasingly characteristic. The question arises as to how essential it is to make a definite diagnosis of mycosis fungoides in its initial premycotic stage. Some centers attach much importance to an early histologic diagnosis by reporting favorable response when lesions are treated in their initial stages. Treatment success, however, may be due to inclusion in their series of patients with parapsoriasis en plaques, or exfoliative erythroderma. The list of confusing differential diagnoses includes parapsoriasis en plaques, chronic eczematous dermatitis, especially of the dermal contact sensitivity type, and pseudolymphomas.

The histologic differences between parapsoriasis en plaques of the poikilodermatous or retiform variety and early phases of mycosis fungoides are ill defined.[44,45] In some cases, one can diagnose parapsoriasis en plaques with assurance on the basis of mild and superficial infiltrate with minimal epidermal involvement. On the other hand, cases showing heavy dermal infiltrate with epidermal involvement by individual mononuclear cells and formation of Pautrier abscesses suggest development of mycosis fungoides. The turning point is judged more accurately by the clinical features of thickening of the plaques and onset of severe pruritus. Dermal contact

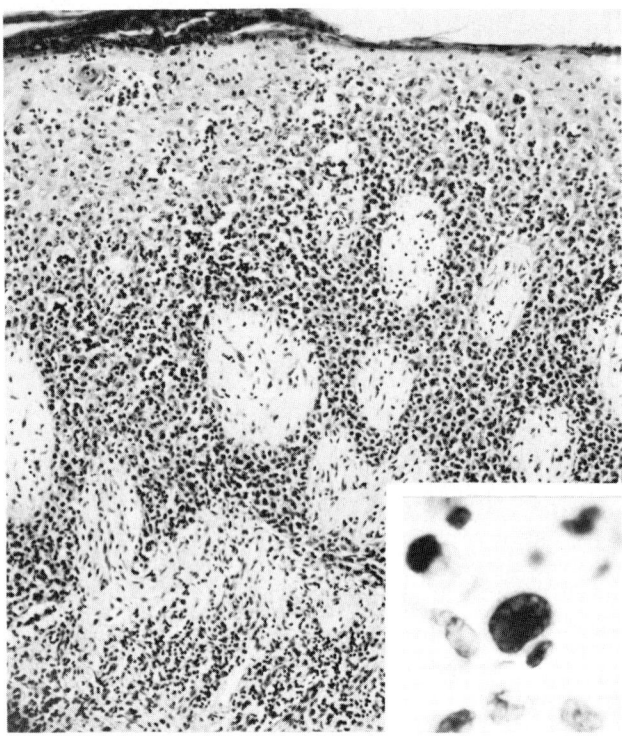

Figure 45–8.
Epidermotropic form of mycosis fungoides. Acanthotic and papillomatous epidermis is diffusely invaded by hyperchromatic mononuclear round cells. H&E. X135. Inset shows mycosis fungoides cell in the dermal infiltrate. H&E. X800.

sensitivity reaction may easily be confused with early mycosis fungoides since the epidermis shows acanthosis, parakeratosis, and round cell invasion but no spongiosis or vesiculation, whereas the dermal infiltrate is heavy and mixed and extends into the pars reticularis. This type of contact dermatitis should be mentioned in every applicable case, and the clinician should be asked to rule it out, if necessary, by intradermal testing.

Alopecia mucinosa was discussed in Chapter 19. In some cases, the mixed infiltrate may become so heavy as to suggest mycosis fungoides. In other cases follicular mucinosis has been found associated with true mycosis fungoides, and in still others the transition from benign alopecia mucinosa to lymphoblastoma has been observed clinically as well as histologically. That event is recognizable by the appearance of atypical cells in the infiltrate, and by the dissociation of the infiltrate from the altered follicles and occurring independently, usually in perivascular distribution.

There are documented cases in which psoriasis eventuated into mycosis fungoides. Histologically, this event is indicated by much heavier infiltrate than one usually sees in psoriasis, by its mixed character, and by the presence of Pautrier abscesses rather than of Munro abscesses.

Sézary Syndrome

A leukemic form of T-cell lymphoma with the clinical manifestations of generalized erythroderma, infiltration, and scaling often to the point of exfoliation is known as Sézary syndrome. The erythroderma is pruritic and may be associated with lymphadenopathy, hair loss, palmoplantar hyperkeratosis, and onychodystrophy.[46]

Histologic features of Sézary syndrome are very similar to those of mycosis fungoides.[47] A rather heavy infiltrate of predominantly small lymphocytes with variable mixture of atypical lymphoid cells is observed within the upper dermis. The infiltrate is epidermotropic forming Pautrier microabscesses. The characteristic Sézary cells are present in the peripheral blood in numbers greater than 1000/mm^3.[48] These are large lymphocytes with folded or convoluted nuclei and scanty clear or vacuolated cytoplasms, containing droplets of PAS-positive and diastase-resistant glycoprotein.[49] Enlarged lymph nodes may show a nonspecific lymphadenitis or specific infiltration of T-cell lymphoma.

Lymphomatoid Papulosis

Since Macaulay first insisted that a patient with skin eruption resembling Mucha–Habermann's disease actually had repeated periodic accumulations of malignant lymphoid cells in epidermis and dermis and therefore applied the name lymphomatoid papulosis to this continuing self-healing eruption, a number of cases and several large series have been reported.[50–52] Macaulay's disease is now considered a T-cell affection in which, apparently, clones of abnormal lymphoid cells proliferate in the dermis and are probably destroyed by an inflammatory cell reaction.[53,54]

Two clinical forms are recognized. Most commonly, trunk and extremities are involved by crops of inflammatory papular lesions that soon are covered with superficial pustules or develop into necrotic lesions that gradually heal with formation of superficial scars.[55] The second clinical form is characterized by appearance of larger and more persistent papulonodular lesions and small plaques with minimal surface changes.

The predominant histologic feature of lymphomatoid papulosis (Fig. 45–11) is the presence of

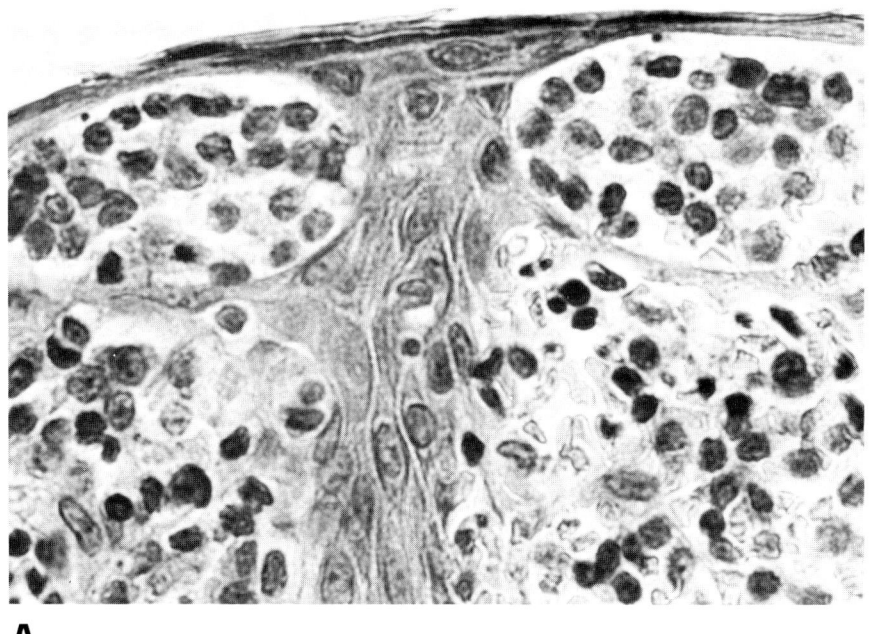

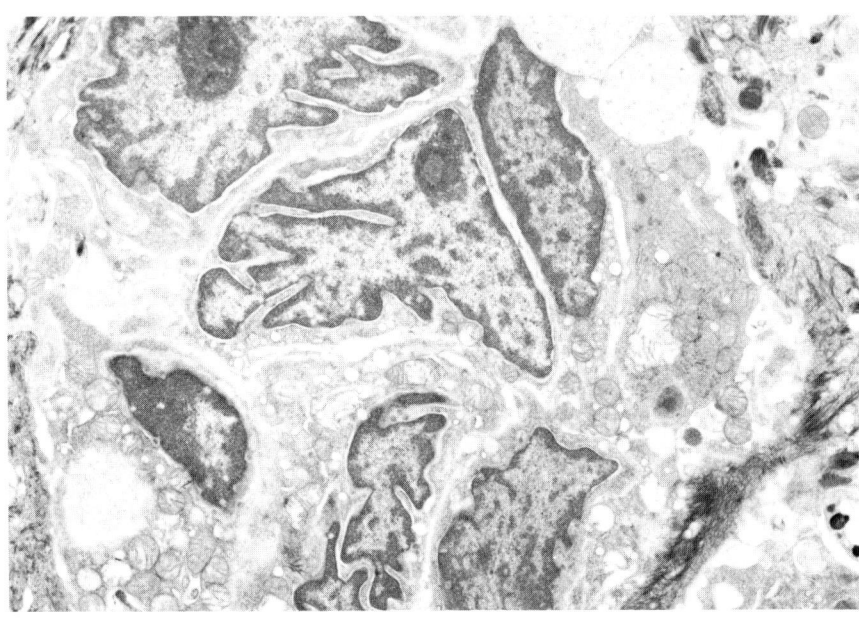

Figure 45–9.
Pautrier abscesses and Lutzner cells. **A.** Accumulations of large mononuclear cells, presumably T lymphocytes, in epidermis. H&E. X800. **B.** Electron micrograph of Lutzner cells with indented nuclei in a Pautrier abscess. (Courtesy of Dr. M. Taylor.)

atypical T lymphocytes in pars reticularis and secondary invasion of the overlying epidermis resembling a malignant lymphoma (Fig. 45–12). The degree of epidermal involvement corresponds with the stage of the lesion ranging from mild spongiotic edema and transmigration of lymphoid cells to variable degrees of epidermal cell necrosis, superficial erosion, and crusting. Dermis is involved by a wedge-shaped superficial and deep perivascular infiltrate, which rarely extends into the fat tissue (Fig. 45–13).[56,57] The composition of dermal infiltrate fits into two categories: in A type there are numerous atypical cells up to 35 μm in diameter with large bizarrely shaped nuclei, prominent nucleoli and abundant cytoplasms, and multinucleated giant cells resembling Reed–Sternberg cells. Other cells present are lymphocytes, histiocytes, neutrophils, and eosinophils. B-type shows predominantly lymphocytic infiltrate with many large cells having hyperchromatic and hyperconvoluted nuclei and a

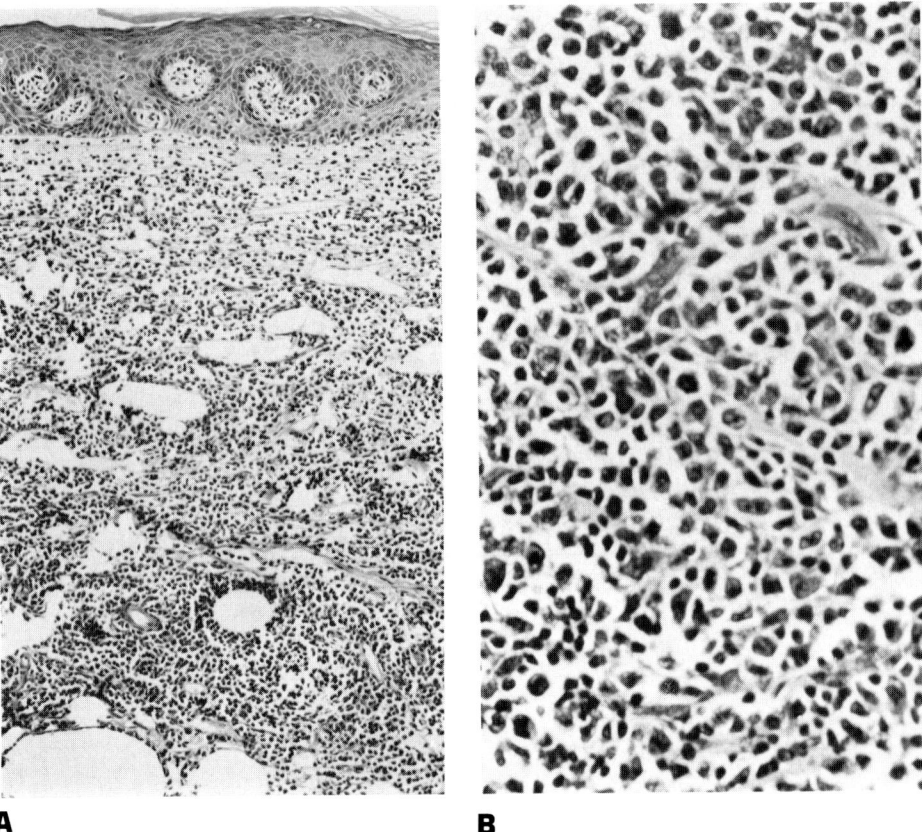

Figure 45–10.
Mycosis fungoides, tumor stages. **A.** Epidermal changes are minimal. Dermal infiltrate is heavy and deep. H&E. X125. **B.** Infiltrate consists mainly of atypical lymphocytes with hyperchromatic and convoluted nuclei. H&E. X400.

minor population of histiocytes. The large cells express pan-T-cell antigens (Leu-4 and/or Leu-5) and helper T-cell antigen (Leu-3). Other cells present include small lymphocytes and eosinophils. Malignant transformation into various lymphoproliferative diseases such as mycosis fungoides, malignant lymphoma, and Hodgkin's disease occur in 10 to 20 percent of cases.[58–60]

Pagetoid Reticulosis

Woringer–Kolopp's disease is a localized, chronic form of cutaneous T-cell disease, originally described as a single plaque on the forearm of a 13-year-old boy in 1939.[61] It was rediscovered in 1970, and a large number of cases and several series have been reported.[62] The skin lesions occur at any age as a single, asymptomatic, circinate, or hypertrophic scaly plaque often localized to the distal portion of the extremities.

The histologic picture (Fig. 45–14) of Woringer–Kolopp's disease is very characteristic. The epidermis is markedly acanthotic and shows diffuse cell infiltrate in pagetoid fashion. The infiltrating cells show large hyperchromatic and sometimes convoluted nuclei and abundant vacuolated cytoplasms.[63] Scattered mitotic figures and necrotic epithelial cells forming eosinophilic bodies are present. The infiltrate appears to be heterogeneous. Helper T cells, cytotoxic–suppressor T lymphocytes, histiocytes, and Langerhans cells have been identified.[64,65]

The clinical course is benign, and the lesion is curable by total surgical excision.[62]

Crosti's Reticulohistiocytoma of the Back

Nodules or tumors are usually localized in the back area.[66] The histologic picture is dominated by heavy infiltration of histiocytes, lymphocytes, and monocytic cells, all situated in the mid-dermis. Tumors are radiosensitive. Progression into lymphocytic lymphoma or Hodgkin's disease have been reported.[67]

Benign Lymphoplasia

Benign cutaneous lymphoplasia, lymphocytoma cutis, and lymphadenosis cutis benigna are synonymous. The clinical manifestation is that of single or multiple erythematous nodules of face, chest, or

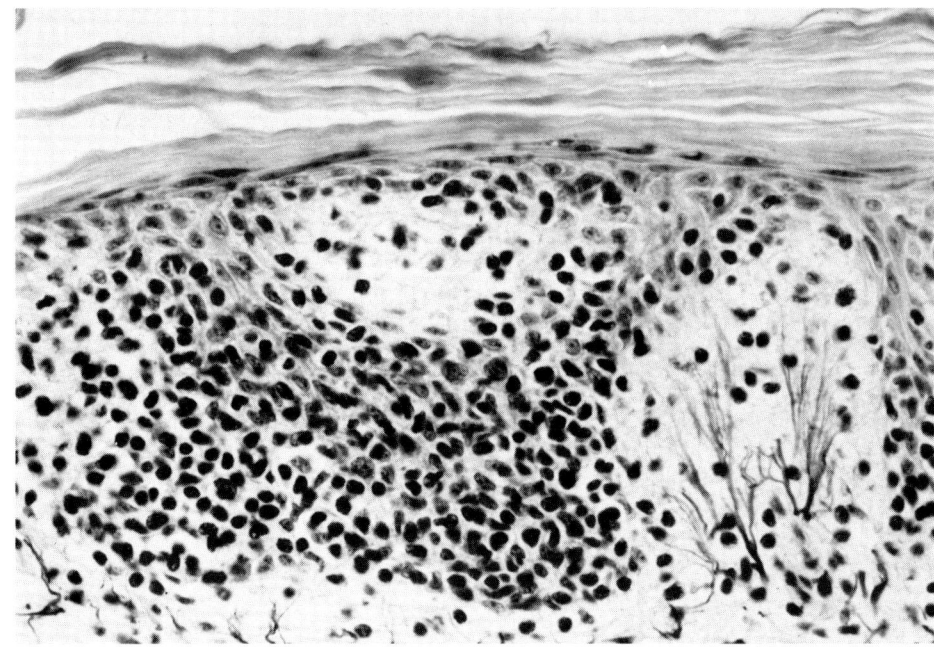

Figure 45–11.
Lymphomatoid papulosis. Early lesion of Macaulay's case. Bizarre hyperchromatic cells have invaded epidermis, which shows no evidence of acanthotic reaction (compare Fig. 45–7). O&G. X225. (From Macaulay. Arch Dermatol 97: 23, 1968.)

back (Fig. 45–15).[68] Histologic features are characterized by heavy dermal infiltrate, which may be diffuse but often is nodular or multilobulated.[69–71] The infiltrate consists predominantly of helper T lymphocytes. Macrophages, plasma cells, and Langerhans cells have also been identified.[72,73] Other features include the presence of a few eosinophils, multinucleated giant cells, and scattered mitotic figures. Some lesions show multiple foci of small lymph follicle-like structures. The epidermis and Grenz zone are intact. The pilosebaceous structures may be involved with edema and cell infiltration.

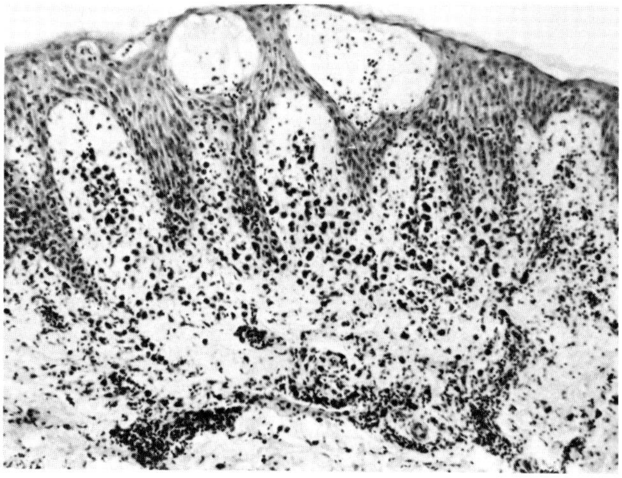

Arthropod Bite Reaction

Solitary lesions with histologic features resembling lymphoma may be unusual chronic reactions to arthropod bite (Fig. 45–16). The epidermis is often acanthotic. The dermis shows increased vascularity and massive infiltrate of lymphocytes, histiocytes, plasma cells, and eosinophils.[74] A similar histopathology may be observed in the persistent inflammatory nodular lesions following scabies.[75]

Actinic Reticuloid

Actinic reticuloid is a chronic and persistent tissue reaction to sun exposure. Infiltrated papules and plaques occur predominantly over the light-exposed skin and may spread into nonexposed areas.[76,77] Tissue sections show deep-reaching dermal infiltrate of T lymphocytes predominantly of the suppressor/cytotoxic subset mixed with some histiocytes, a few plasma cells, and eosinophils. The infiltrate may extend to involve the overlying epidermis.[78] The clinical restriction to light-exposed areas and proof of hypersensitivity to UVB, UVA, and visible light will lead to correct diagnosis.

Figure 45–12.
Lymphomatoid papulosis. Fully developed lesion shows large T cells in upper dermis, associated with inflammatory infiltrate. Epidermis is acanthotic and exhibits inflammatory and degenerating cells in vesicles. H&E. X125.

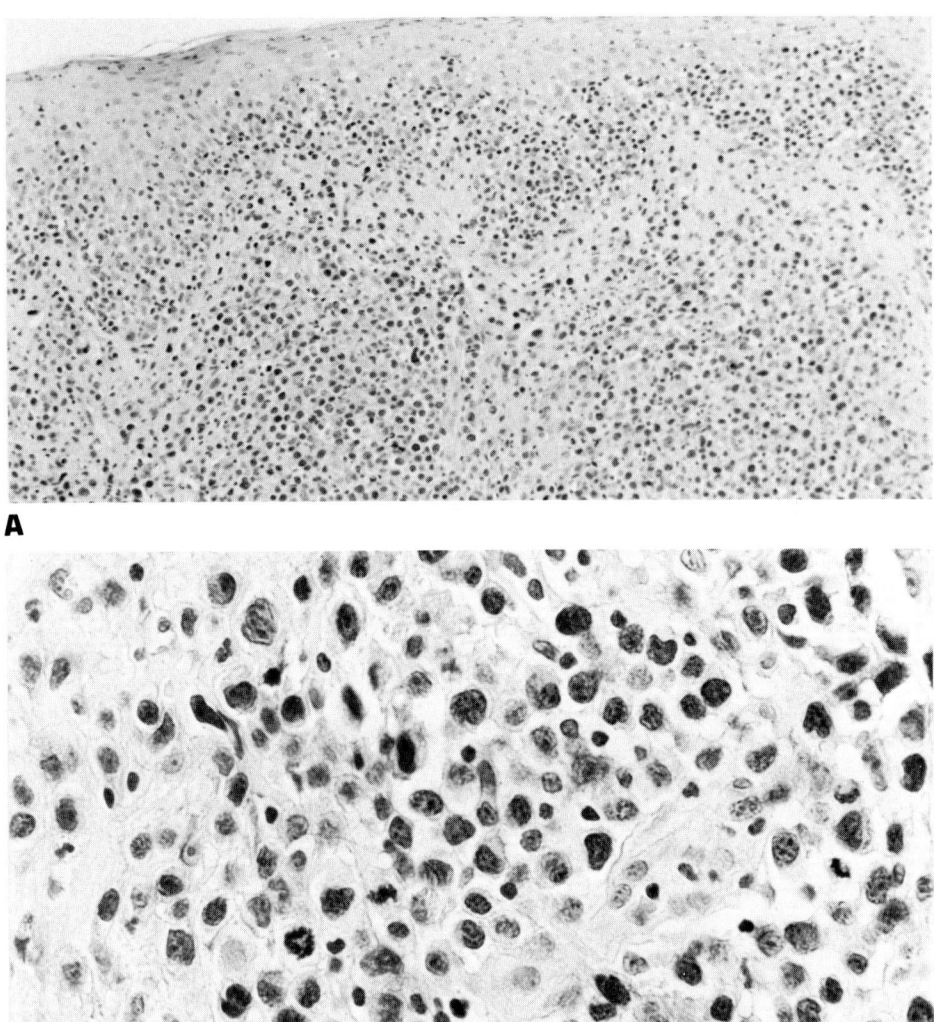

Figure 45–13.
Lymphomatoid papulosis. **A.** Diffuse involvement of the epidermis and heavy dermal infiltrate. H&E. X125. **B.** Numerous atypical cells with large and hyperchromatic nuclei. H&E. X600.

Angioimmunoblastic Lymphadenopathy

Recognized since 1975, and until then often mistaken for Hodgkin's disease, a disease of lymph nodes has been described as angioimmunoblastic lymphadenopathy.[79–81] It is considered to be a benign lymphoproliferative process, possibly due to faulty stimulation of the immune system by medication, and presents a characteristic triad of vascular neogenesis, polymorphous cellular proliferation of lymphocytes, immunoblasts, plasma cells and plasmocytoid cells, and deposits of acidophilic intercellular substances in the affected lymph nodes. In more than half of the cases, maculopapular or papulonodular skin lesions may precede development of lymph node enlargement.[82] There is also enlargement of spleen and liver associated with fever, anemia, and polyclonal gammopathy. Patients with angioimmunoblastic lymphadenopathy may go on to develop malignant lymphoma usually of immunoblastic type.

Sinus Histiocytosis with Massive Lymphadenopathy

Rosai and Dorfman[83] identified a benign self-limiting disease characterized by cervical lymphadenopathy associated with fever, elevated erythrocyte sedimentation rate, leukocytosis with neutrophilia, and polyclonal hypergammaglobulinemia. Approximately 10 percent of the patients have red-brown papular or nodular skin lesions (Fig. 45–17).[84–88] Histologically, heavy dermal infiltrate consists of histiocytes with large vesicular nuclei and abundant pale-staining cytoplasms. Mixture of histiocytes and

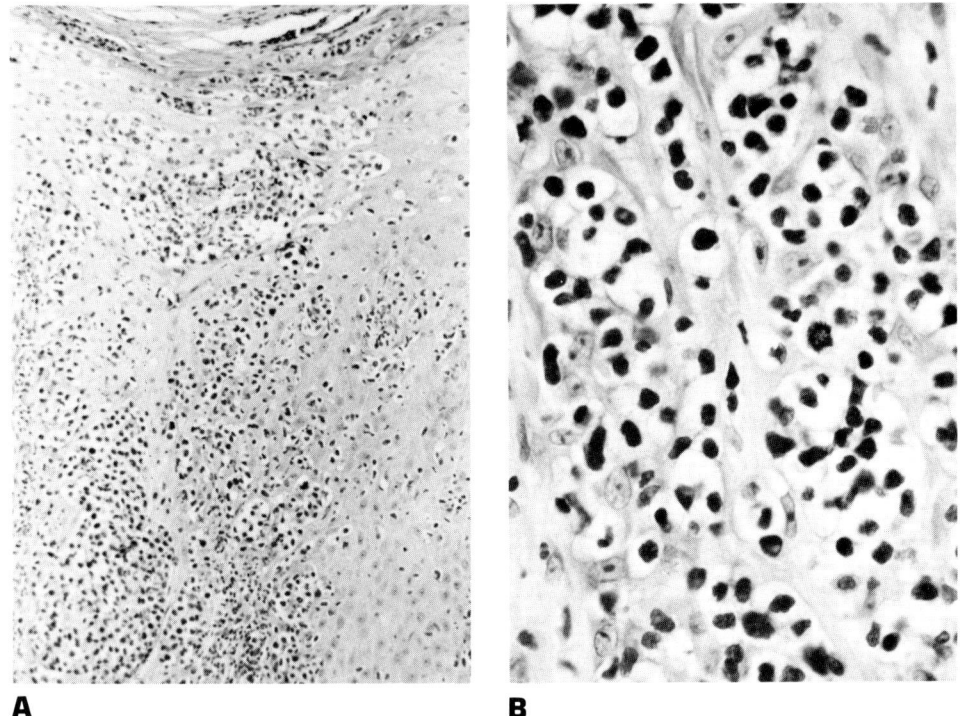

Figure 45–14.
Woringer-Kolopp disease. H&E. **A.** X135. **B.** X600.

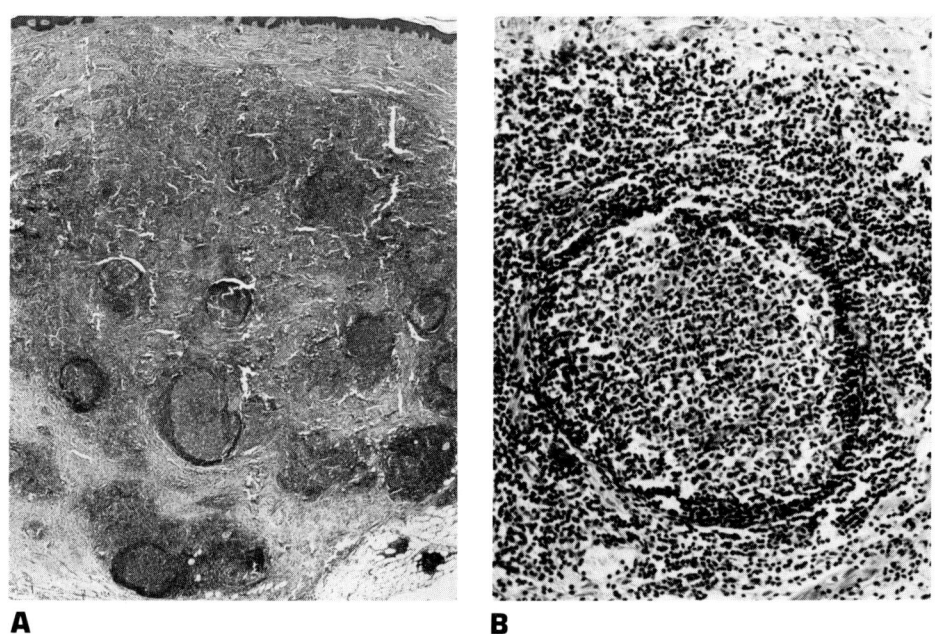

Figure 45–15.
Lymphocytoma cutis (lymphadenosis cutis benigna). Well-delineated germinal centers surrounded by small lymphocytes in lymphadenoid pattern. **A.** H&E. X30. **B.** H&E. X135.

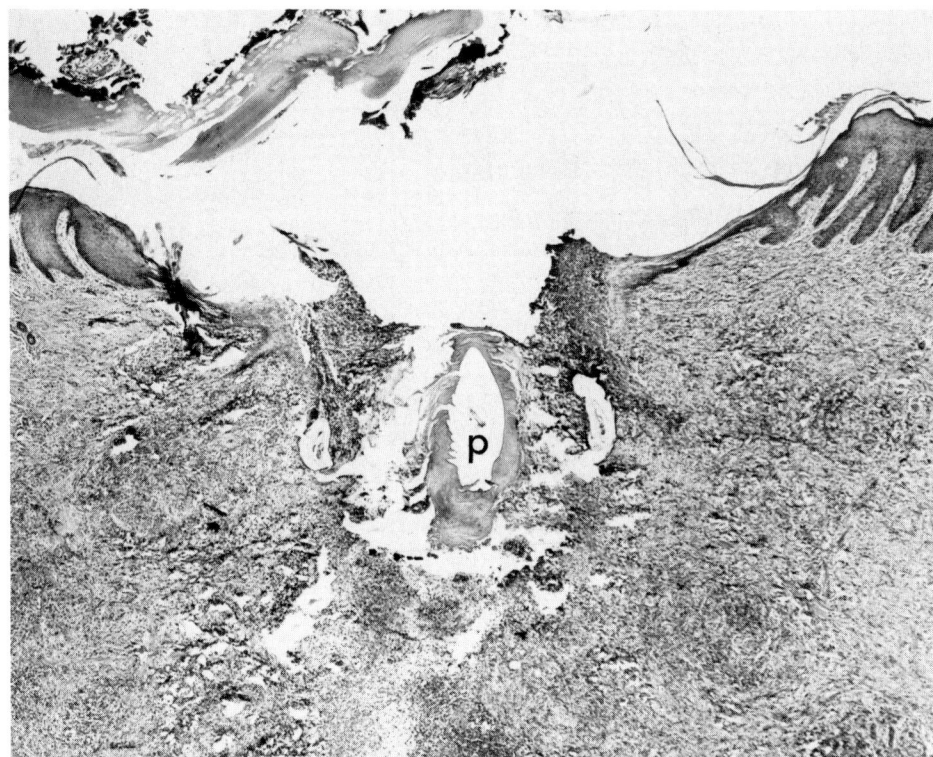

Figure 45–16.
Arthropod bite reaction. Proboscis of tick (p) is embedded in heavy granulomatous infiltrate in dermis which contains many eosinophils, while parts of chitinous shell of engorged body are visible near upper rim of picture. H&E. X30.

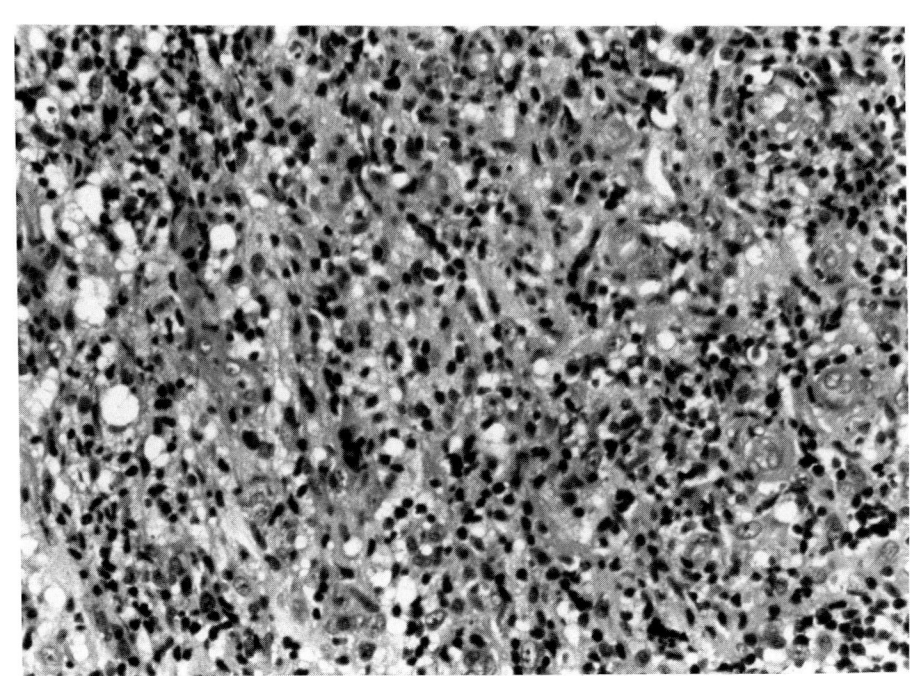

Figure 45–17.
Sinus histiocytosis with massive adenopathy. Large lipid-laden histiocytes are embedded in an infiltrate of lymphocytes and plasma cells. H&E. X225.

lymphocytes may form lymphoid structures. Histiocytes are rich in phagosomes and may contain comma-shaped bodies.

Cutaneous Malignant Histiocytosis

Another condition in which cutaneous involvement is a prominent feature is malignant histiocytosis.[89] Fever, weight loss, and inflammatory subcutaneous nodular lesions are major clinical features (Fig. 45–18). Histologic sections show involvement of deep dermis and subcutaneous fat tissue with atypical large histiocytes with hyperchromatic nuclei and folded nuclear membrane.[90] Some of these cells may show erythrophagocytosis. Multinucleated cells, lymphocytes, foamy histiocytes, and plasma cells are also present.

Lymphomatoid Granulomatosis

Lymphomatoid granulomatosis, described by Liebow et al. in 1972 is an angiocentric and angiodestructive infiltrative process affecting the lung in all cases and the skin and nervous system in one third of the patients.[91] The cutaneous lesions may appear before pulmonary or nervous system manifestations and range from maculopapular eruption to nodular and ulcerative lesions (Fig. 45–19).[92,93] Histologically, there is a distinctive angiocentric infiltrate involving both the superficial and deep vessels and involvement of cutaneous appendages and the subcutaneous fat tissue. The infiltrate is highly polymorphous and consists of dysplastic lymphoid cells exhibiting multiple nuclear indentations and clefts.

Urticaria Pigmentosa and Mastocytosis

Mast cells are normal components of the dermis and are found in small numbers mainly in the surroundings of the capillary blood vessels and cutaneous adnexa (Fig. 45–20). Larger numbers occur without pathologic significance in the stroma of benign tumors and basal cell epitheliomas. Heavy dermal infiltrate of mast cells is almost pathognomonic of urticaria pigmentosa. Papules and nodules composed of mast cells are usually benign and often self-healing skin lesions. In some cases, however, they are part of systemic mastocytosis.[94–96] The histologic picture of urticaria pigmentosa (Fig. 45–21) varies from massive accumulations of mast cells in the entire dermis to a moderate increase in perivascular arrangement.[97] The former is more often found in children and the latter in adults. Cutaneous lesions may contain 9 to 160 times more mast cells than normal skin.[98]

Because the granules do not stain specifically in H&E sections, mast cells may be overlooked or mistaken for histiocytes. Special stain (toluidine blue–alcian blue–PAS) are necessary. Routine use of O&G

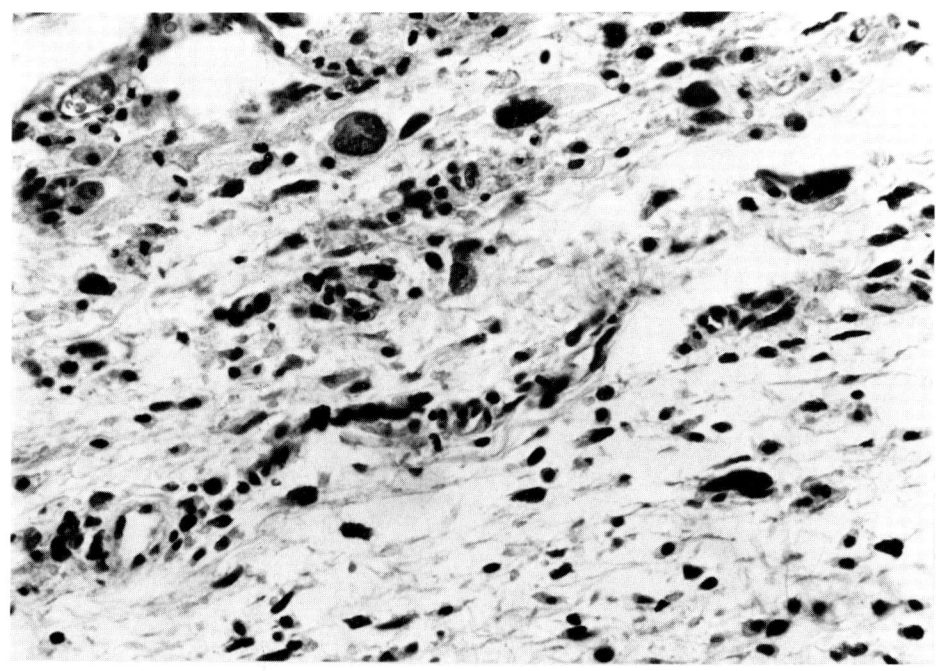

Figure 45–18.
Malignant histiocytosis. Deep dermal infiltrate of atypical histiocytes with hyperchromatic and multilobulated nuclei. H&E. X600.

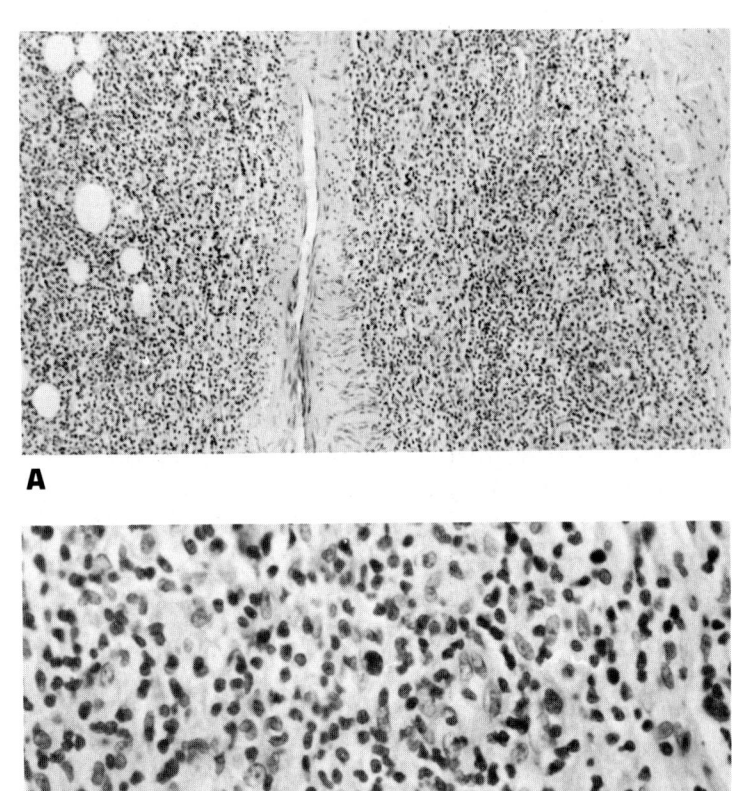

Figure 45–19.
Lymphomatoid granulomatosis. **A.** Dense granulomatous infiltrate surrounds a thick-walled artery in fat tissue. H&E. X125. **B.** Details of mixed granulomatous infiltrate at higher power. H&E. X400.

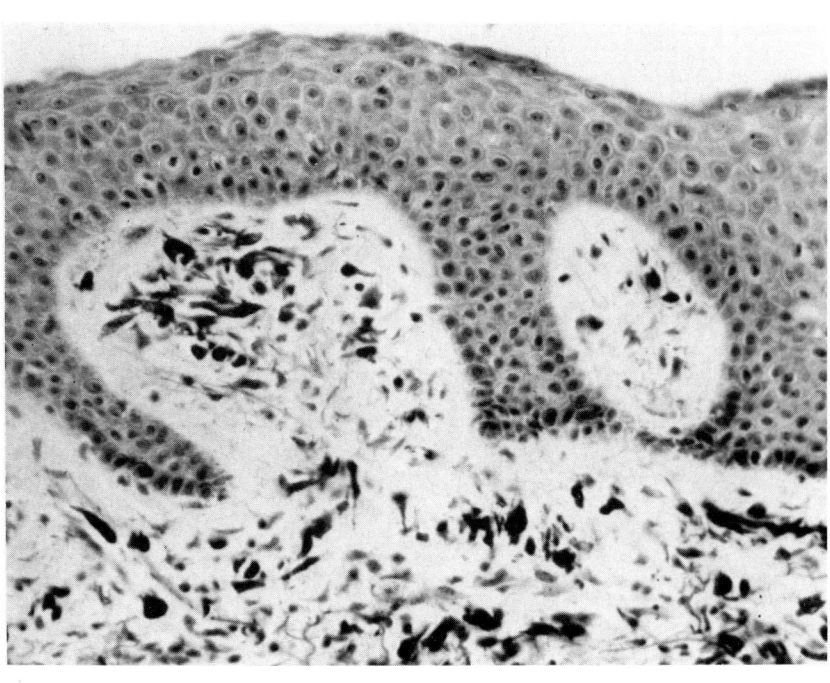

Figure 45–20.
Urticaria pigmentosa. Dark-staining mast cells are gathered around superficial capillary blood vessels. O&G. X400.

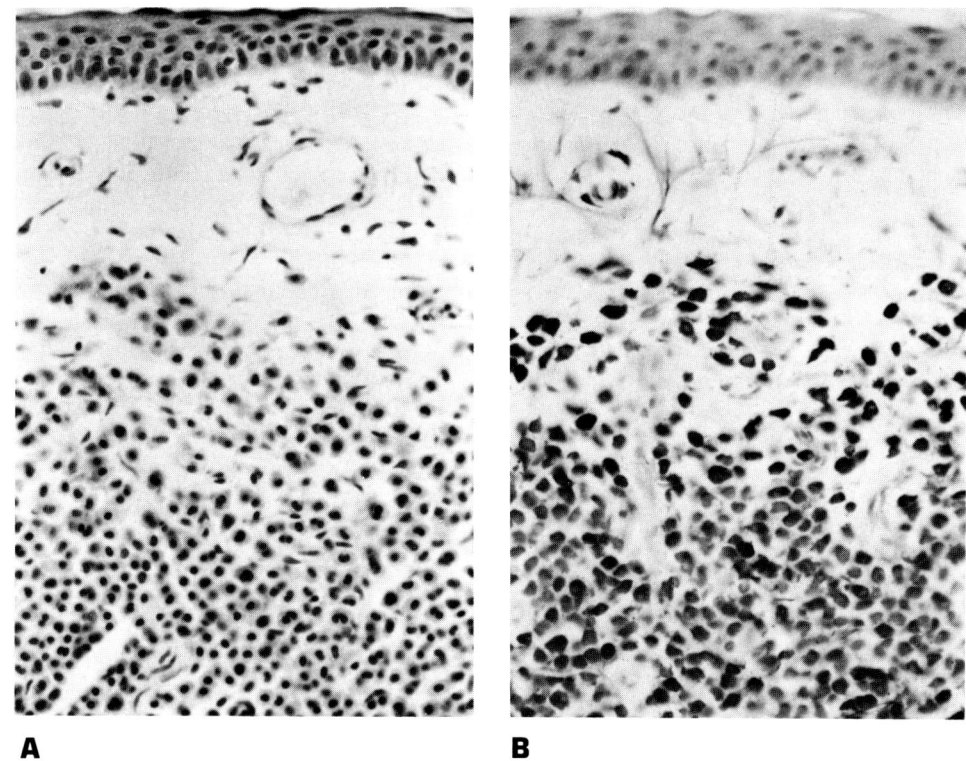

Figure 45–21.
Urticaria pigmentosa. **A.** Dense dermal infiltrate of cells that have moderate amount of stainable cytoplasm. H&E. X250. **B.** Similar section stained with O&G shows dense cytoplasmic granulation of mast cells. O&G. X250.

stain obviates this difficulty. Mast cells granules are stained purple by this method.

Bullous urticaria pigmentosa observed mainly in infancy shows marked papillary edema and subepidermal blister formation.[99–100] An adult variant called telangiectasia macularis eruptiva perstans needs special attention since it shows only a relative increase in the number of mast cells.[101]

REFERENCES

1. Rappaport H: Tumors of the Hematopoietic System. Atlas of Tumor Pathology, Sec 3, Fascicle 8. Washington, DC: Armed Forces Institute of Pathology, 1966
2. Foon KA, Schroff RW, Gale RP: Surface markers on leukemia and lymphoma cells: Recent advances. Blood 60:1, 1982
3. Wright JE: Immunoperoxidase in dermatopathology. J Assoc Mil Dermatol 9:46, 1983
4. Wick MR, Hagen KA, Frizzera G: Three immunostaining techniques for the localization of leukocyte common antigen in formalin-fixed paraffin-embedded dermatological biopsy specimens. Am J Dermatopathol 9:250, 1987
5. Murphy GF, Mihm MC Jr : Lymphoproliferative disorders of the skin. Stoneham MA: Butterworths, 1986
6. Van Vloten WA, Willemze R, Lange Vejlsgaard G, Thomsen K: Cutaneous lymphoma. In: Current Problems in Dermatology, Vol. 19. Farmington, Conn: S. Karger, 1990
7. Burg G, Braun-Falco O: Cutaneous lymphomas, pseudolymphomas, and related disorders. Berlin: Springer-Verlag, 1983
8. Lukes RJ, Collins RD: Immunologic characterization of human malignant lymphomas, Cancer 34:1488, 1974
9. Dorfman RF: Pathology of the non-Hodgkin's lymphomas: New classifications. Cancer Treat Rep 61: 945, 1977
10. Henry K, Bennett MH, Farrer-Brown G: Morphological classification on non-Hodgkin's lymphomas. Recent results. Cancer Res 64:38, 1978
11. Mathé G, Rappaport H, O'Connor GT, et al: Histological and cytological typing of neoplastic diseases of hematopoietic and lymphoid tissues. In WHO International Histological Classification of Tumors, No. 14. Geneva: World Health Organization, 1976

12. Gerard-Marchant R, Hamlin I, Lennert K, et al: Classification of non-Hodgkin's lymphomas. Lancet 2:406, 1974
13. Lennert K, Mohri N: Histopathology and diagnosis of non-Hodgkin's lymphomas. In Uehlinger E (ed): Malignant Lymphomas Other than Hodgkin's Disease. New York: Springer-Verlag, 1978, pp 111–469
14. The Non-Hodgkin's Lymphoma Pathologic Classification Project. National Cancer Institute sponsored study of classification of non-Hodgkin's lymphoma: Summary and description of a working formulation for clinical usage. Cancer 49:2112, 1982
15. Buechner SA, Li C-Y, Su DWP: Leukemia cutis. A histopathologic study of 42 cases. Am J Dermatopathol 7:109, 1985
16. Sun NCJ, Ellis R: Granulocytic sarcoma of the skin. Arch Dermatol 116:800, 1980
17. Foldes C, Vignon-Pennamen M-D, Rostoker G, Cottenot F: Plasmocytome cutané. Ann Dermatol Venereol 115:1217, 1988
18. Burke WA, Merritt CC, Briggaman RA: Disseminated extramedullary plasmacytomas. J Am Acad Dermatol 14:335, 1986
19. Kois JM, Sexton FM, Lookinbill DP: Cutaneous manifestations of multiple myeloma. Arch Dermatol 127:69, 1991
20. Patterson JW, Parsons JM, White RM, et al: Cutaneous involvement of multiple myeloma and extramedullary plasmocytoma. J Am Acad Dermatol 19:879, 1988
21. Baer MR, Barcos M, Farrell H, et al: Acute myelogenous leukemia with leukemia cutis. Eighteen cases seen between 1969 and 1986. Cancer 63:2192, 1989
22. Smith JL, Butler JJ: Skin involvement in Hodgkin's disease. Cancer 45:354, 1980
23. Gordon RA, Lookingbill DP, Abt AB: Skin infiltration in Hodgkin's disease. Arch Dermatol 116:1038, 1980
24. White RM, Patterson JW: Cutaneous involvement in Hodgkin's disease. Cancer 55:1136, 1985
25. Torne R, Umbert P: Hodgkin's disease presenting with superficial lymph nodes and tumors of the scalp. Dermatologica 172:225, 1986
26. Hait WN, Farber L, Cadman E: Non-Hodgkin's lymphoma for the nononcologist. JAMA 253:1431, 1985
27. Knobler RM, Edelson RL: Cutaneous T-cell lymphoma. Med Clin North Am 70:109, 1986
28. Mukai K, Sato Y, Watanabe S, et al: Non-Hodgkin lymphoma of the skin excluding mycosis fungoides and cutaneous involvement of adult T-cell leukemia/lymphoma. J Cutan Pathol 15:193, 1988
29. Sterry W, Korte B, Schubert C: Pleomorphic T-cell lymphoma and large-cell anaplastic lymphoma of the skin. A morphological, immunophenotypical and ultrastructural study of two typical cases. Am J Dermatopathol 11:112, 1989
30. Armitage JO, Greer JP, Levine AM, et al: Peripheral T-cell lymphoma. Cancer 63:158, 1989
31. Nagatani T, Kim ST, Baba N, et al: Phenotypic heterogeneity of lymphoma of the skin. J Dermatol Tokyo 16:443, 1989
32. Weinstock MA, Horn JW: Mycosis fungoides in the United States. JAMA 250:42, 1988
33. Zackheim HS: Cutaneous T-cell lymphomas. A review of the recent literature. Arch Dermatol 117:295, 1981
34. Van Scott EJ, Clendenning WE, Brecher G: Mycosis fungoides. Relationship to malignant cutaneous reticulosis and the Sézary syndrome. Arch Dermatol 89:785, 1964
35. Eng AM, Blekys I, Worobec SM: Clinicopathologic correlations in Alibert-type mycosis fungoides. Arch Dermatol 117:332, 1981
36. Lindae ML, Abel EA, Hoppe RT, Wood GS: Poikilodermatous mycosis fungoides and atrophic large-plaque parapsoriasis exhibit similar abnormalities of T-cell antigen expression. Arch Dermatol 124:366, 1988
37. Edelson RL: Cutaneous T-cell lymphoma: Mycosis fungoides, Sézary syndrome, and other variants. J Am Acad Dermatol 2:89, 1980
38. Buechner SA, Winkelmann RK, Banks PM: T cell and T-cell subsets in mycosis fungoides and parapsoriasis. A study of 18 cases with anti-human T-cell monoclonal antibodies and histochemical techniques. Arch Dermatol 120:897, 1984
39. Norris DH: The pathogenesis of mycosis fungoides. Clin Exp Dermatol 6:77, 1981
40. Hashimoto K, Iwahara K: Immunoelectron microscopy related to T-cell monoclonal surface antigen in mycosis fungoides. Am J Dermatopathol 5:129, 1983
41. Hashimoto K: Electron microscopy for diagnosis of selected dermatoses. Semin Dermatol 3:36, 1984
42. Hantanyapong Y, Iwahara K, Zhuan KG, et al: Comparison of the nuclear contour index (NCI) and T-cell subsets of erythematous, plaque and tumor lesions in patients with mycosis fungoides (MF). J Dermatol Tokyo 14:43, 1987
43. Tosca AD, Varelzidis AG, Economidou J, Stratigos JD: Mycosis fungoides: Evaluation of immunohistochemical criteria for the early diagnosis of the disease and differentiation between stages. J Am Acad Dermatol 15:237, 1986
44. Lazar AP, Caro WA, Roenigk HH Jr, Pinski KS: Parapsoriasis and mycosis fungoides; The Northwestern University experience 1970 to 1985. J Am Acad Dermatol 21:919, 1989
45. Everett MA: Early diagnosis of mycosis fungoides: Vacuolar interface dermatitis. J Cutan Pathol 12:271, 1985
46. Wieselthier JS, Koh HK: Sézary syndrome: Diagnosis, prognosis and critical review of treatment options. J Am Acad Dermatol 22:381, 1990
47. Sentis HJ, Willemze R, Scheffer E: Histopathologic studies in Sézary syndrome and erythrodermic mycosis fungoides: A comparison with benign forms of erythroderma. J Am Acad Dermatol 15:1217, 1986
48. Buechner SA, Winkelman RK: Sézary syndrome. A

clinicopathologic study of 39 cases. Arch Dermatol 119:979, 1983
49. Whang-Peng J, Lutzner M, Edelson R, et al: Cytogenetic studies and clinical implications in patients with Sézary's syndrome. Cancer 38:861, 1976
50. Macaulay WL: Lymphomatoid papulosis. A continuing self-healing eruption, clinically benign–histologically malignant. Arch Dermatol 97:23, 1968
51. Sanchez NP, Pittelkow MR, Muller SA, et al: The clinicopathologic spectrum of lymphomatoid papulosis: Study of 31 cases. J Am Acad Dermatol 8:81, 1983
52. Thomsen K, Wautziu GL: Lymphomatoid papulosis: A follow-up study of 30 patients. J Am Acad Dermatol 17:632, 1987
53. Wood GS, Strickler JG, Deneau DG, et al: Lymphomatoid papulosis expresses immunophenotypes associated with T-cell lymphoma but not inflammation. J Am Acad Dermatol 15:444, 1986
54. Weiss LM, Wood GS, Trela M, et al: Clonal T-cell populations in lymphomatoid papulosis. Evidence of a lymphoproliferative origin for a clinically benign disease. N Engl J Med 315:475, 1986
55. Wantzin GL, Thomsen K, Hou-Jensen K: Lymphomatoid papulosis: A follow-up study. Acta Derm Venereol 64:46, 1984
56. Willemze R, Scheffer E: Clinical and histologic differentiation between lymphomatoid papulosis and pityriasis lichenoides. J Am Acad Dermatol 13:418, 1985
57. Sina B, Burnett JW: Lymphomatoid papulosis. Case reports and literature review. Arch Dermatol 119:189, 1983
58. Wantzin GL, Thomsen K, Brandrup F, Larsen JK: Lymphomatoid papulosis. Development into cutaneous T-cell lymphoma. Arch Dermatol 121:792, 1985
59. Harrington DS, Braddock SW, Blocher KS, et al: Lymphomatoid papulosis and progression to T-cell lymphoma: An immunophenotypic and genotypic analysis. J Am Acad Dermatol 21:951, 1989
60. Lederman JS, Sober AJ, Harrist TJ, Lederman GS: Lymphomatoid papulosis following Hodgkin's disease. J Am Acad Dermatol 16:331, 1987
61. Woringer F, Kolopp P: Lésion érythémato-squameuse polycyclique de l'avant-bras évoluant depuis 6 ans chez un garçonet de 13 ans. Histologiquement infiltrat intraépidermique d'apparence tumorale. Ann Dermatol Syphiligr 10:945, 1939
62. Mandojana RM, Helwig EB: Localized epidermotropic reticulosis (Woringer-Kolopp disease). A clinicopathologic study of 15 new cases. J Am Acad Dermatol 8:813, 1983
63. Deneau DG, Wood GS, Beckstead J, et al: Woringer–Kolopp disease (pagetoid reticulosis). Four cases with histopathologic, ultrastructural, and immunohistologic observations. Arch Dermatol 120:1045, 1984
64. Mielke V, Wolff HH, Winzer M, Sterry W: Localized and disseminated pagetoid reticulosis. Diagnostic immunophenotypical findings. Arch Dermatol 125:402, 1989
65. Natarajan S, Wilson PD: Pagetoid reticulosis (Woringer–Kolopp disease): Histiocyte marker (lysozyme) study and ultrastructural observations. Dermatologica 171:332, 1985
66. Gamby T, Chaudon J-P, Dor J-F, et al: La réticulose de Crosti. A propos de 3 cas dont un avec étude ultrastructurale. Ann Dermatol Venereol 105:821, 1978
67. Brizido E, Themido RB, Menezes-Brandao F, et al: Reticulose de Crosti Revisao de quinze casos. Med Cutan ILA 15:17, 1987
68. Lange-Wantzin G, Hou-Jensen K, Nielsen M, et al: Cutaneous lymphocytomas: Clinical and histological aspects. Acta Derm Venereol 62:119, 1982
69. Geerts ML, Kaiserling E: A morphologic study of lymphadenosis benigna cutis. Dermatologica 170:121, 1985
70. Van Hale HM, Winkelmann RK: Nodular lymphoid disease of the head and neck: Lymphocytoma cutis, benign lymphocytic infiltrate of Jessner, and their distinction from malignant lymphoma. J Am Acad Dermatol 12:455, 1985
71. Iwatsuki K, Yamada M, Takigawa M, et al: Benign lymphoplasia of the earlobes induced by gold earrings: Immunohistologic study on the cellular infiltrate. J Am Acad Dermatol 16:83, 1987
72. Smolle J, Kaudewitz P, Aberer E, et al: Immunohistochemical classification of cutaneous lymphomas and pseudolymphomas. Hautarzt 38:461, 1987
73. Medeiros JL, Picker LJ, Abel EA, et al: Cutaneous lymphoid hyperplasia. Immunologic characteristics and assessment of criteria and recently proposed as diagnostic of malignant lymphoma. J Am Acad Dermatol 21:929, 1989
74. Aoki K, Mori M, Kamata H, Suzuki H: Tick bites: A study using scanning electron microscopy. J Dermatol Tokyo 9:79, 1982
75. Konstantinov D, Stanoeva L: Persistent scabious nodules. Dermatologica 147:321, 1973
76. Ive FA, Magnus IA, Warin PP, et al: "Actinic reticuloid." A chronic dermatosis associated with severe photosensitivity and the histological resemblance to lymphoma. Br J Dermatol 81:469, 1969
77. Toonstra J, Henquet CJM, Van Weelden H, et al: Actinic reticuloid. A clinical photobiologic, histopathologic and follow-up study of 16 patients. J Am Acad Dermatol 21:205, 1989
78. Norris PG, Morris J, Smith NP, et al: Chronic actinic dermatitis: An immunohistologic and photobiologic study. J Am Acad Dermatol 21:966, 1989
79. Lukes RJ, Tindle BH: Immunoblastic lymphadenopathy: A hyperimmune entity resembling Hodgkin's disease. N Engl J Med 292:1, 1975
80. Lessana-Leibowitch M, Mignot L, Bloch C, et al: Manifestations cutanées des lymphoadénopathies angioimmunoblastiques. Ann Dermatol Venereol 104:603, 1977
81. Matloff RB, Neiman RS: Angioimmunoblastic lym-

phadenopathy. A generalized lymphoproliferative disorder with cutaneous manifestations. Arch Dermatol 114:92, 1978
82. Seehafer JR, Goldberg NC, Dicken CH, Su WPD: Cutaneous manifestations of angioimmunoblastic lymphadenopathy. Arch Dermatol 116:41, 1980
83. Foucar E, Rosai J, Dorfman RF: Sinus histiocytosis with massive lymphadenopathy. Current status and future directions. Arch Dermatol 124:1211, 1988
84. Lazar AP, Esterly NB, Gonzales-Crussi F: Sinus histiocytosis clinically limited to the skin. Pediatr Dermatol 4:247, 1986
85. Lorette G, Garand G, Monegier du Sorbier C, et al: Histiocytose sinusale avec manifestations cutanees. Ann Dermatol Venereol 114:1430, 1987
86. Aso M, Hagari Y, Shimao S, et al: A case of cutaneous involvement by sinus histiocytosis with massive lymphadenopathy. J Dermatol Tokyo 14:253, 1987
87. Berti E, Alessi E, Caputo R, et al: Reticulohistiocytoma of the dorsum. J Am Acad Dermatol 19:259, 1988
88. Olsen EA, Crawford JR, Vollmer RT: Sinus histiocytosis with massive lymphadenopathy. J Am Acad Dermatol 18:1322, 1988
89. Ducatman BS, Wick MR, Morgan TW, et al: Malignant histiocytosis: A clinical, histological and immunohistochemical study of 20 cases. Hum Pathol 15:368, 1984
90. Chen M, Takemiya M, Miyauchi S, et al: Malignant histiocytosis. J Dermatol Tokyo 15:420, 1988
91. Katzenstein A-L A, Carrington CB, Liebow AA: Lymphomatoid granulomatosis. A clinicopathologic study of 152 cases. Cancer 43:360, 1979
92. Bender BL, Kapadia SB, Synkowski DR, et al: Lymphomatoid granulomatosis preceded by chronic granulomatous dermatitis. Arch Dermatol 114:1547, 1978
93. Kessler S, Lund HZ, Leonard DD: Cutaneous lesions of lymphomatoid granulomatosis. Comparison with lymphomatoid papulosis. Am J Dermatopathol 3:115, 1981
94. Stein DH: Mastocytosis: A review. Pediatr Dermatol 3:365, 1986
95. Lo W-L, Wong C-K: Systemic mastocytosis. Case report and literature review. J Dermatol Tokyo 14:483, 1987
96. Redondo Mateo JR, Vaquero Perez M, Guinea Esquerdo L: Mastocitosis sistemica. Med Cutan ILA 18:162, 1990
97. Akiyama M: A clinical and histological study of urticaria pigmentosa: Relationships between mast cell proliferation and the clinical and histological manifestations. J Dermatol Tokyo 17:347, 1990
98. Kasper CS, Freeman RG, Tharp MD: Diagnosis of mastocytosis subsets using a morphometric point counting technique. Arch Dermatol 123:1017, 1987
99. Allison J: Skin mastocytosis presenting as a neonatal bullous eruption. Aust J Dermatol 9:83, 1967
100. Miller RC, Shapiro L: Bullous urticaria pigmentosa in infancy. Arch Dermatol 91:595, 1965
101. Francés C, Boisnic S, Belaiche J, et al: Mastocytose systemique maligne de l'adulte avec manifestations cutanées, A type de telangiectasia eruptiva macularis perstans. Ann Dermatol Venereol 114:1379, 1987

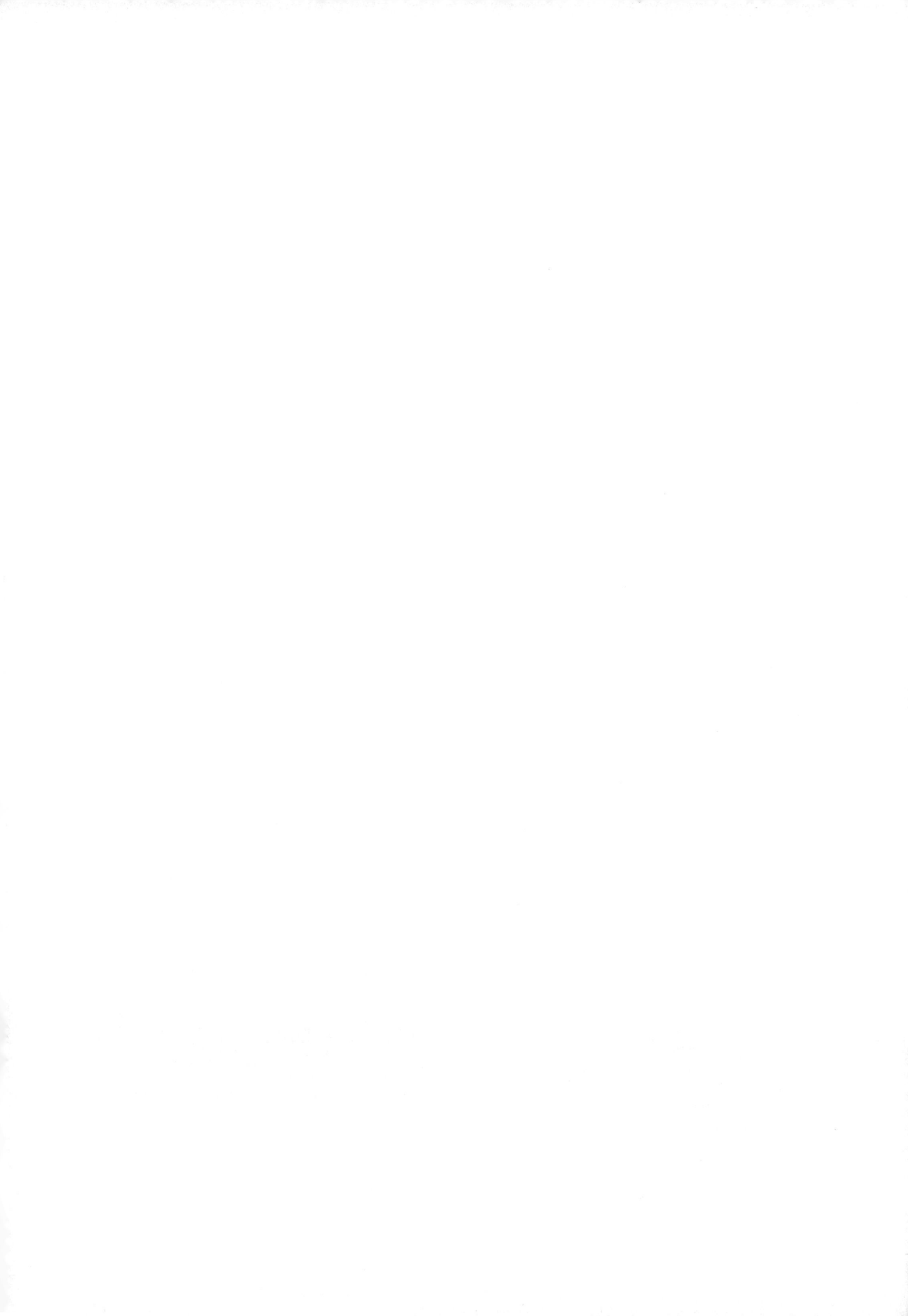

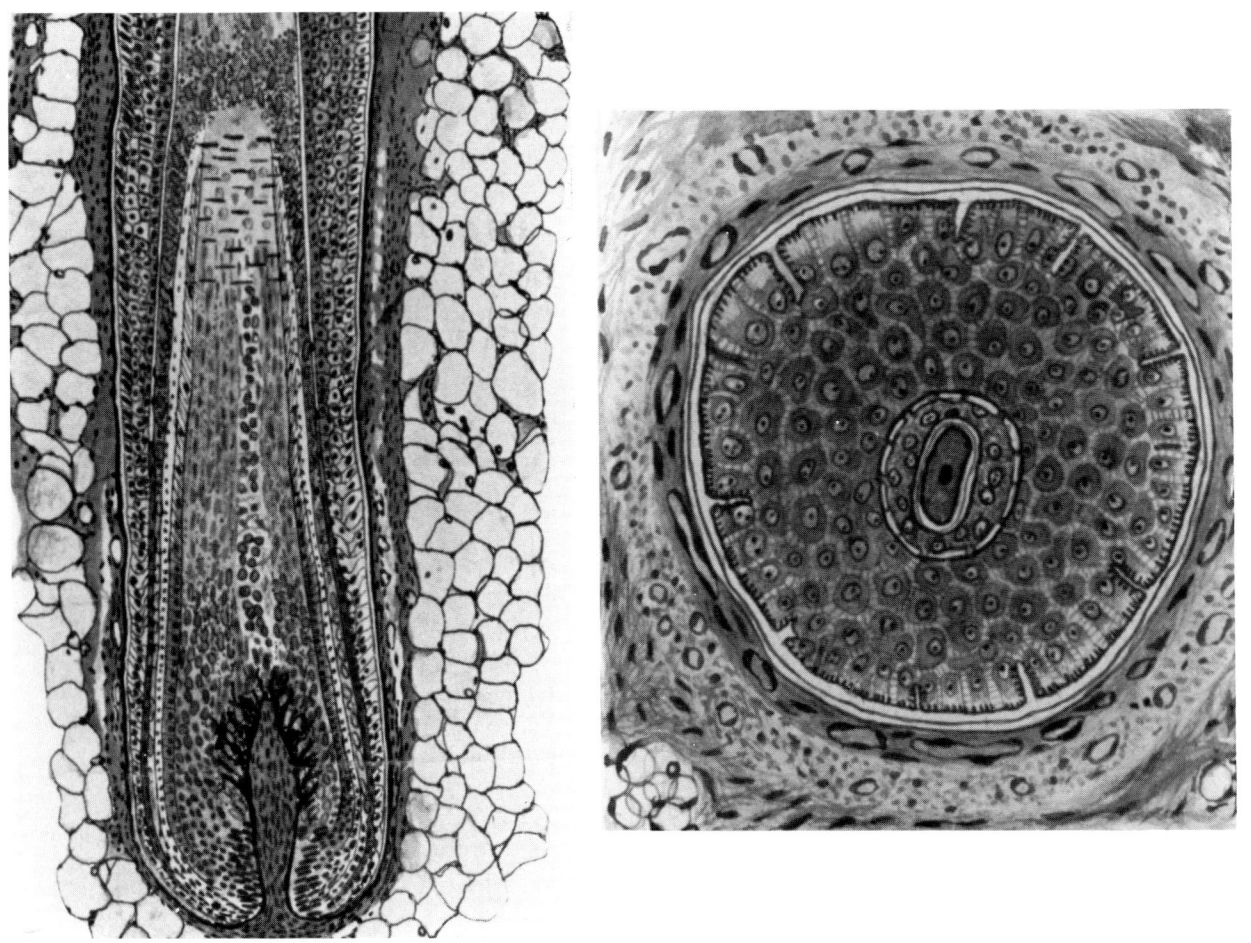

Hair follicle in longitudinal (*left*) and transverse sections (*right*).

SECTION VIII

MUCOUS MEMBRANES, HAIR, AND NAIL

After discussing histopathology of the skin, we feel there are three portions of the body surface left that have their peculiarities and need special techniques and knowledge for adequate examination. The plan of the *Guide* brings together changes that enter differential diagnosis in the examination of a tissue section or other microscopic material. The accessible mucous membranes of mouth, nose, eye, and anogenital area have features that do not lend themselves to exact comparison with those of the diseases of the skin proper but have similarities to each other. The hair and nail are tissues that require special handling and special knowledge of their structure under normal and pathologic circumstances. Thus, we decided to unite mucous membranes, hair, and nail in one section.

Details of the histology of oral mucosa has been reviewed by Squier et al.[1] In addition, three recent publications[2–5] and a color atlas cover diseases of the mucous membranes.[6] In this section we shall restrict discussion to dermatoses and some neoplastic lesions of the mucosa that are apt to come to the attention of dermatologists.

The hair has attracted considerable attention in the past decade. An international congress[7] on hair research in 1979 dealt with many aspects of normal and pathologic hair, and two comprehensive books were published in 1990.[8,9] Two other publications in 1987 have covered diseases of the hair and recent advances.[10–11] The nail was also treated in several books.[12–15] Our discussion will be somewhat short and will pay attention only to some features of diagnostic interest.

REFERENCES

1. Squier CA, Johnson NW, Hopps, RM: Human oral mucosa. Development, Structure and Function. Oxford, London: Blackwell, 1976
2. Cawson RA, Eveson JW: Oral Pathology and Diagnosis. Philadelphia: WB Saunders, 1987
3. Rogers RS III: Diseases of the mucous membranes. In: Dermatologic Clinics. Philadelphia: WB Saunders, 1987
4. Novick NL: Diseases of the mucous membranes. In: Clinics in Dermatology. Philadelphia: J.B. Lippincott, 1987
5. Tovell HMM, Young AW Jr: Diseases of the vulva in clinical practice. Elsevier Science Publishing Co. New York, 1990
6. Laskaris G: Color Atlas of Oral Diseases. New York: Thieme-Stratton, 1988
7. First International Congress of Hair Research. Hamburg, 1979
8. Orfanos CE, Happle R: Hair and hair diseases. Springer-Verlag, Berlin 1990
9. Rook A, Dawber R: Disease of the hair and scalp. 2nd edition. Blackwell Scientific Publisher, 1990
10. Baden HP: Diseases of the Hair and Nails. Chicago: Year Book Medical Publishers, 1987

11. Mitchell AJ, Krull EA: Hair disorders. In Dermatology Clinics, Philadelphia: WB Saunders, 1987
12. Zaias N: The Nail in Health and Disease. New York: SP Medical and Scientific Books, 1980
13. Beaven DW, Brooks SE: Color Atlas of the Nail in Clinical Diagnosis. Chicago: Year Book Medical Publishers, 1984
14. Baran R, Dawber RPR: Diseases of the Nails and Their Management. London: Blackwell Scientific Publications, 1984
15. Scher RK, Daniel CR III: Nails: Therapy, Surgery, Diagnosis. Philadelphia: WB Saunders, 1990

46
LESIONS OF MUCOUS MEMBRANES

In this chapter, affections of the vermilion of the lips, the oral mucosa, the glans penis, and the non-hair-bearing portions of the vulva are considered. Conjunctiva and anus will be mentioned as occasion arises. Although some of these tissues are not true mucous membranes, they have the common features of weak or parakeratotic keratinization above a stratified epidermis-like epithelium and absence of the cutaneous adnexa, except free sebaceous glands. They are frequently involved in some dermatoses, rarely in others, and they have some diseases of their own. They also are subject to neoplasia of various types. The following discussion is divided broadly into inflammatory, bullous, ulcerative, and neoplastic conditions. White- or dark-appearing lesions are grouped together.

INFLAMMATORY LESIONS

Like the skin, mucous membranes can become inflamed as the result of physical or chemical trauma or contact allergic mechanisms.[1,2] They then present a histologic picture of noncharacteristic, acute, subacute, or chronic inflammatory infiltrate in the membrana propria. The epithelium may become hyperplastic and edematous but more often becomes necrotic or separated from its base, with the formation of fleeting bullae followed by erosion. It is the frequent and far from easy task of the pathologist to discern such nonspecific *stomatitis, balanitis,* or *vulvitis* from the changes of specific dermatoses, which we shall now enumerate. It must be kept in mind that, with the exception of the hard palate and the tongue, a granular layer is normally absent or very thin on mucosal surfaces, a nucleated horny layer usually represents the normal condition, and a thick granular layer with compressed keratin is, in fact, abnormal. It is also true, especially in the mouth, that inflammatory infiltrate may contain many plasma cells without special significance.

Plasmocytosis Mucosae

Plasma cell balanitis is a benign lesion of unknown origin.[3,4] Clinical manifestation is a shiny, orange-red macular area. Histologically a plasma cell-rich dermal infiltrate is covered by a thin layer of mucosal epithelium (Fig. 46–1). The surface epithelium shows low-grade spongiotic edema and loss of granular layer but is not dysplastic. Similar lesions have been observed on the female genitalia, oral mucosa, and conjunctiva (*plasmocytosis mucosae*).[5–8]

Psoriasis, Geographic Tongue, Balanitis Circinata

Psoriasis of the oral mucosa does exist but is extremely rare.[9] The mucosa being normally para-

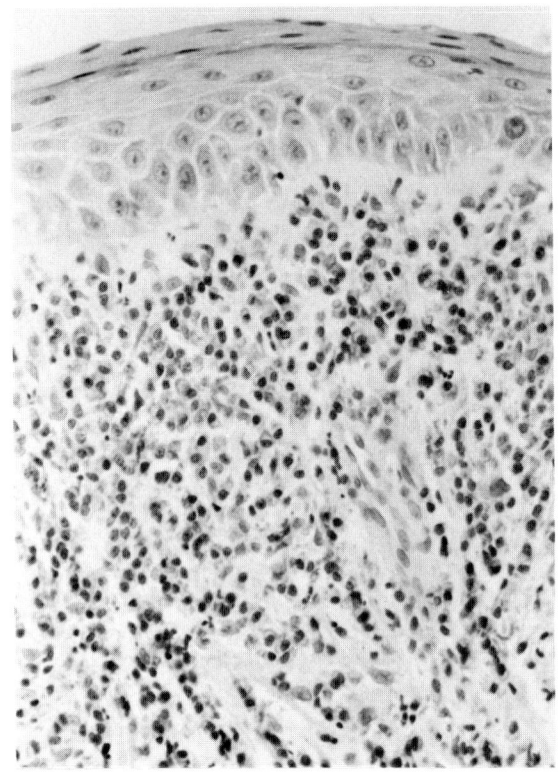

Figure 46–1.
Plasma cell balanitis. The epidermis is parakeratotic but not as thin and atrophic as it sometimes is. There is almost pure plasma cell infiltrate in the dermis. H&E. X400.

keratotic and having fairly high mitotic counts, spongiform edema and leukocytic invasion of the epithelium produce a psoriasiform histologic picture, and the diagnosis must be supported by continuity of oral and cutaneous plaques and response to therapy. The histologic picture of geographic tongue or migrating glossitis (Fig. 46–2) is indistinguishable from that of psoriasis.[10–12] Nosologic relation with psoriasis and atopic dermatitis has been suggested. The histologic picture of psoriasis of the vulva and the glans penis does not differ in principle from that on other parts of the skin, although pronounced acanthosis is uncommon. The changes are very similar to balanitis circinata and related lesions on the vulva,[13] which are manifestations of Reiter's disease in the group of psoriasiform tissue reactions.

Lichen Planus and Lupus Erythematosus

The oral mucosa is much more commonly involved by lichen planus than by lupus erythematosus. Either may produce whitish streaks or, less frequently, ulceration, and the histologic picture may be even more convergent than that of skin lesions (Fig. 46–3). The epithelium consists of large cells (hypertrophy) and develops multiple granular and orthokeratotic horny layers. Basal cells show degenerative changes,[14,15] and the lower strata are invaded by

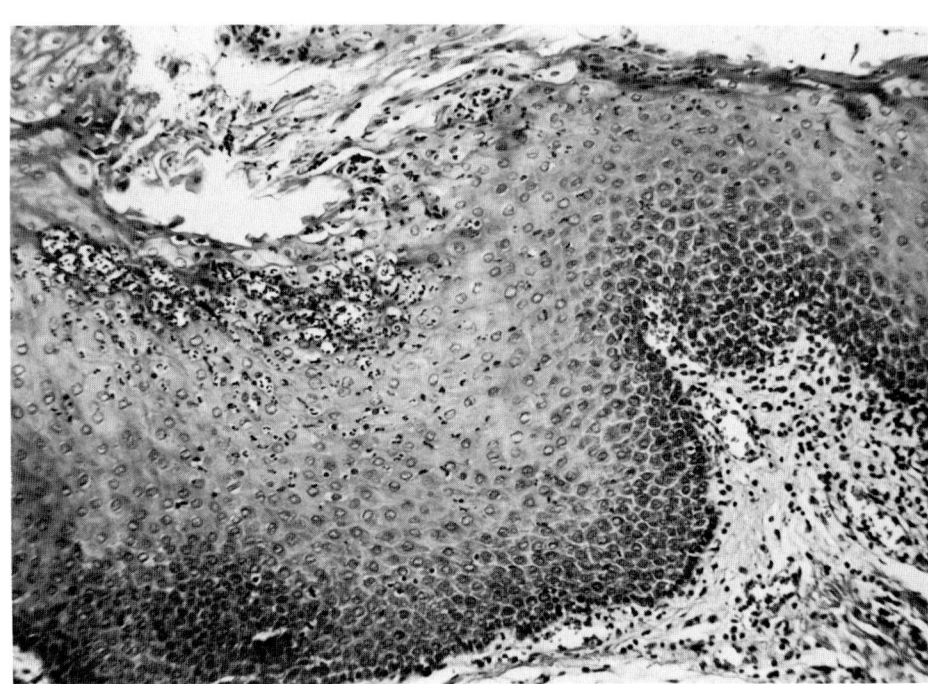

Figure 46–2.
Benign migratory glossitis (geographic tongue). Note remarkable similiarity to a psoriasiform lesion (see Figs. 8–9 and 8–16). H&E. X135.

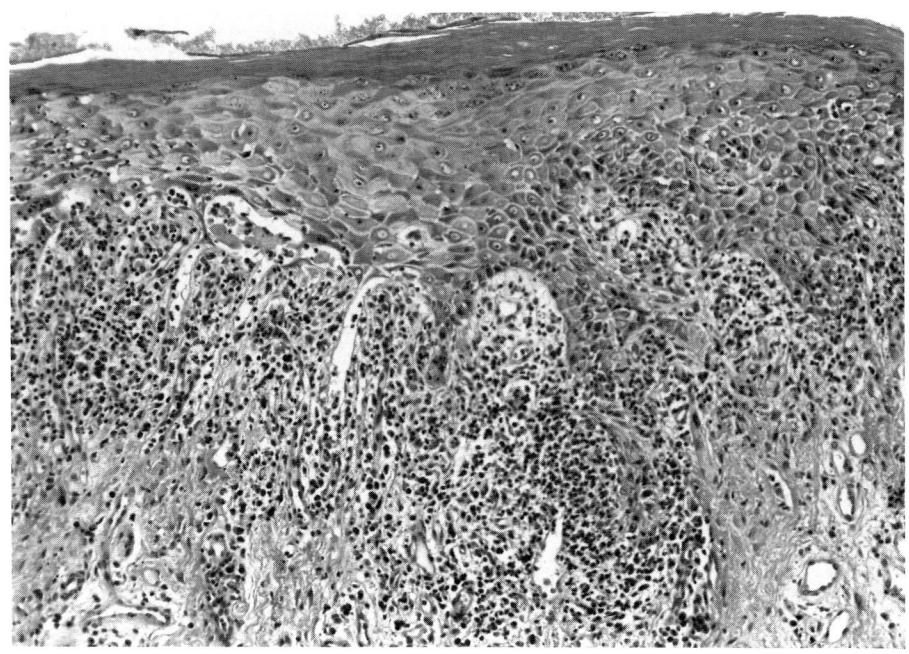

Figure 46–3.
Oral lichen planus. Note development of granular and orthokeratotic keratin layers, foci of liquefaction degeneration of basal cells and lympho-plasmocytic infiltrate. H&E. X225.

round cells from the dense lymphocytic–plasmacytic infiltrate[16] that is present subepithelially. The picture must be differentiated from precancerous leukoplakia by paying attention to cytologic details. In erosive lichen planus[17] and similar lesions due to lupus erythematous, one must try to find diagnostic features in the edge of the ulcer. Histologic diagnosis of lichen planus on the glans and other genital areas offers no special difficulties.

Lichen Sclerosus et Atrophicus

Lichen sclerosus et atrophicus (LSA) (see Chapter 26) deserves special mention here because this benign dermatosis has a predilection for the female genitoanal region and has been confused with *leukoplakic vulvitis* and *kraurosis vulvae*. Without entering into clinical differential diagnosis, we state that the combination of epithelial atrophy with hyperkeratosis, an edematous homogeneous band of connective tissue and perivascular lymphocytic infiltrate characterizes LSA and that the condition is benign and in many cases amenable to dermatologic therapy and cure.[18] It is only when LSA persists for many years and the pruritic atrophic lesions are injured by long continuous excoriation that secondary leukoplakic changes and squamous cell carcinoma may supervene.[19] LSA involving glans penis has been called "balanitis xerotica obliterans," a term that may be eliminated without loss.

Syphilis

Syphilis has a preference for mucous membranes in all of its stages, but biopsy material will come to the pathologist's attention more often by mistake than by intent. Such instances have become more frequent through a combination of unusual sexual habits of patients and lack of suspicion on the part of clinicians. Chancres of tonsil and rectum have been biopsied on the suspicion of carcinoma. Mucous plaques of the secondary stages may be mistaken for leukoplakia. Late *gummatous syphilis* and especially *interstitial syphilitic glossitis,* with its great tendency to malignant transformation, are genuine objects of biopsy. The syphilitic hallmarks of endovasculitis and plasma cell infiltrate or fibrosis following tuberculoid granulomatous infiltration should rouse the pathologist's attention.

BULLOUS LESIONS

The greater fragility of mucous membrane epithelium makes it more difficult to obtain specimens of unbroken blisters. The patient should be watched carefully, and biopsy should be done at the earliest possible moment, preferably by an oral surgeon who is more apt to have the proper instruments and skill for this task. Proper procedures, which should include immunofluorescent and ultrastructural studies, are particularly important in cases in which no skin lesions are present.

Pemphigus, Pemphigoid, Erythema Multiforme

The acantholytic process of pemphigus vulgaris can still be recognized in a deroofed lesion if the basal layer remains adherent to the membrana propria (Fig. 46–4). The bulla of mucous membrane pemphigoid (Fig. 46–5) is subepithelial, and the stratified epithelium is well preserved in the roof, in contrast to the situation with erythema multiforme, where it is apt to be more or less necrotic. Late lesions of mucous membrane pemphigoid show adhesions and scarring, which as such are noncharacteristic but do not occur in other bullous diseases. Scarring does take place in Behcet's syndrome. *Desquamative gingivitis*[20] often develops into cicatricial pemphigoid. An extensive review of the entire field of erosive, ulcerative, and bullous lesions of the oral mucosa was given by Rogers.[1]

Darier's and Hailey–Hailey's Diseases

Rare but well-documented occurrence of Darier's disease and warty dyskeratoma on the oral mucosa[21] and other mucous membranes shows that the name "keratosis follicularis" is a misnomer. The disease of Hailey–Hailey also has been observed in mucosal localization.[22] The expression of these disorders is similar to that on the skin but is even more difficult to differentiate from pemphigus vulgaris. Presence of corps ronds and absence of degenerating acantholytic cells are to be looked for. In addition, proliferative epithelial budding often is found in the diseases of Darier and Hailey–Hailey and does not occur in pemphigus vulgaris. Tzanck smears may be helpful.

ULCERATIVE LESIONS

Any of the bullous lesions just mentioned may lead to denudation and superficial ulceration. Erosive lichen planus and lupus erythematosus may cause painful ulcers. There are, in addition, several diseases that are primarily ulcerative, ranging from tiny aphthae to large granulomatous defect. We can give only some directions for their histologic differentiation.

Aphthae and Aphthosis

Corresponding to the clinical picture, simple aphthae show superficial erosion with partial necrosis of the surface epithelium, edema, and variable degrees of acute inflammatory cell infiltrate (Fig. 46–6).[23] More severe lesions will show complete necrosis and loss of the mucosal epithelium and a very heavy perivascular infiltrate (Fig. 46–7). *Behçet syndrome* is characterized by recurrent ulcers of oral and genital mucosa very similar to aphthosis.[24] Favorable sections may reveal vascular changes in the form of hyalinization, endarteritis, and an infiltrate predominantly of lymphocytes.[25,26] Mast cells have been reported to be increased. Other cutaneous manifestations of Behçet syndrome include erythema nodosum and necrotizing vasculitis.[27,28]

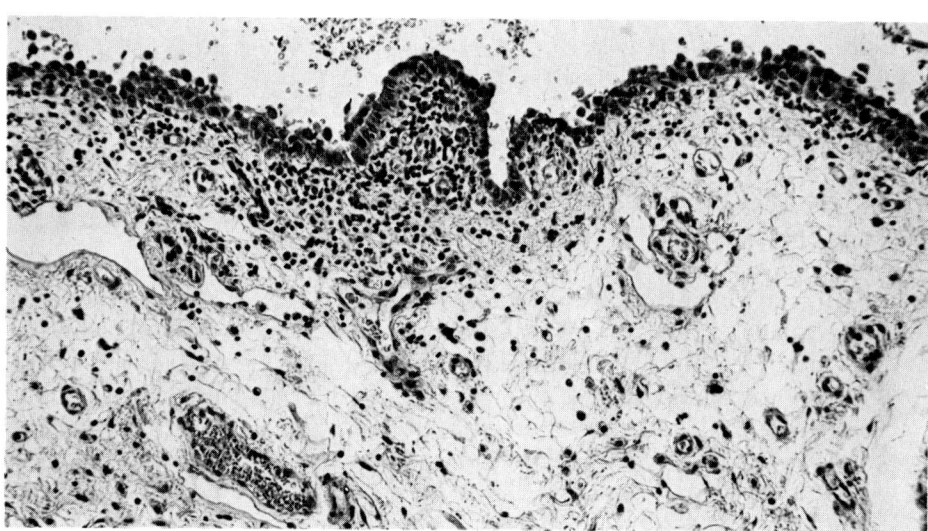

Figure 46–4.
Pemphigus vulgaris of buccal mucosa. Acantholytic cells above the adherent layer of basal cells. H&E. X185.

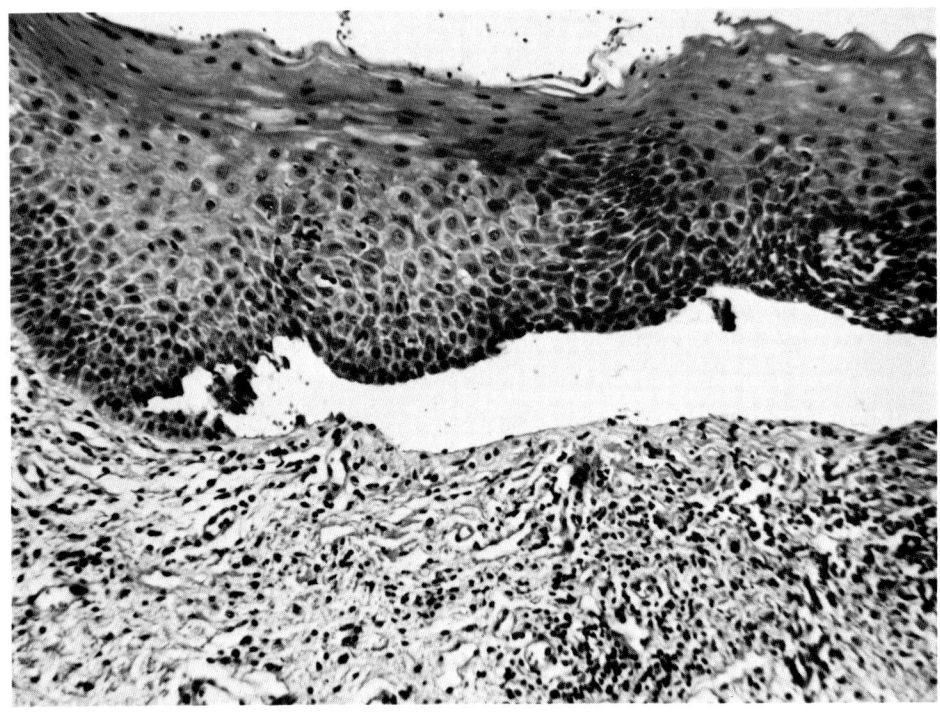

Figure 46–5.
Benign mucous membrane pemphigoid. Complete separation of viable epithelium from membrana propria. Oral lesion. H&E. X180.

Perlèche

We mention here perlèche (angulus infectiosus), an erosive lesion of the commissure of the lips that may be due to maceration in edentulous or excessively salivating patients with or without infection with streptococci or *Candida*. In the latter case,[34] numerous hyphae (Fig. 46–8) are easily seen in the keratin layer by PAS stain. Otherwise, there is subacute inflammatory infiltrate and edema or loss of epithelium without characteristic features.

Cheilitis Glandularis

In cheilitis glandularis, one or both lips are markedly edematous and are covered by a layer of crust.

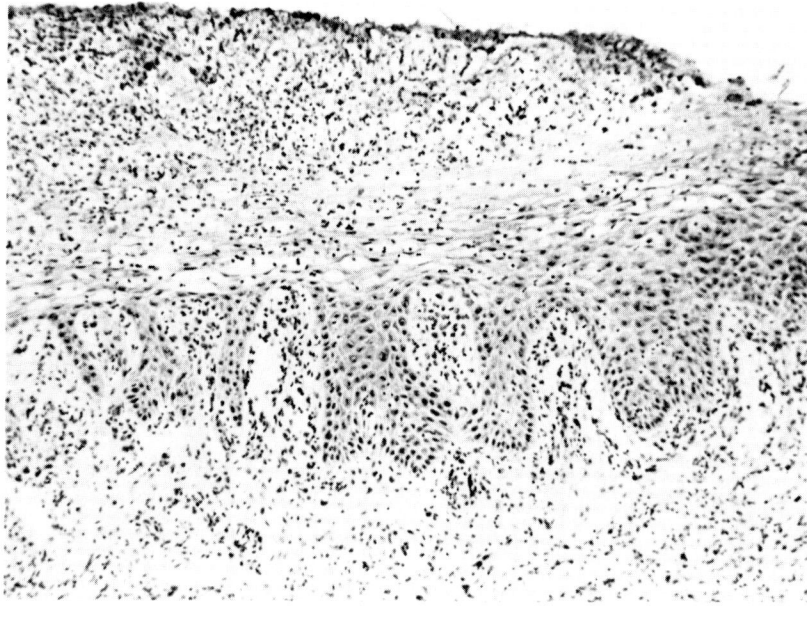

Figure 46–6.
Aphthous ulcer. Superficial necrosis of the mucosal epithelium associated with edema and acute inflammatory cell infiltrate. H&E. X125.

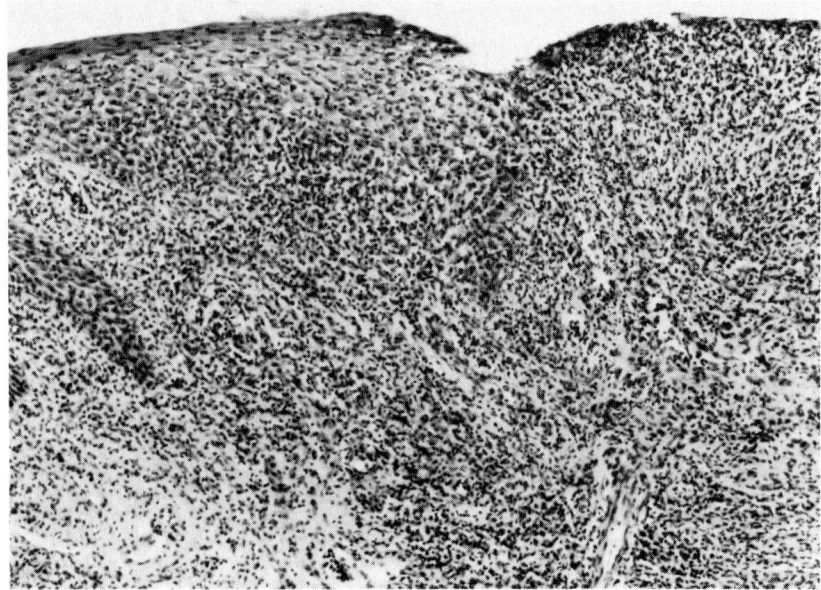

Figure 46–7.
Aphthous ulcer. Edge of an ulcerated lesion shows complete necrosis of the surface epithelium and heavy perivascular inflammation. H&E. X125.

Histologic sections show diffuse edema with minimal chronic inflammatory cell infiltrate but no increase in the volume or number of salivary glands.[29]

Eosinophilic Ulcer of the Tongue

A trauma-induced ulcer of the tongue shows extensive and predominantly eosinophilic infiltrate within the entire submucosa and extending in between the bundles of striated muscles.[30,31]

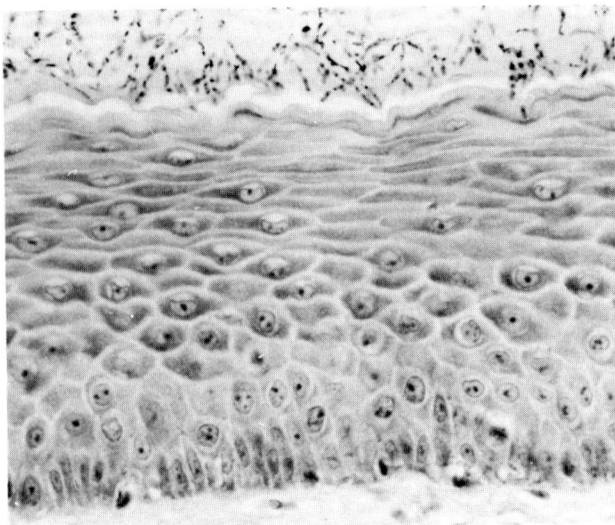

Figure 46–8.
Candidiasis of oral mucosa. Epithelium preserved and regular. Hyphae and spores in horny layer but not penetrating living tissue. O&G. X400.

Another trauma-induced, reactive oral lesion is *atypical histiocytic granuloma* characterized by extensive submucosal lymphohistiocytic infiltrate with some of the histiocytes exhibiting pleomorphism and mitotic figures resembling a malignant lymphoid process.[32]

Mucous Retention Cyst

Mucous retention cyst or *mucocele* is another lesion most likely of traumatic origin. It probably results from the rupture of a duct which lets mucous secretion enter the tissue. Although remnants of an epithelial lining are sometimes found, the cyst usually has a thick wall of granulation tissue (Fig. 46–9) that may be mistaken for an infectious granuloma.[33,34] The presence of mucous secretion may be demonstrated by alcian blue stain. The lesion is benign, although it may recur. In other cases, secondary squamous metaplasia may take place in the surviving remnants of the gland and may simulate squamous cell carcinoma (*necrotizing sialometaplasia*).[35]

Infectious Granulomas

Tuberculosis orificialis of the oral and anal mucosa was discussed in Chapter 21 as a now rare affection of marasmic individuals with waning immune response. It is due to implantation of mycobacteria stemming from an open lesion in lung or bowel. Syphilitic chancre, secondary mucous plaques, and

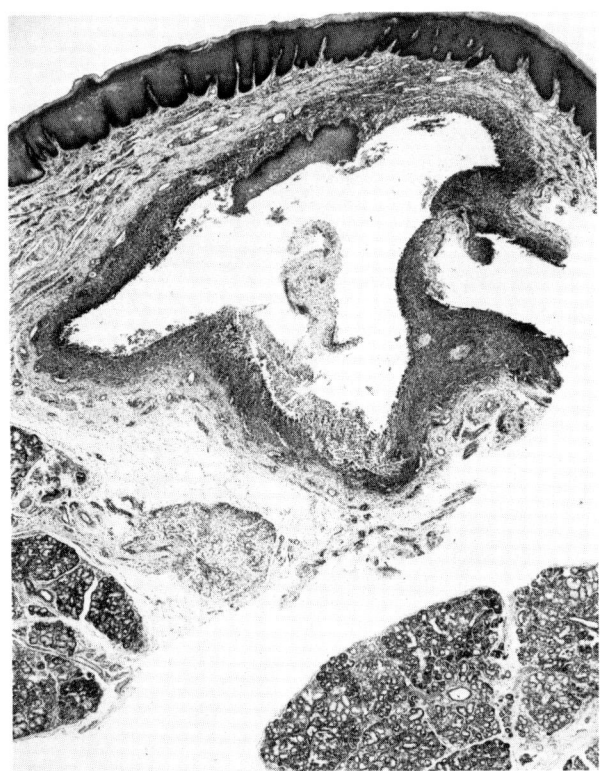

Figure 46-9.
Mucocele. Oral epithelium above, mucous glands below cystic lesion which is only partly lined with stratified epithelium. Most of wall consists of granulation tissue. H&E. X14.

late interstitial glossitis were mentioned. *Tertiary syphilis* may also produce severely destructive gummatous lesions of bone and soft tissues around the nose and mouth, and on the genitalia the so-called *chancre redux*, which has the histologic characteristics of a gumma. *South American leishmaniasis* and *histoplasmosis* commonly produce stubborn ulceration at mucocutaneous junctions or in the mouth and must be diagnosed by the demonstration of the respective organisms in a predominantly mononuclear granuloma (Chapter 21). One should not forget that *granuloma inguinale* may occur in the oral mucosa.

Noninfectious Granulomas

Langerhans cell granuloma (Chapter 25), in manifestations of the Hand–Schüller–Christian type, may produce severely destructive lesions in the genitoanal area and in the mouths of children as well as adults.[36] The presence of large and often foamy histiocytes and variable numbers of eosinophils leads to histologic diagnosis. *Wegener's granulomatosis* may present as gingivitis and frequently produces oral ulcers. The histologic picture shows a combination of necrotizing vasculitis, which may involve small and larger vessels, and a mixed granulomatous infiltrate usually including multinucleated giant cells of the foreign-body type. The *lethal midline granuloma* of the face sooner or later causes destruction of the palate. It presents a mixed infiltrate without specific characteristics. Finally, it should be mentioned that manifestations of *Crohn's disease* of the gut may be found in the mouth, where they present a sarcoid type of tissue reaction.

WHITE LESIONS

The term "leukoplakia" is another of the old descriptive names that have changed in interpretation from clinical to histologic.[37,38] Although the word means nothing but white plaque, many clinicians consider it as synonymous with precancer, and the pathologist should use it only in this connotation. It must be understood that leukoplakia can be used only for lesions of mucous or semimucous membranes not normally possessing a layer of keratohyaline granules which reflect and diffuse incident light and modify the red color of vascularized tissue. Inasmuch as the skin normally has a granular layer, any excessive whiteness due to its thickening is attributable to specific cutaneous disease, such as lichen simplex, lichen planus, or lichen sclerosus et atrophicus. It never is leukoplakia.

Leukoplakia

In proper use, pathologists refer to leukoplakia as a lesion of oral or genital mucous or semimucous membrane that exhibits abnormal keratinization in the form of a more or less prominent granular layer in association with cellular evidence of dysplasia or carcinoma in situ.[39,40] If the living epithelium is not dysplastic, other terms should be employed. Cytologic expression of precancerous change in the oral mucosa can vary from the relatively mild derangement of the basal layer shown in Figure 46–10B, with occasional dyskeratotic cells, to pronounced bowenoid pictures. The granular layer may be thick or may be represented by only a few cells, but the keratin layer always is dense and different from the normal appearance of swollen bulky cells. Presence of reactive inflammatory infiltrate below the epithelium is essential[50] but is not pathognomonic because

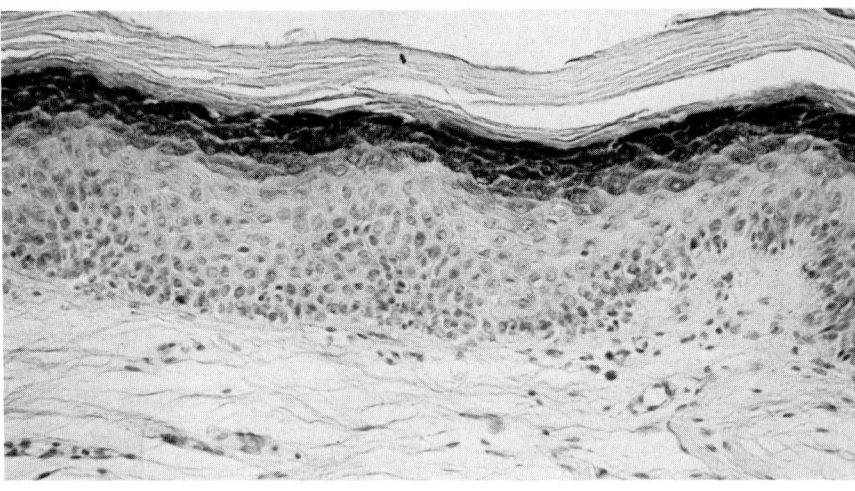

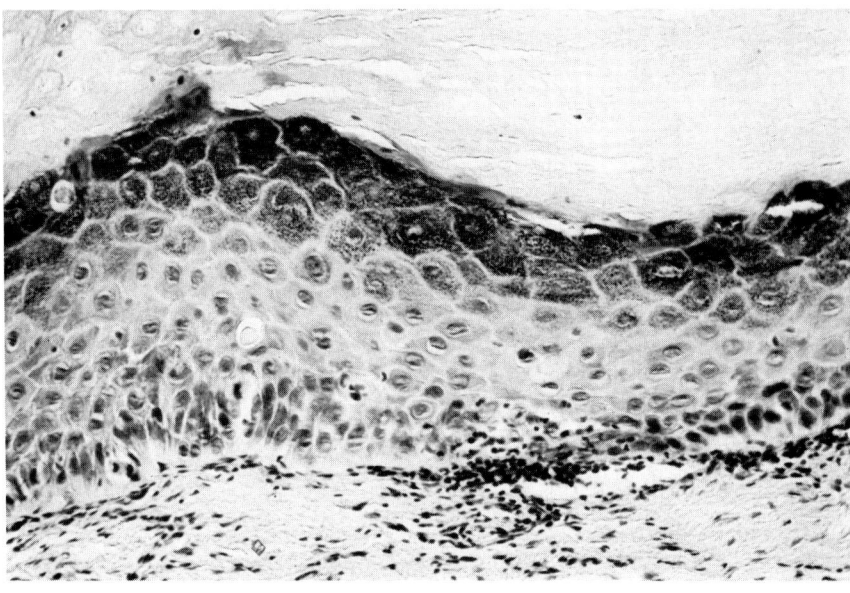

Figure 46–10.
A. Benign leukokeratosis (epidermization) of buccal mucosa. Note regular basal layer and orderly configuration of upper strata. Absence of inflammatory infiltrate. H&E. X135. **B.** Leukoplakia of buccal mucosa. This is a minimal-lesion but exhibits a disturbed basal layer, larger size of cells with hyperchromatic nuclei and increased mitotic activity, individually keratinizing cells, and some inflammatory infiltrate. H&E. X135.

it is shared with lichen planus and other inflammatory lesions. If the lower epithelial surface shows atypical budding, this is a danger signal, and the presence of horny pearls usually signifies beginning invasion. Precancerous leukoplakia may occur as the result of chronic irritation, especially in smokers, in the course of late syphilis, and in the rare familial condition *dyskeratosis congenita*.[41]

Benign White Plaques

Lichen planus, lupus erythematosus, secondary syphilis, and lichen sclerosus et atrophicus were already mentioned as causes of white discoloration. In children and debilitated persons, infection with *Candida* may produce adherent white plaques (thrush). Histologic examination reveals a pseudomembrane consisting of desquamating epithelium, debris, and possible necrotic tissue matted together by numerous fungal hyphae.

Oral Hairy Leukoplakia

This condition occurs exclusively in individuals infected with human immunodeficiency virus (HIV) and is a reliable clinical indication of AID syndrome.[42] White plaques involve the lateral aspects of the tongue (Fig. 46–11). Histologically there is acanthosis with columnar hairlike parakeratotic emanations.[43,44] Epstein-Barr virus particles have

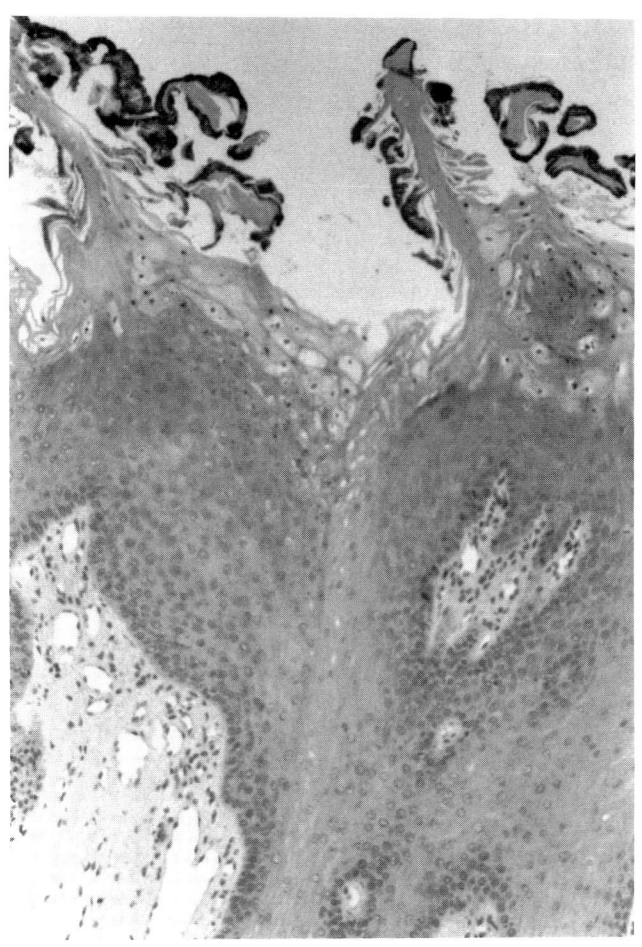

Figure 46–11.
Oral hairy leukoplakia. H&E. X125.

been demonstrated in the majority of lesions. A few show human papillomavirus infection.[45]

Other circumscribed white plaques on oral mucosa result from chronic trauma of ill-fitted dentures, ragged teeth, and so on. Their histologic expression is *epidermization* (Fig. 46–10A) of the oral epithelium, and either this term or *benign leukokeratosis* may be used for diagnosis.

A special form is the condition described as *stomatitis nicotina,* also known as smoker's palate. Small or larger white papules usually have a red center, which corresponds to a keratinized mucous gland duct[46,47] associated with glandular hyperplasia.[48] The epithelium is orthokeratotic and not dysplastic, and the condition is usually benign. A peculiar diffuse bluish whiteness of pigmented buccal mucosa is not infrequently seen in blacks and has been given the name *leukoedema*.[49] The clinician should not confuse it with the opalescent mucous plaques of secondary syphilis or with leukoplakia. Histologically, it exhibits only thickened epithelium without inflammation or dysplasia.

Nevoid and Verrucous White Lesions

Occasionally, a viral wart (Fig. 46–12) resembling those seen in the skin appear on the lips or in the oral mucosa. *Condyloma acuminatum,* however, has been proved to be caused by the human papillomavirus type 6 and 11. A number of human papillomaviruses have been identified in the lesions of bowenoid papulosis.

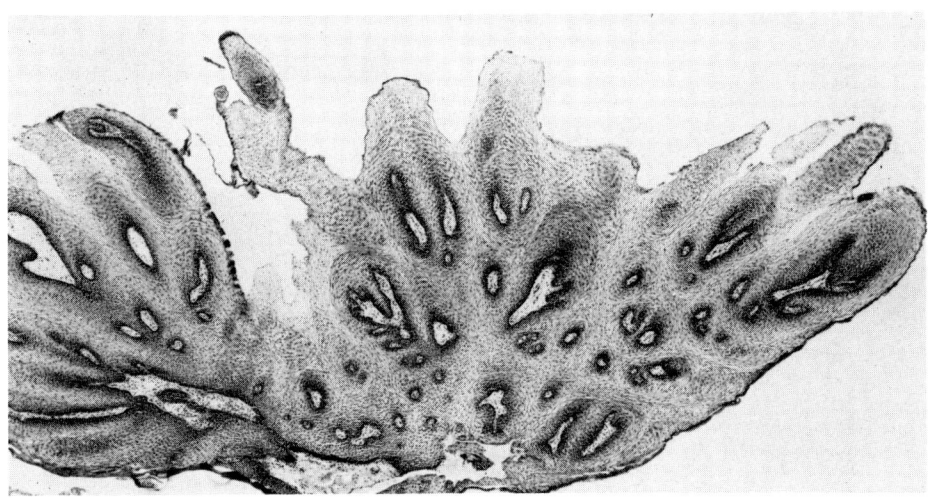

Figure 46–12.
Verruca vulgaris of tongue. Small amount of connective tissue in relation to bulky epithelium differentiates this lesion from condyloma acuminatum. H&E. X29.

Heck's Disease

Familial focal epithelial hyperplasia was first described in American Indians but has now been found in various parts of the world.[50] The crowding of cases in families and schools makes infection likely (see Chapter 32). Human papillomavirus type 13 and 32 have been identified.[51,52] Single or often multiple well-defined elevated and white lesions appear in oral mucosa. The lesions show markedly acanthotic epithelium with a few vacuolated cells but no cellular atypicalities.

Fordyce's Condition

It was mentioned in Chapter 2 that free sebaceous glands occur on mucous membranes. They were described in the mouth by Fordyce as a "disease" in the nineteenth century but are an almost normal feature and have a slightly yellow tinge. Sebaceous glands also occur on the labia minora, sometimes in great numbers, and rarely on the glans and inner prepuce.

White Sponge Nevus

A familial condition, Cannon's white sponge nevus (Fig. 46–13) may produce small wartlike lesions or large soggy protuberances. It causes white color without keratohyalin through the piling up of swollen parakeratotic cells.[53] Favorable response to penicillin has been reported.[54] Similar lesions occur in *pachyonychia congenita* (Chapter 47). These are benign affections but may simulate in their clinical and pathologic features florid oral papillomatosis.

Uremia

In uremic patients, parakeratotic thickening of the oral epithelium may produce white lesions without inflammatory infiltrate (erythematopultaceous form), which regress when the patient's condition improves.[55]

DARK LESIONS

Melanin Pigmentation

We group together several disparate lesions because they may be submitted for microscopic exclusion of malignant melanoma. Benign pigmented nevi and malignant melanomas do occur on conjunctiva, oral mucosa, and the other membranes occasionally and do not offer any special diagnostic difficulty. Epidermal melanin pigmentation is very rarely encountered in normal Caucasian buccal or gingival mu-

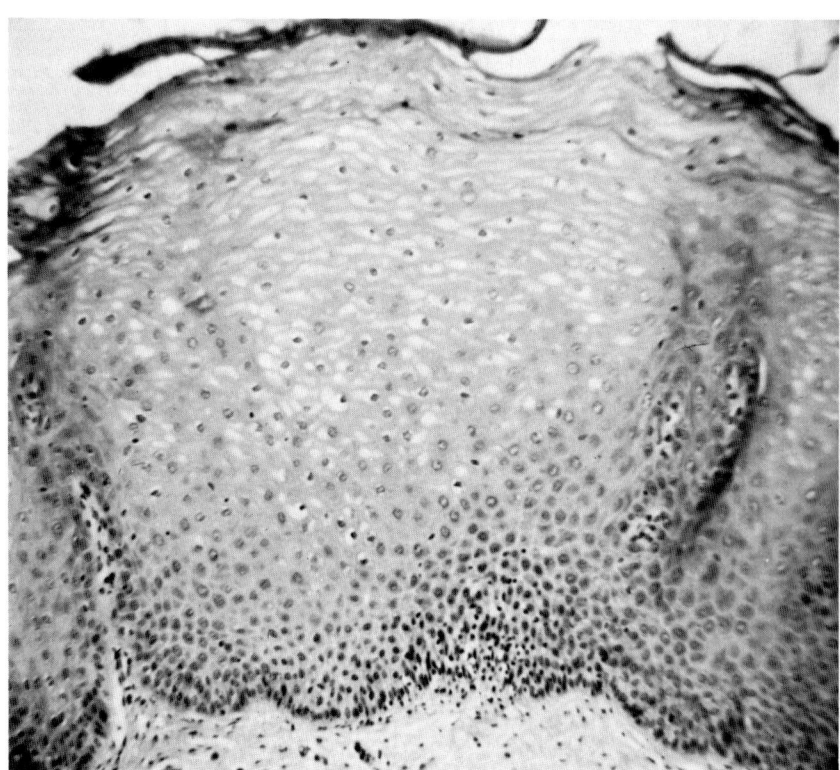

Figure 46–13.
White sponge nevus. Exaggeration of physiologic parakeratosis of buccal mucosa without cellular atypy. H&E. X135.

cosa but is common in more pigmented races. A Swedish study[56] revealed a considerable incidence of pigmentation of the attached gingiva in heavy smokers (*smoker's melanosis*) (Fig. 46–14). Pigmented macular spots similar to those of labial lentigo in oral mucosa have been reported as melanoacanthomas.[57,58] These show moderate thickening of the surface epithelium, hyperpigmentation, and some increase in the number of dendritic melanocytes.[59,60] Pigmentation of the tongue is much rarer and is said to be diagnostic of Addison's disease in Orientals. In blacks, subepidermal bluish pigmentation of the tongue occurs in large plaques, but epithelial melanin is uncommon and usually is restricted to individual fungiform papillae.

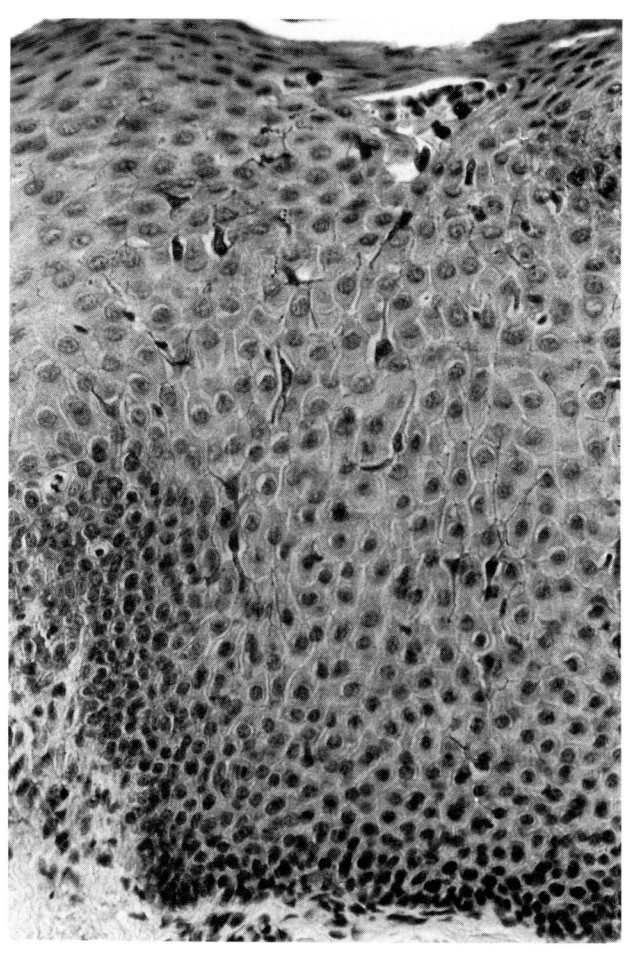

Figure 46–14.
Melanoacanthoma of oral mucosa shows number of dendritic melanocytes within an acanthotic epithelium. H&E. X400.

Vascular Lesions

Varicose widening of veins is not uncommon in elderly people near the lateral ends of the lower lips, and thrombosis may occur. Similar processes may be found on the female genitalia, and scrotal angiokeratomas (Chapter 43) also may look so dark that histologic examination is requested.

Tattoos

Very dark macules may be produced in the mouth by the slip of a dentist's drill that carries silver or mercury into the mucosa.[61] These metals are preferentially deposited on elastic fibers (see Fig. 31–2A) and can be tentatively identified by darkfield examination.

NEOPLASMS

Epithelial Neoplasms

Viral warts and some congenital conditions (white sponge nevus, dyskeratosis congenita) were already mentioned. Extramammary Paget's disease was treated in Chapter 41. We shall not deal with tumors of salivary, mucous, or other glands of the mucous membranes because they are in the field of general pathology. It remains to discuss here epidermoid neoplasia.

Squamous Cell Carcinoma

By far the most common epithelial tumor in the mouth, as well as on the lips and on male and female genitalia, is squamous cell carcinoma. It has a much higher tendency to early metastasis and is relatively immature more often than tumors on the skin proper. It is, therefore, more important to note and report even minor evidence of invasion in a precancerous leukoplakia than it would be in an actinic keratosis.

Verrucous Carcinoma

A peculiarly deceptive variant (Fig. 46–15) is verrucous carcinoma,[62] which is most common in the mouth but may be found on the genitalia. It shows little evidence of dysplasia, often has an intact basement membrane, and invades deeper tissue by pushing solid masses of epithelium downward rather than by growing in an infiltrating manner. Florid oral papillomatosis (Fig. 46–16)[63] and the Buschke–Loewenstein variant of giant condyloma acuminatum occurring on the genitalia are examples of ver-

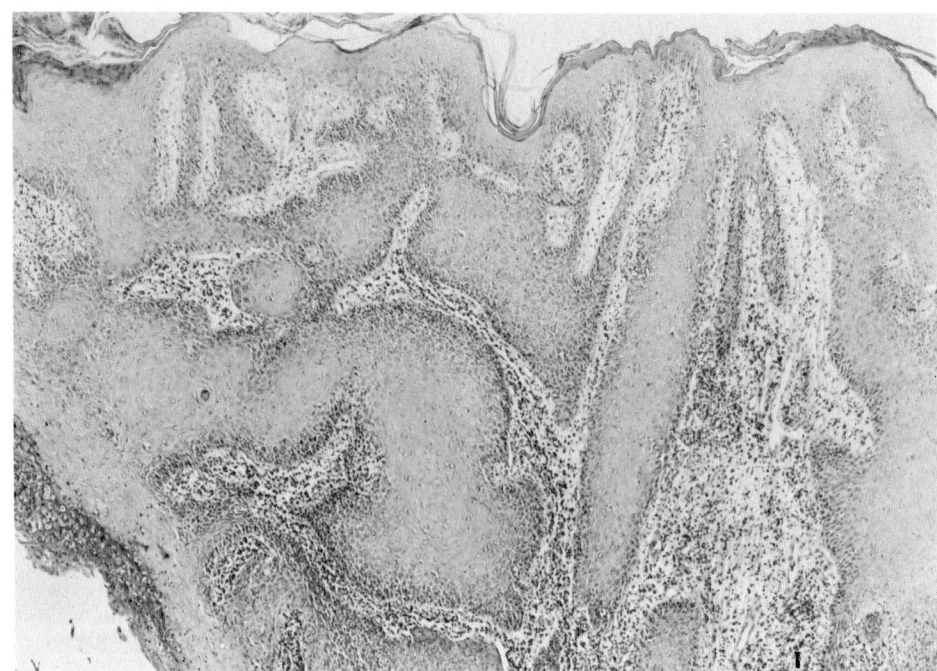

Figure 46–15.
Verrucous carcinoma of oral mucosa. Portion of a large tumor, which protruded above the surface and extended down to striated muscle. The picture illustrates the deceptively benign histologic structure. H&E. X70.

rucous carcinoma. Another variant is epithelioma cuniculatum of the sole of the foot (Chapter 35). All these lesions do not metastasize readily, but complete excision may meet great technical difficulties.

Malignant Mucoepidermoid Tumor

Malignant mucoepidermoid tumor originates from salivary glands in the form of a well-defined neoplasm made up of solid masses of polygonal squamous cells, mucin-producing neoplastic cells, and small cystic spaces containing mucoid material (Fig. 46–17).[64]

Carcinoma in Situ

Of precancerous conditions, leukoplakia was discussed earlier in this chapter. It is to be stressed that

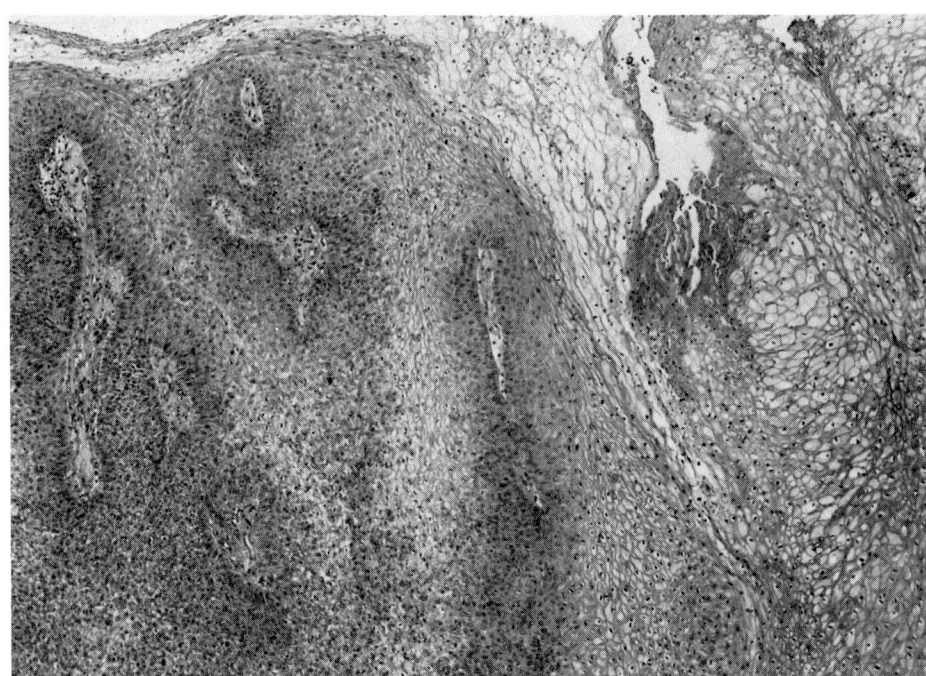

Figure 46–16.
Florid oral papillomatosis exhibiting physiologic type of oral keratinization in exaggerated degree. Extremely bulky acanthosis and retarded maturation of the epithelial cells. Specimens of this type must be carefully examined for evidence of epithelial downgrowth in the manner seen in verrucous carcinoma. (see Fig. 46–15). H&E. X70.

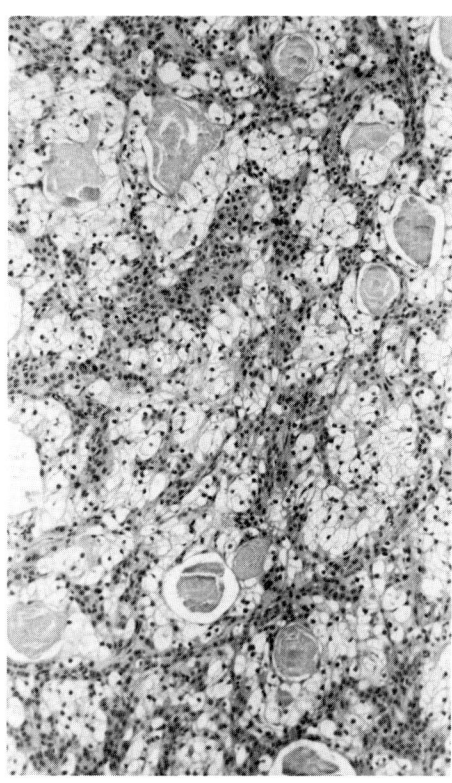 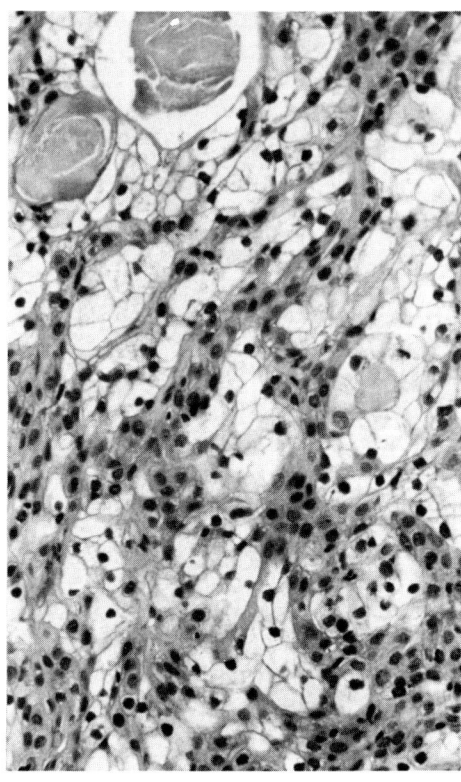

Figure 46–17.
Malignant mucoepidermoid tumor of salivary glands. A mixture of squamous cells, anaplastic mucin-producing cells, and mucin-filled cystic spaces. **A.** H&E. X125. **B.** H&E. X250.

the superficial epidermal layers need not show atypical cells and that high-power examination of the basal layer is essential. In contrast to lichen planus and lupus erythematosus, there is no liquefaction or other loss of basal cells. On the contrary, the lowest epithelial layers consist of somewhat irregular cells with large nuclei and nucleoli in spite of inflammatory cells being present among them (see Fig. 46–10B). This feature also differentiates precancerous leukoplakia and the invasive verrucous carcinoma from benign papillomas in which one basal row of cells underlies the prickle cell layers (see Fig. 46–10A). Marked atypicality of cells and dyskeratosis is the expression of Bowen's disease, a name that dermatologists are not apt to abandon in favor of carcinoma in situ.[65] The reason for this statement is that epithelium exhibiting the characteristic bowenoid changes may at low power have all kinds of configurations, from a thin atrophic epidermis to acanthosis to papillomatosis. The horny layer may be orthokeratotic or parakeratotic. Bowenoid papulosis is discussed in Chapter 32.

Actinic Cheilitis

Another important lesion is actinic cheilitis, which shares many features with keratosis senilis of the skin (Chapter 35) but usually has a much heavier inflammatory infiltrate, consisting of lymphocytes and plasma cells, and often has a rather inconspicuous and even fragmentary, parakeratotic, and uneven epithelium.[66,67] The absence of adnexal structures on the lip vermilion probably is responsible for the fragility of the epithelial cover. Multiple sections should be examined with care in order to identify any invasive cords or nests of epithelial cells, which usually are nonkeratinizing.

Keratoacanthoma

A number of solitary keratoacanthomas of the oral cavity[68,69] and one on the inner surface of the prepuce[70] have been reported. These instances make the relationship of keratoacanthoma to the hair follicle questionable.

Basaloid Carcinoma of the Anus

True basal cell epitheliomas are extremely rare in oral mucosa[71] and are uncommon in the genitoanal area. The anal mucosa, however, gives rise to a specific malignant tumor called either *basaloid carcinoma*[72] or *cloacogenic carcinoma*.[73] These nonkeratinizing neoplasms are apt to metastasize

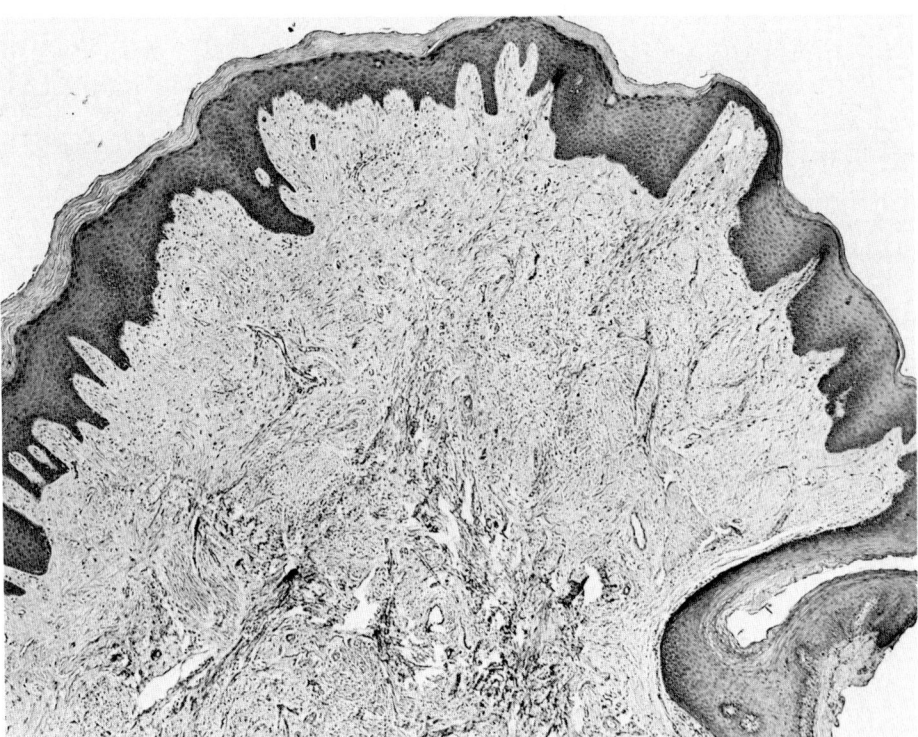

Figure 46–18.
Angiofibroma of buccal mucosa. Epidermization of buccal epithelium above a protruding papule consisting of fairly mature vascular connective tissue. H&E. X14.

and have a cure rate of less than 50 percent in spite of a deceptive histologic appearance simulating that of basal cell epithelioma. The epithelial cells have little cytoplasm and dark-staining nuclei. There may be peripheral palisading and central necrosis with the formation of pseudocysts. Mitotic activity is fairly high.

Mesodermal and Neural Neoplasms

Of very common occurrence are small, often sessile, papular lesions of the tongue or labial mucosa, which may be reactions to trauma rather than true neoplasms. These *angiofibromas* (Fig. 46–18) are usually covered with keratinizing epidermoid epithelium and have a core of vascular collagenous tissue. They are benign. Much rarer are *granular cell myoblastomas* (Chapter 44), which may have pseudocarcinomatous epithelial covering.[74] *Neuromas* are encountered as solitary reaction to trauma and as multiple lesions in the oral mucosal neuroma–medullary thyroid carcinoma syndrome.[75] *Verruciform xanthomas* of oral mucosa[76–78] and the vulva[79] have been described in which the xanthomatous cells are overlaid by a papillomatous epithelium.

REFERENCES

1. Rogers RS III: Diseases of the mucous membranes. In: Dermatologic Clinics. Philadelphia: WB Saunders, 1987
2. Novick NL: Diseases of the mucous membranes. In: Clinics in Dermatology, Vol 5, Philadelphia: J.B. Lippincott, 1987
3. Souteyrand P, Wong E, MacDonald DM: Zoon's balanitis (balanitis circumscripta plasmacellularis). Br J Dermatol 105:195, 1981
4. Murray WJG, Fletcher MS, Yates-Bell AJ, et al: Plasma cell balanitis of Zoon, Br J Urol 58:689, 1986
5. Tenenbaum H, Amar S, Klewansky P: Un cas de plasmocytose orificielle a localisation parodontale. Ann Dermatol Venereol 115:479, 1988
6. White JW Jr, Olsen KD, Banks PM: Plasma cell orificial mucositis. Report of a case and review of the literature. Arch Dermatol 122:1321, 1986
7. Morioka S, Nakajima S, Yaguchi H, et al: Vulvitis circumscripta plasmacellularis treated successfully with interferon alpha. J Am Acad Dermatol 19:947, 1988
8. Aiba S, Tagami H: Immunoglobulin-producing cells in plasma cell orificial mucositis. J Cutan Pathol 16:207, 1989
9. Sklavounou A, Laskaris G: Oral psoriasis: Report of a

case and review of the literature. Dermatologica 180:157, 1990
10. Banóczy J, Szabo L, Csiba A: Migratory glossitis: A clinical-histologic review of seventy cases. Oral Surg 39:113, 1975
11. Kullaa-Mikkonen A: Geographic tongue: An SEM study. J Cutan Pathol 13:154, 1986
12. Kuramato Y, Tadaki T, Hatchome N, Tagami H: Geographic tongue in two siblings. Dermatologica 174:298, 1987
13. Thamba IV, Dunlap R, Thin RN, et al: Circinate vulvitis in Reiter's syndrome. Br J Vener Dis 53:260, 1977
14. Shklar G, Flynn E, Szabo G: Basement membrane alterations in oral lichen planus. J Invest Dermatol 70:45, 1978
15. Shklar G, McCarthy PL: Histopathology of oral lesions of discoid lupus erythematosus. Review of 25 cases. Arch Dermatol 114:1031, 1978
16. Bouquat JE, Gorlin RJ: Leukoplakia, lichen planus, and other oral keratoses in 23,616 white Americans over the age 35 years. Oral Surg Oral Med Oral Pathol 61:373, 1986
17. Pelisse M: Vulvo-vaginal-gingival syndrome. A new form of erosive lichen planus. Int J Dermatol 28:381, 1989
18. Rahbari H: Histochemical differentiation of localized morphea-scleroderma and lichen sclerosus et atrophicus. J Cutan Pathol 16:342, 1989
19. Hart WR, Norris HJ, Helwig EG: Relation of lichen sclerosus et atrophicus of the vulva to development of carcinoma. Obstet Gynecol 45:369, 1975
20. Rogers RS III, Sheridan PJ, Jordan RE: Desquamative gingivitis: Clinical, histopathologic, and immunopathologic investigations. Oral Surg 42:316, 1976
21. Tomich CE, Burkes EJ: Warty dyskeratoma (isolated keratosis follicularis) of the oral mucosa. Oral Surg 31:798, 1971
22. Botvinick I: Familial benign pemphigus with oral mucous membrane lesions. Cutis 12:371, 1973
23. Dolby AE: Mikulicz's recurrent oral aphthae: Histopathological comparison with two experimentally induced immunological reactions. Br J Dermatol 83:674, 1970
24. Wong RC, Ellis CN, Diaz LA: Behçet disease. Int J Dermatol 23:25, 1984
25. Arbesfeld SJ, Kurban AK: Behçet disese. New perspectives on an enigmatic syndrome. J Am Acad Dermatol 19:767, 1988
26. Jorizzo JL: Behçet's disease. An update based on the 1985 international congress in London. Arch Dermatol 122:556, 1986
27. Lee SH, Chung KY, Lee WS, Lee S: Behçet's syndrome associated with bullous necrotizing vasculitis. J Am Acad Dermatol 21:327, 1989
28. Chun S II, Su DWP, Lee S: Histopathologic study of cutaneous lesions in Behçet's syndrome. J Dermatol Tokyo 17:333, 1990
29. Swerlick RA, Cooper PH: Cheilitis glandularis: A re-evaluation. J Am Acad Dermatol 10:466, 1984
30. Rongioletti F, Nunzi E: Traumatic eosinophilic ulcer of the oral mucosa. Cutis 43:357, 1989
31. Borroni G, Pericoli R, Gabba P, et al: Eosinophilic ulcers of the tongue. J Cutan Pathol 11:322, 1984
32. Eversole LR, Leider AS, Jacobsen PL, Kidd PM: Atypical histiocytic granuloma. Light microscopic, ultrastructural and histochemical findings in an unusual pseudomalignant reactive lesion of the oral cavity. Cancer 55:1722, 1985
33. Cataldo E, Mosadomi A: Mucoceles of oral mucous membrane. Arch Otolaryngol 91:360, 1970
34. Lattanand A, Johnson WC, Graham JH: Mucous cyst (mucocele) Arch Dermatol 101:673, 1970
35. Rangi GJ, Kessler S: Necrotizing sialometaplasia. A condition simulating malignancy. Arch Dermatol 115:329, 1979
36. Cavender PA, Bennett RG: Perianal eosinophilic granuloma resembling conduloma latum. Pediatr Dermatol 5:50, 1988
37. Sibuya H, Amagasa T, Seto K-I, et al: Leukoplakia-associated multiple carcinomas in patients with tongue carcinoma. Cancer 57:843, 1986
38. Gupta PC, Bhonsle RB, Muti PR, et al: An epidemiologic assessment of cancer risk in oral precancerous lesions in India with special reference to nodular leukoplakia. Cancer 63:2247, 1989
39. Banoczy J: Oral leukoplakia and other white lesions of the oral mucosa related to dermatological disorders. J Cutan Pathol 10:238, 1983
40. Shklar G: Modern studies and concepts of leukoplakia in the mouth. J Dermatol Surg 7:996, 1981
41. Sirihavin C, Trowbridge AA: Dyskeratosis congenita: Clinical features and genetic aspects. Report of a family and review of the literature. J Med Genet 12:339, 1975
42. Fraga Fernandez J, Chaves Benito MA, Burgos Lizaldez E, Aragues Montanes M: Oral hairy leukoplakia: A histopathologic study of 32 cases. Am J Dermatopathol 12:571, 1990
43. Winzer M, Gilliar U, Ackerman AB: Hairy lesions of the oral cavity. Clinical and histopathologic differentiation of hairy leukoplakia from hairy tongue. Am J Dermatopathol 10:155, 1988
44. Kanitakis J, Zambruno G, Marchand C, et al: La leucoplasie orale chevelue du SIDA. Etude histologique et ultrastructurale de 8 cas. Ann Dermatol Venereol 117:345, 1990
45. Lupton GP, James WD, Redfield RR, Brown C: Oral hairy leukoplakia. A distinctive marker of human T-cell lymphotropic virus type III (HTLV-III) infection. Arch Dermatol 123:624, 1987
46. Forsey RR, Sullivan TJ: Stomatitis nicotina. Arch Dermatol 83:945,1961
47. Laugier P, Extermann J-C, Michau C, et al: L'ouranite glandulaire. Dermatologica 142:344, 1971
48. Pindborg JJ, Reibel J, Roed-Petersen B, Mehta FS:

Tobacco-induced changes in oral leukoplakic epithelium. Cancer 45:2330, 1980
49. Duncan SC, Su DWP: Leukodema of the oral mucosa. Possibly an acquired white sponge nevus. Arch Dermatol 116:906, 1980
50. Samson J, Fiore-Donno G, Avizara N: L'hyperplasie epitheliale focale: Premiers cas Suisse et revue de la litterature. Dermatologica 171:308, 1985
51. Beaudenon S, Praetorius F, Kremsdorf D, et al: A new type of human papillomavirus associated with oral focal epithelial hyperplasia. J Invest Dermatol 88:130, 1987
52. Mahe A, Blanchereau P, Gaulier A, et al: Etude histologique ultrastructural et virologique d'un cas d'hyperplasie epitheliale focale ou maladie de Heck. Ann Dermatol Venereol 116:840, 1989
53. Jorgenson RJ, Levin LS: White sponge nevus. Arch Dermatol 117:73, 1981
54. Alinovi A, Benoldi D, Pezzarossa E: White sponge nevus: Successful treatment with penicillin. Acta Derm Venereol 63:83, 1983
55. Jaspers MT: Unusual oral lesions in a uremic patient: review of the literature and report of a case. Oral Surg 39:934, 1975
56. Hedin CA: Smoker's melanosis. Occurrence and localization in the attached gingiva. Arch Dermatol 113:1533, 1977
57. Matsuoka LY, Barsky S, Glasser S: Melanoacanthoma of the lip. Arch Dermatol 118:290, 1982
58. Sexton MF, Maize JC: Melanotic macules and melanoacanthomas of the lip. A comparative study with census of the basal melanocyte population. Am J Dermatopathol 9:438, 1987
59. Tomich CE, Zunt SL: Melanoacanthosis (melanoacanthoma) of the oral mucosa. J Dermatol Surg Oncol 16:231, 1990
60. Horlick HP, Walter RR, Zegarelli DJ, et al: Mucosal melanotic macule, reactive type: A simulation of melanoma. J Am Acad Dermatol 19:786, 1988
61. Crippa D, Casazza R, Calcinati M, et al: Pigmentazione della mucosa orale de amalgama. Chron Dermatol 18:999, 1987
62. Ackerman LV: Verrucous carcinoma of the oral cavity. Surgery 23:670, 1947
63. Grinspan D, Abulafia J: Papilomatosis florida bucal. Med Cutan ILA 13:43, 1985
64. Spiro RH, Huvos AG, Berk RY, Strong EW: Mucoepidermoid carcinoma of salivary gland origin. A clinicopathologic study of 367 cases. Am J Surg 136:141, 1978
65. Bender ME, Katz HI, Posalaky Z: Carcinoma in situ of the genitalia. JAMA 243:145, 1980
66. Picascia DD, Robinson JK: Actinic cheilitis: A review of the etiology, differential diagnosis, and treatment. J Am Acad Dermatol 17:255, 1987
67. Stanley RJ, Roenigk RK: Actinic cheilitis: Treatment with the carbon dioxide laser. Mayo Clin Proc 63:230, 1988
68. Scofield HA, Werning JT, Shakes RC: Solitary intraoral keratoacanthoma. Oral Surg 37:889, 1974
69. Svirsky JA, Freedman PD, Lumerman H: Solitary intraoral keratoacanthoma. Oral Surg 43:116, 1977
70. Lejman K, Starzycki Z: Giant keratoacanthoma on the inner surface of the prepuce. Br J Vener Dis 53:65, 1977
71. Peters RA, Gingrass RP, Teyes CN, et al: Basal cell carcinoma of the oral cavity: report of case. J Oral Surg 30:73, 1972
72. Pang LSC, Morson BC: Basaloid carcinoma of the anus. J Clin Pathol 20:128, 1967
73. Kheir S, Hickey RC, Martin RG, et al: Cloacogenic carcinoma of the anal canal. Arch Surg 104:407, 1972
74. Dixter CT, Konstat MS, Ginnta JL, et al: Congenital granular cell tumor of alveolar ridge and tongue; report of two cases. Oral Surg 40:270, 1976
75. Walker DM: Oral mucosal neuroma-medullary thyroid carcinoma syndrome. Br J Dermatol 88:599, 1973
76. Shafer WG: Verruciform xanthoma. Oral Surg 31:784, 1971
77. Zegarelli DJ, Zegarelli–Schmidt E, Zegarelli EV: Verruciform xanthoma; further light and electron microscopic studies with the addition of a third case. Oral Surg 40:246, 1976
78. Cobb CM, Holt R, Denys FR: Ultrastructural features of the verruciform xanthoma. J Oral Pathol 5:42, 1976
79. Santa Cruz DJ, Martin SA: Verruciform xanthoma of the vulva. Am J Clin Pathol 71:224, 1979

47
LESIONS OF HAIR AND NAIL

In the formation of the epidermis, every basal germinative cell appears to be equivalent to its neighbors, and the horny layer seems to be a diffuse mass of cells the origin of which is of no great significance. That there is order in epidermal keratinization and that individual basal cells are distinctly different from their neighbors becomes obvious only in precancerous keratoses and some benign tumors, where sharp boundaries separate normal and abnormal cells and their progeny.

In the formation of hair and nail, sharp boundaries between adjoining basal cells are the obvious rule which gives rise to these multilayered structures.

In the nail, the limits of proximal matrix, nailbed, anterior matrix, and nailfold are absolutely sharp (Fig. 47–1), and each type of basal cell (although it is practically indistinguishable from its neighbor across the line of division) forms its predetermined end product—nail, horn of the sole, cuticle—and will continue to do so even after surgical or incidental trauma and disruption.

In the hair, the boundaries are even more defined in the formation of three layers of internal root sheath and three layers of hair out of an immature and indistinguishable mass of pilar matrix cells. They are surrounded by the trichilemma (outer root sheath) with its specific and peculiar type of keratinization. In tumors of pilar nature, the specificity of individual cells becomes even more obvious.

It is therefore not surprising that hair and nail exhibit a variety of pathologic changes closely related to minor and major disturbances of their matrix cells, and a detailed knowledge of their normal anatomic structure is essential to interpret these changes correctly. Knowledge of the normal and abnormal chemistry and metabolism of the tissues of hair and nail has progressed much in recent years. It has already contributed to our understanding and can be expected to do much more.[1]

DISTURBANCES OF HAIR

It may seem arbitrary to separate inflammatory and keratotic lesions of the hair follicle from lesions of hair itself, and a strict separation, admittedly, is not feasible. We do, however, describe in this chapter mainly those changes seen if one puts an entire hair or portions of one under the microscope and will refer to pictures seen in embedded tissue sections only secondarily.

Microscopic Examination of Hair

Elaborate methods have been devised for examination of hair, but we outline here only a relatively simple routine that does not use special equipment. A single hair or a few hairs may be put lengthwise

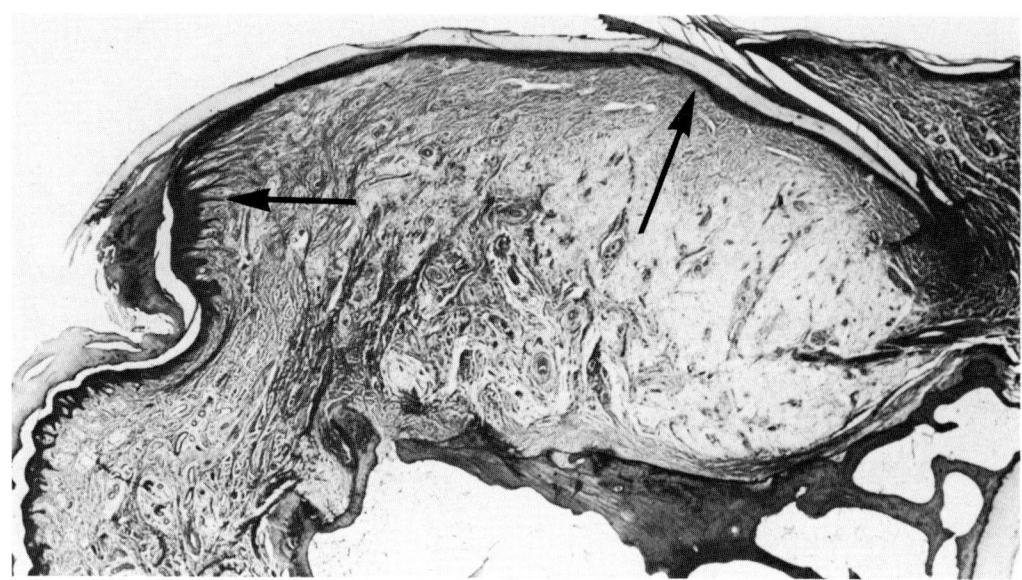

Figure 47–1.
Longitudinal section of toe illustrating the anatomy of the nail. Terminal phalanx with cartilage of interphalangeal joint at bottom of picture. The distance between phalanx and nail is increased, and the tissue shows hypervascularity and edema as evidence of a mild case of pulmonary osteoarthropathy. The nailplate emerges from the posterior nailfold at right and increases in thickness while moving over the matrix, the anterior border of which is indicated by an arrow. The nail then moves over the nailbed, which does not add appreciable substance to it, and emerges free on the left. Beneath the free end of the nail is thick keratin furnished by epidermis with long rete ridges (second arrow). This part is the horn of the sole, and corresponds to the main portion of the horse's hoof. It is the distal matrix of the nail that adds considerable material and binds the distal end of the nail firmly to the underlying tissues. At the lower end of the distal matrix is a shallow anterior groove and below this the epidermis of the tip of the phalanx, which carries eccrine glands (not illustrated). The posterior nailfold is covered with keratin, which projects beyond its anterior end (eponychium) and produces on its lower surface a thin layer of keratin, which is bound to the surface of the nail and lifts up a short distance anterior to the nailfold. This is the cuticle of the nail, which can be pushed back except in some persons where it is tightly bound to the nail as pterygium unguis. H&E. X8. (From Pinkus. In Andrade et al. (eds). Cancer of the Skin, 1976. Courtesy of W.B. Saunders Co.).

on a glass slide if they are relatively short. For a quick preliminary orientation, we find it convenient to put a number of hairs into a folded sheet of plastic and to examine them under the microscope. After that, individual hairs can be selected. Longer hairs should be cut into convenient pieces. For some purposes, for example, examination of pili torti, it is preferable to cut the hair into 1- to 1.5-cm lengths. One may soak the hairs in xylol and then place them on a slide, add several drops of covermount, and seal the slide with a long coverglass. This will provide a permanent slide for teaching and is also suitable for photomicrography. After bright-light examination, one should use polarizing equipment. For most purposes, two pieces of Polaroid film, one below and one above the preparation, are adequate.

Examination should take into account the diameter of the shaft and possible local variations, condition of the cuticle, pigment content of cortex, pigment or gas content of medulla, condition of the hair root (anagen, catagen, telogen), twists and other abnormalities of the shaft, and condition of the free end (natural tip, cut, broken, or frayed). One should examine many normal hairs in order to be able to differentiate truly abnormal states from artifacts or insignificant variations.

Individual variations of hair diameter are great.[2] In order to assess decreased diameter, one should compare hairs from the balding area with those from the patient's occiput, which may be assumed to be normal. Two other types of examination are recommended. According to the method of

Pinkus (hair count),[3] one asks the patient to collect assiduously all combed-out hair, even short pieces, for 24 hours into a dated envelope and to repeat the procedure every day for 1 week. No shampooing is permitted during this time. By counting the hairs in each envelope, one can get a good idea of the severity of hair loss. Up to 100 hairs are lost daily from a healthy scalp. While counting, one separates hairs representing less than 1 year's growth (approximately 12 cm) from longer ones, or if the hair has been trimmed to less than 12 cm into those with cut ends and those with natural tips. If more than about 20 percent of short hairs (or hairs with natural tips) are present, it is an indication of severe chronic weakening of hair growth and most likely of pattern alopecia, if other diseases of the scalp can be ruled out. The newer method, pioneered by Van Scott et al. (telogen count),[4] is somewhat traumatic but less complicated. One grasps approximately 20 hairs in a padded hemostat and pulls them out with a quick jerk. The roots are then trimmed off for examination. If more than about 20 percent are telogen hairs, this speaks for increased hair loss (*telogen effluvium*)[5] but does not differentiate between acute and chronic loss.

Pattern Alopecia

We discussed various types of hair loss associated with more or less inflammation in Chapters 18 and 19. The gradual thinning and disappearance of hair in male and female pattern alopecia[6] is expressed in decrease of diameter of hair follicle and hair and shortening of the hair root.[7] Simultaneously, there is hyperplasia of sebaceous glands. Inflammation may be minor or absent. It takes a good knowledge of size and length of normal hair follicles to appraise early stages of the process. Looking at a biopsy from the scalp of a woman who shows appreciable clinical thinning of hair, one may be surprised to find a practically normal histologic picture until one realizes that every follicle and its hair are reduced in size and no longer penetrate into the subcutis. In a really bald male, the hair roots are mere appendages to the large sebaceous glands, but they do persist (Fig. 47–2). Examination of shed or plucked hairs under the microscope reveals no conspicuous abnormalities.

There is one specific change in biopsy sections that when present is diagnostic.[8] It was mentioned in Chapter 2 that many growing hairs form a small cluster of elastic tissue in the neck of the papilla (the Arao–Perkins body) and that these fibers are clumped in catagen and stay behind at the lowest point to which the papilla extended in anagen (Fig.

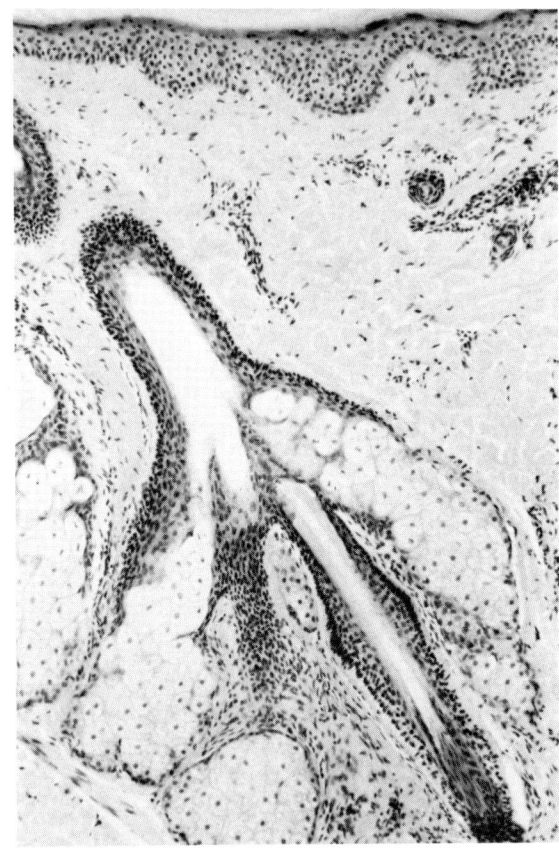

Figure 47–2.
Short, small anagen hair root among large sebaceous glands in advanced male pattern alopecia. H&E. X125.

47–3). In male pattern baldness, the next anagen hair is a little shorter than the previous one, and its Arao–Perkins body will be left behind a distance above the first one. Eventually, in scalps that form good elastic fibers, there will be a row of elastic clumps stacked within the remnants of collapsed fibrous root sheath like the rungs of a ladder. This picture is absolute proof of male or female pattern alopecia.

Acute Hair Loss

Although much less frequent than in times past, acute loss of hair telogen effluvium continues to be observed after febrile illness, surgical procedures, childbirth, and other sudden systemic impairment of health. In these cases, the mortally affected hair will go into telogen and will fall out 60 to 90 days later, while less severely affected hairs will show a temporary local constriction and loss of medulla. Plucked anagen hairs (preferentially white ones be-

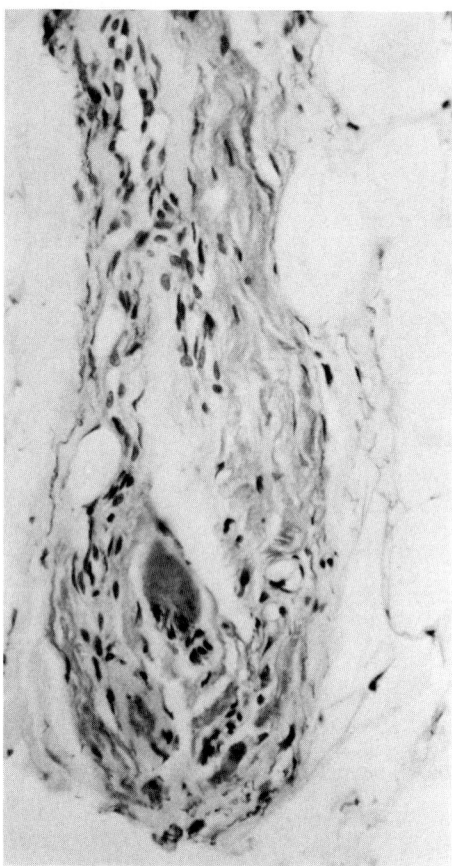

Figure 47—3.
Collapsed fibrous root sheath forms a persistent streamer in the subcutis, indicating the extent of the previous hair growth. Near its lower end, a clumped Arao–Perkins elastinlike body (Chapter 2). O&G. X250.

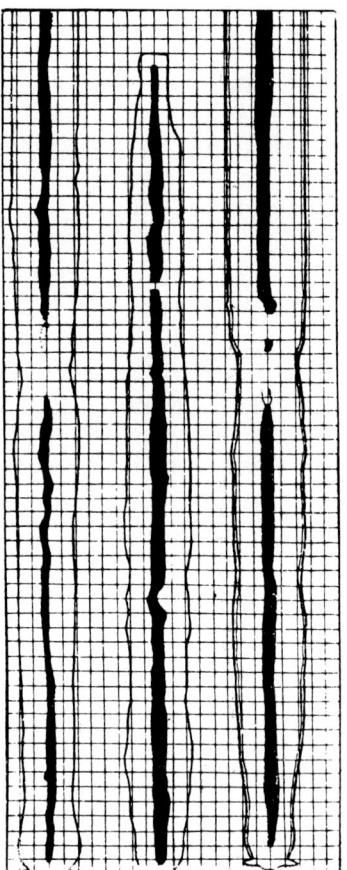

Figure 47—4.
Shown are graphs of three hairs obtained by measuring diameter of cortex and medulla from mm to mm along their length and entering values on a scale exaggerated 1000X for width. Hairs had been plucked from a patient's head 98 days after he fell ill with pneumonia and show Pohl–Pincus' mark. Young hair in center was least affected and grew faster than two older hairs, only bottom halves of which are shown. While older hairs show constriction and loss of medulla (black) beginning 37 and 39 mm from the base and extending for 5 to 7 mm, the vigorous young hair has only a slight constriction and loss of medulla at 41 mm. At average growth rate of 0.4 mm a day, 98 days correspond to 39.2 mm, a value confirming connection of Pohl's mark with febrile illness. (From Pinkus. Die Einwirkung von Krankheiten auf das Kopfhaar des Menschen, 2nd ed, 1928. Courtesy of S. Karger.)

cause their medulla is more conspicuous) should be examined either by simple microscopic inspection or by the more accurate methods developed by Pinkus (Fig. 47–4). The transient decrease in diameter and spindle-shaped tapering of hair shaft (bayonet hair) can also be found following the administration of antimitotic drugs, immunosuppressive drugs, and other drugs,[9] and following x-ray therapy.[10] The common denominator is decrease or cessation of mitotic activity in the hair root. If the hair matrix recovers, temporary thinning of shaft and disappearance of the medulla in a circumscribed zone will result, and this is pushed outward as *Pohl–Pincus's mark*. If the insult was too severe, the hair undergoes precipitous catagen and exhibits a fusiform end instead of a club (Fig. 47–5).

The effect of oral administration of thallium salts,[14] which leads to diffuse hair loss, has some special features consisting of dyskeratotic and necrolytic changes with parakeratosis and spongiform abscesses in the hair follicles and induction of telogen.

Hypertrichosis

The most spectacular form of generalized hypertrichosis is congenital *hypertrichosis lanuginosa,* which in fact represents an arrest of hair differentiation so that silky hair resembling fetal lanugo grows to

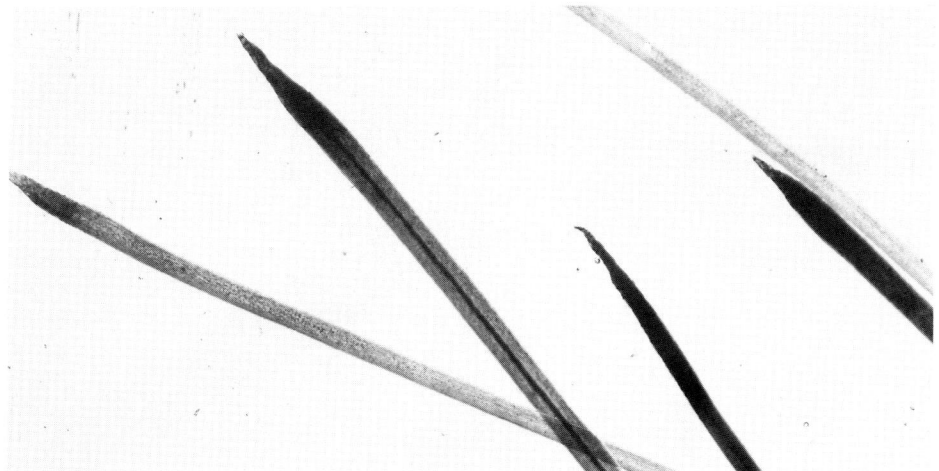

Figure 47–5.
Filiform hair roots in x-ray effluvium. H&E. X30.

great length, but the specific forms of scalp and terminal hair are not developed. On the other hand, *acquired hypertrichosis lanuginosa* (or vellosa), a rare skin manifestation of internal malignancy,[11] results from the conversion of preexisting vellus follicles on face and other areas. Their roots grow longer, often bending sideways (Fig. 47–6), and they form long, soft, and usually colorless hairs.[12,13] A relation to carcinoembryonic antigen was suggested inasmuch as this substance is found in fetuses between the second and sixth months and was elevated in several patients. Other forms of hypertrichosis, whether in porphyria, secondary to hypertensive medications, or in virilizing syndromes (*hirsutism*), are due to conversion of small hair follicles into stronger ones.[14] No new hair roots are formed.

Rhythmic and Discontinuous Disturbances—Hair Shaft Abnormalities

Several amply illustrated reviews on structural abnormalities of the hair shaft have been published.[15–18] They testify to the value of scanning electron microscopy and the application of polarized light, which provide detailed and instructive pictures.

Trichorrhexis nodosa (Fig. 47–7A) is a fracture,

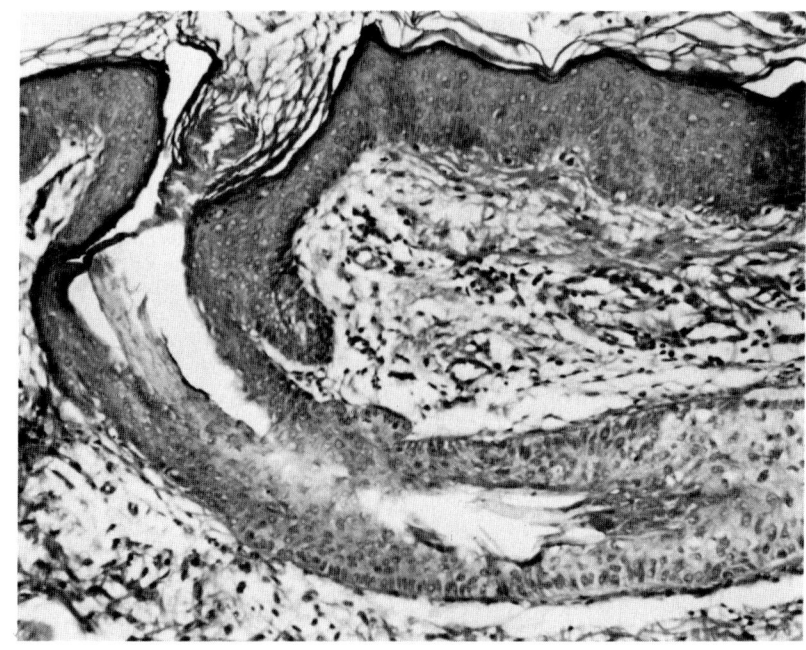

Figure 47–6.
Hypertrichosis vellosa (acquired hypertrichosis lanuginosa) in a case of internal cancer. Lateral deviation of hyperplastic root of a vellus hair. H&E. X100. (From Hegedus and Schorr. Arch Dermatol 106:84, 1972.)

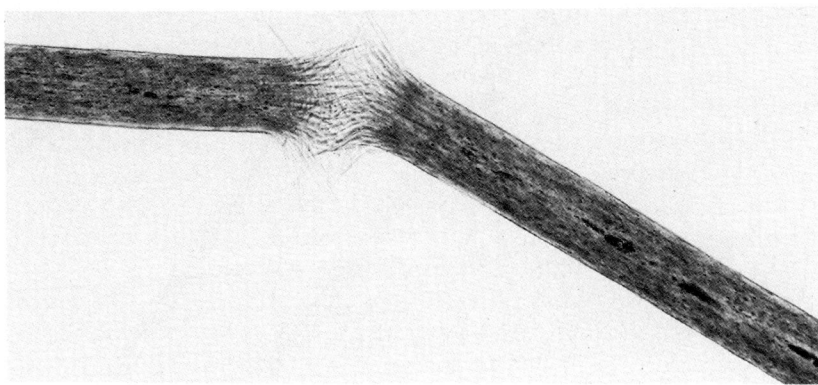

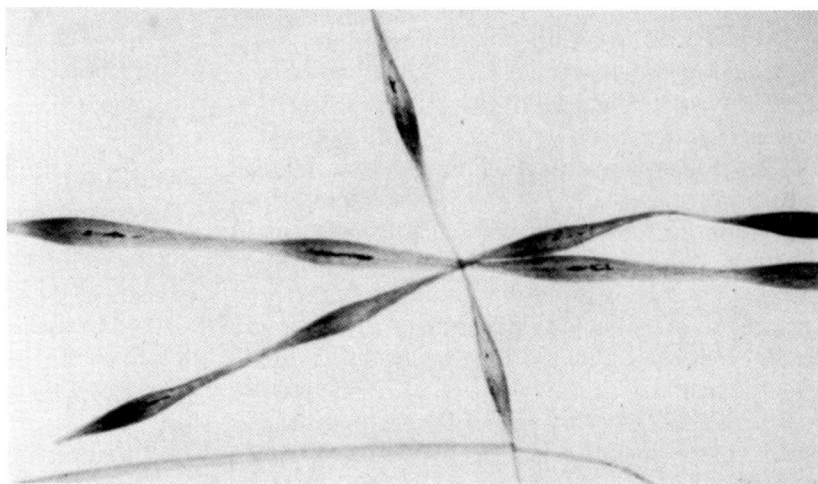

Figure 47–7.
Abnormal hairs. **A.** Trichorrhexis nodosa. **B.** Monilethrix. **C.** Pili torti.

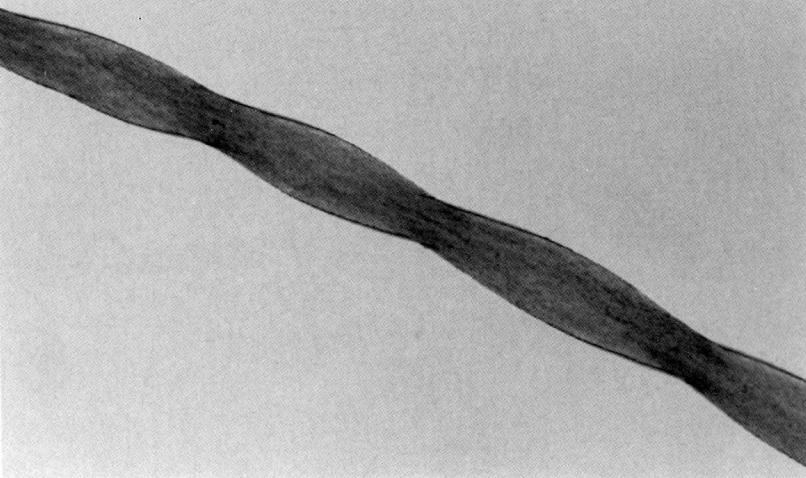

usually trauma-induced, of a hair shaft that is either mechanically or chemically weakened. *Monilethrix* (Fig. 47–7B) shows beaded appearance of hair shaft with elliptical enlargements in 1 mm intervals. The hair breaks within the thin internodes, which usually shows no medulla.[19–20] In *pili torti* (Fig. 47–7C) the hair shaft is flattened and is twisted 180 degrees on its axis. Five or more twists are found in irregular intervals.

Trichorrhexis invaginata (bamboo hair) (Fig. 47–8) shows a ball and socket joint-type swelling of the hair shaft.[21] The club-shaped distal hair is surrounded by a cup-like alteration of the proximal hair shaft. Trichorrhexis invaginata is usually associated with ichthyosis linearis circumflexa in the netherton syndrome.[22]

Pili annulati (ringed hair) (Fig. 47–9A) shows alternating bright and dark bands in microscopic examination due to the presence of air-filled spaces in the abnormal areas,[23] while pili pseudoannulati are due to partial twists of hairs having elliptical cross section. Another finding is twisted hairs that may not be of any diagnostic significance (Fig. 47–9C). Loose anagen hair refers to an idiopathic type of hair loss in children in which tufts of hairs can be pulled out easily.[24,25] Histologic sections show cleft formation between the hair shaft and regressively altered inner root sheaths.

Unmanageable Hair

Several other abnormalities have been described in recent years and accounts may be found in review articles.[15–17]

One of these abnormalities has attracted considerable attention. It was first described as "spun glass" hair[26] because of the refractoriness of the surface of the hairs, each one of which protrudes from the scalp in its own direction and does not lie down. This has led to the appellation "cheveux incoiffables" (unmanageable hair) (Fig. 47–10). Biopsies and electron microscopy have shown that the hair shafts are triangular or fluted[27] and are surrounded in the follicle by inner root sheath of the same configuration. The papilla and matrix appear normal. Unmanageable hair is a purely cosmetic defect which seems to regress as the children get older. It occurs in siblings with an autosomal dominant mode of inheritance.[28–30]

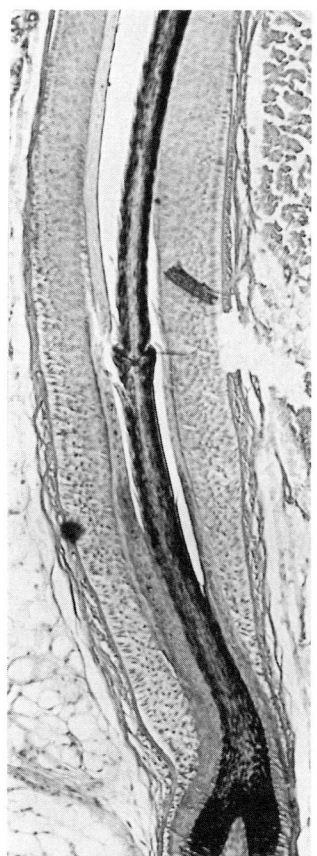
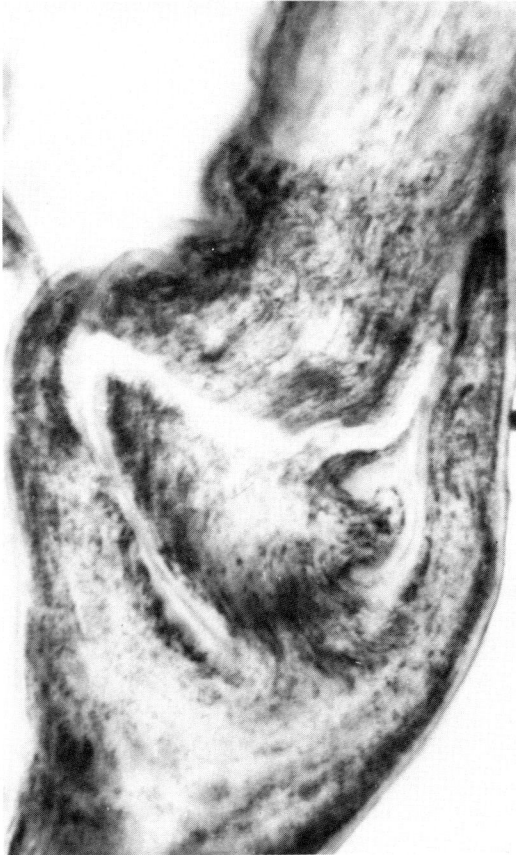

Figure 47–8.
Abnormal hairs. Trichorrhexis invaginata (bamboo hair) in a patient with Netherton syndrome.

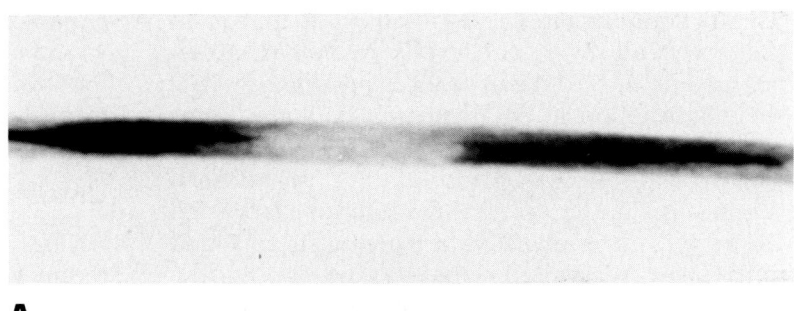

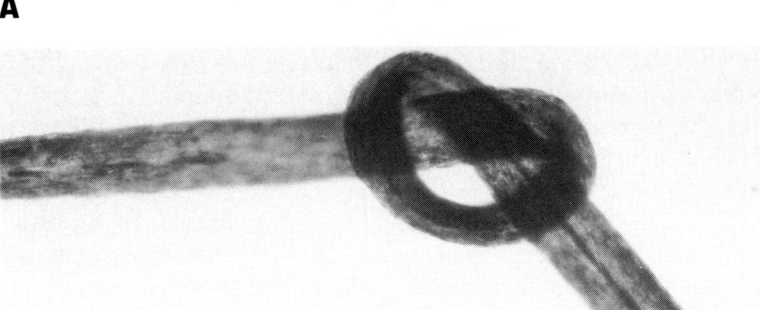

Figure 47–9.
Abnormal hairs. **A.** Pili annulati. **B.** Trichonodosis. **C.** Twisted hairs.

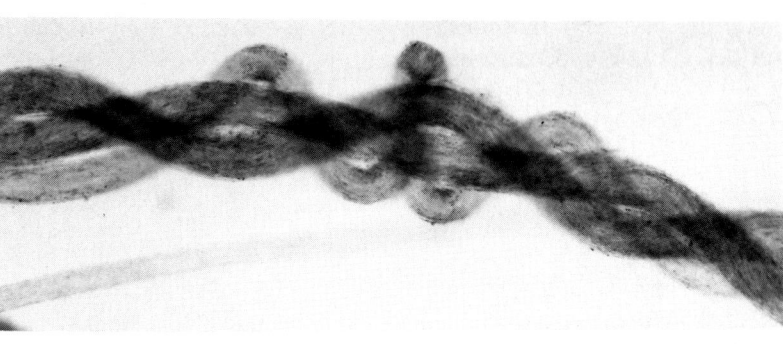

Hair in Congenital Disorders

Hair is a good genetic marker,[31] and many peculiarities of hair growth and color are visible to the naked eye and do not require microscopic examination. Hair dysplasia often is associated with dysplasia of other cutaneous adnexa, such as various forms of hypohidrotic ectodermal dysplasia.[32,33] In some of these long-known disorders, microscopic examination of scalp biopsies and hair can add interesting new findings. We mention the Marie Unna type of hereditary hypotrichosis,[34,35] in which fluting and twisting of hair shafts and unusual epithelial outgrowths on hair follicles may be seen, and Menkes' disease[36] in which copper metabolism is deranged and kinky hairs are a prominent manifestation. Such experiences should encourage dermatologists to take biopsies in cases of macroscopic abnormality of hair more often. It can be expected that missing links in the spectrum of follicular malformation may be thus discovered. A case in point is the discovery of generalized follicular hamartomas where alopecia totalis had been diagnosed on clinical examination.[37]

Circumscribed Abnormalities

Occurrence of abnormal hairs in circumscribed areas was mentioned in Chapter 37. In *congenital triangular alopecia* one-sided or bilateral involvement of the frontotemporal region is present at birth. Small vellus-like follicles are present instead of the normal hair follicles in the area.[38] Another abnormality is woolly hair nevus, which may occur in generalized, localized, and acquired forms.[39–41] The localized form may be limited to an area of verrucous epidermal nevus.[42] The term "woolly" in connection with human hair is confusing. Many authors refer to

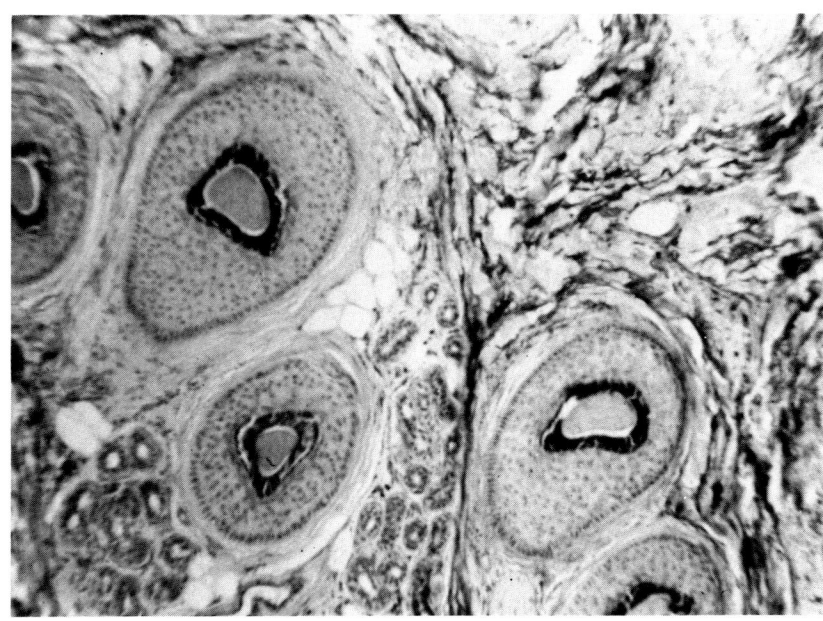

Figure 47–10.
Unmanageable hair. Triangular and kidney-shaped hair shafts. O&G. X125.

the hair of blacks as woolly, but wool of sheep has quite different structural and histochemical characteristics, which are not found in human hair.[43] The hair follicle of blacks has a regular semicircular curve, and the hair continues the curl imposed on it during its keratinizing phase after it leaves the skin. Most authors do not define exactly what they mean by woolly hair, and it is likely that measurements of hair and biopsy of scalp would reveal different anomalies in different cases. It would be better to refer to localized abnormalities of hair as "curly" or "kinky hair nevi" than as woolly hair nevi.

Pili Multigemini

Scattered abnormal hairs may be found on close examination, especially in the beard, and rarely cause symptoms. These abnormalities vary from fluted hairshafts to hair with double medulla, bifurcate,[38] and other monstrous hairs (pagothrix), and in the fullest expression multiple hairs (pili multigemini[44,45]), in which up to seven asymmetric hairs (Fig. 47–11) each with its own inner root sheath, arise from a single multiheaded papilla (Fig. 47–12). The papilla is unusually large, and the total diameter of the divided hair is much thicker than normal, causing difficulties in shaving.

Trichostasis Spinulosa

The occurrences described above must be sharply differentiated from the condition trichostasis spinulosa, in which several to dozens of dead vellus hairs are retained in a follicle (see Fig. 47–13A), each formed successively from the normal matrix.[46,47]

Trichonodosis

Trichonodosis, the formation of true knots (Fig. 47–9B) is easily recognized under the microscope and is

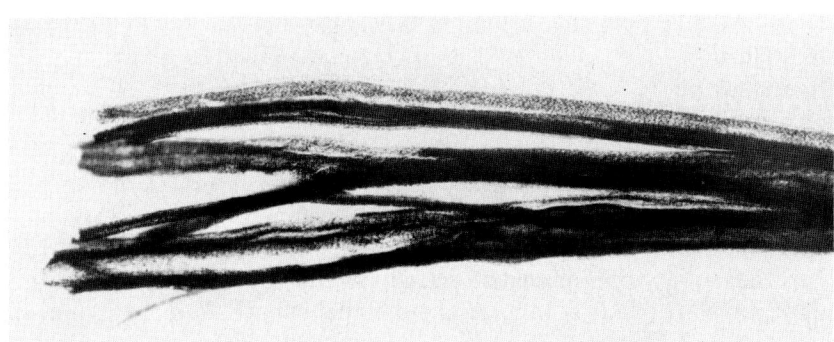

Figure 47–11.
Pili multigemini. Upper end of multiple hair formation consisting of several branching and reuniting asymmetrical shafts (pagothrix). Formations of this type can be differentiated from trichoptilosis (longitudinal splitting of a single hair) by the much greater combined volume of the several hairs, each of which has its own cuticle.

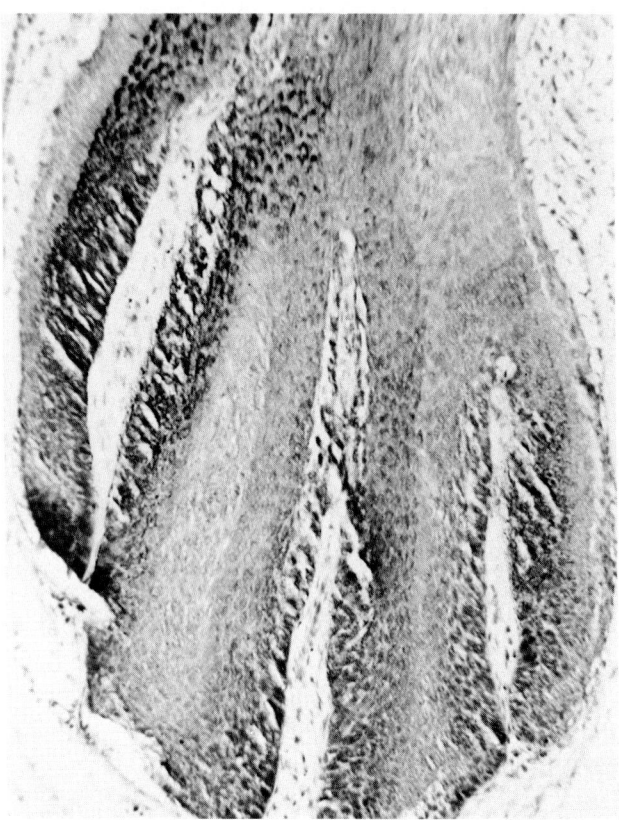

Figure 47–12.
Pili multigemini. Hair bulb showing subdivision of dermal papilla into several lobes, each surrounded by matrix and keratinizing cells which partly unite higher up into a very thick shaft that will break up into multiple hairs (Fig. 47–11). H&E. X135. (From Mehregan and Thompson. Br J Dermatol 100:315, 1979.)

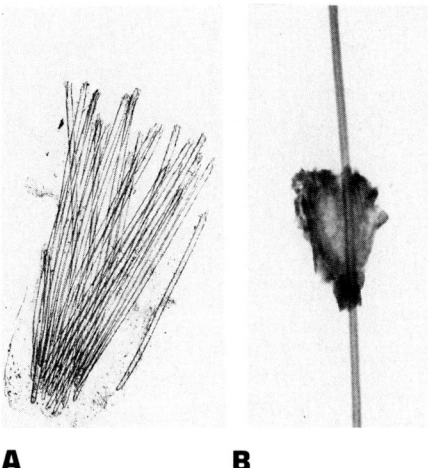

A   B

Figure 47–13.
A. Trichostasis spinulosa. Bundle of hairs expressed from a small hair follicle. X30. **B.** Hair cast. X125.

more common than generally believed, especially in kinky scalp hair.

Disturbances of Hair Due to External Causes: Traction Alopecia and Trichotillomania

The alterations of hair due to common cosmetic procedures cannot be discussed here. Definitely pathologic changes, however, are produced by those manipulations leading to traction alopecia. These include tight braiding and attachments of nurse's caps.[48] Affected follicles enter telogen and become surrounded by inflammatory cells and dermal fibrosis and may even undergo irreversible atrophy. The histologic picture may imitate pseudopelade. A different picture, so-called *trichomalacia* (Fig. 47–14), is produced by compulsive pulling at hair, trichotillomania.[49,50] Here the number of hair follicles is not decreased. There are a number of normal anagen follicles, but many are also found in catagen, a stage rarely seen in other conditions because of its short duration. Strong follicles may contain peculiar deformed hairs or just pigmented keratinous debris. Other histologic findings include longitudinal wrinkling of the affected hair follicles, empty follicles, and perifollicular hemorrhage.

Trichosporosis and Trichomycosis

Changes of the hair due to dermatophytic infection were mentioned in Chapter 18. Spores and mycelia around and in the shaft can be seen in plucked hairs suspended in oil, crushed in xylene,[51] or cautiously treated with 10 percent potassium hydroxide. PAS stain, as illustrated in Figure 47–15A, is rarely necessary. Other organisms, such as *Trichosporon Beigelii* (*cutaneum*) causing *white piedra*[52,53] and *Corynebacterium tenue* causing *trichomycosis axillaris*[54,55] (Fig. 47–15B,C), also attack hair of axillae and pubic region. White, brown, or greenish nodules adhere to the hair shaft and may coalesce into sleeve-like concretions.

Extraneous Material on Hair

In the microscopic examination of shed or plucked hair, extraneous matter is often seen. Commonly, adherent dirt or hair dye is of no consequence except in forensic medicine. The growing anagen hair, when plucked, usually is enveloped in the soft portions of inner and outer root sheath, forming a semi-

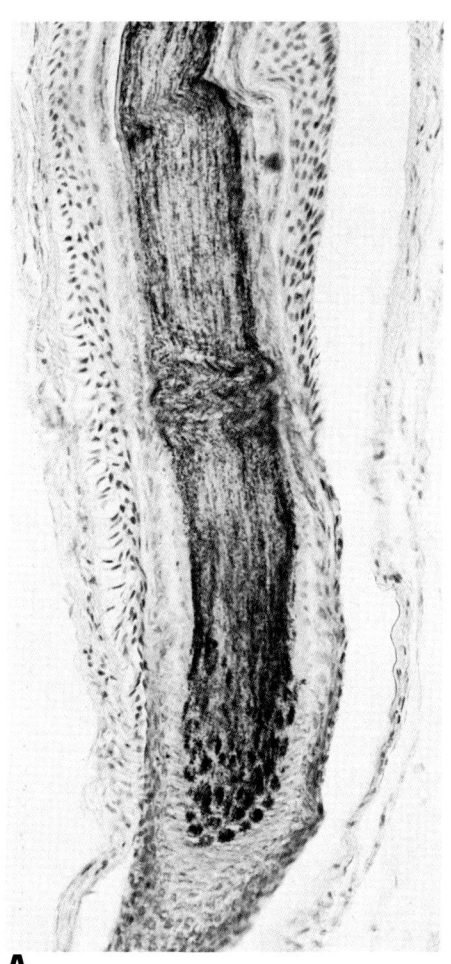 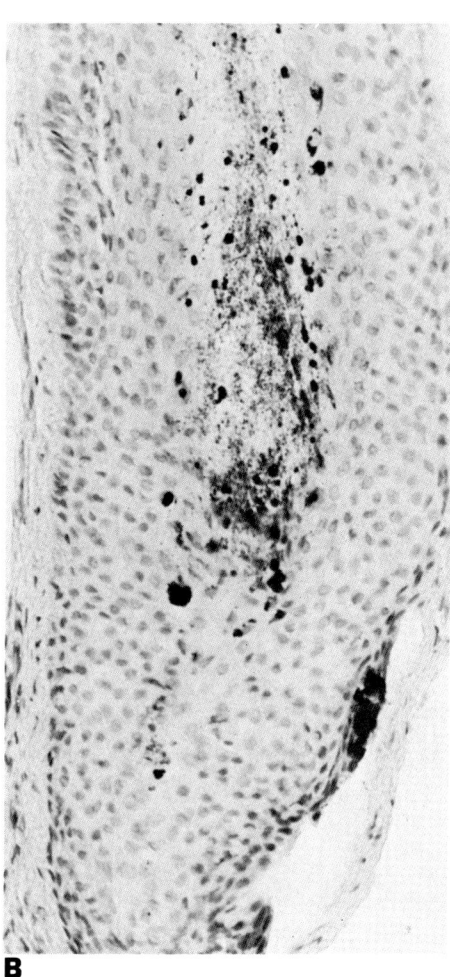

Figure 47–14.
Trichomalacia in a case of trichotillomania. **A.** Deformed hair in fairly normal follicle. **B.** Pigmented debris in another follicle. H&E. X135.

transparent coat around the lower end. This is absent in catagen and telogen hairs. Nits in pediculosis capitis is demonstrated in Fig. 47–15D.

Hair Casts

Hair casts also called peripilar keratin casts are keratinized remnants of inner and outer root sheathes and may be found as sliding whitish rings (Fig. 47–13B) around hair shafts.[56–59] They sometimes are mistaken for nits (see Fig. 47–15D) on naked-eye examination but are movable and can easily be distinguished under the microscope, where they resemble napkin rings of keratotic material.

DISTURBANCES OF NAIL

Punch biopsy specimens of nail and nailbed can be obtained without permanent deformity if the matrix region is avoided.[60] If the matrix must be biopsied, two longitudinal incisions should be made about 2 mm apart and the gap sutured in order to obtain a strip of tissue with minimal scarring.[61] Small punch biopsies can also be taken of the matrix after it is exposed by incising and reverting the posterior fold. Skillful surgery is a prerequisite. Otherwise specimens are of little value, and the nail may remain deformed.

Various Dermatoses

Pathologic changes of the soft tissues under the nail-plate do not differ materially from those of other regions in many inflammatory and neoplastic conditions and need little specific discussion.[62] Nailbed changes in pustular psoriasis[63] are shown in Figure 47–16, those of lichen planus[64,65] in Figure 47–17. Some cases with twenty-nail dystrophy are most likely ungual manifestation of lichen planus. Others developing in childhood may be a separate

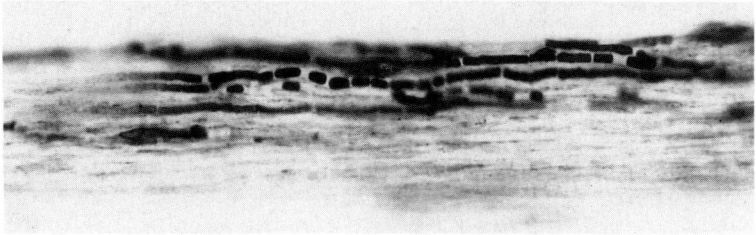

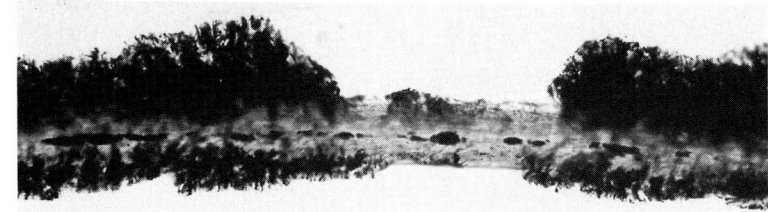

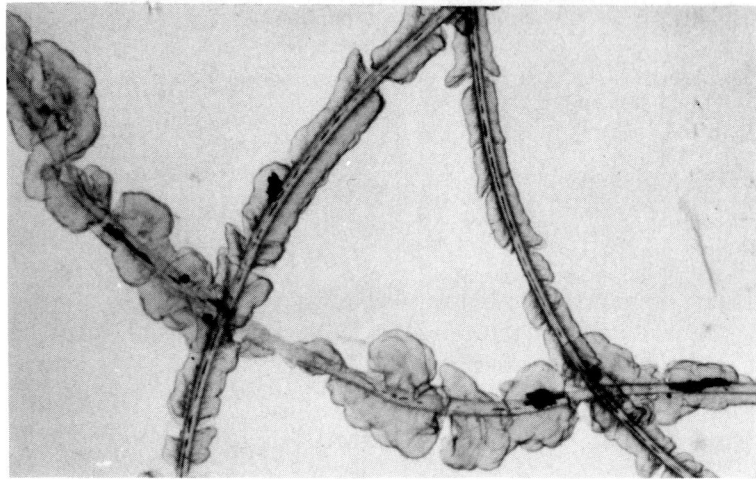

Figure 47–15.
A. Endothrix fungus in a hair shaft. PAS: X225. **B.** Trichomycosis axillaris (black piedra). X225. **C.** White piedra (Trichosporon Beigelii). X125. **D.** Nits in pediculosis capitis. X75.

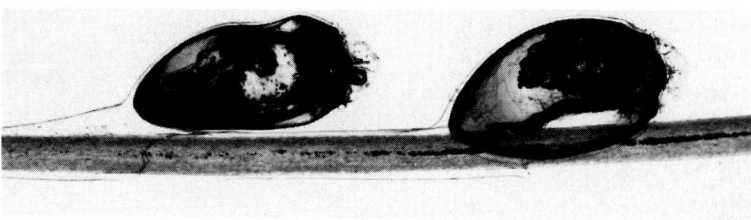

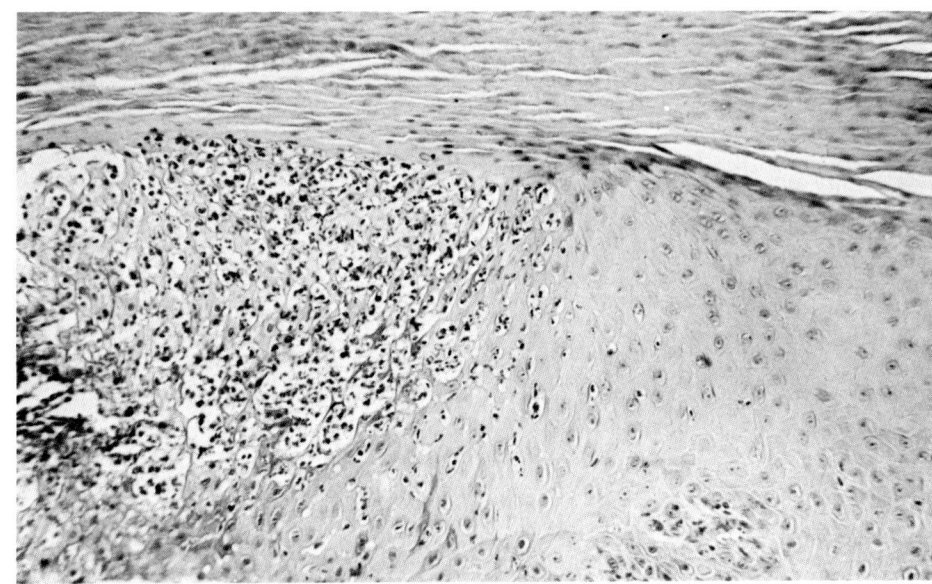

Figure 47–16.
Pustular psoriasis of nailbed. Spongiform pustule and excess formation of parakeratotic material are similar to the processes seen in other areas (see Figs. 8–11 and 8–12).

condition.[66–68] Zaias and Ackerman[69] described characteristic dyskeratotic changes of the soft tissues around the nail in Darier's disease and multinucleated giant cells in the cornified portions of nailplate and nailbed. Scabies mites may occasionally affect the nail and surrounding keratinized tissue.[70]

Bowen's disease and keratoacanthoma may affect the nail matrix and nailbed and may require differential diagnosis from squamous cell carcinoma and from verruca vulgaris. The latter can involve the nailbed for a considerable distance from the distal or lateral margins. These diagnoses require res-

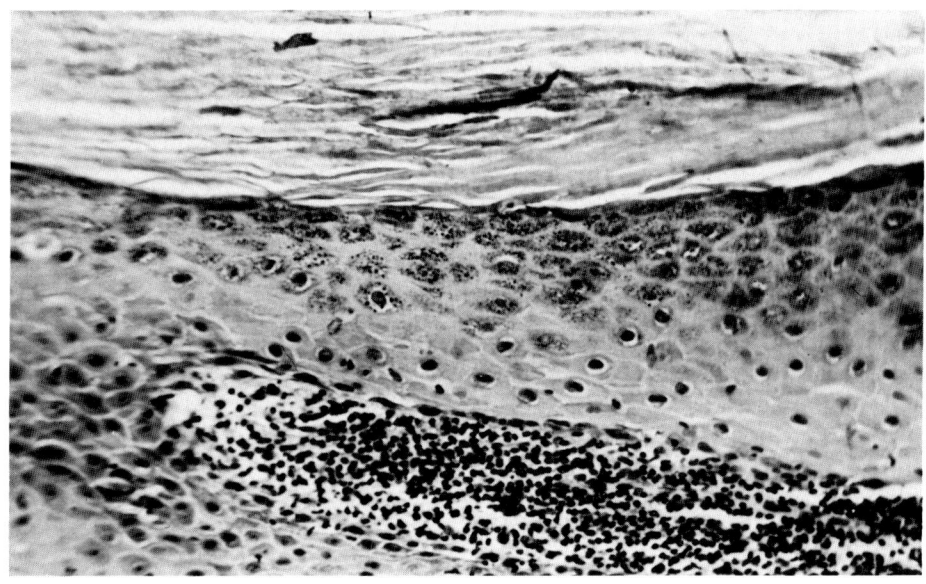

Figure 47–17.
Lichen planus of nailbed. Loss of basal layer and formation of granular layer, not normally present in the bed of the nail. Dense lymphocytic infiltrate. H&E. X180.

olute measures for adequate biopsy. The nailplate must be avulsed in order to inspect the underlying tissues and to obtain a sufficiently large and deep specimen.

Discolored nailplate is rarely submitted for pigment identification as hemosiderin or melanin and its examination is often unsatisfactory. Thickened dystrophic nails and subungual hyperkeratotic material can be processed for paraffin embedding and PAS stain when diagnosis of onychomycosis is suspected and the results are usually superior to the KOH examination (Fig. 47–18). Longitudinal melanonychia has many causes including chronic friction, drugs (azidodeoxythimidine), dermatoses, and the rare Laugier–Hunziker syndrome.[71–74] These are due to either a focal increased melanogenesis or an increase in the number of melanocytes such as in lentigo simplex or junction nevus.[75]

A decision to whether such a lesion is a lentigo simplex, a junction nevus, or an acral lentiginous melanoma can only be made by adequate incisional biopsy after removal of the nailplate.[76] Leukonychia striata characterized by transverse bands of pigmentation has been reported in patients with systemic lupus erythematosus.[77]

Hemorrhage

Hemorrhages involving the nail matrix (Fig. 47–19) will be incorporated into the nailplate as it forms and keratinizes and will either make it so abnormal that it disintegrates or will appear on the surface as the nail moves forward. On the other hand, hemorrhages into the nailbed distal to the lunula will remain below the nailplate but will be moved forward with it.

Pachyonychia Congenita

In pachyonychia congenita[78] (Fig. 47–20), in spite of its name, the nailplate and the proximal nail matrix from which it arises are quite normal.[79–81] The normally semisterile nailbed epithelium, however, and the distal matrix, which normally forms only a small amount of keratin (horn of the sole, hyponychium), are hyperplastic and papillomatous and produce large quantities of abnormal horny material mixed with hyaline masses (*colloid keratosis*). Each of the deformed nails resembles a miniature horse's hoof histologically as well as clinically.[82]

Pterygium Inversum Unguis

A minor deformity of the distal matrix that may occur as a congenital or acquired phenomenon is pterygium inversum unguis.[83,84] Here, the keratin formed by the distal matrix adheres tightly to the lower surface of the nail and is pulled forward.

The monographs on diseases of the nails mentioned in the introduction to Section VIII should be consulted for more detailed discussion.

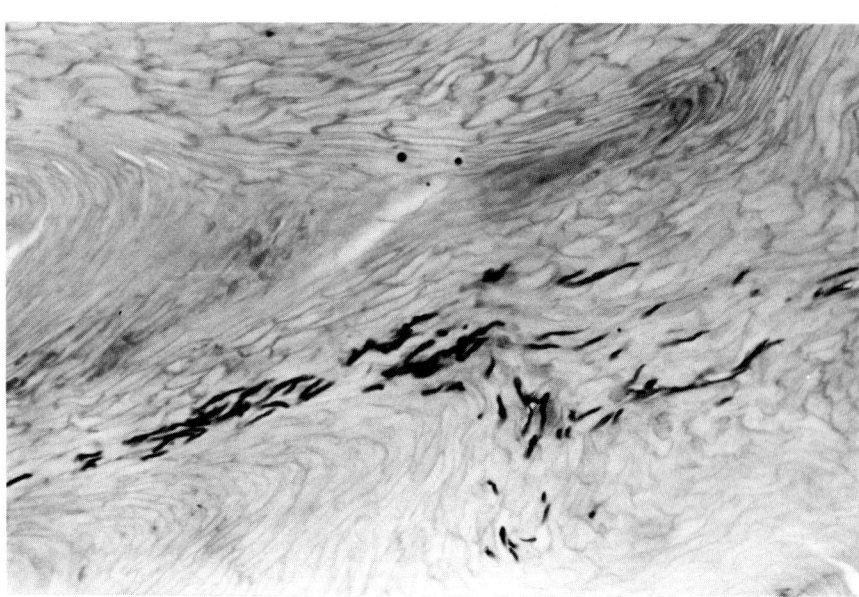

Figure 47–18.
Onychomycosis. Spotty involvement of nailplate with fungus mycelia. PAS. X400.

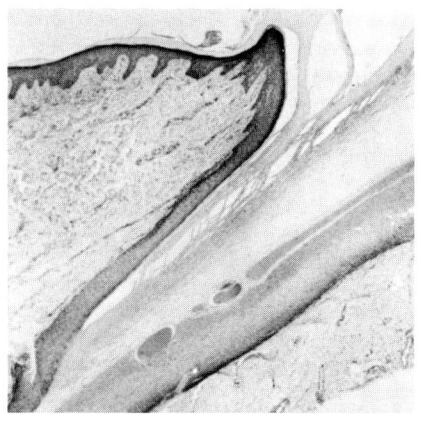 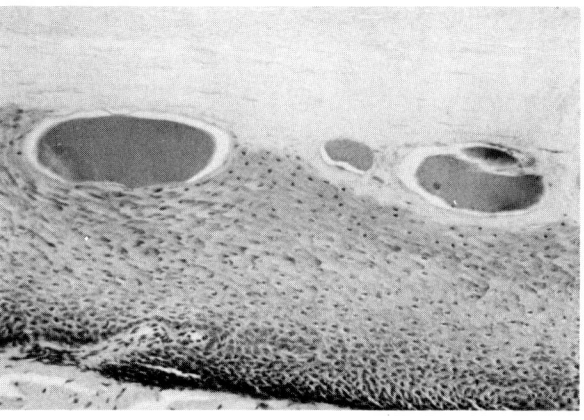

Figure 47-19.
Subungual hemorrhage. **A.** The blood is deposited as several coagulated masses between the nail matrix and the forming nail plate. H&E. X125. **B.** At higher power, it is seen that the clot at the left indents the nail matrix, while the clot at the right has been incorporated into the nail (a form of transepithelial elimination). H&E. X250. Note also in **A** the obvious division of the keratin of the posterior nailfold into eponychium and cuticle (see Fig. 47-1).

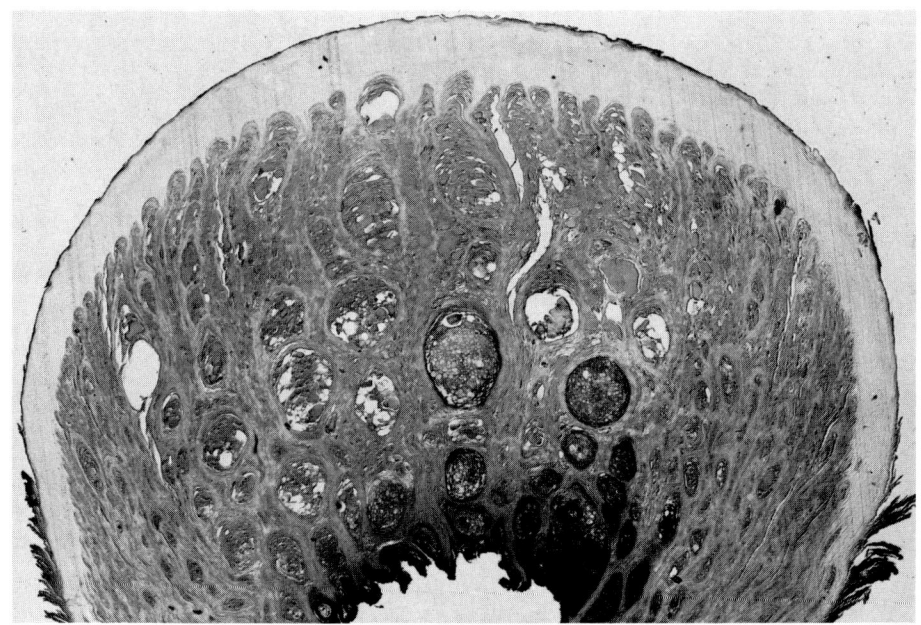

Figure 47-20.
Cross section of nail in pachyonychia congenita shows well-formed sturdy nailplate and papillomatous distal matrix tissue producing abnormal keratin honeycombed with coagulated PAS-positive material (colloid keratosis). Configuration resembles a horse's hoof. Compare with Figure 47-1. H&E. X21.

REFERENCES

1. Orfanos CE, Montagna W, Stuttgen G: Hair research. Berlin: Springer-Verlag, 1981
2. Barth JH: Normal hair growth in children. Pediatr Dermatol 4:173, 1987
3. Pinkus F: Die Einwirkung von Krankheiten auf das Kopfhaar des Menschen, 2nd ed. Berlin: Karger, 1928
4. Van Scott EJ, Reinertson RP, Steinmuller R: The growing hair roots of the human scalp and morphologic changes therein following amethropterin therapy. J Invest Dermatol 29:197, 1957
5. Kligman AM: Pathologic dynamics of human hair loss. I. Telogen effluvium. Arch Dermatol 83:175, 1961
6. Venning VA, Dawber RPR: Patterned androgenic alopecia in women. J Am Acad Dermatol 18:1073, 1988
7. Lattanand A, Johnson WC: Male pattern alopecia. A histopathologic and histochemical study. J Cutan Pathol 2:58, 1975
8. Pinkus H: Differential patterns of elastic fibers in scarring and non-scarring alopecias. J Cutan Pathol 5:93, 1978
9. Levantine A, Almeyda J: Drug-induced alopecia. Br J Dermatol 89:549, 1973
10. Van Scott EJ, Reinertson RP: Detection of radiation effects on hair roots of the human scalp. J Invest Dermatol 29:205, 1957
11. Valda Rodriguez L, Torrico Velasco J, Zaballos Vasconcellos R: Hypertrichose lanugineuse acquise paranéoplasique associée a une sclerodermie. Ann Dermatol Venereol 117:605, 1990
12. Kassis V, Kassis E, Keiding L, et al: Hypertrichosis Lanuginosa acquisita associated with multiple malignancies. J Am Acad Dermatol 12:1106, 1985
13. Hovenden AL: Acquired hypertrichosis lanuginosa associated with malignancy. Arch Intern Med 147:2013, 1987
14. Prigent F, Gantzer A, Romain O, et al: Hypertrichose diffuse acquise au cours d'un traitement par diazoxide chez un nouveau-ne. Ann Dermatol Venereol 115:191, 1988
15. Whiting DA: Structural abnormalities of the hair shaft. J Am Acad Dermatol 16:1, 1987
16. Caserio RJ, Hordinsky MK: Disorders of hair. J Am Acad Dermatol 19:895, 1988
17. Comacho-Martinez F, Ferrando J: Hair shaft dysplasias. Int J Dermatol 27:71, 1988
18. Van Neste D: Dysplasies pilaires congenitales: Conduite a tenir et interet de diverses methodes de diagnostic. Ann Dermatol Venereol 116:251, 1989
19. Comaish S: Autoradiographic studies of hair growth and rhythm in monilethrix. Br J Dermatol 81:443, 1969
20. Comacho-Martinez F: Localized trichorrhexis nodosa. J Am Acad Dermatol 20:696, 1989
21. Ito M, Ito K, Hashimoto K: Pathogenesis in trichorrhexis invaginata (bamboo hair). J Invest Dermatol 83:1, 1984
22. Greene SL, Muller SA: Netherton's syndrome. Report of a case and review of the literature. J Am Acad Dermatol 13:329, 1985
23. Lalevic-Vasic B, Polic DJ: Pili annulati. Etude en microscopie electronique a balayage. Ann Dermatol Venereol 115:433, 1988
24. Hamm H, Traupe H: Loose anagen hair of childhood: The phenomenon of easily pluckable hair. J Am Acad Dermatol 20:242, 1989
25. Price VH, Gummer CL: Loose anagen syndrome. J Am Acad Dermatol 20:249, 1989
26. Stroud JD, Mehregan AH: "Spun glass" hair. A clinicopathologic study of an unusual hair defect. In Brown AC (ed): The First Human Hair Symposium. New York: Medcom, 1974
27. Rest EB, Fretzin DF: Quantitative assessment of scanning electron microscope defects in uncombable-hair syndrome. Pediatr Dermatol 7:93, 1990
28. Shelley WB, Shelley ED: Uncombable hair syndrome: Observations on response to biotin and occurrence in siblings with ectodermal dysplasia. J Am Acad Dermatol 13:97, 1985
29. Mortimer PS: Unruly hair. Br J Dermatol 113:467, 1985
30. Matis WL, Baden H, Green R, et al: Uncombable hair syndrome. Pediatr Dermatol 4:215, 1987
31. Muller SA: Alopecia: Syndromes of genetic significance. J Invest Dermatol 60:475, 1973
32. Sybert VP: Hypohidrotic ectodermal dysplasia: Argument against an autosomal recessive form clinically indistinguishable from X-linked hypohidrotic ectodermal dysplasia (Christ-Siemens-Touraine syndrome). Pediatr Dermatol 6:76, 1989
33. Micali G, Cook B, Blekys I, Solomon LM: Structural hair abnormalities in ectodermal dysplasia. J Pediat Dermatol 7:27, 1990
34. Solomon LM, Esterly NB, Modenica M: Hereditary trichodysplasia: Marie Unna's hypotrichosis. J Invest Dermatol 57:389, 1971
35. Hutchinson PE, Wells RS: Hereditary hypotrichosis (Marie-Unna type). Two cases. Proc R Soc Med 68:534, 1975
36. Enjolras O, Lessana-Leibowitch M, Hewitt J, et al: Maladie de Menkes. Anomalies ultrastructurales cutanéophanériennes nouvelles. Ann Dermatol Venereol 105:493, 1978
37. Mehregan AH, Baker S: Basaloid follicular hamartoma. Report of three cases with localized and systematized unilateral lesions. J Cutan Pathol 12:55, 1985
38. Tosti A: Congenital triangular alopecia: Report of fourteen cases. J Am Acad Dermatol 16:991, 1987
39. Stavrianeas N, Katsambas A, Stratigos J: Naevus laineux. Ann Dermatol Venereol 114:1447, 1987
40. Esterly NB, Lavin MP, Garancis JC: Acquired progressive kinking of the hair. Arch Dermatol 125:813, 1989
41. Reda AM, Rogers RS, Peters MS: Woolly hair nevus. J Am Acad Dermatol 22:377, 1990
42. Peteiro C, Oliva NP, Zulaica A, Toribio J: Woolly-hair nevus: Report of a case associated with a verrucous

epidermal nevus in the same area. Pediatr Dermatol 6:188, 1989
43. Histology of wool and hair and of the wool follicle. In Proceedings of the International Wool Textile Research Conference, Australia 1955, Vol F. Melbourne: Commonwealth Scientific and Industrial Research Organization, 1956
44. Pinkus H: Multiple hairs (Flemming-Giovannini). J Invest Dermatol 17:291, 1951
45. Mehregan AH, Thompson WS: Pili multigemini. Report of a case in association with cleidocranial dysostosis. Br J Dermatol 100:315, 1979
46. Nakamura S, Gotoh M: Trichostasis spinulosa. J Dermatol 11:181, 1984
47. Young MC, Jorizzo JL, Sanchez RL, et al: Trichostasis spinulosa. Int J Dermatol 24:575, 1985
48. Renna FS, Freedberg IM: Traction alopecia in nurses. Arch Dermatol 108:694, 1973
49. Muller SA: Trichotillomania: A histopathologic study in sixty-six patients. J Am Acad Dermatol 23:56, 1990
50. Oranje AP, Peereboom-Wynia JDR, De Raeymaecker DMJ: Trichotillomania in childhood. J Am Acad Dermatol 15:614, 1986
51. Shelley WB, Wood MG: New technic for instant visualization of fungi in hair. J Am Acad Dermatol 2:69, 1980
52. Kalter DC, Tschen JA, Cernoch PL, et al: Genital white piedra: Epidemiology, microbiology, and therapy. J Am Acad Dermatol 14:982, 1986
53. Avram A, Buot G, Binet O, et al: Etude clinique et mycologique concernant 11 cas de trichosporie noueuse (Piedra blanche) genito-pubienne. Ann Dermatol Venereol 114:819, 1987
54. Levit F: Trichomycosis axillaris: A different view. J Am Acad Dermatol 18:778, 1988
55. Wilson C, Dawber R: Trichomycosis axillaris: A different view. J Am Acad Dermatol 21:325, 1989
56. Taieb A, Surleve-Bazeille JE, Maleville J: Hair casts: A clinical and morphologic study. Arch Dermatol 121:1009, 1985
57. Keipert JA: Hair casts. Review and suggestion regarding nomenclature. Arch Dermatol 122:927, 1986
58. Zhu W-Y, Xia M-Y, Wu J-H, Do A-A: Hair casts: A clinical and electron microscopic study. Pediatr Dermatol 7:270, 1990
59. Held JL, Bernstein RM: Hair casts or pseudonits acquired following psychological trauma. Cutis 43:780, 1989
60. Sher RK: Onychomycosis: Examining, diagnosis and treatment. Mycol Observ 4:1, 1984
61. Hanno R, Mathes BM, Krull EA: Longitudinal nail biopsy in evaluation of acquired nail dystrophies. J Am Acad Dermatol 14:803, 1986
62. Zaias N: The Nail in Health and Disease. 2 ed. Norwalk, Conn: Appleton and Lange, 1989
63. Lewin K, DeWit S, Ferrington RA: Pathology of the fingernail in psoriasis; a clinicopathologic study. Br J Dermatol 86:555, 1972
64. Kanwar AJ, Govil DC, Singh OP: Lichen planus limited to the nails. Int J Dermatol 32:163, 1983
65. Tosti A, DePadova MP, Fanti P: Nail involvement in lichen planopilaris. Cutis 42:213, 1988
66. Jeanmougin M, Civatte J: Ongles greses at "twenty-nail dystrophy of childhood." A propos de 2 cas. Dermatologica 168:242, 1984
67. Colver GB, Dawber RPR: Is childhood idiopathic atrophy of the nails due to lichen planus. Br J Dermatol 116:709, 1987
68. Fenton DA, Samman PD: Twenty-nail dystrophy of childhood associated with alopecia areata and lichen planus. Br J Dermatol 119 (Suppl 33): 63, 1988
69. Zaias N, Ackerman AB: The nail in Darier-White disease. Arch Dermatol 107:193, 1973
70. Saruta T, Nakamizo Y: Usual scabies with nail infestation. Arch Dermatol 114:956, 1978
71. Baran S: Frictional longitudinal melanonychia: A new entity. Dermatologica 174:280, 1987
72. Tosto A, Gaddoni G, Fanti PA, et al: Longitudinal melanonychia by 3-azidodeoxythymidine. Dermatologica 180:217, 1990
73. Grau-Massanes M, Millan F, Febrer MI, et al: Pigmented nail bands and mucocutaneous pigmentation in HIV-positive patients treated with zidovudine. J Am Acad Dermatol 23:687, 1990
74. Baran R, Barriere H: Longitudinal melanonychia with spreading pigmentation in Laugier–Hunziker syndrome: A report of two cases. Br J Dermatol 115:707, 1986
75. Baran R, Kechijian P: Longitudinal melanonychia (Melanonychia striata): Diagnosis and management. J Am Acad Dermatol 21:1165, 1989
76. Kato T, Usuba Y, Takematsu H, et al: A rapidly growing pigmented nail streak resulting in diffuse melanosis of the nail. Cancer 64:2191, 1989
77. Friedman SJ: Leukonychia striata associated with systemic lupus erythematosus. J Am Acad Dermatol 15:536, 1986
78. Su DWP, Chun SI, Hammond DE, Gordon H: Pachyonychia congenita: A clinical study of 12 cases and review of the literature. Pediatr Dermatol 7:33, 1990
79. Clementi M, Cardin de Stefani E, Dei Rossi C, et al: Pachyonichia congenita Jackson–Lawler type: A distinct malformation syndrome. Br J Dermatol 114:367, 1986
80. Tidman MJ, Wells RS, MacDonald DM: Pachyonychia congenita with cutaneous amyloidosis and hyperpigmentation—A distinct variant. J Am Acad Dermatol 16:935, 1987
81. Feinstein A, Friedman J, Schewach-Millet N: Pachyonychia congenita. J Am Acad Dermatol 19:705, 1988
82. Kelly EW Jr, Pinkus H: Report of a case of pachyonychia congenita. Arch Dermatol 77:724, 1958
83. Odom RB, Stein KM, Maibach HI: Congenital, painful, aberrant hyponychium. Arch Dermatol 110:89, 1974
84. Catteral MD, White JE: Pterygium inversum unguis. Clin Exp Dermatol 3:437, 1978

INDEX

AA protein, 388
Abscess(es). *See also* Microabscess; Munro abscesses; Pautrier abscess(es)
  of acne, 250
  in blastomycosis, 306
  intraepidermal, 89f
  in maduromycosis, 307, 310f
Acantholysis, 83, 86, 86f
Acantholytic acanthoma, 494
Acantholytic disorders, 157–162
  differential diagnosis, 158t, 161–162, 396t
Acantholytic squamous cell carcinoma.
  See Squamous cell carcinoma, acantholytic
Acanthomas, 501. *See also* Acantholytic acanthoma; Clear cell acanthoma
  basosquamous, 489
  clear cell, 490, 492f
  large cell, 492–493, 495f
  pilar sheath, 533, 535f–536f
Acanthosis, 80f, 81, 101
  in atopic dermatitis, 107–108
  in chronic contact dermatitis, 105–106, 106f
  in contact dermatitis, 104, 105f
  definition of, 80
  nigricans, 419, 482, 484f
  psoriasiform, 115
  in sensitization dermatitis, 103–104
Acetylcholinesterase, in apocrine and eccrine apparatuses, 33t
Acid alcohol solution, 57
Acid formaldehyde hematin, 54
Acid mucopolysaccharides, staining, 46t, 59–60
Acid orcein–Giemsa stain, 32, 46t, 55–58, 60
  advantages of, 96
  for amyloid, 388
  of eosinophils and elastic fibers, 278f
  fixation with, 57

Page numbers followed by t or f indicate tables or figures, respectively.

  in lichen sclerosus et atrophicus, 357f, 358
  solutions, 57
  staining procedure, 57–58
  staining reactions of tissue constituents, 58
  substances staining purple with, 58
Acid phosphatase, in apocrine and eccrine apparatuses, 33t
Acne
  conglobata, 275
  fulminans, 251
  keloidalis, 253–254
  miliaris necrotica, 253
  pustule of, 250
  rosacea, 202f
  vulgaris, 385
    cystic lesion of, 251, 251f
    folliculitis of, 249–251, 250f–251f
Acquired (tufted) angioma *See* Angioma
Acquired digital fibrokeratoma, 624, 624f
Acquired immunodeficiency syndrome
  cutaneous manifestations of, 182t
  histoplasmosis in, 298
  Kaposi's sarcoma in, 655
  oral hairy leukoplakia in, 704–705, 705f
  Reiter's syndrome in, 127
  seborrheic dermatitis in, 116
  tuberculosis in, 281
  ulcerations in, 244
Acral lentiginous melanoma, 460–463, 466f–468f
  differential diagnosis, 466t
Acro-angiodermatitis, 227
Acrochordon, 623, 624f
  strangulated, 645
Acrodermatitis
  chronica atrophicans, 355
  continua, 124
    differential diagnosis, 117t
  enteropathica, 162, 163f
    vesicullobullous eruptions of, 158t
Acrokeratoelastoidosis (Costa), 374
Acrokeratosis
  paraneoplastica, 109
  verruciformis of Hopf, 482

Acromelanosis albo-punctata, 415
Acroosteolysis, 353
Acropigmentation of Dohi, 415
Acrosclerosis
  fingertip ulcers of, 247
  immunopathology, 77
Acrosyringeal cell(s), 15, 16f
Acrosyringium, 15–16, 16f, 35–36, 36f
  definition of, 9t
  development, 8
  rupture of, 273, 274f
Acrotrichium, 15–16, 27
Acrylic fiber granuloma, 297
Actinic cheilitis, 709
Actinic elastosis, 373–374, 377f, 383, 418
Actinic granuloma, 321, 324–325
Actinic keratosis, 387, 502–507, 503f–508f, 509
  architecture of, 502f, 502–503
  atrophic, 504, 505f, 506
  bowenoid, 506, 507f
  combined with lentigo senilis, 506, 508f
  Darierlike form, 505, 506f
  differential diagnosis, 502
  lichenoid, 507
  pigmented, 506, 507f
  progression to invasive cancer, 512, 512f
Actinic reticuloid, 212, 683
Actinomycosis, 305, 307
Acute febrile neutrophilic dermatosis, 150–151, 152f
Adamantinoma, 586
Addison's disease, 415, 707
Adenoacanthomas, 514
Adenocarcinoma, 512. *See also* Apocrine adenocarcinoma; Eccrine carcinoma
  apocrine, 607, 611f
  of meibomian glands, 603, 604f
  and organoid nevi, 523
  sebaceous, 603, 604f
  of sweat apparatus, 603–615
Adenoma
  papillary eccrine, 570, 573f
    malignant transformation of, 606

731

Adenoma (cont.)
  sebaceous, 526, 527f
  sebaceum, 621
  tubular, 398f
Adnexa, cutaneous, development, 7–8
Adnexal basal cell, definition of, 9t
Adnexal carcinoma, 585
  and organoid nevi, 523
  pilary complex, 613f, 614
  undifferentiated, 614
Adnexal cell(s), modulation, in wound healing, 16, 17f
Adnexal epithelium, definition of, 9t
Adnexal histology, terminology, 9t
Adnexal keratinocyte, definition of, 9t
Adnexal matrix cell(s), 17f
  definition of, 9t
Adnexal tumors, classification of, 437
Adrenoleukodystrophy, 38
Adult linear IgA bullous dermatosis
  clinical presentation, 75
  diagnosis, immunofluorescence in, 75
Adventitial dermis, 19
AEI-3, immunostaining reactive patterns, 70t
Aggressive digital papillary adenoma, 576–577, 579f
Aging, skin changes due to, 373
AIDS. See Acquired immunodeficiency syndrome
AK, formalin fixed, paraffin embedded sections, immunohistochemical staining pattern for, 66t
AL amyloid, 387–388
Albinism
  partial, 413, 443
  total, 413
Albright's hereditary osteodystrophy (Albright syndrome), 385, 442
Alcian blue stain (Mowry), 19, 46t, 56, 59
  combined with periodic acid–Schiff and picric acid, 59
Alcoholic eosin solution, 57
Alcoholic fixatives, 53
Aldehyde fuchsin stain (Gomori), 46t, 58, 60
Alizarin red stain, 46t, 61
Alkaline phosphatase, in apocrine and eccrine apparatuses, 33t
Allergic granulomatous angiitis, 220
Allergic vasculitis, biopsy in, 45
Alopecia, 29. See also Pattern alopecia; Scarring alopecia
  areata, 265, 266f
  with breast cancer metastasis to scalp, 616
  congenital triangular, 720
  with inflammation, 265–271
  mucinosa, 265–267, 267f–268f, 680
  neoplastica, 268
  traction, 722
Alpha$_1$-antitrypsin deficiency, panniculitis with, 235
Alpha-galactosidase deficiency, 647
Alternaria spore, as tissue contaminant, 61f, 62
Alternariosis, 312
Aluminum-induced granuloma, 296
Amiodarone, discoloration of sun-exposed skin and, 417
Ammoniacal silver nitrate staining technique (Fontana–Masson), 60
Amputation neuromas, 663
Amylase, digestion of specimens, 60
Amyloid
  skin-limited types, 386–387
  staining, 46t, 58–60, 386–388
Amyloid K, 386, 388
  in basal cell epithelioma, 588

Amyloidosis
  of auricular concha, 386–387
  lichenoid, 386, 389f
  multiple myeloma-associated, 387–388
  nodular, 387–388
  secondary systemic, 388
  systemic, 387–388
Amylophosphorylase, in apocrine and eccrine apparatuses, 33t
ANA. See Antinuclear antibodies
Anagen (phase of hair cycle), 25, 30, 33–34, 35f. See also Hair follicle(s), anagen
Anaplasia, 87
Anchoring filaments, 10
Andrews' pustular bacterid, 125
Anetoderma, 372–373, 376f
Aneurysmal fibrous histiocytoma, 652, 653f
Angiitis. See also Necrotizing angiitis
  allergic granulomatous, 220
  definition of, 217
Angioblastoma, 649–650, 650f
Angiofibroma(s), 621
  of mucous membranes, 710
Angioimmunoblastic lymphadenopathy, 684
Angiokeratoma, 647, 648f
  neviforme, 647
Angioleiomyoma(s), 621, 634, 636f
Angiolipoma(s), 637, 638f
Angiolupoid, 295
Angiolymphoid hyperplasia with eosinophilia, 652, 654f–655f
Angioma
  acquired (tufted), 649–650, 650f
  serpiginosum, 646
Angiomatoid fibrous histiocytoma, 652, 653f
Angiosarcoma, 652, 654–655, 657f–658f
Anthrax, 243
Antibody(ies). See also Antinuclear antibodies; Autoantibodies
  antibasement membrane, in bullous pemphigoid, 157
  anticentromere, 77
  antiintercellular, 67
  antinuclear ribonucleoprotein, in mixed connective tissue disease, 76
$α_1$-Antichymotrypsin, immunostaining reactive patterns, 70t
Anticoagulation, and biopsy, 50
Antifibrinogen, in direct immunofluorescence, 65
Antifibrohistiocyte, in direct immunofluorescence, 66t
Antihypertensives, lichenoid drug eruption caused by, 141
Antikeratin, in direct immunofluorescence, 66t
Antimelanoma, in direct immunofluorescence, 66, 66t
Antinuclear antibodies
  in scleroderma, 77
  in systemic lupus erythematosus, 76
$α_1$-Antitrypsin, immunostaining reactive patterns, 70t
Anus, basaloid carcinoma of, 709–710
Aphthae, 700, 701f
Aphthosis, 700
Aphthous ulcer, 701f–702f
Aplasia cutis congenita, 356f, 356–357
Apocrine adenocarcinoma, 607, 611f
  epidermotropic, 608
Apocrine apparatus, enzyme activities in, 33t
Apocrine cystadenoma(s), 418, 523, 564–565, 565f
Apocrine gland(s), 24f, 31, 32f
  apical cap, 31
  development, 25
  distribution of, 31
  inflammation involving, 274–276

Apocrine nevus, 564
Apocrine secretory epithelium, 32f
Apocrine tumors, 564–569
Apoeccrine glands, 273
Apoptosis, 88
Apoptotic cells, 132, 132f
Aqueous light green counterstain, 0.5 percent, 58
Aralen. See Chloroquin hydrochloride
Arao–Perkins body, 29, 715, 716f
Areolae, nevoid hyperkeratosis of, 482, 483f
Argyria, 417, 418f
Arrector muscle, 24f, 26–27, 28f, 31–32
  development, 25
  hypertrophy, 31
Arrector pili
  hamartoma, 480
    congenital, 634
  and leiomyoma, 633–636
Arterial spiders, 646
Arteriosclerosis, leg ulcer with, 245
Arteriovenous fistula(s), vs. Kaposi's sarcoma, 656
Arteriovenous hemangioma, 647, 648f
Arteriovenous malformation, leg ulcer with, 245
Arthropod bite reaction, 683, 686f
Arthropods, foreign body granuloma caused by, 315–316
Arthus phenomenon, 224
Aspergillosis, 312
Asteatotic dermatitis, 119, 120f
  differential diagnosis, 117t
Asteroid bodies, in multinucleated giant cells, 93, 93f
Atopic dermatitis, 101, 107–108, 108f
  follicular involvement in, 254
Atopic disease, and infantile seborrheic dermatitis, 119
Atrophie blanche, 221, 227, 418
Atrophoderma(s), 351
  biopsy in, 46
  of Pasini and Pierini, 354, 356f
  vermicularis, 536–537, 544f
Auriasis, 417
Auricular calcification, 385
Auspitz phenomenon, 133
Autoantibodies, 69
  in bullous pemphigoid, 162
  indirect immunofluorescence, 66–67
Autoimmune progesterone dermatitis of pregnancy, 165
Avidin–biotin immunoperoxidase technique, 68, 68f

B-15, immunostaining reactive patterns, 70t
Bacillary angiomatosis, 651
Bacteria, staining, 46t, 58–59, 61–62, 85
Bacterial infections, ulcers in, 243–244
Balanitis, 697
  circinata, 127, 698
  plasma cell, 697, 698f
  xerotica obliterans, 358, 699
Balloon cell nevus, 451–452, 453f
Ballooning degeneration, 181, 182f, 186
Bamboo hair, 719, 719f
Barbiturate coma, bullous eruptions associated with, 176, 176f
Barium granuloma, 295
Bartonellosis, 645
Bart's syndrome, 173
Basal cell(s), 7f–8f, 9–10, 14f, 18f, 713. See also Adnexal basal cell; Epidermal basal cell
  biology of, 8t
  definition of, 9t, 85
  disintegration, 83

Basal cell(s) (cont.)
  epidermal
    damage, cascade of histobiologic events associated with, 133, 135f
    definition of, 9t
    mitotic division of, 8
  germinal, 85
  glycogen in, 11
  hyalinization, 86
  liquefaction degeneration of, 86
    in subacute lupus erythematosus, 207f, 208
  morphology, 9, 86
  nucleus, 9–10
Basal cell carcinoma(s), 512. See also Basal cell epithelioma(s)
Basal cell epithelioma(s), 335, 385, 509–510, 583–598
  adamantinoid pattern, 585f, 586
  adenoid, 587, 588f
  aggressive (infiltrating), 590, 595f
  bowenoid pattern, 587, 591f
  cell-mediated inflammatory reaction with, 588
  cells of, 10
  with clear cells, 587, 591f
  curette biopsy, 51
  development of, 583–585, 584f
  epithelial portion, 584f, 585–587
  formalin fixed, paraffin embedded sections, immunohistochemical staining pattern for, 66t
  histogenesis, 583–585
  intraepidermal, 596–598
  keratotic, 585f, 586
  mesodermal portion, 587–588, 592f
  metastatic, 596
  morphea-like, 591–596, 598f
  and organoid nevi, 523
  pigmented, 587, 592f
  pilar differentiation in, 586, 586f
  plexiform, 587, 589f
  pseudocystic, 586, 587f
  reticulated, 587, 590f
  retraction spaces in, 588, 592f
  sclerotic, 591, 596f–597f
  with sebaceous differentiation, 527
  squeezing effect on, 51, 52f
  superficial, 589–590, 593f–594f
  terminology for, 583
  versus trichoepithelioma, 536
  with tumor of follicular infundibulum, 534
Basal cell tumor(s), with eccrine differentiation, 606
Basalioma(s), 335, 337f, 437. See also Basal cell epithelioma(s)
Basalioma cell(s), 10
  definition of, 9t
Basal lamina, 17, 18f
Basal layer, disturbances in, 85–86
Basaloid carcinoma, of anus, 709–710
Basaloid cell(s), 10, 85–86
  clonal nests of, 489–490, 490f
  definition of, 9t
Basaloid eddies, 598
Basaloid follicular hamartoma, 536, 543f
Basement membrane, 510
  breaks in, 88
  PAS-positive, 88
  staining, 59, 88
  in tumors, 18
Basement membrane zone, 16–18
  components of, 19f
Basosquamous acanthoma, 489
Bathing trunk nevus, 457–458
  excessive hair in, 531
Bayonet hair, 716
Bazex syndrome, 109
Bazin's disease, 233, 286
Behçet disease, 218

Behçet syndrome, 700
Bejel, 293
Benign (term), definition of, 435–438
Benign cephalic histiocytosis, 340
Benign chronic bullous dermatosis of childhood, diagnosis, immunofluorescence in, 75
Benign familial pemphigus. See Hailey–Hailey disease
Benign juvenile melanoma, 452–454, 454f–456f
Benign leukokeratosis, of buccal mucosa, 704f, 705
Benign lymphoplasia, 682–683, 685f
Benign mucous membrane pemphigoid. See Cicatricial pemphigoid
Beryllium granuloma, 295, 299f, 321
  differential diagnosis, 282t
Beta-glucuronidase, in apocrine and eccrine apparatuses, 33t
Biopsy. See also Curette biopsy; Excisional biopsy; Punch biopsy; Specimen(s)
  and anticoagulation, 50
  artifacts, 48, 62–63
  clinical information accompanying, 45
  deep, 49–50
  dermalepidermal separation in, 48, 50f, 62f
  forceps injury, artifacts due to, 48, 49f–50f
  ideal specimen, 51f
  lesion for, selection of, 45–46
  of nails, 723
  procedure, 47–50
  site, selection of, 45–46
  with subcutaneous inflammation, 229
  superficial, 48–49
  in systemic sclerosis, 352
  of ulcer, 241
Biphasic ichthyosiform dermatosis, 405t, 408f, 409
Birbeck granules, 39, 40f, 343, 345
Birt–Hogg–Dubé syndrome, 544f, 545
Bizzozero's nodule, 10f
Black heel, 419, 419f
Black piedra, 724f
Blacks
  disorders affecting hair of, 253–254
  melanocytes in, 39
Blastomyces dermatitidis, 306
Blastomycosis
  North American, 89f, 244, 305–306, 307f
  South American, 305–306
  Lobo's type (keloid type), 306, 308f
Blepharochalasis, 373
Bloch–Sulzberger's disease, 416
Blood, extravasation of, 388
Blood cells, on skin surface, 85
Blood eosinophilia, 354
Blood vessels
  in dermis, 19, 21
  in inflammatory disease, 96
  pathologic changes of, 94
Blue nevus, 449, 459, 461f
  cellular, 459, 461f
  giant, 459, 461f
  malignant, 459, 462f–463f
    differential diagnosis, 466t
Blue rubber bleb nevus, 654
B lymphocyte(s)
  definition of, 91
  morphology, 672
BMZ. See Basement membrane zone
Bodnar tumor, 631–633, 633f
Boeck's sarcoid, 295
Bone, extracellular deposits of, 385
Bone formation
  with pilomatricoma, 535
  in skin, 627
Bone tumor(s), 385
Borrelia burgdorferi, 355
  in pityriasis rosea, 188

Borst phenomenon, 597–598, 599f
Botryomycosis, 307–308, 310f
Bowel-associated dermatosis–arthritis syndrome, 218
Bowenoid keratoses, 509
Bowenoid papulosis, 429–430, 430f, 705
Bowen's disease. See Bowen's precancerous dermatosis (Bowen's disease)
Bowen's precancerous dermatosis (Bowen's disease), 86–87, 387, 503–504, 507–509, 508f–510f, 597–598, 709
  differential diagnosis, 502, 611–613
  formalin fixed, paraffin embedded sections, immunohistochemical staining pattern for, 66t
  in nails, 725
  progression to invasive cancer, 512, 513f
Bizzozero's nodule, 10
Bramble bush fibers, 372, 374f–375f
Branching enzyme, in apocrine and eccrine apparatuses, 33t
Breast cancer
  cutaneous metastasis of, 615, 615f
  and Paget's disease, 607
Brocq phenomenon, 133
Bromoderma, 244, 314, 315f
Bronchogenic cyst, 559f, 560
Brown recluse spider bite, necrosis of, 245
Bullae, 82–83
  disorders with, 157, 158t
  in incontinentia pigmenti, 416, 417f
  intradermal, 83
  intraepidermal, 82–83
  in systemic sclerosis, 352
Bullous congenital ichthyosiform erythroderma, 404
Bullous dermatosis. See Adult linear IgA dermatosis; Chronic bullous dermatosis of childhood; Juvenile linear IgA dermatosis
Bullous disease, 148, 157–179
Bullous impetigo, 158t, 174, 175f
Bullous pemphigoid, 157, 162, 164f, 175–176
  autoantibodies, localization, 72–73
  clinical presentation, 71
  coexistence with Hailey–Hailey's disease, 399
  diagnosis
    immunoelectron microscopy in, 72–73
    immunofluorescence in, 67, 67t, 71–72, 73f
  vesiculobullous eruptions of, 158t
Burn(s)
  bullae due to, 176
  epidermal regeneration after, 414
  vesiculobullous eruptions of, 158t
Buruli ulcer, 243
Buschke–Ollendorf syndrome, 370, 621, 622t
Butchers' warts, 284

Café au lait spots, 442
Calcinosis cutis, 384f, 385
  metastatic, 385
  of scrotum, 385
Calcium
  extracellular deposits of, 383–385, 384f
  staining, 46t, 57, 61, 383–385
Callosities, 495
Cancer family syndrome, 528
Candida, 189
  and acrodermatitis enteropathica, 162
Candidiasis
  chronic granulomatous, 312
  of oral mucosa, 701, 702f, 704
Cantharidin, artifacts introduced by, 63
Capillaries, intrapapillary, descriptive terminology for, 89
Carbon, 416
Carbon monoxide poisoning, bullous eruptions associated with, 176

Carbuncle, 249
Carcinoembryonic antigen (CEA)
  immunostaining, 70t, 563
  in Paget's disease, 613
  in sweat gland neoplasms, 603
Carcinoma, 629. *See also* Adenocarcinoma; Adnexal carcinoma; Basal cell carcinoma(s); Basaloid carcinoma; Eccrine carcinoma; Squamous cell carcinoma; Verrucous carcinoma
  cloacogenic, 709–710
  comedo-type, 610
  ichthyosis vulgaris-like skin with, 403
  internal, cutaneous metastasis of, 615f, 615–616
  meibomian, 603, 604f
  Merkel cell, 614f, 614–615
  metastatic, 615f, 615–616
  neuroendocrine, 614f, 614–615
  scirrhous, 616
Carcinoma in situ, 87, 502, 509, 597
  of mucous membranes, 708–709
  progression to cancer, 510–512
Cardiac drugs, discoloration of sun-exposed skin and, 417
Carotinemia, 419
Catagen (phase of hair cycle), 33–35, 34f–35f. *See also* Hair follicle(s), catagen
Cat-scratch disease, 321, 328
Cauliflower ear, 361
Cellular angioma of infancy, 649, 649f
Cellulite, 238
Cellulitis, 151
  eosinophilic, 151, 153f, 321
Cementosome(s), 12, 14f, 15
Cerebriform intradermal nevus, 458
Ceruminous gland(s), of ear canal, 31
Chanarin–Dorfman syndrome, 404
Chancre
  redux, 703
  syphilitic, 291, 292f
  tuberculous, 283
Chancroid, 243, 243f
Chediak–Higashi syndrome, 414
Cheilitis. *See also* Actinic cheilitis
  glandularis, 701–702
  granulomatosa, 297, 300f
Chemotherapy, neutrophilic eccrine hidradenitis associated with, 274
Cheveux incoiffables, 719, 721f
Cheveux pseudopeladiques, 268
Chlamydia trachomatis, 317
Chloasma, 415
Chloroquin hydrochloride (Aralen), dermatosis caused by, 141
Chlorothiazide, lichenoid drug eruption caused by, 141
Cholesterosis, extracellular, 383
Cholinergic urticaria, 145
Chondrodermatitis nodularis, 88
  chronica helicis, 245–246, 246f, 361
Chondroid syringoma, 575–576, 578f
Chondroitin sulfate, staining, 59–60
Chondroma, 627, 628f
Chromoblastomycosis, 307
Chromomycosis, 305, 307, 309f
Chronic bullous dermatosis of childhood, 164, 167f
  vesiculobullous eruptions of, 158t
Chronic eczematous dermatitis, 10, 10f, 679
  epidermis in, 80, 80f
Chronic renal failure
  calcium deposits in, 385
  perforating lesions in, 358, 360f
Chronic superficial dermatitis, 194
Chronic x-ray dermatitis, 138, 222, 225f

Page numbers followed by t or f indicate tables or figures, respectively.

Churg–Strauss syndrome, 220, 321
Cicatricial pemphigoid
  clinical presentation, 73
  diagnosis, immunofluorescence in, 67, 67t, 73, 74f
  localized (Brunsting–Perry type), 73, 162–163, 165f
  vesiculobullous eruptions of, 158t
Cinnabar, 416
Cirsoid aneurysm, 646–647, 648f
Civatte bodies, 87, 132, 132f, 134f
Cladosporium, 190, 307
Clavus, 258, 495, 496f
Clear cell acanthoma (Degos), 490, 492f
Clear cell eccrine carcinoma, 606, 609f
Clear cell hidradenoma, 575, 577f
Clear cells of Masson, 38, 38f, 413
Clear cell syringoma, 572, 574f
Clefts, 83
  subepidermal, 86, 86f
Clinicopathologic coordination, in diagnosis, 96–97
Cloacogenic carcinoma, 709–710
Coccidioides immitis, 305
Coccidiomycosis, 305, 306f
Collagen
  changes in, 351–367
  in keloids, 621
  staining, 46t, 57–58
  type IV, immunostaining reactive patterns, 70t
  type VII, in transient bullous dermolysis of newborn, 173
Collagen bundle(s), 19–20, 20f
Collagen fibers, 20f–21f, 369
Collagenoma, 621
  familial cutaneous, 622t
Collagenosis, 88
Collagenous fibers, in epidermis, 89f
Collastin, staining, 58
Collodion baby, 404, 406
Colloidal iron stain, 46t, 59
Colloid droplets, staining, 59
Colloid keratosis, 85, 726
Colloid milium, 375–376, 379f
Colon cancer, cutaneous metastasis of, 615f, 615–616
Comedo, 257
  closed, 251
  open, 251
Comedo-type carcinoma, 610
Complement C3, antibodies, in direct immunofluorescence, 65–66
Compound nevus, 445–446, 447f, 448
Condyloma acuminatum, 424, 428, 429f, 705
  Buschke–Loewenstein variant of, 428, 707
  differential diagnosis, 428–429
Condylomata lata, 291
Congenital arrector pili hamartoma, 634
Congenital nevi, 457–458
Congenital poikiloderma of Thomson, 138
Congenital self-healing reticulohistiocytosis, 345, 345f–346f
Congenital self-healing (transient) mechanobullous dermatosis, 173
Congo red stain, 46t, 60
Connective tissue, lesions with unusual differentiation of, 624–627
Connective tissue disease, panniculitis in, 235–236
Connective tissue nevi, 621, 622t
  zosteriform, 622t
Contact dermatitis, 101–106. *See also* Dermal contact sensitivity reaction; Sensitization dermatitis
  acute, 104–105, 105f
  chronic, 105–106, 106f
  primary irritant type, 101–103, 102f
    epidermal regeneration in, 102f, 102–103

Contact sensitivity reaction, 679–680
  dermal, 106, 107f
  See also Dermis
Corium. *See also* Dermis
Corneocyte(s). *See also* Keratinized cell(s)
  morphology, 13
Cornified cell, cellular envelope of, 12
Corps ronds, 86, 86f, 395, 396f, 700
Corticosteroid atrophy, 355
Corynebacterium, 496
Corynebacterium acnes, 250
Corynebacterium minutissimum, 190
Corynebacterium tenue, 722
Cotton dyes, 46t
  for amyloid staining, 46t, 60
Coumarin necrosis, 222, 223f, 245
Cowden's disease, 534–535
Coxsackie virus, 181, 184–186
Crohn's disease, in oral mucosa, 703
Crosti's reticulohistiocytoma of the back, 682
Crow–Fukase syndrome, 651
CRST syndrome, 77, 385, 646
Crust, parakeratotic, 85, 85f
Cryptococcosis, 308, 311f
Cryptococcus, 305
Cryptococcus neoformans, 308
  staining, 61
Crystal violet, 46t, 60
Curette biopsy, technique, 51
Cutaneous ciliated cyst, 557, 558f
Cutaneous cylindroma, 569, 570f
  malignant, 569
Cutaneous horn, 434f, 509
Cutaneous nerve corpuscles, 23, 23f
Cutaneous papilloma, definition of, 88
Cutaneous plasmacytoma, 91f
Cutaneous sarcoidosis, 295
Cutis. *See also* Dermis
  hyperelastica. *See* Ehlers–Danlos syndrome
  laxa, 370–371, 372f
  marmorata, 221
  marmorata telangiectatica, 646
  rhomboidalis nuchae, 383
Cylindroma. *See also* Cutaneous cylindroma
  malignant transformation of, 606
Cyst(s)
  bronchogenic, 559f, 560
  classification of, 549, 550f
  cutaneous ciliated, 557, 558f
  definition of, 549
  dermoid, 557, 558f
  epidermoid, 385, 509, 552f, 553
  epithelial, 418
  eruptive vellus hair, 553, 553f
  glandular, 549–551
  hybrid, 555, 556f
  keratinous, 551–560
  median raphe, 557
  myxoid, 360–361, 364f
  pilosebaceous, 551
  sebaceous, 549
  thymic, 560, 560f
  trichilemmal, 554–555, 555f–556f
    proliferating, 555–557, 557f–558f
Cystadenoma. *See also* Apocrine cystadenoma(s)
  papilliferous, 398f
Cysticercus cellulosae, 312
Cytokeratin, immunostaining, 563
Cytokeratin CAM 5.2 synaptophysin, immunostaining reactive patterns, 70t
Cytophagic histiocytic panniculitis, 235
Cytoplasm, staining, 57–58
Cytoplasmic viruses, vesiculobullous eruptions with, 158t

DAKO antikeratin, immunostaining reactive patterns, 70t
Darier–Roussy sarcoid, 236, 295, 296f

Darier's disease, 86f, 86–87, 162, 393, 395–398, 396f–398f, 482, 483f
 differential diagnosis, 396, 396t, 398f
 of mucous membranes, 700
 nails in, 725
Dark cells, in eccrine glands, 36–37
Darkened skin, histologic substrates of, 413, 414t
Decubitus ulcers, 247
Deep dermis, pathology, descriptive terminology for, 79
Deep inflammatory processes, 203
Degenerative collagenous plaque of hands, 374, 378f
Degos' disease, 222, 224f
Demodex folliculorum, 26f, 30
 and rosacea, 260, 261f–262f
Dendritic cell(s), 8f
 definition of, 9t
 intraepidermal, 37–40
Dendrocyte(s). *See* Dermal dendrocytes
Denudation
 definition of, 241
 epidermal regeneration after, 414
Depigmentation, 413–414
Dermal contact sensitivity reaction, 106, 107f
Dermal dendrocytes, 331
Dermal duct tumor, 569, 572f
Dermalepidermal separation, due to biopsy trauma, 48, 50f, 62f
Dermal papilla, 15, 25, 29
Dermatitis
 definition of, 99
 exfoliativa neonatorum, 166
 herpetiformis, 46, 157, 163–164, 166f
  in children, 164
  clinical presentation, 75
  diagnosis, immunofluorescence in, 67, 67t, 75, 75f
  and pemphigus, mixed cases of, 161
  vesiculobullous eruptions of, 158t
 papillaris capillitii, 255f
Dermatofibrosarcoma protuberans, 333–334, 630–631, 632f
 pigmented, 631–633, 633f
Dermatofibrosis
 disseminata with microcysts, 622t
 lenticularis disseminata, 370, 622t
Dermatoglyphics, 15
Dermatomegaly, 371
Dermatomes, development, 7
Dermatomyositis, 138, 194, 213, 213f
 juvenile, 385
 myositis of, 213, 213f
 panniculitis in, 236
 poikilodermatous features, 212f, 213
 type Wong, 260
Dermatopathology, 45
Dermatophilus congolensis, 496
Dermatophytes, skin changes caused by, 189
Dermatophytic folliculitis, 251–252
Dermatosis
 cenicienta, 137
 papulosa nigra, 490
Dermis, 7f. *See also* Adventitial dermis
 descriptive histopathology of, 88–94
 development of, 6–7
 noncellular components, 93–94
 normal structure of, 18–23
 pathology, descriptive terminology for, 79
Dermoepidermal interface, 15, 15f, 17f
Dermoepidermal junction, 16–18, 18f
Dermographism, 145
Dermoid cysts, 557, 558f
Dermoject anesthesia, artifacts with, 48f
Desmin, immunostaining reactive patterns, 70t
Desmoplastic nevus, 454

Desmoplastic trichoepithelioma, 536, 542f
Desmosine, 21, 369
Desmosome(s), 10, 10f–12f
 in acantholytic disease, 157
Desquamative gingivitis, 700
Diabetes mellitus
 bullae in, 176
 and granuloma annulare, 323
 and necrobiosis lipoidica, 325
 ulcers in, 247
Diaminobenzidine, in immunohistochemical methods, 68
Diaper dermatitis, 106
Diastase digestion, 59
Dichromism, 531
Differential diagnosis, 97
Differentiation (term), definition of, 437
Digested PAS stain, 46t
Digital fibrokeratoma, acquired, 624, 624f
Digital fibrous tumor of childhood, recurrent, 633, 635f
Digital myxofibromas, 624, 625f
Digital papillary adenoma, aggressive, 576–577, 579f
Digitate dermatosis, 194
Dilated pore, 533, 534f
Diphtheria, 243–244
Direct immunofluorescence, 65–66
 application of, 68–69
 indications, 67t
 modification of, 66
 patterns, 67t
Dirofilariasis, granulomatous inflammation caused by, 312
Discoid lupus erythematosus, 202f
 butterfly lesion of, 76
 chronic, 205–206
 clinical presentation, 75–76
 diagnosis, immunofluorescence in, 67, 67t, 76
 versus Jessner's lymphocytic infiltration, 209
 lower surface of epidermis in, 81f
Dissecting cellulitis of scalp, 254
Disseminated intravascular coagulation, 222
DLE. *See* Discoid lupus erythematosus
Donovan bodies, 316, 318f
Donovania granulomatis, 316, 318f
Dopa-oxidase. *See* Tyrosinase
Dowling-Degos disease, 496, 497f
Down syndrome, syringomas associated with, 574
Drug eruptions, 99, 145, 148
 lichenoid, 131, 141, 142f
 lymphocytic vasculitis of, 217
 toxic erythema due to, 150f
Drug exanthem, 184
Duhring's disease, 163, 166f
Dyschromatosis, universal, 86
Dyshidrosiform dermatitis, 101, 106–107, 107f, 124
Dyskeratosis
 benign versus malignant, 86–87
 congenita, 138
 definition of, 86
Dyskeratosis congenita, 704
Dysplasia, 87
Dysplastic nevi, 450, 450f–452f

Ear cartilage, affections of, 361, 364f
Eccrine angiomatous nevus, 563, 564f
Eccrine apparatus, 15–16
 enzyme activities in, 33t
Eccrine carcinoma, 605–606
 clear cell, 606, 609f
 microcystic, 606, 608f
 mucinous (adenocystic), 606, 609f
 tubular (adenoid cystic), 605–606, 607f
Eccrine duct(s), 16f
 cysts, 37, 37f

 intraepidermal, 35–36, 36f. *See also* Acrosyringium
 subepidermal, 35, 36f
Eccrine epithelioma, 606
Eccrine gland(s), 35–38
 abscesses, 273–274
 ampulla, 36
 components, 35
 development, 7–8, 35
 inflammation involving, 273–274
 mucoid granules, 37
 PAS-positive material, 37
Eccrine nevus, 563, 564f
Eccrine porocarcinoma, 598, 605, 605f–606f
Eccrine poroma, 569, 571f–572f, 598
 malignant transformation of, 606
Eccrine spiradenoma, 574–575, 576f
 malignant transformation of, 606, 610f
Eccrine syringofibroadenoma, 569, 573f
Eccrine tumor(s), 569–577
 malignant transformation of, 606–607
Ecthyma, 243–244
 contagiosum, 181, 183–184, 185f–186f
Ectoderm, 5
Ectodermal cell(s)
 adult, 17f
 fetal, 17f
Ectodermal derivatives, 5, 6f
Ectodermal epithelium, definition of, 9t
Ectodermal modulated cell, definition of, 9t
Ectodermal pluripotentiality, 16, 17f
Ectothrix, 251
Eczema
 herpeticum, 182
 vaccinatum, 182
Eczematous dermatitis, 38f, 99. *See also* Chronic eczematous dermatitis
 follicular involvement in, 254
 vesiculobullous eruptions of, 157, 158t
Eczematous tissue reactions, 101–112
 definition of, 101
Edema. *See also* Epidermal edema; Spongiotic edema
 in sensitization dermatitis, 103–104
Ehlers-Danlos syndrome, 351, 358, 372
 classification of, 361t
 clinical manifestations, 361t
 genetics of, 361t
 syringomas associated with, 574
 types of, 361t
Elacin, staining, 58
Elastic fiber(s), 19f, 21f, 28f
 absence of, 94
 components of, 369
 of dermis, 17, 20–21
 disorders of, 369–382
  acquired, 370t, 372
  congenital, 370t, 370–372
 in epidermis, 89f
 fragmentation of, 93–94
 in inflammatory disease, 96
 normal properties of, 369
 pseudofragmentation of, 93, 93f
 staining, 46t, 57–58, 60, 278f, 369
 stains for, 55–58. *See also* Acid orcein–Giemsa stain
Elastin, 21, 369
Elastofibrils, 21
Elastolysis, 94
Elastosis. *See also* Actinic elastosis
 perforans serpiginosa, 372, 373f–374f
Elaunin fibers, 19
 staining, 58
Electric current, artifacts introduced by, 63
Embedding, of biopsy specimens, 54, 55f
 angles of, 54, 55f
Embolism, 221
Endometriosis, in skin, 560
Endothelial cells, morphology, 672
Endothrix, 251, 252f

Enzyme digestion, of specimens, 60
Eosinophilia, 151–152
Eosinophilic cellulitis, 151, 153f, 321
Eosinophilic fasciitis, 353–354, 355f
Eosinophilic granules, staining, 58
Eosinophilic granuloma, 343
Eosinophilic pustular folliculitis, 256, 256f
Eosinophilic spongiosis, associated with pemphigus, 161, 162f
Eosinophils
 in erythema multiforme, 148
 in inflammatory infiltrates, 279–280
 in skin disease, 145, 152
 staining, 278f
 in vesiculobullous eruptions, 158t
Ephelis, 415, 441
Epidermal basal cells. See Basal cell(s), epidermal
Epidermal cell(s)
 death, 87–88
 intercellular bridges, and intracellular edema, 82–83, 83f
 life span, in psoriasis versus lichen planus, 133
 necrosis, in erythema multiforme, 147, 149f
Epidermal dysplasia, 403
Epidermal edema, in erythema multiforme, 147, 148f
Epidermal germinal cell. See Epidermal matrix cell
Epidermal keratinocyte, definition of, 9t
Epidermal malignant transformation, 502, 502f
Epidermal matrix cell(s), 17f
 definition of, 9t
Epidermal melanin unit, 39
Epidermal nevus, 479–483, 509
 definition of, 479
 verrucous, 479, 480f
  linear, 479, 481, 481f. See also Inflammatory linear verrucous epidermal nevus
Epidermal nevus syndrome, 481–482
Epidermal ridges, 15
Epidermal symbiosis, 15–16
Epidermal turnover, 13–14
Epidermal unit, 19
Epidermis, 7f–8f, 15f–16f
 acanthotic. See also Acanthosis
  glycogen in prickle cells of, 81–82, 82f
 architecture of, 15
 atrophy, 80, 81f
 biology of, 13–14
 definition of, 9t
 development of, 5–6
 downgrowth of, 516
 general configuration, terminology for, 80–84
 hyperplasia, 80, 80f
  in lichen simplex chronicus, 111
 hypertrophy, 80, 80f
 hypoplasia, 80, 81f
 layers of, 8
 lichenified, versus psoriatic, 111
 mitotic index, 14
 multinucleated giant cells in, 87, 87f
 nonneoplastic epithelial and pigmentary disorders of, 393
 normal structure of, 8–16
 pathology, descriptive terminology for, 79
 pseudocarcinomatous proliferation, 18
 psoriatic, 120, 121f
 regeneration, in contact dermatitis, 102f, 102–103
 in vesiculobullous eruptions, 158t
Epidermodysplasia verruciformis, 424, 430, 430f
Epidermoid cyst(s), 385, 509, 552f, 553

Page numbers followed by t or f indicate tables or figures, respectively.

Epidermoid epithelium, definition of, 9t
Epidermoid inclusion cyst, 553
Epidermoid tumor(s)
 benign, definition of, 479
 malignant, definition of, 479
Epidermolysis bullosa, 74, 83, 168–173
 acquisita
  clinical presentation, 74
  diagnosis, immunofluorescence in, 67, 67t, 74–75
  pathophysiology, 74
 classification, antibodies and ultrastructural changes useful for, 170t
 dystrophica, 170–172, 174f
  dominant, 171
   antibodies and ultrastructural changes useful for classification of, 170t
   variant type, 171
  inversa type, 171
  recessive, 171
   antibodies and ultrastructural changes useful for classification of, 170t
   generalized type, 170–171
   localized type, 171
 et albopapuloidea, 621, 622t
 herpetiformis, of Dowling–Meara type, 169–170, 172f
 junctional, 170
  antibodies and ultrastructural changes useful for classification of, 170t
  lethalis, 170, 173f
 simplex, 168–170, 169f–172f
  antibodies and ultrastructural changes useful for classification of, 170t
  localized form, 168–169
 vesiculobullous eruptions of, 158t
Epidermolysis dystrophica, vesiculobullous eruptions of, 158t
Epidermolytic hyperkeratosis, 83, 404, 405t, 407f
 vesiculobullous eruptions with, 158t
Epithelial cells, 92–93
Epithelial cyst(s), 418
Epithelial membrane antigen (EMA)
 immunostaining, 70t, 563
 in sweat gland neoplasms, 603
Epithelial tumors, diagnosis, 96
Epithelioid angiomatosis, 651
Epithelioid cell(s), in inflammatory infiltrate, 279–280
Epithelioid (histiocytoid) hemangioma(s), 652–656
Epithelioid sarcoma, 629, 630f
Epithelioma. See also Basal cell epithelioma(s)
 adenoides cysticum, 535
 cuniculatum, 515, 708
 eccrine, 606
 sebaceous, 30, 527, 528f
Epithelium. See also Adnexal epithelium; Ectodermal epithelium; Epidermoid epithelium; Mucosal epithelium; Squamous epithelium; Stratified epithelium
 acantholytic, downward budding of, 397, 397f
 sebaceous, atrophic, 30, 32f
Equestrian cold panniculitis, 238
Erosion, definition of, 241
Erosive adenomatosis of nipple, 568f, 568–569
Eruptions, circular, biopsy of, 45–46
Eruptive nevi, 449
Eruptive vellus hair cysts, 553, 553f
Erysipelas, 151
Erythema
 ab igne, 373, 378f
 annulare centrifugum, 149
 chronicum migrans, 149–150
 definition of, 145
 dyschromicum perstans, 131, 137, 137f

 elevatum diutinum, 223–224, 226f, 383
 exudativum multiforme, 99, 146–148, 147f, 166
  bullous phase, 148
  epidermal edema in, 147–148, 148f
 gyratum repens, 150
 induratum, 232–233, 286
 marginatum, 148
 multiforme, 157. See also Erythema, exudativum multiforme
  epidermal type, 148, 149f
  of mucous membrane, 700
  vesiculobullous eruptions of, 158t
 nodosum, 232–233, 235f–236f
  biopsy in, 48, 51f
  chronic, 233
  etiology, 233
  subacute, 233
 nodosum leprosum, 289
 perstans, 149
 pustular, 273
 toxic, 149–152
 toxicum neonatorum, 109, 109f, 273
Erythrasma, 190–191
Erythrocytes, in epidermal cells, 94
Erythroderma, 676
 psoriatic, 125–126
Erythrokeratodermia variabilis, 405t, 409
Erythromelanosis follicularis
 colli, 138
 faciei et colli, 415
Erythroplasia of Queyrat, 509, 511f
Erythropoietic protoporphyria, 386, 387f
Eschar, with tick bite, 146
Essential telangiectasia, 646, 647f
Esthiomène, 317
Exanthem(s), differential diagnosis, 184
Excisional biopsy, technique, 48
Excoriation(s), 46, 47f, 62
 in eczematous tissue reaction, 108
Exfoliative dermatitis, 101, 109–110
Exocytosis, 98f, 101
 in atopic dermatitis, 107–108
 in sensitization dermatitis, 103–104
Extramedullary plasmacytoma, 675

Facial milia, 553
Factor VIII (-related antigen), immunostaining, 70t, 331
Factor XIII, immunostaining, 331
Familial cutaneous collagenoma, 622t
Familial focal epithelial hyperplasia, 706
Familial hemorrhagic telangiectasia, 646
Familial Mediterranean fever, 151
Fasciola hepatica, 313, 314f
Fascioliasis, 313, 314f
Fat
 proliferating atrophy of, 229, 232f, 297f
 subcutaneous. See Subcutaneous fat
Fat cells, 22, 22f
Fat embolisms, 221
Febrile nonsuppurative nodular panniculitis, 233–234
Feet. See also Soles
 inflammatory vesiculobullous eruption on, 191
Fetal biopsy, in epidermolysis bullosa, 168
Fiberglass dermatitis, 389
Fibrillin, 21
Fibrin, staining, 58
 in thrombi, 59
Fibrinoid substances, staining, 58
Fibroblast(s), 629
 giant, in chronic x-ray dermatitis, 222, 225f
 versus histiocytes, 92
Fibrocyte(s), 19, 21
 morphology, 672
Fibroepithelial tumor of Pinkus, 387

Fibrofolliculoma, 544, 544f, 622t, 623
Fibrokeratoma. *See also* Acquired digital fibrokeratoma
 acral, 621
Fibroma, 621–622, 634
 durum, 333
 pendulum, 623–624
 perifollicular, 622t, 622–623, 623f
 periungual, 621, 624
Fibrosarcoma(s), 629
 infantile, 629f
Fibrous hamartoma of infancy, 626
Fibrous histiocytoma, 629. *See also* Histiocytoma(s)
 aneurysmal (angiomatoid), 652, 653f
 formalin fixed, paraffin embedded sections, immunohistochemical staining pattern for, 66t
 malignant, 630, 631f
Fibrous papule of the nose, 622, 622f
Fibroxanthoma, atypical, 630, 632f
 formalin fixed, paraffin embedded sections, immunohistochemical staining pattern for, 66t
Filaggrin, 11, 15
Filiariasis, granulomatous inflammation caused by, 312
Finger(s). *See entries under* Digital
Fish tank granuloma, 290
Fite method (staining), 46t, 61
 of Hansen's bacilli, 289, 289f
Fixation, of biopsy specimens, 51–54
Fixed-tissue-type cell(s), 19, 92, 672
 morphology, 672
Flame figures, 151, 153f
Flegel's disease, 409, 409f
Flexures, reticulated pigmented anomaly of, 496, 497f
Florid oral papillomatosis, 707, 708f
Florid papillomatosis of nipple ducts, 568f, 568–569
Fly larvae, granulomatous inflammation caused by, 312
Foam cell(s), 92, 233, 383
 in xanthomas, 331–332
Focal dermal hypoplasia, 638–639, 639f
Focal epithelial hyperplasia, 424, 430–431
Fogo selvagem, 159–161
Follicular inflammations, 249
Follicular infundibulum, tumor of, 533–534, 537f
Follicular keratoses, 249, 256–260. *See also* Inverted follicular keratosis
Follicular mucinosis, 254–256, 265–267
Follicular poroma, 534, 538f
Folliculitis
 decalvans, 256, 267
 dermatophytic, 251–252
 eosinophilic pustular, 256, 256f
 et perifolliculitis suffodiens et abscedens, 253–254, 275
 necrotizing, 253, 254f
 perforating, 252–253, 253f
 pityrosporum, 253
 staphylococcal, 249
 with superficial lesions, 254–256
Fonsecaea, 307
Fordyce's condition, 706
Foreign bodies, 237–238, 389–390
 in tissue sections, 62
Foreign body granuloma(s), 280, 315–316
 differential diagnosis, 282t
 sarcoidal, 295–297
Formaldehyde, neutral buffered solution, 52
Formalin
 alcoholic, 53
 10 percent solution, 52
Formalin fixation, artifacts, 53f
Formalin pigment, 54, 61f, 62
Fox–Fordyce disease, 274f, 274–275

Frambesia, 293
Francisella tularensis, 300
Freckles, 415, 441
Freezing, artifacts introduced by, 63
Friction
 artifacts introduced by, 62–63
 bullae due to, 176
Friction amyloidosis, 387
Frisch bacilli, 301
Fucosidosis, 647
Fullmer's orcinol new fuchsin stain, 58
Fungal granulomas, 305–312
Fungi
 hyphae, as tissue contaminant, 61f, 62
 opportunistic, 312
 staining, 46t, 58–59, 61, 85
Fungous infections
 deep, 232, 236, 280
 superficial, 189–191
Furuncle, 249, 250f, 275
Furunculosis, 249

Ganglioneuroma(s), 668
Gastrointestinal malignancy, and seborrheic verruca, 490
GCDFP-15. *See* Gross cystic disease fluid protein-15
Generalized elastolysis, cutis laxa, 370–372, 372f
Generalized eruptive histiocytoma, 340
Genitalia, pigmented macules of, 441–442
Genital touch corpuscle, 23f
Genital warts, 428, 429f
Genodermatoses, 349, 403
Geographic tongue, 698, 698f
German measles, 184
Germinal layer, 85–86
Gianotti–Crosti syndrome, 181, 187
Giant cell arteritis. *See* Temporal arteritis
Giant cell fibroblastoma, 627
Giant cell tumor of tendon sheath, 626, 626f
Giant condylomata acuminata (Buschke–Loewenstein type), 428, 707
Giemsa stain, 415
Glial fibrillary acidic protein, in neural tumors, 663
Glioma(s), 667
Glomangioma, 654, 656f
Glucagonoma, dermatosis with, 175
Glucagonoma syndrome, vesiculobullous eruptions of, 158t
Glycogen
 in eccrine glands, 37
 in epidermal regeneration, 103
 in prickle cells, 11
 of acanthotic epidermis, 81–82, 82f
 removal, 59–60
 staining, 46t, 59
Gnathostoma spinigerum, larva, granulomatous inflammation caused by, 312–313, 313f
Gold
 demonstration of, 61
 in skin, 417
Goltz syndrome, 638–639
Gomori's stain. *See* Aldehyde fuchsin stain (Gomori); Methenamine silver stain
Gonococcemia, 221
 skin eruption of, 218
Gougerot–Blum's lichenoid purpuric eruption, 197
Gouty tophi, 385–386, 387f
Graft-vs-host reaction, 131, 138, 140f
 sclerodermoid, 353
Graham–Little syndrome, 135
Grains, 395, 396f
Gram stain, 46t, 61–62

Granular cell(s), 8, 10–12, 13f–14f
 biology of, 8t
 edema and rupture of, 83
Granular cell myoblastoma. *See* Myoblastoma, granular cell
Granular cell tumor, 667f–668f, 668–669
Granular layer, loss of, 84, 84f
Granulation tissue, 242, 242f, 279, 620f
 components of, 620
 origin of, 620
Granuloma, 279, 673
 annulare, 88, 286, 321–324, 322f–324f
  perforating, 324, 325f
  subcutaneous, 323, 324f
 atypical histiocytic, oral, 702
 eosinophilic, 343
 faciale, 223–224, 226f
 fissuratum, 246, 247f
 gluteale infantum, 314
 infectious, of mucous membranes, 702–703
 inguinale, 305, 316, 317f–318f, 703
 microorganisms found in, 290t
 mixed cell, 305–320
 multiforme, 324
 noninfectious, of mucous membranes, 703
 palisading, 321–330
 in syphilis, 292–293
 predominantly histiocytic, 331–341
 predominantly mononuclear, 281–303
  differential diagnosis, 282t
  microorganisms found in, 290t
 pyogenicum, 242, 650–651, 653f
  atypical, 652, 654
  telangiectaticum, 651
Granulomatosis disciformis (Miescher), 321, 324–325, 326f
Granulomatous halogen eruptions, 280
Granulomatous inflammation, 90, 279, 516
 development of, 279–280
Granulomatous proliferation, 280
Granulomatous slack skin, 321, 326
Grenz zone, 224, 226f, 373
Grocott methenamine silver stain, 46t, 61
Gross cystic disease fluid protein (GCDFP), in sweat gland neoplasms, 603
Gross cystic disease fluid protein-15, immunostaining, 563
Ground substance, 21. *See also* Mucin
 changes in, 351–367
Grover's disease, 395, 399, 400f
 differential diagnosis, 396t
Guarneri bodies, 183
Gumma, syphilitic, 292–293, 294f
Gummatous syphilis, 699

Haarscheibe, 24f, 32–33, 544–545
Haber syndrome, 537
Haemophilus ducreyi, 243, 244f
Hailey–Hailey disease (Benign familial pemphigus), 161, 395, 396t, 396–399, 399f
 differential diagnosis, 396, 396t
 of mucous membranes, 700
 vesiculobullous eruptions of, 158t
Hair, 695
 circumscribed abnormalities of, 720–721
 in congenital disorders, 720
 diameter of, 714
 disturbances of, 713–723
 epithelial outer root sheath, 25
 extraneous material on, 722–723
 formation of, 713
 germ cells, 24f, 24–25
 grouped arrangements of, 23
 layers of, 713
 microscopic examination of, 713–715
 pigmentation, 25–26
 woolly, 720–721
Hair apparatus germ, 8

Hair canal, 24, 24f
Hair casts, 722f, 723
Hair cone, 24
Hair cortex, 24
Hair count, 715
Hair cycle, 33–35, 34f. *See also* Anagen; Catagen; Telogen
Hair disk, 24f, 32–33, 33f, 392f, 544–545
Hair follicle(s), 24f, 694f
 adult, structure of, 25–30
 alarm reaction, 112f
 anagen, 29f, 34f
 bulge area of, 26–27, 28f–29f
 catagen, 26, 29f, 35f
 fetal, 24f
 fibrous root sheath, 26f, 29–30
 in inflammatory disease, 96
 inner root sheath, 26f, 26–27, 27f
  staining, 58
 isthmus, 26–27
 keratogenous zone, 27f
 matrix region (bulb), 25–27, 26f
 mesodermal component, 622
 outer root sheath. *See* Trichilemma
 telogen, 34f
 upper, 29f
 vellus, 31f
Hair follicle nevus, 531, 532f
Hair follicle tumors, 531–535
Hair loss. *See also* Pattern alopecia
 acute, 715–716
Hair nevi, 531
Hair papilla, 25. *See also* Dermal papilla
Hair shaft, 27
 abnormalities of, 717–719, 718f
 cortex, 27f–28f
 cuticle, 24, 27, 27f–28f
 medulla, 27, 27f–28f
Halogen eruptions, 314
Hamartoma, 436. *See also* Basaloid follicular hamartoma; Fibrous hamartoma of infancy; Multiple hamartoma syndrome
 arrector pili, 480, 634
 pilar smooth muscle, 480
Hamartomatous conditions, 385
Hand-foot-and-mouth disease, 184–186
Hands. *See also* Palms
 degenerative collagenous plaque of, 374, 378f
Hand–Schüller–Christian disease, 343, 703
Hansen's bacilli, staining, 61, 289, 289f
Hansen's disease. *See* Leprosy
Hard nevus of Unna, 479, 480f
Harlequin fetus, 405t, 406–409, 408f
Harris' hematoxylin solution, 56–57
Hartnup's disease, 212
H&E. *See* Hematoxylin and eosin
Heck's disease, 706. *See also* Focal epithelial hyperplasia
Hemangioma(s)
 arteriovenous, 647, 648f
 capillary, 645, 646f
 cavernous, 645
 epithelioid (histiocytoid), 652–656
 sclerosing, 333
Hemangiopericytoma, 649
Hematoxylin and eosin, 46t, 55–57, 60–61
 fixation with, 56
 ground-glass appearance of nuclei stained by, 181, 182f
 solutions, 56–57
 specimen technique for, 56
 staining procedure, 57
 staining reactions of tissue constituents, 57

Page numbers followed by t *or* f *indicate tables or figures, respectively.*

Hemidesmosome(s), 17, 18f
 as target of bullous pemphigoid autoantibodies, 72–73
Hemochromatosis, 415, 553
Hemorrhage, intrakeratinous, 419
Hemosiderin, 389
 skin color change caused by, 416
 staining, 46t, 58, 197
Henle's layer, 24, 26–27, 27f–28f
Heparin, staining, 59
Heparin therapy, necrosis after, 222
Hereditary sclerosing poikiloderma, 138
Herpes gestationis, 164–166, 167f
 clinical presentation, 73
 diagnosis, immunofluorescence in, 73–74
 vesiculobullous eruptions of, 158t
Herpes gestationis factor, 74, 165
Herpes simplex, 181, 183f
 superinfection, in atopic dermatitis, 182
Herpes zoster, 181, 243
Herxheimer spirals, 10
HGF. *See* Herpes gestationis factor
Hibernoma, 639–640
Hidradenitis suppurativa, 274–275, 275f
Hidradenoma, 523
 clear cell, 575, 577f
 definition of, 563
 nodular, 575, 577f
 papilliferum, 567f, 568
 terminology for, 563
 of vulva, 567f, 568
Hidroacanthoma simplex, 569, 571f, 598
 malignant forms of, 598
Hidrocystomas, 549, 550f
 apocrine, 549
 eccrine, 549, 550f
Hirsutism, 717
Hirsutoid papillomas, 622
Histiocyte(s), 19, 21, 279, 629
 definition of, 92
 in granulomatous inflammation, 331–341
 morphology, 672
 multinucleated. *See* Multinucleated giant cells
Histiocytoma(s), 331, 333–338, 621, 629, 634. *See also* Fibrous histiocytoma
 associated epithelial changes, 334–338
 cartwheel pattern, 334, 336f
 generalized eruptive, 340
 hemosiderotic, 334, 337f
 histology, 333–334, 335f–336f
 nature of, 333
 regressive changes of pilar complexes above, 335, 338f
 variants, 334
 xanthomatized, 334
Histiocytosis X, 39, 84, 280, 332, 343–347, 383
 histopathology, 343–345, 344f
 skin manifestations, 343, 344f
Histologic diagnosis, 3
Histologic section, preparation, 54–55
Histology, terminology, 9t
Histopathologic interpretation
 systematics of, 95–97
 technique, 95
Histoplasma capsulatum, 297
Histoplasmosis, 280, 297–298, 703
 African, microorganisms found in, 290t
 differential diagnosis, 282t
 microorganisms found in, 290t
HLA (human leukocyte antigen(s)), in subacute cutaneous lupus erythematosus and neonatal lupus erythematosus, 76–77
HMB-45, immunostaining reactive patterns, 70t
Hodgkin's disease, 673, 675, 676f, 682
 in mycosis fungoides, 676

Hoffmann's disease, 253–254, 275
Hookworm, granulomatous inflammation caused by, 312
Horny cell(s), 8, 13, 14f, 15. *See also* Keratinized cell(s)
Horny layer, changes in, skin color changes due to, 418–419
HPV. *See* Papillomaviruses
Hunter syndrome, 360
Hurler syndrome, 359
Hutchinson's angioma serpiginosum, 197
Huxley's layer, 24, 26–27, 27f–28f
Hyalin
 extracellular deposits of, 386, 387f
 staining, 386
Hyalinosis cutis et mucosae, 386
Hyaluronic acid
 removal from tissue sections, 60
 staining, 60
Hyaluronidase, digestion of specimens, 60
Hybrid cyst, 555, 556f
Hybridoma, 69
Hydroa vacciniforme, 212
Hydrochloric acid solution, normal, 58
Hydroquinone bleaching creams, 418
Hydroxyurea, artifacts introduced by, 63
Hypereosinophilic syndrome, 151–152
Hypergranulosis, 84
Hyperkeratosis, 84. *See also* Epidermolytic hyperkeratosis
 follicularis et parafollicularis in cutem penetrans, 253, 258, 258f
 lenticularis perstans, 409, 409f
 multiple minute digitate, 482–483, 485f
Hypernephroma, cutaneous metastasis of, 615
Hyperparathyroidism, 385
 leg ulcer with, 245
Hyperpigmentation, 415
Hypertrichosis, 716–717
 lanuginosa, 716–717
  acquired, 717, 717f
 vellosa, 717, 717f
Hypervitaminosis D, 385
Hypoderm, 18, 21
Hypogranulosis, 84
Hypomelanosis of Ito, 414, 443
Hypotrichosis, Marie Unna type of, 720

Ichthyosiform dermatoses, 403–411
 histology, 403, 404t–405t
 inheritance, 405t
 major forms of, 405t
 rare types of, 405t
Ichthyosiform erythroderma
 bullous form of, 83
 congenital
  bullous, 404
  nonbullous, 404
Ichthyosis, 419. *See also* Lamellar ichthyosis
 acquired, 405t, 409
 definition of, 403
 hystrix, 396, 404–406, 407f, 479–480, 482, 509
  Curth–Macklin. *See* Biphasic ichthyosiform dermatosis
 linearis circumflexa with bamboo hairs, 405t, 409
 psoriasiform, 405t
 vulgaris, 403, 405t, 406f
Ichthyotic dry skin, 108
Idiopathic guttate hypomelanosis, 414
Idiopathic macular atrophy, 372–373
ILVEN. *See* Inflammatory linear verrucous epidermal nevus
Imbibitio lipoidica telae elasticae, 383
Immunity, disturbances of, ulcers with, 244–245

Immunofluorescence, 65. *See also* Direct immunofluorescence; Indirect immunofluorescence
Immunoglobulin(s), in direct immunofluorescence, 65–66
Immunopathology, 65–77
Immunoperoxidase, 68
  application of, 68–69
Impetiginization, 174
Impetigo, 174–175. *See also* Bullous impetigo
  Bockhart, 249, 250f, 256
  contagiosa, 174, 175f
  herpetiformis, 124, 164–166
    differential diagnosis, 117t
    vesiculobullous eruptions of, 158t
  vesiculobullous eruptions of, 158t
Incision(s), 47f, 51f
  vertical, 50, 51f
Incontinentia pigmenti, 90, 206f, 415–416, 417f
  achromians, 414
  bullous, vesiculobullous eruptions with, 158t
  Naegeli type of, 416
Indirect immunofluorescence, 66–67
  application of, 68–69
  indications, 67t
  patterns, 67t
Indoxyl esterase, in apocrine and eccrine apparatuses, 33t
Infantile acropustulosis, 108f, 108–109
Infantile fibrosarcoma, 629f
Infarction, 222
Inflammation
  alopecia associated with, 265–271
  of eccrine or apocrine glands, 273–276
  granulomatous, 279
  in pilosebaceous complex, 249–263
  subcutaneous, 229–239
Inflammatory, definition of, 99
Inflammatory cell(s), in vesiculobullous eruptions, 158t
Inflammatory dermatophytosis, 189–190, 190f
Inflammatory disease(s), diagnosis of, 69–77
Inflammatory lesions, categorization of, 96
Inflammatory linear verrucous epidermal nevus, 480, 481f, 482
Inflammatory processes, deep, 203
Inflammatory virus diseases, 181–188
Infundibulofolliculitis, disseminated and recurrent, 256, 257f
Injury, reaction to, 99
Insect bites
  allergic reaction to, 145
  foreign body granuloma caused by, 315–316
  middermal reaction to, 146
  reaction to, 348f
Insect stings, foreign body granuloma caused by, 315–316
Interstitial glossitis, 703
  syphilitic, 699
Intradermal nevus, 447–449, 447f–449f
Intranuclear viruses, 181–182
  vesiculobullous eruptions with, 158t
Intravascular papillary endothelial hyperplasia, 652, 653f
Inverted follicular keratosis, 509, 523, 534, 538f
Involucrin, 12
Iris lesion, of erythema exudativum multiforme, 146, 147f
Iron, staining, 46t, 60
Iron pigment, in biopsy specimen, 54
Islet cell carcinoma of pancreas, dermatosis with, 175
Isodesmosine, 369

Jadassohn–Lewandowsky's law, 283
Jadassohn phenomenon, 598

Jessner's lymphocytic infiltration, 149, 207, 209–210, 211f
Juliusberg's disease, 193
Junctional epidermolysis bullosa, 170
Junction nevus, 445–446, 446f
  nails in, 726
  recurrence after removal, 455, 457f
Juvenile aponeurotic fibroma, 626, 628f
Juvenile colloid milium, 386
Juvenile dermatomyositis, 385
Juvenile elastoma, 370, 370f, 621
Juvenile hyaline fibromatosis, 386, 626, 627f
Juvenile linear IgA dermatosis
  clinical presentation, 75
  diagnosis, immunofluorescence in, 75
Juvenile xanthogranuloma, 332, 334f

Kamino bodies, 454
Kaposi's sarcoma, 225–227, 389, 652, 655–656, 659f
Kaposi's varicelliform eruption, 182
Kawasaki's disease, 184, 220
Keloid(s), 333, 619–621, 621f
Keratin amyloid, 386
Keratinization, 86–87
  in basal cell epithelioma, 585f, 586
  disorders of, 403
  fetal genetic disorders of, 6
Keratinized cell(s), 12
  biology of, 8t
  definition of, 9t
Keratinocyte(s), 38. *See also* Adnexal keratinocyte; Epidermal keratinocyte
  acrotrichial, 15
  biology of, 8t
  definition of, 9t
  life span of, 14
  maturation, 8
  modulation, in wound healing, 16, 17f
  neoplastic, 501
  shape, 14f
  size, 14f
Keratinosome, 12
Keratin products, 15
Keratoacanthoma, 509, 517–519, 518f–519f
  Ferguson–Smith type, 518
  Grzybowski type, 518
  of mucous membranes, 709
  in nails, 725
  subungual, 518
Keratoderma
  blennorrhagicum, 126–127, 126f–127f
    differential diagnosis, 117t
  palmare, 418–419
  palmare at plantare, 494–495, 495f
  palmare et plantare, 260
  palmare punctatum, 495, 496f
  palmoplantar, 404–406
  striate, 495
Keratoelastoidosis marginalis of hands, 374, 378f
Keratohyalin, 15, 419
  staining, 57–58
Keratohyalin cells. *See* Granular cell(s)
Keratohyalin granule(s), 11–12, 14f, 27
Keratosis. *See also* Bowenoid keratoses
  definition of, 501
  follicular, 249, 256–260
  follicularis, 700. *See also* Darier's disease
  lichenoides chronica, 139, 141f
  pilaris, 257f, 257–258, 403–404
  pilaris rubra, 257
  precancerous, 501–507
  recurrence after removal, 512
  senilis, 502–505, 503f, 508f, 597. *See also* Actinic keratosis
Keratotic plugs, 256–257
Kerion, 251

Kimura's disease, 652
Klebsiella rhinoscleromatis, 301
Knife blade, artifacts, 56f
Koenen tumors, 624
KOH fungus mount, 13
Kraurosis vulvae, 358, 699
Kveim test, 295, 297f
Kyrle's disease, 253, 258, 258f

Lacunae, 83, 399
Lamellar bodies, 12, 15
Lamellar ichthyosis, 393, 404, 405t, 406f
Lamina densa, 17
Lamina lucida, 17
Laminated bodies, 14f
Langerhans cell(s), 39–40, 40f, 92, 343
  definition of, 9t, 440t
  identification of, 39
Langerhans cell granulomas, 673. *See also* Histiocytosis X
  of mucous membranes, 703
Lanugo hair, 25
Large cell acanthoma, 492–493, 495f
Large-plaque parapsoriasis, 194, 195f–197f
Larvae, granulomatous inflammation caused by, 312–313
Larva migrans, 312
Laugier–Hunziker syndrome, 726
Leg ulcer(s), 245
  chronic, malignant angioendothelioma of, 654
Leiomyoma(s), 333, 633–636, 636f
  papular, 621
Leiomyosarcoma(s), 636, 637f
Leishman bodies, 51
Leishmania braziliensis, 298
Leishmania donovani, 298
Leishmaniasis, 280, 298–300
  American, 298–299
    microorganisms found in, 290t
  early, differential diagnosis, 282t
  late, differential diagnosis, 282t
  Oriental, 298–299, 301f
    microorganisms found in, 290t
  post-kala-azar, 298–299
    microorganisms found in, 290t
  South American, 703
Leishmania tropica, 298, 301f
Lentigines, inherited patterned, 443
Lentiginosis, with atrial myxomas, 443
Lentigo, 415
  maligna, 460–462, 464f
    differential diagnosis, 466t
  senilis, 443–444, 444f, 484, 487f
    combined with actinic keratosis, 506, 508f
  simplex, 443, 443f
    nails in, 726
Lentigo maligna melanoma, 463–465, 465f
  differential diagnosis, 466t
Leopard syndrome, 443
Lepra cells, 287
Lepra reaction, 289
Leprosy, 280, 287–290
  borderline lesions of, 288–289
  histoid, 288f, 289–290
  lepromatous, 279, 287–288, 289f
    differential diagnosis, 282t
    microorganisms found in, 290t
  tuberculoid, 287–288, 288f, 295
    differential diagnosis, 282t
Lesion(s), categorization of, 96
Lesser–Trélat sign, 490
Lethal midline granuloma, 703
Letterer–Siwe disease, 343
Leucine aminopeptidase, in apocrine and eccrine apparatuses, 33t
Leukemia(s)
  definition of, 674

Leukemia(s) (cont.)
  involvement in dermal strata, 672, 673f
  lymphocytic mass of, 90
  in mycosis fungoides, 676
Leukemia cutis, 674
  involvement in dermal strata, 672
Leukocyte common antigen, immunostaining reactive patterns, 70t
Leukocytoclasia, 90
Leukocytoclastic vasculitis, 217–218, 218f–219f
Leukoderma acquisitum centrifugum, 456, 458f
Leukoedema, 705
Leukonychia striata, 726
Leukoplakia, 12, 703–704, 704f
  definition of, 703
  of mucous membranes, 419
Leukoplakic vulvitis, 699
Lewandowsky's disease, 260
Lichen amyloidosus, 386, 388f
Lichen aureus, 197
Lichenification, 101
  in chronic contact dermatitis, 105–106, 106f
Lichenified dermatitis, 87, 87f
Lichen invisible pigmenté de Gougerot, 136
Lichen myxedematosus, 360
Lichen nitidus, 96, 131, 139–141, 142f
Lichenoid benign keratosis, 138
Lichenoid melanodermatitis, 137
Lichenoid tissue reactions, 131–144, 415
  definition of, 131
Lichen pigmentosus, 137
Lichen planopilaris, 135, 136f
Lichen planus, 12, 99, 131–137, 242
  actinicus, 137–138, 138f
  annular form, 134–135
  atrophic form, 134–135, 135f
  bullous form of, 135
  Civatte bodies in, 87
  clinicohistologic correlation in, 133–134
  epidermal hypertrophy in, 80, 80f
  follicular, 135, 136f
  follicular plug in, 208f
  healing, 136–137
  histology, 131–133, 132f–134f
  hypertrophic, 516
  hypertrophic form, 135, 136f
  infiltrate of, 133, 134f
  versus lichen nitidus, 140–141
  lower surface of epidermis in, 81f
  versus lupus erythematosus, 141–143, 208
  mitotic activity in, 132–133
  of nailbed, 723, 725f
  of oral mucosa, 698, 699f, 703–704
  pemphigoides, 135
  pigmented, 136–137
  tropicus, 137–138, 138f
  verrucous form, 135
Lichen purpuricus, 197
Lichen ruber verrucosus et reticularis, 139
Lichen sclerosus et atrophicus, 49f, 351, 357f, 357–358, 415, 418–419
  epidermal atrophy in, 80, 81f
  of genitoanal region, 699
  of oral mucosa, 703–704
Lichen scrofulosorum, 221, 257, 285, 285f
Lichen simplex, epidermal turnover in, 14
Lichen simplex chronicus, 101, 110–111, 111f–112f, 516
  circumscriptus, 110f
  hypertrophic, 47f, 112f. See also Picker's nodule
  lower surface of epidermis in, 81f
Lichen spinulosus, 257, 258f
Lichen striatus, 198f, 198–199
Lichen urticatus, 145–146, 147f, 184, 348f
Light cells, in eccrine glands, 36–37

Page numbers followed by t or f indicate tables or figures, respectively.

Lightened skin, histologic substrates of, 413, 414t
Light sensitivity eruption, 210–213, 212f
Linear and whorled nevoid hypermelanosis, 415
Linear IgA dermatosis. See also Adult linear IgA dermatosis; Juvenile linear IgA dermatosis
  diagnosis, immunofluorescence in, 67, 67t
Linear melorheostotic scleroderma, 353
Linear scleroderma, 353
Lingua plicata, 297
Lip, pigmented macules of, 441–442
Lipids
  extracellular deposits of, 383
  staining, 60
Lipodystrophia centrifugalis abdominalis, 356
Lipodystrophy, 351, 355–356
Lipofibroma(s), pedunculated, 623
Lipoid proteinosis, 383, 386
Lipoma(s), 637
  pleomorphic, 637
  spindle cell, 637, 638f
  subcutaneous, 637
Lipophage(s), 92
Liposarcoma, 637
Liquefaction degeneration, 138
  of basal cells, 86
  in lichen planus, 131
  in subacute lupus erythematosus, 207f, 208
Liquefying panniculitis, 233–234, 236f
Livedo
  racemosa, 219f, 221, 221f
  reticularis, 219f, 221, 221f
Livedoid vasculitis, 221, 221f
Liver flukes, 313, 314f
Loaisis, granulomatous inflammation caused by, 312
Loboa loboi, 306
Local anesthesia, for biopsy, 47–48
Localized nodular tenosynovitis, 626, 626f
Loxosceles reclusa. See Brown recluse spider bite
Lucio phenomenon, 289
Lupus anticoagulant, 209
Lupus band test, 71, 72f, 76
Lupus erythematosus, 96, 131, 138, 194, 415. See also Discoid lupus erythematosus; Systemic lupus erythematosus
  acute, 205, 207f
  bullous, diagnosis, immunofluorescence in, 67, 67t
  chronic, 205, 206f
    hypertrophic, 208
    spotty absence of elastic fibers in, 208
    variants, 208–209
    verrucous, 208
  diagnostic features of, 209t
  edema in, 207–208
  epidermal changes in, 205
  follicular changes in, 205
  follicular plug in, 206, 208f
  histology of, 205–209
  versus lichen planus, 208
  lymphocytic infiltrate in, 90, 206f, 206–208, 207f
  maternal, and erythema annulare centrifugum in infants, 149
  neonatal, 76–77
  of oral mucosa, 209, 698–699, 703–704
  papular and nodular mucinous lesions in, 360
  poikilodermatous form, 213, 213f
  of scalp, 209
  sebaceous atrophy in, 205
  subacute, 205, 206f
    diagnosis, immunofluorescence in, 67, 67t
Lupus erythematosus profundus, 208–209, 209f–210f, 235

Lupus miliaris disseminatus faciei, 286–287f
Lupus miliaris disseminatus faciei, rosacea-like tuberculid of, 286–287, 287f
Lupus panniculitis, 208–209, 235
Lupus pernio, 295
Lupus tumidus, 284, 293
Lupus vulgaris, 283–284, 284f, 293, 295, 298
Lutzner cells, 678, 681f
Luxol fast blue, 621
Lyell syndrome, 166, 168f
Lyme disease, 149–150
Lymphadenosis cutis benigna, 682–683, 685f
Lymphangioendothelioma, 648
Lymphangioma, 647–648
  circumscriptum, 647–648, 649f
Lymphedema, 93, 351, 359
  verrucous, 359, 362f
Lymphoblastoma, 267
Lymphocyte(s), 279
  definition of, 90–91
  identification of, 91
  in vesiculobullous eruptions, 158t
Lymphocytic vasculitis, of pityriasis lichenoides acuta, 217
Lymphocytoma
  cutis, 682–683, 685f
  versus Jessner's lymphocytic infiltration, 209
Lymphogranuloma venereum, 305, 317
Lymphoma(s), 126, 267
  angiotropic, 650
  cutaneous, 212
  diagnosis, 671
  epidermotropic, 673, 677, 679f–680f
  histiocytic, 92
  ichthyosis vulgaris-like skin with, 403
  involvement in dermal strata, 672–673
  large cell (histiocytic), 675, 677f
  lymphocytic, 149
    and seborrheic verruca, 490
  lymphoplasmocytic, 675–676
  small and large (mixed) type, 675
  small cleaved cell, 675
  small lymphocytic, 675
  T-cell, 672–673, 677. See also Mycosis fungoides
Lymphomatoid granulomatosis, 220, 687, 688f
Lymphomatoid papulosis, 680–682, 683f–684f
  malignant transformation, 682
Lymphoplasmacytic cells, morphology, 672
Lymphoproliferative neoplasms, 671–689
  classification of, 674, 674t
  cytologic interpretation with, 671–673
  infiltrate in, quantity of, 673
  involvement of dermal strata in, 672–673
  involvement of epidermis and adnexa, 673–674
  morphology of cells with, 671–672
  polymorphism versus monomorphism in, 673
  structural interpretation with, 673–674
  terminology for, 674
Lymphosarcoma, in mycosis fungoides, 676
Lysozyme, immunostaining reactive patterns, 70t

MA-902, immunostaining reactive patterns, 70t
MA-904, immunostaining reactive patterns, 70t
Macaulay's disease, 680
Macrophage(s), hemosiderotic, 224–225, 227f
Macrosporum, 251
Maduromycosis, 307, 310f
  granules in, 307–308, 310f
Majocchi granuloma, 251
Majocchi's disease, 197
MAK-6, immunostaining reactive patterns, 70t
Malakoplakia, 297
  microorganisms found in, 290t

Malenodermatitis toxica, 138
Malformation(s)
 definition of, 435
 melanocytic, 439–473
Malherbe's calcifying epithelioma, 535
Malic dehydrogenase, in apocrine and eccrine apparatuses, 33t
Malignancy
 bullous eruptions with, 175–176
 definition of, 435–438
 erythema gyratum repens with, 150f
 of melanocytic tumors, criteria for, 470–473
 and seborrheic verruca, 490
Malignant angioendothelioma, 654–655, 657f–658f
Malignant atrophic papulosis of Degos, 222, 224f
Malignant fibrous histiocytoma, 630, 631f
Malignant histiocytosis, cutaneous, 687, 687f
Malignant lymphoma, 675–676, 677f, 682
Malignant melanoma, 449–450, 464–468. *See also* Acral lentiginous melanoma; Lentigo maligna; Nodular melanoma
 amelanotic, 471, 512
 and bathing trunk nevus, 458
 biology of, 459–462
 Clark's classification of, 460–462
 Clark's grading of dermal invasion, 473, 473f
 desmoplastic, 471, 472f
 development above benign congenital nevus, 471, 471f
 differential diagnosis, 466t
 diffuse melanosis secondary to, 416
 formalin fixed, paraffin embedded sections, immunohistochemical staining pattern for, 66t
 histologic grading of, 473
 metastatic, differential diagnosis, 466t
 in mucous membranes, 706–707
 neurotropic, 471
 ocular, 459
 pagetoid, 469
 prognosis, 473
 in situ, 462
 superficial spreading, 467–469, 469f–470f
  differential diagnosis, 466t, 613
  pagetoid features, 613
 tumor thickness, measurement of Breslow, 473
Malignant mucoepidermoid tumor, 708, 709f
Malignant proliferating angioendotheliomatosis, 650, 651f
Malpighian cells. *See* Prickle cell(s)
Mantle hair, 30–31, 31f–32f
Marfan syndrome, 372
 syringomas associated with, 574
Marginal band, 12, 14f, 15
Masson's ammoniacal silver nitrate stain, 46t
Masson's neuronevus, 450
Masson's trichome stain, 46t
Mast cell(s), 687, 688f
 in dermis, 90
 morphology, 672
Mast cell granules, staining, 58–60, 687–689
Mastocytosis, 687–689
Matrix cells, pluripotential, 437
Max Joseph spaces, 131, 132f–133f
MCTD. *See* Mixed connective tissue disease
Measles. *See* Rubella
Mechanobullous dermatosis, congenital self-healing (transient), 173
Mechanobullous disease, 168
Median raphe cyst, 557
Meibomian carcinoma, 603, 604f
Meissner's corpuscle(s), 19, 23f, 663, 664f
Melanin, 38–39, 86
 epidermal, decrease and increase of, 413–415
 pigmentation of mucous membranes, 706–707
 staining, 46t, 58, 60–61, 413
 subepidermal, increase of, 415–416
Melanin block, 415
Melanin granules, in basal cell epithelioma, 587, 592f
Melanin unit, epidermal, 39f
Melanization, disturbances of, 86
Melanoacanthoma, 490, 491f
 of oral mucosa, 707, 707f
Melanoblast(s), 439
 definition of, 440t
Melanocyte(s), 8f, 38f, 38–39, 439, 444–445, 445t
 amelanotic, 28f
 definition of, 9t, 440t
 dendritic, 38f
 dermal, 458
  lesions involving, 458–459
 descriptive terminology for, 86
 epidermal, 38f
  identification of, 439–441
  lesions involving, 441–444
Melanocytic nevus, 436
Melanocytic tumor(s), 439–473
 criteria for malignancy, 470–473
 neural crest derivation of, 466f
Melanoma. *See* Malignant melanoma
Melanophage(s), 90, 90f, 92, 279
 identification of, 439
 in lupus erythematosus, 207f, 208
Melanophore(s), definition of, 440t
Melanosome(s), 39
 definition of, 440t
Melasma(s), 415, 441–442
Meleney's synergistic gangrene, 243
Melkersson–Rosenthal syndrome, 297, 300f
Membrane coating granule, 12
Meningioma(s), cutaneous, 666f, 667
Meningococcemia, 221
 chronic, 218
Menkes' disease, 720
Mercury
 demonstration of, 61
 in skin, 417
Mercury-induced granuloma, 295–296
Merkel cell carcinoma, 614f, 614–615
Merkel cells, 33, 40
 definition of, 9t
 staining, 41
Mesoderm, 5–6, 18
Mesodermal nevi and tumors, 619–640
Metabolic dermal diseases, 349
Metachromasia, 59–60
Metal pigmentation, 416–417
Metastasis, 437
Methenamine silver stain (Gomori), 60
Methotrexate, artifacts introduced by, 63
Methoxsalen, 415
Methyldopa, lichenoid drug eruption caused by, 141
Mibelli's disease, 491–492, 494f
Michaelis–Gutmann bodies, 297
Microabscesses. *See also* Munro abscesses
 in psoriasis, 120, 122f
Microfibrils, 21, 369
Microsporon, 251
Microsporum, 251
Microsporum audouini, 252
Microsporum canis, 252
Middermis, pathology, descriptive terminology for, 79
Migrating glossitis, 698, 698f
Mikulicz cell, 300–301
Miliaria, 273
 apocrine, 274f, 274–275
 crystallina, 273
 rubra, 273, 274f
Miliary tuberculosis, 221
 of skin, 287
Milker's nodule, 183, 184f–185f
Minocycline, discoloration of sun-exposed skin and, 417
Mitotic index, epidermal, 14
Mixed cell granulomas, 305–320
Mixed connective tissue disease, 209
 clinical presentation, 77
 immunopathology of, 76–77
Mixed tumor of skin, 575–576, 578f
 malignant, 576
Moll's glands
 cyst, 549
 of eyelids, 31
Molluscum bodies, 423
Molluscum contagiosum, 423, 424f
Mondor's disease, 221, 232
Mongolian spot, 439, 458
 persistent, 458
Monilethrix, 718f, 719
Monoblasts, 92
Monoclonal antibodies, 672t
 in diagnosis of lymphoproliferative disorders, 671
Monoclonal antibody technique, 66t, 69, 70t
Monocyte(s), 92
Monocytes-macrophages, morphology, 672
Mononuclear giant cells, 93
Morphea, 77, 352–353, 352f–354f
 profunda, 353
Morphea-like epithelioma, 591–596, 598f
Morton's neuroma, 668
Mucha–Habermann disease, 193
Mucicarmin, 61
Mucin, staining, 58–60
Mucinosis. *See* Follicular mucinosis
Mucinous syringometaplasia, 549, 551f
Mucin substances, accumulation of, 360
Mucocele, 702, 703f
Mucocutaneous lymph node syndrome, infantile acute febrile, 220
Mucolipidoses, 359
Mucopolysaccharides, staining, 59
Mucopolysaccharidoses, 359–360
Mucormycosis, 312
Mucosal epithelium, definition of, 9t
Mucous membranes, 695
 bullous lesions of, 699–700
 dark lesions of, 706–707
 inflammatory lesions of, 697–699
 lesions of, 697–710
 melanin pigmentation of, 706–707
 mesodermal and neural neoplasms of, 710
 neoplasms of, 707–710
 ulcerative lesions of, 700–703
 vascular lesions of, 707
 white lesions of, 703–706
Mucous retention cyst, 702, 703f
Muir–Torre syndrome, 528, 528f
Multinucleated giant cells, 92f
 asteroid bodies in, 93, 93f
 definition of, 93
 in epidermis, 87, 87f
 foreign body type, 92f, 93
 formation, with herpes infections, 181, 182f–183f
 in granuloma annulare, 323, 323f
 in histiocytoma, 333, 336f
 in inflammatory infiltrate, 279–280
 Langerhans type, 93
 Langhans type, 92f
  in epidermis, 89f
 Touton type, 92f, 93
 in tuberculosis, 278f
Multiple endocrine neoplasia syndrome, 663
Multiple hamartoma syndrome, 534–535
Multiple myeloma, cutaneous manifestation of, 675
Multiple myeloma-associated amyloidosis, 387–388
Munro abscesses, 84, 119, 123f
Muscle fibers, staining, 57

Musculus arrector pili. *See* Arrector muscle
Mycelia, in inflammatory dermatophytosis, 191, 191f
Mycetoma, 307
Mycobacteria, atypical, 290
Mycobacterium balnei, 290
Mycobacterium marinum, 290, 291f
Mycobacterium ulcerans, 243, 290
Mycosis cells, 678, 681f
Mycosis fungoides, 84, 138, 192–193, 267, 672–673, 682
  definition of, 676
  differential diagnosis, 678–680
  histologic features of, 676–678, 678f
Myelin basic protein(s)
  immunostaining reactive patterns, 70t
  in neural tumors, 663
Myoblastoma, granular cell, 667f, 668–669, 710
  malignant, 668f, 669
Myofibroblast(s), 620, 635f
Myxedema, 93, 351, 359, 362f
Myxoid cysts, 360–361, 364f
Myxoid fibromas, digital, 624, 625f
Myxoid neurofibroma(s), 624, 625f
Myxoma(s), 624, 625f. *See also* Nerve sheath myxoma(s)

Naevus sur naevus, 449
Nail(s), 695. *See also* Keratoacanthoma, subungual
  anatomy of, 713, 714f
  biopsy of, 723
  disturbances of, 723–726
  formation of, 713
  hemorrhages involving, 726, 727f
Nailplate, discolored, 726
Necrobiosis, in palisading granulomas, 321
Necrobiosis lipoidica, 321, 325–326, 327f, 383
  and granuloma annulare, 323
Necrobiotic xanthogranuloma, 321, 328, 328f, 383
Necrolytic migratory erythema, 175
Necrotizing angiitis, 217–220
Necrotizing fasciitis, 235
Necrotizing folliculitis, 253, 254f
Necrotizing sialometaplasia, 702
Necrotizing vasculitis, 217
  classification of, 218t
Neonatal lupus erythematosus, 76–77
Neoplasm(s)
  benign versus malignant, 435–438
  classification of, 437, 438f
  definition of, 435
  of mucous membranes, 707–710
Nerves, pathologic changes of, 94
Nerve sheath myxoma(s), 625f, 663–667
Netherton's syndrome. *See* Ichthyosis linearis circumflexa with bamboo hairs
Neural tumors, 663–669
Neurilemmoma, 666f, 667
Neuroblastoma(s), 668
Neurodermatitis, 110
Neuroectoderm, 5
Neuroendocrine carcinoma, 614f, 614–615
Neurofibroma, 663–667, 665f
Neurofibromatosis, 442
Neurofilament antibody, 32
Neurologic disorders, bullae in, 176
Neuroma(s), 663, 664f
  of mucous membranes, 710
Neuromyoarterial glomus of Masson, 21f, 22
Neuronevus, 450–451, 453f

Neuron-specific enolase
  immunostaining reactive patterns, 70t
  in neural tumors, 663
Neurothekeomas, 663–667
Neutrophilic eccrine hidradenitis, 274
Neutrophilic leukocytes, in inflammatory infiltrates, 279–280
Nevoid basal cell epithelioma syndrome, 491, 493f, 596
Nevoid hyperkeratosis, of nipples and areolae, 482, 483f
Nevoid tumors, 436
Nevoxanthoendothelioma, 332
Nevus/nevi. *See also* Apocrine nevus; Connective tissue nevi; Epidermal nevus; Junction nevus; Mesodermal nevi and tumors; Sweat gland nevi; Vascular nevi and tumors
  anemicus, 418, 645
  angiolipomatosus, 639, 640f
  araneus, 646
  of Becker, 480–481, 482f
  benign, biopsy of, 48
  cerebriform intradermal, 458
  comedonicus, 531, 532f
  congenital, 457–458
  definition of, 435–436
  depigmentosus, 414, 443
  desmoplastic, 454
  dysplastic, 450, 450f–452f
  eccrine angiomatous, 563, 564f
  elasticus, 621, 622f
  elasticus en tumeurs disséminés, 370
  elasticus regionis mammariae (Lewandowsky type), 370
  epitheliomatosus capitis, 523, 525f
  eruptive, 449
  fibroepithelial, classification of, 437, 438f
  flammeus, 646
  formalin fixed, paraffin embedded sections, immunohistochemical staining pattern for, 66t
  hair follicle, 531, 532f
  ichthyosiform, 404–406
  incipiens, 445, 445f, 466
  inflammatory reaction with, 471
  intradermal, 447–449, 447f–449f
  of Ito, 459
  lipomatosus superficialis, 637–639, 642f
  melanocytic, 436
  minus, 370
    definition of, 436
  nevus cell, 436, 621
    with blue nevus, 449
    papillomatous, 448, 448f
    pigmented, 444–445
    regression of, 455–456
  of Ota, 458–459, 460f
  pilosus, 531
  plus, 370
  porokeratotic eccrine ostial and dermal duct, 492
  recurrence after removal, 455, 457f
  sebaceus of Jadassohn. *See* Organoid nevus
  sebaceus, definition of, 436
  spilus, 415, 442–443
  sudoriparus, 563, 564f
  unius lateris, 479
  vascular, 646t
Nevus cell(s), 444–445, 445t
  derivation of, 439, 440f
  identification of, 439
  types of, 448
Nevus sebaceus syndrome, 524
Newborn
  subcutaneous fat necrosis of, 234, 237f
  transient bullous dermolysis of, 172–173
    antibodies and ultrastructural changes useful for classification of, 170t
Nicotinamide deficiency, 212

Nipple. *See also* Supernumerary nipple
  erosive adenomatosis of, 568f, 568–569
  nevoid hyperkeratosis of, 482, 483f
Nits, in pediculosis capitis, 723, 724f
NLE. *See* Neonatal lupus erythematosus
Nocardiosis, 307
Nodular calcinosis of children, 384f, 385
Nodular elastosis with cysts and comedones, 374–375
Nodular fasciitis, 633, 634f
Nodular hidradenoma, 575, 577f
Nodular melanoma, 460, 469–470, 470f
  differential diagnosis, 466t
Nodular migratory panniculitis, 233
Nodular vasculitis, 232–234, 234f
Nonbullous congenital ichthyosiform erythroderma, 404
Non-Hodgkin's lymphomas, classification of, 674, 674t
Noninflammatory dermal diseases, 349
Nonkeratinocytes, definition of, 9t
Nonvenereal sclerosing lymphangitis, of penis, 221
Non-X histiocytic tumors, formalin fixed, paraffin embedded sections, immunohistochemical staining pattern for, 66t
North American blastomycosis. *See* Blastomycosis, North American
Norwegian scabies, 199, 199f
Nose, fibrous papule of, 622, 622f
Nuclear antigen, extractable, antibodies against, in mixed connective tissue disease, 76
Nuclear contour index, 678
Nuclear dust, 90, 217, 218f–219f
Nuclei
  hyperchromatic, 654, 658f
  hyperconvoluted, 678
  polarization of, 51, 52f
  staining, 57–58
Nucleic acids, staining, 60
Nummular eczema, 116, 127f, 127–128
Nylon fiber granuloma, 297

Oblique section(s), 15, 16f
Occupational vitiligo, 414
Ochronosis, 417–418, 418f
Ocular pemphigoid. *See* Cicatricial pemphigoid
Odland body, 12
Ofuji's disease, 252, 256, 256f
O&G. *See* Acid orcein–Giemsa stain
Oil red O, 60
Older hair germ, 8
Omphaloenteric polyp, 557–560, 559f
Onchocerciasis, granulomatous inflammation caused by, 312
Onychomycosis, 726, 726f
Oral hairy leukoplakia, 704–705, 705f
Oral mucosa, 695
  benign white plaques, 704
  lichen planus of, 698, 699f
  lupus erythematosus of, 209, 698–699
  melanoacanthoma of, 707, 707f
  precancerous change in, 703–704, 704f
  psoriasis of, 697–698
  sebaceous glands of, 27, 30f
Orf, 183–184, 185f–186f
Organoid nevus, 523–524
  adnexal tumors developing in, 523
  apocrine hyperplasia within, 564
  life history of, 523, 524f–525f
  of scalp, 524f
    infantile form of, 523, 525f
Original nevus of scalp, 202f
Orthokeratosis, 84
Orthokeratotic cell(s), definition of, 9t
Osteogenesis imperfecta, 372

Osteoma, 627
Osteoma cutis, 384–385, 385f
Osteomyelitis, 385
Ovary, dermoid cyst of, 558f
Oxytalan fibers, 19

Pachydermoperiostosis, 353
Pachyonychia congenita, 706, 726, 727f
Pacinian neurofibromas, 663, 665f
Paget cells
  origin of, 607
  staining, 608, 612f
Pagetoid reticulosis, 682, 685f
Paget phenomenon, 597
Paget's disease, 509, 597
  areolar, 608–613, 612f
  and breast cancer, 607
  differential diagnosis, 608–613
  extramammary, 607–613, 612f
Pagothrix, 721
Palisaded encapsulated neuroma, 663
Palmar and plantar fibromatosis, 626
Palmar pits, 491, 493f
Palmoplantar keratoderma, 404–406
Palms
  keratoderma of, 494–495
  psoriasis of, 124–125, 125f–126f
  true pustular psoriasis of, differential diagnosis, 117t
  vellus hair on, 531
  vesiculopustular lesions of, 107
Palpable purpura, 217
Panatrophy of Gower's, 356
Pancreatic carcinoma, elastolysis with, 373
Pancreatic disease, fat necrosis in, 383
Pancreatic panniculitis, 234–235, 237f
Panniculitis, 22, 229, 233f, 233–235, 243, 383.
  See also Lupus panniculitis
  with alpha1-antitrypsin deficiency, 235
  in connective tissue disease, 235–236
  differential diagnosis, 229–232
  factitial, 237
  liquefying, 233–234, 236f
  secondary to pancreatitis, 234–235, 237f
Papillae, 8f, 15f. See also Dermal papilla
  descriptive histopathology of, 88–90
  elastic fibers of, 20f
  pathology, descriptive terminology for, 79–80
Papillary eccrine adenoma, 570, 573f
  malignant transformation of, 606
Papilloma(s), 425, 623
  cutaneous, definition of, 88
  hirsutoid, 622
Papillomatosis
  cutis carcinoides, 517
  definition of, 88
  florid oral, 707, 708f
  of Gougerot and Carteaud, 482, 484f
  of nipple ducts, florid, 568f, 568–569
  reticulated and confluent, 482, 484f
Papillomavirus, 424, 705–706
  in Bowen's disease, 509
  cutaneous and mucosal manifestations of, 424t
  immunostaining, 424, 425f
Papilloma virus common antigen, immunostaining reactive patterns, 70t
Papular acrodermatitis of childhood, 187
Papular dermatitis of pregnancy, 165
Papular eruptions of pregnancy, 148
Papular leiomyoma(s), 621
Papular mucinosis, 360, 363f
Papular urticaria, 46, 145
Papulonecrotic tuberculids, 221, 285–286, 286f
Papulosquamous disorders, 189
Papulosquamous lesions, 99
Paracoccidioides braziliensis, 306
Paraffin, for embedding, 54

Paraffinoma, 296–297
  differential diagnosis, 282t
Parakeratosis, 84, 84f, 87, 101
  in atopic dermatitis, 107–108
  focal, in psoriasiform tissue reactions, 115
  in sensitization dermatitis, 104, 104f
Paraplast, 54
Parapsoriasis, 138, 192–194
  en plaques, 194–197, 195f, 676–677, 679–680
  large-plaque, 194, 196f–197f
  lichenoid, and poikiloderma, 193–194
  retiform, 193–194
  small-plaque, 194, 195f
Paravaccinia, 148, 181, 183, 184f–185f
Parkinson's disease, seborrheic dermatitis in, 116
Pars papillaris, 18–19, 369, 620
  descriptive histopathology of, 88–90
Pars reticularis, 18–22, 620
  descriptive histopathology, 90–94
PAS. See Periodic acid–Schiff reaction
Pathologists' warts, 284
Pathology, descriptive terminology for, 79
Pattern alopecia, 715, 715f
Pautrier abscess(es), 194, 195f, 673, 677–680, 678f–679f, 681f
Paving stone nevus, 622t
Pearly penile papules, 622, 623f
Pediculosis capitis, nits in, 723, 724f
Pellagra, 212–213, 257
Pemphigoid. See also Bullous pemphigoid
  gestationis, diagnosis, immunofluorescence in, 67, 67t
  mucous membrane, 700, 701f
Pemphigus
  and dermatitis herpetiformis, mixed cases of, 161
  endemic Brazilian, 159–161
  eosinophilic spongiotic, 152, 161, 162f
  erythematosus, 70–71, 157, 159, 161f, 162
    immunohistology, 71
  foliaceus, 157, 159, 161f, 174, 398
    clinical presentation, 71
    diagnosis, immunofluorescence in, 67, 67t, 71
    vesiculobullous eruptions of, 158t
  vegetans, 157, 159, 160f, 161, 395
    clinical presentation, 70
    diagnosis, immunofluorescence in, 67, 67t, 70
    differential diagnosis, 396t, 397
    Hallopeau type, 70
    Neumann type, 70
    vesiculobullous eruptions of, 158t
  vulgaris, 157–159, 159f, 161, 395
    acantholytic cells in, 159, 160f
    clinical findings, 69
    diagnosis, immunofluorescence in, 67, 67t, 69–70, 71f
    differential diagnosis, 396t
    epidemiology, 69
    of oral mucosa, 700, 700f
    vesiculobullous eruptions of, 158t
Penicillamine therapy, cutaneous complications of, 162, 370, 372, 374f–375f
Penis. See also Pigmented penile macules
  median raphe cyst of, 557
  nonvenereal sclerosing lymphangitis of, 221
  pearly penile papules, 622, 623f
Pentazocine injection, cutaneous complication of, 353
Perforating collagenosis, 89f
Perforating dermatoses, 246
Perforating elastosis, 88
Perforating folliculitis, 88, 252–253, 253f
Perforating granuloma annulare, 88
Periarteritis nodosa, 219f, 219–220
Periderm, 5–6, 7f
Periderm cells, 7f

Perifollicular connective tissue, tumors of, 537–545
Perifollicular elastolysis, 373
Perifollicular fibroma(s), 537–544, 622t, 622–623, 623f
Periocular dermatitis, 119
Periodic acid–Schiff reaction, 46t, 56
  of Hotchkiss and McManus, solutions, 58–59
  staining of basement membrane, 88
  staining of microorganisms, 85
  staining procedure, 59
  staining reactions of tissue constituents, 59
Periodic acid solution, 0.5 percent, 58
Perioral dermatitis, 119, 119f, 254
Periporitis, 273
Perlèche, 701
Pernio, 222, 222f
Peroxidase(s), cellular, 68
Peroxidase–diaminobenzidine reaction, 68
Peutz–Jeghers syndrome, 443
Phaeohyphomycosis, 312
Phakoma, 436
Photoaging, 373
Photoallergic dermatitis, 210–212
Photocontact dermatitis, 210–212
Photosensitivity dermatitis, 106
Photosensitivity reactions, 210–213
  in neonatal lupus erythematosus, 76–77
  in subacute cutaneous lupus erythematosus, 76–77
Phototoxic eruption, 210, 211f
Photoxic bullae, 176
Phrynoderma, 257
Picker's nodule, 111, 112f
Picric acid, 56
Piezogenic papules, 238
Pigmentary disorders, 12, 393, 413–421
  histologic substrates of, 413, 414t
Pigmentatio maculosa multiplex, 416
Pigment block, 39f, 86
Pigmented dermatofibrosarcoma protuberans, 631–633, 633f
Pigmented follicular cyst, 554, 554f
Pigmented hairy epidermal nevus, 480–481, 482f
Pigmented macules, 441, 442f
Pigmented moles, excessive hair in, 531
Pigmented penile macules, atypical, 441
Pigmented purpuric eruptions, 197–198
  differential diagnosis, 197–198
Pigment-forming cells, malformations and tumors of, 440t
Pilar apparatus, 23–35, 24f
  development, 7–8, 21–25
Pilar complex, 32f
  intraepidermal portions of, 15
Pilar smooth muscle hamartoma, 480
Pilar tumors, 555–557, 557f–558f
  malignant, 557, 557f
Pili annulati, 719, 720f
Pili multigemini, 721, 721f–722f
Pili pseudoannulati, 719
Pili torti, 718f, 719
Pilomatricoma, 384–385, 535, 540f
  malignant, 535
Pilomatrix carcinoma, 613–614
Pilonidal sinus, 254, 255f
Pilosebaceous canal, 27, 30
Pilosebaceous complex, inflammation in, 249–263
Pilosebaceous cysts, 551
Pinta, 138, 293, 295f
Pitted keratolysis, 190, 496, 496f
Pityriasis lichenoides, 192–194
  acute, 192–193, 193f, 286
    lymphocytic vasculitis of, 217
  chronic, 192, 192f–193f
    scale in, 85
  et varioliformis acuta, 242–243
  scale in, 192, 192f–193f

Pityriasis lichenoides (cont.)
  subacute, 192–193, 193f
  types of, 192–194
  varioliform, 192–193, 194f
Pityriasis rosea, 106, 184, 187f, 187–188
  herald patch, 188
Pityriasis rubra pilaris, 31, 259f, 259–260
Pityrosporum
  folliculitis, 253
  in seborrheic dermatitis, 116
Pityrosporum orbiculare, 482
Plantar warts, 424, 427–428, 428f
Plant hairs, as tissue contaminant, 61f, 62
Plasma cell(s), 91, 91f, 279
  morphology, 672
  in syphilis, 290
Plasma cell balanitis, 697, 698f
Plasma cell leukemia, 675f
Plasmacytoma(s), 675
  cutaneous, 91f
Plasmacytosis mucosae, 697
Pleomorphic lipoma, 637
Plexiform neurofibroma, 663
PMN. See Polymorphonuclear leukocytes
Podophyllin, artifacts introduced by, 63
Podophyllin cells, 429f
Pohl–Pincus's mark, 716, 716f
Poikiloderma, 131, 138–139, 415. See also Congenital poikiloderma of Thomson
  acrokeratotic, 138
  atrophicans, 676
  atrophicans vasculare, 138, 140f, 194, 197
  of Civatte, 138
  and dermatomyositis, 213, 213f
  hereditary sclerosing, 138
  and lupus erythematosus, 213, 213f
  and parapsoriasis, 193–194
Poikilodermatous tissue reactions, 137f, 138–139, 140f
Polarization, of cells, by electrodesiccation, 51, 52f
Polarization microscopy, 61
Poliosis, 531
Polyarteritis nodosa, 219–220
Polymorphonuclear leukocytes
  accumulations, in epidermis, 83
  dermatoses associated with, 176t
  in vesiculobullous eruptions, 158t
Polymorphous light eruption, 207, 210, 212f
Polythelia, 564
Polyvinyl pyrrolidone, cutaneous infiltration by, 297
Porgeria, 354–355
Porocarcinoma. See Eccrine porocarcinoma
Porokeratosis, 491–492, 494f
  of Mibelli, 491–492, 494f
  plantaris discreta, 492
Porokeratotic eccrine ostial and dermal duct nevus, 492
Poroma. See Eccrine poroma; Follicular poroma
Porphyria cutanea tarda, 166–167, 169f, 353
  vesiculobullous eruptions of, 158t
Postinflammatory pigmentation, 416
Practolol, dermatosis caused by, 141
Prayer's nodule, 246
Precanceroses, 437, 501–502
Precancerous lesion, progression to cancer, 510–512
Pregnancy
  dermatoses of, 164–166
  papular eruptions of, 148
  pruritic papules of, 165
Premalignant fibroepithelial tumors, 589, 593f
Premelanin, staining, 60
Premelanosome, definition of, 440t
Prickle cell(s), 7f, 8, 10f, 10–12, 11f, 14f

Page numbers followed by t or f indicate tables or figures, respectively.

atrophic, 81
biology of, 8t
configuration, terminology for, 81–84
definition of, 9t
in epidermal atrophy or hypoplasia, 80, 81f
in epidermal hyperplasia, 80, 80f
in epidermal hypertrophy, 80, 80f
glycogen in, 11, 81–82, 82f
intracellular edema, 82, 82f. See also Spongiosis
membrane thickening in, 12
nucleoli, 11, 11f
nucleus, 11, 11f
  size of, 81
perinuclear halos, 82, 82f
staining, 81
Primary epithelial germ, 8
Pringle's disease, 623f
Pringle tumors, 621, 622t
Proliferating atrophy, of fat tissue, 229, 232f
Proliferating trichilemmal cyst, 555–557, 557f–558f
Prototheocosis, 312, 313f
Proud flesh, 242
Prurigo, 101, 110
  Besnier, 110
  ferox, 110
  hiemalis, 110
  nodularis, 111
  simplex, 110
Pruritic disease, 46
Prussian blue, 46t, 60
Psammomas, 666f, 667
Pseudoacanthosis, 80, 80f, 133
Pseudoatrophoderma colli, 416
Pseudocancers, 437
Pseudocarcinoma, 516–519
Pseudochromidrosis, 419, 419f
Pseudocyst(s), 50f
  of the auricle, 361
Pseudoepitheliomatous hyperplasia, 242, 245, 293
  in blastomycosis, 306, 307f
Pseudoepitheliomatous proliferation, 516
  in Darier's disease, 397, 397f
  with granular cell tumor, 668–669
Pseudofolliculitis, of beard, 253–254, 255f
Pseudolymphoma(s), 679
Pseudomembrane, of diphtheria, 244
Pseudopelade of Brocq, 256, 268, 269f–271f
Pseudosarcomatous fasciitis, 633, 634f
Pseudosclerodermatous artifact, 353
Pseudosclerodermatous changes, in deep dermis, 48, 49f
Pseudosinus, 48, 49f
Pseudoxanthoma elasticum, 94, 370, 371f, 385, 418
Psoralen. See also PUVA therapy
  bullae associated with, 176
Psoriasiform ichthyosis, 405t
Psoriasiform tissue reactions, 111, 115–128
  differential diagnosis, 117t
  vesiculobullous eruptions of, 158t
Psoriasis, 11, 99. See also Palms, psoriasis of; Soles, psoriasis of
  acute guttate, 120, 122f
  basal cells in, 9
  biopsy in, 48
  classic, 119–122
  coexistence with Hailey–Hailey's disease, 399
  cyclic suprapapillary exudate in pathogenesis of, 122, 123f
  early, 259
  differential diagnosis, 117t
  epidermal turnover in, 14
  fully developed, differential diagnosis, 117t
  generalized pustular of von Zumbusch type, 123, 124f, 174
  lower surface of epidermis in, 81f

mitotic speedup in, 122
mycosis fungoides secondary to, 680
of oral mucosa, 697–698
petechial threshold in, 121–122
plaque, 120f
pustular, 123, 124f
  of nailbed, 723, 725f
  versus pustulosis palmaris et plantaris, 124–125, 125f–126f
pustulosa, differential diagnosis, 117t
scale in, 85
seborrheic, 123
with spongiform pustule, 123, 123f
ultrastructural changes in, 122
variants, 123–126
volar, 125
of vulva and glans penis, 698
Psoriatic erythroderma, 125–126
Pterygium inversum unguis, 726
Punch biopsy
  artifacts, 48, 49f
  technique, 48
Purpura, 389
  pathologic changes in, 94
Pustular vasculitis, 218
Pustulosis palmaris et plantaris, 124–125, 125f–126f
  vesiculobullous eruptions of, 158t
PUVA therapy
  cutaneous complications of, 506–507
  hyperpigmentation with, 415
Pyknosis, 87–88
Pyknotic cells, with sunburn, 63
Pyknotic nuclei, 28f
Pyoderma gangrenosum, 244–245, 245f
Pyodermite végétante, 70

Radiation therapy, malignant angioendothelioma of, 654
Reactive perforating collagenosis, 351, 358, 359f
Red blood cells
  in epidermis, 90
  extravasation of, 90, 388
  staining, 58
Reed–Sternberg cells, 675
Refsum's disease, 405t
Reiter's disease, 126–127, 126f–127f, 698
  differential diagnosis, 117t
Reiter syndrome, on glans penis, 127
Relapsing polychondritis, 361, 364f
REM syndrome, 360
Rete malpighi, 10
Retention milia, 553
Rete pegs, 15, 16f
Rete ridges, 14, 15f
  configuration, terminology for, 80–81, 81f
  downgrowth of, 80, 516
  exaggerated, 80
  sawtooth-shaped, 131–132
Reticular erythematous mucinosis syndrome, 360
Reticular pigmented dermatosis, 416
Reticulate acropigmentation of Kitamura, 415, 496–497
Reticulated pigmented anomaly of flexures, 496, 497f
Reticulate hyperpigmentation, zosteriform, 415
Reticulating degeneration, 83, 181, 182f–183f, 186
Reticulin, staining, 59
Reticulohistiocytic granuloma, 279, 338
Reticulohistiocytoma, 338, 339f. See also Crosti's reticulohistiocytoma of the back
Reticulum, staining, 46t, 60
Reticulum cell(s), 92
Retraction spaces, in basal cell epithelioma, 588, 592f

Rhabdomyosarcoma, 637
Rheumatic nodules, 321, 326
    and granuloma annulare, 323
Rheumatoid nodules, 321, 326, 327f
Rhinophyma, 260, 261f
Rhinoscleroma, 300–301
    differential diagnosis, 282t
    microorganisms found in, 290t
    Russell bodies in, 91f
Rhizopus, 312
Ribonuclease, digestion of specimens, 60
Rickettsial disease, 146
Rickettsioses, 186
Riehl's melanosis, 138
Ringed hair, 719, 720f
Ritter's disease, 166
RNA, removal from tissue sections, 60
Rocky Mountain spotted fever, 146
Rosacea, 260
    granulomatous, 260, 260f
    tuberculoid, 260
Round cell(s), in inflammatory infiltrate, 279–280
Rubella, 181, 184
Rubeola, 181, 184
Rupial psoriasis, differential diagnosis, 117t
Russell bodies, 91, 91f, 301

Sand fleas, granulomatous inflammation caused by, 312
Sarcoid. *See also* Boeck's sarcoid
    Darier–Roussy, 236, 295, 296f
    definition of, 293–294
    Spiegler–Fendt type, 236
Sarcoid granuloma, 389
Sarcoidosis, 89f, 232, 280, 283, 293–297
    differential diagnosis, 282t
    ichthyosis vulgaris-like skin with, 403
Sarcoid reactions, 293–297, 296f
Sarcoma(s), 627–629
    epithelioid, 629, 630f
    spindle cell, 629, 629f
Satellite cell necrosis, 138
SC-170, 77
Scabies, 152, 198f, 199, 297f, 683
    in nails, 725
Scabies mites, 85
Scale, descriptive terminology, 84–85
Scalp
    breast cancer metastasis to, 616
    lupus erythematosus of, 209
Scar
    hypertrophic, 620–621
    normal, 619–620
Scarring alopecia, 267–268. *See also* Pseudopelade
Scarring pseudofolliculitis, of beard, 253–254, 255f
Scars, color of, 418
Schamberg–Majocchi eruption, 197–198, 1963f
Schamberg's disease, 197
Schiff's leucofuchsin solution, 58
Schistosomiasis, 324
    granulomatous inflammation caused by, 312, 315f
Schönlein–Henoch purpura, 217
Schwann cell(s), nucleus, 31–32
SCLE. *See* Subacute cutaneous lupus erythematosus
Scleredema, 351
    adultorum, 358–359
    neonatorum, 234
Sclerema neonatorum, 383
Scleroderma
    clinical presentation, 77
    generalized, 351–352, 352f
    immunopathology of, 77

localized, 351–353, 352f–354f
    panniculitis in, 236
Sclerodermoid disorders, 353
Sclerodermoid processes, 351
Scleromyxedema, 360, 363f
Sclerosing hemangiomas, 333
Sclerosing lipogranuloma, 296–297, 299f
Scrofuloderma, 284–285
Scrotal tongue, 297
Sebaceous adenoma, 526, 527f
Sebaceous cysts, 549
Sebaceous duct, 27, 30
Sebaceous epithelioma, 30, 527, 528f
Sebaceous epithelium, atrophic, 30, 32f
Sebaceous follicle(s), facial, 25, 25f
Sebaceous gland(s), 30–31
    adenocarcinoma, 603, 604f
    chronic alarm reaction, 111, 111f–112f
    of oral mucosa, 27, 30f
    of pilar apparatus, 24f
    subcorneal displacement of, 51, 53f
Sebaceous trichofolliculoma, 526, 526f
Sebaceous tumors, 523–528
    origin of, 523
Seborrheic dermatitis, 98f, 106, 115–119, 116f, 123, 162
    cycle of suprapapillary exudate in, 116, 118f
    differential diagnosis, 117t
    follicular form, 116, 116f, 254
    parakeratotic crust in, 85f
    scale in, 85
    Unna's petaloid form, 115–116, 116f
Seborrheic keratosis, 387
    formalin fixed, paraffin embedded sections, immunohistochemical staining pattern for, 66t
Seborrheic psoriasis, 123
Seborrheic verruca, 334–335, 419, 483–490, 509
    acanthotic, 485
    activated, 485–489, 489f
    biopsy of, 48
    clonal, 598
        and intraepidermal nests, 489–490, 490f
    deeply pigmented, 485, 488f
    flat type, 485, 488f
    papillomatous, 483, 486f
    reticulated, 483–484, 487f
    solid, 483, 485f
Senear–Usher syndrome. *See* Pemphigus erythematosus
Senile angioma(s), 645
Senile atrophy, 354
Senile elastosis, 373
Senile sebaceous hyperplasia, 525, 526f
Sensitization dermatitis, 103f, 103–104
Sex-linked ichthyosis, 405t
Sézary cells, 680
Sézary syndrome, 680
Shagreen patch, 622t
Shagreen plaques, 621
Sheep pox, 183–184, 185f–186f
Sialidase, digestion of specimens, 60
Sialomucin
    in Paget cells, 610
    removal from tissue sections, 60
    staining, 59–60
Sickle cell ulcer, 245, 246f
Signet-ring cells, 615, 615f
Silica, 62, 389–390
    demonstration of, 61
Silica granuloma, 295, 298f
    differential diagnosis, 282t
Silicone, augmentation mammoplasty, scleroderma after, 353
Silicone granuloma, 297
Silver
    in skin, 417, 418f
    staining, 61
Silver nitrate, 60

Sinus histiocytosis with massive lymphadenopathy, 684–687, 686f
Sister Marie-Joseph nodule of umbilicus, 616
Sjögren–Larsen syndrome, 405t
Sjögren's syndrome, subacute cutaneous lupus erythematosus and, 76
Skin
    development, 5–8
    embryology, 5–8
    normal, 6f
    specimens. *See* Skin section(s); Specimen(s)
Skin color
    blood flow changes and, 418
    disturbances of. *See* Pigmentary disorders
    horny layer changes and, 418–419
Skin section(s)
    descriptive terminology for, 79
    examination of, 95
    foreign bodies in, 61f, 62, 62f
    formalin fixed, paraffin embedded, immunohistochemical staining pattern for, 66t
    preparation, for immunofluorescence, 65
Skin tag, 623
SLE. *See* Systemic lupus erythematosus
Small-plaque parapsoriasis, 194, 195f
Smallpox, 182
Smith antibody, in SLE, 76
Smoker's melanosis, 707, 707f
Smoker's palate, 705
Smooth muscle, versus nerve, 31
Sneddon–Wilkinson's disease, 174
Solar keratosis, 131, 502f, 509
Soles
    keratoderma of, 494–495
    piezogenic papules of, 238
    psoriasis of, 124–125, 125f–126f
    vesiculopustular lesions of, 107
Solitary labial lentigo, 441, 441f
Solitary lichen planuslike keratosis, 138, 139f
Solitary pigment spots, 415
South American blastomycosis. *See* Blastomycosis, South American
Specimen(s). *See also* Skin section(s)
    clinical information that should accompany, 96–97
    contamination from waterbath, 56f
    cutting, artifacts, 56f
    defatting, 54
    dehydration, 54
    embedded, cutting, 54–55, 56f
    embedding, 54
        angles of, 54, 55f
    enzyme digestion, 60
    fixation, 51–54
    foreign bodies in, 62
    histologic section, preparation, 54–55
    identification, 54
    stains for. *See* Stains
    tissue processing, 54–55
    trimming, 54
Speckled lentiginous nevus, 443, 449
Spicules, dermatitis due to, 104–105
Spider bite, necrotic, 245
Spider nevus, 646
Spindle cell lipoma(s), 637, 638f
Spindle cell melanoma, diagnosis, immunofluorescence techniques in, 66
Spindle cell sarcoma, 629, 629f
Spinous cell, definition of, 9t
Spiradenoma. *See also* Eccrine spiradenoma
    definition of, 574
Spitz nevus, 452–454, 454f–456f, 466
Split skin preparation(s), 81, 81f
Spongiform pustule(s), 83, 123, 123f
Spongiosis, 82–83, 83f, 98f, 101
    eosinophilic, associated with pemphigus, 161, 162f
    in sensitization dermatitis, 103–104, 104f
Spongiotic dermatitis, 101
Spongiotic dermoepidermitis, 101

Spongiotic edema, 101
Spongiotic vesicles, 82
Spontaneous keloids, 621
Sporotrichosis, 293, 308–312, 311f
Sporotrichotic gumma, 321
Sporotrichum, 305
Sporotrichum schenckii, 312f
Spotted fever, 186
S-100 protein
  in eccrine glands, 37
  immunostaining, 70t, 563
  in neural tumors, 663
Spun glass hair, 719
Squamous cell, definition of, 9t
Squamous cell carcinoma, 509, 512f, 512–516
  acantholytic, 505, 513–514, 515f
  formalin fixed, paraffin embedded sections, immunohistochemical staining pattern for, 66t
  histologic grading of, 512
  immature tumors, 514, 515f
  keratinizing, 512, 513f
  of lower lip, Borst phenomenon in, 599f
  of mucous membranes, 707
  and organoid nevi, 523
  self-healing, 516–517
  small-cell, 514
  spindle cell, 514–515, 516f
  well differentiated, 512, 514f
Squamous eddies, 489
  in inverted follicular keratosis, 534, 538f
Squamous epithelium, definition of, 9t
Squirting papilla, 115
SSA (Ro), in subacute cutaneous lupus erythematosus and neonatal lupus erythematosus, 76–77
SSB (La), in subacute cutaneous lupus erythematosus and neonatal lupus erythematosus, 76–77
Stains, 55–62
Staphylococcal infections, folliculitis in, 249
Staphylococcic follicular keratosis, 267
Starch granule(s), 62f, 389
  staining, 59
  as tissue contaminant, 61f, 62
Stasis dermatitis, 197, 224–227
  hypertrophic, 227f
Steatocystoma multiplex, 549–551, 552f, 556
Steatocystoma simplex, 549
Stellate spontaneous pseudoscars, 375, 379f
Steroid acne, 253
Stewart–Treves syndrome, malignant angioendothelioma of, 654, 657f
Stomatitis, 697
Stomatitis nicotina, 705
Stone pox, 183
Straight-hair nevus, 531
Stratified epithelium, definition of, 9t
Stratum corneum, 8f
  basketweave appearance of, 13, 84
  changes in, skin color changes due to, 418–419
  configuration, descriptive terminology for, 84
Stratum germinativum, 5, 9, 85–86
Stratum granulosum, 8f, 13f
  configuration, descriptive terminology for, 84
Stratum lucidum, 13, 13f
Stratum spinosum, 8f, 13f
Streptomyces, 190
Stria distensa, 376, 380f
Strophulus, 145
Stucco keratosis, 483
Subacute cutaneous lupus erythematosus
  clinical presentation, 76
  immunopathology, 76
  and Sjögren's syndrome, 76

Page numbers followed by t or f indicate tables or figures, respectively.

Subcorneal pustular dermatosis, 174–175, 175f
  vesiculobullous eruptions of, 158t
Subcutaneous fat, 18, 22, 22f
  pathology, descriptive terminology for, 79
Subcutaneous inflammation, 229–239
  differential diagnosis, 229–232
Subcutaneous tissue, 22–23
Subepidermal nodular fibrosis, 333–334
Subpapillary layer
  descriptive histopathology of, 88–90
  elastic fibers of, 20f
Subungual exostosis, 385, 386f
Subungual hemorrhage, 726, 727f
Succinic dehydrogenase, in apocrine and eccrine apparatuses, 33t
Suction, artifacts introduced by, 62
Sudan black stain, 60
Sulzberger–Garbe disease, 128
Sunburn, artifacts introduced by, 63
Suntanning, 415
Superficial, definition of, 99
Superficial granulomatous pyoderma, 244–245
Superficial inflammatory process(es), 99
  definition of, 99
Supernumerary digits, 663, 664f
Supernumerary nipple, 564, 565f
Suprapapillary exudate, in psoriasiform tissue reactions, 115
Suprapapillary plate, configuration, terminology for, 80
Sutton's halo nevus, 456, 458f–459f, 471
Suture material, as tissue contaminant, 61f, 62
Sweat apparatus
  adenocarcinoma of, 603–615
  definition of, 563
  tumors, 563–579
Sweat duct milia, 37
Sweat gland(s)
  cysts. *See* Hidrocystomas
  in inflammatory disease, 96
  necrosis, 274
  tumors, identification of, 563
Sweat gland nevi, 563–564
Sweet syndrome, 145, 150–151, 152f, 218, 223
Swimming pool granuloma, 290
Sycosis vulgaris, 249
Synovial lesions, 360–361, 364f
Syphilis, 232, 280, 290–293
  chancre of, 291, 292f
  gummatous, 233, 321
  juxta-articular nodes of, 321, 326
  late, differential diagnosis, 282t
  lichen planuslike histology in, 143
  in mucous membranes, 699
  plasma cells in, 290
  primary lesion, 291, 292f
  secondary, 291–292, 292f
    differential diagnosis, 285
  tertiary, 292–293, 293f, 703
  ulcerations in, 244
Syphilitic chancre, 702
Syphilitic gumma, 292–293, 294f
Syringadenoma papilliferum, 398, 398f, 565, 566f
Syringoacanthoma, 569, 571f
  malignant, 598
Syringocystadenoma papilliferum, 523. *See also* Syringadenoma papilliferum
Syringofibroadenoma, eccrine, 569, 573f
Syringoma, 570–574, 574f–575f
  chondroid, 575–576, 578f
  clear cell, 572, 574f
Syringoma-like sweat duct proliferation, 268, 271f
Systemic lupus erythematosus, 221
  bullous, 208
  cutaneous lesions, clinical presentation, 76
  diagnosis, immunofluorescence in, 67, 67t

generalized elastolysis in, 371–372
immunopathology of, 76
Systemic sclerosis, 77, 351

Takayasu's arteritis, 220
Talc, 389. *See also* Silica
Tape stripping, epidermal response to, 102f, 102–103
Tattooing, 416, 707
Telangiectasia, 645–646
  macularis eruptiva perstans, 646, 689
Telogen (phase of hair cycle), 33–35, 34f
Telogen count, 715
Telogen effluvium, 34f, 715, 717f
Temporal arteritis, 220, 220f, 232–233
Tenosynovitis, localized nodular, 626, 626f
Terminal hairs, 25
Tetracycline, photosensitization due to, 167
Thallium salts, acute hair loss caused by, 716
Thequocytes, 448
Thromboangitis obliterans, 221
Thrombophlebitis, of legs, 233
Thrombosis, 221
Thrush, 704
Thymic cysts, 560, 560f
Thyroid disease, telangiectasia in, 646
Tick bite(s), 146, 152
  foreign body granuloma caused by, 315–316
  reaction to, 683, 686f
Tinea, 251–252
  circinata, 190
  faciei, 192f
  nigra palmaris, 190
  superficialis, 190–191
  versicolor, 189–190, 190f, 414, 419
    achromians type, 414
Tissue imprints, preparation of, 62
Tissue macrophage(s), 92
Tissue reactions, 99
Tissue section(s). *See* Skin section(s)
T lymphocyte(s)
  cytotoxic–suppressor, 671
  definition of, 91
  development of, 671
  helper–inducer, 671
  morphology, 671
Toe(s). *See also* Aggressive digital papillary adenoma
Toluidine blue–alcian blue–PAS stain, 687
Toluidine blue stain, 46t, 59–60
Tombstone appearance, of basal layer, in pemphigus, 159, 160f
Tongue
  eosinophilic ulcer of, 702
  pigmentation of, 707
Tonofibrils, 10–11
Tonofilaments, 18f
Touch receptor, 33
Touton giant cells, 332, 334f
Toxic epidermal necrolysis, 166, 168f
  adult form of, 148, 149f
    vesiculobullous eruptions of, 158t
  infantile, vesiculobullous eruptions of, 158t
Toxic erythema, 148–150
  differential diagnosis, 150
Toxic hyalin, 223
Toxic shock syndrome, 148
Trabecular carcinoma, 41, 614f, 614–615
Traction alopecia, 722
Tranquilizers, discoloration of sun-exposed skin and, 417
Transepidermal elimination, 84, 88, 89f
Transepidermal perforation, 84
Transepithelial elimination, 88, 89f
Transient acantholytic dermatosis. *See* Grover's disease

Transient bullous dermolysis of newborn, 172–173
  antibodies and ultrastructural changes useful for classification of, 170t
Transmigration, 88
Treponema carateum, 293
Treponemal infection, 293. *See also* Syphilis
Treponema pallidum, 290, 293
Treponema pertenue, 293
Trichilemma, 25–27, 26f–27f, 713
Trichilemmal cysts, 385, 509, 554–555, 555f–556f
  proliferating, 555–557, 557f–558f
Trichilemmal horn, 555
Trichilemmal keratinization, 27, 29f
Trichilemmoma, 523, 534, 539f
Trichoadenoma, 533, 534f
Trichodiscoma(s), 544–545, 545f, 622t, 622–623
Trichoepithelioma(s), 28f, 385, 535–537, 541f–542f
Trichofolliculoma, 532–533, 533f
  sebaceous, 526, 526f
Trichohyalin, 27
  staining, 58
Trichohyaline granules, 28f
Trichoma, 585
Trichomalacia, 722, 723f
Trichomycosis, 722, 724f
  axillaris, 722, 724f
Trichonodosis, 720f, 721–722
Trichophyton, 190, 251–252
Trichophyton rubrum, 251, 252f
Trichophyton violaceum, 252f
Trichorrhexis
  invaginata, 719, 719f
  nodosa, 717–719, 718f
Trichosporon beigelii, 722, 724f
Trichosporosis, 722
Trichostasis spinulosa, 35, 721, 722f
Trichotillomania, 722, 723f
Trophic ulcer, 246–247
Tubercle(s), 93
Tuberculid(s), 285–287
  lichenoid, 285, 285f
  of lupus miliaris disseminatus faciei, 286–287, 287f
  papulonecrotic, 281, 285–286, 286f, 321
Tuberculoderma(s), 283t, 283–285
Tuberculosis, 280–287, 293
  biology of, 281–283
  changing pattern of, 281
  congenital, 283
  cutaneous, 232–233
  cutis colliquativa, 285
  differential diagnosis, 282t
  luposa, 283–284, 284f
  microorganisms found in, 290t
  multinucleated giant cells in, 278f
  orificialis, 244, 287, 702
  primary, 283
  progressive lesions in host with low immunity, 287
  verrucosa cutis, 284
Tuberculous chancre, 283
Tuberous sclerosis, 414, 622, 623f
Tubular apocrine adenoma, 567f, 568
Tularemia, 243, 300
  differential diagnosis, 282t
Tumor(s). *See also* Epidermoid tumor(s), benign
  benign versus malignant, 435–438
  melanocytic, 439–473
Tumoral calcinosis, 385
Tumor cells
  in dermis, 93
  nonkeratinizing, definition of, 9t
Turban tumors, 569
Turnbull's reaction, 46t, 60
Twisted hairs, 719, 720f

Tyrosinase
  and albinism, 413
  staining, 60
Tzanck smear, 181–182
  in herpes simplex and zoster, 62, 181–182
  in pemphigus vulgaris, 159, 160f
  preparation of, 62

Ulcer(s), 241–248
  artifactual, 247
  in bacterial infections, 243–244
  biopsy of, 241
  definition of, 241
  generic features of, 242
  with immune dysfunction, 244–245
  of mucous membranes, 700
  in secondary syphilis, 291–292
  versus wounds, 241–242
Ulerythema ophryogenes, 257–258
Undetermined etiology, 95
Universal erythroderma, 110
Unmanageable hair, 719, 721f
Uremia, oral plaques with, 706
Uric acid, extracellular deposits of, 385–386
Urticaria, 145–146
  acute, 145
  cholinergic, 145
  chronic, 145, 146f, 148
  pigmentosa, 152, 687–689, 688f–689f
    bullous, 889
Urticarial vasculitis, 217

Vaccinia, 181–182
Vacuole(s), 41f
  artifactual, in biopsy specimen, 53, 53f
Vagabond's disease, 415–416
Van Gieson stain, 46t
Varicella, 181, 183f
Varicella-herpes virus, 181
Varicose veins, in mucous membranes, 707
Variola-vaccinia virus, 181–182
Vascular lesions, of mucous membranes, 707
Vascular nevi and tumors, 645–659
  consisting of vessels, 645–648
  with proliferation of vessel-associated cells, 648–652
Vascular response, entities involving
  differential diagnosis, 145, 146f
  morphologic relations of, 145, 146f
Vascular stasis
  versus Kaposi's sarcoma, 656
  leg ulcer with, 245
Vasculitis, 243. *See also* Leukocytoclastic vasculitis; Necrotizing vasculitis
  allergic, biopsy in, 45
  definition of, 217
  entities involving
    differential diagnosis, 145, 146f
    morphologic relations of, 145, 146f
  livedoid, 221, 221f
  lymphocytic, of pityriasis lichenoides acuta, 217
  pustular, 218
  urticarial, 217
Vater–Pacini corpuscle(s), 23, 23f, 663, 665f
Vellus hair, 25, 30, 31f
Venous lake, 645, 647f
Verhoeff's iodine–iron hematoxylin, 58
Verocay bodies, 666f, 667
Verruca
  digitata, 424, 426–427
  filiformis, 424, 426–427
  plana, 84, 424, 426, 426f
  plana juvenilis, 424, 426, 427f
  plantar type, 424, 427–428, 428f
  vulgaris, 424–426, 425f–426f, 509

  digitate, 434f
  of lips or oral mucosa, 705, 705f
  in nails, 725
  vulgaris plana, 426, 426f
  vulgaris plantaris, 427–428, 428f
Verruciform xanthoma(s), 332, 333f
  of mucous membranes, 710
Verrucous carcinoma
  of mucous membranes, 707–708, 708f
  of oral mucosa, 515
  of skin, 515, 517f
Verrucous epidermal nevus, 479, 480f
Verrucous lymphedema, 359, 362f
Verruga peruana, 645
Vesicular disease, 157–179, 158t
Vesiculation, 82–83, 101
  in contact dermatitis, 104, 105f
  intraepidermal, 82–83
  intragranular, 82
  in sensitization dermatitis, 103–104
  subcorneal, 82
  subepidermal, 82–83
Vesiculobullous dermatitis, biopsy in, 45
Vesiculobullous eruption(s), 157, 158t
Vimentin, immunostaining reactive patterns, 70t
Viral disease(s). *See also* Inflammatory virus diseases; Intranuclear viruses
  epidermoses, 393, 423–432
  Tzanck smear, 62
  warts, 424–431
    of lips or oral mucosa, 705, 705f
Viral exanthem, 184, 186f
Virchow cells, 287, 289f
Virus elementary bodies, 423
Vitiligo, 413–414
  repigmenting, 414
Vitreous membrane, of hair follicle, 26, 26f–27f, 29
  staining, 58
Vogt–Koyanagi syndrome, 414
Volar keratoderma, 495
Volar skin, pigmented macules of, 441–442
Von Kossa stain, 46t, 61
von Recklinghausen's disease, 442, 663, 665f
Vulvitis, 697
  leukoplakic, 699

Wart(s). *See also* Verruca
  flat, biopsy of, 48
  viral, 424–431
    of lips or oral mucosa, 705, 705f
Warty dyskeratoma, 398, 398f
  of mucous membranes, 700
Warty tuberculosis, 284
Wegener's granulomatosis, 220
  in oral mucosa, 703
Weigert's resorcin fuchsin stain, 58
Wells syndrome, 151, 153f
Werner syndrome, 353
White forelock, 531
White piedra, 722, 724f
White sponge nevus, 481, 706, 706f
Wickham's striae, 12, 133
Wilder's stain, 46t
Winchester syndrome, 353
Winer's dilated pore, 533, 534f
Winter eczema, 119
Wiscott–Aldrich syndrome, 175
Wood splinter, foreign body granuloma caused by, 315, 316f
Woolly hair, 720–721
Woolly-hair nevus, 531, 720
Woringer–Kolopp's disease, 682, 685f
Worms, granulomatous inflammation caused by, 312–313
Wound(s), 241–242
Wucheratrophie, 229, 233

Xanthelasma of eyelid, 331, 332f
Xanthoma, 280, 331f, 331–332, 383
　disseminatum, 332
　eruptive, 331
　tuberous, 331
　verruciform, 332, 333f
　　of mucous membranes, 710

Xeroderma pigmentosum, 509–510
X-linked ichthyosis, 403–404
X-ray damage. *See also* Chronic x-ray dermatitis

Yaws, 293

Ziehl–Neelsen's carbofuchsin and methylene blue stain, 61
Zinc deficiency, 162
Zirconium granuloma, 295
　differential diagnosis, 282t
Zoster. *See* Herpes zoster
Zosteriform connective tissue nevus, 622t

Page numbers followed by t *or* f *indicate tables or figures, respectively.*